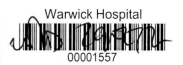
Surgical Nursing

For Churchill Livingstone:

Commissioning Editor: Ninette Premdas
Project Manager: Gail Murray
Project Development Manager: Valerie Dearing
Page make-up: Gerard Heyburn

Surgical Nursing
Advancing Practice

Edited by

Kim Manley MN BA RGN DipN (Lon) RCNT PGCEA
Acting Head of Practice Development, Royal College of Nursing Institute, London, UK

Loretta Bellman BSc(Hons) PhD RGN RCNT RNT CertEd
Programme Director, Royal College of Nursing Institute, London, UK

Foreword by

Judy Lumby BA MHPEd PhD RN FCN(NSW) FRCNA
Executive Director, New South Wales College of Nursing; Emeritus Professor, Faculty of Nursing, University of Technology Sydney, Sydney; Honorary Professor, Faculty of Nursing, University of Sydney, Sydney; formerly EM Lane Chair of Surgical Nursing, Faculty of Nursing, University of Sydney and Concord Repatriation Hospital, Sydney, Australia

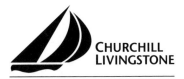

CHURCHILL
LIVINGSTONE

EDINBURGH   LONDON   NEW YORK   PHILADELPHIA   ST LOUIS   SYDNEY   TORONTO   2000

CHURCHILL LIVINGSTONE
An imprint of Harcourt Publishers Limited

First published 2000

ISBN 0 443 05421 5

British Library Cataloguing in Publication Data
A catalogue record for this book is available from the British
Library.

Library of Congress Cataloging in Publication Data
A catalog record for this book is available from the Library of
Congress.

Note
Medical knowledge is constantly changing. As new information becomes available, changes in treatment, procedures,
equipment and the use of drugs become necessary.
The author and the publishers have, as far as it is possible,
taken care to ensure that the information given in this text is
accurate and up to date. However, readers are strongly
advised to confirm that the information, especially with
regard to drug usage, complies with current legislation and
standards of practice.

The Body Mass Index Ready Reckoner on p. 567 is
reproduced by kind permission of Servier Laboratories
Limited.

The
publisher's
policy is to use
**paper manufactured
from sustainable forests**

Printed in China

Contents

Contributors

Helen Allan BSc RN RNT PGDE
Lecturer in Nursing, RCN Institute, London, UK

Gosia Brykczynska BA BSc DipPH CertEd RN RSCN RNT
Lecturer in Ethics and Philosophy, RCN
Institute, London, UK

Julia Cambitzi BSc(Hons) RGN
Clinical Nurse Specialist, Pain Management,
University College Hospitals, London, UK

Ailsa Cameron BA(Hons) MSc
Research Fellow, School for Policy Studies,
University of Bristol, Bristol, UK

Mark Edward Collier BA(Hons) RGN ONC RCNT RNT
Nurse Consultant/Senior Lecturer – Tissue
Viability, Centre for Research and
Implementation of Clinical Practice, Wolfson
Institute of Health Sciences, London, UK

Ruth Davies MSc BSc(Hons) RGN RMN RNT
DipCouns Dip Therapeutic Community Practice
Programme Director, RCN Institute, London,
UK

Sarah Dawson BSc(Hons) MSc RGN DipN (Lon) RNT
Senior Nurse – Special Projects, Quality and
Nursing, St Thomas' Hospital, London, UK

Sharon L. Edwards RGN DipN (Lon) MSc PGCEA
Senior Lecturer, Department of Nursing and
Paramedic Science, University of Hertfordshire,
Hatfield, UK

Hilary Fanning BSc(Hons) RGN
Renal Senior Lecturer-Practitioner, St Mary's
NHS Trust Renal Services and Thames Valley
University, London, UK

Debbie Field SRN ENB249 DipN (Lon) BSc(Hons) MSc
Respiratory Specialist Nurse, Centre for
Anaesthesia, Middlesex Hospital, London, UK

Lesley Fudge MA(Hons) MSc RGN ONC DipEur HJM
Clinical Nurse Manager – Theatres, Critical Care
Directorate, Frenchay Hospital, North Bristol, UK

Deena Graham BSc MSc DipNurs(Lon) RGN ENB176
Senior Lecturer, Wolfson Institute of Health
Sciences, Thames Valley University, London, UK

Mark Harries BPharm MSc
Paediatric Directorate Pharmacist, UCL
Hospitals NHS Trust, The Middlesex Hospital,
London, UK

Agnes Hibbert BSc(Hons) MSc PhD CertEd RGN
Senior Lecturer in Applied Physiology and
Programme Director of Short Courses, RCN
Institute, London, UK

Danielle Holmes RGN ONC RNT
Consultant in Safe Patient Handling for D.R.H.
Associates, London, UK

Rozila Horton MPhil RN
Director, Edhitec Health Systems, Harrogate, UK

Michael Lyon BA(Cantab) PhD PGCert
Senior Research Fellow, Centre for Nurse
Practice Research and Development, School of
Nursing and Midwifery, The Robert Gordon
University, Aberdeen, UK

Michèle Malster BA(Hons) RGN
Lecturer, Florence Nightingale Division of
Nursing and Midwifery, Kings College,
University of London, London, UK

Abigail Masterson BSc MN PGCEA RGN
Director, Abi Masterson Consulting Ltd,
Southampton, UK

Rhona Meek BA MA RGN RCNT RNT
Senior Lecturer, University of Greenwich,
London, UK

Carolyn Mills BSC (Hons) MSc RGN PGCEA
Assistant Director of Nursing, Hillingdon
Hospital, Uxbridge, UK

David Morris MSc CertEd DipHE(Lon) RGN
RCNT RNT
Senior Lecturer, Anglia Polytechnic
University, South Chelmsford, UK

Angela Parry BSc(Hons) MSc DipN DipNEd
JBCNS100 RGN
Lecturer and Adult Pathway Leader,
Florence Nightingale Division of Nursing
and Midwifery, Kings College, University
of London, London, UK

Kristin Dina Plowes ENB176 ENB998 Diploma in
Professional Studies of Nursing, RGN
Lead 'G' Grade, Heygroves Theatres, Bristol
Royal Infirmary, Bristol, UK

Ella van Raders BSC RGN PGCEA
Research Nurse, Anaesthetic Laboratory,
St Bartholomew's Hospital, London, UK

Jane E. Schober MN RGN RCNT RNT DipN(Lon)
DipNEd
Principal Lecturer, School of Nursing and
Midwifery, De Montfort University, Leicester, UK

Christine Spiers BSc(Hons) RN DipN DipNEd RNT
Senior Lecturer – Cardiac Courses, Faculty of
Healthcare Science, St George's Hospital,
London, UK

Karrie Ward MSc DipN(Lon) CertEd(FE) RGN RMN RNT
Senior Lecturer, Anglia Polytechnic University,
Chelmsford, UK

Bernice West MA(Hons) PhD RGN PGCert
Director, Centre for Nurse Practice Research and
Development, School of Nursing and Midwifery,
The Robert Gordon University, Aberdeen, UK

Foreword

Surgical texts have a history of being fairly dry and technical. However, as any surgical nurse knows, nursing people undergoing and recovering from surgical procedures is far from dry or technical. It is filled with the challenge of ensuring the highest quality of care to patients who are so often feeling frightened and vulnerable. They may well be the older, more physically frail person, and increasingly we are caring for the patient who may become confused following surgery. But care does not stop with the patient. There are the carers waiting anxiously for news during and after the operation, and requiring support and education if they are to be the main support post-operatively. Such complex management of care requires a nurse who knows more than the facts and more than the latest techniques. It requires a nurse who is wise enough to critically reflect on her or his own practice, curious enough to follow a path of inquiry for better outcomes, sensitive enough to know when to be there for a patient or colleague, and confident enough to work in collaboration with all health care professionals.

This text covers essential knowledge about nursing in a surgical environment. It covers contemporary surgical practices such as optimum nutrition, pain control and wound management, along with a plethora of techniques, knowledge and innovations required across the contexts in which surgical nurses work. For this reason the text is of immense value to both pre-registration and undergraduate courses as well as to post-registration and graduate courses in surgical nursing. But what makes this text stand out from others is its attention to contemporary issues which impact on surgical nurses and the health care system. The issues are wide-ranging and include values and beliefs; ethical, socio-economic and political perspectives; and the changes in models of care which are all part of the world of the surgical nurse. Global professional issues are also presented within an extremely well informed and critical text.

In an era when the textbook is being questioned as a contemporary information tool *Surgical Nursing: Advancing Practice* defies the trend. It would be an asset to any nurse on entering nursing as a career, choosing to specialise in surgical nursing on registration, and contributing to the lifelong learning of experienced practitioners. It is a must for libraries, practitioners, and students, whether they are in universities, clinical areas or professional organisations. The book is engaging, thoughtfully constructed and thorough in every sense of the word. I congratulate the editors, Loretta and Kim, for what must have been a massive task. The outcome is well worth it and should certainly advance the practice of surgical nursing.

Judy Lumby

Preface

How may surgical nurses within current health-care settings be enabled to develop, update and advance their practice? This text does not provide all the answers but its chapters contain a wealth of knowledge to inform, challenge and advance current thinking about adult surgical nursing practice.

The practice of surgical nursing encompasses a lifelong developmental process of caring. The book reflects the need to care holistically for oneself, and one's patients and peers. It also advocates the view that the quality of surgical nursing care is enhanced through critical and reflective thinking, and the integration of research, practice development and education in practice.

To advance surgical nursing there must be recognition of the value and uniqueness of each nurse's practice knowledge, together with an awareness of the need for both self- and collaborative development. Also, an understanding of the political context will enable wider appreciation of the possibilities and challenges for advancing surgical nursing care initiatives.

Surgical Nursing: Advancing Practice evolved from an invitation to comment on a proposal to publish a new edition of a traditional adult surgical nursing text, written by a surgeon. We felt that surgical texts for nurses seemed to be descriptive and prescriptive, and were not designed to reflect on current practice or advance nurse-led initiatives.

Our initial ambitious proposal for this book also included a focus on surgery in childhood. We are grateful to Pat Rose for her caution regarding the complexities of encompassing the needs of both adults and children in one text. We decided therefore to focus on adults alone.

This book has five parts which are structured around the metaparadigm of nursing: nursing, person, environment, health and patient care, rather than medical specialties, for example orthopaedic surgery. Part 1 addresses the personal and professional development of the surgical nurse. Part 2 considers the patient as a person undergoing surgery. Whilst we acknowledge the many terms for the word patient, for example client/user/consumer/participant in care, we chose to remain with patient, our focus being the person rather than the label. The focus of Part 3 is an exploration of diverse surgical settings, and the role of the surgical nurse in maintaining a safe and conducive environment. Part 4 explores, describes and challenges approaches to determining the health outcomes of surgery. Finally, Part 5 encompasses key concepts in caring for patients undergoing surgery. Each concept is explored in depth and contributes both to the art of surgical nursing practice and to its scientific knowledge base.

The contributors were chosen because of their surgical background and/or their continuing links with surgical nurses. We provided all contributors with general chapter guidelines but encouraged them to write what they felt was most relevant for understanding and advancing surgical nursing practice. There is therefore recognition of different writing and learning styles. Consequently, some readers will find that some chapters can be read from beginning to end, while others will be a resource to return to on many occasions.

We would like to thank Angela Parry for her extensive critical reading and insightful feedback for many of the chapters. We also gratefully acknowledge Agnes Hibbert's physiological critique of three chapters, as well as feedback by Colin Torrance.

As the surgical nursing context is dynamic and the world of health care ever changing, we would very much value feedback from readers on the content of this book, for the purpose of developing nurses' knowledge, advancing clinical practice, and ultimately for the benefit of patients experiencing surgical intervention.

London 2000   Loretta Bellman and Kim Manley

PART 1

The surgical nurse and the nature of surgical nursing

PART CONTENTS

1

The surgical nurse and the advancement of surgical nursing

Kim Manley

AIMS

The aims of this chapter are:

- to explore the reasons for increasing specialisation within society and consider the nature of surgical nursing as a specialism
- to understand different concepts of expertise within surgical nursing and link this to a clinical career pathway
- to appreciate the role of leadership in advancing surgical nursing and mechanisms for developing leadership potential
- to provide insight into exploring one's own values and beliefs about surgical nursing
- to explore guided structured reflection and clinical supervision as mechanisms that enable surgical nurses to continue to develop their effectiveness in the context of lifelong learning
- to consider surgical nursing's knowledge base for practice in relation to different ways of knowing, therapeutic nursing and evidence-based practice.

INTRODUCTION

This opening chapter is about clarifying the concept of surgical nursing and exploring how to advance it. To advance surgical nursing requires more than demonstrating expertise in the practice of nursing, although this has to be the first essential component. For, however much expertise in practice a surgical nurse may possess, only the recipient of that care and immediate observers will benefit unless surgical nurses are committed to enabling others to learn, and contribute to public knowledge and understanding about surgical nursing through research, publication, and the sharing and dissemination of knowledge. Therefore advancement of surgical nursing also requires expertise in: enabling others to learn, in creating a conducive learning environment that will benefit all health care providers; and also in diverse approaches to research

2

which will contribute to the many facets of knowing in nursing, from personal knowing which is effective, to practice-based research methodologies, as well as more traditional approaches to knowledge generation. All of this requires more than educational and research expertise in practice – it requires skills in leadership to create a culture of empowerment for all practitioners, and also an attitude towards lifelong learning which focuses on providing a climate of continued challenge and support for oneself, as well as for others. Self-mastery and personal knowing require active understanding of one's own values and beliefs about surgical nursing and one's own role within the health care team at all levels from clinical through to strategic level. Integral to personal knowing is knowing one's own vision, mission and values and beliefs. Through knowing self one can then help others to develop their personal visions which in turn is a powerful mechanism in developing a shared vision. Having a shared vision is a characteristic of learning organisations. Learning organisations are effective organisations where quality is truly everyone's business. The ability to develop a shared vision will underpin the successful implementation of shared clinical governance, and ensure that surgical services are both responsive to and appropriate for contemporary health care settings, where staff will be increasingly recognised as the greatest resource for providing quality services. This chapter is therefore about the qualities required by surgical nurses who aspire to advancing surgical nursing, their own and their team's practice, now and in the future. This book is about considering and identifying key skills and knowledge – the foundations on which to build such a vision – an exciting opportunity for surgical nurses in these times where facilitating effective change, both personal and professional, has to become a way of life. This is both challenging and daunting to surgical nurses working in today's highly pressurised dynamic environment where there are fewer qualified nurses than ever before; a constant increasing demand for greater productivity, efficiency and effectiveness; and the demand for quality and personalised services, where patients, their families and other members of the health care team are partners in the care process working to a common vision of health gain for all.

INCREASING SPECIALISM AS A SOCIAL MOVEMENT

What does it mean to be a specialist practitioner? Before exploring the terms it is important to understand the broader social context in which increasing specialism has become prevalent. Increasing specialism is a social movement which pervades all activities within a growing technological society, one where there is also an explosion of knowledge. Gallessich (1982) recognises this in relation to the growth of, and need for, consultants within society. Consultants can be viewed in three ways: those who have a specific expert knowledge base, those who have expertise in diagnostics and problem solving; those who have expertise in processes and developing others (Schein 1987). Gallessich argues that the use of consultants is generally linked to an increasing focus on specialism within society, owing to two factors:

- increasing need for social and technical knowledge
- corresponding demand from institutions and organisations to keep abreast of a growing number of changes in knowledge and technology.

Within nursing, the International Council of Nurses (ICN 1992) identify three major forces underpinning the nursing specialisation movement:

- new knowledge
- technological advances
- public needs and demands.

This trend is reflected in the pace of specialisation and the myriad and diverse nursing specialties and sub-specialties identified by the ICN proliferating throughout the world (ICN 1992). The ICN recognise that although there are advantages resulting from the specialist movement there is also the fear that the holistic nature of the profession of nursing may be weakened.

> **Reflective point**
>
> What are the advantages and disadvantages of increasing specialisation for surgical nursing?
> Is there a place within nursing for generalists and specialists, can specialists also be holistic (see Ch. 7)?

Your thoughts will reflect your own values and beliefs about surgical nursing's purpose; what you consider your role is in developing and enabling others, be they patients, colleagues or students; and how you believe you should interface with other members of the interdisciplinary team. If holism, humanism and the therapeutic relationship are central to effective nursing practice (this reflects my own belief system), then nurses within any specialism can still practise holistically but their specialist knowledge and skills will be deeper and more refined than would be expected of the newly registered nurse, although this would always need to be applied to a specific client group, within or across different settings and contexts. In relation to surgical nursing this client group could be considered to be all those people who potentially experience and/or are experiencing surgical intervention regardless of the context, whether in the community or the hospital. Increasingly there will be cross-boundary working where initiatives such as 'Hospital at home' and liaison teams try to address issues of improving both the continuity and consistency of care (Bacharach 1993, Beddar & Aiken 1994, Lampe & Stempel 1994, McHugh et al 1996). But even within surgical nursing there are currently sub-specialisms.

Reflective point

What would you consider to be sub-specialisms within surgical nursing? Do such specialisms have to run in parallel with medical specialisms or can they cross them? Think about the number of medical specialisms with which surgical nursing currently interacts – does this suggest that surgical nursing therefore crosses over several medical specialisms rather than running in parallel with them?

Contextual factors influential on the development of increasingly narrower specialisms include changes in the working conditions of medical practitioners (Calman 1993), and the freeing up of professional activity enabling nurses to expand their role (UKCC 1992). The latter development emphasises individuals' accountability and responsibility for their own practice and encompasses providing evidence of competence and its maintenance, justifying clinical decision-making, and informed risk management. Educational opportunities for competence become a support mechanism for practice rather than guaranteeing a standard of practice – the onus is on individuals to demonstrate how and what they do has an impact on patient care. Thus understanding and defining the specialism of surgical nursing involves incorporating fundamental values about nursing which do not define nursing in terms of medical interventions, although medical interventions may well be incorporated into the care provided by the surgical nurse. Such core fundamental values may define the uniqueness of nursing to be about a specific combination of skills and knowledge used in practice. Such skills and knowledge may not necessarily be unique in

their own right, but when used in partnership with patients and clients for the purpose of health gain they are unique in their combination, for example combining:

- caring values
- focusing on the relationship with individuals/groups and populations
- managing the context of care
- enabling coordination and continuity of care
- using knowledge of patients as people with concepts and implications of health and illness to inform interventions, patient education and health promotion.

For example, a general surgical nurse may be a complete novice in performing an endoscopy, when compared with the specialist 'endoscopy' nurse. Although all surgical nurses may be skilled in expertly preparing patients and caring for them following the procedure – they may have detailed theoretical knowledge (know-that) of anatomy, pathology, patients' experiences post-endoscopy, and anxiety and coping mechanisms, and pharmacological understanding of the sedatives used during the procedure – they would not have the practical skill (know-how) to undertake such a procedure. Extensive training and support in the development of new skills and decision-making concerned with the use of those skills would be required. Competence and maintaining competence are tied up with practise that is sufficiently frequent to maintain one's skill – that is, assuming that there is a well-demonstrated need for developing such skills in terms of enhancing the quality of the services patients receive. For example, there are many opportunities for surgical nurses to develop skills in venepuncture and cannulation. But before deciding to spend valuable time and resources in learning these skills, it is necessary for the surgical nurse to consider several points:

1. How will developing expertise in this skill benefit the quality of care the patient receives? This involves looking at both the risks and the benefits.

2. Am I the best person to develop this skill in terms of providing better quality of care for the patient? This also relates to Question 3 and evidence covering frequency of performance and maintenance of competence.

3. Having learnt the skill, will I actually be practising it enough to remain competent? For example, one could argue that if someone is only practising the skill of cannulation every 4 months, competence cannot be maintained and, hence, it may be inappropriate for that person to develop the skill in the first place.

From both the endoscopy nurse's point of view and the cannulation example it can be argued that the nurse is performing what was previously a medical procedure and that this is not nursing. Others would argue that the procedure may be undertaken within nursing frameworks and that the quality of patients' experience is the determining factor – this includes considering aspects of continuity, holism, and whether receiving more personalised care from a small number of caregivers who know their patients and are multi-skilled results in better care than that received from many different caregivers who may have great in-depth expertise in one or two skills but are task focused. To explore the validity of such an argument one would need to know the nurse's perception in relation to their role and nursing. It is still possible to undertake what can be perceived as a medical inter-vention but perform it in relation to nursing values. The endoscopy nurse or indeed the breast care nurse or the total parenteral nutrition (TPN) nurse (unfortu-nate titles because they emphasise the task and part rather than holistic nursing; see Ch. 7) may be excel-lent nurses in a holistic sense and also highly compe-tent at using such interventions within a nursing value system. Indeed, there will increasingly be new inter-ventions and narrowing of specialisms or an increase in sub-specialisms if Gallessich's argument in the first part of this chapter is accepted. So it is important that surgical nurses always have 'an eye to the future' in anticipating new developments and services – an aspect of leadership which will ensure that surgical nurses are at the forefront of meeting changing health care needs but in a way that is experienced as holistic and personalised by patients and clients. It is essen-tially the values and beliefs held by the nurse and operationalised every day which determine whether nursing practice or medical practice is being advanced (Manley 1996a). Nursing values will be further explored later in the context of different types of nursing expert and also in relation to clarifying one's own values and beliefs.

What does it mean to be a specialist practitioner?

There has been much comment about the confusion different nursing titles have caused, particularly to the public (UKCC 1999). Within the profession also there has been confusion over the use of different terms for different roles and their inconsistent applica-tion. It is important to recognise that just as different specialisms develop, so do knowledge and new techniques and that new labels are applied in order to discriminate subtly between different phenomena. Sometimes there has to be confusion before greater clarity results. For example, many nurses relate the concept of 'clinical supervision' to managerial control and monitoring because of the use of the word 'super-vision', rather than its intended purpose of enabling practitioners to become more effective in their practice through a professional trusting relationship aimed at providing high support and high challenge whilst reflecting on real experiences. Related concepts to supervision are those of mentorship and preceptor-ship but they are not exactly the same and have subtly different meanings and intentions. An expectation of all surgical nurses working at post-diploma or gradu-ate level would be the academic skill of being able to separate the label given to concepts from the meaning. Alongside this skill is the recognition that multiple realities and perceptions exist about the meaning of different concepts, and that it is not until there is a willingness to share different perceptions that a new consensus can evolve (Guba & Lincoln 1989). Only when there is greater clarity can nurses then articulate this in simple language that both the public and col-leagues from other disciplines, as well as new entrants to the profession, can easily understand. These so-called 'academic skills' are also argued as being central to quality nursing, in the sense that we need to be able to see the world through patients' eyes and to under-stand their reality, which involves getting to know each patient as a person (Jenny & Logan 1992, Tanner et al 1993), and spending time with them, being avail-able for them (Johns 1994) to explore their understand-ing of the situation. This understanding will be unique to each individual.

The terms and concepts most relevant to this dis-cussion therefore are specialism/specialty, specialist, expert, advanced. Analysing these terms, they imme-diately fall into two areas:

• The domain or focus of care – specialism or spe-cialty, ideally defined by client group or sometimes by setting, e.g. the GP unit, the community, the minor injuries setting, etc.
• The person providing care – the specialist, novice, expert, advanced. All terms except specialist reflect a level of practice rather than a role, whereas specialist, e.g. clinical nurse specialist, is a role that implies a specific level of expertise within a specific specialism. This is where much of the confusion has lain with many new roles being given a title that implies expertise. So what is a specialist surgical nurse a specialist in?

Specialists in what?

The answer to this question will reflect the nurse's values. For example, if the answer were 'I am a specialist in stomas', the implication is that the nursing focus may only be on the 'stoma' and its technical aspects in which the nurse may be an expert. The response 'I am a specialist in caring for people with stomas' implies a more holistic answer and possibly more holistic values, although one must always be aware that one can articulate strong nursing values, and write about them, but may not actually demonstrate them in practice. This challenge is something that those who make judgements on practice outcomes are always aware of. Excellent practice portfolios may only convey an individual's excellence in writing, rather than actualising such approaches in practice. Individuals may be able to articulate their values and beliefs, but may not practise them even though they think they are. This is a common phenomenon, one that as individuals we may be unaware of in relation to our own practice. Argyris & Shon (1989) recognise this phenomenon and term it 'espoused theory' versus 'theory-in-action'. Espoused theory is what we say we do, but actually do not do: theory-in-action is what we actually do in practice. We may therefore be unaware of the gap between what we say and what we do, but there may also be many factors within the environment that prevent us doing what we want to do. There are increasing opportunities to help us identify these contradictions through mechanisms such as professional/clinical supervision and guided structured reflection. Their purpose is to enable us to become more effective practitioners through developing insight into our own practice as well as understanding how the context in which we operate influences us, or has socialised us into operating as we do. These approaches enable us to make changes supported and challenged by colleagues formally and informally through individual, peer and group supervision and/or action learning.

Specialty or specialism would therefore need to be defined in terms of client group if nurses are to emphasise their nursing role as holistic practitioners, caring for the whole person. Client groups may consist of those with specialist needs or those residing within a specific geographical area, e.g. caring for all postoperative surgical patients within a community setting. Specialist roles such as a clinical nurse specialist in surgical nursing imply an expert working within the specialism, but many nurses working within a specialism may be working anywhere on the novice to expert continuum (Benner 1984), hence the confusion: 'there is a

clear difference between practising within a specialty and being a nurse specialist' (UKCC 1994).

Therefore, when focusing on the person providing care, although surgical nurses may be working within a specialism which focuses on people undergoing surgical intervention, they will not necessarily be specialists.

[Although] ... Specialist Practitioner intervention and leadership are likely to be needed in most areas of clinical practice ... This will not require everyone to become a specialist.

(UKCC 1996)

Although much of this chapter is about identifying the sort of skills and qualities necessary to proceed along a career pathway in surgical nursing, it is recognised that many practitioners within surgical nursing may feel because they are working part time and are caring for a family that there is little opportunity to advance themselves and their practice without moving along the career pathway. Within the context of lifelong learning, the assumptions underpinning the concept of 'advancement' are that all nurses can develop their leadership potential and their effectiveness as practitioners through the processes of clinical supervision, and that all nurses working within a specialism at whatever level can both advance their own practice and enable the advancement of others' practice.

The UKCC have tried to address the difference between any nurse working within a specialism and the specialist by refusing to use any role-based terms; instead they have chosen to focus only on 'Higher Level Practice' (UKCC 1999) and the evidence necessary to demonstrate that nurses are working at a higher level. Formal recognition on the register will then protect the public in terms of assuring them that nurses accorded this recognition have demonstrated *all* the specific outcomes in practice at this higher level. However, all nurses, be they specialists or not within their specialism, will be working towards developing aspects of their practice, and hence advancing their own practice.

Level of practice

The UKCC's stance on higher level practice is that this is practice at a significantly deeper, broader and more complex level than that seen at registration (UKCC 1999). But what does this mean in terms of the depth of decision-making and/or the scope/breadth of the practice? Does the scope/breadth of the practice relate to increasing medical interventions or broader responsibility regarding service provision, practice development and development of others?

Reflective point

When considering higher level practice within surgical nursing what would your perceptions be that such nurses were doing? What decision-making characteristics would they be demonstrating?

Would the focus only be on direct client-centred care or would it also encompass leadership, political development, development of others? How many nurses will be operating at this level?

The UKCC's role (and that of the body that takes over from them) is primarily about protecting public safety, which means that the standards they identify at both registration and at any higher level will need to be at a minimum threshold standard. The UKCC (1999) have chosen to focus on higher level practice from a generic rather than a specialist perspective – this means that each specialism will need to customise the UKCC's descriptor for its own area of practice. Demonstration of higher level practice will probably involve presenting a range of different sources of evidence, through practice portfolios and profiles. Judgements will need to be made, through peer review, that the evidence identifies the nurse as working at the higher level, and mechanisms to corroborate written profiles with evidence from other sources will need to be explored. The breadth, depth and complexity of higher level practice is alluded to within the UKCC's draft descriptor (1999) which is structured around seven areas, each of which has between three and eight further criteria:

1. Providing effective health care
2. Improving quality and health outcomes
3. Evaluation and research
4. Leading and developing practice
5. Innovation and changing practice
6. Developing self and others
7. Working across professional and organisational boundaries.

From viewing the seven areas it is evident that to be recognised as practising at a higher level will involve much more than practising surgical nursing; it will require demonstration of leadership, change facilitation, expertise in research and evaluation and a strong focus on improving services to patients.

In the past, entrance to a particular specialism has been through undertaking a specialist course of study. However, the focus of the study may have had differing emphases in terms of the ratio of theory to practice and the promotion of traditional educational or radical approaches to the integration of theory and practice. Little consistency has existed nation-wide, courses have been run at different academic levels, and also the purpose of the courses has varied in relation to enabling consolidation of past practice or preparation for practice within a new specialism (Scholes et al 1999). Needless to say, having successfully completed a course of preparation within a specialism, e.g. surgical nursing, and achieved the course outcomes, one can not be considered an expert but one would be competent to practise independently and safely for patients/clients within the specialism. There is now increasing emphasis on demonstrating practice outcomes reflecting different levels of practice (Manley 1996b). Higher level practice focuses on 'how' and 'what' practitioners do rather than their qualifications; education is perceived by the UKCC as a support to practice rather than a determinant of it (UKCC 1999). Increasingly, the focus on what nurses do, how they do it and what they achieve in practice will have greater emphasis than their qualifications. This is not to say that academic qualifications are not necessary – they will be as important as ever in supporting nurses in the development of their cognitive, reflective and logical development skills, but in the future there will be much more focus on the changes that result in practice as a result of education, than on the academic qualifications per se.

The use of the word 'specialist' within the past could therefore be ambiguous in that it could mean that one was competent to work within the specialism, or one was working at a specific level of expertise. There has been an explosion of different titles with the increasing use of titles such as clinical nurse specialist, emergency nurse practitioner, nurse practitioner surgical nursing, etc. Within the UK, also, the use of similar terms to those used in the USA implied a similar role description, which was not the case (Manley 1993, 1997a). This has identified the need for the UKCC to undertake their work, and also the increasing focus on what people do in practice rather than what they can achieve academically. Although one can argue that there is a link between the two, academic outcomes and practice outcomes are as yet only crudely correlated in nursing (Manley 1996b).

This discussion introduces the next concept in terms of level of practice, that of expertise in surgical nursing. How would an expert in the specialism of surgical nursing be recognised?

EXPERTISE IN THE PRACTICE OF SURGICAL NURSING

As stated earlier (p. 5), the academic expectation of the graduate nurse is the ability to unpack concepts, to separate their labels from their meanings and to identify the assumptions underpinning different meanings. So what does having expertise actually mean? Such concepts evolve over time, through their use. It is accepted now because of arguments within the philosophy of science that concepts are socially constructed and, although it may be appropriate when considering natural concepts to develop operational definitions, it is inappropriate to develop these for social phenomena (Morse 1995, Rodgers 1989). The concept of expertise is one such concept. What does it actually mean to demonstrate expertise? Such concepts are value laden. This can be demonstrated in the work of Conway (1996) who identified four types of experts in British nursing practice, each of which had different orientations to eight factors, one of which was the philosophy and values held by the practitioner (Box 1.1).

These eight points emphasise the influence of the organisation in which expert practitioners of nursing work, again supporting the role of clinical/professional supervision as a mechanism for helping practitioners recognise how organisational as well as local

contexts may frustrate or enable their own actions, or how one may be socialised into taking for granted certain aspects of practice.

The four types of experts are identified by Conway (1996) as:

- traditionalists
- technologists
- specialists
- humanistic existentialists.

The four different types of experts have different underlying values and goals, but also value-different knowledge bases, and have other characteristic skills in relation to, for example, teaching style. These are outlined in summary in Table 1.1.

You may be able to relate to all four of the types of expert that Conway outlines; certainly I can. Although Conway does not state this, one way to make sense of this is as a continuum and a personal journey. For me, humanistic nursing values have always been central to my practice but I have not always had expertise from the technological and specialist perspective to enable my nursing approach to be developed to its optimal potential. Humanistic existentialists draw from eclectic knowledge bases and skills; they also have expertise from the perspectives of the technologist and specialists but they integrate this expertise within a strong nursing value system based on humanism and a commitment to the therapeutic potential of nursing. They also have a highly developed reflective ability and are committed to developing a culture for development of others. It is also important to note the influence of the organisation in which all experts work. This is a powerful factor that is recognised as influential in trying to operationalise any advanced nursing role (Manley 1997a).

Conway (1996) demonstrates, then, that expertise within nursing is influenced by different values, but what are the specific attributes and enabling factors of expertise? Remembering the role of concept analysis raised earlier, Figure 1.1 has drawn on the literature extensively and portrays the concept of expertise from a concept mapping exercise undertaken by Manley & McCormack (1997).

Table 1.1 Four different types of experts and their characteristics (after Conway 1996)

	Traditionalists	Technologists	Specialists	Humanist-existentialists (H-Es) ('a holistic patient-centred nurse')
Goal	Survival. Preoccupied with getting the work done and managing care with scarce resources	Diagnosis	Prescribing treatment regimes, recommending medication and extending their roles. Many have extended practice into doctors' previous territory	Strong nursing focus, view patients holistically and humanistically
Knowledge-base	Monitoring knowledge, based on medical model. Overseer based on experience	Wide variety of different knowledge, including technical knowledge which extends into the province of the doctor. Monitoring knowledge of patients' conditions, junior doctors, machinery. Anticipatory knowledge – being prepared and being able to deal with all eventualities, quick at picking up cues	Comfortable with their knowledge and able to identify treatment regimes, etc. Have knowledge in assessment of health and diagnosis. Well-developed communication and counselling abilities. Remember the various complications that might arise in relation to diagnosis and medication	Complex, underpinned by theories in social sciences and nursing. Practice an amalgam of different types of theoretical knowledge, values, experience and subject matter knowledge – enabling them to be proactive. Integrate theory into practice, able to deconstruct processes used so as to provide a rationale for their approach. Reflection and reflective abilities are the hallmark. Use both deductive and reflection-in-action modes in patient assessment
Processes and skills	Monitor actions of patients and nurses. Medical model guides practice. Task-focused. Experience strongly influences actions, scant evidence of theoretical frameworks being used to guide care. Operate as overseers and assistants to doctors. Present themselves as powerless, lacking in awareness of own worth. Subservient to the doctor. Largely non-assertive and reactive – view doctors' time as more important than their own. Interpret medical jargon for the patient. Lack ability to bring about change, struggle to maintain standards. Professionalism equated to etiquette	Able to anticipate situations. Trust own judgement. Expertness apparent in degree of autonomy. Constantly diagnosing. Assess complex variety of cues – which factors are significant – when and where significant? Healthy distrust of equipment – always monitoring it in relation to own judgement which they trust	Have distinctive roles, e.g. breast care nurses, stoma therapists, infection control nurses. Used as consultants by other nurses. Early detection of warning signals. Proactive and autonomous. Give consideration to and estimation of patients' quality of life. Have a transformative ability, i.e. they are able to listen and transform a difficult situation to a more manageable one. Specialists may be further divided into technologists, traditionalists and humanistic existentialists	Dynamic and passionate about nursing practice. View the nursing role holistically. Politically aware, devise strategies to develop their practice. Used devolved hierarchy, e.g. primary nursing. Risk takers – have supportive management and good resources. Educationally well developed. High level of self-awareness as well as reflective ability. Critically aware of self and others. Exert considerable power and influence – see themselves as setting the culture of their unit. Artistry – can enter into the 'real world' of the patient. Transformative ability where apparently intractable problems can be turned into positive situations. Approach patient with open mind. Use therapeutic interventions which may include complementary therapies

Table 1.1 (Contd.)

	Traditionalists	Technologists	Specialists	Humanist-existentialists (H-Es) ("a holistic patient-centred nurse")
Teaching/education	An optional extra Value attached to 'doing' and not to 'reflecting' 'Papering over the cracks' was what nursing was about and this is what others had to learn to do Dispossess the dispossessed	Tend to be didactic, using images and in-depth questioning		Contribute to a nurturing environment which creates a breeding ground for expertise development Aware of the influence they have on others. Foster reflection in others

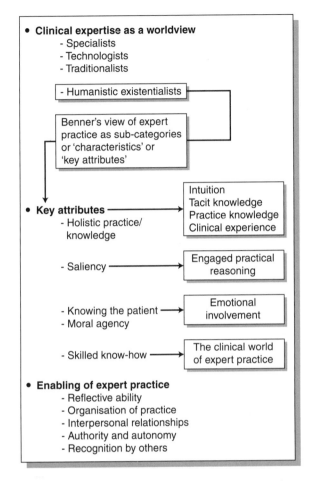

Figure 1.1   Derived categories from the concept map of expertise (reproduced by kind permission from Manley & McCormack 1997).

The five attributes of expertise, derived from Benner & Tanner (1987) and Benner et al (1996), are identified as:

- *Holistic practice and holistic knowledge:* synthesising different types of knowledge and different ways of knowing and practising holistically. For example, using knowledge of the individual person combined with extensive experience in caring for postoperative thoracotomy patients, with skill and knowledge of pain control from both a physiological and a psychological perspective, to identify, skilfully implement, and evaluate a number of strategies helpful to a particular patient within a specific situation.
- *Saliency:* seeing the most pertinent issues in a situation and ways of responding to them. This, therefore, involves being able to identify, prioritise and act

appropriately on problems identified. For example, experts through pattern recognition and many hours of caring for patients undergoing similar experiences can identify a problem quickly without needing to use an extensive array of assessment tools. They also can put into practice immediate solutions. Therefore saliency has two integrated components – identifying the priority problem and taking appropriate action.

- *Knowing the patient:* as a person with a typical pattern of responses as a prerequisite to skilled judgement. Knowing the patient has been linked with, for example, reduced length of stay – an outcome indicator in the critical care environment (Jenny & Logan 1992).
- *Moral agency:* a concern for responding to patients as persons, respecting their dignity, protecting their personhood in times of vulnerability, helping them feel safe, providing comfort and maintaining integrity in the relationship.
- *Skilled know-how:* performance is fluid, seamless and highly proficient. Actions reflect attunement to the situation which is shaped by patient responses, and does not rely on conscious deliberation.

Other attributes identified in experts as a result of the RCN Expert Practitioner Project (RCN 1998) include:

- the assessment and management of risk
- welcoming challenge from patients, colleagues and peers alike about professional actions and judgements
- even experts require facilitation and support through supervision to enable them to demonstrate their expertise.

For the attributes of expertise to be developed and demonstrated there are also a number of enabling factors necessary. The enabling factors derived from the literature, highlighted by Manley & McCormack (1997), are:

- *Reflective ability:* a highly developed reflective ability implies the ability to describe one's practice, analyse it and synthesise new practice insights in one's own practice. Developing such ability would be expected of the graduate nurse, although others may have achieved such ability through other mechanisms such as skilled group/individual supervision and action learning.
- *Authority and accountability:* official sanction to do what they do. Accountable for what they do to the patient, employer, colleagues and the law.
- *Interpersonal relationships:* with patients, clients and significant others as well as with other colleagues and members of the interdisciplinary team.

- *Organisation of practice:* this has a direct effect on whether nurses are enabled to get to know their patients. An organisation of care in which nurses are repeatedly caring for different rather than the same patients/clients may work against the development of expertise in practice, through the mechanism of not knowing the patient.
- *Recognition by others:* experts are recognised by others.

The concept map outlined above has been used as the basis for developing the RCN Recognised Expert Practitioner Project (RCN 1998), a national project aimed at achieving three main purposes:

- to recognise, value and celebrate expert practitioners in client-centred nursing
- to understand the nature of expertise within different specialisms within British nursing
- to begin to explore the links between expertise and patient outcomes.

Reflective point

Consider an experience that you handled well in practice. Analyse your practice against the attributes and enabling factors mentioned. To what extent did the experience go well in light of these attributes and enabling factors?

KEY ROLES IN SURGICAL NURSING: INDIVIDUAL AND PROFESSIONAL ADVANCEMENT
Specialist practitioner

The UKCC argued that advancing practice was something that all nurses were involved in doing (UKCC 1997). However, to advance the practice of nursing requires the development of others and/or contributing to the body of knowledge. One can be an expert in the practice of nursing but only the recipient of that care, and possibly observers, will vicariously gain from this. To advance the profession of nursing requires the development of others and/or adding to the public knowledge base and understanding of the profession. To achieve this means one may not be practising clinical nursing 100% of the time, although one may be totally practice-focused and practice-based. The two new roles considered here have a specific purpose concerned with advancing nursing through the practice of nursing, fostering practice development, and enabling others to develop, as well as contributing to the knowledge base and understanding of nursing.

The consultant nurse

'Nurse consultant' are the words used by Tony Blair in his speech at the Nursing Standard Nurse of the Year Awards (Blair 1998). But what does this actually mean? Does it mean that consultant nurses parallel consultants in medicine, or are they consultants in nursing rather than medicine? It has been argued reasonably that such posts parallel roles in medicine, such as consultant physician and consultant surgeon, where the practice of one's discipline – in this case surgical nursing – is just as important at the pinnacle of the career ladder. Consultant nurse is associated then with an internal model and suggests that the post-holder is a consultant in *nursing*. In the literature, *nurse consultant* has subtly different connotations (Manley 1996c). It is more associated with a business model where nurses may be independent consultants, contracted as external agents to provide consultancy on some aspect of nursing to health care providers (Keane 1989), rather like management consultants – they may not actually be practising nursing, or have a caseload of patients. Semantics maybe, but nursing cannot afford to promote an unclear picture of what is meant by a consultant nurse and such posts need to ensure that they are positioned strongly within the nursing camp and not the medical camp. The only research which has been undertaken within Britain on this role involved the operationalising of an advanced practitioner/consultant nurse post (Manley 1997a). The consultant nurse role is presented as multidimensional and centres around four interdependent sub-roles, as well as leadership. The conceptual framework illuminates this in more detail (Fig. 1.2).

The consultant nurse is an expert practitioner as either a specialist or generalist in nursing a specific client-centred group. Additionally, consultant nurses have expertise in education and providing learning opportunities in the practice environment, and thus the development and enablement of others. They have expertise in the use of practice-based research methodologies, i.e. research and development methodologies directly relevant to the world of practice *with* practitioners, rather than *on* practitioners as with traditional, technical and 'ivory tower' research. They act as a consultant at all levels of the organisation from clinical to strategic; and finally, as leaders, they are skilled in helping everyone to become a leader on some aspect of care provision/innovation, subsequently enabling cultural change towards becoming a true learning organisation akin to the 'magnet hospitals' within the USA (Bellman 1996, Manley 1997a). Nursing, unlike medicine, is not just concerned with specific interventions but is also concerned with the context in which care

and supervisors are fully aware of the purpose and benefits of supervision. This includes stating how issues are raised, discussed or recorded and how confidentiality is dealt with.' (UKCC 1996, p. 4).

Skilled supervision is the cornerstone of good clinical supervision, as is the need for supervision of the supervisors. Skilled supervision is also guided by structured tools which help supervisees to remain focused on specific clinical experiences. One such tool is outlined in Box 1.8 – Johns' ninth model for guided structured reflection (Manley & McCormack 1997). Johns uses Carper's (1978) different ways of knowing

to identify the interrelated ways of knowing pertinent to nursing practice.

Although it is difficult to capture holistic knowing, Box 1.9 begins to illustrate this for the endoscopy nurse referred to earlier, working within a nursing value system. It shows the different knowledge, skills and diversity that it is necessary to integrate for effective nursing practice to occur.

The work of Carper (1978) has long been used to demonstrate the integrated ways of knowing necessary for informing effective nursing practice. Knowledge is not just a static collection of dry facts ('know-that'), it also encompasses understanding and skill ('know-how') (Manley 1997b) and is influenced in turn by the values and beliefs we hold about what

---

Box 1.8   Model of structured reflection: ninth edition, July 1993

The following cues are offered to help practitioners access, make sense of, and learn through experience:

1. **Description**
1.1   Write a description of the experience
1.2   What are the key issues within this description that I need to pay special attention to?
2. **Reflection**
2.1   What was I trying to achieve?
2.2   Why did I intervene as I did?
2.3   What were the consequences of my actions:
   • for the patient and family?
   • for myself?
   • for the people I work with?
2.4   How did I feel about this experience when it was happening?
2.5   How did the patient feel about it?
2.6   How do I know how the patient felt about it?
3. **Influencing factors**
3.1   What internal factors influenced my decision-making and actions?
3.2   What external factors influenced my decision-making and actions?
3.3   What sources of knowledge did or should have influenced my decision-making and actions?
4. **Alternative strategies**
4.1   Could I have dealt better with the situation?
4.2   What other choices did I have?
4.3   What would be the consequences of these other choices?
5. **Learning**
5.1   How can I make sense of this experience in light of past experience and future practice?
5.2   How do I now feel about this experience?
5.3   Have I taken effective action to support myself and others as a result of this experience?
5.4   How has this experience changed my ways of knowing in practice?
   • empirics
   • ethics
   • personal
   • aesthetics   (Carper 1978)

Box 1.9   Different types of knowing used by an endoscopy nurse

Empirical knowing
• Detailed anatomy and pathology
• Radiography
• Pharmacology
• Risks and hazards
• Evidence underpinning all interventions
• Nursing knowledge: factors conducive to developing therapeutic relationships, knowing the patient, interpersonal skills
• Audit and evaluation strategies

Aesthetic knowing
• Detailed holistic assessment skills and interpretation
• Skill in manipulation and dexterity in handling the endoscope and technique in minimising the time span involved
• Radiographic skills
• Skills in patient positioning and recognition of nonverbal and physiological indicators of discomfort and distress
• Skills in risk assessment and management
• Skills in developing a therapeutic relationship with the patient
• Skill in collaborative working with the interprofessional team

Ethical knowing
• Handling of in situ ethical dilemmas which directly relate to specific patients undergoing specific investigations and the implications of the treatment and results for them

Personal knowing
• Active development of self-mastery and personal knowing to enable greater personal effectiveness as a nurse in the care and interventions used with patients experiencing endoscopy

counts as knowledge. Understanding and skill does not come from books: it comes from our own experience of practice through examining our own actions using the tools of 'critique' and 'reflection', thus enabling our practice to be further refined and developed. Greater insight into the relationship between 'knowing' and 'action' can be achieved through guided reflection and skilled supervision. All surgical nurses need to tap into and become aware of the knowledge informing their own practice, as well as the impact the context in which they work has on their own actions. Only through becoming enlightened about this will surgical nurses be able to take the first steps to advancing their own practice. Enlightenment, that is, awareness of our actions and why we act as we do is a prerequisite for empowerment – the motivation to act. Empowerment in turn is a prerequisite of emancipation – actually acting (Fay 1987).

Johns (1994), through the Burford Nursing Development Unit Model, demonstrates an understanding of what nursing is about in a framework which has been derived from practitioners' own reflections on practice and their values and beliefs about their role and purpose as nurses. The development of this model from practitioners' reflections demonstrates how practitioners can contribute to the professional understanding of nursing, as well as enabling themselves to become more effective as practitioners. The Burford NDU model reflects a number of learning domains that practitioners need to focus on to be therapeutic, thus further endorsing the therapeutic nature of nursing. These are outlined in Table 1.3.

Other models of nursing will provide other frameworks to guide nursing actions; however, models are only tools to help guide practitioners in the implementation of their purpose and values. Surgical nurses must first be clear of their own purpose, values and beliefs before either selecting a model that reflects these values or developing their own frameworks from reflection.

CONCLUSION

A number of frameworks and tools have been identified to enable surgical nurses to advance their practice. It has been emphasised that all surgical nurses can contribute to and advance nursing through knowing their values and beliefs, through participating in clinical/professional supervision, through critiquing and reflecting on the knowledge informing their practice, through sharing and refining that knowledge, through developing their leadership potential and enabling others, and finally, through contributing to the knowledge base underpinning surgical nursing. Thus, all surgical nurses can advance their own practice and the practice of others. Much of the knowledge, skills and values necessary for advancing surgical nursing have been alluded to within this chapter; much more will be developed and emphasised in the later chapters of this book.

Table 1.3 Learning domains in becoming more effective at work (adapted from Johns, 1994)

Focus of experience		Aim of work	Learning domain
Intrapersonal	Self in the context of the environment	'Knowing' self	1. Becoming patient-centred
Interpersonal	Self in the context of the patient/client	'Knowing' therapeutic work	2. Becoming therapeutic with patients and families: – ethical decision-making – involvement with patients – responding with appropriate and skilled action
Intrapersonal	} Self in the context of therapeutic work with others	'Knowing' responsibility	3. Giving and receiving feedback
Interpersonal		'Knowing' others	4. Coping with work in ways that sustain therapeutic work

REFERENCES

Argyris C, Schon D A 1989 Theory in practice: increasing professional effectiveness. Jossey-Bass, San Francisco

Bacharach L L 1993 Continuity of care and approaches to case management for long-term mentally ill patients. Hospital and Community Psychiatry 44: 465–468

Bass B M 1985 Leadership and performance beyond expectations. Free Press, New York

Beddar S M, Aiken J L 1994 Continuity of care: a challenge for ambulatory oncology nursing. Seminars in Oncology Nursing 10: 254–263

Bellman L 1996 Changing nursing practice through reflection on the Roper, Logan and Tierney model: the enhancement approach to action research. Journal of Advanced Nursing 24: 129–138

Benner P 1984 From novice to expert: excellence and power in clinical nursing practice. Addison-Wesley, Menlo Park, California

Benner P, Tanner C 1987 Clinical judgement: how expert nurses use intuition. American Journal of Nursing 87(1): 23–31

Benner P, Tanner C, Chesla C 1996 Expertise in nursing practice: caring, clinical judgement and ethics. Springer Publishing, New York

Bennis W, Nanus B 1997 Leaders: strategies for taking charge. HarperCollins, New York

Blair T 1998 Prime Minister's speech at the Nurse 98 Awards ceremony, Tuesday 8 September, 1998. Internet address: http://www.number10.govuk/public/info/releases/speeches

Blake R R, Moulton J S 1985 The managerial grid iii: the key to leadership excellence, 3rd edn. Gulf Publishing, Houston

Borders L, Leddick G 1987 Handbook of counselling supervision. Association of Counsellor Education and Supervision, Virginia

Butterworth T 1997 It is good to talk: an evaluation of clinical supervision and mentorship in England and Scotland. School of Nursing, Midwifery and Health Visiting, University of Manchester, Manchester

Calman K (Chair) 1993 Hospital doctors: training for the future. The report of the working group on specialist medical training. DoH, London

Carper B A 1978 Fundamental patterns of knowing in nursing. Advances in Nursing Science 1(1): 13–23

Carroll M 1996 Workplace counselling: a systematic approach to employee care. Sage Publications, London

Clinical Nurse Specialism Conference 1999 4th Professional Nurse Conference on Clinical Nurse Specialism: a framework for higher levels of practice. March 17th & 18th, Kensington Town Hall, London

Community Psychiatric Nurses' Association (CPNA) 1992 Clinical practice issues for community psychiatric nurses. CPNA Publications, London

Conway J E 1996 Nursing expertise and advanced practice. Quay Books, Dinton

Dilts R B 1994 Effective presentation skills. Meta Publications, Capitola, California

Dilts R B, Bonissone G 1993 Skills for the future: managing creativity and innovation. Meta Publications, Cupertino, California

Faugier J, Butterworth T 1992 Clinical supervision: a position paper. University of Manchester, School of Nursing Studies, Manchester

Fay B 1987 Critical social science: liberation and its limits. Polity Press, Oxford, pp 27–41

Fitzpatrick J J 1989 The empirical approach to the development of nursing science. In: Fitzpatrick J J, Whall A O Conceptual models of nursing, 2nd edn. Appleton and Lange, Norwalk

Gallessich J 1982 The profession and practice of consultation. Jossey-Bass, San Francisco

Gardner J W 1986 The nature of leadership: introductory considerations. The Independent Sector, Washington, D.C.

Guba E G, Lincoln Y S 1989 Fourth generation evaluation. Sage, London

Hawkins P, Shohet R 1989 Supervision in the helping professions. Open University Press, Milton Keynes

Hinshaw A S, Atwood J R 1984 Nursing staff turnover, stress and satisfaction: models, measures and management. In: Werley H H, Fitzpatrick J J (eds) Annual Review of Nursing Research 1(part II): 133–153

International Council of Nurses 1992 Guidelines on specialisation. ICN, Geneva

Jenny J, Logan J 1992 Knowing the patient: one aspect of clinical knowledge. Image: Journal of Nursing Scholarship 24(2): 254–258

Johns C (ed) 1994 The Burford NDU Model: caring in practice. Blackwell Science, Oxford

Johns C 1995 Achieving effective work as a professional activity. In: Schober J E, Hinchliff S M (eds) Towards advanced practice: key concepts for health care. Arnold, London, pp 252–280

Keane B 1989 Independent nurse-consultants: the lateral leap. In: Pratt R, Gray G (eds) Issues in Australian Nursing 6: 277–287

Kouzes J M, Posner B Z 1987 The leadership challenge. Jossey-Bass, San Francisco

Lampe G S, Stempel J E 1994 Nurse case management from the client's view: growing as insider-expert. Nursing Outlook 42: 7–13

Lancaster J, Lancaster W 1982 The nurse as a change agent. CV Mosby, St Louis, pp 24–38

Loganbill C, Hardy E, Delworth U 1982 Supervision: a conceptual model. Counselling Psychologist 10(1): 3–42

McHugh M, West P, Assatley C et al 1996 Establishing an interdisciplinary patient care team: collaboration at the bedside and beyond. Journal of Nursing Administration 26: 21–27

Manley K 1992 Quality assurance: the pathway to excellence in nursing. In: Jolley M, Brykczynska G (eds) Nursing care – the challenge to change. Edward Arnold, London, ch 7

Manley K 1993 Clinical nurse specialist. Surgical Nurse 6(3): 21–25

Manley K 1996a Advanced practice is not about medicalising nursing roles. Nursing in Critical Care 1(2): 56–57

Manley K 1996b Developing practice: the contribution of the Master's prepared nurse. Journal of Clinical Nursing 5(6): 339–340

Manley K 1996c Consultancy. MSc in Nursing. Distance Learning Module. RCN Institute, London

Manley K 1997a A conceptual framework for advanced practice: an action research project operationalizing an advanced practitioner/consultant nurse role. Journal of Clinical Nursing 6(3): 179–190

Manley K 1997b Knowledge for nursing practice. In: Perry A (ed) The knowledge base for nursing, 2nd edn. Arnold, London, ch 10

Manley K 1998 A clinical career ladder for nursing and more on consultant nurses. Editorial. Nursing in Critical Care 3(6): 265–266

Manley K, McCormack B 1997 Exploring expert practice. Study Guide MSc in Nursing. Distance Learning. RCN Institute, London

Marquis B, Huston C 1996 Leadership roles and management functions in nursing: theory and application, 2nd edn. Lippincott, Philadelphia

Mezirow J 1981 A critical theory of adult learning and education. Adult Education 32(1): 3–24

Morse J M 1995 Exploring the theoretical basis of nursing using advanced techniques of concept analysis. Advances in Nursing Science 17(93): 31–36

Munhall P L 1993 'Unknowing': toward another pattern of knowing in nursing. Nursing Outlook 41(3): 125–128

National Health Service Management Executive (NHSME) 1993 A vision for the future: the nursing, midwifery and health visiting contribution to health and healthcare. HMSO, London

Platt-Koch L M 1986 Clinical supervision for psychiatric nurses. Journal of Psychological Nursing 26(1): 7–15

RCN Institute 1999 Realising clinical effectiveness and clinical governance through clinical supervision. An open learning programme. Radcliffe Medical Press, Oxford

Rodgers B L 1989 Concepts, analysis and the development of nursing knowledge: the evolutionary cycle. Journal of Advanced Nursing 14(4): 330–335

Royal College of Nursing (RCN) 1997 Ward leadership project: a journey to patient-centred leadership. Executive summary. RCN, London

Royal College of Nursing (RCN) 1998 RCN expert practitioner project. Fringe event, RCN Congress, Bournemouth

Sashkin M, Burke W W 1990 Understanding and assessing organisational leadership. In: Clark K, Clark M B (eds) Measures of leadership. Leadership Library of America, West Orange, New Jersey, pp 297–325

Sashkin M, Rosenbach W E 1993 A new leadership paradigm. In: Rosenbach W E, Taylor R L (eds) Contemporary issues in leadership, 3rd edn. Westview Press, Boulder, Colorado, pp 87–108

Schein E H 1987 Process consultation volume II: lessons for managers and consultants. Addison-Wesley, Reading, Mass

Scholes J, Endacott R, Chellel A 1999 Documentary analysis and literature review of critical care nursing. English National Board, London

Schon D A 1983 The reflective practitioner: how professionals think in action. Jossey-Bass, San Francisco

Senge P M 1990 The fifth discipline: the art and practice of the learning organisation. Currency Doubleday, New York

Senge P M, Kleiner A, Roberts C, Ross R B, Smith B J 1994 The fifth discipline fieldbook: strategies and tools for building a learning organisation. Nicholas Brealey, London

Tanner C A, Benner P, Chesla C, Gordon D R 1993 The phenomenology of knowing the patient. Image: Journal of Nursing Scholarship 25(4): 273–280

United Kingdom Central Council for Nursing, Midwifery and Health Visiting (UKCC) 1992 The scope of professional practice. UKCC, London

United Kingdom Central Council for Nursing, Midwifery and Health Visiting (UKCC) 1994 The future of professional practice: the Council's standards for education and practice following registration. UKCC, London

United Kingdom Central Council for Nursing, Midwifery and Health Visiting (UKCC) 1996 Clinical supervision. UKCC, London

United Kingdom Central Council for Nursing, Midwifery and Health Visiting (UKCC) 1997 PREP – the nature of advanced practice, CC/97/06. UKCC, London

United Kingdom Central Council for Nursing, Midwifery and Health Visiting (UKCC) 1999 A higher level of practice: draft descriptor and standard 29/3/99. UKCC, London

Warfield C, Manley K 1990 Developing a new philosophy in the NDU. Nursing Standard 4(41): 27–30

2

The surgical nurse as independent and collaborative practitioner

Loretta Bellman

AIMS

This chapter aims to:

- explore and develop the role of the surgical nurse as both an independent and a collaborative practitioner
- value the therapeutic interventions that may be developed within these roles
- promote critical reflection on strategies for independent and collaborative practice.

INTRODUCTION

The surgical nurse's role is dynamic and multifaceted and continues to evolve as a result of changes from within nursing, national and local service policies, and as a consequence of rapidly changing technology. The surgical nurse of the 21st century therefore needs to be a flexible, confident, professional practitioner who is able to articulate nursing values and effectively innovate caring practices for the benefit of patients and carers, in collaboration with the interprofessional team. A contradiction appears to exist between the need for the surgical nurse to act as both an independent and also a collaborative practitioner. Yet, incorporating these two dimensions of the surgical nurse's role into practice will not only demonstrate the provision of high-quality care, it will enhance effective interprofessional relationships as well as contribute towards the advancement of both personal and clinical practice development.

Within the nursing strategy document entitled 'The Challenges for Nursing and Midwifery in the 21st Century'(DoH 1994) nurses are viewed as 'more independent, alone or working in teams, coping with rapid changes in a quasi-market setting, coming to terms perhaps with new forms of accountability and changed perceptions across society' (p. 23).

Surgical nurses need to be cognisant of changes in health care provision; they need to consider how nursing changes will affect others and reflect on how these changes will affect them personally. For this to occur: 'There must be an open collaborative approach to managing this, with nurses helping shape the agenda and make the choices' (DoH 1994).

Independent and cross-boundary working have also been emphasised within the 'Working for Patients' document (DoH 1989). It is essential therefore to explore the nature of both the independent and collaborative practitioner roles to enable surgical nurses to work in collaboration with patients and their carers, and to be at the forefront of nursing practice change and developments.

This chapter is loosely divided into two sections – the independent practitioner and the collaborative practitioner. Yet, it is recognised that the boundary between the two roles is arbitrary and often invisible. Indeed, although nurses may pursue professional autonomy within independent roles, the opportunity for collaborative practice should also be nurtured between nurse and patients; nurse and carers; nurse and nurse; nurse and interprofessional teams; nurse and managers.

INDEPENDENT NURSE PRACTITIONER

The concept of the independent nurse practitioner may conjure up different meanings and images. These differing perceptions may include a self-employed nurse acting as a consultant; a nurse practitioner; a nurse in a specialist role, for example a stomatherapist, a breast care nurse, an infection control nurse; a nurse in an expanded role, for example a surgeon's assistant, a nurse anaesthetist; a research nurse; a lecturer–practitioner; a practice nurse in a community health centre/GP clinic. An exploration of the nursing literature reveals fascinating insights into the diverse meaning of the concept of independent nurse practitioner for each nurse and also its significance in relation to therapeutic nursing interventions.

THERAPEUTIC NURSING

According to Wright (1991), independent practice is linked to therapeutic nursing which is operationalised through holistic healing and humane approaches. He asserts that each individual nurse's expressive skills demonstrate therapeutic nursing. Examples of independent therapeutic skills may be reflected, for example:

- in the preoperative phase:
  - providing psychological comfort to an anxious person
  - a ward visit from the theatre nurse

- postoperatively:
  - anticipating, assessing and effectively relieving a person's pain
  - implementing and evaluating individual ways of helping patients regain their independence
  - discharge planning.

Wright (1991) asserts that independent therapeutic actions are often viewed as 'basic, menial tasks', yet, they each are actually complex and intricate. They encompass both personal and professional values and beliefs about nursing and a wealth of nursing knowledge. Lumby (1991, p. 468) acknowledges the art of nursing through the nurse's creative use of light, space, sound, words, movement and touch. The nurse is busy 'creating' the day and appropriate environment for another person.

Snyder (1992) states that nurses have been using independent nursing interventions, but little attention has been given to identifying and describing those activities that foster creativity in practice. Kubsch (1996), in her exploratory, grounded theory study, identified psychomotor and affective as well as cognitive interventions (see Table 2.1). Psychomotor interventions were tangible and observable in that they involved 'hands-on' care. Affective interventions were used to support or change various emotional states. Cognitive interventions were used to increase abilities in problem-solving, prevention and adaptation. The hospital setting was found to be the most difficult in which to practice therapeutic nursing interventions. However, Scholes (1996) produced evidence from observational data, nurses' interviews and video footage to demonstrate the ways in which critical care nurses use self as a therapeutic tool (see Box 2.1).

According to Allsopp (1991, p. 86) the identification and application of independent nursing interventions significantly advanced the surgical unit's professional practice of nursing. The independent nursing interventions implemented in Allsopp's surgical unit included:

- advanced and diverse wound care
- alternative temperature-taking regime
- therapeutic massage
- music and relaxation
- natural juice therapy.

Each nurse may therefore be considered an independent therapeutic practitioner. However, in order to develop the role effectively the surgical nurse needs to be able to:

Table 2.1 Examples of independent therapeutic nursing interventions (adapted from Kubsch 1996)

Psychomotor interventions	Affective interventions	Cognitive interventions
Breathing strategies	Presencing – 'being there'	Problem-solving
Positioning	Touch	Teaching
Bowel/bladder training	Reminiscence	Distraction
Sensory stimulation	Active listening	Journal writing

Box 2.1 The use of self as a therapeutic tool (adapted from Scholes 1996)

Bringing comfort by:
- relieving fear and anxiety
- relieving pain
- reorienting the patient who is confused
- reaching a patient whom others could not
- facilitating a death which is dignified, pain-free, peaceful
- establishing trust
- managing complex care situations that bring great comfort

Bringing comfort to the relatives by:
- establishing a special bond and trust

Advocating:
- speaking up on behalf of patients and ensuring that their wishes are fulfilled

Reflective point

Which independent nursing interventions, including those already mentioned, have you used in practice? Which would you consider implementing for your client group? How would you elicit more information including research evidence regarding these strategies?

- demonstrate in practice personal values and beliefs about surgical nursing therapeutic interventions
- identify and value personal, aesthetic, ethical, and evidence-based knowledge
- feel confident to articulate this aspect of the surgical practitioner's role to a wider audience, (including to non-nurse managers and other health care professionals).

Equally important is the need to determine gaps in personal knowledge which may be identified through reflection on practice within the enlightening process of clinical/professional supervision (Johns 1993).

Advancing one's knowledge results in increased personal and professional confidence and its application in practice enhances the quality of patient care. Snyder (1992) suggests that one reason that many nurses seek advanced education is to function in a more autonomous manner. However, to be able to use independent therapeutic nursing interventions Kubsch (1996) asserts that nurses need to function within work cultures that are tolerant of nursing autonomy and intervention.

AN AUTONOMOUS PRACTITIONER?

Implicit within the independent nurse practitioner role is the notion of autonomy. Yet, there are perceived differences in operationalising these two concepts. Mitchinson (1996) suggests that autonomous practice is 'professional practice which is defined, negotiated and developed by individual practitioners who are solely responsible and accountable to the patient and to their professional body for their actions and omissions' (p. 34). Independent practice is slightly different as professionals have less freedom to define their practice but are able to negotiate a degree of freedom within their prescribed role without direct supervision or monitoring from any other practitioner or manager, i.e.: 'Practice which is assigned to and developed by individual practitioners who are then responsible and accountable for their actions which are undertaken without direct supervision or monitoring from any other practitioner or manager' (Mitchinson 1996, p. 34).

However, according to Batey & Lewis (1982), the various uses of the concept of autonomy do include self-direction, independence, and not being controlled.

Gray & Pratt (1991) assert that autonomy cannot be considered in isolation from responsibility and authority in nursing. If authority is defined as the rightful power to fulfil responsibility, it would be derived from two sources. Firstly, the organisational structure should provide for the exercise of autonomy. However, Clifford (in Lorentzon 1993) argues that preoccupation with measurement has been taken up by managers as a way of controlling health professionals and denying them autonomy. Indeed, this is certainly the case when auditing tools are produced which do not reflect the qualitative nature of surgical nursing practice. For example, to what extent are the following skilled nursing practices valued?

- 'being there' for a highly anxious patient prior to forthcoming surgery
- comfort and support for a recently bereaved family
- patient participation in the development, testing, implementation and evaluation of operation-specific patient information leaflets
- exploration and understanding of the behaviour of the 'unpopular patient' (Stockwell 1972).

Many surgical nurses will be able to identify with the following – intuitively knowing that a patient's condition has changed, for better or worse, before there is any explicit clinical evidence. Although this significant aspect of nursing knowledge and skill can not be 'captured' within an audit tool, it needs to be recognised and valued equally amongst audit criteria.

Reflective point

Do you consider that the audit tools that are used in your surgical area are appropriate? To what extent have nurses in your area been included in the creation/selection of clinical audit tools? What creative approaches to audit can you identify to attempt to accommodate the above nursing examples?

The second factor, according to Gray & Pratt (1991), which restricts nursing autonomy is when accountability to the patient is viewed as being less important than accountability to the agency in which the nurse operates. This may happen as professional boundaries become blurred, in particular, when taking on duties once performed by a junior doctor. Indeed, the UKCC (1996) states that in exercising your professional accountability, there may be conflict between the interests of a patient or client, the health or social care team and society … 'Whatever decisions you take and judgements you make, you must be able to justify your actions' (p. 8).

Reflective point

To whom are you accountable?

Walsh (1997) discusses the heavy burden of accountability. The nurse is accountable to:

- the UKCC code of professional conduct
- the employer, including compliance with the employer's policies and protocols
- the law of the land
- the patient, to whom the nurse clearly has a duty of care
- herself or himself, as the nurse's own conscience normally induces a desire to ensure that she or he has done the best for the patient.

Some surgical nurses may also be accountable to a medical practitioner and/or the Surgical Directorate. Indeed, Øvretveit (1997, p. 15) identifies the need for interprofessional team accountability. The burden of accountability is therefore not only heavy but complex. Consequently, to address the complexity of accountability for evolving surgical nursing roles, central combined action from the UKCC, the General Medical Council and the NHS Executive is required. In the development of nursing expertise Conway (1996) states that expert practice does not develop in a vacuum and issues to do with autonomy and authority, advocacy, assertiveness and empowerment all need to be considered (see Box 2.2).

Indeed it could be argued that nurses may only achieve independent practitioner status when they are empowered to define their role and the parameters of their practice. To advance this process the surgical

---

Box 2.2 Issues of autonomy and authority (Conway 1996, pp. 25–26

We were very busy … on ITU [with] lots of critically ill patients … one of the patients coned … and was going down to theatre for organ harvesting and there is a lot of organising in that. My manager thought that once the patient was brain dead, then they would not require much care and the nurse could be cancelled for the following shift. I was told to cancel a bank nurse that we had booked for the late shift and I refused to do so … When the manager came down and saw the bank nurse, I was pulled up again for it, but I felt I justified my position. I felt that as the clinical expert I was there to tell the manager the needs of my patients, which would reflect on the number of staff at the time … It seemed as if all the manager could see was this patient who was not moving, going on a bed to theatre for his life to be ended and she did not seem prepared to see beyond that. There is an awful lot of care needed for the relatives. Had I not had the bank nurse I feel I would have taken the incident further, but as it happened the incident fizzled out.

nurse would need to explore power relationships, recognise disempowerment feelings and situations, and initiate or elect to participate in collaborative practice to enable the discrete, sometimes invisible, value of nursing to be recognised and rewarded.

POWER AND INFLUENCE

Within the context of surgical nursing practice, power relationships and imbalances exist between nurse and patient, nurse and nurse, nurse and doctor and associated health care professionals, nurse and manager. Hawks (1991) maintains that power has two main meanings, 'power to' and 'power over'. 'Power over' is a struggle for dominance or to rise from an inferior to a superior position. It encompasses control, competitiveness, authority and some forms of leadership. 'Power to' relates to effectiveness and includes the ability to achieve objectives, the means of attaining them and the capacity to do so. Power as an interpersonal process involves participation. This definition equates with the power released through collaboration and commitment to one's peers, patients and professional colleagues.

Nurses often tend to believe that they have little power and consider the concept from a negative perspective. They feel that they are unable or lack the authority to make decisions or to effect change. This can lead to a self-fulfilling prophecy by undervaluing one's worth and the status of nursing. Street (1995, p. 25), a sociologist, asks nurses to analyse the control myths in nursing. She encourages nurses to create new rituals to replace the traditional ones of dependence and oppression:

Together nurses are discovering the power to disbelieve the control myths that disempower nurses and patients ... We are discovering the subtleties of disempowering language ... We hear ourselves say:

No, he is not a doctor. He is **just** a nurse!

It is the job of the primary nurse to ask the doctor what **he** wants done with **his** patients.

Let's ask **the girls** if they want to change the format for the nursing care plans.

(Street 1995, p. 17)

Reflective point

In your clinical area listen closely to the way that language is used by nurses. In particular note derogatory expressions such as comments and exchanges which demonstrate an undermining of nurses' self-worth and ability. How may this situation be rectified?

Surgical nurses function in both powerful and powerless positions. They may not recognise the extent of their power that may be used over patients. Disempowering routine practices may be employed, for example telling patients to change into night attire on admission to hospital, withholding information, removing and locking away medications and cigarettes, offering patients few choices or little opportunity to participate in their care.

Taken for granted cultural norms and traditional practices enable both nurses and patients to participate willingly in their own domination without even recognising it. For surgical nurses to function in an independent way they need to feel and to be empowered. They need to analyse critically and, where appropriate, question, challenge and change the status quo.

Nurse–doctor relationships reveal a paradox of power differentials. Within the interprofessional team there should be equal recognition of each member's contribution. Stein et al (1990), three doctors, explored the political and social changes which surround the (revisited) doctor–nurse game. They concluded: 'Physicians and nurses can both benefit if their relationship becomes more mutually interdependent. Subservient and dominant roles are both psychologically restricting. When a subordinate becomes liberated, there is potential for the dominant one to become liberated too' (Stein et al 1990, p. 549).

Yet, Warelow (1996, p. 34) states: 'it is well documented that issues of medical dominance within health care settings are manifold with, in some cases, nursing staff allowing this situation to be maintained by remaining silent.' The author also believes that nurses often undermine or sabotage in a passive/aggressive way decisions made by the (medical) team rather than individually or collectively confronting and/or challenging the power base of medicine. The status quo is therefore maintained.

For all the above reasons and 'to reclaim and regenerate nursing, the profession must be looked at with a fresh sense of vision and from new points of view' (Ford & Walsh 1994). Many authors (Bellman 1997, Crane 1991, Warelow 1996) now advocate an understanding by all nurses of critical social theory. Critical social theory entails exposing the contradictions, oppressions and power imbalances that inhibit both nurses' individual freedom and autonomy and those of patients. Key concepts which reflect the application of this theory to practice are reflection, understanding, action. Ford & Walsh (1994) assert: 'The notion of social critical theory ... has striking relevance for nursing, so much so that we might usefully talk of empowerment as liberation nursing.'

The application of this theory in practice underpins the approach to adult learning and education advocated by Mezirow (1981). This theoretical perspective is the basis of the guided structured reflection process for exploring expert practice proposed by Manley & McCormack (1997). Critical social theory, when operationalised within an action research study, is an empowering problem-solving approach to change, undertaken on either a micro or macro scale. The process involves nurses identifying and exploring current political influences which constrain and even oppress their current practice and the sociocultural context in which they work.

'In this sense a critical social science will provide the kind of self-reflective understanding that will permit individuals to explain why the conditions under which they operate are frustrating and will suggest the sort of action that is required if the sources of these frustrations are to be eliminated' (Carr & Kemmis 1986).

Examples of this approach include: transformative cultural shifts in nursing (Robinson 1995); the development of advanced clinical roles (Manley 1997, Sutton & Smith 1995); a nurse curriculum revolution (Hendricks-Thomas & Patterson 1995); changing nursing practice (Bellman 1996); advancing practice development (Bellman 1997); researching nursing culture (Street 1995).

According to Murrell (1985), two factors which really determine a person's power in an organisation are:

- information and knowledge
- interpersonal competence or the ability to work with other people in order to accomplish tasks.

A conceptual framework has been developed for empowering individuals by managers. The six key concepts to be adopted by managers are:

1. educating
2. leading (sometimes from behind)
3. structuring – creating structures in which people can become powerful and not alienated
4. providing – the provision of resources for people to get their job done or for them to feel and act powerful
5. mentoring
6. actualising – the summation of all the five previous methods put together.

Murrell (1985, p. 37) asserts that empowerment is a positive use of power to create more power and to energise an organisation. This cannot be done without risk, and it cannot be done under total control.

To empower requires a great deal of trust and confidence in those with whom you are working. It also means that there needs to be a more enlightened and less traditional, entrenched approach regarding the nature of the nursing, medical, and management hierarchy. Health service leaders, within NHS trusts and the independent sector, at both local and executive level of the organisation should consider the adoption of a transformational leadership approach. Sashkin (1988, cited in Antrobus 1997) identifies five specific charismatic behaviours to achieve organisational transformation:

- Focus attention on specifics
- Take risks that create opportunities
- Employ two-way skilful communication that incorporates active listening and feedback
- Demonstrate consistent trustworthy behaviour, with follow-through on commitment
- Have active, expressed concern for people that reinforces the worth of others and self.

The decision to empower staff assumes that employees are able to make appropriate decisions. However, nurses often fail to question who holds or acquires power and underestimate their potential as a group to exercise power (Gray & Pratt 1991, p. 360). Indeed the importance of collectively working together to effect change is of great significance. This enables the surgical nurse to act as a change agent and interrelate the roles of independent and collaborative practitioner.

CHANGE AGENT

The knowledge base for the nurse as change agent encompasses knowledge of the environment for change, change theories, empowering and collaborative strategies for change, skills of facilitating change, methods of evaluating/auditing the change. Change agents must have the ability, the commitment and the support to question the status quo; to challenge outmoded nursing practices; to be a clinical leader. Five interrelated factors which are considered essential to the accomplishment of change are:

- the innovation itself
- the environment
- the users
- change agent/s
- change strategies (ENB 1987).

Wright (1989) believes that the potential to be a change agent lies, to a greater or lesser extent, in every nurse. Change is a complex, continuous process. There needs to be 'protected time' in practice to explore the change process and develop a shared commitment to developing action plans, implementation and evaluation. Six attributes for an effective change agent have been identified by Lancaster (1982):

1. Be accessible to all who are involved in the change process.
2. Develop trust among participants.
3. Be honest and straightforward about goals, plans, priorities, and problems.
4. Keep the goals clearly in mind and assist others to do so and not get diverted by side issues or activities.
5. Define (jointly) the responsibilities of others; enable the participants the freedom to do their part.
6. Listen.

To this list the nurse change agent should add the need to share personal values and beliefs with peers about surgical nursing. This will help to build a trusting relationship, the foundation on which to develop the change process. This approach is two-way; colleagues' values and beliefs about surgical nursing should also be clarified. Manley (1992) advocates the use of a values clarification exercise. This strategy should enhance a 'bottom-up' approach to change. Also, power issues need to be identified. From personal reflection, when surgical nurses meet together they often cite critical incidents which involve, in many instances, perceived conflict with doctors and managers. Feelings of (perceived) powerlessness need to be aired in a supportive environment where each individual situation may be analysed with one's peers. The need to highlight the conflict in relation to both personal values and beliefs about nursing and the role of the surgical nurse are paramount. Rogers (1989) notes that for many nurses, having an opportunity to discuss the meaning of nursing and to talk about their beliefs, values and assumptions is a new experience.

The practitioner, to be an effective change agent, needs to demonstrate self-worth, and value and respect for her peers. Speedy (1989) claims that nurses think of themselves as second-class citizens and lack self-esteem. Rogers (1989) asserts that many nurses are not consciously aware of nor do they value their nursing knowledge and their capacity to affect the health of people. Nurses tend to value medical knowledge more highly. However, Fry et al (1994) believe that nurses are no longer submissive powerless people; nursing is learning to value itself as its own best resource. Indeed, a significant change that has been implemented which demonstrates the value of independent and collaborative nursing practice is that of primary nursing.

PRIMARY NURSING

Primary nursing is a system of organising care. The primary nurse functions in both independent and collaborative roles and has achieved a level of competence to use her authority (the power to act) and autonomy (the freedom to act) to benefit the patient. Other key concepts which reflect the role include accountability, continuity, coordination of care and comprehensiveness of care.

When considering whether to adopt this system of organisation the surgical nurse should firstly consider the philosophical perspectives that underpin the approach. Manley (1994, p. 45) has cited her beliefs about primary nursing:

- The nurse–patient relationship is therapeutic
- The central focus of nursing is the patient (and the patient's family) not the task
- The development of the personal knowledge of practitioners is essential to the successful practice of primary nursing
- Decentralised decision-making can improve the job satisfaction of nurses, if this takes place within a supportive and nurturing environment
- Improved job satisfaction indirectly improves the quality of care for patients.

Allsopp (1991) believes that the introduction and implementation of primary nursing created the chance to give more individualised care and a greater level of continuity of care. As a result of implementing primary nursing:

- the use of the nursing process improved dramatically
- nursing audit revealed an improvement in the quality of care particularly in the areas of individual psychosocial care, communication and initiative
- personal motivation and job satisfaction were found amongst the nurses
- patients seemed to appreciate the individualised approach to care (p. 85).

McCormack (1992) evaluated primary nursing following implementation in a general surgical ward

---

Reflective point

When considering adoption of primary nursing, a philosophical shift in thinking about the nature and purpose of nursing is required. To what extent are your personal beliefs about surgical nursing practice congruent with those of primary nursing?

in a district general hospital over a 2-year period. Ethnographic methods were employed and data collection was by diary-keeping and semi-structured interviews. McCormack (1992) identified 13 key issues which demonstrate the nurses' feelings regarding the change to primary nursing (see Box 2.3).

The extent to which primary nursing has had an impact on patient satisfaction was explored by Thomas et al (1996). The authors suggest that their findings hold some surprises for advocates of primary nursing. The data analysis revealed that wards using primary nursing did not generate more positive experiences of nursing care or higher levels of patient satisfaction.

Box 2.3 Key issues in primary nursing (McCormack 1992)

- Nurses on the ward feel more directly involved in patient care on a continuous basis than in previous posts.
- The nurses feel they have an increased knowledge of this system, thereby leading to more accurate individualised care planning and caregiving.
- The role of the nurse as patient advocate appears to be made more explicit in this organisational framework.
- There are indicators that these nurses have an increased sense of accountability and responsibility while remaining unclear about their distinctions.
- The nurses feel more autonomous in their work but find the restrictions on and interruptions to their autonomy frustrating and restrictive.
- There is evidence that there is a relationship between the number of patients each primary nurse has responsibility for and the resulting quality of care.
- There is evidence that these nurses experience an increase in level of stress and that knowledge and experience have some relationship in coping with this.
- These nurses feel satisfied in their work and the greatest satisfaction comes from the nurse–patient relationship.
- The nurses indicate that they have an increased knowledge of fewer patients but experience role conflict between this and the 'in charge' role.
- There is evidence that there is a poor relationship between doctors and nurses in this particular organisation.
- Student nurses appear to develop role conflict in this particular setting and this appears to cause problems in the ward team.
- The nurses appear to feel a heightened sense of responsibility for students' learning and devote a lot of energy towards it.
- There is evidence that these nurses appear to feel a sense of ownership over patients and have difficulty letting go.

The most significant problem, according to Allsopp (1991), was the increase in stress within the primary nurse role, as nurses take on more responsibility. The recognition and management of the potential for increased stress within a primary nursing system is acknowledged by Manley (1994). However, her extensive critical exploration of primary nursing encompasses many positive perspectives.

Indeed, a forum for open discussion where staff feel supported in their role needs to be created and maintained. Creating a psychologically safe environment where staff can share their anxieties and plan for change should be a priority before primary nursing is implemented; it will facilitate the change process and subsequently should be ongoing.

Johns (1992) discusses the stresses of both primary and associate nurse and the need to create an harmonious therapeutic team. He cautions that the emphasis on developing autonomy within primary nurses may be misguided if it results in these nurses perceiving themselves as independent from their colleagues, with a reliance on self-coping methods of working rather than mutual working and sharing methods of working. Indeed, Rafferty (1992) previously noted that primary nursing may also be detrimental to the cohesiveness of the ward team. Yet, primary nursing may strengthen collaboration with the interprofessional team.

In spite of some acknowledged problems, the move to primary nursing may be viewed as an innovative and empowering process for nurses, which demonstrates continuity and enhancement of patient care. The role of the primary nurse may be further developed within a system of case management.

CASE MANAGEMENT

Hale (1997) acknowledges that case management is expanding and broadening its scope to encompass acute care areas and to manage the hospital–community interface. In acute care areas the case managers are frequently nurses. According to Lamb (1995), nurse case managers appear to work with individuals, families, and populations at high risk of adverse health outcomes; they are responsible for applying the nursing process in ways that potentially enhance both quality and cost outcomes; they have access to individuals and families in more than one localised setting.

Case managers in hospital-based models work across units; case managers in continuum-based models work across multiple settings (Lamb 1995). Common to all case management models are the following service components:

- client identification and outreach
- individual assessment and diagnosis
- service planning and resource identification – linking clients to needed services
- service implementation and coordination
- monitoring service delivery
- advocacy
- evaluation (Allred et al 1995).

The key aspects of the role appear to be: the nurse as clinical expert in the management of complex illnesses; the nurse as a caring and accessible partner in patients' health experiences; the nurse as coordinator of care through the use of managed care tools such as multidisciplinary pathways of care (see p. 37 and Ch. 20) and by the facilitation of a collaborative interprofessional team communication network. Yet, Lamb (1995, p. 133) concludes from her literature review that as the number of professions and individuals with a stake in the future of case management expands, it is increasingly difficult to cut through the debate and rhetoric to get to some basic questions, such as: What is case management? Who needs it? Who provides it? For how long? What are its outcomes? What are its costs?

Ignatavicius & Hausman (1995) describe case management as a practice model which uses a systematic approach to identify specific patients and to manage patient care to ensure optimum outcomes. Hale (1997, p. 69) cites two basic models of case management which originated in the USA:

1. From Boston – nursing case management is seen as an extension of the primary nurse's role. High-risk patients are identified; the primary nurse initiates the relationship before admission whenever possible, is involved in the implementation of care, actively engages in discharge planning and follows up the patient for 2 weeks or more after discharge.

2. The Arizona model sets selection criteria for high-risk patients in each clinical area. These patients are then referred to a nursing case manager (a separate role) who monitors and coordinates the patient's case with the primary nurse, physician and other health professionals. He or she may be a direct caregiver. In this model, the role of case manager may transcend the boundary between hospital and community.

Jones (1995) has reservations regarding this system of organisation for UK nurses. The author explores how case management appears to have evolved within the American and British literature from an initial cost-containment focus to an approach that also addresses quality issues. Latterly, there is an emphasis on empowerment of the patient and family to make choices within a coordinated care framework. Whilst

acknowledging that case management has its genesis in the philosophical age of humanism (with the extension of primary nursing and the nursing process), Jones (1995) proposes that this is incongruent with the pragmatic values of consumerism. In particular, there may be conflict between the case manager and the interprofessional team; having responsibility for effective outcomes for both the patient and the organisation may prove problematic; the process of case management re-establishes quality of care as a product rather than a service.

Lamb (1995) highlights the dearth of nursing research on case management. Yet Smith (1993) believes that case management is essential to the transformation of health care for the 21st century. She believes that the integration of nursing theory (e.g. the Newman and Watson theories of nursing) with case management systems results in true professional nursing practice.

Reflective point

What do you envisage as the costs and benefits for nurses, patients, the interprofessional team, the organisation, of implementing a case management system of care in your practice area?

TEAM NURSING

Team nursing encompasses collective responsibility; it views the team leader and team members as collaborative caregivers. According to Rafferty (1992) the method assumes the premiss that nurses working in small groups with a team leader provide better care than when working as individuals. There is no one way of practising team nursing but Kron (cited in Waters 1985) cites three prerequisites:

1. Each team is led by a registered nurse, who must have leadership and management skills.
2. There must be effective communication, both written and spoken.
3. The style of ward management must ensure the role of the team leader can be practised.

These requisites reflect two underlying philosophical beliefs: that every patient has the right to receive the best care that can be provided, and that all workers have the right to receive help in doing the best work they are capable of doing.

The ward manager's role is one of overall coordinator and expert support for each of the teams (usually two or three per ward). Each team has a team leader who assumes a leadership role, yet there is shared responsibility for patient care within the team. This approach advocates both collective accountability and power-sharing. However, nurses are accountable for their own practice whatever system of organisation is implemented.

To develop both as an independent and collaborative practitioner whether it be within a primary nursing, case management or team nursing system, the surgical nurse must identify her unique function and role. Rafferty (1992) has highlighted that although there is increased collaboration when primary nursing is used, accountability to doctors is still a view which is widely held. This view values dependence and subservience to the doctor, and may also reflect surgical nursing practice within team nursing and case management systems too. An exploration of the concept of collaboration should enable surgical nurses to value their knowledge, skills, clinical judgements alongside those of their peers and medical colleagues.

THE CONCEPT OF COLLABORATION

Collaboration is a complex phenomenon in which nurses engage with others as a means of enabling surgical patients' goals to be realised and improving workplace relationships and practice. Henneman et al (1995) suggest that the concept of collaboration is being heralded as the solution to many of the problems arising from the more traditional, hierarchical workplace. Indeed, Strumpf & Asimos (1996) assert that collaborative practice, although largely misunderstood, rarely valued by academic institutions ... 'is a necessary ingredient in accountable advanced nursing practice and for solutions to (America's) continuing health care crisis' (p. 173).

Although the emphasis on collaboration is strong, there is still little information available that provides direction for accomplishing this formidable task (Oie & Recker 1992). Indeed, the study of collaboration is, according to Henneman et al (1995), in its infancy. The literature does, though, provide some useful information regarding the nature of collaboration as well as strategies for the surgical nurse to consider.

A concept analysis of collaboration was undertaken by Henneman et al (1995). They identified nine specific attributes (see Box 2.4). To enable sharing of knowledge and collective responsibility, certain individual and environmental factors need to be in place:

- an individual's readiness to collaborate
- an understanding of one's own role and expertise
- confidence in one's ability

- excellent communication skills
- respect and trust for collaborative partners.

The working context requires a team orientation with effective group dynamics; recognition of the boundaries of one's discipline; visionary leaders supportive of autonomy; organisational values which include participation and interdependence. These antecedents reflect a nursing leadership approach for the 21st century, which includes connective leadership.

CONNECTIVE LEADERSHIP

'The style of leadership which connects individuals creatively to their tasks and visions, to one another, to the immediate group and the larger network, empowering others and instilling confidence, represents a crucial set of strategies for success, not only in the workplace, but in our interdependent world community' (Lipman-Blumen, cited in Klakovich 1994, p. 187).

According to Klakovich (1994) this new leadership paradigm will effectively address health care reform while preserving caring practice. The outcomes of connective leadership are identified as:

- a caring, professional practice environment with empowered nursing staff
- collaboration among health care disciplines
- an increase in the contributions that nursing makes to health care policy and delivery system changes.

Yet, although she asserts that nurse practitioners and nurse managers must be aligned and working toward the accomplishment of mutual goals, she asks: 'How do we rid our profession of the elitism that has systematically devalued nursing practitioners and begin to value what everyone contributes?' (p. 52).

Box 2.4 The defining attributes of the concept of collaboration (Henneman et al 1995)

- Joint venture
- Cooperative endeavour
- Willing participation
- Shared planning and decision-making
- Team approach
- Contribution of expertise
- Shared responsibility
- Non-hierarchical relationships
- Power-sharing – on the basis of knowledge and expertise not role or title

Interestingly, she equates the qualities of connective clinical nursing leaders with those of effective change agents. These leaders have mastered interdependence by creating strategic alliances, discouraging competition, and encouraging cooperation among all stakeholders in the change process.

Reflective point

Is collaboration a valued concept in your practice area? Reflect on the previous discussion, on the antecedents and attributes of the concept of collaboration and consider the extent to which you believe that you engage in collaborative practice with peers, students, patients, carers, health care professionals, managers.

THE ELEMENTS OF COLLABORATION

According to Spross (1989), three elements essential to collaboration emerge from the literature. These are:

- common purpose
- diverse and complementary skills and contributions
- coordinating and communicating processes.

Common purpose

The need for a common purpose may seem straightforward yet when this is not clearly stated its absence can compromise patient care. A common shared sense of purpose should lead to cohesive and valued working relationships. Street (1995, p. 36) provides examples of how nurses work together to understand and restructure their clinical practices so as to care for the interests of ill people and their families rather than responding to the competing demands of clinical rituals, or medical and administrative interests. She states that the nurses were both courageous and supportive of each other as they put their clinical practices under scrutiny and began to discover that caring actions were actions which empowered people and that to do this required the restructuring of their workloads to prioritise time spent with people. The nurses in the group were challenged to think about how they could collaborate to help each other meet the needs of the families in their care.

Collaborators want to work together. They believe that their combined efforts are synergistic – that the sum of their combined efforts is greater than independent efforts. They trust each other and acknowledge interdependence (Spross 1989).

Complementary skills and contributions

The existence and recognition of divergent and complementary skills and contributions is the second essential element to enable collaboration to emerge. Valuing and seeking individual contributions from peers and health care professionals enables greater team cohesion and insight into service colleagues' roles. Open communication, group problem-solving and consensus enable this to occur. In an action research study (Bellman 1996), diverse professional skills and contributions were elicited from surgical nurses and interprofessionals at the group meetings:

The group sessions were very, very useful. Things that you think are silly then you find out that other people have the same problems. I think we gave each other a lot of confidence. We all got together and found ways round the problems whereas one person probably wouldn't have been able to do it ... everyone had their say.

(Lorraine, Staff Nurse)

I felt that once they got used to the group idea it brought out people who might normally have said nothing. I thought that some quite good ideas came out of it. They all agreed to do things and they actually did it.

(Mary, Ward Manager)

They were especially good for a moan. We looked into how to solve problems ... everybody's input was considered.

(Fiona, Staff Nurse)

Yet the study by Mackenzie (1993) revealed that a quarter of the sisters/charge nurses ($n = 93$) did not feel free to make autonomous decisions on clinical and professional matters. Likewise, East & Robinson (1993) found that many ward sisters who wanted to make changes seemed blocked at every turn: 'they felt like victims of organisational forces over which they had no control'. However, the knowledge and skills of expert nurses are acknowledged within 'The Scope of Professional Practice' (UKCC 1992), complementing those of medical colleagues, and increasingly receiving recognition in many NHS trust and independent sector clinical settings.

Coordinating and communicating processes

Webb (1989) asserts that a collaborative and supportive atmosphere is the essential foundation for motivation and commitment to change. For this to occur and for the provision of quality care, effective coordination and communication is crucial. Yet Spross (1989) presents many timely reminders regarding the obstacles to collaboration. These particularly reflect the lack of coordination and communication and the conflicts that occur in clinical practice. The nature of collaborative practice within an interprofessional team does not just happen, it evolves. It is naive to expect individuals from different professional groups to work as a collaborative team without an investment of time to develop relationships.

Obstacles to coordinating and communicating

Increased acuteness of illness in both inpatient and outpatient settings has resulted in nurses and health care providers becoming 'one-minute managers' (Spross 1989). There appears to be less time to communicate or team build. This problem is exacerbated if there is an inappropriate nursing skill/grade mix and also by alternative shift patterns which reduce contact time between peers. Lip service may be paid to collaboration whereby managers, nurses, link-lecturers, consultants may provide verbal support for a team initiative but no effort or overt behavioural commitment is evident. Goren & Ottoway (1985, cited in Spross 1989) refer to collusion whereby there is either a conscious or unconscious commitment to maintain the status quo.

Lack of acknowledgement amongst nurses and doctors regarding shared ideas and knowledge can result in conflict. For example, a surgical nurse may have specialist wound care knowledge which when offered is ignored by the surgeon. This lack of collaboration and devaluing of nurse's knowledge on the doctor's part can lead to a nurse feeling frustrated and even humiliated.

McEniery (1992) asserts that there is a need for recognition of each other's competence, and a willingness to behave in ways which provide for the interpersonal support which will assist in buffering against the organisational pressures and stresses that both groups encounter in their professional lives. Experienced, knowledgeable and confident nursing leaders are required to initiate and sustain collaborative practice. They need to facilitate a common purpose, recognise and value diverse professional skills and contributions, and enable effective coordinating and communicating processes. There must be an overt commitment by all members of the team to engage in collaboration.

COLLABORATIVE STRATEGIES

Collaborative/group reflection

One strategy which 'helps isolate the disempowering potential of rituals that nurses subscribe to' (Street 1995) is that of collaborative reflection. This approach to group reflection can be adopted by nurse practitioners, educators, managers and researchers. Group reflection can be undertaken within any surgical setting. It requires sensitive facilitation skills and managerial support to empower nurses to explore current issues and to effect change. Indeed, from group reflection on practice, surgical nurses challenged structured processes of social control and decision-making and changed the status quo (Bellman 1996).

Street (1995) believes that collaborative reflection will undo the myth that the modern nurse has no time for writing, talking, researching or reflecting on clinical practice. Titchen & Binnie (1993) found that people only become involved when they are ready and that it requires sustained investment in individuals to help them to reach a point where they are ready to move from being reflective practitioners to becoming researchers of their own practice.

Multiprofessional collaboration

Strategies to promote nurse–doctor collaboration are required. Nurse–doctor problems and potential conflict result in non-collaboration. Yet Keenan et al (1990) state that while conflict may be perceived as a disconcerting process by many nurse managers and nurses, it should also be viewed as the first step toward developing collaboration among staff members.

In the USA a National Joint Practice Commission (NJPC) was established in 1977, and comprised representatives from both nursing and medicine. The NJPC identified five elements it deemed essential to the enhancement of nurse–physician collaboration and the implementation of collaborative practice within the acute care setting. These factors were:

- primary nursing
- encouragement of nurse decision-making
- a joint practice committee
- integrated user/patient records
- a joint record review.

The role of the primary nurse/independent practitioner has previously been discussed. Primary nursing is also viewed as a major contributor to improving nurse–physician communication. There is certainly the potential for collegial sharing of knowledge and mutual respect. Nurse decision-making is defined as any decision within the scope of nursing practice that may be made using both nursing and medical consultations.

The NJPC provides a mechanism where gaps in the knowledge and understanding of each other's role and functions could be filled (Crowley & Wollner 1987). Strategies to achieve this include the integrated patient record (which is akin to the collaborative care plan) where nurses and medical staff document observations, judgements and actions. The joint user/patient care record review is also viewed as an educational experience where each discipline learns the other's rationale for care. It is, though, significant to note that there is no mention of patient involvement/participation in care.

Crowley & Wollner (1987) describe the implementation process and evaluation of the NYPC's approach to collaborative practice; the desire for change is the most important factor necessary for the implementation of the concept of collaborative practice (p. 60). However, management support is critical to its success.

Reflective point

Which strategies do you adopt to promote collaborative practice in your clinical area?

Lenkman & Gribbens (1994) provide insight into a generic process for building interdisciplinary teams. The authors advocate exploring the culture of organisations based on their goal directedness, human resource perspective, political interests, and values and beliefs of the members. In particular the authors outline factors which promote and those which militate against collaboration.

To engage in multiprofessional collaboration:

1. Establish an environment for change. This would encompass group rather than individualistic professional behaviour and should include group reflection on a shared philosophy of care for the surgical area.

2. Choose the organisational framework in which care will be given through teamwork, for example, primary nursing (see p. 31), team nursing (see p. 32), case management (see p. 33).

3. Determine barriers against successful teams. Identify the criteria for a successful team; explore the concept of collaboration and the extent to which the consequences can be identified in practice (see Box 2.5).

4. Establish opportunities and strategies for successful change. Try to reach a consensus for a change in practice. Also, explore the change literature, the action research literature and develop an action plan.

5. Embark on the educational and developmental phase of team building necessary for effective team work. Each team should pass through the following stages:
   - orientation – developing trust, open communication, defining boundaries

---

> **Box 2.5** Consequences of collaboration (Henneman et al 1995)
>
> - Supportive and nurturing environment
> - Reinforces confidence, self-worth and importance
> - Promotes win–win attitude and sense of success and accomplishment
> - Esprit de corps
> - Interprofessional cohesiveness
> - Improved productivity and effective use of personnel
> - Increased employee satisfaction
> - Improved patient outcome

- adaptation – the formation of a team identity, understanding of one another's contribution
- emergence – the ability to negotiate through resolution of power and conflict issues.

It may be appropriate to engage an 'outside' facilitator to advance this process. However, the role of facilitator must be clearly defined. A nurse and doctor as co-facilitators may be an innovative way forward.

6. Develop techniques to involve and support all staff as they learn to work in an interprofessional context. For example, regular team meetings will be required where each member in turn could chair the meeting. When the meetings are co-chaired by a nurse and doctor, 'true collaboration begins' (Kerfoot 1989).

The best way to guarantee success is to start with a project that has great possibility for success and that is uniquely suited to a practice area. One example, Kerfoot (1989) suggests, may be a quality issue which interests both professions. A joint nurse–physician collaboration project examining quality issues on a unit is a useful starting point. The purpose of the collaboration must be clearly defined, communicated and structured. Successful collaborative practice goals must have a clearly defined vision or outcome accompanied by a collaboratively devised action plan and evaluation strategy.

Positive outcomes for the interprofessional team following the implementation of the five elements of the National Joint Practice Commission (Crowley & Wollner 1987, see p. 36) are to be found in Box 2.6. Overall, achieving positive outcomes involves creating the appropriate culture in which collaboration can be nurtured and flourish.

Interprofessional/multidisciplinary pathways of care

An interprofessional approach to collaborative practice includes the development of multidisciplinary

Box 2.6 Positive outcomes of collaborative practice (adapted from Crowley & Wollner 1987)

- Improved communication, trust, respect
- Increased understanding of each other's roles and responsibilities
- Greater consideration of each other's time and effort when developing changes in practice
- A more collegial atmosphere with greater job satisfaction and feelings of self-worth
- More consistent policies and standards of practice developed
- Everyone's participation in proactive rather than reactionary change
- Reduced tensions amongst medical, nursing and administrative staff at all levels
- Patients experience a more friendly and relaxed environment

pathways of care (MPCs). MPCs have a variety of synonyms, for example anticipatory recovery pathways, critical paths, clinical paths, collaborative care plans, integrated care pathways.

The success of the MPC development process depends on the interprofessional/multidisciplinary team working collaboratively with good team spirit and sharing of responsibilities. NHS trusts have cited the outcomes of using MPCs as improved quality of care, reduced morbidity, better cost per case information, and higher patient and staff satisfaction (Wilson 1997, p. 23). MPCs also provide a catalyst for integrated care delivery, clinical research and change management.

An example of a devised MPC (Nelson 1997) is to be found in Figures 2.1–2.4. This example appears to demonstrate the nature of collaboration in action.

Reflective point

Have all appropriate aspects of surgical nursing care been included in the MPC for transurethral resection of prostate gland in Figures 2.1–2.4?

Why are psychological, spiritual and sexuality needs omitted from the MPC? This may be acceptable if a nursing care plan is also being used. However, if an MPC alone is to be used, this approach undervalues and renders invisible many aspects of holistic surgical nursing care (see also Ch. 7). There are significant and serious limitations to the use of MPCs if they only reflect a medical model framework. The need for collaboration in the development of MPCs is evident (see also Ch. 20).

Research and practice development

Sims (1991) advocates collaborative research, for example action research, for the integration of theory, research and practice. Other innovative ways of creating research and practice links include the development of nursing research liaison roles and the creation of nursing research and development units.

The main work of the research liaison nurse comprises:

- research and educational activities aimed at increasing practitioner research knowledge and skills
- research awareness
- the implementation of research findings.

Sims (1991) acknowledges that the research liaison nurse may work independently, but preferably, he or she is part of a nursing research and practice development unit. The philosophy and practice of the members of the unit should demonstrate an overt commitment to an integrated approach to practice development, research initiatives, and clinical effectiveness.

Lorentzon (1993) has suggested that little collaboration exists between nurse researchers and nurse managers; indeed there is 'evidence of disunity' between the different branches of nurses. 'Co-operation and collaboration between nurse managers, clinical nurses, researchers and educators is not optional, but a necessity in order to achieve optimum health care for patients.' (Lorentzon 1993, p. 43).

Innovative approaches should demonstrate increased cooperation and collaboration between management, research and education, for example an increase in joint-appointment posts such as the lecturer–practitioner role, the clinical professor of nursing, based in practice. A practice-based professor of surgical nursing (who I had the privilege to meet in Australia) would:

- support and initiate collaborative patient-centred practice-focused projects
- substantially raise the visibility of nursing
- demonstrate the interrelationship and value of nursing practice development, nursing research, nursing education
- demonstrate the outcomes of effective surgical nursing practice
- enable the application of surgical nursing knowledge in practice and the generation of new nursing knowledge from practice.

McEniery (1992) reinforces the need for collaboration between nursing education and nursing practice

MULTIDISCIPLINARY PATHWAY OF CARE
CHEVIOT AND WANSBECK NHS TRUST
TRANS URETHRAL RESECTION OF PROSTATE GLAND (TURP)

Patient Name: . . . .   Day & Date admitted: . . . .   Unit No: . . . .

	ADMISSION		PRE OP DAY 1		PRE OP DAY 2		OP DAY / PRE OP		OP DAY /POST OP	
M **E** **D** **I** **C** **A** **L**	HISTORY AND EXAMINATION CONSENT INCLUDING EXPLANATION OF RISKS BLOODS PSA U&E, RBG, FBC GP & SAVE ECG IF REQUIRED CXR IF REQUIRED PRESCRIBE DRUGS ANAESTHETIST ASSESSMENT		S.H.O TO REVIEW NOTES AND DISCUSS OPERATION WITH PATIENT OBTAIN BLOOD RESULTS INSTRUCTIONS AS ISSUED BY ANAESTHETIST				WARD ROUND PRIOR TO LIST IF MONDAY ANAESTHETIST ASSESSMENT		WARD ROUND	
P **H** **Y** **S** **I** **O** **T** **H** **E** **R** **A** **P** **Y**	PRE-OP ASSESSMENT TEACH BREATHING EXERCISES TEACH FOOT/ANKLE/ QUADS EXERCISES EXPLAIN NECESSITY FOR VARIOUS EXERCISES									

Figure 2.1   Multidisciplinary pathway of care for transurethral resection of prostate gland: medical and physiotherapy – pre- and perioperative periods (reproduced with kind permission from Nelson 1997).

settings. She believes that the two key reasons for this are the provision of the best quality of care for patients and a suitable learning environment for nurse students. To achieve these outcomes it is necessary that the practice environment should support questioning, enquiry, flexibility, and independence of thought rather than rigidity, conformity, dependence on rules and regulations, and adherence to long-standing practices which lack an established knowledge base.

Action research

Action research is a collaborative nursing research strategy. Hart & Bond (1995, p. 37) have identified seven criteria which distinguish action research from other methodologies. Action research:

1. is educative
2. deals with individuals as members of social groups
3. is problem-focused, context-specific and future-oriented
4. involves a change intervention
5. aims at improvement and involvement
6. involves a cyclic process in which research, action and evaluation are interlinked
7. is founded on a research relationship in which those involved are participants in the change process.

The criteria reflect the assertion of Fry et al (1994): 'The complexities of conducting a research project in the "real world" clinical setting of a busy surgical ward presents challenges to be faced and resolved.'

Action research would appear to be an appropriate collaborative approach for the challenges ahead. Indeed, action research has resulted in innovative approaches to care and role development. For example, nurses (co-researchers) in a surgical ward initiated, developed action plans, implemented and evaluated in collaboration with patients and the interprofessional team, patient self-administration of drugs, patient controlled analgesia (via a wristwatch device), patient operation-specific and drug information leaflets (Bellman 1996).

The action research process, as with any change process in clinical practice, is complex and messy.

MULTIDISCIPLINARY PATHWAY OF CARE
CHEVIOT AND WANSBECK NHS TRUST
TRANS URETHRAL RESECTION OF PROSTATE GLAND (TURP)

Patient Name: .... Day & Date admitted: .... Unit No: ....

		POST OP DAY 1		POST OP DAY 2		POST OP DAY 3		POST OP DAY 4		POST OP DAY 5	
M E D I C A L		WARD ROUND U&E FBC		WARD ROUND PRESCRIBE DISCHARGE DRUGS (AS REQUIRED)		WARD ROUND DISCHARGE LETTER TO GP WITHIN 48 HOURS					
P H Y S I O T H E R A P Y		RE-ASSESS CHEST REINFORCE BREATHING EXERCISES REINFORCE FOOT/ANKLE/ QUADS EXERCISES CHECK MOBILITY		CHECK MOBILITY							

Figure 2.2 Multidisciplinary pathway of care for transurethral resection of prostate gland: medical and physiotherapy – postoperative period (reproduced with kind permission from Nelson 1997).

However, the factors which contribute towards a positive outcome include continuous management support, a known and credible facilitator/change agent, endorsement of the change by patients and the multidisciplinary team, a knowledge of the change process, a commitment to group shared reflection, learning and action.

Collaboration with patients

How may surgical nurses work in a collaborative partnership role with patients? McEniery (1992) states that if a collaborative relationship is to be established, health care professionals will need to redefine the form of the encounter from exercising influence and decisional control to one of joint decision-making; and redefine the role activities from active–passive to an active–active interaction. The guiding principles include:

- consideration of the power relationship – ensure a 'power to' rather than a 'power over' approach

- the patient's right to autonomy and self-determination
- creating an appropriate environment to enable patients to articulate their needs and their views
- the provision of clear explanations and information to enable the patient to participate in joint decision-making.

Patient participation is encompassed within collaborative practice. This approach is advocated by Roper et al (1996, p. 52). Two of the philosophical assumptions upon which the model is based are:

• Within a health care context, nurses work in partnership with the patient who, except for special circumstances, is an autonomous, decision-making person.

• Nurses are part of a multiprofessional health care team who work in partnership for the benefit of the patient, and for the health of the community.

Øvretveit (1997) provides a framework for health care professionals to audit patient and carer participation (see Box 2.7).

MULTIDISCIPLINARY PATHWAY OF CARE
CHEVIOT AND WANSBECK NHS TRUST
TRANS URETHRAL RESECTION OF PROSTATE GLAND (TURP)

Patient Name: . . . . Day & Date admitted: . . . . Unit No: . . . .

	ADMISSION	PRE OP DAY 1	PRE OP DAY 2	OP DAY / PRE OP	OP DAY /POST OP	
N U R S I N G	INTRODUCTION TO WARD NURSING ASSESSMENT TPR & WEIGHT WATERLOW SCALE URINALYSIS MSU IF REQUIRED UROFLOMETRY IF REQUIRED DISCHARGE PLANNING ORDER DRUGS FROM PHARMACY CHECK X-RAYS ON WARD INFORM PHYSIO	REINFORCE INFORMATION AND PREPARATION SHAVE R. THIGH MEASURE FOR TED STOCKINGS EXPLAIN FASTING ARRANGEMENTS TPR PREPARE NOTES, X-RAYS CHECKLIST & BLOOD RESULTS FOR ANAESTHETIST		HIBISCRUB SHOWER/BATH TED STOCKINGS PREPARE BED/COTSIDES COMPLETE CHECK LIST REMOVE CATHETER IF REQUIRED PRE MED TRANSFER TO THEATRE	TRANSFER TO WARD TPR & BP BP & P UNTIL NORMAL RANGE NORMAL SALINE BLADDER IRRIGATION UNTIL URINE CLEAR ENSURE INTAKE – OUTPUT OBSERVE I.V. THERAPY & SITE DRUGS FOR SPASM OFFER MEAL	
P H A R M A C Y	DISCUSS MEDICATIONS WITH PATIENT REVIEW PRESCRIBED MEDICATION	DISCUSS MEDICATIONS WITH PATIENT REVIEW PRESCRIBED MEDICATION	DISCUSS MEDICATIONS WITH PATIENT REVIEW PRESCRIBED MEDICATION			

Figure 2.3 Multidisciplinary pathway of care for transurethral resection of prostate gland: nursing and pharmacy – pre- and perioperative periods (reproduced with kind permission from Nelson 1997).

Patient participation in decision-making is perceived not only as a collaborative approach but also as an empowering anxiety-relieving strategy (Teasdale 1993). To enhance the decision-making process and enable patients to have some control over their lives, they need appropriate information.

Reflective point

Do you subscribe to this approach? Indeed, if you say you use the Roper et al model, and it is cited in your ward/unit philosophy, to what extent is your practice underpinned by the philosophical assumptions (bearing in mind that not all patients would wish or be able to participate in their care)?

The two widely cited studies of Hayward (1975) and Boore (1978), have attempted to demonstrate how giving relevant information to patients preoperatively would reduce postoperative pain. Yet Teasdale (1993)

Box 2.7 A framework to audit patient and carer participation in their service (Øvretveit 1997)

To consider where more patient influence and involvement would be of benefit, a team needs to ask:
• What are the key types of decisions in which they should participate in the care of an individual, in service operations and in planning future services?
• What are the decision-making processes and steps? Who is responsible and what is that person's authority and accountability?
• How do, or can, patients or carers influence each of these types of decisions?
• What could, or do, patients do for themselves? What could we do to help them?
• What are the limits to increased influence or involvement? Where is it not helpful or not wanted?

has argued that this hypothesis is an oversimplification. Whilst relevant information giving is an essential requisite for most surgical patients, specific empowering strategies, for example patient-controlled analgesia,

MULTIDISCIPLINARY PATHWAY OF CARE
CHEVIOT AND WANSBECK NHS TRUST
TRANS URETHRAL RESECTION OF PROSTATE GLAND (TURP)

Patient Name: .... Day & Date admitted: .... Unit No: ....

		POST OP DAY 1	POST OP DAY 2	POST OP DAY 3	POST OP DAY 4	POST OP DAY 5	
N U R S I N G		DISCONTINUE BLADDER IRRIGATION BEFORE 09.00hrs	PATIENT TO DRINK MINIMUM 180 MLS HOURLY AND CHART INPUT &OUTPUT	REMOVE CATHETER BY 0700 HRS MSU IF NITRATES PRESENT	COMPLETE DISCHARGE CHECK LIST		
		DISCONTINUE I.V. THERAPY DISCONTINUE BP & P RECORDING	BATH/SHOWER	DISCONTINUE SPASM DRUGS	PATIENT INFORMATION DISCHARGE LIST OF CONTACTS		
			TEMPERATURE 1800 HRS	BATH/SHOWER & REMOVE TEDS	VERBAL POST OP INFORMATION & REFER TO TURP BOOKLET		
		ASK PATIENT TO DRINK MINIMUM OF 180 MLS FLUID HOURLY	DRUGS FOR SPASM	PATIENT TO USE URINAL EACH VOIDING			
			ORDER DISCHARGE TRANSPORT IF REQUIRED		DRUGS TO TAKE HOME		
		RECORD INTAKE & OUTPUT		RECORD INTAKE & OUTPUT	GP LETTER TO TAKE HOME		
		TEACH PATIENT TO EMPTY CATHETER BAG		PATIENT TO DRINK MINIMUM 180 MLS EVERY 2 HOURS			
		BATH/SHOWER		TEMPERATURE AT 1800 HRS			
		TEMPERATURE 1800 HRS		MAKE FINAL DISCHARGE ARRANGEMENTS			
		DRUGS FOR SPASM		DISCHARGE SCRIPT TO PHARMACY			
P H A R M A C Y		DISCUSS MEDICATIONS WITH PATIENT	DISCUSS MEDICATIONS WITH PATIENT	DISCUSS MEDICATIONS WITH PATIENT			
		REVIEW PRESCRIBED MEDICATION	REVIEW PRESCRIBED MEDICATION	REVIEW PRESCRIBED MEDICATION			

Figure 2.4 Multidisciplinary pathway of care for transurethral resection of prostate gland: nursing and pharmacy – postoperative period (reproduced with kind permission from Nelson 1997).

would more appropriately reduce postoperative pain and anxiety. Surgical nurses need to network and share strategies which enable patients to have more control over their care. Yet, it is important to heed the cautionary advice provided by Elliott & Turrell (1996) regarding the potential conflicts of patient empowerment. These encompass:

• power conflicts and misunderstandings due to a lack of clarity regarding the patient's role in interdisciplinary decision-making about his or her care
• enabling patients to be passive if they so choose, within the practice of individualised care
• the potential for intrusion and insensitivity regarding obtaining patients' views
• the relationship between the degree of acute physical illness and the level of involvement in decision-making.

Many patients should be enabled to become more active participants in surgical settings. 'The Patient's Charter and You' (DoH 1995) states: 'You have the right to have any proposed treatment, including any risks involved in that treatment and any alternatives, clearly explained to you before you decide whether to agree to it.'

The balance of power between patients and professionals is slowly changing. Surgical nurses need to consider the extent to which there is collaboration in practice between patients' expectations and needs, and the goals of the nursing and interprofessional team.

Developing collaborative relationships with patients

The reasons why surgical nurses need to consider building on their current knowledge of collaborative practice is succinctly identified by Wilson (1997, p. 17) and, to a greater extent, reflects current UK social policy (see Box 2.8). When exploring the process of collaboration with patients the characteristics of a therapeutic relationship should be realised (Hobbs 1994, cited in Whyte et al 1997):

• respect for the patient

> **Box 2.8** Social and political determinants for advancing collaborative practice (adapted from Wilson 1997)
>
> **Why change clinical practice?**
> - Integrated quality care
> - Research/evidence-based practice
> - Increasing health expectations
> - The Patient's Charter
> - Demographic changes
> - Technological changes
> - NHS reforms
> - Health of the nation
> - Strategies for health care
> - Reprofiling of skill mix
> - Educational changes
> - Patients' increased expectations
> - Working in a more litigious environment

- genuine interest in the patient as a person
- emotional warmth
- tolerance and non-judgemental acceptance of the patient as a person
- receptivity, especially the capacity to listen attentively
- empathy, the capacity to feel one's way into what the patient is experiencing
- realistic confidence in one's skills and resources
- awareness of one's limitations
- adherence to an appropriate ethical code.

> **Reflective point**
>
> Consider how you may demonstrate each of the above characteristics in your day-to-day practice. What gaps in knowledge can you identify and how will these be rectified?

Peplau (1988) states that there is nothing new about the kind of nursing she is advocating as she believes that good nurses everywhere practise it in varying degrees. However, the purpose of her work is to enable practitioners to deepen their understanding of interpersonal relations in nursing situations in order that their work will be more effective and socially useful. Insight into surgical nursing practice may be elicited by considering the nursing roles that Peplau has identified: stranger, resource person, teacher, leader, surrogate, counsellor.

In the first instance, nurse and patient meet as strangers. The guiding principles within this role are:

- to accept the patient as he is
- to treat the patient as an emotionally able stranger and relate to him on this basis until evidence shows him to be otherwise.

As a resource person, the nurse provides specific answers to questions usually formulated in relation to a larger problem. In other words, nurses learn to make discriminating judgements in practice about questions that require direct, straightforward, factual answers and about those that involve feelings and may require application of the principles of counselling (Peplau 1988, p. 48).

The teaching role is operationalised most often by learning through experience. Teaching always proceeds from what patients already know and it develops around their interest in wanting and being able to use additional (medical) information (Peplau 1988, p. 48). A democratic leadership style is advocated:

Democratic leadership roles require attitudes of respect for the dignity and worth of each human being encountered and these attitudes can not be assumed; they operate or they don't and the patient knows by way of his feelings what the attitudes of others are towards him.

(Peplau 1988, p. 50)

Nurses are often cast in the role of surrogate. Surrogate roles are determined by psychological needs. Often the surgical nurse may be unaware that the patient views her as someone else, for example his mother, daughter, teacher. The patient's behaviour towards her will reflect his relationship with the person the nurse reminds him of. Once the patient says, 'You remind me of my ...', the nurse can say, 'I wonder what she is like,' providing the opportunity to understand the patient's feelings towards her. In surrogacy situations, Peplau (1988, p. 60) asserts that facilitating changes, and improvements in understanding, and resolving the difficulty faced by the patient, with professional help, requires collaboration based upon attitudes of trust in and respect for the capacity of each to grow and change.

The final role is that of counsellor. Counselling in nursing has to do with helping patients to remember and to understand fully what is happening to them in the present situation, so that the experience can be integrated with, rather than disassociated from, other experiences in life (Peplau 1988, p. 64). Patients, whenever possible, and within the constraints of the organisation, need to work through feelings concerning surgery. This is especially so in relation to operations to do with the erogenous zones – oral, anal and genital areas. The guiding principle implies that a tonsillectomy, circumcision, haemorrhoidectomy, etc. could be considered minor operations from a physical perspective, but are major ones when acknowledging the psychological meaning to the patient (see also Ch. 9).

Reflective point

Can you identify the extent to which you fulfil the roles described by Peplau? Which roles do you feel require further development?

CONCLUSION

This chapter has attempted to critically analyse some of the current challenging developments related to the surgical nurse as an independent and collaborative practitioner. Independent and collaborative practice development must encompass not only convincing others of the value of nurses' knowledge and skills within individual therapeutic interventions, but, also, of the nurse's central role in collaborative interprofessional coordination, teamwork and change strategies. Significant change cannot be accomplished without protected time, personal and team commitment and management support. Creative collaborative strategies are required for the closer integration of nursing practice, education and research. Research and development monies should be made available for nurses to undertake collaborative action research studies which focus on quality care improvement, role and knowledge development. This collaborative approach should result in power shifts between nurses, health care professionals, patients, and managers. Indeed, to start to realistically explore power issues, Mitchinson (1996) suggests a possible agenda for change including: 'Consideration of the hierarchical relationship between health service managers, nurse managers and clinical nurses and a review of the effects of this relationship on independent and autonomous nursing practice'.

An exploration of some key strategies to enable independent and collaborative role development has been undertaken. Some of the strategies advocated have been and are being implemented in practice within a shared clinical governance approach (DoH 1999, Ch. 7). Yet, all surgical nurses should consider the extent to which the quality of patient care that they provide could be enhanced by the advancement of both their independent and collaborative roles.

REFERENCES

Allred C A, Arford P H, Michel Y, Veitch J S, Dring R, Carter V 1995 Case management: the relationship between structure and environment. Nursing Economics 13(1): 32–41, 51

Allsopp C 1991 Primary nursing in a surgical unit. In: Ersser S, Tutton E (eds) Primary nursing in perspective. Scutari, Royal College of Nursing, Oxford

Antrobus A 1997 Nursing leadership. MSc in Nursing, Distance Learning, Royal College of Nursing, London

Batey M V, Lewis F M 1982 Clarifying autonomy and accountability in nursing service. Journal of Nursing Administration 12(9): 13–18

Bellman L 1996 Changing nursing practice through reflection on the Roper, Logan and Tierney model: the enhancement approach to action research. Journal of Advanced Nursing 24: 129–138

Bellman L 1997 Do not believe a word that I say: a critical science approach to advancing nursing practice. Managing Clinical Nursing 1(2): 70–74

Boore J R P 1978 Prescription for recovery. Royal College of Nursing, London

Carr W, Kemmis S 1986 Becoming critical: education, knowledge and action research. Falmer, London

Conway J 1996 Nursing expertise and advanced practice. Quay Books, Cheltenham

Crane S 1991 Implications of the critical paradigm. In: Gray G, Pratt R (eds) Towards a discipline of nursing. Churchill Livingstone, Melbourne

Crowley S A, Wollner I S 1987 Collaborative practice: a tool for change. Oncology Nursing Forum 14(4): 59–63

Department of Health (DoH) 1989 Working for patients. DoH, London

Department of Health (DoH) 1994 The challenges for nursing and midwifery in the 21st century; the Heathrow debate. DoH, London

Department of Health (DoH) 1995 The patient's charter and you. DoH, London

Department of Health (DoH) 1999 Making a difference. Stengthening the nursing, midwifery and health visiting contribution to health and health care. DoH, London

East L, Robinson J 1993 Attitude problem. Nursing Times 89(48): 42–43

Elliott M, Turrell A 1996 Understanding the conflicts of patient empowerment. Nursing Standard 10(45): 43–47

English National Board (ENB) 1987 Managing change in nursing education: Section 3 The process of innovation. ENB, London

Ford P, Walsh M 1994 New rituals for old. Butterworth-Heinemann, Oxford

Fry A, Mortimer K, Ramsey L 1994 Clinical research and the culture of collaboration. Australian Journal of Advanced Nursing 11(3): 18–25

Gray G, Pratt R (eds) 1991 Towards a discipline of nursing. Churchill Livingstone: Melbourne

Hale C 1997 The development and implementation of case management and managed care in an orthopaedic unit of a major U.K. teaching hospital: a nursing-led approach. In: Wilson J (ed) Integrated care management: the path to success? Butterworth-Heinemann, Oxford

Hart E, Bond M 1995 Action research for health and social care. Open University Press, Buckingham

Hawks J 1991 Power: a concept analysis. Journal of Advanced Nursing 16: 754–762

Hayward J 1975 Information: a prescription against pain. Royal College of Nursing, London

Hendricks-Thomas J, Patterson E 1995 A sharing in critical thought by nursing faculty. Journal of Advanced Nursing 22: 594–599

Henneman E A, Lee J L, Cohen J I 1995 Collaboration: a concept analysis. Journal of Advanced Nursing 21: 103–109

Ignatavicius D, Hausman D 1995 Clinical pathways for collaborative practice. W B Saunders, Philadelphia

Johns C 1992 Ownership and the harmonious team: barriers to developing the therapeutic nursing team in primary nursing. Journal of Clinical Nursing 1: 89–94

Johns C 1993 Professional supervision. Journal of Nursing Management 1(1): 9–18

Jones A 1995 An analysis of case management – the efficient utility of human resources, but to what end? Journal of Nursing Management 3: 143–149

Keenan M J, Hurst J B, Dennis R S, Frey G 1990 Situational leadership for collaboration in health care settings. Health Care Supervisor 8(3): 19–25

Kerfoot K 1989 Nurse/physician collaboration: a cost/quality issue for the nurse manager. Nursing Economics 7(6): 335–336

Klakovich M D 1994 Connective leadership for the 21st century: a historical perspective and future directions. Advances in Nursing Science 16(4): 42–54

Kubsch S M 1996 Conflict, enactment, empowerment: independent therapeutic nursing intervention. Journal of Advanced Nursing 23: 192–200

Lamb G S 1995 Case management. Annual Review of Nursing Research 13: 117–136

Lancaster J 1982 Change theory: an essential aspect of nursing practice. In: Lancaster J, Lancaster W (eds) The nurse as a change agent. Mosby, London

Lenkman S, Gribbens R 1994 Multidisciplinary teams in the acute care setting. Holistic Nurse Practice 8(3): 81–87

Lorentzon M 1993 Research for health: managing the nursing input. Journal of Nursing Management 1: 39–46

Lumby J 1991 Threads of an emerging discipline: praxis, reflection, rhetoric and research. In: Gray G, Pratt R (eds) Towards a discipline of nursing. Churchill Livingstone, Melbourne

McCormack B 1992 A case study identifying nursing staffs' perception of the delivery method of nursing care in practice on a particular ward. Journal of Advanced Nursing 17: 187–197

McEniery M 1992 Collaborating for health care. In: Gray G, Pratt R (eds) Issues in Australian nursing 3. Churchill Livingstone, Melbourne

Mackenzie J 1993 Effects of change on sisters/charge nurses. Nursing Standard 7(36): 25–27

Manley K 1992 Quality assurance: the pathway to excellence. In: Jolley M, Brykczynska G (eds) Nursing care: the challenge to change. Edward Arnold, London

Manley K 1994 Primary nursing and critical care. In: Millar B, Burnard P (eds) Critical care nursing. Baillière Tindall, London

Manley K 1997 A conceptual framework for advanced practice: an action research project operationalising an advanced practitioner/consultant role. Journal of Clinical Nursing 6: 179–190

Manley K, McCormack B 1997 Exploring expert practice. MSc nursing distance learning study guide. Royal College of Nursing, London

Mezirow J 1981 A critical theory of adult learning and education. Adult Education 32(1): 3–24

Mitchinson S 1996 Are nurses independent and autonomous practitioners? Nursing Standard 10(34): 34–38

Murrell K L 1985 The development of a theory of empowerment: rethinking power for organisational development. Organisation Development Journal (Summer): 34–38

Nelson S 1997 Improving urological flow through multidisciplinary pathways of care. In: Wilson J (ed) Integrated care management: the path to success? Butterworth-Heinemann, Oxford

Oie M, Recker D 1992 Empowerment through collaboration: implementing a team quality assurance model. Journal of Nursing Care Quality 6(2): 32–40

Øvretveit J 1997 How patient power and client participation affect relations between professions. In: Øvretveit J, Mathais P, Thompson T (eds) Interprofessional working for health and social care. Macmillan, London

Peplau H 1988 Interpersonal relations in nursing, 2nd edn. Macmillan, London

Rafferty D 1992 Team and primary nursing. Senior Nurse 12(1): 31–34

Robinson A 1995 Transformative cultural shifts in nursing: participatory action research and the 'project of possibility'. Nursing Inquiry 2(2): 65–74

Rogers E M 1989 Creating a climate for the implementation of a nursing conceptual framework. Journal of Continuing Education in Nursing 20(3): 112–116

Roper R, Logan W, Tierney A 1996 The elements of nursing, 4th edn. Churchill Livingstone. Edinburgh

Scholes J 1996 Therapeutic use of self. Nursing in Critical Care 1(1): 60–66

Sims S E R 1991 The nature and relevance of theory for practice. In: Gray G, Pratt R (eds) Towards a discipline of nursing. Churchill Livingstone, Melbourne

Smith M C 1993 Case management and nursing theory-based practice. Nursing Science Quarterly 6(1): 8–9

Snyder M 1992 Independent nursing interventions, 2nd edn. Delmar, Albany

Speedy S 1989 Theory–practice debate; setting the scene. Journal of Advanced Nursing 6(3): 12–20

Spross J A 1989 The CNS as collaborator. In: Hamric A B, Spross J A The clinical nurse specialist in theory and practice, 2nd edn. W B Saunders, Philadelphia

Stein L, Watts D, Howell T 1990 The doctor–nurse game re-visited. New England Journal of Medicine 322(8): 546–549

Stockwell 1972 The unpopular patient. Croom Helm, Beckenham

Street A 1995 Nursing replay: researching nursing culture together. Churchill Livingstone, Melbourne

Strumpf N E, Asimos K 1996 Accountability: the covenant between patient and nurse practitioner. In: Hickey J V, Ouimette R M, Venegoni S L (eds) Advanced practice nursing: changing roles and clinical applications. Lippincott, Philadelphia

Sutton F, Smith C 1995 Advanced nursing practice: new idea and new perspectives. Journal of Advanced Nursing 21: 1037–1043

Teasdale K 1993 Information and anxiety: a critical appraisal. Journal of Advanced Nursing 18: 1125–1132

Thomas L, McColl E, Priest J, Bond S 1996 The impact of primary nursing on patient satisfaction. Nursing Times 92(22): 36–39

Titchen A, Binnie A 1993 Research partnerships: collaborative action research in nursing. Journal of Advanced Nursing 18: 858–865

United Kingdom Central Council for Nursing, Midwifery and Health Visiting (UKCC) 1992 The scope of professional practice. UKCC, London

United Kingdom Central Council for Nursing, Midwifery and Health Visiting (UKCC) 1996 Guidelines for professional practice. UKCC, London

Walsh M 1997 Accountability and intuition: justifying nursing practice. Nursing Standard 11(23): 39–41

Warelow P J 1996 Nurse–doctor relationships in multidisciplinary teams: ideal or real? International Journal of Nursing Practice 2: 33–39

Waters K 1985 Team nursing. Nursing Practice 1: 7–15

Webb C 1989 Action research: philosophy, methods and personal experiences. Journal of Advanced Nursing 14: 403–410

Whyte L. Motyka M, Motyka H, Wsolek R, Tune M 1997 Polish and British nurses' responses to patient need. Nursing Standard 11(38): 34–37

Wilson J 1997 Introduction to integrated care management – introducing multidisciplinary pathways of care into an organisation through project, risk and change management. In: Wilson J (ed) Integrated care management: the path to success? Butterworth-Heinemann, Oxford

Wright S 1991 Facilitating therapeutic nursing and independent practice. In: McMahon R, Pearson A (eds) Nursing as therapy. Chapman and Hall, London

Wright S 1989 Changing nursing practice. Edward Arnold, London

FURTHER READING

Fetterman D M, Kaftarian S J, Wandersman A 1996 Empowerment evaluation: knowledge and tools for self-assessment and accountability. Sage, London

Henneman E A 1995 Nurse–physician collaboration: a poststructuralist view. Journal of Advanced Nursing 22: 359–363

Johnson M, Webb C 1995 Rediscovering unpopular patients: the concept of social judgement. Journal of Advanced Nursing 21: 466–475

King K B, Parrinello K M, Baggs J G 1996 Collaboration and advanced practice nursing. In: Hickey J V, Ouimette R M, Venegoni S L (eds) Advanced practice nursing: changing roles and clinical applications. Lippincott, Philadelphia

McFayden J, Farrington A 1997 User and carer participation in the NHS. British Journal of Health Care Management 3(5): 260–264

Patronis Jones R A 1994 Conceptual development of nurse–physician collaboration. Holistic Nurse Practitioner 8(3): 1–11

Scott E, Cowen B 1997 Multidisciplinary collaborative care planning. Nursing Standard 12(1): 39–42

Tiffany C R, Lutjens L R J 1998 Planned change theories for nursing. Sage, Thousand Oaks

Walsh M 1997 Will critical pathways replace the nursing process? Nursing Standard 11(52): 39–42

Warelow P J 1996 Nurse–doctor relationships in multidisciplinary teams: ideal or real? International Journal of Nursing Practice 2: 33–39

3

The surgical nurse as teacher and health promoter

Christine Spiers

AIMS

This chapter aims to:

- encourage surgical nurses of the 21st century to adopt an enquiring and critical stance in the promotion of their clients' and the nations' health
- explore the historical, theoretical and practical foundations of health education, health promotion and patient education
- provide heath education strategies for surgical nurses to adopt within their practice area.

INTRODUCTION

The surgical nurse needs to ask the following questions:

- To what extent does health promotion form part of my practice?
- How do I integrate health education within my clinical role?
- Do I believe that health promotion is only an issue for practice nurses, occupational health nurses and community nurses?

This chapter enables you to explore these key questions.

Research suggests that health promotion by hospital nurses is disjointed and inconsistent (Gott & O'Brien 1990, Wilson-Barnett & Macleod Clarke 1993). However, research studies have also shown that hospital nurses are keen to take up the challenge of integrating health promotion into their practice (McBride 1994, Mitchinson 1995). Indeed, literature suggests that nurses value health promotion and are capable of fulfilling many roles in health promotion, but are prevented from developing this role by constraints in the clinical environment (Close 1988, King 1994, Mitchinson 1995). Conversely, whilst a health promotion role is acknowledged, the credence and priority nurses give to this role is not always congruent with their observed activities (Wilson-Barnett & Macleod Clark 1993, Mitchinson 1995).

Many nursing authors advocate the health promotion role for surgical nurses (Dobson 1992, Millar 1994, New 1995), and yet the Royal College of Nursing (1993) in its response to the 'Health of the Nation' (DoH 1992) addresses the issues for community-based nurses with little reference to hospital health care professionals. The challenge would appear to be to translate health promotion concepts into surgical nursing practice in both hospital and community settings.

Health promotion needs to be seen as a complete strategy with hospitals and communities working in partnership. A recent report, 'The Challenges for Nursing in the 21st Century' (DoH 1994) predicts an important coordinating role for nurses in bridging the hospital–community gap as the desire for a 'seamless approach' to health care develops.

Perhaps these dichotomies and inconsistencies can be explained by exploring the terms – 'health education' and 'health promotion'. These terms are difficult to define and often cause confusion; however, brief definitions are offered here. Health education is a communication activity aimed at enabling individuals and groups to achieve positive health in social and lifestyle issues. Empowerment is a fundamental concept and health education addresses physical, mental, spiritual and social well-being. Health promotion, on the other hand, may be seen as an umbrella term encompassing political, societal, and environmental activities in which health education is a composite part.

Surgical nurses should ask the question: 'To what extent am I involved in promoting health?' Professional nurses should consider health promotion as an absolute basic concept of nursing. Indeed the Strategy for Nursing (DoH 1989) states that health education and health promotion should be a recognised part of health care; all practitioners should develop their skills in, and use every opportunity for health promotion.

The use of a second question (McBride 1995) should promote a more positive response: 'How could I integrate patient education within my clinical role?' Many nurses working in acute settings recognise patient education as part of the daily nursing activity (Wilson-Barnett & Macleod Clark 1993). Indeed it is interesting to note that 'patient education' has been included in the nursing curriculum since 1944 (General Nursing Council 1944).

Health promotion is a complex concept and difficult to define (Tones et al 1990, Yeo 1993). However, health promotion is emerging as a politically directed health care strategy in which the nursing function is

implicit (DoH 1992, Wilson-Barnett & Macleod Clark 1993, King 1994). Client responsibility for health and client choice in health care decisions are proposed in current health reforms. At the same time, the clients are seen as the consumers of health care and, paradoxically, quasi-controllers of their health status (Naidoo & Wills 1994, North 1993).

Health is therefore on the political agenda. There is a current shift in emphasis away from disease-oriented health care towards a realisation that education for health is essential in society today. It has been argued that the greatest benefit to the nation's health would be achieved by optimising both the community and hospital services to achieve a 'seamless approach' to health care provision (McBride 1994, p. 93). Demographic trends, economic considerations and the emphasis on health consumerism (healthism) confirm this stance.

Surgical patients often have a short hospital stay and a desire for health-related knowledge. Increasingly it is recognised that many of the causes of current mortality and morbidity are lifestyle related and potentially preventable. Similarly, many of today's illnesses are largely chronic and incurable and hence there is a need for patients and their families to become involved, and to manage their own treatment and care (Latter et al 1992, Millar 1994, Salvage 1990). However, Waterworth & Luker (1990) caution that including clients and carers in health decisions may be financially driven; having people accept responsibility for their health care may be one way of reducing costs in the current health care market.

Many authors have argued that nurses are in the best position to instigate health education because of the nature and duration of the nurse–patient relationship and the method of nursing delivery employed (Close 1988, Maben et al 1993, Tones 1993). Both the named-nurse method and primary nursing offer appropriate opportunities for nurses and clients to develop a therapeutic relationship which is a prerequisite of effective health education. McBride (1994) suggests that whilst a hospital admission may be potentially stressful, it may also act as a catalyst to change by increasing motivation and readiness to learn.

Health promotion is thus a developing paradigm in nursing (King 1994, Wilson-Barnett & Macleod Clark 1993). It is also politically constructed and emerging as a health care strategy. Nurses are being urged to take up the gauntlet to incorporate health promotion in their arena of practice. In the current context of a health service which is politically led and economically driven, health promotion has much to offer nurses and most importantly their clients and carers.

The key areas therefore that need to be explored in this chapter include:

- the relationship of patient education to health education and health promotion
- the extent to which health education is the same as or different from health promotion, and
- how these concepts translate into practice with surgical patients and their families.

There is, therefore, a continued need to address the potential for health promotion in surgical settings. In this chapter, an evolutionary approach has been adopted to explore these issues as well as the identification of health promotion strategies for surgical nursing practice.

HISTORICAL DEVELOPMENT

Much of nursing's historical tradition is rooted in health promotion approaches. Florence Nightingale's (1859) view of health as an essential aspect of nursing is well known: 'The very elements of what constitutes good nursing are as little understood for the well as for the sick. The same laws of health or of nursing, for they are in reality the same, obtain among the well as among the sick'. (Nightingale 1859, p. 6 of 1970 edition).

Similarly the concepts of health education and health promotion may also be traced back to the mid-19th century. Bunton & MacDonald's (1992) typology clearly depicts this evolution, as shown in Figure 3.1, and suggests that the public health movement of the late 19th century led to the development of health education in the early 20th century, which in turn informed the emerging disciplines of the New Public Health and health promotion.

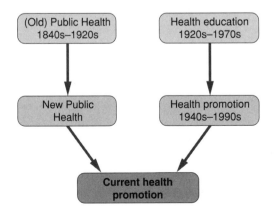

Figure 3.1 Health promotion typology (adapted from Bunton & MacDonald 1992).

The industrialisation of Britain during the 19th century led to overcrowded and insanitary working conditions. Diseases such as smallpox, tuberculosis and cholera were not new, but the insanitary working and living environments provided conditions for these diseases to flourish. The need for municipal reform and the efforts of protagonists such as Edwin Chadwick and Jeremy Bentham, from which stemmed much social and environmental reform, are often cited (Ross 1991, Naidoo & Wills 1994).

There is no doubt that the public health legislation of the 1840s and 1850s led to a considerable reduction in epidemics associated with poor sanitation and ventilation. The discovery of inoculation as a method of preventing infectious diseases was also a significant medical advance in reducing mortality from infectious disease.

Thus the changing patterns of mortality led to a concentration upon biomedical aspects of disease and a shift in emphasis towards lifestyle issues and personal behaviours. By the early 20th century, health had become an individual concern, although alongside this philosophy the Liberal Government (1906–1911) developed social reforms such as national insurance and pensions provision.

World wars

The Central Council for Health Education was established in 1927 and its essential remit was the establishment of an educational programme based upon coercion, propaganda and individualism. The evidence that 10–20% of soldiers in the First World War had contracted venereal disease led to a series of mass media approaches including lectures and posters aimed to shock. Health education at this time emphasised temperance and moderation in individual behaviours (Blythe 1986).

The intervening Second World War and the inception of the National Health Service in 1948 gradually moved the philosophy of health education towards a medical model of health and illness. This was emphasised when the Health Education Council was established in 1967 as a quango (quasi-autonomous nongovernmental organisation) under the auspices of the Department of Health and Social Security. The Health Education Council became synonymous with mass media campaigns based upon an individualistic and behavioural approach which laid responsibility for health (and ill health) firmly at the door of the individual. These notions, although well meaning, endorsed a philosophy of culpability and liability, primarily aimed at individuals, which has since been recognised as 'victim blaming' and deemed unacceptable (Crawford 1980, Fahlberg et al 1991).

Politics, social policy and current trends

Yet, the 'victim blaming' approach appears to have been emphasised within the political and social reform. It has been suggested that the health education approaches in the 1970s and 1980s constructed health and ill health as individually determined. 'Prevention and Health: Everybody's Business' published by the Department of Health and Social Security in 1976 is a classic example of this. The emphasis and responsibility for health in this document was placed entirely with the individual.

In 1987 the Health Education Council was disbanded and the Health Education Authority was established as a special health authority in the NHS in England. Similar changes took place in Wales and Scotland. Almost overnight health education units were renamed health promotion units and professionals working within these units became health promotion officers. This reorganisation appears to have occurred merely as part of the general reorganisation inherent in the NHS at this time.

In 1990 the NHS and Community Care Act introduced the principle of the internal market to the provision of health care. The Act divided health authorities into 'purchasers' and 'providers'. The purchasing authority assesses and determines health needs and commissions services from provider units. The Act also introduces the concept of client choice and participation, principles engendered within the Patient's Charter (DoH 1991), which establishes the patient as a consumer of health care. Current health and social policy also places greater emphasis upon primary care in the community. Technological and therapeutic advances have reduced surgical hospital stays and enabled an expansion of minimally invasive surgical techniques and day care facilities. Consequently health care resources are being diverted from acute sector to community care provision (Masterson 1995).

Health for all by the year 2000

These approaches are consistent with the World Health Organization's strategy 'Health for All by the Year 2000' (WHO 1984). This strategy provides a framework for the development of broad-based health programmes which aim to help individuals to achieve a level of health which enables them to lead socially and economically productive lives.

The principles of health promotion are outlined in the Ottawa Charter (WHO 1986) and key areas for action include:

- building a healthy public policy
- creating supportive environments
- developing personal skills
- strengthening community action
- reorienting health services.

'Health for All by the Year 2000' and the Ottawa Charter also discuss three ways in which health may be promoted: by advocacy, enablement and mediation.

Advocacy

Knowledge and understanding of factors which may affect health need to be improved. It has been suggested that health promoters need to empower individuals and communities to argue for their health rights and for access to appropriate resources.

Enablement

Health promotion aims to reduce inequalities in health status by promoting equal opportunities and resources to enable all people to achieve their health potential.

Mediation

Health promotion involves coordination of resources by many agencies and not merely the health care sector. Governments, health care, social services, nongovernmental and voluntary organisations all have a role to play in the pursuit of health. Health promotion aims to mediate between all sectors in society to achieve effective collaboration and action.

The basic tenets of 'Health for All by the Year 2000' and thus current health promotion activity strive to promote empowerment of individuals and communities, eradication of health inequalities and intersectoral collaboration.

The Government's response to 'Health for All by the Year 2000' was the publication of 'The Health of the Nation' (DoH 1992) and a commitment to global ecology as outlined at the Rio Conference in 1992.

HEALTH OF THE NATION

The 'Health of the Nation' strategy aims to address health 'in its widest sense' and borrows much of its introductory rhetoric from 'Health for All by the Year

2000'. 'The Health of the Nation' discusses 'adding years to life and life to years'. It recognises the contribution that needs to be made by many organisations and agencies, including the Government, health care professionals and families and individuals themselves and refers to this collaboration as 'healthy alliances'.

To this extent 'The Health of the Nation' therefore seems to follow the underlying philosophies of 'Health for All by the Year 2000'. The strategy focuses on five main key areas for action including:

- coronary heart disease and stroke
- cancer
- mental illness
- accidents
- HIV/AIDS and sexual health.

These key areas were chosen because they represent the main causes of mortality and morbidity in the country and are thus deemed amenable to action. Hence, targets for reduction of mortality and morbidity have been set within each key area and progress is being monitored. According to the 'Health of the Nation: One Year On ...' (DoH 1993a), the first year of the strategy has been successful with considerable progress made towards each target.

The strategy is not without its critics and it has been variously pronounced that the strategy is too risk factor oriented and individualistic and avoids a commitment to eradicating health inequalities. It gives only token acknowledgement to social, ecological and community issues and focuses too strongly on the concepts of 'individualism' and 'healthism' within the current consumer culture (Bunton 1995, North 1993, Rogers & Whyms 1995).

The internal market is now well established in the NHS and, similarly, health promotion is seen as a legitimate and key role for health care professionals. Many authors suggest that nursing has a fundamental role to play in promoting health whilst at the same time caring for the sick. It is therefore essential that if nurses intend to embrace health education/promotion as an activity, then they need to be clear about what they have to offer and how they are able to rationalise their contiguous roles (Gallagher & Burden 1993, Tones et al 1990).

Within this new culture, surgical nurses have an opportunity to develop their health promotion role to give better quality of care to clients. The concepts of empowerment, autonomy, self-care and partnership are central to this provision and are essential to health promotion practice.

THEORETICAL FOUNDATIONS OF HEALTH, HEALTH EDUCATION AND HEALTH PROMOTION

These concepts are complex and difficult to define – indeed many authors are unable to agree precise definitions. What is relevant, however, is not so much the way that concepts are defined, but how the concepts may be used in practice. Previous discussion in this chapter has clearly identified a role for surgical nurses in 'health promotion' within the current perspectives of the NHS. What is therefore important here is how theories may be useful for practice.

Health

Yeo (1993) states that to some extent the multiplicity of meanings ascribed to health promotion is a function of the multiplicity of meanings of the concept of health. King (1994) suggests that health is a relative, highly individualistic perception that is always evolving, and Zola (1978) asserts that 'health is socially constructed yet experienced at an individual level'.

The World Health Organization has been responsible for furthering the discussion of the concept of health by offering a variety of definitions. Their current definition suggests that health is the extent to which an individual or a group is able to achieve their potential, meet their needs and cope with changes in the environment. Health is seen as a positive concept encompassing social, personal and physical issues (WHO 1984).

This is a very broad definition which encompasses a variety of issues. It establishes a social as well as an individual focus for health, it views health as both dynamic and positive and offers a broad range of activities designed to promote health. Its major criticism is the expansive nature of the definition, making it difficult to apply in practical situations.

From these definitions it is clear that health can means different things to different people at different stages in their lives. There is also an individual as well as a collective perspective on health. Health is a fundamental issue in all our lives, and no more so than when one is confronted with a position of poor health. Surgical nurses are in a potentially unique position to develop a professional stance to participate in health promotion by providing patients with information and support. The contiguous roles of caring for sick individuals whilst enabling them to reach their health potential requires immense skill and provides a challenge for the surgical nurse.

Surgical nurses work in a variety of environments: acute hospital wards, perioperative departments, hospital-at-home schemes and continuing care in the community. Health education and patient education are relevant and applicable in all settings.

Reflective point

What is the current position of health promotion in your area of practice? From where has it evolved and why?

Health promotion or health education?

Health promotion is a relatively new concept. It rose to prominence in the 1980s and appeared to emerge out of the somewhat discredited health education. Indeed nearly all authors agree that health education should be considered within an overall framework of health promotion.

On reviewing the position of academics and practitioners of health promotion, the issues become a little blurred. Tones (1990) sees a clear distinction between health education and health promotion. He sees health education as:

Any planned activity which promotes health or illness related learning, that is, some relatively permanent change in an individual's competence and disposition.

(Tones 1990, p. 2)

This definition emphasises health education as a systematic, planned, educational process aimed at producing changes in attitudes, beliefs, values, knowledge or even behaviour. For Tones et al (1990) health promotion operates at a broader global level involving policy-planning, politics and multisectoral collaboration.

However, Tones et al's (1990) essentially educational approach has been criticised as being too narrow and simplistic. Downie et al (1990) suggest that health education is more than planned education. It is:

communication activity aimed at enhancing positive health and preventing or diminishing ill health in individuals and groups through influencing the beliefs, attitudes and behaviours of those with power and of the community at large.

(Downie et al 1990, p. 28)

This definition emphasises two-way communication and collective (as well as individual) responsibility for health and it implies empowerment as a cardinal principle of health education.

French (1990) also centres upon empowerment in his definition:

health education is about enabling and supporting people to set their own agendas, agendas that that they can then implement in ways decided by themselves, collectively or as individuals.

(French 1990, p. 9)

In these definitions both Downie et al (1990) and French (1990) seem to impinge upon what Tones et al (1990) see as fundamental issues in health promotion: social policy and politics.

Tones (1993) more recently proposes another way of viewing the relationship between health education and health promotion by offering a simple formula:

Health promotion = Health education × Healthy public policy

(Tones 1993, p. 3)

This formula encapsulates the two main strands or themes which are considered fundamental to health promotion strategy: individual (lifestyle) and structural (fiscal/ecological) issues. As Bunton & MacDonald (1992) suggest, health promotion is currently concerned with these two principal themes which are aimed at reducing ill health and premature death. They go on to state that these two principal functions form the bulk of current health promotion activity.

Within Tones' (1993) formula, empowerment is considered to be the major tenet of health education. Tones (1993) sees empowerment as the key health-promoting activity for nurses working with patients, families and groups.

Health education is therefore concerned with facilitating learning and empowering people to put change into practice. It is concerned with promoting positive aspects of health, encouraging collaboration and participation and enabling free choice and effective decision-making (Wilson-Barnett & Macleod Clark 1993).

Reflective point

Does the discussion encompassed within this section reflect your approach to the concept of patient education?' The next section addresses this question.

Health education or patient education?

A semantic discussion also exists in defining the differences between the terms health education and patient education. One approach is that patient education is a planned, systematic process which may help the patient to learn health-related information. Simonds

(1979, cited in Close 1988) sees patient education as: 'the process of influencing patient behaviour, producing changes in knowledge, attitudes and skills required to maintain and improve health'.

The similarity with Tones' (1990) definition of health education is very apparent, as it takes a primarily educational stance.

Toms (1993) suggests that the aim of patient teaching is the promotion of health which may contribute towards patient independence, adaptation to new situations and reduction of stress in hospitals. She too accepts education as the primary focus of this process.

Bellman (1994) also believes that patient education incorporates provision of information, promotion of patient independence and helping patients feel in control. She suggests that if the nurse motivates the client to seek information, this will create a shift from patient dependence to patient independence.

Many authors agree that it is beneficial to enable patients to exert greater control over their condition as it may overcome factors which may hinder recovery (Bridge & Nelson 1994, Wilson-Barnett & Fordham 1982). For example, counselling a woman before and after breast cancer surgery and encouraging her to verbalise her fears and concerns is a prerequisite for enabling her to participate more fully in her postoperative care and recovery. Secondly, it may influence long-term survival by encouraging a positive attitude to health

Surgical patient education is often linked to patient outcomes including reduction in postoperative symptoms, recovery from the surgical problem and coping with stress and medical crises more effectively (Dutton 1994, Farrelly & Lakeman 1993/1994, Leino-Kilpi et al 1993).

Patient education therefore benefits both the client and the organisation by helping to improve physical recovery and psychological coping and by helping to reduce health care costs by minimising postoperative complications and length of hospital stays.

Much of the literature on patient education should lead the surgical nurse to consider communication as a fundamental issue. The need for nurses to focus upon patients' informational needs and also upon their role in the educational process is apparent (Wilson-Barnett & Batehup 1988). Similarly, questions regarding which information, how much, which way, when and by whom also need to be addressed.

HEALTH PROMOTION THEORIES FOR PRACTICE

The preceding discussion reflects the knowledge base which underpins health education, health promotion and patient education. The following statement represents the value of that knowledge to practice: 'In a practice discipline such as nursing, knowledge for knowledge's sake is useful, but knowledge for practice is paramount' (Walker & Avant 1995, p. 207). These authors also believe that models are a means of depicting the views expressed in a theory and can be used to describe, explain and predict aspects of the discipline. A model therefore demonstrates one author's view of a number of interrelated concepts to provide a systematic view of a situation (Fawcett 1989, Meleis 1991). Put more simply, models are a comprehensive analogue of reality (Tones 1990).

Using a model may therefore help surgical nurses to think systematically, to prioritise interventions, and to consider alternative approaches to care. It may also form a foundation upon which to evaluate care and to advance professional knowledge within the profession. It is also useful to reflect upon one's value position in relation to theory as this will inevitably enhance one's practice. Many of the models and approaches to health promotion are compatible with nursing models and philosophies, e.g. the model of Tones et al (1990) promotes self-empowerment and fits well with Orem's (1985) self-care philosophies.

In recent years there has been a proliferation of models in health promotion, reflecting considerable overlap in views but with differences in emphasis. The diversity of health issues leads, not surprisingly, to a variety of methods or approaches to promote health. These approaches, widely attributed to Ewles & Simnett (1995), address a number of aims and methods which can be used to promote health in a number of settings.

The approaches include:

- medical
- behavioural
- educational
- client-centred
- social change.

Most nurses will recognise their practice in at least one approach and most of the health promotion models are underpinned by at least one major approach. Each approach has a distinct aim and method of delivery and evaluation. Each approach offers a useful philosophical basis for health promotion in at least one practice setting.

Medical approach

The medical approach is founded upon activities aimed towards reducing mortality and premature morbidity. It is predicated upon the absence of disease, not the promotion of positive health, and tends to involve medical activities aimed at populations or high-risk groups.

There are many examples of 'success' with this approach, particularly the previously mentioned immunisation and vaccination campaigns, which have virtually eradicated diseases such as smallpox, polio and diphtheria.

Screening is another example of a medical approach to health promotion. High-risk groups such as sexually active women (cervical screening), menopausal women (breast screening) or middle-aged men (cholesterol screening) are targeted to receive the intervention (Naidoo & Wills 1994).

Screening may, however, be criticised for a number of reasons. It encourages dependency on medical personnel, it augments the power of the medical hierarchy, and it removes control over health decisions from individuals.

For screening to be effective it must fulfil a number of criteria:

• The 'disease' being screened for must have a well-defined treatment which would improve the outcome.
• The 'disease' should have a long preclinical phase, so that screening would not miss the early signs.
• The test must be safe and socially acceptable.
• The test must be specific – it should detect only those with the disease.
• The test should be sensitive – it should detect all those with the disease.
• The test should be cost-effective (adapted from Naidoo & Wills 1994).

Reflective point

Given current publicity surrounding breast and cervical screening, to what extent do you consider these 'national' programmes fulfil the above criteria?

The Cancer Research Campaign (1990) has demonstrated that there has been no reduction in mortality from cervical cancer since many of those at risk from developing the disease do not attend for screening. Other factors may include faults in the recall system, inadequate training of laboratory personnel and a more virulent virus (Naidoo & Wills 1995).

The medical approach is best evaluated by using epidemiological data (mortality and morbidity statistics) or by evaluating the increase in uptake of the

screening by the identified target population. Recent changes to GP contracting include offering incentive payments for achieving cervical screening targets of women on practice lists.

Behaviour change

This approach aims to encourage individuals to adopt a change in behaviour – such as to change to a 'healthy diet' or to stop smoking.

Reflective point

Consider how many of your patients were referred to you as a result of self-assessment or screening by a GP and/or a practice nurse. To what extent do you consider that self-assessment/screening in these patients was a successful outcome to health promotion? How does this relate to 'The Health of the Nation' (DoH 1992, p. 18) target for breast cancer: 'To reduce the death rate for breast cancer in the population invited for screening by at least 25% by the year 2000'?

It works on the premiss that it is an individual's choice to make such a change; the health care professional's role is to facilitate such a change by providing information and support. Ultimately, however, the responsibility lies with the individual, and hence, unless extreme care is taken, a victim-blaming, guilt-inducing scenario may develop.

The 'Health of the Nation' strategy (DoH 1992) essentially adopts such an approach, by setting targets related to individual lifestyle behaviours. The document, however, has been criticised for adopting such an individualistic approach whilst ignoring the social, economic and environmental context in which individuals attempt to make such changes. Hence, the Government demonstrates a commitment to 'health promotion' but without providing a supportive framework for action to take place.

Behaviour change thus assumes that individuals can and wish to make changes and attempts to achieve compliance whilst laying responsibility for success (or failure) at the door of the individual.

However, behaviour change has received a recent boost to its image via the 'Helping people change' project (DoH 1993b). This project offers a training programme to primary health care professionals involved in one-to-one counselling. It helps professionals identify how people change and how to respond to individuals according to their readiness to change. The programme is founded upon four key areas; smoking,

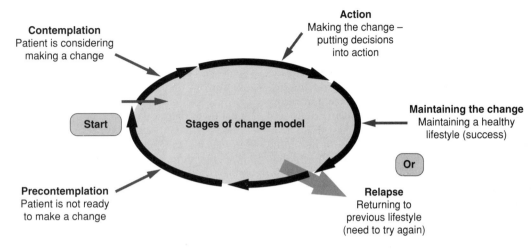

Figure 3.2   The stages of change model (adapted from Prochaska & DiClemente 1984).

alcohol, eating and physical activity, and uses Prochaska and DiClemente's (1984) model as its action framework. This model primarily encompasses a skills-based programme (see Fig. 3.2). It recognises the need to identify whether an individual is ready to change before instituting a compliance programme.

Many nurses may recognise their patient education approach in such a scenario and may find the Prochaska and DiClemente model a useful framework to assess, plan and evaluate care. It can be used pre- or postoperatively when giving advice to a patient attempting a behaviour change such as giving up smoking.

Evaluation of behaviour change relates to the length of time needed to evaluate such a change. Whilst many surgical nurses offer very useful lifestyle advice to clients as inpatients or as part of their discharge planning, how many nurses are able to follow up patients to assess the long-term efficacy of their intervention?

Educational approach

The educational approach may appeal to nurses and surgical nurse educators. The approach aims to provide knowledge, support and the necessary skills to enable an individual to make an informed choice. It differs essentially from the behaviour change approach in that it does not require compliance with a predetermined outcome, but is underpinned by the essential principle of voluntarism. Voluntarism is concerned with individuals making informed choices and thus taking responsibility for their health. It is also about allowing the individual the right to take personal risks. Tones (1990)

suggests that this is difficult for health care professionals to accept – allowing people to make the 'wrong' or 'unhealthy' choice is a difficult path to follow.

Tones (1986) questions whether an 'educative' approach is sufficient to facilitate informed choice and decision-making, as education is not value or belief free. Similarly, McKenna (1993) suggests that access to knowledge, access to resources and respect for individuals and their beliefs are essential prerequisites of free choice.

An educational programme is usually led by a professional (educator or nurse) and may thus be perceived as 'expert-led' and 'top-down'.

Whilst educational approaches are proven to be effective in terms of raising awareness and improving knowledge, their efficacy in assisting behaviour change is doubtful. Most people in society are aware of the risks of cigarette smoking. Indeed, prior to surgery the nurse should ensure that the patient is aware of the increased risks to recovery. However, a reduction or cessation of smoking behaviour does not always correlate with this knowledge.

Client-centred approach

The client-centred approach essentially differs from previously mentioned approaches in the nature of its 'bottom-up' approach. The health promoter acts as a facilitator, working with a client or groups to help them identify what they want to know, and to help them gain the necessary knowledge and skills to make effective decisions.

This approach is primarily underpinned by the concept of empowerment, whereby the health care professional respects people as equals, and strives to share and transfer power to other individuals, who are assumed to have the right to make decisions and choices about their health care.

Caring for patients with chest drains demonstrates an excellent example of how nurses may use empowerment to promote patient independence and recovery. If the surgical nurse offers the patient advice and information about the importance of chest drain management (i.e. which includes the reason for not lifting the drainage bottle above the level of the chest), then the patient is enabled to self-care and become independent of the nurses' care in this respect.

Empowerment is perceived as a fundamental tenet of health promotion practice (Rissell 1994, Yeo 1993) and as an emerging paradigm in nursing (King 1994, Rodwell 1996). However, relinquishing the expert role may prove difficult for both the health care professional and also the patient. Problems also exist with evaluation of such methods, as by their nature the process tends to be long term and its outcome perceivably vague.

Societal change

This approach, which is occasionally referred to as radical health promotion, aims to address the socioeconomic and environmental issues that contribute to the health status of society. It tends to involve groups and communities and, whilst a top-down approach, requires the commitment of members of society in order to be successful. It involves such activities as policy-planning, social control, media activities, political lobbying and campaigning.

Health promotion is not just about helping individuals to change aspects of their lifestyle but involves the society in which we live and the policies which help to create a healthy environment. Referring back to Tones' (1993) definition – 'Health promotion = Health education × Healthy public policy' – this approach refers specifically to the healthy public policy involved in 'making healthy choices easy choices'. Examples of activities regarding this approach would include active involvement in a hospital healthy eating policy, developing a ward-based display of advice for stopping smoking, or running a stress workshop.

Excellent discussion regarding hospital health promotion and examples of such activity are included in the handbook by McBride (1995) to which the reader is referred.

Within the health promotion models to be discussed in the next section, aspects of these approaches tend to emerge and the core beliefs of the theorists tend to direct the emphasis. For example, Tones et al's (1990) model reflects empowerment as its major aim and Tannahill (1985) emphasises prevention, education and protection as overlapping spheres of activity, whereas Beattie (1991) emphasises political issues within his model.

A consideration of diverse models for practice enables the surgical nurse to be analytical and discriminative about more and less desirable ways of promoting health. Judgements about what is preferable and possible will contribute to the effectiveness and efficiency of health promotion (Naidoo & Wills 1994).

Tannahill's model of health promotion

Tannahill's (1985) model is frequently acknowledged by health care professionals as a most useful model for practice. It depicts three overlapping spheres of activity; health education, prevention and health protection (Fig. 3.3).

Health education

Tannahill sees health education as:

Communication activity aimed at enhancing positive health and preventing or diminishing ill-health in individuals and groups, through influencing the beliefs, attitudes and behaviour of those with power and of the community at large.

(Tannahill, cited in Downie et al, p. 28)

He is therefore emphasising issues to do with health beliefs, power, control, attitudes and behaviour in this definition. A central assumption is that health education is a communication activity.

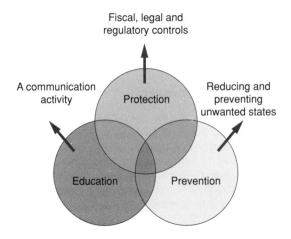

Figure 3.3 Tannahill's model of health promotion (adapted from Tannahill 1985).

Prevention

Prevention refers to the notion of reducing the risk of occurrence of a disease process, illness, injury or some other unwanted state. It is proposed that the usual classification of primary, secondary and tertiary prevention is unsatisfactory and a framework which moves beyond merely the prevention of disease is suggested; positive health promotion is emphasised.

Health protection

Health protection stems from the old public health measures previously alluded to and is defined as:

Health protection comprises legal or fiscal controls, other regulations and policies and voluntary codes of practice, aimed at the enhancement of positive health and the prevention of ill health.

(Downie et al 1990)

These authors suggest that health protection is about making healthy choices, easier choices through reducing environmental hazards, and increasing opportunities for a healthy lifestyle.

Surgical nurses frequently care for diabetic patients, for whom health promotion to enhance foot care is an important issue. Using Tannahill's (1985) model, all three spheres of education, prevention and protection can be used. Preventive services include the provision of free chiropody services, diabetic clinics and access to these services for all diabetic patients. Positive health education involves nurses augmenting chiropodists' advice on effective foot care (e.g. well-fitting shoes, toenail and skin care), and health protection includes the most effective health awareness activities undertaken by such groups as The British Diabetic Association and dissemination of information by diabetic nurses.

Beattie's model of health promotion

Beattie (1991) describes his model as a structural map which demonstrates the different strategies which are present in contemporary health promotion. The map demonstrates four quadrants of activity divided by two bipolar dimensions: 'mode of intervention' and 'focus of intervention' (Fig. 3.4). Both poles depict the enduring debate which exists in social policy, namely the top-down/bottom-up dimensions and the individual versus the collective debate.

Beattie's map may prove useful in orienting us to the diversity of activity available to the health promoter and may help us to understand the relationship of these activities to the approaches previously

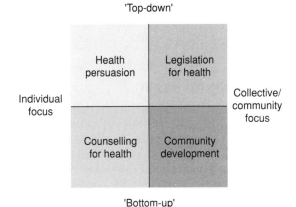

Figure 3.4 Strategies of health promotion (adapted from Beattie 1991).

described, namely empowerment (community development), behaviour change (health persuasion), and medical model (legislation for health).

Health persuasion

Connotations of control and compliance have given this approach a 'bad name' yet its historical roots in health education are impressive. This activity encompasses activities derived by health promoters aimed at individuals and is often underpinned by an educational or behavioural change approach. Health persuasion aims to get health messages to the people. Examples of such activity include media health promotion campaigns and targeting of high-risk groups with leaflets and educational workshops.

The current high-profile AIDS awareness and drink–driving campaigns and the implementation of the 'Health of the Nation' demonstrate this strategy. 'Commit to get fit', the Health Education Authorities' exercise and fitness campaign, is another example of an awareness-raising activity. However, raising awareness does not always result in lifestyle change.

Legislation for health

This strategy also has strong historical roots – striking health benefits achieved through public health policies formed the basis of this health promotion activity in the 19th century.

Legislative action includes interventions led by health care professionals aimed at protecting communities and promoting positive health by policy development. Examples include professionals lobbying Parliament to develop seat belt policies and the implementation of healthy eating policies (such as food labelling). At the hospital level the implementation of a non-smoking hospital policy is an example of legislative action.

Counselling for health

This activity grants the client group an active role and focuses upon helping individuals to identify their needs and to develop skills and knowledge to enable them to make changes to their life. It therefore seeks to empower the individual and the professional aims to act in a facilitative role within the client–professional encounter.

An example would be enabling an overweight young mother admitted with an acute episode of cholecystitis to identify her needs (dietary reform), working with her to set realistic goals and referring her to appropriate agencies to help her develop the necessary skills and knowledge to achieve the changes.

Community development

Community activities involved in empowering groups in society are currently promoted as a most effective way of achieving consistent long-term change. Health promotion workers, in conjunction with community leaders aim to enable the group to identify their own needs, determine their own actions and set their own agendas. The professional's role in such an endeavour is to act in a way that is primarily facilitative.

Nurses who act in a supportive, facilitative role with self-help groups such as diabetic-support or cardiac-support groups are functioning within a community development approach. Similarly, charitable organisations such as the Mastectomy Association work within this approach.

The Tones, Tilford & Robinson model

Tones et al (1990) view health promotion as an amalgam of policy development and health education and offer a somewhat complex map of the issues involved in promoting health. Essentially the model depicts the two-pronged approach required to promote positive health and absence of disease (Fig. 3.5). These two approaches include promoting health choices and social engineering to achieve this aim.

This model is underpinned by an empowerment philosophy, the central premise being that social change can occur only by empowering individuals or groups to modify their environment. This change may be augmented by agenda setting and the raising of critical consciousness (the process of generating public consciousness about health issues), professional education (the contribution made by health care personnel) and lobbying, advocacy and mediation (the process of influencing the decision-making process through liaising with powerful individuals or pressure groups).

Nurses may see roles for themselves in a variety of settings and contexts and may feel comfortable with the notion of empowerment, which is essentially a client-centred process enabling patients to identify and set their own agenda, to make their own health choices and decisions and to implement change by addressing the people with power. Nurses themselves have immense political power and may see a

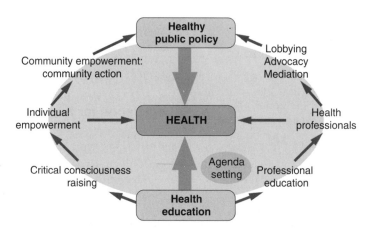

Figure 3.5 Health promotion = Health education × Healthy public policy (adapted from Tones et al 1990).

role for themselves as patient advocates. Examples of nurses working in a lobbying role include committee work in developing healthy workplace initiatives such as healthy eating in hospital policies or smoking in the workplace policies. The reader is once again directed to the excellent text by McBride (1995) for further examples of ways in which nurses might become involved in health promotion initiatives in hospitals.

PATIENT EDUCATION AND THE PRINCIPLES OF ADULT LEARNING

The aim of patient education is to promote health, to prevent health breakdown or to augment post-recuperative recovery.

Traditionally patient education developed from a need to translate doctors' advice to patients, where the nurses' role incorporated amplification and explanation of health-related information. Surgical nurses have always recognised the need for information-giving to influence pre- and postoperative outcomes. Contemporary criteria against which such interventions are measured include earlier patient discharge, and reduced postoperative medication and complications.

Nurses are frequently cited as valued patient educators owing to their credibility, experience and relationship with patients and their families (Clarke 1991). However, research also shows that whilst patients want information about their illness and treatment, many have immense difficulty remembering the information given and do not comply with their treatment regimes (Ley 1990).

Redman (1993) sees similarities between the patient education process and the nursing process and contends that nurses are best placed to perform this activity with patients and their families. Bellman (1994) suggests that in preparation for this role, nurses may wish to perform some form of self-assessment to identify their strengths and weaknesses in this area and to recognise any professional development needs. She suggests a self-assessment tool (see Box 3.1).

Adult learning

The process of helping adults to learn incorporates some basic tenets which may also be applied to helping patients to learn (Knowles 1973). It should, however, be remembered that certain physiological, psychosocial and pathological conditions may inhibit the education process; if a patient is distressed or in

---

> **Box 3.1** Nurses' self-assessment patient education tool (Bellman 1994)
>
> - How confident do I feel about teaching patients?
> - Do I have the appropriate knowledge and skills?
> - Am I familiar with contemporary issues in adult learning?
> - How can I apply these to my patients?
> - Which factors will create a good learning environment for patients?
> - Which factors may hinder patient teaching?
> - What further knowledge and skills do I need to facilitate patient education?
> - How will I gain these?

---

pain, it is clearly not appropriate to embark upon a learning encounter.

Knowles (1973), the 'father' of adult learning, identifies the following issues as important in the learning process:

- self concept of the learner
- previous life experiences
- readiness to learn
- preferred learning style
- motivation to learn.

Kolb (1984) suggests that individuals learn in different ways, dependent upon past experiences, preferences and environmental issues. Kolb (1984) identified four styles of learning – convergent, divergent, assimilative and accommodative – and suggests that individuals will gravitate towards their preferred learning style. It is therefore useful for nurses to understand the possible models of learning which may be used by their clients in order to develop effective teaching strategies.

Convergent

Convergent learners are essentially practical learners, they prefer to apply knowledge, see results and participate in learning activities. Convergent learners essentially learn by 'doing'. Nurses can encourage patients with this learning style to practise skills or to take a very active role in theoretical learning.

Divergent

Divergent learners prefer to understand the knowledge and assimilate this into their existing knowledge base. Nurses should ensure that they identify what the patient already knows from past experience and then build upon this in the learning activities they provide for the patient.

Assimilative

The assimilative learner focuses upon facts and knowledge. The emphasis is upon thinking and the patient will essentially see the surgical nurse as 'expert'. The nurse may therefore adopt the role of 'expert giver' and allow the patient time to assimilate given information and reflect upon what has been learnt.

Accommodative

Accommodative learners place the emphasis on feeling as opposed to thinking. They tend to learn by trial and error and risk-taking. They are intrinsically intuitive but tend to rely upon others for information and support. The nurse should encourage this patient to explore the variety of options available and to practise these options within the context of a safe environment.

The teaching–learning process

The teaching–learning process is an integral part of the nursing process. Meeting the learning needs of patients and their families through effective use of the principles of learning and effective teaching strategies is best considered within the context of the nursing process.

Assessment

An assessment of education needs is carried out to identify the patient's beliefs and values, to explore relevant issues and to raise awareness of learning needs.

It is important to identify how much a patient already knows in order that previous knowledge and experience can be built upon. It also enables any gaps or inaccuracies in the knowledge base to be identified and acted upon. This is also important to ensure clarification of teaching content; any discrepancy between the nurse's and patient's perceptions will affect the learning process.

The patient's readiness to learn is often related to the need to know or to do things and hence if a subject seems relevant, this will increase motivation. Similarly, ability to learn may be hindered by a number of factors such as pain, distress, or metabolic or neurological disorders. Visual, hearing, speech or language impairments should also be assessed and the patient's cognitive, intellectual and physical ability should be identified to ensure individualisation of the educational encounter and to avoid stereotyping (Bellman 1994).

> **Reflective point**
>
> Consider the information you have just read and reflect upon the methods you use to effectively assess your patients' existing knowledge base and readiness and motivation to learn. Also consider how you might include the client's family and friends in this assessment process.

Planning

The assessment discussion should form the basis for the goal-setting exercise. The nurse and the patient and family should work together to set realistic, achievable goals, the aims of which are mutually agreed.

The Patient's Charter (DoH 1991) actively encourages patients' involvement and emphasises patients' rights to partnership in care decisions. 'Owning' the goals encourages patients to learn (Redman 1993), and Wallerstein (1992) confirms that participation in care decisions will enhance the patients' self-esteem and belief in the mutability of situations.

The agreed goals of health education should be documented in the care plan which will facilitate continuity of teaching and will also provide reinforcement for both the nurse and the patient.

At this stage it may help to ask the question: 'Am I teaching the patient what *he* wants to know or what *I* want to teach him?'

Intervention/implementation

Benner (1984) suggests that the nurse's role at this stage is a 'teaching–coaching' function. She suggests that the ability to enable patients to interpret their illness and integrate the implications of that experience into their lifestyle is a skilled nursing activity. Similarly, Wilson-Barnett (1988) says that helping individuals to make sound decisions about their health is the ultimate goal of health education.

The ability to stimulate and motivate the patient may be improved by adopting a problem-solving approach and using a variety of teaching methods. The use of videotapes, tape–slide programmes, leaflets and models is encouraged within an interactive process. Having knowledge and skill does not necessarily ensure that it is passed on; one needs to engage the patient in the learning process as well.

Time is often cited as an inhibitory influence at this stage. Finding time to sit down with patients is frequently identified as an inhibitory factor in hospital ward settings (Mitchinson 1995). With this in mind it is also important to note, however, that a patient's attention span and ability to retain information may limit any encounter to no more than a 10-minute teaching episode. Similarly, factors such as environmental temperature, noise level, lighting and the time of day may affect a patient's ability to concentrate. The constant interruptions and distractions of a busy surgical ward make the use of a teaching or seminar room invaluable (Bellman 1994).

Recent research has linked the method of organising and performing nursing to effective patient education. Maben et al (1993) noted that primary nursing was associated with more effective health education in hospital practice. This suggests that if nurses were empowered and autonomous in their practice, they would be more likely to empower their patients and include them in health care decisions.

Evaluation

It is vital to document patient teaching, in order to evaluate its effectiveness and improve its quality. It may also serve to enable nurses to demonstrate their effectiveness and to facilitate earlier patient discharge and reduced postoperative complications. It is important that nurses demonstrate these issues by documenting outcomes in the care plan and evaluating care using quality audit tools to monitor patients' progress.

Less formal methods of patient evaluation include quizzes and games, which some patients find fun and enjoyable (Burnard 1988). Beware, however, as others do not.

Self-evaluation

Burnard (1988) states that whilst self-evaluation can enable us to clarify what is still to be learned, it is also essential to identify how past learning can be incorporated with the present. Reflection on one's strengths and limitations is also a useful beginning and endpoint to patient education. Many nurses are now seeing the value of undertaking post-registration courses in teaching and assessing as a valuable addition to their nursing skills.

COMMUNICATION

Fundamental principles of teaching and learning should be followed by nurses involved in patient education. Similarly, basic communication skills should be employed to ensure that the educational process is as effective as possible.

Basic educational and communication principles identified by Redman (1993), Bellman (1994), Lowry (1995) and Vahabi & Ferris (1995) for the surgical nurse to employ include:

- Check the patient's understanding of the issues.
- Give important information first – as it is more likely to be remembered.
- Use short words, brief sentences and avoid medical jargon.
- Repeat and reinforce key issues, several times.
- Give specific advice rather than vague general advice, i.e. 'take your medication every morning before breakfast'.
- Support issues with relevant leaflets (see p. 62).
- Record what has been said in the nursing notes and encourage other professionals to reinforce the information. This should ensure consistency and avoid confusion.
- Check that the patient has understood by asking relevant questions. Avoid using closed questions, e.g. 'do you understand?' It is preferable to say, 'Tell me what you don't understand'.

Working with clients who do not speak/read English

When English is not the patient's spoken language, other strategies are needed to ensure understanding (see Box 3.2).

A number of patients will come through the surgical wards every day, and many of these patients will

---

Box 3.2 Strategies to be considered when English is not the patient's spoken language

- More time may need to be allocated to patient education in order to ensure sufficient understanding.
- Speak slowly and clearly, using the same words each time – using a variety of words to mean the same thing may cause confusion.
- Avoid slang, medical jargon and complicated terminology.
- Pictures, word cards and specialist literature may be very useful and are often available from the local health promotion unit or the Health Education Authority.
- Use an interpreter if available – some hospitals have a list of suitable interpreters.
- Use a member of the family or visitor to interpret, but beware that in some cultures this may cause embarrassment or be inappropriate.
- Endeavour to check that the patient has understood.

have limited or no English. These patients are likely to be extremely frightened and anxious and need additional support. Reliance on interpreters and leaflets written in the more common minority languages may help, but specific needs should be identified according to your patient demographic profile and the local health promotion unit should be able to offer you various resources to support patient education with these client groups (Farrelly & Lakeman 1993/1994).

Health promotion materials

Current health legislation and reform is constructing patients as active participants and consumers of health care who are at the same time required to accept greater responsibility for their health (Grace 1991). There is, therefore, a need to develop health promotion materials to communicate health messages. It is imperative that given the apparent diminishing resources available, materials which are used need to be evaluated as appropriate, effective and accurate. Earlier hospital discharge, increased patient awareness, and the need for self-care in the community, also require the need for effective health promotion materials to supplement and augment the health messages in the recuperative period.

Communication is the means by which all information and knowledge is transmitted, and in essence the communication event is to do with the conveyance of meaning (MacDonald 1992). Different forms of communication are used in health promotion activity, from mass media interventions to one-to-one interactions; the way the ideas are expressed, however, is of vital importance, particularly when the message is being communicated in the absence of the health promoter (Wilson-Barnett 1993).

The mass media are an integral part of our society and a powerful method of communicating health messages. Tones (1994) has stated that whilst the mass media should not be considered a panacea for health promotion, it is nevertheless part of the armamentarium of the health promoter.

The objective of effective patient education is to encourage patients' active participation in their treatment and recovery and this process can be aided by effective good-quality patient education materials. Leaflets and posters are extensively used in health promotion practice and their use in surgical ward areas will be considered.

Alderson (1994) states that clearly written health information is essential to keep the patient informed and that poorly written information is not only unhelpful but is likely to make people feel more worried. Comprehensible information may motivate patients to seek knowledge about even frightening and uncomfortable health issues. Schwalb & Crosson (1988) and Ley (1990) assert that providing clients with information enables true informed consent and increased patient understanding and satisfaction. Client choice is also important as it is the prerequisite of informed decision-making (McKenna 1993).

Leaflets

Leaflets play an increasingly important part in patient education, partly because of increased demands from patients for relevant knowledge and partly owing to earlier hospital discharge. Murphy & Smith (1993), however, have identified that too much activity centres on the use of leaflets, but that currently there is nothing to replace them.

Ley (1990) states that those who receive written information express favourable attitudes to it, whereas Ewles & Simnett (1995) state that leaflets may end up as waste paper unless the educator actively involves the patient in using the material. The leaflet should aim to translate the health education message into practice for people (Murphy & Smith 1992).

Encouraging client participation and active use of the leaflet (perhaps by personalisation of the leaflet) may enhance its use (Dougherty & Stuttaford 1993).

Health promotion leaflets have many advantages; they are relatively cheap to produce, portable, and have reusable references which offer flexibility to clients in terms of self-pacing and self-teaching. Information can also be shared with family and friends, and patients can use the leaflet to 'revise' the content of health teaching at their leisure (Bernier & Yasko 1991, Ewles & Simnett 1995, Murphy & Smith 1992).

It is important, therefore, that nurses examine the patient education leaflets in use in their surgical settings to ensure that they are of high quality and appropriate for the client group. Leaflets may be analysed using specific criteria including design considerations, readability and comprehensibility, and content issues.

Reflective point

Have the patient education leaflets in your practice area been evaluated by your patients?

Design considerations

General design considerations include visual impact, use of colour, size and style of print, texture of paper and use of illustrations.

Visual impact is essential to generate interest and motivate individuals to read the text. A simple title has best impact if presented as white letters on a solid colour background (Lohr et al 1989). Colours have unique relationships to each other and to the viewer. In general the perception of colour is a culturally learned value, hence the adage in western society 'orange and green should never be seen'. Colours clash when they are similar in saturation or hue – red and orange clash as they are adjacent colours on the spectrum. Opposite spectrum colours, however, complement each other. Some colours have certain associations: red – danger; purple – death; green and blue are perceived as cool or soothing; and yellow is bright and cheerful. Colours used should be congruent with the health message (Bushy 1991, Duchin & Sherwood 1990).

Layout and format has also been shown to be important. Legibility of the text is enhanced by good paper texture and size and style of text. The Royal National Institute for the Blind recommend the use of a minimum of 12 point print size and the avoidance of italic and bold type (Petterson 1994).

Information should be organised so that only the most important and necessary information is included in the leaflet – to ensure that patients are not overloaded with unnecessary information (Vahabi & Ferris 1995).

Conversational style is recommended and a narrative style often personalises the message and makes the text easier to read. It is also important that any health messages are written in the active (rather than the passive) voice. The use of 'you' rather than 'we' or 'one' personalises the message and is more likely to result in encouraging change and a sense of positivity. For example:

'You should not combine this drug with alcohol' is more likely to be effective than:

'It is recommended that this drug should not be taken with alcohol' and is more likely to result in a compliant response by the patient.

It is also important to remember that health education leaflets do not need to be lengthy to be effective, and that messages which appear to be personalised for the patient are perceived as being important to read and remember (Vahabi & Ferris 1995).

Illustrations can be invaluable in helping people with reading difficulties comprehend the health education messages. 'A picture is worth a thousand words' and illustrations, if used effectively, can aid recall and should augment the written material. Any illustrations used should be simple and demonstrate only one concept (Rohret & Ferguson 1990, Vahabi & Ferris 1995).

Readable and comprehensible

As Petterson (1994) states, whilst attention to details such as paper texture, illustrations and the use of colour are admirable, they must come second to the clear presentation of the information in the leaflet. If communication is to be effective, the language used in the leaflet should be clear, concise and simple.

The use of short words, short sentences and short paragraphs will produce more readable leaflets and will be more easily understood by people with poor literacy skills.

It is important to remember that the average reading age of an adult in the UK correlates with that of a 10–14-year-old and hence many studies suggest that written materials are aimed at the reading level of a 10–11-year-old (Vahabi & Ferris 1995).

Readability formulae can help to assess the reading level of written materials and the Gunning Fog (frequency of gobbledegook) is recommended here (see Box 3.3).

As a general rule, the lower the score achieved for a text, the easier the passage is to read, and a score greater than 12 may represent the upper level of readability for the general population (Ewles & Simnett 1995). Petterson (1994) suggests that a novel by James Herbert would achieve a score of 9, a *Daily Mirror* Leader would achieve a score of 12, an *Independent* Leader a score of 19 and an Insurance Policy – 20.

A practice exercise example of readability assessment is given on a passage taken from a leaflet on post-haemorrhoidectomy care:

Box 3.3 Gunning Fog test (Petterson 1994, p. 14)

Select a passage of 100 words, ending in a full stop. The passage selected should be considered representative of the language and layout of the document. The average sentence length is determined by dividing 100 by the number of sentences. The number of long words (defined as those of three syllables or more) is recorded. This definition excludes (a) proper nouns (b) combinations of easy words (e.g. photocopy), (c) verbs that have become three syllables when 'es', 'ing' or 'ed' are added (e.g. committed) and (d) jargon which the reader would recognise easily. The reading score is obtained by adding the average sentence length to the number of long words and multiplying this value by 0.4.

This formula should be repeated on at least three 100-word passages to gain a mean score.

Discharge Information for Patients who have undergone haemorrhoidectomy or cryotherapy to haemorrhoids.
Haemorrhoids occur when veins beneath the skin of the anal canal become dilated, they then fill up with blood during straining at stool and may burst following passage of the stool. They may be associated with pain. Haemorrhoids may sometimes be injected, but if they are large they are treated by surgical excision or cryotherapy (freezing). If your haemorrhoids have been treated by cryotherapy, you may expect a watery discharge for at least two weeks. This is however quite normal and shows that the haemorrhoid is disappearing.

This passage clearly illustrates an example of patient education literature in which the readability level is too high.

The average sentence length is 16 (six sentences in a 100 word passage).

The number of difficult words is 19 (includes haemorrhoids, cryotherapy, injected, anal canal and surgical excision).

16 (average sentence length) + 19 (number of difficult words) = 35 × 0.4 = 14.0

This leaflet is only used as an example to illustrate readability levels, and most patient education leaflets have good readability scores.

Whilst the Gunning Fog test is considered simple and reliable in assessing texts, its use is considered more valid when used in conjunction with other general design considerations. As previously discussed these include visual impact, use of colour, size, and style of print and use of illustrations.

Content

The content of any leaflet should clearly be accurate and up to date and should aim to act as a resource for patients and families and friends. Given current technology, leaflets should be updated regularly and their content reviewed.

The accuracy of information presented can be assessed by other health care professionals, other patients, voluntary agencies and support groups.

Language. Issues related to patients for whom English is not the primary spoken or written language have already been considered. Many leaflets are now available in a variety of minority languages and your local health promotion unit should be able to advise you on gaining the appropriate resources for your ward. It is important not to assume, however, that all patients are able to read.

There are numerous health education/patient education leaflets available; however, Murphy & Smith (1993) have suggested that they may serve many purposes from crutches, to confetti, to useful tools. In

---

Box 3.4 A tool to analyse the usefulness of a patient education leaflet

Analysis of patient education leaflets
- Who is the target audience: is the material appropriate to the target group?
- What are the stated messages: are they clear?
- Consider design issues such as colour, print size and type, illustration, layout: do these issues enhance or detract from the health education message?
- Is the text readable and comprehensible to your target audience? Conduct a gobbledegook test: does it achieve an appropriate reading level for your target audience?
- Overall, how would you evaluate this leaflet (marks out of 10)?

---

order to assess the value of the leaflets in current use on your ward, the analysis tool shown in Box 3.4 is suggested. Alternatively, it may be used as a framework for designing a new leaflet for use with your own patient group.

Health education displays

An effective way to encourage patients to read health education leaflets is to develop a media display on your ward. This display could relate to a specific theme, e.g. stoma care, wound care or medications, and could be changed weekly to maintain interest. Use of corridor space or the day room would ensure that patients and their families and friends would be effectively targeted.

A media display could include posters and leaflets and would also include contact addresses and other pertinent resources to encompass the whole theme.

Posters

Posters are frequently used, independent sources of information which may be used to support other health promotion activities. They are relatively inexpensive and have the potential to transmit messages to a large population.

A good poster is visually dynamic and eminently interactive, and should attract people to stop and read, possibly even re-read, its contents and stimulate them to seek further information.

The setting of the poster may impact on its effectiveness and hence it should be appropriately placed and consideration should be given to lighting, eye-level or picture-level placement and the presence of any distractions (Bushy 1991, Duchin & Sherwood 1990).

Keep it simple smarty – KISS

Bushy (1991) advocates the use of the KISS principle (keep it simple smarty) which recognises that most viewers will not read a lengthy or detailed display. The message should be straightforward and the meaning clear. The use of an active verb in the title invites the viewer to participate. A picture or illustration is especially pertinent and it should impart a lasting image and support the message presented (Duchin & Sherwood 1990).

Colour influences previously discussed in relation to leaflets enhance the aesthetic appeal of a poster. Whilst a poster should not be too wordy, it is important that any text is easily readable from a distance of 4–6 feet.

An effective poster is concise, readable and has a clear message. It should be eye-catching and cheerful and should appeal to the target audience. Used in conjunction with leaflets and augmented by a health professional, it should prove an effective medium for providing health messages.

Posters and leaflets are readily available from the local health promotion unit, specialist agencies (such as Cancer Research) or the Health Education Authority.

CONCLUSION

One cannot tell what the future will hold for surgical nursing in the millennium. However Macleod Clark (1993) recommends that nursing needs to shift its focus away from what she terms 'sick nursing'

towards a philosophy of 'health nursing' in order to respond to future health needs. She states that 'sick nursing' is founded upon medical diagnosis and care which is largely prescribed and administered by health care professionals and similarly health care decisions are dominated by professionals (p. 256).

Consequently for the millennium 'health nursing' must be emphasised to accommodate a change in the balance of power between clients and carers. Principles implicit in a health promotion approach will need, in particular, to include the concept of empowerment to enable people to accept responsibility for health care based upon the notions of collaboration and partnership.

Nurse education now has its Project 2000 curriculum firmly rooted in health nursing and future research will be founded upon health indicators rather than medical diagnoses. The way is therefore open for surgical nursing to develop upon the same basis and to incorporate the concepts and principles of health promotion into its philosophy of nursing.

Health promotion has been high on the health service agenda since the publication of 'The Health of the Nation' (DoH 1992). The aim of this chapter has been to enable surgical nurses to become more involved in health promotion in their day-to-day practice. Surgical nurses may develop this practice by using a variety of health promotion approaches and models and by a more thoughtful use of patient education literature in the clinical settings. It is the responsibility of all nurses to ensure that the health promotion needs of their clients are met.

REFERENCES

Alderson P 1994 As plain as can be. Health Service Journal 104(5403): 28–29

Beattie A 1991 Knowledge and control in health promotion: a test case for social policy and social history. In: Gabe J, Calnan M, Bury M (eds) The sociology of the health service. Routledge, London

Bellman L 1994 Principles of educating patients. Surgical Nurse 7(1): 7–10

Benner P 1984 From novice to expert: excellence and power in clinical nursing practice. Addison Wesley, California

Bernier M J, Yasko J 1991 Designing and evaluating printed education materials: model and instrument development. Patient Education and Counselling 18(3): 253–263

Blythe M 1986 A century of health education. Hygiene 7: 105–115

Bridge C, Nelson S 1994 A deficit in care: the educational needs of thoracic patients. Professional Nurse 10(1): 8–13

Bunton R 1995 Health off the shelf? Health Matters 21(Spring): 8–9

Bunton R, MacDonald G 1992 (eds) Health promotion: disciplines and diversity. Routledge, London

Burnard P 1988 Self evaluation methods in nurse education. Nurse Education Today 8(4): 229–233

Bushy A 1991 A rating scale to evaluate research posters. Nurse Educator 16(1): 11–15

Cancer Research Campaign 1990 Fact sheets: Cervical cancer screening 13.1–13.5. CRC, London

Clarke A C 1991 Nurses as role models and health educators. Journal of Advanced Nursing 16(10): 1178–1184

Close A 1988 Patient education: a literature review. Journal of Advanced Nursing 13(2): 203–213

Crawford R 1980 Healthism and the medicalisation of everyday life. International Journal of Health Services 10(3): 365–387

Department of Health (DoH) 1989 A strategy for nursing. A report of the Steering Committee. Department of Health Nursing Division, London

Department of Health (DoH) 1991 The patient's charter. HMSO, London

Department of Health (DoH) 1992 The health of the nation. HMSO, London

Department of Health (DoH) 1993a The health of the nation one year on, a report on the true progress of the health of the nation. HMSO, London

Department of Health (DoH) 1993b Better living, better lives. HMSO, London

Department of Health (DoH) 1994 The challenges for nursing in the 21st century. DoH, London

Department of Health and Social Security (DHSS) 1976 Prevention and health: everybody's business. HMSO, London

Dobson F 1992 Health promotion: a role for perioperative nurses. Journal of Clinical Nursing 1(5): 253–258

Dougherty L, Stuttaford J 1993 Turning over a new leaflet. Nursing Times 89(45): 10, 46–48

Downie R S, Fyfe C, Tannahill A 1990 Health promotion: models and values. Oxford Medical Publications, London

Duchin S, Sherwood G 1990 Posters as an education strategy. Journal of Continuing Education in Nursing 21(5): 205–208

Dutton K E A 1994 Patient education in a day surgery unit. Journal of One Day Surgery 3(4): 22–24

Ewles L, Simnett I 1995 Promoting health: a practical guide, 3rd edn. Scutari Press, London

Fahlberg L L, Poulin A L, Girdano D A, Dusek D E 1991 Empowerment as an emerging approach in health education. Journal of Health Education 22(3): 185–187, 189–193

Farrelly H, Lakeman D 1993/1994 Patient education in day care. Journal of One Day Surgery 3(3): 18–20

Fawcett J 1989 Analysis and evaluation of conceptual models and nursing, 2nd edn. Davis, Philadelphia

French J 1990 Boundaries and horizons: the role of health education within health promotion. Health Education Journal 49(1): 7–9

Gallagher U, Burden J 1993 Nursing as health promotion: a myth accepted? In: Wilson-Barnett J, Macleod Clark J (eds) Research in health promotion and nursing. Macmillan, Basingstoke

General Nursing Council for England and Wales 1944 Revised syllabus of subjects for the preliminary examination. GNC, London

Gott M, O'Brien M 1990 The role of the nurse in health promotion: policies, perspectives and practice. Open University, Milton Keynes

Grace V M 1991 The marketing of empowerment and the construction of the health consumer: a critique of health promotion. International Journal of Health Services 21(2): 329–343

King P M 1994 Health promotion: the emerging frontier in nursing. Journal of Advanced Nursing 20(2): 209–218

Knowles M 1973 The adult learner: a neglected species. Gulf, Houston

Kolb 1984 Learning style theory and patient education. Journal of Continuing Education in Nursing 21(1): 28–31

Latter S, Macleod Clark J, Wilson-Barnett J, Maben J 1992 Health education in nursing: perceptions of practice in acute settings. Journal of Advanced Nursing 17(2): 164–172

Leino-Kilpi H, Iire L, Suominen T, Vuorenheimo J, Valimaki M 1993 Client and information: a literature review. Journal of Clinical Nursing 2(6): 331–340

Ley P 1990 Communicating with patients. Chapman and Hall, London

Lohr G, Ventura M R, Crosby F, Burch K, Todd K 1989 An experience in designing patient education materials. Journal of Staff Nursing Development 5(Sept/Oct): 218–224

Lowry M 1995 Knowledge that reduces anxiety: creating patient information leaflets. Professional Nurse 10(5): 318–320

Maben J, Latter S, Macleod Clark J, Wilson-Barnett J 1993 The organisation of care: its influence on health education practice on acute wards. Journal of Clinical Nursing 2(6): 355–362

McBride A 1994 Health promotion in hospital: the attitudes, beliefs and practices of hospital nurses. Journal of Advanced Nursing 20(1): 92–100

McBride A 1995 Health promotion in hospital: a practical handbook for nurses. Scutari Press, London

MacDonald G 1992 Communication theory and health promotion. In: Bunton R, MacDonald G 1992 (eds) Health promotion: disciplines and diversity. Routledge, London

McKenna G 1993 Voluntarism: is it a useful concept for health education in the accident and emergency department? Journal of Advanced Nursing 18(10): 731–736

Macleod Clark J 1993 From sick nursing to health nursing: evolution or revolution. In: Wilson-Barnett J, Macleod Clark J (eds) Research in health promotion and nursing. Macmillan, Basingstoke

Masterson A 1995 Why nurses need to know about social policy. Surgical Nurse 8(2): 4–6

Meleis A I 1991 Theoretical nursing: development and progress. Lippincott, Philadelphia

Millar B 1994 Promoting patient self-management-cooperative care. Surgical Nurse 7(4): 33–35

Mitchinson S 1995 A review of the health promotion and health beliefs of traditional and Project 2000 student nurses. Journal of Advanced Nursing 21(2): 356–363

Murphy S, Smith C 1992 An examination of the use of health education leaflets by health promotion officers. Health Education Journal 51(4): 166–170

Murphy S, Smith C 1993 Crutches, confetti or useful tools? Professionals' views on and use of health education leaflets. Health Education Research 8(2): 205–215

Naidoo J, Wills J 1994 Health promotion: foundations for practice. Baillière Tindall, London

New H 1995 Health promotion role of the surgical nurse in cancer care. Surgical Nurse 8(3): 28–30

NHS and Community Care Act 1990 HMSO, London

Nightingale F 1859 Notes on nursing: what it is, and what it is not. Reprinted 1970, Duckworth, London

North N 1993 Empowerment in welfare markets. Health and Social Care 1(3): 129–137

Orem D E 1985 Nursing concepts of practice, 3rd edn. McGraw Hill, New York

Petterson T 1994 How readable are the hospital information leaflets available to elderly patients? Age and Ageing 23(1): 14–16

Prochaska J O, DiClemente C C 1984 The transtheoretical approach: crossing traditional boundaries of therapy. Dorsey Press, Homewood, Illinois

Redman B K 1993 The process of patient education. Mosby, St Louis

Rissell C 1994 Empowerment: the holy grail of health promotion? Health Promotion International 9(1): 39-47

Rodwell C M 1996 An analysis of the concept of empowerment. Journal of Advanced Nursing 23(2): 305–313

Rogers A, Whyms D 1995 A broader horizon for health promotion. Health Matters 21(Spring): 12–13

Rohret L, Ferguson K J 1990 Effective use of patient education illustrations. Patient Education and Counselling 15(1): 73–75

Ross E 1991 The origins of public health. In: Draper P (Ed) Health through public policy. Green Print, London

Royal College of Nursing (RCN) 1993 Agenda for action. A response to the Health of the Nation. RCN, London

Salvage J 1990 The theory and practice of the new nursing. Nursing Times 86(4): 42–45

Schwalb E, Crosson K 1988 Helping you help your patients. The patient education program of the National Cancer Institute. Oncology Nursing Forum 15: 651–655

Tannahill A 1985 What is health promotion? Health Education Journal 49(1): 7–10

Toms E 1993 Patient teaching: a neglected area of nurse practice? Senior Nurse 13(1): 37–39

Tones B K 1986 Health education and the ideology of health promotion: a review of the alternative approaches. Health Education Research 1(1): 3–12

Tones B K 1990 Why theorise? Ideology in health education. Health Education Journal 49(1): 2–6

Tones B K 1993 The theory of health promotion: implications for nursing. In: Wilson-Barnett J, Macleod Clark J (eds) Research in health promotion and nursing. Macmillan, Basingstoke

Tones K 1994 Marketing and the mass media: theory and myth: reflections on social marketing theory. Health Education Research 9(2): 165–169

Tones B K, Tilford S, Robinson Y K 1990 Health education: effectiveness and efficiency. Chapman and Hall, London

Vahabi M, Ferris L 1995 Improving written patient education materials: a review of the evidence. Health Education Journal 54(1): 99–106

Walker L O, Avant K C 1995 Strategies for theory construction in nursing, 3rd edn. Appleton and Lange, Norwalk

Wallerstein N 1992 Powerlessness, empowerment and health: implications for health promotion programs. American Journal of Health Promotion 6(3): 197–205

Waterworth S, Luker K 1990 Reluctant collaborators: do patients want to be involved in decisions concerning care. Journal of Advanced Nursing 15(8): 971–976

Wilson-Barnett J 1988 Patient teaching and patient counselling. Journal of Advanced Nursing 13(2): 215-222

Wilson-Barnett J 1993 Health promotion and nursing practice. In: Dines A, Cribb A (eds) Health promotion: concepts and practice. Blackwell Scientific Publications, Oxford

Wilson-Barnett J, Batehup L 1988 Patient problems: a research base for nursing care. Scutari Press, London

Wilson-Barnett J, Fordham M 1982 Recovery from illness. Wiley Medical Publications, UK

Wilson-Barnett J, Macleod Clark J 1993 (eds) Research in health promotion and nursing. Macmillan, Basingstoke

World Health Organization (WHO) 1984 Health promotion: a discussion document on concepts and principles. WHO, Geneva

World Health Organisation (WHO) 1986 The Ottawa charter for health promotion: an international conference on health promotion. The move towards public health. November 17–21. WHO, Ottawa

Yeo M 1993 Towards an ethic of empowerment for health promotion. Health Promotion International 8(3): 225–235

Zola I K 1978 Pathways to the doctor – from person to patient. In: Tuckett D, Kaufert J M (eds) Basic readings in medical sociology. Tavistock Publications, London

FURTHER READING

Dodds F 1993 Access to the coping strategies: managing anxiety in elective surgical patients. Professional Nurse 9(1): 45–46, 48, 50

Draper P 1991 Health through public policy. Green Print, London

Jones P S, Meleis A I 1993 Health is empowerment. Advances in Nursing Science 15(3): 1–14

McAllister G, Farquhar M 1992 Health beliefs: a cultural division? Journal of Advanced Nursing 17(12): 1447–1454

4

Ethical issues in surgical nursing

Gosia Brykczynska

AIMS

The aims of this chapter are:

- to introduce surgical nurses to ethical and legal concepts that are intrinsic to surgical nursing and underpin practice
- to present an overview of the current legal and ethical position that represents contemporary practice
- to challenge traditional methods of moral reasoning and suggest some creative forms of moral behaviour and integrity.

INTRODUCTION

In today's world of fast moving technological and medical improvements, it seems almost inevitable that moral issues will abound. Some of these issues result from demands for surgical interventions outstripping resources to more profoundly moral concerns, such as addressing the very nature and purpose of medical, surgical and nursing interventions. This chapter will present some classic ways in which people have morally argued and will show how the many ethical issues that arise in practice can be approached using these moral guidelines or patterns of reasoning. Ethical problems will always be with us, but it is our responsibility to address the issues sensitively and sensibly. This chapter will not magically sort out ethical problems, but it will indicate ways of approaching and appreciating ethical issues, within the surgical nursing context.

THEORETICAL FOUNDATIONS

In this section a review of some of the major theories, or ways of morally arguing a case, will be presented. The five major moral philosophy movements, or ethical theories, that will be discussed are:

- Utilitarianism
- Deontology
- Social contractarianism
- Existentialism
- Dualism.

Some texts refer to ethics and moral philosophy using the terms synonymously. *Ethics* is the study of 'moral ways' with a Greek derivation to the word. *Moral philosophy* is probably a more descriptive term, derived from the Latin language, describing the type of philosophy, i.e. about morality, that is, ways of moral being, behaviour, issues etc.

Utilitarianism

Utilitarianism is a particular form of consequentialism. Consequentialism is a type of moral theory that describes and determines the rightness and wrongness of moral acts according to the consequent results of those acts. Consequentialist theories are all those theories of ethics (including utilitarianism) that determine correct moral conduct according to the beneficial results of those acts. It is the results of the acts or the consequence of the moral rules which govern the acts that determine the moral status of the moral conduct. Thus, for a consequentialist nurse, it is morally *more important* to enquire when a patient would like a bed-bath (as bad timing could cause distress to the patient) than to fulfil her duty to provide a bed-bath even if there is no indication that the bed-bath is either necessary or wanted at that time.

There is a big push currently, to refocus much of traditional surgery to a minimal intervention approach which could be adapted for day surgery. Thus, renal calculi can now be blasted by laser treatment on a day surgery basis; this otherwise positive surgical progress has a typical consequentialist ring to it. If the majority of patients would benefit from this approach, then it is a good surgical approach to adopt. The fact that it is not appropriate for *all* patients, or that some patients may not wish it, would be of secondary significance. What counts for utilitarians is that a particular action appears to promote happiness in the majority of people; that is, the greatest amount of happiness, satisfaction, etc. is generated by pursuing a particular course.

Utilitarianism has its origins in the writings of the philosopher David Hume (1711–1776); Jeremy Bentham (1748–1832), who is generally regarded as the father of utilitarianism; and in the writings of the son of his good friend and disciple John Stuart Mill (1806–1873). John Stuart Mill can be considered the most famous populariser of utilitarianism and his famous tract on 'Utilitarianism' is still read and disputed today. There are several forms of utilitarianism, and it is generally regarded as a more complex set of theories than it superficially appears to be. All utilitarians believe that it is possible and indeed desirable to ascertain the moral worth of an action using non-moral criteria or values, such as pleasure or happiness. Hence the utilitarian dictum that it is morally desirable to perform those acts which maximise pleasure and one should avoid those acts which increase pain/displeasure/distress etc.

There are two main problems with this approach, namely:

1. In spite of efforts to minimise the significance, criteria for pleasure and happiness are highly subjective.
2. Utilitarianism at its worst can appear to be tyrannical rule of the majority wishes, and, at its more acceptable levels, accepts that because of democratically considered preferences, a certain percentage of minority preferences will have to be disregarded.

In a health care setting these problematic areas of utilitarianism can be seen when a government decides to ring-fence money for health care projects which will maximise the happiness, pleasure or the health status of a particular group of patients, over the expressed displeasure of a few 'minority' patients, e.g. with rare syndromes. Correcting and replacing arthritic joints has become a commonplace surgical intervention for the elderly; however, this is often done at the cost of limiting access to other surgical or medically indicated procedures, such as cardiac bypasses. More patients are potentially satisfied by having knee or hip joints replaced than the numerically few who would benefit from cardiac surgery. Since maximising their health and pleasure will yield overall smaller positive results than maximising the pleasure and health of a sizeable group of patients, trusts opt for what pleases the majority, e.g. those recovering from hip replacements. Utilitarianism is closely related to theories of democracy and apart from its moral significance has a place in the writings of political philosophers and political scientists (Smart & Williams 1973).

Deontology

Deontologists believe that apart from the results of an action (and the positive pleasure, happiness, health, etc. that it can promote), an action in order to be morally acceptable needs to be intrinsically good, that is, possess inherent moral merit. Deontology asserts that some actions have moral value independent and in addition to their consequences. It would be wrong to claim that deontology is totally unconcerned with the consequences of an act; rather, it claims that it is precisely because an act has moral worth, e.g. not lying to patients, that the consequences cannot be all negative or considered totally immoral. The most famous deontologist, who proposed the most unambiguous theory of non-consequentialism, is Immanuel Kant (1834–1804). He claimed that by utilising a totally rational approach, devoid of preferences and inclinations, and following a series of moral rules (imperatives) it is possible to know (that is reason through) what sort of conduct would be morally acceptable.

The result of his moral theory has become the claim that one 'ought' to perform certain acts, whether or not one would like to or feels that they will promote much good, e.g. one ought to keep secrets, maintain confidentiality, etc. even though it is not too difficult to envisage instances when it may be better to divulge secrets or share a confidence.

For the health care worker deontological theories are quite important, as all the major health care codes of ethical conduct are deontological in nature. They are prescriptive rules of moral conduct pertinent to specific professions. Like the categorical imperatives of Immanuel Kant, their major drawback is their abstractness and generality. Individual patients and their needs, individual cases and individual problems of health care workers all take on a secondary importance to the overall insistence that rationality, impartiality and duty must be seen to govern the rules of our moral conduct. Additionally, for the health care worker there may be a clash of moral perspectives as the nurse is obliged to act according to the code of professional conduct (UKCC 1992) but the patient may be expressing individualistic needs much more in keeping with a philosophy that emphasises personal moral responsibility and choice (Tschudin 1994). Thus, a nurse may feel he ought to help a patient mobilise, but the patient does not wish to be moved or to cooperate. The patient is prepared to take responsibility for her actions and the nurse is aware of the patient's right to self-determination; but nurses are also bound by a ruling that as advocates they promote the patients' best interests (perceived by the nurse as health) at all times. This stand can also be interpreted as demonstrating paternalism. Beauchamp & Childress (1994) spend some time in their classic textbook on defining paternalism, specifically so-called 'weak paternalism'. In weak paternalism it can be argued that it is the *duty* of nurses to at least present their professional perspective to the patient. Immobility is seen by health care workers

as detrimental to the health interests of a patient. A conflict of interest arises which deontological theories do not particularly respond to (Korner 1955).

Deontological theories tend to address what *ought* to be done, rather than argue for realistic compromise or take into account conflicting perspectives. By definition, a deontological approach is one governed by a rule or maxim that is binding at all times. It does not allow for exceptions to the rule.

Social contract theories

Another group of ethical theories addresses the issues of justice and often go under the general heading of social contract theories.

Some of these theories are very old and are reflected in the political philosophies of Socrates (e.g. *The Republic* and in some of the Dialogues of Plato) and in the writings of Aristotle. In various forms theories of justice have been around for 3000 years.

In recent times the social contract theory of John Rawls, explained and presented in his classic work *A Theory of Justice* (1971), is considered the most influential theory of justice. John Rawls posits that given the current intransigent social–cultural and economic inequalities in society, the only way that a new form of justice can be achieved is if there occurs an equal distribution of common goods/wealth to all, *unless* an unequal distribution would benefit *all*, especially those who are currently disadvantaged. John Rawls' theory of justice is provocative and creative in its justification. For the nurse the significance of his theory is that it has profoundly influenced political thinking both in the USA and the UK (Brown 1986). Much of the thinking on the political, social and moral implications of distributive justice and resource allocation can be traced to the influence of this contemporary theory. Since the moral implications of resource allocation are high on the list of concerns of health care workers, it is a theory that needs closer investigation by senior health workers.

Apart from John Rawls' theory of justice, there are several other forms of social contract theories reflected in modern social life. Social contract theories underlie much of egalitarian thinking and much of the thinking of rights advocates. If citizens of a country are entitled to certain rights, e.g. the right to health care, then that implies at least a minimum acknowledgement of the existence of a state which has corresponding responsibilities with regards to that society. Advocates of theories of rights believe in the interaction of the state and the individual, even if for some rights theorists a perfect state is one where the individual has maximum individual rights and minimum social responsibility, that is where the state is minimally intrusive. A country where the state is attempting to be minimally intrusive could be the USA; a country traditionally considered maximally intrusive would be the People's Republic of China. On the other end of the spectrum are those rights theorists who place their theory comfortably among social contract theories. The whole of society and the state is seen as a fluid interactive organism based on rights and responsibilities, social contracts and moral sensitivity. Thus, if any one part of the system falters there may be social problems – and the theories of rights look more attractive theoretically than they are in practice, since it is very difficult to maintain all parts of the system in equal harmony. Often they argue for maximum state intervention and minimum individual dissatisfaction, e.g. all members of society need to be vaccinated for the overall health of everyone. Thus it is the responsibility of everyone to be vaccinated and the state provides the means by which this is achieved. The problem with some of the outcomes of social contract theories, as they are practically applied, is that individuals can be disadvantaged and the state needs to acknowledge a far greater responsibility on its part to compensate and protect society if the demands it puts on society turn out to be detrimental, or simply to maintain some form of covenant contract. The state expects citizens to pay taxes and defend the country in times of war, but in return, it is obliged to provide health care coverage and compensation for injuries, medical accidents and so on. The present National Health Service (NHS) system of health care delivery in the UK reflects a profound belief in the beneficial aspects of social contract theories as they are applied in health care settings but also highlights the lack of commitment in some areas to a true acknowledgement of rights and responsibilities, both of members of society and of the government. The publication of the Patient's Charter (DoH 1991) and, more recently, of the Children's Charter (DoH 1995) demonstrates a growing awareness by the government that patient's rights form part of the overall moral social contract (Brown 1986, Rawls 1971).

Existentialism

Existentialism and phenomenology are fairly recent moral and philosophical theories. They are particularly relevant to nurses since contemporary nursing theories explicitly refer to existentialism and phenomenology as underpinning the theoretical base of nursing. The existentialist most cited as influencing nursing theory is the French philosopher Jean-Paul Sartre (1905–1980). Jean-Paul Sartre espoused a particular form of atheistic humanism, where his most profound statement was, that 'Man is nothing else but that which he makes himself.' (Sartre 1989). As this theory was never intended to be adopted by health care workers, taken at face value, there are two main areas of concern. Firstly, Sartre does not sufficiently account for the all-pervasive determinants of fate, such as genetic disposition/constitution, pathophysiological influences, on the make-up of an individual, and so, thus far, we can only be responsible for creating our essence (that is our being) to the extent that we are physically and mentally capable of doing so. Whereas he does not negate this fact, it is all too obvious that many individuals cannot create (and therefore be responsible) for their 'being' as this 'being' has been created and is dependent on a host of variables and accidents surrounding the individual. That is, individuals reflect society's influence and expectations more than their own individual preferences and convictions.

Profoundly physically handicapped individuals will in all probability more closely reflect in their thinking the result of their environment and society, than the end result of a personally thought-through self-determined individualistic self-expression in the form of a unique essence. 'Essence' for existentialists is those characteristics of an individual that make that person precisely who they are. Whereas one is first born *into* existence (a physiological state), a person's 'essence' is something that the individual him- or herself contributes to and determines only later. Thus the problem may be due not to lack of intellectual ability or absence of concerted effort but because such individuals are so heavily dependent on society for their physiological existence and all that surrounds them. This is an extremely relevant point as many of the clients and patients that nurses see are indeed victims of accidents and fate, either from birth or acquired subsequently, and Sartre's insistence that we have no real essence or true being until we have created it for ourselves and that we alone are responsible for our true beings and our lives, may be difficult to accommodate for many people who are highly dependent on others for their very existence. A theory that only comfortably applies to a certain percentage of people is a theory lacking universability, and therefore lacks strength of conviction. Sartre's theory is interesting and provocative but difficult to apply to all people and still in need of creative adaptation in a nursing context (Brykczynska 1995a).

Secondly, Sartre is sufficiently atheistic in his humanism that many nurses and patients would feel quite uncomfortable to take on board all of his theories. For Sartre it is precisely because 'God is dead' that man is creator of his destiny. As he notes: 'Atheistic existentialism, of which I am a representative, declares with greater consistency that if God does not exist there is at least one being whose existence comes before its essence ... that being is man ... thus there is not human nature, because there is no God to have a conception of it. Man simply is.' (Sartre 1989, pp. 27–28).

Phenomenology is also a recent theory of philosophy, that can be, and has been, applied to general theories of ethics. Soren Kirkegaard (1813–1855) is generally regarded as the founder of the philosophical movement but it is the writings of Edmund Husserl (1859–1938) and Martin Heidegger (1889–1976) that seem to be most applicable and cited by nurses. Phenomenologists posit that rather than a philosophical analysis of an abstract nature, philosophers should occupy themselves with an investigation of *perceived* phenomena. Since everything is seen and perceived and therefore 'known' and understood individualistically, no two people can 'see' and therefore understand something (or experience something) the same way. Phenomenologists have created a paradoxical philosophy of internal conflict, that is, a rigorous philosophical investigation of the subjective experience. There are many aspects of phenomenology but the philosophical aspects of phenomenology adopted by nurses are most likely to be felt in forms of qualitative research with surgical patients. Thus nurses are currently conducting phenomenological research into how patients feel after myocardial infarcts or following cardiac transplants, trying to elicit the personal, non-repeatable experiences of these patients which are only expressible by someone who has gone through the experience. No-one can 'imagine' what it is really like, and any one patient can only feel a unique tale. However, the collection of 'tales' may reveal a story with common threads.

Additionally, Heidegger's theory of caring (1962, originally 1926), based on his description and analysis of the human individual's true 'essence' and significance is another area much discussed by nurses. For Heidegger, one of the pivotal properties of individuals who are aware of, and content in the knowledge of, their own self-determined essence is the capacity of human individuals to care for and about themselves and others. Most caring theories refer to the work of Martin Heidegger, but whereas much subsequent writings by philosophers are readable and practically accessible, the original writings of Heidegger himself are, like the writings of Kant, difficult for the non-philosopher to wade through in the first instance, and

subsequently to understand and apply to practice. These are important criticisms of important theories of the philosophy of nursing and ethics which claim to underpin *nursing* practice (Danto 1985, Macquarrie 1972, Steiner 1978).

Reflective point

As mentioned above, Heidegger's writings are complex and so it will take considerable persistence to explore and critique how his work has been used in nursing. However, to begin such an exploration you may wish to consider a nursing model with which you are familiar, which uses Heidegger's work, and explore how Heidegger's concept of caring as implied above is used, and whether it is congruent with Heidegger's theory.

Dualism

Dualism, strictly speaking, is not a theory of philosophy directly concerned with morality and human conduct or the nature of being as understood by ontologists, such as the existentialists. Dualism is interested in the *nature of man* but not so much his essence as his total presentation of self in life, that is the total nature of man, body, mind and soul.

Dualism is concerned with the fundamental types of entity that make up an individual – namely, material and mental: hence the body–soul divide debate encouraged by Descartes (1596–1650). Nursing and medicine have both been influenced by dualism, because it is dualism that states that man has these two irreconcilable aspects of his nature, namely, body and soul. Health care is mainly about healing the 'body', and religion, art and the humanities are about 'healing' the 'spirit' or the 'soul'. The recent introduction of art and music into hospitals puts emphasis on psychology training for nurses and illustrates the increasing rejection of hard dualism, in favour of a more holistic integrated approach to the human individual. Moral problems can arise when greater emphasis is placed on either aspect of the human nature, at the cost of ignoring the essentially indivisible nature that a person possesses. Surgical nurses cannot emphasise the body to the extent that they risk ignoring the human spirit, as this would probably lead either to efficient clinical care which is short of 'caring' or even to totally ignoring the main issues that a patient presents with. More often than not it is not the need for surgical intervention that is primarily bothering patients but some aspect of their 'spirit' or soul, such as family ties, unfinished business, incomplete ambitions, etc. Ignoring one area at the cost of another can be counter-productive. This body–soul division has therefore profoundly influenced science and medicine, and it is only in recent times that the more holistic integrated nature of the human individual has begun to be recognised (Nagel 1987).

ETHICAL PRINCIPLES

Apart from ethical and philosophical theories, there are ethical principles that influence our values and our moral conduct.

Moral principles are those moral positions (statements) that, everything else being equal, have a morally binding capacity and are universally relevant and absolute. Thus principles of ethics are, according to Tom Beauchamp and James Childress, authors of the most popular text book on *Principles of Biomedical Ethics* (1994), as follows:

- autonomy
- beneficence
- non-maleficence
- justice.

Figure 4.1 illustrates the relationship of ethical principles to theories and codes of conduct, rules and finally actions.

Veracity, that is, truthfulness, is also an important principle of moral conduct, regarded as a sub-category of either beneficence, that is, the principle that advocates 'doing good', or autonomy, which is about a healthy presentation of self and responsibility for personal actions and lifestyle. In fact, although principles of ethics are referred to as discrete 'units', they often overlap and their boundaries blur. Veracity is a principle of moral conduct that speaks not only to the imperative to tell the truth and not to lie, but also to the necessity to live and behave with integrity and honesty, that is, not to cheat, fiddle taxes, pretend to be more important than you are, and so on. This principle of veracity is universal, in that it holds true in all cultures. Most cultures recognise the difference between an honest and a corrupt or cheating person. There may be varying cultural responses to swindling, lying and/or cheating, but all societies know that it is possible to lie and that it is possible to tell the truth. How they culturally adapt to this principle, however, will vary enormously.

There are several major ethical principles, and many secondary or subservient principles, such as promise-keeping. Promise-keeping is an ethical principle secondary and integral to the major principle of fidelity. Of the major ethical principles relevant to health care work, Beauchamp & Childress (1994) identify the four highlighted earlier as the most relevant, namely, autonomy, non-maleficence, beneficence and the principle of justice. There has been some recent criticism of principle-based ethics, but approached with understanding and necessary reflection, a principle-based approach to bioethical issues is no more problematic than employing one of the traditional ethical theories. The main objection to principle-based ethics is that it is too prescriptive in nature, a fundamentally deontological approach to ethical issues. Certainly the popularity of this method of

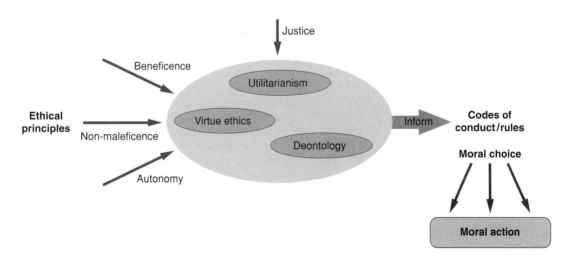

Figure 4.1   Interrelationships of ethical principles with moral theories and codes of conduct that shape moral choices.

analysing ethical issues in health care and the positive influences that it has had on health care workers and bioethicists alike is quite astounding (Beauchamp & Childress 1994, Edwards 1996).

Autonomy

Autonomy, a word derived from the Greek, meaning self-governance, originally had political connotations, e.g. an autonomous state. It is also considered an ethical principle in the sense of claiming self-determination and self-governance with concomitant responsibility for one's actions. This principle is extremely important in health care work and for surgical nurses, as no-one has the legal right to impose their will (however well intended) upon another, and it is a *right* of all people to determine their own actions and what is done to and for them. Any surgical interventions or delivery of nursing care, in a legal or ethical sense, is solely possible because the client or patient has consented to this intervention. In the principle of autonomy, legal and ethical issues meet and merge but in places they clearly differ. The principle of autonomy underlies the concerns about informed consent for surgical, medical and nursing interventions. It is the principle of autonomy that underpins the moral approach to surgical interventions and is the justification for much of the current emphasis on patients' rights, reflected in the Patient's Charter (DoH 1991). Precisely because patients have a right to be respected as autonomous beings, capable of making decisions for themselves and responsible for their own actions, they need to know their health care rights and responsibilities and what to expect from the Department of Health, NHS, local health services and even individual nurses and surgeons whom they may encounter.

Non-maleficence

The principle of non-maleficence, which literally means 'the not-doing-of-harm', derived from the Latin *male* harm and *facere* to do, is of great importance to all moral agents but specifically health care workers. Indeed, it is so important in health care work that it is the very first point in the ancient script of the Hippocratic Oath. Whatever else health care workers do, they should not inflict harm or be contributory to harm occurring. This principle has been varyingly interpreted, both at the straightforward level of primary obligation, encompassing such directives as being competent to perform the job at hand (otherwise there is the increased risk of inflicting harm), and at the more distant level of a legal obligation on the part

of the employer to provide a safe working environment, so that harm is not done to employees and is not likely to occur, e.g. the provision of adequate numbers of hoists on surgical units, adequate safety training for the use of orthopaedic equipment, etc. Recently, the recommendations of the Clothier Report, published at the conclusion of the Allitt Inquiry, have re-emphasised the obligation of non-maleficence on health care workers to include aspects of safety and security of *patients and their families* while under the care and protection of health care workers (Clothier 1994). This obligation to uphold the principle of non-maleficence, that is, that harm is not done to patients, refers therefore not only to what nurses directly do to patients, but also the total health care environment which they provide for patients and the imperative of deliberate avoidance of harm and potentially harmful situations.

Beneficence

Beneficence, also a word with a Latin root, means 'doing good'. There is an obvious ethical obligation to do good. The obligation to do good (that is, the right and correct act) is important so as not to do harm. Surgical nurses, as with all health care workers, are obliged to do good as regards their patients. This is, however, a very general global imperative that can appear quite subjective and problematic at times. Thus it is not always clear what will promote good in a specific circumstance. Is health and promotion of health always to be seen as a clearly defined 'good'? Are there times when prolonging life, or trying to enhance a failing health situation, e.g. by surgical intervention, should be considered harmful or at least of dubious benefit to the patient, and thus to the promotion of patient-centred goodness? Beneficence is theoretically a contentious principle. Although it would appear that the promotion of good and beneficial acts is straightforward, it is around this single ethical principle that most moral distress clusters. Thus moral distress is that moral feeling which one has when there is a realisation that something is not quite right or ethically 'sound' but does not necessarily involve an immediate solution or intervention from the moral agent. It is neither obvious nor clear that what constitutes goodness for one party should signify goodness for someone else. Additionally, well-motivated nurses, intent on demonstrating beneficence towards their patients are quite likely to fall into the trap of benevolent (or weak) paternalism, possibly tolerated legally, but potentially quite offensive to some patients and therefore at times of questionable ethical status. The nurse who slips dissolvable vitamin tablets into the drinks of postoperative patients (to aide their healing process) may be behaving benevolently, but it is also a paternalistic act if she does not inform patients of what she is doing for fear of angering them. Some patients do not like vitamin supplements and are under no obligation to take these – or any other medicines – but that is no reason to behave paternalistically. Such behaviour is in the authoritative, benevolent mode, of a father. Much deceit and the frequent breaching of the principle of autonomy are due to paternalistic acts. The only real justification for paternalism is where it obviously belongs, that is, in familial relationships, and in those health care situations where, precisely because doctors or nurses not only know better but are obliged to also protect the patient, they *must* behave in a particular way. For example, if a patient asked for a poisonous drink, because she had heard that 'it is good for you', it would be wrong in this instance to abide by the patient's wishes. A benevolent but also paternalistic stance would demand that the health care professionals refuse this request. In some instances this is where placebos could be supplied instead, and of course the use of placebos themselves is fundamentally a paternalistic approach, which is on the whole difficult to justify morally.

Lastly, there is the issue of the *doctrine of double effect*. Since the imperative to do good and the imperative to do no harm can at times conflict, or at best be hard to combine, there has arisen in health care ethics, as a result of the thinking of moral theologians in combination with bioethicists, the doctrine of double effect. This doctrine states that if the primary intention of an act is to promote good and the accomplishment of this good is not possible without serious negative side-effects or the possibility of serious negative side-effects, then the occurrence of harm, should it occur, is justified. Thus, this doctrine is often invoked when there are problems with the administration of potent analgesics, or performing surgical or medical interventions on a pregnant woman or treating a child or adolescent who has cancer, and either all the long-term negative side-effects are not known, or they are known, but like the decreased respirations after potent analgesics, they are predictably but largely unavoidable. Obviously there is an obligation to try to minimise negative side-effects of treatments, but at least the doctrine of double-effect accounts for the possibility of a serious clash of primary ethical principles, and re-emphasises the importance of motivation.

Justice

The principle of justice addresses several issues. It is one of the more fundamental principles governing our reasoning in respect to equity, equality, fairness, resource allocation and societal retribution (including punishment, reward, compensation and liability). Beauchamp & Childress (1994) identify several distinct but at times overlapping and always interconnecting aspects of justice, namely distributive justice, social justice, fairness and entitlement.

Distributive justice

This looks at how common goods can be most fairly distributed. The theory in its oldest version is traditionally attributed to Aristotle in the formula: equals must be treated equally and unequals must be treated unequally. Obviously there are many problems with this approach, mostly surrounding the issue of what constitutes equality and what constitutes inequality. What characteristics are 'common' to all to justify equality and which characteristics – of social origin, disease type, age, sex or cultural allegiance – constitutes a significant difference so that we are considering 'unequals'? The recent controversy among transplantologists, as to whether or not *a child's* organs should be used for *adult* patients is a good example of this problem. The patients' needing cardiac transplants are all considered in one general group, adults and children, with histological compatibility accounted for. When a suitable organ becomes available, some argue that it should go to the person, whether an adult or child, who is most in need of it and most closely related on an HLA (human lymphocytic antibodies) compatibility basis. This approach disregards three important differences or variables, opting for HLA compatibility as the most important unifying and equalising factor. The three main differences are, that:

1. The person who needs the transplant *most* is probably the sickest, with most systemic disease. All other factors being equal, this patient is most likely therefore to reject the organ and/or not survive the treatment process. This can be seen as a 'waste' of a precious resource. Morbidity is an important variable.

2. There are far more adult organs available than children's organs and, whereas an adult can comfortably accommodate an adult-size organ, a child cannot do so. Thus, there are *more* chances of locating an organ suitable for an adult than for a child. To give a child's organ to an adult, where this is sometimes seen as a temporary measure, can at best be seen as depriving a child of a far more reasonable chance of survival. It is also unfair in that adults stand a greater chance than children of being allotted 'an organ'.

3. Most significantly, the parents of the child donor often stipulate or believe that the organ will be used

another *child*. They can be quite upset when they realise that it is intended for an adult, who, in their opinion, has already had a chance at living, or in some cases has already rejected a donor organ. Here the difference is one of intention – the non-intended receipt of an organ being seen as a form of 'usurpation'.

To avoid all these problems, transplant nurse coordinators try to assure the anonymity of both donor and recipient, but this is not always possible or even desirable. The central problem remains – does the diagnosed necessity of a heart transplant make all such patients equal in respect to donated organs, or are age and disease severity sufficiently important variables to make some patients 'unequal'?

Social justice

In the context of health care, social justice is that aspect of justice that looks at societal provision for the maintenance of fairness. Under social justice are concerns for equal tax burdens (proportional to income); equal access to social amenities, such as education, transport, health care, etc.; equal treatment under the law and so on. It is aspects of equal access to health care provision that interests health workers most, as this aim of justice is often unrealisable. There are simply not the resources in personnel and finances to guarantee all citizens *equal* fair access to equally good and appropriate health care. The result is the need for some form of overt or covert rationing and prioritisation of health care resources. Usually a society structures health care provision in a two-tier system (Fig. 4.2).

There is a universal coverage of health care in some carefully defined areas (Area 'A' on the diagram) and a more selective coverage in a more particular (and harder to provide) area (Area B). Thus, in the UK, regardless of whether people are homeless, or affluent,

live in a middle class area of town or in inner-city high-rise flats, they can always gain access to a GP's surgery or the services of a nurse practitioner and be advised about their lifestyle and associated health risks. This is the absolute bare minimum that we as a society can guarantee to all people in the UK. The more expensive the necessary treatment, however, and the more it is dependent on expert knowledge, skills and available personnel, the more likely that the health care provision will be selective, rationed or unequally distributed in the country. Additionally, how the health care budget is distributed in regards to individual cases is also unequal. Thus, although the Department of Health statistics quote a single average figure for the amounts of monies which are allotted to each citizen of the UK, this is a totally hypothetical figure. Not only do individual needs for sums of money vary, but at any one time, the needy individual does not receive an average sum or an unlimited health care provision as required, but receives health care provision which is dependent upon the resources available within a particular health care budget, some of which is geographically based and some of which might be disease-modality ring-fenced. This type of chaotic distribution of health care resources leads to various societal injustices. Patients attending hospital 'A' might have access to community stoma nurses but patients attending hospital 'B', even if they live on the same street and have exactly the same needs, may be deprived of this service. Some people have access to district nurse services, some do not. There is much controversy currently surrounding apparently unjust distribution of health care packages according to disease orientation; thus ring-fenced monies available for cancer patients only serve to highlight the lack of resources available for patients with neurodegenerative problems and so on. Of all the issues in the area of justice, equitable resource allocation and its underlying justification in social justice is the single biggest problem and one that confronts all of society, that is, providers of health care and health care recipients.

Justice as entitlement (rights theories)

Justice can also be seen as a form of social dues, that is equitable distribution of what is owing and due to one by virtue of a moral or legal claim to that good. Many people argue that a society ought to provide for adequate health care, that it is a people's basic right. Such rights-based arguments consider concepts of justice as something to which, as members of society, we are entitled. The government paper, 'The Patient's Charter' (DoH 1991), is a form of health care Bill of

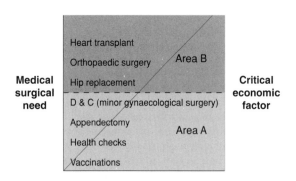

Figure 4.2 Areas of health care coverage in a two-tier system.

Rights. In the interest of fairness and justice it spells out the main points that a patient in an NHS hospital is entitled to, that is, those aspects of health care provision to which a patient can lay moral and/or legal claim.

The writings of philosophers and ethicists on theories of rights go back to the political tracts of John Locke (1632–1704) and the writings of the founding fathers of the Independent States of America, culminating in the Declaration of Independence in 1776. The preamble to the Declaration of Independence is still considered a powerful and meaningful statement of entitlement rights, even today. The French revolutionary writers also contributed to the debate on civil rights. Today, health care rights are considered one of several categories of rights to which an individual can lay claim, and both governmental declarations such as The Patient's Charter and non-governmental international statements, such as those by the United Nations Human Rights Convention, and the statements made in the European Court of Human Rights, such as the European Human Rights Charter, all stipulate the minimal health care rights a person can expect. Some areas of rights and obligations in the health care context are not particularly clear, and clarification is often sought in the courts, both domestically and in Strasburg. Thus, it is not clear whether or not it is a woman's right to be assisted in achieving a pregnancy. The argument used most often is that of easy availability of access to assisted conception clinics. In other words, a woman has the right to expect access to the services of gynaecological experts, but these would be considered weaker health care rights than rights to emergency services, intensive care units, etc. Even access to health care as a rights-based issue is seen to have a hierarchy of values, if not by the patient then certainly by health care administrators.

Few rights are considered universal and immutable. Most rights are seen as dependent on many variables. If the acknowledgement that it is the right of everyone to have surgery when it is medically needed were adhered to, we may be enforcing rights on people which they would rather not have, or would not particularly benefit from. Everyone in the UK can expect the right of surgical intervention to fix a fracture, but some patients may benefit more, in the life left to them, if they do not have the surgery to which they are entitled. Thus, we can possess rights which we do not take up, and conversely we may have rights which society is reluctant to acknowledge, e.g. many handicapped and disabled members of society have to labour hard to convince health care providers of their claim to equitable health care, even though, were they

not disabled, their requests would be granted; indeed, it would be considered their right to have equal access to health care or welfare or education.

Finally, there are some rights which, on penalty of transgressing the law and/or being considered unethical, we are bound to respect. Thus, it is the moral and legal right of every sentient and competent individual to *refuse treatment*. It is additionally *illegal* to provide a treatment if this is not desired, requested or in some clear form consented to. It is considered the basic right of all individuals to have the final say about what happens to their body, how they are to be medically and surgically treated, and so on. This fundamental right is invoked as much under the auspices of justice as that of the principle of autonomy. Of all the health care rights, it is probably the most important, problematic and also the most contentious. We are as much entitled to refuse treatment as we are to receive treatment; however, it is considerably harder for the right to refuse treatment to be upheld than it is to insist on the right to receive treatment. Thus, although the law courts upheld Cambridgeshire Health Authority's right to refuse treatment of Child 'B', in the recent case of *Child 'B'* v. *Cambridge Trust* (1995), at the expense of the father who wanted further treatment, most such cases brought to court have centred on the patient refusing treatment and the physicians and surgeons uncertain how to proceed, since to treat against someone's wishes is a criminal offence. To treat against someone's wishes can be considered unjust towards that individual, since the person's right to autonomy and self-determination is fundamentally infringed. Additionally, it could be considered illegal, since not to treat someone can be considered negligent and harmful. It can also be considered a violation of the Hippocratic Oath, and a lack of beneficence on the part of the health care worker towards the patient. Few areas of health care work and nursing evoke as much moral distress as the problem of refusal of treatment, as it is one of the few true examples of undisputed ethical dilemmas, since whatever course of action is taken, the result is less than satisfactory for one or the other interested parties. It is also one of the few areas of health care work where ensuing unease and distress is the normal response of sensitive, caring health care workers (Brykczynska 1995b).

There are, of course, the problems of unconscious patients and those who are deemed incompetent to provide a clear and binding decision as to what they would wish done. In such cases, decisions may have to be made by proxy. Increasingly, there is talk about living wills and prior medical directives; however, they do not have the binding force of law and at present only serve to give a rough idea about how the patient might feel about certain issues.

ETHICAL DECISION-MAKING

Whichever system of moral reasoning is employed, whether it be according to a developed ethical theory or considering various ethical principles, and how these may shape and influence our perspectives on the issues and problematic areas of practice, a simple, systematic and logical approach to decision-making is both useful and beneficial. An ethical decision-making framework is useful, because it can be applied and analysed by all members of the health care team at the same time and a consistency of approach is useful at such times. It is also useful and beneficial in terms of understanding how one makes ethical decisions. If the approach is haphazard and rather chaotic, it is difficult to keep track of *how* decisions were arrived at and to see if there are any patterns of moral persuasions or conclusions emerging; that is, the absence of an ethical framework may not seriously alter decisions undertaken at the time, but neither can the decision-making process serve in any capacity as a guide to further decision-making or to highlight changes in thinking or to throw light on aspects of one's moral development.

There are many decision-making models, all of them to some extent following a sequential and logical approach to examining impinging factors and determining variables that influence the case. Leah Curtin's (1978) ethical decision-making model has stood the test of time and, in its broadness and all-inclusiveness, is one of the most universally applicable, relevant to all areas of health care work, not only clinical and surgical nursing (see Fig. 4.3).

When making an ethical decision, the first point is to determine what is known and to gather as much background information on the case as is possible. This approach ensures that whatever decision is eventually reached, it is based on the best knowledge at that time. It also ensures that problematic issues that are not strictly speaking of an ethical nature are addressed separately.

Having determined the nature of the case, it should be possible to identify the main *ethical issues* at hand, e.g. problems of truth-telling, equitable distribution of health care resources, etc. The ethical component may be of a macro- or micro-perspective, that is, it could be about the nature of truth in general, when it comes to disclosing unpleasant news, or concrete problems with informing patients about diagnosis, when relatives are asking the doctors and nurses to withhold information.

The third stage involves determining who are the relevant people (ethical agents) involved in the case. This information is necessary in order to determine who should be involved in discussions concerning the issues, who might have something to contribute, who might legitimately be hurt if they were not included in discussions and debates. Certain important issues can even be debated nationally or in parliament, via special committees and specifically convened ethical inquiries, as was the case following the judicial permission to withhold nutrition from the patient, Tony Bland, who was in persistent vegetative state following the Hillsborough disaster. Initially, however, moral disquiet is experienced by health care workers who then, sometimes, take their concerns to the public – or indeed the public find out about an ethical problem and choose to debate the wider issues nationally.

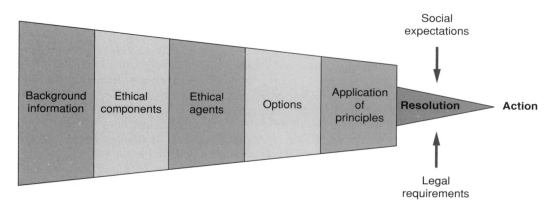

Figure 4.3 Leah Curtin's ethical decision-making model (reproduced by kind permission from Curtin 1978).

Whatever course of action is taken, there will always be a selection of options available for the moral agent to choose from. Sometimes these options are not pleasant or are rejected as ridiculous, but they are, nonetheless, possible ways of reacting morally to the problem. By considering as many options as possible, it is easier to see that several alternatives were considered and the best option chosen *given the circumstances*.

Once our caring approach suggests a particular option, this course of action can be viewed in the light of ethical principles, that is, does it promote the patient's interests, does it promote the maximum good, and so on. There have been critiques of principle-based approaches to health care, on the grounds that the principles can appear too rigid and that health care workers desperately try to fit all moral actions into the artificial boxes that the principles represent. Nonetheless, whether or not nurses are aware of ethical principles, the corresponding moral conduct does already exist, e.g. telling the truth, respecting people, trying to be fair to everyone, etc. Applying an ethical option against an ethical principle simply implies that these underlying ethical justifications are acknowledged and in trying to address one ethical issue another more significant moral problem is not produced. An attempt is made to avoid a clash of principles.

When the decision to implement the resolution is finally reached, this moral response needs to be weighed up in the light of societal expectations, which involves also the health care system and, additionally for nurses, the requirements of the UKCC, but also the legal position. It is not sufficient to claim a moral victory but legal ignorance. It was for this reason that Tony Bland's physicians took his plight to the courts – for whereas they may have felt that it was morally correct to withdraw nutrition from the patient, they were aware that it could be seen as an illegal act. Often morality and the law overlap, but this is not always the case. Most laws are attempting to uphold a universally recognisable ethical position, but occasionally the law allows certain acts to occur and refrains from prosecution – but this does not necessarily mean that it either condones the acts or considers them, of themselves, good acts, as in the case of termination of pregnancies, granting divorces, or removing children from problematic families.

The moral solution itself need not necessarily 'feel good'. The object of moral deliberation is to review all data and material evidence, consider various perspectives and to finally reach a decision that is primarily based on a caring approach to patient care, supported by ethical theory and moral reasoning. Moral reasoning

without a caring approach can be callous and rigid, while an uninformed caring approach can lead to much needless distress for the moral areas of human life. Wisdom and discernment lie at the centre of moral peace and acceptance.

Applying ethical theory to practice

So far we have looked at many different aspects of ethical theory and decision-making and how moral thinking underpins much of our societal, cultural, legal and professional behaviours. Recently, under the influence of post-war humanistic and phenomenological writings of Buber (1947), Heidegger (1962), Meyeroff (1971), Gaylin (1976), etc., nurse–ethicists such as Lanara (1981), Fowler (1986), Fry (1989), Bradshaw (1995), and health care (applied) philosophers such as Seedhouse (1988), or ethicists such as J Blumstein (1994) or Van Hooft (1995), have striven to integrate moral development, professional conduct, personal responsibilities and caring approaches to patient interactions in an essentially virtue-based ethical approach (Brykczynska 1992, Kitson 1993).

Virtue-based ethics is that approach to moral philosophy which is primarily based on a personal conscience-based perspective to decision-making, assuming an approach which calls for self-discipline and a concerted effort to be 'a good person'. Proponents of virtue-based ethics range from Aristotle through Thomas Aquinas and Kant to Kirkegaard and, in recent times, MacIntyre (1984) and nurses Lanara (1981), Roach (1984) and Bradshaw (1995).

Caring theories and the philosophical underpinnings of caring theories owe much of their power and energy to an applied approach to moral conduct that puts a heavy emphasis on personal moral development and integrity. Nurse ethicists are stating that it is the increased awareness and sensitivity of nurses' caring attitudes and behaviours that make the single greatest difference in moral conduct. They base their arguments on the works of Heidegger and Sartre, and contemporary philosophers such as MacIntyre (1984), Blumstein (1994) and Van Hooft (1995) have added to the intellectual debate surrounding caring theories. Van Hooft (1995), in his latest monograph, explains why he considers caring to be the core quality that determines morality, and Blumstein (1994), in his analysis of commitment, challenges health care workers to consider the level of commitment that the profession can realistically expect from its practitioners, and compels nurses to consider the nature of their commitment to their chosen profession and the patients they are working with and serving. In the early 1980s, Canadian Nurse, Sister Simon Roach, launched her theory of nurse caring at the 1st International Conference of Law and Ethics, in 1984 in Tel Aviv. Subsequently, this has been addressed by several other nurse ethicists and nurse theorists. Simon Roach described caring as 'the human mode of being', that is, as the natural, normal state of being that humankind is best suited for. She saw caring as consisting of five basic (later amended to six) constructs, which, although discrete, can also be seen as overlapping and interlocking (Roach 1984). These are competence, confidence, confidentiality, commitment, conscience and compassion.

Competence and integrity

Few constructs of caring and ethical professional conduct are so basic and un-negotiable as the demand and expectation that health care workers will be skilled and competent at the work that they are performing. However, arguments and debates about levels of competence, skills mix, student rights versus patients' requirements, remuneration for clinical expertise and providing adequate finances for maintenance of professional competence are all ethicolegal issues that are anything but straightforward. Whereas it is an obligation of nurses to be competent at the task they are doing, and they can only be truly caring towards patients if they are competent, it still remains questionable how to define and specify levels and types of competence. Managers, especially from a non-health-care background, may be sceptical of the skills required to provide adequate care, and surgical nurses may need to defend not only their professional skills but the very existence of their nursing specialty. Thus with encroachments on their field of work from theatre assistants, orderlies and ward-based health care assistants, on one end of the scale, and surgeons' assistants and products specialists, such as non-nurse stoma consultants, on the other end, surgical nurses' competences are called into question. Certainly it is a measure of the level that surgical nurses care about their specialty and their patients, the extent to which they are prepared to develop their own clinical expertise and field of knowledge. This, according to Roach (1984), would appear to be a moral imperative and integral to a caring, ethical stance.

Confidence and confidentiality

In order to be effective in a caring capacity, there is the requirement to share a confident attitude toward the health care profession (and surgical nursing) and to keep in confidence certain issues. Confidence is not an easily understood moral characteristic, and is dependent on fidelity and trust for its ethical legitimacy. A nurse exudes confidence because she is competent; she can share this confidence with patients in the form of hope, a moral quality closely associated with trust. In order to promote the patient's trust in the surgical procedure and the healing process, the nurse needs to impart hope, which in turn is dependent on competence. Confidence is not aloofness or even self-assuredness, although the latter may be sometimes present; rather, it is a very gentle quality that is present and manifestly visible to patients and others because the nurse, upon sound evidence, truly believes that there is something to trust, and something to hope for. In order to assure this, and precisely because there is an all-important element of trust to consider, the nurse, as part of the quality of confidence, keeps confidential information about patients to herself. Confidentiality is a particular manifestation of confidence, stemming from an understanding of trust, hope and fidelity. The nurse wishes to *gain* the patient's confidence and trust, and therefore in her own behaviour demonstrates confidence, keeps information 'in trust', that is, confidential, and as part of the nurse–patient relationship attempts to promote hope and maintain a faithful contract with the patient.

Usually there are not many problematic aspects of the theory of confidence, confidentiality or aspects of fidelity. Problems stem not from awkwardness of theory, but from the chaotic and disorganised nature of human lives and human nature. It is not always easy to keep information in confidence, or indeed possible. It is clear in law and in moral theory that the utterings of patients as they recover from surgery have no value or significance, and that in all probability what is told to a nurse in an accident and emergency department while the patient is still under the stress of trauma, is of no moral or legal relevance. But what of the confidences of a sentient, reasonably calm patient about to go to surgery? From a legal and ethical perspective, the only information given by a patient that *needs* to be shared, and at times *must* be shared, is that information relevant to the delivery of safe, competent, holistic care in the first instance, and information of reasonable significance to the law. The latter issue is not straightforward either, as, should the nurse inform the police (even with the patient's knowledge), the patient can deny all such allegations, and indeed turn around and sue the nurse for libel. Whatever the outcome, for the nurse, it may be a rather nasty experience.

Nonetheless it is clear that certain information may need to be shared. It may be a legal requirement or it may be part of the social contract that the nurse has with the rest of society of which she is a member. Just as the patient is not living in isolation, both parties have not only certain rights but also social obligations. It is unethical to tell other patients on a surgical ward a person's diagnosis – but presumably on an oncology or HIV ward all of the patients already know or are aware of their own diagnosis and of the diagnosis of those around them. The visiting public also realise the nature of the ward and the diagnosis of all the other patients, and here the question arises whether the patients' privacy is invaded or a breach of confidentiality has occurred, or neither, or both? In any other circumstances, this clear demonstration of diagnosis to all the public would be considered an invasion of privacy and a breach of confidentiality. Why should a speciality ward be an exception to this rather clear moral and legal expectation? The areas delineating privacy from confidentiality are hard to demonstrate, and whereas it is within the realms of custom and practice that certain surgical patients are nursed together, e.g. orthopaedic patients or cancer patients and so on, this approach to their care demonstrates the lack of consistency in our approach to aspects of privacy and confidentiality. It is somewhat paradoxical that nurses have been known to be reluctant to share with *colleagues* diagnosis and nursing matters relevant to patient care, especially in the area of AIDS and AIDS-related cases, and yet disregard one of the most obvious and often embarrassing aspects of a person's life, i.e. that the person is ill, or in hospital, or on a particular ward, etc. Breaking confidences may take place therefore, not only as a result of verbal messages and communication, but even by virtue of context, care and location.

In conclusion, the nurse may have to share information about a patient, but, if she has won the trust and confidence of the patient, she should be able to explain to the patient why something told in confidence, or discovered about a patient, needs to be shared. No information should be shared without the patient being informed of the intention. This is part of the faithful contract with the patient, based on fidelity. To do otherwise would demonstrate lack of confidence on the part of the nurse that she can trust the patient with this prospect. Clearly, in real life, issues are not so easy or clear cut. Lastly, health care workers should always ask themselves why a certain piece of information was shared. The old adage, a secret shared is a secret no longer, has a powerful message. Of a significantly more complex nature is the problem of 'discovered' and accidentally acquired information resulting from surgical procedures, medical interventions and/or diagnostic tests. The woman discovered to be

pregnant during an operation, whose husband claims that they cannot have children and all their married life assumed that they were an infertile couple, poses a classic case of do we tell the spouse or do we not. A clear ethical rule of thumb is that if the knowledge is not strictly relevant to the present admission or delivery of care, then there is no compulsion to divulge information and certainly *not* against a patient's wishes. For nurses, this approach can be quite problematic, as it is a rather dualistic and 'medical' model that compartmentalises a patient's life and affairs. The nurse building up a relationship with the surgical patient and approaching her work holistically may have difficulties distinguishing levels of relevance, not to mention loyalties, or disentangling conflicts of interests.

Commitment

According to Roach (1984), nurses ought to feel and demonstrate a certain amount of commitment to their chosen profession and patients. Whereas in the past, commitment to the profession was rewarded with some societal respect, the prospect of work for life, and for the most part some assured comforts of life, such as a place to live, a pension and/or the security of a sisters' home, in the present changes in the NHS all this has changed. The almost feudal (and certainly hierarchical) professional structure that this entailed has given way to far more professional independence and freedom for the practitioners, but with it job insecurity and a lack of any significant commitment on the part of the health care system towards individual members working within it. Thus, although the caring commitment to the profession and health care structure/system is important, there is no corresponding level of commitment on the part of society towards health care workers and nurses in particular. In such an unequal moral context it is difficult to expect junior surgical nurses to demonstrate commitment to the profession unless senior nurses demonstrate respect for them and encourage their professional development and clinical progress. The same of course could be said for NHS managers. Unless they demonstrate commitment towards their staff, it is difficult to expect loyalty in return.

Commitment to patients is slightly easier to discuss, since it is possible for patients to feel some allegiance to nurses, as literature pertaining to primary nursing has demonstrated. Within the surgical nursing context there have been examples of nurses structuring their work such that it reflects a perioperative commitment to patients (Cox 1987, Robert 1988, Swatton 1991). Thus the same nurse is present at outpatient appointments, checks the patient in when he or she is admitted to the surgical ward, liaises with theatre nurses and is present with the patient postoperatively. This type of work-related patient commitment is of course possible to organise for day surgery cases but also, with creative planning, for elective major surgery cases, especially so if the surgical cases are grouped according to type of surgery, e.g. ENT or gastroenterology, etc.

Commitment to patients, however, is not only about how one structures one's work. The commitment that Roach is referring to, in addition to some form of allegiance to one's profession (perhaps membership of the relevant nursing society), and demonstrated in a striving to maintain competence and credibility with one's colleagues and with patients, refers also to an internal approach towards patients that centres around the covenant relationship with the patient. Because the nurse has entered into a relationship with the patients, he has both declared a commitment towards them and bound himself by some ethical and social expectations. Modern managerial labour-market approaches towards work deny the existence of what Pam Smith and Ellen Egaard call the emotional labour of nursing (Smith & Egaard 1996). Yet it is this emotional labour and the ethical 'baggage' which constitute a significant burden for nurses, and makes up a high proportion of the moral distress experienced by nurses. The more committed one becomes towards patients the more likely that there will be some degree of emotional labour.

It is not clear that distancing themselves from patients and deliberate non-involvement would make nurses feel any better or prove more efficacious in the long run. It is not the pains of caring that perturb nurses so much as unsupported commitment towards patients and lack of demonstrable concern from colleagues and managers. In order to care in a committed, creative and structured way, the commitment itself must be recognised, supported and appreciated.

Conscience, whistle-blowing and accountability

Moral developmentalists and ethicists who are concerned with the moral integrity of the person put a heavy weighting on the personal moral reasonings and convictions of the individual. Traditional philosophers such as John Stuart Mill and Immanuel Kant assumed a certain amount of moral development to be already present and their theories did not negate the importance of personal moral asceticism or development. In fact, a total understanding of their approach to morality must include the realisation that they took

it for granted that a developed conscience and moral maturity will already be in place, hence Kant's insistence on moral asceticism and Mill's famous dictum: 'Better to be a human being dissatisfied than a pig satisfied; better to be a Socrates dissatisfied than a fool satisfied.'

For those modern ethicists who place much weight on conscience-based approaches to moral development and discernment, virtue and the cultivation of virtues is of prime importance. Increasingly, modern nurse ethicists and nurses concerned with the ethical, philosophical and spiritual aspects of nursing care are advocating a re-look at and re-evaluation of virtue ethics and conscience-based ethical decision-making. Conscience-based decision-making and ethical reflection is not a rejection of established forms of moral reasoning, or need not be; rather, it is putting greater emphasis on personal knowledge and moral integrity than would otherwise be the case. Additionally, conscience-based ethics assumes a thorough understanding and acknowledgement of other ways of moral reasoning, but prioritises those approaches to moral discernment which are based on moral convictions stemming from moral asceticism and self-discipline, if not self-awareness. This form of morality is far from the orderless parameters of situational ethics advocated by some applied philosophers such as Peter Singer (1993).

Roach (1984), when she refers to conscience as a construct of caring in nursing, is considering those qualities of personal maturity and moral development which inform our moral make-up, and therefore construct our moral selves. Our consciences are those parts of ourselves which most closely reflect our cultural, social, religious and personal values; they constitute our unique, personal heritage. Their collective values impinge on our being – formulating our 'true' selves; hence the significance of the folk adage, 'you can fool many people but not your own conscience.' In the professional context of caring, our consciences are needed to intelligently inform and morally prioritise ethical demands and problems. One can understand and know all the ethical theories ever devised, which would be quite a feat, but still not be able to make wise ethical decisions and sound, caring, professional judgements. In fact it is possible to be a professional ethicist and yet behave quite unethically, as if without a conscience. Those individuals who appear to function in society as if they had no developed conscience are often deemed by psychiatrists to be psychopaths, that is, individuals whose psychological make-up is so 'diseased' that there is an absence of a recognisable conscience. Such individuals occur in all walks of life and come from all backgrounds. They can also function within nursing and health care, such as the young nurse Beverley Allitt, who was employed on a children's ward in an NHS hospital in the early 1990s (Clothier 1994). Between the highly developed consciences of those people who Lawrence Kohlberg (1986) refers to as operating at Level 6 of his stages of moral development, and Abraham Maslow (1970) refers to as self-actualised individuals, and those members of society who seem to operate without a recognisable conscience at all, lies the range of consciences of most individuals.

Nursing, to be truly empathetic and caring, needs to be informed by a sensitive, knowledgeable conscience. It is the nurse's conscience which will guide and determine future actions and present deliberations. An informed conscience will actually help highlight what needs to be done. In the Christian tradition, the gospel story of the Good Samaritan is not only memorable because it emphasised the point that caring for others may mean caring for strangers, outsiders, enemies and so on, a point often emphasised in modern health care work and clearly demonstrated in the disinterested work of international health care agencies, emergency relief organisations and the Red Cross, but it wonderfully pointed out that an informed conscience is crucial for *effective* caring.

Thus, first one needs to see the need for intervention. Many a nurse rushes round a ward and does not 'see' the elderly patient slumped on the chair. Caring intervention, here, is based on the requirement to see the need for assessing the patient's condition. Secondly, the care delivered needs to be skilled, thorough and appropriate (a recognition of the need for competence). A leaking stoma bag may need to be changed but this requires knowledge and expertise. And finally, any intervention needs evaluation of its effectiveness, a closure and promise of future help – should this be needed. Jean McFarlane (1988) in her essay on caring recalls the story of the Good Samaritan as illustrative of the conscience-based (caring) approach of nurses to patient care. Ann Bradshaw (1995) is even more emphatic, stating that if modern nursing in the European context loses touch with its cultural and religious heritage, it will lose its conscience. Just as practical skills can become jaded and, if not used, forgotten, so the 'soul' of nursing can be lost, and this she states could have serious repercussions for the profession.

In our present multicultural society many nurses and patients will reflect values coming from religions and traditions other than those of western European, but all individuals in society need to be sensitive to the

profound effect that consciences can have on our moral thinking. Nurses need to respect those decisions made by patients based on their moral convictions and conscience, e.g. decisions made by Jehovah's Witnesses. In turn, members of the public need to remember that nurses have consciences of their own, and therefore may not wish to comply with all the wishes of patients, e.g. for supplies of drugs or hospital equipment. In such an instance the nurse's conviction that this would constitute stealing may lead him to refuse cooperation with the patient's wishes; it would also be illegal, as it would/could represent theft. Some decisions of conscience are far more serious and complex. Sally Hutchinson (1990) in a fascinating article looking at the morally inspired conscience-based decisions of nurses to break rules and laws in order to be true to their personal convictions, noted that it is the qualified, competent, committed nurse who, based on her conscience, *knows* when to break rules and transgress regulations in the best interest of the patient.

Sometimes nurses and health care workers, frustrated with ongoing malpractice or unsafe practice and having exhausted existing management structures, feel that the only way they can move forward to improve matters is by letting 'outsiders' know what is going on. Whereas the nurses in Sally Hutchinson's (1990) survey never professionally endangered their patients' lives by their actions or their colleagues' reputations, or even put their own professional integrity under question in so-called whistle-blowing, this is not always the case. Whistle-blowing is a term borrowed from industry, where unsafe, illegal or dubious practices are often taking place, and one of the employees of the firm or company, 'blows-the-whistle' on their colleagues or employer or company, in order to alert the public. In the fierce competitive market of private enterprise, blowing-the-whistle on one's firm or colleagues could mean financial losses, certainly bad publicity and possibly police investigations. A very similar situation arises in the health care context.

Recently nurses, in an attempt to improve the poor service offered to patients in NHS hospitals, have resorted to going to the press in order to force managers to implement changes that would benefit the patients. This was the case with Mr Graham Pink, a senior nurse on a care of the elderly ward. Invoking the nurses' Code of Conduct, he proceeded to approach the local press about conditions on his ward. Although this occurrence of whistle-blowing resulted in a long-drawn-out legal dispute, it is interesting that the UKCC did not consider his actions harmful to the point of removing him from the register and certainly did not consider that he had 'breached' the confidentiality clause (Clause 9 of the UKCC Code of Professional Conduct). The NHS managers rested their case primarily on aspects of breach of confidentiality and creating an environment where people will lose trust in the service provided. The case of Mr Graham Pink is important as it serves as an example both of the level of staff frustration and the expected response of the managers. Geoff Hunt (1995) in a study of whistle-blowing considers that its occurrence will increase. Certainly, with increasing cost consciousness within the NHS, there is even more scope for cutting corners, covering-up, and an aura of 'secrecy', which only fosters the mentality of deception. Where such a climate is prevalent, to improve or change dubious and unsafe practices can be hard, and managers of NHS trusts will feel, understandably, that they need to invoke the breach of confidentiality clause – even though transgressions of the clause in its medical and nursing context does not primarily relate to general breaches of 'public trust'. In fact Mr Pink found that most nurses supported his actions. Professional accountability for one's action and practice was the prime reason why Mr Pink, having exhausted all other avenues, proceeded to approach the local press. Often the local community already know that a hospital or unit is under-resourced and unsatisfactory, but when this is confirmed by a professional working within the system, this information takes on even greater weight and significance.

Discussions concerning whistle-blowing must therefore include such related issues as conscience, accountability for practice, confidentiality and breach of trust. It is hard to envisage the NHS or any health care managers demanding a 'secrecy-oath' prior to employment and yet the very moral integrity of health care workers may be challenged should they sign such an oath or decline to sign such an oath. This is an example of a true moral dilemma – resolvable only with careful recourse to an informed conscience.

Compassion

Of all the constructs of caring, compassion seems to be the most straightforward and yet, in spite of its universal humanitarian appeal, in a professional context it is hard to achieve and even harder to sustain. Creative, fruitful compassion is dependent on professional competence and commitment; a confident interpersonal attitude contingent on an informed and active conscience.

Compassion is clearly called for in an appreciation of pain control, a major problem in surgical nursing. Some philosophers and psychologists consider compassion to include empathy, and certainly to understand another's pain may call for feelings of empathy, hence the expression to empathise with a patient or relative's pain. Compassion is not just limited to aspects of empathy, however; it is a much broader human trait. It may be difficult for individual nurses to empathise with *all* their patients, but compassion as an informed attitude of the moral agent demands that we *see* and respond to the vulnerable human being in the patient. It is not a purely affective emotion dependent on our mood; rather it is something we can learn to control, develop and foster.

The UKCC Code of Professional Conduct (1992) demands of the nurse a caring compassionate stance. How could this be a reasonable expectation from every nurse, if it were merely a mood or pleasant personality trait? Sometimes, compassion towards patients and others can call for acts of heroism, such as nurses looking after disaster victims without thought to their own safety or comfort. Sometimes it may take the form of going to a very dangerous and unsafe area, e.g. a war zone, an area devastated by an earthquake and so on. It can also call for acts of heroism on a much longer and sustained basis, e.g. a heroism that is only apparent in retrospect. A nurse because of a caring commitment to a patient group, may decide to stay with certain decisions and forgo certain personal pleasures in order to maintain the patient covenant relationship, e.g. work longer hours, stay with a patient in specialism, etc. Such altruistic acts are not rare – but neither can they be imposed upon someone. Altruism and courageous acts must be totally voluntary in nature to be considered truly altruistic. Managers cannot *demand* acts of heroism and altruism on the part of their staff; compassion, however, at least in its most basic value, can be expected from all staff. Altruistic acts and courageous acts are sometimes called supererogatory acts and all moral theories have to accommodate and acknowledge their occurrences.

The nurse may well respond to most colleagues, patients and members of the public she meets, with a caring compassionate approach, but have real difficulties with a compassionate attitude towards certain *types* of patients – that is, certain members of the public. Some of the earliest nursing research to be conducted in the UK was Felicity Stockwell's study on so-called difficult patients (Stockwell 1984). It would be untrue to say that there is no such thing as a difficult patient, or that the 'problem' always lies with nurses and their attitudes towards patients. Just as nurses reflect the public at large, so patients in a hospital reflect a cross-section of the public. Some patients are frightened, angry, insecure and demanding; others are quite uncooperative, devious or simply unpleasant and, increasingly, simply violent. The call for a caring approach to patients – to demonstrate compassion – may mean to go more than the proverbial 'half way' to recognise in 'difficult' patients the vulnerability of their position in the health care context. With the increase in academic studies of social psychology and the emotional responses of patients, nurses should be better able to cope with such problematic patients and their families. This does not account, however, for developing a compassionate approach to the criminal or social outcast or person who is on the margins of society. Rather than pretend that these patients do not pose a problem, or try to ignore the issues that can arise when looking after them, a caring response on the part of the management and senior nursing staff would entail deliberately *addressing* the issues. Open communication and freedom to vent fears and concerns can go a long way to rekindling flagging compassion. Nonetheless there will always be some patients whom a particular nurse cannot bring herself to care for, e.g. a rapist. Usually this is because of deep psychological wounds and much emotional turmoil. Here a sensitive management would not demand that the nurse look after that particular patient. Caring, as understood by Roach and caring ethicists, is not limited to clinical nurses – it is a general human mode of being. It is for this reason that nurses themselves need to be cared for; they require a sensitive, growth-promoting environment in which to work. The more caring the employer will be towards the staff, the more loyalty and commitment the staff will have towards the health care system and patients. Burnout, frustration and negligence are more likely to occur where there is a lack of staff support than where such support is present and nurtured, not just tolerated. Care generates more care and a reasonable amount of sensitivity and caring support of staff can go a long way to promoting a caring and compassionate attitude towards patients, even difficult and violent patients.

SELECTED ETHICAL ISSUES

This section will address some specific issues that might and do arise in the course of work on surgical units, and they will be analysed as to their ethical significance.

Responsibility for health

Moral philosophers have always recognised that sentient adults are responsible for their actions, including moral acts. It is a fundamental principle of ethics that the moral agent is responsible for consciously choosing to act in a particular way. As noted with the problems about personal responsibility for the events of one's life as discussed by Sartre, responsibility for choices and actions is not always totally within our control.

Among many of the moral issues that present health care workers face is the issue of the extent of personal responsibility for health and, contingent on that understanding, society's obligation to intervene when health suffers or collapses. The problem is posed, if I insist on taking part in dangerous sports, without reasonable safety precautions, to what extent am I entitled to health care services if I suffer an injury? Society is deeply divided on such issues, reluctant to condone reckless behaviours, but even more hesitant to withhold treatment. Withholding treatment is seen as a form of punishment, additional to 'punishment' of injury.

Part of the problem with human behaviours is that for many of our actions, the consequences of our acts are not immediately evident, and our present society creates a way of thinking that promotes short-term gratification at the cost of long-term benefit. Thus, if cigarette smoking makes you feel better, more important, sophisticated or simply ensures group acceptance, that is considered all right and sufficient legitimacy to continue smoking. It is considered almost outmoded to think about the long-term consequences of one's actions. Additionally, especially youth and young adults defend one questionable action by pointing out the hazards of another action, e.g. increased cigarette smoking among young people is defended by the existence of car and city pollution or alcohol abuse. They claim that the latter forms of harm are *more* detrimental and accuse society of inaction on these other matters.

If personal lifestyles are not considered significant enough for debate, there are the problems of scarce resources. If health care has to be justified, how come an alcoholic with cirrhosis of the liver can get a liver transplant and can be put on a waiting list for a liver transplant, like all other patients, while patients ill with non-infectious congenitally determined hepatitis, whose disease was beyond their control, are likewise put on the same waiting list, without recognition of 'apparent injustice'? After all, say some people, the alcoholic contributed to his ill health. Obviously, nothing is so clear cut or straightforward. If one starts to list contributing factors to ill health, one can reach quite absurd conclusions; nonetheless, the problem of contribution to ill health is an ethical issue that will not go away. The health care system in the UK, as the NHS is currently structured, has addressed the issue by not considering personal responsibilities for ill health as a liability. However, there have already been instances of physicians refusing treatment *until* a patient agrees to change a particularly unhealthy or unhelpful practice, on the grounds that the proposed treatment will not benefit the patient unless the patient stops the offensive habit, e.g. goes on a diet, stops smoking and so on.

Usually when considering responsibility for personal health, society has in mind carelessness, offensive behaviours and so on; however, little attention is paid in the discussions to the practical consequences of neglecting one's health. These consequences are often seen by nurses and cause them much moral distress, such as the practical nursing difficulties of care for the obese patient. Personal autonomy and responsibility for health-related actions so far rests with the individual, but with these rights for self-determination, including self-harm, come the duties and obligations of a citizen, e.g. people with contagious conditions do not donate blood. There is some accountability therefore towards society for what they are doing. In some instances society can and does intervene if the accountability is found wanting and it will prevent abuses of autonomy and freedom of action, e.g. limiting access to medications for other than medicinal purposes and so on. The problem of personal responsibility for health status and subsequent access to the health care system is not just a straightforward issue of health care consequentialism; rather it represents the complex nature of justice and social contract that exists in our society (French 1993).

Health and safety

Increasingly, nurses are asked to consider their responsibilities in relation to the environment in which they work, and for the actual safety of the work which they do.

Individual nurses need to be aware of safety precautions, but management may need to physically protect nurses also. Two examples will suffice to demonstrate some of the ethical issues inherent in a practical approach to health and safety concerns. The surgical nurse who often has to come in close contact with body fluids and/or blood products may wish to be protected from viruses and bacteria that can breed in this medium. In the recent past, nurses have insisted on access to protective gloves, goggles and vaccinations, especially against hepatitis B, but not all health authorities and trusts have seen the priority for such protection in the same way as nurses. Employers have a duty to provide a safe working environment, but

what constitutes a safe environment can differ enormously from individual to individual and legislation can be surprisingly vague and unhelpful.

In spite of the recent publication of guidelines for universal precautions against contagious diseases, some nurses are still not using gloves when administering blood products, phlebotomising, touching open wounds, etc. Such nonchalant professional behaviour is irresponsible, and should the nurse contract a disease, the managers would have a good argument against financial compensation. The UKCC Code of Professional Conduct (1992) is clear that nurses, upon obtaining their nursing registration, cannot choose not to care for someone with a contagious disease because they are afraid of succumbing to the disease themselves, or because of some other unrelated sociocultural reasons. The health care authority or hospital trust must, however, do all it can and all that is within its power to protect its employees. To put its employees at needless risk when measures can be taken to protect them is unethical and could be illegal.

In the second example, nurses are told to use a hoist to move, lift and transfer patients who are immobile. It is important to change patients' positions and to ensure a range of postures and positions to prevent bed sores, contractures and wasting. Some patients, however, refuse to be put into/onto a hoist for the purposes of moving them or to transfer them. Patients are afraid of hoists for many reasons and the equipment used can be quite frightening for many people. Nonetheless, if after explanations and persuasions the patient still refuses to use the hoist, the nurses have an ethical problem. In order to promote the patient's welfare the nurse needs to move/transfer the patient, on the other hand the patient refuses to use the hoist, which is the only permissible method of moving a patient. Some nurses faced with such a problem ignore the rules and transfer the patient manually. There are several problems here. Firstly, the patient does not have the right to dictate to a nurse how to deliver professional care, as this is outside the sphere of competence and knowledge of the patient. The patient can always refuse care, but then must be prepared to take the consequences of that refusal. It is highly unethical to demand of another sacrifices beyond the call of duty, i.e. to do things against the rules and potentially ruining one's health. For the sake of one patient's wishes a nurse may find herself disabled, unemployable and without recourse to compensation. A patient cannot impose such a demand on a nurse, but neither should the nurse be so easily swayed by the patient's demands. If the hoist is particularly unpopular among patients, perhaps there could be an argument to look around for a hoist that does suit the patients' needs more closely.

Organ donations, transplants

As surgical technology improves the chances of healthy survival for many people, the problems faced by one group of patients is not whether technology can help them, but how they are going to get access to the technology in the absence of a donated organ. The need for various organs for transplants has never been so great. Improvements in keeping seriously ill patients alive on respirators, dialysis machines and on medicines has resulted in enormous numbers of individuals waiting for organs for transplants. Coincidentally, with the success of the seat belt campaign and more careful driving, the number of cadaver organs suitable for transplants has dwindled. There is a lot of pressure to either procure organs for transplant or to obtain organs from known individuals (under considerable duress). With the exception of bone marrow transplants, no other organ donation can be said to be without lasting implications and of physiological significance. Additionally, there is much evidence that psychological damage can occur both to donor and recipient after a transplant, regardless of whether or not it is accepted by the host. Donating organs is not without physiological and psychological risks. Most non-cadaveric kidneys are donated within the family context, but here much care is needed to make sure that no undue pressure has been put on family members to feel 'obliged' to donate the kidney (see Case study 4.1).

On the whole, the paediatric community is reluctant to condone children being organ donors and in some countries this has been made illegal. The international health care community for the most part does not condone organs for sale. To buy an organ in the UK or to use an organ obtained in this manner is illegal.

Reflective point

You may like to consider the following three questions in relation to Case study 4.1:
1. What are the ethical issues involved here?
2. To whom does Mr T owe primary responsibility for his actions?
3. What might be the role of surgical nurses in such a case?

Physicians and surgeons who 'trade' in bought kidneys face professional sanctions and criminal prosecution. It may be that occasionally these organs were 'fairly' bought, but the evidence seems to show that it is poor and illiterate citizens of developing countries who sell their kidneys to rid themselves of debts, not fully understanding what is involved and often very poorly paid for their 'priceless gift'. Once the operation is performed, it is impossible, by definition, to rectify the situation. Nurses involved in the field of transplantology need to be vigilant and careful that the organs which they use are obtained legally and that there is no evidence of pressure involved.

Once the organs are available, the next question often is, how many of these organs should be transplanted and made available to whom. This is a very specific debate stemming from the advances in multiple organ transplant techniques. Thus, is it just to give a heart–lung transplant to one young man with cystic fibrosis, or should two patients benefit, a patient needing a heart transplant and a patient needing a lung transplant? Some of these questions are answered by the nature of the medical conditions and by an understanding of the relevant pathophysiology, but the question of when to stop offering transplants is considerably more difficult to answer. Traditionally, once the medical profession had invested energy and money in treating a patient, it was reluctant to give up treatment, causing the embarrassing position of one patient having two or three kidney transplants while other patients were still waiting for a first transplant.

Occasionally a patient makes surgical history and becomes the topic of much controversy. Thus, when Baby Laura was flown to the USA for a total organ transplant, that is, a transplant of all the internal organs, she was, together with the preceding 18 child patients, making surgical history and pushing the boundaries of the possible ever further forward. When, after several months she started to reject the transferred organs the hospital surgeons suggested to the parents another such multiorgan operation. It was at this stage that many individuals in the health care

---

Case study 4.1   Mr T

Mr T is a 25-year-old teacher who has been recently diagnosed with acute renal failure. He is on the list awaiting a kidney transplant. He has a fraternal twin who is keen to help his brother. His twin brother is married and has a daughter, and his wife is expecting their second child. The nurses are concerned that Mr T is unaware of the emotional problems involved with transplants, especially as he is heavily influenced by his mother, who is urging her married son to donate a kidney.

profession thought that the parents should request a halt to all further procedures. There were many complex issues at stake here, not the least of which was the desire of the parents to offer the child any last chance of survival which they could. Health care workers additionally were concerned that with the notable lack of success with this procedure, to offer yet another such operation to the child was wasteful of precious resources and cruel to the child (Brykczynska 1995b).

When heart transplants were surgical novelties, a moratorium was called on the procedures until the pharmacological possibilities of significantly affecting donor rejection and infections were addressed. There are some members of the public who are calling for a similar moratorium as far as multiple transplants are concerned. The latest medical technology, however, is focusing not on human-to-human transplants, but rather on non-human-to-human organ donations. The evidence so far is that primed non-human organs may be of some use, but it is not clear to what extent all organs will be equally acceptable. Thus animal lungs and kidneys may be accepted with the same understanding as animal tissue is today, but non-human hearts may not be seen as so readily acceptable to all. Animal-to-human organ transplants may solve some ethical problems, but will undoubtedly create new ones.

Living wills, advanced directives, withholding and withdrawing treatment, alternative treatments

One of the consequences of surgical advances is that it is possible to do quite major surgery with very ill patients and/or fairly elderly patients. Surgeons and health care workers do not like to 'let a patient die' or go without surgical interventions. The principle of beneficence is very strong and health care workers can act with much paternalism. The prevailing argument seems to be that if we can intervene surgically, that is, if we can possibly do something, then we ought to do something. Surgery is seen as the correct moral act, regardless of patient preferences and underlying indications that might pose a query as to the suitability of the patient for surgery.

In 1994, the press noted the story of an athlete (Mr Ian Hudson), who was left handicapped after an accident. He repeatedly requested surgeons to amputate his injured leg, as it was the cause of much pain and discomfort to him. The man was prepared to have an amputation and to literally rid himself of the cause of his pain, rather than undergo yet another operation 'to save his leg'. When it became clear that the surgeons were not listening to him, he decided to amputate his own leg, by placing it on the railway tracks and allowing a high speed train to sever it. This is a harrowing story of how far some patients will go, if dissatisfied with surgical care (Gorman 1994).

Other patients also have great difficulties in assuring that their wishes will be respected, and so these patients draw up living wills or advanced medical directives which they hope will guide surgeons and health care workers as to their wishes. The patients presume that since no-one can intervene in their care or perform surgery without their expressed consent (or the consent of those designated as having the right of proxy), if they let people know in advance how they feel about potential medical or surgical intervention, this declaration will have the force of 'informed opinion' if not refusal to consent.

There are several legal problems with advanced directives and at the present time they do *not* carry the same legal weight as traditionally obtained informed consent or refusal at the time of surgery or need for medical intervention. The problem, as health care workers and lawyers perceive the issue, is that consent or directives for refusal of care and/or intervention, expressed when we are relatively healthy, do not mean that we really would desire to refuse treatment should we be left neurologically damaged after a procedure or as the result of a deteriorating illness. The health care workers are most likely to listen to the consistent, repeated opinion of someone suffering from a neurodegenerative disorder or fatally progressive chronic disease such as cancer or cystic fibrosis than feel bound by the advanced directive of an individual they do not know, who is now presented to the hospital following a sudden massive stroke or road traffic accident. The general ethos of the health care system is to err on the side of caution, and to treat patients aggressively in the absence of any *consistent* and recent indications as to preferences to the contrary.

Finally, there is the problem that, whereas health care workers have a large scale of reference both in terms of potential consequences and outcomes of treatments and disease processes, and also in terms of the spectrum of possible disabilities that one can learn to live with and adapt to, individual patients may have no such reference points, and base their judgement of preferences on inadequate, inaccurate or even outmoded data. These are problems extremely difficult to resolve in a hurry and often time is needed to obtain a truly accurate estimation of a patient's informed wishes. Time can be quite a luxury in today's fast-moving impersonal health service, and often, of course, it is irrelevant if decisions have to be made *for* a patient who is presented in a coma or post-stroke or after massive cerebral damage.

Withholding active treatment is always an acceptable option for health care workers, but as noted, the principle of beneficence coupled with a strong paternalistic perspective skews most health care workers to opt for treatment modalities rather than palliative care options. There are of course two problems here: first the problem of defining what would constitute 'good' for any one individual and, secondly, the enormous difficulty that palliative care workers face in convincing colleagues that palliative care is a legitimate form of treatment option, not a 'non-option'. Many of the horrendous stories concerning needless health care interventions centre round these two problems (see Case study 4.2).

Case study 4.2   Mrs P

Mrs P is an 85-year-old lady, recently widowed. She has been suffering from diabetes for the last 30 years. She has congestive heart failure and has been blind for the past 10 years.

Mrs P is now on a surgical ward, but does not wish to be in hospital for surgery or any medical treatment. Her daughter, however, is insisting that she undergo a below-the-knee amputation for complications due to her diabetes.

The medical and surgical team are also insistent that Mrs P should have the amputation to improve the quality of her life. The surgical nurse on the ward, who is preparing Mrs P for the surgery, is worried about the validity of Mrs P's consent form and the overall readiness of Mrs P for such major surgery.

Reflective point

In relation to Case study 4.2 consider the following three questions:

1. What are the ethical issues raised in this case?
2. How might the nurse approach the issues identified?
3. What might be the reaction of the surgical team to the nurse's concerns?

Sometimes physicians and surgeons opt to withhold treatment very early on in the course of a disease or disability, usually when there are many uncorrectable or very complex additional underlying disorders and/or abnormalities. Not all members of the public agree with surgeons' decisions to withhold interventions, but on the whole, the courts do not like to intervene and, when cases are taken to court, the vast majority of cases uphold the physicians and surgeons' decision on the basis that these decisions are taken on clinical grounds and the law courts do not have this level of expertise. Recently, in the case of Child 'B' where physicians refused to administer a new course of chemotherapy to treat a second cancer which developed as a result of treatment for an unrelated oncological condition, the trust executives defended the move on the basis that it would be wasteful of resources to treat a child who was not expected to survive the treatment. They claimed that the monies and human resources could be used more profitably elsewhere. This public announcement of financial and human resource implications of health care rationing and prioritisation put the issue on the ethicolegal and social map in a significant way, as many individuals in the UK consider their National Insurance monies and taxes as forming a type of health care insurance scheme – but in fact this is not strictly the case. So long as the decisions made are based on clinical grounds, few people have problems understanding the reasoning behind decisions to withhold treatment, but few people are prepared to consider the possibility of a rationing system or a system of prioritisation of health care.

Issues concerning withdrawal of treatment are even more emotive. Surgeons and physicians are obliged to evaluate the efficacy of their work and if the disease progress is such that further intervention in the disease process will not benefit the patient, then according to the principle of non-maleficence active treatment should be ceased. Withdrawing medical and surgical treatment is difficult for some health care workers, as it is seen as evidence of failure. Withdrawing established treatment is considered a public manifestation of medical and surgical failure to halt morbidity or stop mortality. Nonetheless, there are times when to withdraw treatment is the most caring thing that health care workers can do. It is part of the expertise of health care specialists that they can state with authority and compassion when active treatment should be withdrawn. Just as in cases of authorisation for treatment, there are many problems connected with withdrawal of treatment – not the least being that there are no definitive criteria for what constitutes active treatment, what is considered routine care, what is considered treatment that is solely prolonging life and treatment that is improving the quality of life. These are not academic debates among bioethicists but routine clinical issues on surgical wards in district general hospitals. Case study 4.2 reinforces this point. Surgical nurses can and should join in the interdisciplinary discussions, in order to feel included in the debates and part of decision-making and to present the perspective of the patient and family should this be required.

Increasingly health care workers are including the family in decision-making processes and acknowledging the inherent rights that family members have to be included in the 'health care team'. Most of the time, family members are important contributors to the recovery of the patient, but this is not always the case. A good rule of thumb is to ask patients who they consider as a significant person in *their* life and who ought to be included in the health care team. Neglecting family and friends can be hurtful and even short-sighted, but assuming that spouses or relatives matter can be equally awkward or occasionally devastating (see below).

It is at this stage that patients and families sometimes turn towards alternative therapies. Alternative, or complementary therapies are considered to be all those therapies which operate alongside but are independent of traditional western medical and surgical practice. Some of these therapies are truly complementary to established clinical practices and have beneficial influences on patient morbidity while some of them are of an unproven nature. Unfortunately, some are at best of doubtful benefit and at worst harmful. Included in the calculation of any harmful effects on the patient from the alternative treatment itself must be the amount of harm that accrues from opting for alternative treatment *instead of* traditional clinical approaches. As more members of the public are looking at complementary therapies and considering withdrawing from traditional clinical options, nurses need to become familiar with these other treatment options, to understand their risks and benefits and be prepared to work with those therapies that are beneficial to the patient, and have the courage to explain why they would discourage the patient from opting for other types of treatment. There is rather a facile modern philosophy currently in vogue that considers much of traditional western science and medicine as wrong and harmful and most of the alternative therapies, alternative lifestyles and New Age thinking as unquestionably good. Among the many health education roles of the surgical nurse must surely be the explanation and briefing of patients and the public of the genuine progress and advances of modern surgery which is minimally invasive and dependent on technology and informatics to an extent that the average member of the public is unaware of. The short hospital stays, day

surgery and keyhole surgery are all results of modern advances that have revolutionised modern surgical wards beyond recognition. However, these advances must serve the perceived interests of the public and potential patients – or patients will turn to alternative therapies for all the wrong reasons. Complementary therapies need to be explored, promoted and incorporated into clinical practice, but they need to be working in tandem with other health care disciplines, not against them.

Patients' and relatives' rights in the surgical context

As already mentioned, all patients have certain health care rights and these have been recently enshrined in the Patient's Charter. Of all the patients' rights, the rights to informed consent and informed refusal of health care services are the most known and well publicised. Whether it is possible to inform patients adequately, such that their ensuing decisions are truly based on comprehensive information, is a well-debated point among health care workers and bioethicists. It is certain, however, that the knowledge differential and power inequality between the health care professional and member of the public, should not become the excuse for mal-information or inadequate information-giving. It is still quite surprising how many patients are not *sufficiently* informed about their procedures – the risks involved and amount of expected pain or inconvenience. With the expected shorter stay of patients in hospital, it is even more important than ever to ensure that patients and their families are aware of what to expect and are adequately briefed.

The families and friends of the patients have rights too. As care of patients is being increasingly focused on the community, relatives living in the community are involved in care provision, and therefore should be consulted at all stages of the surgical procedure. This is not just a social nicety supported by the Patient's Charter but a moral obligation stemming from the contractual arrangement between the NHS and trusts and the public. Families have a right to visit the patient, be consulted and kept informed about care and should be treated as integral members of the health care team. When these fairly obvious social relationships break down, however, patients and their families can seek redress, initially at the hospital trust level, and if this is unsatisfactory, then via the NHS Ombudsman. The Ombudsman's yearly reports make interesting reading and the increasing number of complaints against nurses is fairly disquieting.

All patients have a right to know what information is kept about them; however, the hospital records as such are considered NHS property. Recently, the tendency to keep records on computers has complicated the position, as computer-held information is subject to the Data Protection Act 1984. Whereas, most of the time, information about a patient is highly innocuous and/or strictly of a medical and nursing nature, sometimes implications derived from the notes can have serious social implications, hence the need for confidentiality and accuracy of reporting. Information about a patient can be shared with relevant members of the health care team and family (when this is appropriate), but not with other members of the medical or nursing profession that just happen to work in the same hospital. Recently, district nurses have found that it can be difficult for them to gain access to information concerning patients who are about to be discharged into their care, in the community. Sharing patient information in such circumstances is not only appropriate professional behaviour, it is the best possible moral behaviour that ensures smooth transfer of patient from hospital to the community.

Some patients choose to discharge themselves from hospital against medical advice, usually because of a perceived conflict of interests between what the patient wants and what health care providers are prepared to offer. Unless it can be proven that they are permanently or temporarily of unsound mind, as the law stands in England, no patients have to stay in hospital or have care/treatment forced upon them unless they are a danger to others, i.e. could harm others as a result of erratic, psychotic behaviours – as in some psychiatric conditions – or as a result of suffering from a highly contagious disease, such as Lassa fever, or more commonly, tuberculosis. Even in cases where they could potentially harm someone, if they can assure the public authorities that they will not go around infecting members of the public, they cannot be forced to accept treatment for themselves. Mature adults *can* choose to resign from treatment options and discharge themselves from hospital – even if such an act will in all probability hasten their death. This is one of the most stressful aspects of health care work, as health care workers often feel that there are aspects of care that they could negotiate with patients, and patients' decisions to discharge themselves from the hospital are seen as both threatening and worrisome. Nonetheless, however painful, such decisions are for others; surgical intervention cannot be forced on mature, sentient adults.

Children and vulnerable adults pose a significantly different problem, but the underlying principle is essentially the same, i.e. we should be attempting to obtain as fully an informed consent as is possible from the patients themselves, not just relatives and third parties. For a more detailed analysis of the problems inherent in proxy consent, please refer to Priscilla Alderson's work (Alderson 1991, 1994).

In order to gain fully informed consent for treatment and in order to gain cooperation from the patient and family in treatment protocols and regimes, it is sometimes necessary to use a translator. In areas where there are large immigrant communities these translators should be full-time members of the hospital staff. It is rather bad practice, violating the principle of confidentiality and fidelity, to attempt to utilise as translators visiting members of the public, family members and/or unconnected members of the hospital trust. Probably the most ethically questionable is the use of children as translators for older relatives. This practice is both professionally unsound and violates the child's right to privacy and an appropriate childhood.

Because hospitals are often also places of medical and nursing education, and because much research is conducted in hospitals, there is often a problem maintaining confidentiality and privacy during consultants' rounds, or surrounding medical photography sessions. In recent times, patients' privacy has additionally been violated by the intrusion of television cameras into the hospital environment. This is a complex problem, which has many good points, but also many negative aspects to it and nurses should try to steer the situation in such a manner that patients' privacy and confidentiality is maximally maintained, while legitimate public interest and concerns are satisfied. Talking directly to the public about problematic cases, however, is not considered ethical and the UKCC may yet sanction a nurse who 'whistle-blows' on a legitimate ethical issue, but in the process risks the loss of privacy of other patients or a particular patient. These are not new concerns, but they are certainly areas of growing concern.

CONCLUSIONS AND RECOMMENDATIONS

It can be seen from this brief overview of moral reasoning, caring approaches, and growing areas of public concern, that improvements in one area often call for a re-examination and re-evaluation of values held in another area. Surgical nurses do not work in isolation, and the more informed and competent they become, the more they will be able to discern moral responsibilities and action. Undoubtedly, the introduction of ethics and ethical decision-making into the pre-registration nursing curriculum must be a useful introduction for junior nurses to the immensity of moral problems that are found in health care work. However, basing ethics solely on such 'problematic' approaches to moral reasoning deprives nurses of the opportunity to manage their moral development proactively, by attending ethics rounds, taking continuing education courses in ethics and specifically health care ethics, and by reading about and discussing

with colleagues difficult ethical cases and dilemmas. The caring theorists, writing from the moral perspective, keep emphasising that the moral issues in health care delivery will not go away – and in fact keep changing. The best response we can have therefore as health care workers is to develop a way of approaching these issues with moral sensitivity and professional discernment, aware that our primary focus must always be the patient or client.

REFERENCES

Alderson P 1991 Parent's consent. Oxford University Press, Oxford

Alderson P 1994 Children's consent to surgery. Open University Press, Milton Keynes

Beauchamp T, Childress J 1994 Principles of biomedical ethics, 4th edn. Oxford University Press, New York City, NY

Blumstein J 1994 Caring and commitment. Oxford University Press, Oxford

Bradshaw A 1995 Lighting the lamp: the spiritual dimension of nursing care. Scutari Press, London

Brown A 1986 Modern political philosophy: theories of the just society. Penguin Books, London

Brykczynska G 1992 Caring: a dying art? In: Jolley M, Brykczynska G (eds) Nursing care – the challenge to change. Edward Arnold, London. pp 1–45

Brykczynska G 1995a Humanism: a weak link in nursing theory. In: Schober J, Hinchliff S (eds) Towards advanced nursing practice. Edward Arnold, London, pp 111–132

Brykczynska G 1995b To do no harm. Journal of Paediatric Nursing 7(3): 6–7

Buber M 1947 Between man and man. Routledge and Kegan Paul, London

Clothier C 1994 The Allitt Inquiry: independent inquiry relating to deaths and injuries on the children's ward at Grantham and Kesteven Hospital. HMSO, London

Cox H 1987 The peri-operative role. NATNews 24(1): 15–16

Curtin L 1978 Nursing ethics: theories and pragmatics Nursing Forum 17(1): 4–11

Danto A 1985 Sartre, 2nd edn. Fontana Press, London

Data Protection Act 1984 HMSO, London

Department of Health (DoH) 1991 The patient's charter. HMSO, London

Department of Health (DoH) 1995 The patient's charter: services for children and young people. HMSO, London

Edwards S 1996 Nursing ethics: a principle based approach. Macmillan, Houndmills, Basingstoke

Fowler M 1986 Ethics without virtue. Heart and Lung 15(5): 528–530

French P 1993 Responsibility matters. Kansas University Press, Lawrence, KS

Fry S 1989 Toward a theory of nursing ethics. Advances in Nursing Science 11(4): 9–22

Gaylin W 1976 Caring. Harper and Row, New York

Gorman E 1994 Gymnast crippled by crash amputates his leg under train. The Times, 18 June

Heidegger 1962 (orig. 1926) Being and time. (trans Macquarrie J, Robinson E) Blackwell, Oxford, ch 6, pp 225–273

Hunt G 1995 Is the whistle-blower right? Health Service Journal (105) 2(4): 4

Hutchinson S A 1990 Responsible subversion: a study of rule bending among nurses. Scholarly Inquiry for Nursing Practice 4(1): 3–17

Kitson A 1993 Formalizing concepts related to nursing and caring. In: Kitson A (ed) Nursing: art and science. Chapman and Hall, London, ch 3, pp 25–47

Kohlberg L 1986 Moral stages and moralization. In: Lickona T (ed) Moral development and behaviour theory: research and social issues. Holt, Rinehart and Winston, New York, pp 31–35

Korner S 1955 Kant. Pelican, London

Lanara V 1981 Heroism as a nursing value. Sisterhood Evniki, Athens

McFarlane J 1988 Nursing: a paradigm of caring. In: Fairburn G, Fairburn S (eds) Ethical issues in caring. Averbury Press, Aldershot, pp 10–20

MacIntyre A 1984 After virtue, 2nd edn. University of Notre Dame Press, Notre Dame, Indiana

Macquarrie J 1972 Existentialism: an introduction, guide and assessment. Penguin Books, London

Maslow A 1970 Motivation and personality, 2nd edn. Harper and Row, New York

Meyeroff W 1971 On caring. Harper and Row, New York

Nagel T 1987 A very short introduction to philosophy: what does it all mean. Oxford University Press, New York

Rawls J 1971 A theory of justice. Harvard University Press, Cambridge, Mass

Robert S 1988 A study of peri-operative patient care. NATNews 25(12): 8–10

Roach S 1984 Caring: the human mode of being – implications for nursing. Perspectives in Caring Monographs 1. Faculty of Nursing, University of Toronto, Toronto

Sartre J P 1989 Existentialism and humanism. (trans Mairet P) Methuen, London

Seedhouse D 1988 Ethics: the heart of health care, J Wiley, Chichester

Singer P 1993 Practical ethics, 2nd edn. Cambridge University Press, Cambridge

Smart J J C, Williams B 1973 Utilitarianism – for and against. Cambridge University Press, Cambridge

Smith P, Egaard E 1996 Care costs: towards a critical understanding of care. In: Brykczynska G (ed) Caring: the compassion and wisdom of nursing. Edward Arnold, London, pp 180–204

Steiner G 1978 Heidegger. Fontana Press, London

Stockwell B 1984 The unpopular patient. Croom Helm, London

Swatton S 1991 Peri-operative documentation. British Journal of Theatre Nursing 1(1): 10

Tschudin V (ed) 1994 Ethics: conflicts of interest. Scutari Press, London

United Kingdom Central Council for Nursing, Midwifery and Health Visiting (UKCC) 1992 The code of professional conduct. UKCC, London

Van Hooft St 1995 Caring: an essay in the philosophy of ethics. University Press of Colorado, Niwot, CO

FURTHER READING

Aristotle 1976 Ethics. (trans Thomson J A K) Penguin Classics, Harmondsworth

Bok S 1978 Lying: moral choice in public and private life. Vintage Books, New York

Brykczynska G 1996 Caring: the compassion and wisdom of nursing. Edward Arnold, London

Descartes R 1970 Philosophical writings. (trans Anscombe E, Grach T) Open University Press, London

Gates B 1994 Advocacy: a nurses guide. Scutari Press, London

Heidegger M 1993 Basic writings revised and expanded. (ed Farrell D K) Routledge, London

Kant I 1959 Foundations of the metaphysics of morals. (trans Beck L W) Bobbs-Merrill, Indianapolis

Mill J S 1991 On Liberty and other essays. Oxford University Press Oxford

Rawls J 1971 A theory of justice. Harvard University Press, Cambridge, Mass

Sartre J P 1889 Existentialism and humanism. (trans Mairet P) Methuen, London

Smith P 1992 The emotional labour of nursing: how nurses care. Macmillan, Houndmills, Basingstoke

Watson R 1994 (ed) Accountability in nursing practice. Chapman and Hall, London

5

Support for the surgical nurse and supporting others

Ruth Davies

AIMS

The aims of this chapter are:

- to explore the concept of support
- to explore the surgical nurse's need for support
- to identify the ways in which surgical nurses can give and receive support
- to examine the challenges of giving and receiving support.

INTRODUCTION

I have deliberately not included in this chapter a list of stressors in the surgical environment and the effects of stress on the body, behaviour and emotions. These are all well documented elsewhere and as it is relatively rare that the unconscious feeling world of the nurse is given much space, this is my attempt to redress that omission. Some basic texts/chapters on stress in nursing are included in the list of further reading at the end of the chapter (Bailey 1985, Bond 1986, Kagan & Evans 1995).

Major changes have occurred over the last few years in the technology of medicine, surgery and nursing and the socioeconomic climate in which we live and work. These have considerable psychological implications for both ourselves and the patients for whom we care. Our own concerns will range from the quality of care which we can offer to whether we will have a job. Patients' concerns will range from fear of diagnosis or procedure to whether they will be seen at all, the length of time awaiting surgery, whether they will survive and what form the outcome of surgery will take. The work of the surgical nurse is emotionally challenging, and nurses often put others' needs before their own. This can and has resulted in stress, strain and burnout, with nurses often feeling that they have nothing left to give, to patients, to their own families and friends and to themselves (Bailey 1985). It is this crucial issue which this chapter seeks to address, as I, and many others, believe that as people we cannot give what we have not or do not receive ourselves. By attending to our own needs, we become able to identify helpful and limiting behaviours and then to open ourselves to concern, pain and also joy and delight. This in turn enables us to be attentive to our patients' needs and emotions in a holistic fashion as we live our own lives more authentically.

The primary focus of this chapter is on the nurse, given that if nurses feel supported, they are in turn more able to support others.

AN EXPLORATION OF THE CONCEPT OF SUPPORT

What is support?

This is not an easy question to answer. We often say or hear 'no-one ever supports me/us here', assuming that our meaning is clear. This is not the case. We all need support in different forms at different times. Support may take the form of agreement with an idea or action, doing something on behalf of someone, being willing and able to listen to someone, or simply noticing someone's presence or mood. This is by no means an exhaustive list, but it is worth noting that sometimes when we say we need support, we are, perhaps unawarely, asking for sympathy and collusion, playing on someone else's compulsion to help. This of course will not serve us in the longer term, although it may temporarily seem to help. It is worth asking ourselves what we really need in various situations, and whether we are able to risk being supported, as this may result in change. It is often easier to perpetuate old patterns of being and working rather than become powerful people. This is one of the challenges of support.

What, then, is support? A dictionary definition includes aspects of the above, 'to bear the weight of, to hold up, to sustain, to endure, to maintain, to keep going, to make good, to back up, to represent in acting, … to supply with means of living, to nourish, to strengthen' (*Chambers Twentieth Century Dictionary* 1972, p. 1357). The same ideas feature in the *Oxford Reference Dictionary* (1995, p. 1450) and they include 'to keep from falling, sinking or failing, to sustain, to endure, to maintain, to keep going, to make good, to back up, to represent in acting'. We may look at aspects of these definitions literally – how many times each day do we actually bear the weight of people, lifting them, helping them to move or walk? More importantly, how many times do we do this without being aware of the burden on our physical body, the actual weight which we are lifting or carrying? We can be

equally unaware of the psychological burden which we may carry – the impact of wounds, of suffering, of daily (though often unexpressed) contact with life and death, the concerns of existence. As we support patients and relatives, we also support each other, carrying, metaphorically, the colleague who is unhappy or has a health problem, or is new to a ward and its ways of working. We might ourselves be the person who is carried or held up while we are unhappy or unwell or new to an area. Lack of support may well result in us sinking, or feeling that we have failed.

The next points in the Oxford definition are more worrying to me – 'to sustain, to endure, to maintain, to keep going, to make good'. There is a myth that the more support people receive, the more they can achieve, the more they can endure, which somehow detracts from the fact that we are human beings, not machines to be given more fuel in order to work without breaks. Some organisations provide counselling in order to help staff deal with work-related stress (often due to major change in the work setting) but fail to look at their own responsibility and systems in the roots of the distress. They perceive that problems are located in the individual rather than the organisation, and it is the individual who may be ill, not the organisation. This is not to say that support does not maintain people – it does – but the aim of such support should not be to maintain people in isolation in a collusive, harmful environment. This making good, or patching up may not serve the individual. We all know the stress caused by working unpaid overtime, stretching ourselves thin, working to a bare minimum because of lack of staff and resources. Some of us will be harmed by this, whilst the organisation continues to function.

By contrast, the definitions improve to include 'to back up, to represent in acting'. These are clear ways of giving and receiving support, to hear or say 'I agree with you', 'I think you're right', both in private over coffee, and more importantly, in public debate or discussion. It is also important to know that your views or situation will be fairly and honestly represented, for example by a senior nurse at a management meeting. One traumatic time which most of us will encounter at some stage will be to be involved in a patient complaint and it is very useful to know that the manager will respond by saying that she or he will investigate, or support you immediately in what you did, without automatically believing the complainant. Equally, another form of support is to know that as a team you all have a consistent way of dealing with difficult situations.

'To supply with the means of living, to nourish, to strengthen' are aspects of support which imply life, development and growth. Surgery may well supply a person with the means of living – some surgery is literally life-saving and heroic. I recall a lady with severe haematemesis who underwent multiple transfusions while investigations were made and ultimately she went for surgery with the source of bleeding undiagnosed. A perforated gastric artery was identified, oversewn and she made a speedy recovery with us on the ward. This was immensely pleasing for those of us involved in her care and we went through the full range of emotions of concern, fear, and ultimately relief and joy, which mirrored her and her family's experiences. The support which we as nurses needed over these few days was mostly practical – the patient needed constant individual care so we had to have extra staff deployed to our ward. At times, nursing her was frightening – she bled so much, we thought that she could have died at any time. Taking her to the X-ray department, where our support would be less, was terrifying. Therefore this had to be acknowledged and we talked about our fears. At times, for this reason, two of us would be with her, for each other as much as for her. It helped also to know that we would all hurt equally if she died and have full sympathy for the nurse involved at the time. When she recovered, we were able to acknowledge great delight, pleasure and satisfaction, and also the need for a break from nursing someone so acutely ill for the next couple of shifts. Later reflection allowed us to understand how much we had learned from this lady and caring for her – how much we had given, how our confidence in the body's striving for growth and healing had increased, how our confidence in our nursing care and in each other had been strengthened.

With reference to strength, it is worth noting that we sometimes erroneously equate strength with stoicism or keeping going. It takes strength not to cry at times and it takes strength to ask for help and to acknowledge our limitations. I prefer to use the word courage in this situation and it is helpful at times to complete the sentence, 'If I had the courage I would …'. This may include offering help or support or asking for help, both of which actions take courage. At times, it may also be courageous to leave a situation which is intolerable.

Support clearly involves specific actions and behaviours and yet it is a complex concept. Sometimes the only way to support someone is to be there for them, to be present. Ersser (1991) writes clearly and evocatively about this concept, which he says is valued by both patients and nurses. There are no actions to do, nothing practical is possible. In this way, the nourishing aspect of support, of supplying with the

means of living, of strengthening, is more spiritual and emotional than behavioural. It is in being there, being present, that we are both most helpful and most challenged. It is not at all easy or comfortable to sit with someone and have no answers for them, to allow people to suffer the emotional pain of hearing unwelcome news or to express their grief and anger at life and death. This is where healing in a different sense can begin or continue, but is where we often get little education, development and time or opportunity to reflect. We rarely see these tender moments being role modelled – they are often both spontaneous and private and then not discussed in a busy surgical nursing setting. I will return to this later.

What support is not

We have so far considered what forms support might take. However, it is also worth exploring what support is not. There is little written about what support is not and generally it is included as part of a definition of support, as if it is an opposite or opposing tendency. Whilst acknowledging the times when support is freely and authentically given, there are times when this may result in collusion with old patterns of denial and behaviour, for example the people who always wait for others to speak on their behalf. At times, the most supportive intervention can be to do nothing for people but to help or challenge them to do it themselves. It would not be supportive to collude with or promote dependency in this instance. Heron (1990) is clear about the nature of supportive interventions, which warmly and authentically affirm the worth of individuals and their characteristics, but do not collude with rigid and defensive behaviour and belief systems. Equally, Culley (1991, p. 14) writes of support as 'being a source of strength to, standing alongside and not colluding with or rescuing'. Both of these authors, then, include support and what support is not in the same context. Culley (1991) goes on to write, similarly to Heron (1990), of support underpinning challenge, and that support without challenge may not result in change.

One phrase which I frequently recall as a tool for analysis when assessing which nursing intervention might be the one of choice is, 'Don't do anything for clients which they can do for themselves'. This is not dismissive, as it may sound, but is empowering in intent, in that the helper's role may be one of enabling someone to develop a skill, or of awareness and being there to provide support during the process. It will promote independence in the client, rather than the unquestioning informing or advising, giving and doing for that so often happens, which may also repeat a pattern. A student who continually asks for help with a procedure will learn from a demonstration and then supervised practice. A patient who must learn to care for a stoma is similar. Neither will be served by continually observing experienced nurses without taking up the challenge of trying the procedure themselves. I remember when I was a Registered Mental Nurse undergoing Registered General Nurse training, one of the staff nurses on a ward said, 'I love watching you work, you never do anything,' by which she meant that I helped patients do everything possible for themselves, including washing and dressing and feeding which she and many other staff unthinkingly did for patients. I believe that I was supporting my own patients in their recovery by strengthening their independence wherever possible. Those observing me also could notice that working with patients rather than doing for them took no extra time – by attending to those activities such as washing, dressing, mouth care, mobilising, eating and drinking, and working together, we achieved all that had to be done.

Support, likewise, is not the same as reassurance which may again serve to maintain patterns of rigid or defensive behaviour without change. A further danger of being reassured that 'you're doing all right' is that we do not hear the underlying message of fear, anxiety or sadness which may be being expressed. This is sad because it means we are incomplete in our caregiving to patients and each other and are not 'present' in any real sense.

The characteristics of support and what it is not can be summarised as follows:

The person who is supportive works with a person rather than does to, is respectful and sensitive to individual needs, builds confidence, promotes independence, challenges rigid behaviours and thoughts, is open to change in herself and others. The non-supportive person does to rather than works with, is reactive rather than reflective, inappropriately provides reassurance and advice, denies or is unaware of rigid and defensive behaviours and thoughts in the other and herself, colludes with and promotes dependency.

Reflective point

Identify and analyse a recent situation when you felt supported, and another in which you supported someone. Consider this also as a mutual activity, i.e. in which you both supported someone and in turn were supported by them.
  Identify a time when you did not feel supported. Consider what you did need in the way of support at the time.

I hope that so far you have begun to realise the breadth of issues which the word 'support' includes, and you might have more sense of what we mean when we say 'no-one ever supports me'. Do we mean no-one takes care of me, no-one offers to help me, no-one carries my weight, no-one notices me, no-one listens to me, no-one gives me the off-duty time I want, no-one sees how miserable I am, no-one does my shopping and laundry? Are we making a true observation or are we repeating a pattern from our past? By using phrases like the ones above we may be putting ourselves in a victim role, waiting to be rescued. How different our lives may be if we can accept our own contribution to our world. Would you ask someone to bear your weight? Do you ask for help, for someone to listen? Do you tell someone you are unhappy? Do you expect anyone to help if you do ask? Sometimes it is easier to moan than to take responsibility for ourselves. The first step of asking for support or to be noticed may be the most difficult one, and asking may not guarantee that you get what you want, but it will improve the chances. The first step in both giving and receiving support is in identifying the need, and this is where self-awareness is central both to this discussion and the practicalities of support.

AN EXPLORATION OF OUR NEED FOR SUPPORT

Self-awareness and support

Self-awareness is a central feature of support, whether we are the giver or the recipient. We must be sufficiently self-aware to recognise our need for support, in whatever form it is required, and, equally, if we are supporting others, we must be able to notice whether or not our interventions are actually the most helpful, whether we are really hearing what is asked for or whether we are colluding with old patterns. Our awareness may also include noticing our resistance to our own vulnerability and our willingness (or not) to ask for support.

Burnard (1995) writes clearly of the role of self-awareness within the counselling relationship and his summary can be used for any therapeutic (helping) relationship, including that of nurse–patient and nurse–nurse. He tells us that self-awareness enables us to:

- differentiate ourselves from others
- know what is our own and what is a patient's problem or difficulty
- work from choice rather than unconscious habit, respond rather than react

- be more sensitive to our own needs and those of others
- prevent exhaustion and burnout (Burnard 1995, pp. 36–37).

There is a great deal in what Burnard writes. It is easy to lose ourselves in our work, to identify with patients, to continually react to need rather than reflect and respond. It can be seen, therefore, that self-awareness is essential if we are to take care of ourselves in order to deliver quality care, relating authentically to all the people we meet (social and family life included). He also makes a clear statement regarding the value of self-awareness, 'Without self-awareness, the person appears merely to have a set of skills 'tacked on' to her: those skills are used neither sensitively nor awarely but in a robotic and automatic way' (Burnard 1995, p. 37). Self-awareness provides the foundation for therapeutic use of self with all those whom we meet.

A framework for support

It is not always easy to identify what we mean when we say we need support. We might at times be aware of a vague discomfort or lack, at others we may know exactly what we need. What follows is a framework which I have found helpful in clarifying these issues.

Hopson (1982) identified six helping strategies, and his work can assist us in identifying the sort of support we need (see Box 5.1). All of the strategies are ways in which we can help people and therefore they may be seen and adapted as forms of support. One key feature is that we as individuals, with awareness, can state the form of help we need. At times we may lack information or skill, at other times we may need someone to listen and help us work out how to relate to a patient, how to address the 'difficult subject' or to deal with our own grief at someone's circumstances. Having identified a need, we may know who to approach to meet that need. It is important to note that one helping strategy is not superior to another, it is the appropriate use of the strategy which is important, i.e. you are meeting the client's needs and not compulsively helping or supporting in either an unwanted or inappropriate fashion. Equally from the first to the fifth strategy, there is a gradient from helper-centred to client-centred in terms of empowerment.

Hopson provides a very useful framework for helping us analyse the form in which we need support. His first helping strategy is that of direct action. Sometimes we do need someone to do something for us or on our behalf. This may be a colleague taking over the care of

---

Box 5.1 Hopson's helping strategies (adapted from Hopson 1982. In: Chapman and Gale Psychology and People). (Reproduced by kind permission of Macmillan Press and The British Psychological Society.)

- Direct action   Helper-centred
- Giving advice
- Giving/providing information
- Education
- Counselling   Client-centred
- Systems change

---

some patients when one becomes acutely ill and needs one-to-one attention for a period. It may take the form of someone buying us a sandwich for lunch, or anticipating that you might want one and buying it without being asked. When we are unable to cope with our workload, the colleague who says 'What can I do to help?' is offering to act on your behalf with some of your patients, including reallocating them. The favours and kindnesses we do one another, willingly given and based in sensitivity rather than habit, are a very concrete way of providing support and are often underestimated in their impact. Smith (1992) refers to these as the 'little things' which are so important in nursing.

The second form of helping strategy described by Hopson is that of giving advice, or prescribing an action. This is a contentious strategy. Sundeen et al (1994) state that advice is anti-therapeutic (and in this context, not necessarily supportive) in that it removes power from clients and can ignore their needs. Advice may be too readily given at times, such as when we really need someone to listen to us explore an issue. There may also be times when we genuinely do want to hear someone's expert opinion and be guided by them. It will help to hear an experienced nurse say, 'I am concerned by this change in … and I advise you to call the doctor now'. Such a statement may give the junior nurse the confidence she needs to call that doctor and not worry about bothering her unnecessarily. She is secure in the opinion she has sought. There are, however, times when our own views must be withheld. It must be the patient's decision to sign a consent form, or to participate in research, and advice would be inappropriate here. Obviously it can be difficult at times to separate giving advice from being overprescriptive – with regard to informed consent it may help a patient to hear the nurse say, 'Yes, I would have it if I needed it', which is quite different from the coercion and manipulation which we must guard against, for example with entry to clinical trials. In this instance, the nurse might support the patient by being an advocate for her. Other times when we might pre-scribe action (give advice) are with instructions for drugs, or exercise, or positioning in bed. Just as we may be willing to heed advice, so we may be able to give it appropriately. We all know, however, that the advice 'Don't worry' is particularly useless. It is unlikely to have ever helped us and equally will not help others.

Hopson's next helping strategy is that of giving information. He tells us that information is power and to inform clients will empower them. In terms of our own support, we may clearly need information, in a variety of forms. One student I met was confused by the term 'hypertensive' and thought it meant 'over-anxious' although this made no sense at handover times. She began to lack confidence and eventually was able to ask me what it meant. When I told her 'high blood pressure' she visibly relaxed, understood her confusion and became more confident again in using nursing terminology. Likewise, a simple expla-nation may suddenly help a client tremendously, or the willingness to say 'surgery can be painful' to the person who is denying analgesia but is immobilised by pain, 'it's normal to feel this way' to a patient who is in tears a few days postoperatively. Much work has been done on the impact which giving information has on anxiety (Hayward 1975, Teasdale 1993, Wilson-Barnett 1978) and this is addressed elsewhere in this book (see Chs 2 and 18).

The fourth helping strategy is that of education or teaching. This follows on from information and includes the process of helping someone learn. This may be from written material or it may be helping someone acquire a skill, such as managing a syringe driver or a Hickman line. It may also take the form of putting theory into practice. Again, this is a way in which we may require support. We may have informa-tion about the principles of postoperative observation of vital signs and wounds. What we then need is someone to help us understand, internalise those prin-ciples, apply them to practice, demonstrate what is being looked for and measured and help us learn to interpret the measurement of vital signs. Ultimately we become experienced in this ourselves; we have confidence in our skills and judgements as a result of this form of being helped. This level of support contin-ues throughout our careers as procedures and ideas and our roles change and we meet the demands of these changes. At one stage we may wish to develop our clinical knowledge and skills through further edu-cation, at another we may wish to explore labour rela-tions issues when we enter a different role. Support is needed throughout our lives and careers, not only when we are novice nurses. If we are lifelong learners, support is a key part of that learning process.

Counselling is the next helping strategy defined by Hopson and by this he means helping others to help themselves. This may be the strategy of choice when individuals are deciding whether to change jobs, to work out what is happening for them or when they feel angry or sad. There will be times when we know that no-one can make our decisions for us, make our lives better for us, but what we do need is the time and space to talk and be listened to. To receive this form of support is rare. We seldom pay enough attention to our own emotions and needs, let alone identify that we need time to talk and be listened to.

The final helping strategy is that of systems change. This happens on a bigger scale than the first five, which all normally occur within a one-to-one setting or relationship. Systems change may involve devising a new rota, moving to primary nursing, building in a new break within a shift. These changes may well be initiated by nurses for the benefit of clients, and might also be introduced for the benefit of colleagues. For example, a system on a ward might be that only one nurse on the staff gets study leave at a time. For two or three to be granted study leave would require a system change. The support we require may take this form, and many may benefit. Likewise, a nurse who wishes to move to part-time work but retain an H grade may find that she challenges the system. A change in the system which would support her needs and acknowl-edge the level of her work is necessary. Some systems changes are of course instigated by management or external bodies for political or economic reasons and in this situation, the support we need might include information, education and counselling.

Hopson's framework may help us identify what form of support we need, whether practical, advisory, informative, educative, counselling or systems change. It can be used to help us clarify a vague need into a request for help. It can be used as a framework for reflection and an increase in self-awareness. If I ask myself 'what do I need?' and the answer is 'infor-mation', I then have clarity about the process (i.e. information-seeking) into which I must enter. I may then consider who or what is the best resource and enter into my own problem-solving process about how to get there. Emotions will play a part here – we might fear looking stupid, we might be reluctant to call on people's time when we know they are busy. As people trying to help and support others, we can be helped by Hopson's framework to work with them to identify what they need when they are unsure.

Reflective point

Review your contact with three patients or colleagues. Using Hopson's (1982) framework, identify the way(s) in which you supported them. Was this the most appropriate way? Provide a rationale for this decision or suggest an alternative more appropriate strategy.

Reflective point

Consider how you like to work and what suits your personality best. Are you lonely or isolated? Do you get enough time to yourself? What could you do to improve your life in these senses?

Why do we need support?

It can be seen from the discussion above that support takes many different forms. If we return to the statement, 'No one ever supports me' and rephrase it as 'I need support in the form of ...' we have (a) become more aware of our need, (b) become able to make a specific request and (c), importantly, taken an active role and responsibility for trying to meet that need. What we have not yet explored is why we need support, and the depth of that cry at times. We can fairly easily identify a lack of knowledge or proficiency in a practical skill, and the support which learning requires, but what of our emotional needs? These have been well documented by Smith (1992) in her research, and she includes many evocative verbatim comments from nurses about their own emotional needs. Intellectual and behavioural support can be relatively simple to find or organise, but emotional support, as Smith (1992) explains, brings in a further dimension. For an appreciation of this latter area, we can now explore the classic psychoanalytic work of authors such as Menzies (1959) and Main (1957) and more recent continuations of this by Hawkins & Shohet (1989) and Dartington (1993).

The emotional demands of nursing

Human beings generally need contact with each other in an affirming and warm relationship in order to maintain psychological health. Some models of mental illness look at how relationships contribute to ill health, and Lindsay & Powell (1994, p. 18) tell us that, 'Lack of social support is frequently believed to contribute to the seeking of professional help by people in distress'. Isolation and loneliness feature highly in people who are unhappy and depressed, and are different from a sense of having space to be oneself or for a period of quiet reflection. We all have preferred ways of working – in close teams, in hospitals or perhaps more individually and separately in community settings, with opportunities for meeting colleagues at set times.

Before looking particularly at the emotional nature of nursing, it is worth identifying some of the reasons why we chose to enter the profession. The more honest we can be with this, the more open we will be to identifying what we might be acting out. Hawkins & Shohet (1989, p. 8) quote Ram Dass and Paul Gorman, who assert, 'Without minimising the external demands of helping others, it seems fair to say that some of the factors that wear us down, we have brought with us at the outset'. Examples of these may be rigid patterns of behaviour and thinking; a need to please others; a need to belong; a need to understand personal or family pathology; a need for respect and esteem, to feel important; a need to control, having not had control previously; a need to be cared for, having not experienced this previously. Somewhere there is likely also to be a genuine wish to help others, and to be involved in the healing process. This is not to be denied, but it is likely that there are other less pure motives, often referred to as shadow or hidden, which can help us understand our behaviour. For example, a need to please at all costs for fear of upsetting someone will rapidly pull us down, whereas a balance will be in pleasing ourselves as well. Nurses often seem to have low self-esteem and may need help to value the contribution they personally make to care and to acknowledge their skills and abilities. It may be that many nurses enter the profession and learn to feel not good enough, which may be compounded by continual performance reviews which identify further learning, goals and targets. We may wonder if we will ever be enabled to work at a level which suits us and not feel we should always be doing more. Sometimes we need to know that we are OK as we are and it is rare that we hear this, from others or ourselves.

Menzies (whose original work was published in 1959 but is now available in a collection of her papers, Menzies-Lyth 1988) writes evocatively of the causes of stress in nursing. She refers to the constant contact with people who are ill, diseased or dying, being confronted with suffering and death as few lay people are, the nature of the tasks we undertake, the intimate contact with patients. She writes, 'The work situation arouses very strong and mixed feelings in the nurse:

pity, compassion and love; guilt and anxiety; hatred and resentment of the patients who arouse these strong feelings; envy of the care given to the patient' (Menzies-Lyth 1988, p. 46). We can, if we are honest, notice these in ourselves at times. Menzies continues to add to the stresses by including the feelings of patients and relatives: 'The hospital, particularly the nurses, must allow the projection into them of such feelings as depression and anxiety, fear of the patient and his illness, disgust at the illness and necessary nursing tasks … Thus to the nurse's own deep and intense anxieties are psychically added those of the other people concerned' (Menzies-Lyth 1988, p. 48). No wonder we feel exhausted at times, drained and saddened by our work, carrying not only our own feelings, but unconsciously those of others too. How do we deal with this in a self-caring manner? It cannot be surprising that nurses deny feelings – how can they begin to explore everything they experience during a span of work? When we give so much to patients how can we give to each other too?

Menzies' (1959) original work identified and explained how the social system of the hospital and task allocation within nursing helped the nurse to manage the anxieties of the role, although she had initially been asked to research into the high wastage rates of trainee and newly qualified nurses. The move to primary nursing and patient allocation has potentially opened the nurse and patient to more holistic and rewarding relationships with each other but paradoxically this may be more stressful and distressing as affection and personal involvement increase. It is even more important then, that the support structures which this requires are part of the development, implementation and evaluation of all such schemes.

Dartington (1993) writes of the ambivalence with which nursing is viewed by society and nurses themselves. This is apparent in the image of angels who at the same time have poor pay and working conditions. Nurses remind people of their vulnerability to illness and death, and one way nurses (and other health care professionals) have of coping is to feel omnipotent or despondent, unable to help. A difficulty here is that when we feel omnipotent (or at least fine) we deny the need for support, and when we feel despondent, we deny that we are worthy of support. Main (1957, p. 9) tells us that 'Cured patients do great service to their attendants' and he also warns of the need to be aware of our hidden motives in caring. He uses the phrase 'heroic surgical attack' and makes the point that 'the sufferer who frustrates a keen therapist by failing to improve is always in danger of meeting primitive human behaviour disguised as treatment'. Primitive

human behaviour in this sense, is impulsive, including attack and defence, persecution, wanting to win, refusing to accept failure. It can be seen at times when the immediate reaction to patients who will not comply or who do not improve is to transfer them, operate again, or discharge them to the care of the general practitioner. Barker (1992) touches on this theme when he writes of the aims of supervision (in psychiatric nursing) as being, 'to protect people from nurses and to protect nurses from themselves' (Barker 1992, p. 66). A moment of reflection may be helpful here, in order to assess our own motivation behind a decision. Also, talking to the patient is likely to result in a more acceptable outcome for all concerned.

All of the above may indicate why we need support in our role as surgical nurses. Hawkins & Shohet (1989, p. 18) summarise this succinctly: 'What happens if you do not have enough support is that you absorb more disturbance, distress and dis-ease from your clients and patients than you are able to process and let go of and then you become overburdened by the work'. This may be when signs of stress and strain become routine, for example always feeling busy, insomnia, overeating, worrying, substance abuse, and we feel out of control. It is of course, desirable to intervene before this happens, which will be explored in the next section. Going back to Burnard (1995), we can see how the self-aware nurse might see and experience these signs happening in herself and ask for support.

WAYS IN WHICH WE CAN GIVE AND RECEIVE SUPPORT

Gestalt psychotherapists (e.g. Clarkson 1989) refer to internal and external support, by which they mean how we support ourselves and how we use our environment to support us. Internal support would include such activities as we know individually serve us well, for example taking physical exercise, having alternative interests, meditation or other spiritual activities, reflection. External support involves another person or agent and this is where it is helpful to know where to go. A search for information may include mobilising internal support and going to a library, it may also include approaching someone perceived as knowledgeable such as a senior nurse or a lecturer. We must not forget that often the person with the most relevant information is the patient and we can learn a great deal from our patients.

Clinical supervision and reflective practice

Much has been written about the role of mentors, preceptors, supervisors, clinical supervisors and the role of supervision. The debate is ongoing and may occupy the profession for a long time yet. Current definitions include those here, although these terms have changed subtly over the years. Mentors may be defined as those nurses who will help students achieve learning objectives and competencies for a clinical area, often working similar shifts and explaining what they are doing as they work, with a period of consolidation, usually during report writing. Butterworth & Faugier (1992, p. 11) define a mentor simply as 'An experienced professional nurturing and guiding the novitiate'. Preceptorship is more structured and Brennan (1993) suggests that preceptors have a specific role in supporting new staff nurses from Project 2000 courses. Supervision in nursing is often seen as a management-led activity where standards can be ensured (practice is supervised) and information exchanged. Clinical supervision, by contrast, is client/case-based, but may mirror supervision if a manager is the supervisor. Counselling is different from all forms of supervision, mentoring and preceptorship, although counselling skills may be used in those activities. The terminology may be confusing and is complicated by the relatively clear definition of the purposes of supervision which mental health and social work professionals use. All these activities (mentoring, preceptorship, supervision) are essentially defined by their purpose, so it is important to ask about and discuss this purpose when someone offers you supervision or mentoring or preceptoring or asks you to carry out the function for someone else.

The United Kingdom Central Council for Nursing, Midwifery and Health Visiting in its position statement on clinical supervision for nursing and health visiting (UKCC 1996) tells us that: 'Clinical supervision assists practitioners to develop skills, knowledge and professional values throughout their careers. This enables them to develop a deeper understanding of what it is to be an accountable practitioner and to link this to the reality of practice more easily than has previously been possible'. They go on to state: 'Potential benefits are not thought to be limited to patients, clients or practitioners. A more skilled, aware and articulate profession should contribute effectively to organisational objectives' (UKCC 1996, p. 2). They make it clear that this definition includes preceptorship for newly qualified nurses.

I am concerned, though, that little mention is made of the emotional nature of nursing. Not all professional values may be healthy for the individual, for example the denial of feeling, the willingness to continually put others first. What assurance is there that a supervisor, mentor or preceptor has the skills or

willingness to address wider issues? People in any of these roles may be able to answer (or help the student to explore) technical or role-related questions as a local, available expert, but can they help a student, new staff nurse or experienced nurse respectively with emotional distress related to patient care or relationships? For example, a student may feel that a person should not be resuscitated, a staff nurse may see similarities between the care of one patient and a close family member, spiritual beliefs might be challenged by a patient or situation. If the mentor, preceptor or supervisor also has a managerial relationship with the student or staff nurse, is it safe to raise such issues? In order to fulfil the roles of mentor, preceptor and supervisor, counselling skills and self-awareness are clearly necessary. However, these skills may be lacking and will be addressed later in the chapter.

The role of mentor would suggest that immediate support (at least at technical level) is possible because of the working patterns, whereas this will not be the case for preceptorship and supervision. Some support may not be immediately available. It is also quite likely that no one person can meet all of another's work-related needs and to presume that someone can may be to perpetuate the myth of the supernurse who as well as being highly knowledgeable, technically brilliant, procedurally skilful and warm, communicative, open and reflective, is able to develop her staff and students to the same level. She will of course also have a fulfilling life outside work. It is far more likely and reasonable that having identified the form in which support is required, people approach those who can meet that need. This will account for a student or patient approaching one nurse for information, another for skills advice and another to cry. Although this may be organisationally difficult, or advised against, there is nothing wrong in this approach – it may well demonstrate responsibility for self on the help-seekers part. It does, however, go contrary to the individualised care approach where one nurse is expected to meet or at least identify all the needs of one patient, and may challenge our own notions of omnipotence and omniscience. I regularly supervise nurses and nurse teachers about the emotional or relationship aspects of their work with clients who comprise patients, students and other staff. We all know that I will not advise on areas about which I know little, for example physical examination or pharmacological regimes. They will approach others for this and I will at times suggest that they do so. What matters is that nurses are supported in all aspects of their work and know where to go for this support. It may be that for student nurses, concentrating on learning practical skills, most support is given in the clinical setting, and they might also approach a link tutor or lecturer–practitioner for information of a different nature or depth. For those who feel that local support is inappropriate or unavailable, the Royal College of Nursing's Nurseline service might be of help or the National Association of Staff Support, which has local groups in some areas.

Having said this, to separate out the intellectual/technical aspects of our role from the emotional aspects is to make a false division and may perpetuate denial of the latter. Some people will be capable of supporting students and colleagues to the required degree in all areas, and it is important that supporters can identify their limits of safe practice. They also need education and support themselves in when to refer elsewhere, particularly for people with emotional difficulties.

It is also unnecessary, in my opinion, to separate out the terms supervision and clinical supervision. All supervision is, by definition, role related, whether this role is ward-based, educational or managerial, and client-focused, whether the client is patient, student or employee. Perhaps what needs exploring and clarifying is the purpose and process of supervision, in order that principles may guide the supervisor, whatever the role. I will use the term supervision to include clinical supervision from now on.

Reflective point

Who do you go to when you need help? Do you approach different people for different forms of support? What do patients ask you for or talk to you about? How might a patient support you?

What is supervision?

In its best sense, supervision provides an opportunity for us to mobilise our internal support structures and to use external support. Supervision provides a structured time, place and relationship in which reflection on action can be facilitated. It is a planned, purposeful activity and its purposes relate to the ground rules for which it was established which will include a client-related focus. Reflection, like supervision, is a structured, purposeful activity. Boud et al (1985) are clear that reflection brings together the intellect and the affect and propose the structure of returning to the experience, attending to feelings and re-evaluating the experience. The outcomes of reflection are described by Boud et al (1985, p. 21) as 'a personal synthesis, integration and appropriation of new knowledge, a new affective state, or the decision to engage in some further activity'. The outcomes of supervision are similar. New understandings and behaviours may be identified, the supervisee may feel free from concern or guilt, new learning goals may be set. It is not, in my view, essential that supervisors are clinical experts. What is important is that they have the skills to enable reflection in the supervisees. These skills include being able to listen, to reflect, to challenge, to support, to confront, to focus and to accept and explore the work-related emotional world of the supervisee. Thus supervision is a structured form of support.

Much has been written in the nursing press recently regarding supervision, and there are several models and theoretical frameworks that underpin the purpose and process of supervision. Some definitions of supervision are fluid, others more precise, and it is important that the supervisor and supervisee are aware of the parameters within which they are working. Hawkins & Shohet (1989) describe three functions of supervision: educative, supportive and managerial. The latter is concerned with quality and standards. They also refer to a fourth, consultancy, where qualified and experienced members of staff retain responsibility for their work but consult with a supervisor who has neither a training nor a managerial relationship with them. This may be the optimal form of supervision. It will include education and support and may well have a quality control aspect but without the fears that may go with trusting a manager. As an experienced nurse, I still need challenge about the quality of my care, or feedback when I seem to be ignoring aspects of my work. I also need praise and acknowledgement of work which has gone well. I may have quite legitimate concerns about discussing some of these areas with a manager when I know I will be applying for regrading. It is, of course, quite appropriate that role competence is addressed, as one purpose of supervision is to protect the best interests of the client. Whilst students and staff nurses may be supervised by mentors and preceptors, it is essential that those mentors and preceptors are themselves supervised, and this may be where the consultancy model can be developed. All nurses, educators and managers could make good use of supervision for their own practice – it is not only an activity for the novice.

Supervision and learner nurses

Using Hawkins & Shohet's (1989) themes of education, support and management (quality and standards) it can be seen that whether we are mentor, preceptor or supervisor, we are addressing the same areas within these relationships. Perhaps the different terms serve no purpose other than to confuse and frustrate those involved and perpetuate rigid role boundaries. It may be that for students the emphasis is mainly on education and support, whereas for the new staff nurse the emphasis may be on support and quality/standards, but this will never be exclusively the case. Students and new staff nurses may find that they have limited choice of who to go to formally (named nurses will be writing their practice assessments for example) but these latter should ideally take any relationship difficulties to their own supervisors.

One approach to this multifaceted nature of supervision is to encourage problem-solving in the moment. If we can learn to develop awareness of what, specifically, we need, who can meet the need, when (immediate or can wait), where (ward, library, outside) and why (is it for reasons of habit or reassurance that I want to refer this to someone else or could I take the challenge of making my own decision?) we can identify a way forward. I often go to my supervisor with specific questions about one client, a vague sense of dissatisfaction about my work with someone else and have in the meantime independently sorted out a clinical issue with another expert. What I will now consider are some of the practicalities of external or consultancy supervision, which some surgical nurses are or will be addressing.

Practical considerations

It is often the case that people write of supervision, or communication or support. but do not discuss what actually happens. I will try to do this here.

To restate the above, supervision (in my view) is a structured purposeful activity in which reflection on action (rather than reflection in action; see Schon 1991) can occur within a warm, trusting, supportive and inquiring relationship. The primary purpose is to enable reflection on role-related issues, which means that the supervisees bring in patient/case material which remains the focus throughout and leave with a way to continue with their client/situation.

Supervision contracts

Supervision is normally a contracted activity, by which I mean that a regular, protected time and place is identified, and the cost and who will bear it is addressed, as are issues of missed sessions, holidays, confidentiality,

etc. This is pertinent when an employer may be paying for supervision and it may be reasonable for that employer to at least be told (if they ask) of your attendance. Whether an employer should be told the content of individual sessions must be explored, and it is possible that a regular global report is provided, signed by both supervisor and supervisee.

Location

Location is an issue which must be addressed. It is often the case that supervision occurs in an office on the ward, with the supervisor coming to the client's setting. Whilst this may make sense on a practical level, it can be very difficult to leave a busy ward, to not be disturbed, to not respond to the sound of bells and buzzers etc. It is preferable, despite the possible inconvenience, to go elsewhere for supervision. This is important for several reasons:

- Distance from the work setting may enable greater reflection and objectivity about what is happening.
- The lack of interruption may enable supervisees to relax.
- It may be easier to trust that the relationship is confidential.
- It is clear that the time is for the supervisee.
- Immediate need gratification may be frustrated with useful effect.

By this last comment I mean that supervisees may reflect on and resolve issues for themselves and then discuss this with the supervisor, rather than immediately call for help on non-urgent issues. They will, in this way, become more self-reliant.

Lateness or non-attendance

These will provide insights into the personal or managerial attitudes to supervision in practice. For example, if a nurse can be told to cancel supervision as the ward is short staffed, this can be taken up with management who have identified the need for supervision in order to maintain quality care. Equally, it may suggest that a nurse considers patients' needs more important than her own. The role of the supervisor is to notice and explore this with the supervisee. (This can of course happen where supervision happens on the ward too.)

Supervision and counselling/personal therapy

The purpose of supervision may not always be clear initially to the supervisee. This will emerge as time and the relationship progress, but one area where confusion sometimes occurs is the relationship between supervision and personal therapy or counselling. Supervision is not the same as personal therapy and the supervisor must hold this boundary. This is not to say that supervision is not therapeutic – being listened to and helped is often experienced this way – but that it is not the place for in-depth personal work. A supervisor may suggest that a supervisee sees a counsellor for unresolved distress, or for deep-rooted issues of low self-esteem for example, or where repeated blocks occur, but if the supervisor's primary responsibility is to the patient, then her role is to equip the supervisee with strategies which serve the patient. If, for example, my supervisor notices that as I talk about my work, I seem to be reproaching myself more than usual, we know from experience and previous reflection that this is a sign for me of tiredness and fatigue. It is her role to point this out, but not to explore my lack of sleep due to domestic problems. This is business for me and possibly my therapist, where I am the client and the primary focus. Yegdich (1998) extends the debate on personal/professional development, stressing that attention to the purposes and boundaries of supervision and therapy is essential. She provides examples of how the supervisee might become a patient rather than a colleague and identifies how, in this way, nursing supervision can lose sight of the patient and can perpetuate the avoidance of anxiety in intimate therapeutic work. It is therefore of paramount importance that supervisors are clear about the purpose and process of supervision, and preparation for the role of supervisor should address this. A 2- or 3-day course is unlikely to be sufficient.

Group or individual?

Supervision can occur in individual (one-to-one) formats or in small groups. For nurses, the latter is often ideal, as the group members will support each other and in so doing, begin to supervise each other. This will serve them well when (if) they wish to develop the supervision aspects of their own work roles. They will also learn from each other's presentations, struggles and successes. This is where the 'tender moments' mentioned earlier can be explored and shared, thereby enhancing learning opportunities. A weekly 1-hour session with two supervisees may work well, in which each person presents a case study and there is time at the end for processing general themes. Group supervision often makes role play or practising difficult situations easier as well as having the advantage of feedback and ideas from people other than supervisors.

It may work also to have supervisees from different areas (perhaps similar levels of seniority) to learn from.

Group supervision will bring up further issues of trust and confidentiality and the boundary must be maintained to ensure that there is no gossiping outside the sessions about patients or supervisees' disclosures. The relationship is central to working well in supervision.

Duration of supervision

As in any helping relationship, the supervisory relationship will evolve over time and it is necessary that trust is established, and that warmth, acceptance, genuineness and empathy feature, at least in the supervisor. This will take time. It is not easy to admit to difficulties with someone who you do not know but will continue to meet. A supervisor is likely to work in annual contracts, but it may be desirable for longer to be possible, perhaps for the duration of training or for 2 years post-qualification. This can be negotiated between supervisor and supervisee, plus whoever is paying.

Who is a supervisor?

The UKCC (1996) delegates this decision to local policy makers. Supervisors should be skilled in supervision, and need not necessarily be nurses. Some psychiatric nurses have as their supervisors social workers or psychologists and act as supervisors themselves to these groups. The UKCC, however, make it clear that where supervision is offered by someone from a different discipline, this 'would normally be in addition to supervision from a fellow practitioner' (UKCC 1996, p. 4). In my experience, a supervisor might not be working in the same area of nursing, but is likely to have a sound understanding and appreciation of the demands of the role and the organisation. The skills needed for supervision, identified earlier, must be evident and supervisors themselves will need supervision on their supervisees. Supervisors must also be able to demonstrate an attitude of inquiry rather than accusation or blame, of willingness to listen before jumping to conclusions or offering solutions. At a sufficiently senior level, peer supervision is appropriate, and this remains structured, contracted and purposeful.

There is a possible role for link tutors in developing their role as supervisors in the sense of which I write. They too would need support and education within this role plus the acknowledgement of its importance and the time required. Nursing practice groups equally might develop which have a supervision focus, particularly for those who work in isolated or specialist areas.

Reflective point

Would you consider someone other than a surgical nurse for a supervisor? Explore the advantages and disadvantages of meeting with a surgical nurse or someone from a different background.

What happens in a supervision session?

I have already suggested that in group supervision each member presents a case or cases. This is a regular format. The supervisor, as well as listening to what is said will be noticing what is not said, any themes which emerge and will enable reflection on the case through skilful use of questioning, reflecting content or emotions, challenging, focusing and summarising. She may ask the supervisee to identify what went well and what could be improved. She may work to a structured model of reflection, such as that suggested by Johns (1995), who suggests writing a description of the experience, followed by asking questions to do with purpose, motivation, awareness of self and other, feelings and emotions, knowledge required and reflection on what has been learnt from the exercise (Johns 1995, p. 227). The supervisor will not necessarily supply information, preferring to help the supervisees explore their own solutions to problems. She will, where appropriate, give information which the group do not seem to have. She will also at times offer the opportunity to practise a skill which is relevant to returning to the client. Generally in group supervision, the major interaction is between each individual and the supervisor, with other members listening and observing initially, and then being asked for comments later. In this way the supervisee gets individual attention rather than a general discussion happening for the whole time. It is my experience that supervision is clearly an activity which supports me in my work with clients and puts back in some of the energy which I have expended during my work. It also provides an outlet for emotion, including humour, which is clearly of beneficial effect as identified by Heron (1990).

Support groups

I remain unclear about the definition of support groups and their value. Many have been, in my experience, misused, provided as a panacea to unhappy staff and with little attention paid to purpose and structure. By contrast, some have worked well and this may be due to members' needs being met. I would suggest that time is well spent identifying need and purpose before establishing any group, the primary purposes of which might then be social, educational, political, supervision/reflection, or therapeutic/counselling (Kagan & Evans 1995 provide a framework for this). Once need and purpose are established, the resources can be identified. It is likely that a social group (e.g. to meet to develop friendships and non-work interests) will be self-led, whereas the others are more likely to require an external facilitator and a regular room for meeting. A supervision group will, of course, meet some social needs, for example contact with other professionals, but this is not the primary purpose. One responsibility of the leader is to retain a focus on purpose. Similarly, if a group meets for educational reasons, e.g. to study for examinations, but spends the time chatting about fashion, some members will feel frustrated. It is my belief (yet to be tested) that when people say they need support, they may be asking for supervision, which will be supportive, reflective and growth-promoting in its purpose and effects.

Developing skills for support and supervision

If you have read through this chapter from the beginning, I hope you will have become aware of the importance of self-awareness and reflection. These are fundamental personal skills which can be developed and enhanced through contact with others and feedback from them. Following on from these comes the ability to relate to others in a manner which will help them. Barker (1992) writes about the difference between being helpful and helping, 'Nurses need to "be helpful" in their everyday work with people in care. Such helpful actions are part and parcel of any social system in which interdependence is the rule and genuine independence is rare. Helpfulness is the support system which characterises all social units … Helping is about arranging ways of promoting growth and development' (Barker 1992, p. 67). Whilst much of nursing is about being helpful to people, this might create or continue to create dependency, whereas by helping, the nurse will promote independence in the client. This is not to say that doing things for someone is automatically wrong, but that we should continually ask ourselves whether there is an alternative.

It may be challenging to become self-aware and to use the opportunities presented during personal and interpersonal skills sessions which are regularly included in most courses. This, however, is the time which can be used to try out listening styles, to practise 'being with' someone, to question, to reflect, to challenge, to focus, to help people reach their own solutions rather than offering advice or information automatically.

The skills of support underpin those required in supervision, where the supervisor will be more experienced in the use of these skills and will also be able to hold the purpose and boundary of the meeting, and have an overview of the whole situation. Some authors (Whitmore 1991) use 'super-vision' in order to denote the overview, the bigger picture, the breadth and depth in the scenario. Supervisors will also need to be aware that they will be seen as powerful, as experts initially, because of their role, and that trust will not be automatic between supervisor and supervisee.

One very useful way to learn the skills of support and supervision is to be a client within such a relationship – to own that you need support and reflect on how you have been helped most, the interventions which were made with best effect, and to own that supervision is necessary and seek it out.

I mentioned earlier that supervisors themselves have supervision. We do not reach a pinnacle of expertise where we no longer need support or supervision. Our roles and relationships change, as might the environments in which we work. Wherever there is change, support and supervision is essential at all levels of an organisation. Part of being a lifelong learner is being continually open to learning and new experience, and supervision can help us work with this in a way which facilitates growth and nurturing.

Reflective point

Identify key skills and qualities which you think a supervisor should have. What would you ask a potential supervisor? Could you be a supervisor?

THE CHALLENGE OF SUPPORT

I have hinted throughout this chapter at some underlying issues regarding the challenges related to the giving and receiving of support. The first must be our own willingness and ability to acknowledge our own needs. It is difficult to accept that we need help, that we are not omnipotent, or even that we are worth helping. Many people leave the profession for a variety of reasons, but contributing to this decision must be the amount of pain and suffering which we see and take on. It may be courageous to leave and the best decision at the time. It may equally be courageous to stay and try to change systems which are not healthy.

One myth in nursing (and indeed all the helping professions) is that the nurse is well and the patient is sick. Therefore, if I am a nurse, I must be well, I must cope. This gives us both high expectations for ourselves and a non-acceptance of illness. Running an experiential therapy group for health professionals over an academic year, it was clearly observable that most struggled with the experience of being a patient or client in this group for at least the first term. Only when acceptance of this role and their needs occurred was there movement and openness to emotional aspects of being alive. It can be very difficult to ask for help on an emotional or relationship level, yet when we can do this and find someone who meets these needs, we can become much more able to help our patients in this way – we have learnt not to be afraid of emotions, we can begin to accept that there are some situations we cannot change but this does not mean we deny them or leave these patients in isolation.

A related challenge is that to ask for help is to take responsibility for oneself, rather than wait to be rescued. In transactional analysis (see Whitton 1993), one drama triangle is that of victim–persecutor–rescuer, where we identify with one or other role. Victims often wait to be rescued, have no sense of power, are done to; rescuers save victims, often without invitation; persecutors challenge, frighten, put down. This is horribly true of nursing at times where patients are victims of persecutors and rescuers (nurses) and, in other settings, nurses are victims at the mercy of persecutors and rescuers (perhaps managers, other compulsive helpers). To come out of this way of relating (which is often relatively safe through its familiarity) challenges us to be adult, authentic, and responsible. A consequence is that we may challenge the status quo or the existing system. If I refuse to stay late again (rescuer) I may be unpopular, blamed, respected and I must cope with this. I may need support during this time and my line manager may not be the person to offer this.

A further challenge is to be able to give the support which is needed. It does take courage to sit with someone who is distressed, or to say 'you look sad, do you want to talk?' A frequently expressed fear is of 'opening a can of worms' with such a comment, but the myth which supervision might unravel is that you caused the can of worms by asking such a question. This is not the case, but it might help you to clarify your sense of responsibility and also skills for containing the can of worms if this is appropriate. Similarly, supervision can support you while you challenge or confront self-limiting behaviours in patients or staff.

Another challenge of support is to be able to say that you do not know, when asked for information. A supervisor must be able to do this, and modelling this will help the nurse say the same to a student. One nurse teacher I worked with used to say 'I can guarantee three things. You and I don't know everything, some things we will be able to work out and some things we won't, but these we'll explore'. This clarity is quite useful at times in accepting what is so. Equally in the context of lifelong learning, the areas where there is a lack of knowledge may indicate a line of inquiry for us.

One major challenge when we look at formalised support and supervision structures is that of economics. We do know that nursing recruitment is often difficult, at all levels, and that many nurses leave the profession, never to return. We also know that we live in a world of tight budgets, with little if any money available for investment. However, formalised supervision arrangements will mean payment for supervisors, and staff being away from their clinical areas which will need cover. Costs may be more than economic as some staff become more assertive in their care of clients and as others become less willing to compulsively be helpful and regularly stay late or work extra unpaid hours. Managers must address their ambivalence to structures which support staff but at the same time will have cost implications. The identification and training of supervisors will in itself require time and financial input. In the longer term, of course, the value of supervision must be fully evaluated, with staff satisfaction, quality of care audit and patient satisfaction all considered. This does require taking a financial risk in the short term.

We must also acknowledge that for some staff supervision alone will not be sufficient. Relatively few employers offer staff counselling services or will contribute towards formal counselling where this is needed. Nurses are human and may at times in their lives need help in a variety of forms. Practical support may also include child care facilities or hours which fit with schools.

CONCLUSION

In this chapter I have addressed the concept of support, both what it is and what it is not. Self-awareness is essential both in identifying what we mean by support and then asking for or giving support. Supervision was introduced as one form of support, which might or might not meet all the needs of a learner but will have a role-related focus in helping the supervisees reflect on their work and identify or reach appropriate outcomes. Future research on the nature of support and supervision must be undertaken in terms of staff and patient outcomes to identify whether or not it is a justifiable investment. I believe it is and hope that you have gained an understanding of the related concepts of support and supervision through reading this chapter.

REFERENCES

Bailey R D 1985 Coping with stress in caring. Blackwell, London
Barker P 1992 Psychiatric nursing. In: Butterworth T, Faugier J 1992 Clinical supervision and mentorship in nursing. Chapman and Hall, London
Boud D, Keogh R, Walker D 1985 Promoting reflection in learning: a model. In: Boud D, Keogh R, Walker D (eds) Turning experience into learning. Kogan Page, London
Brennan A 1993 Preceptorship: is it a workable concept? Nursing Standard 7(52): 34–36
Burnard P 1995 Learning human skills, 3rd edn. Butterworth-Heinemann, London
Butterworth T, Faugier J 1992 Clinical supervision and mentorship in nursing. Chapman and Hall, London
Clarkson P 1989 Gestalt counselling in action. Sage, London
Culley S 1991 Integrative counselling in action. Sage, London
Dartington A 1993 Where angels fear to tread: idealism, despondency, and inhibition in thought in hospital nursing. Winnicott Studies 7: 21–41

Ersser S 1991 A search for the therapeutic dimensions of nurse–patient interaction. In: McMahon R, Pearson A 1991 Nursing as therapy. Chapman and Hall, London
Hawkins P, Shohet R 1989 Supervision in the helping professions. Open University Press, Milton Keynes
Hayward J 1975 Information: a prescription against pain. Royal College of Nursing, London
Heron J 1990 Helping the client. Sage, London
Hopson B 1982 Counselling and helping people. In: Chapman A, Gale A Psychology and people. Macmillan, London
Johns C 1995 Facilitating learning through reflections within Carper's fundamental ways of knowing in nursing. Journal of Advanced Nursing 22: 226–234
Kagan C, Evans J 1995 Professional interpersonal skills for nurses, 3rd edn. Chapman and Hall, London
Lindsay S J E, Powell G E 1994 The handbook of clinical adult psychology, 2nd edn. Routledge, London
Main T 1957 The ailment. Now available. In: Main T 1989 The ailment and other psychoanalytic essays. Free Association Books, London

Menzies I 1959 The functioning of social systems as a defence against anxiety. In: Menzies-Lyth I 1988 Containing anxiety in institutions. Free Association Books, London

Menzies-Lyth I 1988 Containing anxiety in institutions. Free Association Books, London

Schon D 1991 The reflective practitioner. Basic Books, London

Smith P 1992 The emotional labour of nursing. Macmillan, London

Sundeen S J, Stuart G W, Cohen E, Rankin S 1994 Nurse client interaction: implementing the nursing process, 5th edn. C V Mosby, London

Teasdale K 1993 Information and anxiety; a critical reappraisal. Journal of Advanced Nursing 18: 1125–1132

United Kingdom Central Council For Nursing, Midwifery And Health Visiting (UKCC) 1996 Position statement on clinical supervision for nursing and health visiting. UKCC, London

Whitmore D 1991 Psychosynthesis counselling in action. Sage, London

Whitton E 1993 What is transactional analysis? A personal and practical guide. Gale Centre Publications, Loughton, Essex

Wilson-Barnett J 1978 Patients' emotional responses to barium X-rays. Journal of Advanced Nursing 3: 37–46

Yegdich T 1998 How not to do clinical supervision in nursing. Journal of Advanced Nursing 28(1): 193–202

FURTHER READING

Bailey R D 1985 Coping with stress in caring. Blackwell, London

Bond M 1986 Stress and self awareness: a guide for nurses. Heinemann, London

Boud D, Cohen R, Walker D 1993 (eds) Using experience for learning. Open University Press, Milton Keynes

Kagan C, Evans J 1995 Professional interpersonal skills for nurses, 3rd edn. Chapman and Hall, London

6

Career opportunities for nurses working with surgical patients

Jane E. Schober

AIMS

This chapter aims to:

- provide an introduction to the preparation for and development of a career in surgical nursing
- highlight the roles and options specific to surgical nursing
- consider the notion of career progression, for example in relation to ongoing, specialist practice, re-registration and the personal professional profile
- discuss the potential of the process of career guidance as a means of supporting career planning
- explore the mechanisms for 'selling yourself' in a competitive job market.

INTRODUCTION

The successful completion of a course leading to registration as a first-level nurse and subsequent progression to a senior clinical post are significant achievements which raise questions such as 'What next?' Making decisions about our career options and opportunities is complex and many nurses need support and information to make these choices effectively. The quality of careers may be shaped and influenced by a range of personal, social and professional factors, for example the location of a post, family needs and employer demands and expectations.

There is no doubt that career patterns for nurses have changed in recent years. Nursing careers have been influenced by a number of professional developments, e.g. the clinical grading structure introduced in the late 1980s, the United Kingdom Central Council (UKCC) recommendations for post-registration education and practice (PREP) (UKCC 1991, 1997), the English National Board (ENB) framework for continuing professional education and the Higher Award (ENB 1991a) and 'The Scope of Professional Practice' (UKCC 1992a). Higher-level practice and the role development initiatives such as consultant nurse continue to attract much professional debate (NHSE 1998, UKCC 1998) and policy development (DoH 1999).

There is an increasing trend towards nurses taking career breaks, time out and part-time employment. Many change jobs frequently and opt for jobs allied to nursing and health care. In addition, within the job market generally, there are expectations that individuals will offer greater productivity, take on diverse roles and responsibilities and be flexible in their attitudes and approaches to work (Handy 1985). Nurses opting for surgical specialties have the potential to choose career paths from a range of options. The job market is competitive and professional demands are complex, but opportunities are great and wide-ranging. This chapter will explore and explain them. Nurses should not underestimate that to take full advantage of these opportunities means being extremely proactive and organised about all aspects of career planning so as to manage effectively all career-related decisions. These include job applications, continuing education opportunities and the development of a personal professional profile (UKCC 1994, 1995).

Out of the 640 000 registered nurses in the UK, over 300 000 work in the National Health Service (NHS) (RCN 1996). Table 6.1 illustrates the whole-time equivalents, by grade, and it can be seen from these figures, that there appear to be proportionally fewer posts available at F and G grade compared with those at D and E. By implication, the traditional approach to careers being a process of progression into more senior roles is affected for those wishing to remain in the NHS. Despite these details, the recruitment and retention of qualified staff in the public and private sectors are a cause of much concern as there is currently a national nursing staff shortage and opportunities for part-time work have increased. By 1996 the proportion of part-time NHS nurses had risen to 35%.

Many employers of nurses are giving greater consideration to the recruitment of qualified nurses, particularly female nurses, who need to have their needs for employment flexibility recognised to cope with their domestic demands (Smith & Seccombe 1998). Employment patterns of nurses have changed overall in recent years. While females still make up around 90% of the NHS workforce, the numbers employed by doctors in general practice, and working in private hospitals and in nursing homes, have increased. This suggests a general exodus from the acute sector where the majority of surgical nursing care is practised.

From this introduction, it is necessary to explore and analyse the range of career issues as they relate to and impact on nurses working in surgical settings. It is recognised that many activities relating to career planning have commenced during the pre-registration period and been developed further following registration. This is particularly pertinent in relation to portfolio developments, understanding the career options available in the short and long term, being prepared for the competitive aspects of the job market and, probably most importantly, developing skills to self-assess career needs.

TRENDS IN WORKING PATTERNS AND CAREER MANAGEMENT

There are general trends within our society relating to careers and work patterns which are influencing the individual and employers. For the individual, career insecurity has resulted from the impact of a prolonged recessionary period, patterns of redundancy and high unemployment. Self-employment and part-time employment are increasing overall. Part-time employment may facilitate flexible working patterns, but may not result in progression and promotion. Older employees often need updating and retraining as new technologies are introduced, particularly in relation to computing, information technology and communication systems, e.g. e-mail, the Internet. Academic and vocational qualifications are desirable as manual work opportunities decline.

For employers, the growth in the service sector has resulted in the increasing employment of part-time workers, particularly women, which impacts on family life, child care needs and care provision. The steady increase in educational opportunities for young people, particularly in further and higher education, increases the potential competition for employment in some sectors. There is also evidence that the employment of those from ethnic minority groups is increasing.

In recent years we have witnessed significant fluctuations in employment patterns among nurses. In 1993, a third of NHS nurses worked part time (as in

Table 6.1 Nursing posts in the NHS: whole-time equivalents by grade (RCN 1996)

Scale	Whole-time equivalent
D	84 757
E	93 414
F	31 762
G	58 636
H	10 959
I	3 906

1996). However, they tended to be in lower-grade posts, as were those returning after a career break. Seccombe et al (1993) found that 14% of management posts in hospitals were held by men, though only 7% of NHS nurses at that time were men. It was also found that there were significant concerns about job security and redundancy (52% in the NHS). Career breaks are common in the NHS (47%), the main reason being maternity leave. Seccombe et al (1993) suggest that women with family commitments are disadvantaged when it comes to career progression. They found that 75% of women working part time had family commitments (compared with 38% who were full time) and the part-timers were less likely to occupy senior posts. So, while opportunities for part-time work appear to be improving, these opportunities do not necessarily correspond to the range of work and responsibility available. In addition, workload stress is well reported and is greatest among NHS nurses working excess hours – 60% report working an average of 5.8 hours overtime per week (Smith & Seccombe 1998). By 1998, one in three NHS nurses had a second job and there continues to be increasing dissatisfaction with pay. Thus the challenges for a nursing career are great.

Reflective point

Consider the points raised about the trends in work patterns. How do these relate to nurses and their employment, particularly in relation to surgical nursing?

WHAT IS A NURSING CAREER?

The notion of a career being a lifelong commitment characterised by open-ended contracts, job stability, promotion prospects and eventual progression into positions of seniority has changed dramatically in recent years. This is also true in nursing where changes resulting from the development of the clinical grading structure, the introduction of the post-registration education and practice (PREP) project (UKCC 1991) and managerial restructuring are just three examples of developments influencing career opportunities. Nurses are shaping the job market. Attrition rates among registered nurses fluctuate and many nurses choose to change jobs after being in them for less than 12 months (Seccombe & Ball 1992). Nurses are increasingly choosing to work for organisations outside the NHS, for example the private sector, and to develop other roles, for example therapists in homeopathic medicine, social work and researchers in the university sector.

Reflective point

What does a career in nursing mean to you? Aim to express what the main characteristics of such a career are and the positive feelings you hope to experience.

There are two related ways of considering what a career is. There is the personal perspective which is characterised by the need to achieve, succeed and advance in ways relating to professional and work-based roles. With these ambitions come the sense of purpose and personal satisfaction through the contribution which is made through undertaking work activities. A sense of commitment is usually part of this experience and may be regarded as part of an overall sense of purpose and responsibility for the standards of intervention, conduct, service and reputation of the profession for which nurses are accountable (UKCC 1992b).

Secondly, there are the societal and professional perspectives which describe the typical features of a career and usually relate to a sequence of jobs and the requirements necessary to progress, for example periods of experience and educational and professional qualifications.

No matter how long or short a career in nursing is, the quality of the experience will depend on a range of factors. Those pursuing a career in surgical nursing have a great deal of control over the choice of experience.

The pursuit of opportunity is essential at a time when the job market is competitive, where there are fluctuations in job mobility among registered nursing posts and where more senior positions (particularly those beyond F grade) depend on highly developed skills, educational attainment and a range of personal and professional qualities.

Who employs nurses?

For qualified nurses wishing to undertake clinical positions, the main employers are NHS trusts and private hospitals. Most senior surgical nurses have had initial posts based in a hospital unit where systems of preceptorship are generally established and where it is expected that the new member of staff will need supervision, to learn specific practice-based skills and be an active member of the nursing and multidisciplinary team.

The choices associated with these first posts may appear overwhelming, particularly in relation to the range of specialist areas found in surgical units or directorates. Subsequently, those wishing to specialise in surgical nursing may find a far more competitive market.

Knowing what job opportunities exist early in your career is important in shaping your career pathway. Many careers are incremental in as much as experience, the personal and professional profile and educational and managerial skills are built on and developed and may lead you into the position to which you have aspired for some time.

There are many agencies and organisations which may employ nurses with a background in surgical nursing (Box 6.1). Of course, every organisation has its own requirements for employment, and prerequisite experience, qualifications and time in a particular role, for example, may all be identified and clarified in advance. Many require considerable experience and it is vital to know, for example, the details of necessary qualifications and the balance between clinical experience and managerial experience (which may be central to the shortlisting criteria for senior posts).

Choosing to work for a nursing agency or a trust 'bank' in order to gain some experience and income may be useful in the short term but does not usually contribute to the quality of a career. The main reasons for this are:

- there is usually a lack of continuity of experience
- records of experience are difficult to maintain
- the quality of supervision and preceptorship is often lacking and difficult to manage
- education and training opportunities are limited
- the limited control over where the work is undertaken.

Box 6.1 Major employers of nurses and those with a surgical background

- Charitable bodies, e.g. Macmillan nurses
- HM armed forces
- Local authorities
- NHS commissioning authorities
- NHS trusts
- Nursing agencies
- Occupational health services
- Overseas development organisations, e.g. OXFAM
- Primary care authorities
- Private hospitals
- Publishing houses
- Statutory bodies (UKCC and national boards)
- Trade unions and professional organisations
- Universities and colleges of higher education

Roles available to nurses with a surgical background

There is a wide range of posts available to nurses with a surgical background at E grade or above as illustrated in Box 6.2. It is usual for all these posts to demand specific experience within a named clinical field as part of the specifications for the post. In addition, in England it is not uncommon for some E-grade posts, and for the majority of F-grade posts, for a specific English National Board (ENB) course in that speciality to be required also, particularly courses at level 3. Courses of particular interest and relevance to surgical nurses are illustrated in Box 6.3. In the main, the certificated ENB courses, which, historically, were between 6 and 12 months in length, have been integrated into diploma and/or degree courses in nursing in universities and may also be part of the ENB Higher Award. There are similar schemes for post-registration clinical courses in Northern Ireland, Scotland and Wales. Currently, these are regulated by the respective National Board. Most of these schemes are modular in design which means that nurses fulfilling the necessary entry requirements, may complete a menu of *learning modules* which, on successful completion, result in an academic award.

Career pathways – opportunities for surgical nurses

When referring to developing a career in surgical nursing, it would not be unreasonable to consider the notion of promotion through the clinical grades, applying for progressively more senior clinical posts, and considering options such as those relating to management, teaching and research. However, this rather traditional view has changed for many reasons associated with working patterns, particularly of women. It is the nature of career opportunity that has changed and the demand that nurses consider with great care how they are going to manage their working lives. A working life for many bears very different characteristics. These characteristics will include such features as:

- the need for job security
- the need for a stable income
- accessibility and convenience of travel
- job satisfaction
- working hours which fit with family commitments
- contact with patients/clients/peers and other professionals
- opportunities to develop personally, professionally and clinically

---

Box 6.2 Roles for experienced staff nurses relating to patients requiring surgical interventions

E- to F-grade staff nurse posts
- General surgery: primary nurse/senior staff nurse
- Day case unit: primary nurse/senior staff nurse
- High-dependency unit: primary nurse/senior staff nurse
- Intensive therapy unit: primary nurse/senior staff nurse
- Accident and emergency department: primary nurse/senior staff nurse
- Operating theatre and anaesthetic room nurses, e.g. theatre practitioners
- Minor injuries unit: primary nurse/senior staff nurse/practice nurse
- Community staff nurse
- General practice nursing

F- to H-grade posts
- Team leader, e.g. theatres, recovery
- Ward sister/charge nurse/ward manager
- Clinical nurse specialist, e.g. infection control, pain management
- Practice development nurse
- Nurse practitioner
- Lecturer–practitioner posts
- Clinical nurse advisor

Other nursing posts where experience, for example in surgical nursing, is relevant but statutory and educational requirements are also prerequisites for practice
- Public health nursing – health visitor (usually G grade)
- Community nursing in the home – district nurse (usually F or G grades)
- Occupational health nurse
- School nurse
- Lecturer, senior lecturer, principal lecturer in higher education

---

Box 6.3 Examples of English National Board courses of particular interest to surgical nurses

- Accident and emergency nursing – ENB 199, No 3
- Altered body image – A58
- Breast care – ENB A11, No 9
- Burns and plastic surgery nursing – ENB 264, A15
- Cardiothoracic nursing – ENB 160, 249, A13
- Complementary therapy – A49
- General intensive care – ENB 100
- Gynaecological nursing – ENB 225
- Haematology and bone marrow transplant – N14
- Infection control nursing – ENB 329, 910, N26
- Infection control and wound management – N54
- Maxillofacial – A15
- Neuromedical and neurosurgical nursing – ENB 148, N42
- Oncology nursing – ENB A27, 237, 285
- Operating department nursing – ENB 176 and 182
- Ophthalmology nursing – ENB 346, N76
- Orthopaedic nursing – ENB 219
- Pain management – N53
- Perioperative care – A21, N33
- Renal and urological nursing – ENB 136
- Renal transplant – N39
- Research – ENB 850
- Stoma care – ENB 216, 980
- Surgical nursing – A25
- Teaching and assessing – ENB 998
- Trauma care – N52
- Wound management, tissue viability – N49

Key:
Courses numbered 100–870 and with a prefix A, 40 days or more, recordable qualification
Courses numbered 901–998 with prefix N, less than 40 days, ENB Award

---

- the need for a supportive working environment
- the need to develop responsibility
- the need to undertake associated roles.

For many, these features may not result in the need to be promoted, work through until retirement and remain in full-time employment. For others, the nature of personal ambition may result in determined actions to fulfil career aspirations and needs held for many years. These examples illustrate that there is a range of career behaviours and a need to focus on the assessment of career opportunity to maximise the need to match the talents of employees with the needs of employers.

A career pathway is a very personal experience. There is no doubt that it can be shaped by a range of factors. Taking clinical grades and posts for surgical nurses (Box 6.4), you can see that there is an incremental and progressive element to these posts as responsibilities increase, specialisation develops and the range of managerial skills broadens. Within these grades there is a range of roles, e.g. staff nurse and primary nurse (e.g. Grades E and F), clinical nurse specialists, team leaders and nurse managers (e.g. Grades G and H).

In practice, the interpretation and operationalisation of the clinical grading scheme has resulted in the most senior grades adopting a full range of managerial responsibilities within a named clinical specialty, usually a directorate. The opportunities for direct clinical intervention are, therefore, limited both by the relatively few post holders, compared with the number at E grade and the need, in many situations, to provide a nursing leader in relation to clinical matters. Common role specifications for the most senior posts often

Box 6.4 Role specifications through the clinical grades

The role specifications for E-grade posts will usually include:

- previous experience in the specialty (usually 1 year)
- previous experience of teaching and supervising pre-registration nursing students
- qualification with an ENB clinical course relevant to the speciality
- qualification with the ENB 998, Teaching and Assessing course is desirable or essential
- evidence of effective communication and interpersonal skills
- evidence of a commitment to team work, personal and professional development and the development of leadership skills.

The role specifications for F-grade posts will usually include:

- all the E-grade specifications (as listed above)
- evidence of the potential to lead a team
- a period of experience in the specialty (e.g. 2 years)
- evidence of clinical and managerial skills.

The role specifications for G-grade posts will usually include:

- all the E- and F-grade specifications
- a period of experience in the specialty (e.g. 3–5 years)
- evidence of advanced study, e.g. diploma or degree level in a subject relevant to the post
- evidence of research ability and/or experience
- evidence of proven clinical, managerial and leadership skills
- the potential for innovative practice.

The role specifications for H-grade posts will usually include:

- the G-grade specifications
- evidence of the ability to provide leadership, advice and development support across a clinical directorate
- the ability to work as a member of a management team
- evidence of managerial, professional, research and clinical experience relevant to the post
- the ability to initiate and respond to innovations, policies and quality initiatives.

Reflective point

Consider the characteristics of the grades described in Box 6.4. What do they have in common? What are the implications of this for career opportunities?

to the development of higher-level practice and the consultant nurse role (UKCC 1998, Manley 1997).

Historically, nurses have been frustrated by their inability to remain in clinical practice while at the same time maintaining and developing their career. For many, it has been a significant disappointment to reach a level of seniority only to find that further progress necessitates movement away from direct patient care. For surgical nurses, this still appears to be a problem despite the development of clinical specialist posts, particularly in infection control, stoma care and diabetic liaison, for example, which have gone a small way towards facilitating expert practice alongside case management and thus managerial responsibility in surgical settings.

In addition, these care pathways indicate levels of expertise required in relation to teaching, education research and the clinical field itself. A paradox exists here for nurses wishing to pursue a clinical career pathway as it is often the 'expertise' associated with developing managerial, research and educational skills that is rewarded with promotion rather than the development of expertise in clinical practice. Opportunities for expert practice development and the development of practice exist but they tend to be associated with specialist areas of practice and nursing development units, and they are difficult to define, despite the UKCC (1994) definition which states: 'Advanced nursing practice is concerned with adjusting to the boundaries for the development of future practice, pioneering and developing new roles responsive to changing needs and with advancing clinical practice, research and education to enrich professional practice as a whole' (UKCC 1994, p. 20).

The maintenance, control and development of clinical practice comprise one of the most important challenges facing nurses at the present time.

In addition, Manley (1997) sees advanced practice as the means of advancing expert nursing practice. She states: 'This view encompasses expert nursing practice (as a generalist or specialist), but it is more than that, as it also integrates the sub-roles of educator, researcher and consultant.'

It appears that nurses need to be considering their career opportunities both in terms of career pathways

require the applicant to possess skills relating to teaching and research as well as management within that field of practice. It is here that we are beginning to see the high regard being afforded to educational and research activities alongside the more traditional and more obvious profile of experience and managerial responsibility. This is particularly the case in relation and, more specifically, in terms of clinical career pathways. Some nursing roles are beginning to fulfil aspects of the criteria which Manley (1997) suggests are central to the process of advanced practice. These include the lecturer–practitioner and the nurse–practitioner roles. Difficulties arise because role definitions are subject to wide interpretation and there is a tendency for some posts, especially the lecturer–practitioner posts, to function within short-term contracts. Also, these roles tend to place particular emphasis on particular sub-roles, e.g. practice *or* research *or* education.

If, as Manley (1997) recommends, advanced practice embraces the roles of expert practitioner, researcher, educator and consultant and the UKCC supports these dimensions for the development of clinical practice, then the implications for the professional development of nurses will be far-reaching. Career opportunities and challenges for nurses will need frameworks for the educational development and accreditation of nurses. A central tenet will be the judgement of clinical standards of practice, which currently are rarely reviewed and assessed beyond those at F grade who undertake the Higher Award or an ENB clinical course.

Senior nurse opportunities for surgical nurses

Though the number of senior posts may be few, the opportunities exist for surgical nurses to practise in a range of settings and to maintain and extend their clinical skills accordingly.

It is important when considering a senior role that detailed consideration is given to the context of the post, how it relates to the organisation, the short-, medium- and long-term objectives for the trust, directorate and unit, as well as the influence of the 'newness' of the post. If this is an established post, what are the priorities and objectives, what are the expectations of the post, what are the projects requiring attention? For a new post – what are the priorities, expectations and strategic context of the post? Much background information can be gleaned informally in relation to these posts, and key examples are here by way of illustration and example.

Senior clinical nurses

The clinical nurse specialist is an advanced practitioner with leadership potential who will usually have a caseload as well as being expected to offer advice, teaching and supervision relating to the specialism. The grading, range of responsibilities and networking

activities may vary between one post and another. It is not unusual for post holders to be called upon to give advice to directors of nursing within trusts, to be involved with associated professional activities and write for publication. This is a demanding role with nurses progressing into such specialities as stoma care, diabetic liaison and infection control. The management of a caseload alongside more trust-wide activities, e.g. policy and practice development, are common features of this post. A clear role definition and appropriate support networks serve to provide post holders with a clearer perspective for the short- and longer-term management of this role.

The lecturer–practitioner role is one that has grown in recent years and is usually characterised by formal teaching responsibilities and leadership qualities running alongside specific clinical input (Goodman 1998). The operationalisation of lecturer–practitioner posts has been widely interpreted and it is not unusual for posts to reveal emphasis on one or more of the following, i.e. clinical practice, research or teaching. Some lecturer–practitioners work between two organisations, e.g. an NHS trust and a university department of nursing. This arrangement facilitates access to resources necessary for the lecturing and practitioner elements of the role, supports the integration of theory with practice and provides the post holder with formal access to student nurses within the two organisations central to the successful execution of nurse education programmes.

Lecturer–practitioners are often responsible to more than one manager and close liaison, management and support for the post holder are essential. The interpretation of the job description and the management of workload are central to the smooth running of these posts.

The consultant nurse is a relatively new concept which is becoming more associated with those committed to clinical leadership, the development of nursing, the pioneering of nurse-led initiative, usually in practice (Sanderson 1993), as well as teaching and research (Castledine 1998).

Nurse education

With the almost complete integration of schools and colleges of nursing into higher education, those wishing to pursue a career in nurse education will normally need to explore opportunities in the university sector. Those embarking on a career as a nurse lecturer will be expected to have undertaken a significant amount of clinical and educational activity. Applicants are widely expected to be first-level nurses, graduates in nursing or a subject relevant to nursing, with a recent clinical background of 4 years or more. Evidence of teaching experience and teaching qualification are desirable, sometimes essential. Those who are professionally active, have undertaken aspects of research, have publications and have evidence of established professional networks, possess characteristics which often result in being shortlisted. For senior lecturer and principal lecturer posts, relevant qualification at Master's level, research evidence, leadership potential and academic experience are important criteria. Increasingly the need for clinical doctorates will also be required.

Nurse management

A nurse manager is one with significant clinical experience who is appointed to a position of management and leadership over a team of nurses. Nurse managers are concerned with and have responsibilities for a range of activities associated with staff recruitment and support, quality assurance and audit of the nursing services, project developments and the management of innovation and change. The need to team build, motivate staff, and provide support as well as clinical and managerial leadership, are key qualities of this role. Promotion to a nurse manager's post will usually depend on the assessment of a wide range of qualities, including personal and professional qualities to meet the responsibilities of the post as well as necessary clinical, managerial and academic experience to support the application. More nurse managers are graduates and for many posts this is a requirement. Previous clinical, managerial and administrative activities are scrutinised for their relevance and complexity and to assess how the candidate has developed from them.

So far we have considered a range of issues and information relevant to the choices of employers and roles for nurses with surgical experience. In order to understand the implications of career development in nursing and the factors which influence it, it is essential that nurses are in no doubt about their professional responsibilities for practice.

Reflective point

Identify and consider the statutory and professional guidelines and requirements which govern the roles of practising nurses.

STANDARDS FOR PROFESSIONAL PRACTICE AND EDUCATION

The UKCC has the responsibility to protect the interests of the public. The Nurses, Midwives and Health Visitors Acts of 1979 and 1992 make clear what the standards are. As a result, the UKCC set standards for education, training and professional conduct.

The standards required of nurses in terms of responsibility to patients/clients, the public and the profession and in relation to personal accountability for practice are clearly stated in 'The Code of Professional Conduct for the Nurse, Midwife and Health Visitor' (UKCC 1992b) and further explored and discussed in the UKCC 'Guidelines for Professional Practice' (UKCC 1996a). These guidelines provide valuable help in relation to issues which often cause nurses considerable concern and, in many instances, personal and professional conflict. The areas discussed relate directly to the Code of Professional Conduct (UKCC 1992b) and include reference to:

- accountability
- duty of care
- patient and client advocacy and autonomy
- communicating for good practice
- truthfulness
- consent
- making concerns known
- working together, collaborating with other carers
- conscientious objection
- confidentiality
- advertising and sponsorship
- complementary and alternative therapies
- research and audit.

In addition, these guideline replace three UKCC documents, i.e. 'Exercising Accountability' (UKCC 1989), 'Confidentiality' (UKCC 1987) and 'Advertising by Registered Nurses, Midwives and Health Visitors' (UKCC 1985).

The interdependence of standards of practice on education is well recognised in the UKCC (1997) post-registration and practice initiatives and are summarised as follows.

The maintenance of an effective registration

There are four key elements to maintaining registration:
- completing a notification of practice form at the point of re-registration every three years and/or when your area of professional practice changes to one where you will use a different registerable qualification
- a minimum of five days or equivalent of study activity every three years

- maintaining a personal professional profile containing details of your professional development
- a return to practice programme if you have not practised for a minimum of 750 hours or 100 working days in the five year period leading up to the renewal of your registration (from 1 April 2000).

(UKCC 1997, p. 6)

The responsibility for the maintenance and development of professional knowledge and competence is essentially with the individual practising nurse. While resources need to be made available to nurses to support their professional development, the initiative needs to be with the individual nurse to either pursue opportunities available and/or to encourage colleagues to do so. The 'five days' for professional development in 3 years, appears minimal and should be interpreted broadly to maximise the opportunity for and relevance of learning and development for the individual. These are minimal requirements and the imposed time limit has caused much controversy both in terms of how these days may be managed and, for many nurses, the need to capitalise on relevant opportunities. The UKCC (1994) identifies a range of activities to indicate categories of study. These include those associated with:

- reducing risk, e.g. new approaches in practice
- care enhancement, e.g. standard setting, client-centred initiatives
- patient, family, client and colleague support, e.g. leadership and counselling initiatives
- practice development, e.g. research activities, personal study, role developments
- education development, e.g. research activities, personal study.

Notification of practice

Since April 1995 all practitioners are required to submit a personalised notification to practise form to the UKCC detailing qualifications and area of practice.

You will also have to complete a notification of practice form:

- every three years when you apply to renew your registration
- if you change your area of practice to one where you will use a different registerable qualification
- if you return to practice after a break of five years or more.

(UKCC 1997, p. 8)

The personal professional profile

The core components of a profile are:

information on the requirements of the Council for maintaining professional knowledge and competence; summary of key personal and professional details, including

pre- and post-registration education, professional education and employment and career history; record of learning experience with a demonstrable relevance to meeting the Council's requirements for five days study; record of professional development and space for other records.

(UKCC 1994, p. 7)

It is not unusual for reference to be made to maintaining a professional profile and a professional portfolio. The terms are often used interchangeably. However, Brown (1992) makes a distinction. She defines a profile as:

a collection of evidence which is selected from the professional portfolio for a particular purpose and for the attention of a particular audience

and the personal portfolio as:

a private collection of evidence which demonstrates the continuing acquisition of skills, knowledge, attitudes, understanding and achievement. It is both retrospective and prospective, as well as reflecting the current stage of development of the individual.

So the profile is 'a record of career progress and professional development' (UKCC 1997).

The UKCC (1996b) summarises the benefits of using a profile as follows:

to help you assess your current standards of practice

- to develop your analytical skills – these are fundamental to your professional practice and the profiling process will help to sharpen your ability to reflect constructively on and analyse what you do
- to enable you to review and evaluate past experience and learning in order to plan your continuing education and career development
- to provide effective up-to-date information for use in application forms and interviews when you apply for jobs or courses
- to provide evidence of what you have learned from your own experience. This may allow you to obtain credit toward further qualifications from an institution of higher education through schemes such as APEL (accreditation of prior experiential learning) and CATS (credit accumulation and transfer system)'

(UKCC 1996(b), p. 7)

The personal professional profile of information should contain details of your:

- reflections on your professional and work-related experiences – particularly how they have contributed to your learning and competence as a practitioner
- record of experience, learning, professional activities and initiatives, e.g. teaching activities, involvement in managerial and research activities, journals subscribed to, publications and formal study days.

Many nurses have begun the process of portfolio development from the outset of their pre-registration programme. This is a great advantage in terms of understanding how portfolios are maintained, developing reflective skills and for nurses applying for their first posts. It is common for portfolios to be requested as part of the selection process for posts.

Profiles must be:

- clearly structured
- maintained regularly so that relevant details are not forgotten or omitted
- used to record all relevant professional, clinical, educational, managerial and research-related activities
- used as a means to record reflections about practice.

There is a good range of useful portfolios on the market which have proved popular among nurses. Some, for example the ENB Portfolio (ENB 1991b), are clearly structured with guidelines to aid completion and maintenance. Whether you choose such a package or develop your own, there are essential details which should be included – remember that it is a statutory requirement that the profile is completed as part of the process of re-registration every 3 years. The UKCC is going to require details and information relating to the period after 1 April 1995. Finally, under the Welsh Language Act 1992, nurses may complete their profiles in Welsh and the UKCC will pay for translation costs.

The profile may be structured as follows:

Personal details:
- Full name
- Previous surname
- Title
- Date of birth
- Personal index number (PIN)
- Address for correspondence.

Academic qualifications:
- Secondary school: subject, grade, date
- Further/higher education: qualifications, subject, grade, date.

Professional registerable qualifications:
- e.g. RGN, RM, RMN, RNMH, RSCN, EN (G) and, if relevant, the part of the register.
- Qualification, date, college of nursing/university department or faculty.

Professional recordable qualifications:
- e.g. National Board Certificate courses, Occupational Health Nursing
- Qualification, date, college of nursing/university department or faculty.

Professional qualifications:
- e.g. Diploma in Nursing
- Qualification, date, college of nursing/university department or faculty.

Professional employment. Document this chronologically, beginning with your current post.

Other relevant responsibilities and activities. Here is the opportunity to list other activities which you are involved in and may include:

- other previous employment, e.g. prior to commencing nursing course
- membership of professional organisations and interest groups
- voluntary work
- research activities
- publications
- management activities, e.g. membership of working parties.

Record of education and formal learning activities. Aim to give details of:

- courses, study days, conferences, seminars and workshops attended
- personal learning activities undertaken, e.g. teaching activities, use and application of literature/research relevant to your work, developing a learning resource for use by student nurses
- visits to other centres for the purpose of enhancing your work.

The UKCC (1996b) advises that for each of these you need to give details of:

'its relevance to your professional practice
what you hope to achieve from it
your assessment of the outcomes of your activities
the time spent on each event and on any follow-up work'
(UKCC 1996b).

Record of working hours. Hours worked during the 3-year period should be recorded.

Self-assessment and evaluation of performance. This is your opportunity to comment on:

- Your experiences to date, what and how you have learned from them.
- The contribution these experiences have made to your role and development as a registered nurse.
- Specific events which have occurred and are documented in detail on the basis that they were unusual to you and you learnt from that because they were particularly significant. Such events are called critical incidents and may be positive or negative in outcome, e.g. managing a violent patient, managing a patient with acute pain, the first experience of comforting the family of a patient who has died.
- Your perceptions of your skills and competencies and those you feel need further development.

Action planning. This is your opportunity to look ahead and document your plans and objectives for the future. This is often difficult to do as none of us can predict the future. So, aim to have a few statements of intent which may, for example, relate to ideas concerning the development of a specialist skill or undertaking a course of study. It can be helpful to relate details of your own appraisal here thus relating personal and profession development plans to this section of your portfolio.

Remember:

• safeguard confidentiality by not naming individuals in your profile
• the portfolio is yours and may be structured and organised in a number of ways
• seek advice from professional colleagues if you need support and help with its completion.

Despite these strategic plans to clarify nurses' responsibilities for education and practice, nurses still face challenges and conflicts relating to roles and career opportunities.

Nursing roles, specialist practice and the Scope of Professional Practice

Clarifying the role of the professional nurse has been the focus of much debate and analysis over the years. What appears to be part of the difficulty is nurses being able to agree and accept a definition of the nurse's role and the demand to adapt to the range of patient/client needs by maintaining authority but delegating responsibility for certain caring activities to other health care workers. There also appears to be increasing conflict for nurses who, through undertaking pre-registration nursing courses, complete a general education and training programme, only to find that they are called upon to provide specialist nursing activities which they may not have covered. Despite systems of preceptorship and supervision for the newly registered nurse, and the recognition that consolidation and 'new' learning must take place after registration, it remains that registered nurses face a continuing challenge to their roles which is manifested by the need to be able to provide skilled specialist care, fulfil their commitment to the provision of quality patient-focused nursing and the delivery of care alongside a range of health care workers.

The rapid developments in technology, medical practice, pharmacology and genetics, for example, have for decades been a continuing challenge for nurses and their leaders to adapt and extend their roles. Today, as well as the debate about advanced practice, the demand for nurses to become doctors'

assistants has returned the issue once more into the limelight. Previously, the debate focused on the strategy for nurses to extend their roles by undertaking activities that were traditionally the work of doctors (DHSS 1977).

'The Scope of Professional Practice' (UKCC 1992a) has been a useful attempt to facilitate the transition from a system of assessment and certification of post-registration skill development being influenced by medical need, to a system of nurse-led educational initiatives based on the analysis of patient need. The recognition by the UKCC (1994, 1996b) that further specific education is needed for specialist practice is clearly stated. Programmes for the preparation of specialist practitioner posts are available throughout the UK and information is available from the National Boards. It remains that roles within hospital settings are more difficult to define and prepare for. They are reliant on the clinical grading structure, the Higher Award, and specialist courses which are usually conjointly validated by the National Board and an institution of higher education.

Attempts to strengthen the role of registered nurses and to clarify how accountability for care may be operationalised have been seen in the introduction of, and optimism over, such major initiatives as primary nursing, lecturer–practitioner roles, clinical nurse specialists and nurse practitioners.

Castledine (1996) in an attempt to clarify and explain the dynamics of nursing roles, offers the following four categories of practice and definitions for each.

• Generalist nursing practitioner: a nurse who is able to demonstrate a level of knowledge and skill across a wide variety of fields. Nursing practice is based on the knowledge and skill acquired during first-level registration and continuing education. Such generalists are the 'core' of the profession and are staff nurses, some ward and community nurses and sisters.
• Specialist nursing practitioner: a nurse who is able to demonstrate a level of knowledge and skill in one particular field of activity and who has acquired additional specialist education for the role, e.g. some nurse practitioners, clinical nurse specialists and ward and community sisters.
• Advanced nursing practitioner: a specialist or generalist nurse who is able to demonstrate a higher level of nursing knowledge, skill, autonomy, responsibility, consultancy and leadership through research, evaluation and clinical nursing innovation. He/she may have postgraduate qualifications and several years' experience in his/her chosen field of nursing.
• Paramedical nurse: a nurse who is able to demonstrate the necessary knowledge and skill to supplement and support a physician or surgeon in his/her medical work. He/she will have acquired knowledge and skill in the medical field and be accountable to a doctor, e.g. physicians' assistants, nurse clinicians and some nurse practitioners and nurse technicians.

Part of the difficulty some nurses have of accepting nurses who have developed their role is that they are not used to 'rational authority' based on knowledge and skill development. It is time that we did, otherwise the confusion both within and without the profession will get worse.

(Castledine 1996, p. 1338)

These definitions perhaps go some way towards clarifying the current range of roles, though the labels used to describe them are not in common usage.

Nursing and health care literature contains many examples of effective practice, positive patient feedback and clinical developments and research emanating from these roles. However, preparation and education for these roles remain uncoordinated and difficult to assess, particularly in terms of standards of clinical competence. Currently, nursing leaders recognise the need to coordinate developments of roles in clinical practice in order to consider role clarification, educational preparation and competence to practise, particularly beyond first degree level, and the implications for employment and for other professions. The UKCC, and chief nursing officers have considered the implication of current health care needs for the nurse's role. Changes are afoot in relation to role developments and specialist practice (DoH 1996, UKCC 1998). This will inevitably impact on career development for individual nurses. This makes it essential for you to feel confident about your career decisions, knowing from where and how to seek career guidance and information and how to manage employment-related activities.

Career opportunities and the need for education

It is accepted that ongoing education is essential to both the development of the individual nurse and the development of nursing as a whole. All nurses are required to provide evidence of ongoing education for PREP, both formally, through the completion of periods of study, and informally through personal and professional updating, use of journals, professional networking and involvement in clinical and professional initiatives, e.g. local interest groups and ward-based innovations.

The professional requirements for registration are clear. However, there is a range of educational opportunities available, though local provision varies and there are cost implications in terms of time, fees, study leave and the impact on family and social commitments. Increasingly, practitioners are expected to fund their own developments though it is possible to negotiate study leave with managers.

The English National Board Framework for Continuing Education

In an attempt to coordinate continuing professional education for first-level nurses, midwives and health visitors, the English National Board introduced their Framework for Continuing Education and the Higher Award in 1991 (ENB 1991a).

The Framework is:

- 'a flexible system for the organisation and delivery of continuing professional education'
- 'a structure leading to the Higher Award, a professional and academic qualification.' (ENB 1991a, p. 12).

The necessary skill, knowledge and expertise are embraced by the 10 key characteristics which those working in clinical practice should be able to demonstrate to provide quality care. Programmes of study supporting the Higher Award have been set at first degree level (minimum) and some are incorporated into Master's level programmes.

The 10 key characteristics are summarised as follows:

1. Professional accountability and responsibility
2. Clinical expertise with a specific client group
3. Use of research to plan, implement and evaluate strategies to improve care
4. Team working and building and multidisciplinary team leadership
5. Flexible and innovative strategies
6. Use of health-promotion strategies
7. Facilitating and assessing development in others
8. Handling information and making informed clinical decisions
9. Setting standards and evaluating quality of care
10. Initiating, managing and evaluating clinical change (ENB 1991b).

To achieve the Higher Award, practitioners must demonstrate their ability to integrate all these characteristics within their practice. A contract is developed from a tripartite arrangement between the practitioner, the manager and educationalist responsible for the Framework. Following a review, a practitioner may index for the Higher Award in an ENB-approved higher education institution. This institution, usually a university, will have a range of approved courses designed to support practitioners to achieve the Higher Award, e.g. ENB Awards, BA in Nursing, BSc in Nursing courses. The educational elements of the programme will usually include registering for a course or programme of study, e.g. a degree in nursing, an open learning course at degree level and in-service educational activities. The advantage of the Higher Award is that practitioners can negotiate their pathway through a learning contract with their manager and educators. Maintaining a professional profile is a part of the process and provides a record of achievement of previous learning as well as evidence of the achievement of each of the 10 characteristics.

Academic qualification for surgical nurses

There are many opportunities for nurses to study following registration; however, the choice appears overwhelming. In general, there is an expectation that nurses need to study to the equivalent of diploma level (which is now the minimum academic level of the pre-registration nursing course) in order to contend for clinical posts beyond D grade. However, many choose to develop academically and opt for a degree course, often to 'top up' their pre-registration to a degree. This is possible through credit accumulation and transfer schemes (CATS) which have the following characteristics:

CATS Level 1 – Certificate level	120 credits
CATS Level 2 – Diploma level	120 credits
CATS Level 3 – Degree level	120 credits

To be awarded a degree, it is necessary to have completed the equivalent level of study at each level. Therefore, an honours degree has 360 CATS points. If you, as a diplomate, apply for a degree course, your CATS points may mean you gain credit exemption from modules on the course, particularly where your course has similar or complementary subject matter to the one applied for. Assessment of prior learning (ALP) not only considers previous courses and formal learning outcomes but also assessment of prior experiential learning experiences. Universities have systems in place to assess each applicant formally, which usually involves the assessment of a portfolio followed by an interview with staff involved with the professional development and education of nursing staff.

More nurses are choosing to follow Master's programmes, either formally taught MA or MSc programmes or Master by research, MPhil. The first Master's in Nursing by distance learning is now established at the RCN Institute of Nursing (see Useful addresses, p. 128). Undertaking degree-level study is demanding at any level, because most nurses choose part-time study in order to maintain their employment. For surgical nurses it is important to assess carefully the potential contribution of

degree-level study – be that at first degree, Master or doctorate level – to career opportunities. It is vital to scrutinise the course content, applicability to practice, opportunities to study specialist practice as it relates to your roles, especially where opportunities for undertaking a dissertation are part of a course.

Undertaking academic study which directly relates to work roles does much to enhance the decision-making and professional development potential of the individual nurse. We have seen the range of ENB Award courses available which both incorporate ENB Awards as well as exploring nursing and health-related matters in ways which support the development of surgical nursing. It is necessary to explore options by obtaining course details, university prospectuses and seeking advice about the best routes to follow.

MAKING CAREER DECISIONS – THE CASE FOR CAREER GUIDANCE

Few nurses or employers of nurses have explicit responsibility for career guidance provision. The NHS careers service has an established information-giving service and a careers networking facility. This ensures that there are named local professional nurses, usually lecturers or nurse managers, who can be available to offer information about pre- and post-registration opportunities. The information they hold relates to nursing and midwifery courses. The other national boards also have careers services and provide information relating to post-registration courses and the Higher Awards (see Useful addresses, p. 128).

It is the experience of many nurses that career decisions are made on a rather ad hoc basis, often in response to job availability, not least because access to planned career guidance has been limited.

> **Reflective point**
>
> There are many factors which may influence career choices and job selection. Consider your own circumstances – identify the personal factors which would influence your choice of your next post. The needs are likely to reflect personal, family, social and professional issues – it may be helpful to use these to guide your thoughts.

Now examine Box 6.5. Here you will find a range of factors found to be important to nurses making career choices (Schober 1990). In addition it is vital that you

Box 6.5 Factors affecting career choices (Schober 1990)

Personal needs
- Job satisfaction
- Job security
- Status of the role
- Salary
- Reluctance to change roles
- Working hours
- Terms of the contract

Family/social needs
- Family need for income
- Child care availability
- Availability of accommodation
- Travelling distance from home
- House prices
- Support of partner/family members

Work needs
- Need to work
- Promotion
- Motivation and opportunities to learn and develop professionally
- Interest/commitment to the work and role
- Range of responsibility
- Dynamics of the team and management structure

Reflective point

What factors influence your job satisfaction at work? Consider the variables in Box 6.5 and try to elaborate on factors which are particularly important to you at work. Reflect on your current post. What gives you particular satisfaction at work? In addition, what influenced your choice of your current post?

Now consider Box 6.6 which contains a range of factors that influence job satisfaction: Which are of particular priority for you?

---

begin to give serious consideration to these factors which give you job satisfaction. It has been found that job satisfaction is central to the quality of the work experience (Schober 1988).

In considering what motivates nurses at work, a range of issues emerges. As with the variables which influence career choice (Box 6.5), Stechmiller & Yarandi (1992) suggest that personal and work-related variables have significant influence over job satisfaction. Among critical care nurses, they found that the meaningfulness of the work, the quality of supervision and opportunity for advancement were more significant than other factors such as pay, job security and expectations about the work. Other studies have considered the influence of work organisation methods on job satisfaction. Primary nursing has been found to positively influence the job satisfaction of nurses in an intensive care unit (ICU) (Manley et al 1996). The nurse–doctor relationship, when collaborative in nature, also has a positive influence.

Undertaking self-assessment exercises to help you clarify your own needs in relation to career aspirations and needs is to be recommended. There are a number of approaches which may be taken – some of the most useful relate to the self-assessment of work values and general skills (Pedler et al 1986). Undertaking these

exercises provides you with opportunities to gain some insight and understanding of personal needs as they relate to work activities. They are repeatable, user-friendly and provide a useful tool to discuss needs with mentors, supervisors, teachers and colleagues – assuming that they are used in a constructive way. They provide indicators of needs, skills and work-related priorities and should not be regarded as definitive. The work values inventory includes factors associated with recognition at work, achievement, interpersonal relationships, variety and the work environment. The general skills inventory (Pedler et al 1986) seeks to help you identify your strongest assets, the areas where improvements may be made and areas where learning and further experience may be an advantage. The areas covered include problem-solving, leadership, management of people, creativity and communication.

These exercises are useful and revealing but they should be used wisely and in a supportive way. For some, these activities provide confirmation and reassurance of skills already understood, though for others, they may reveal indicators of strengths and needs not previously realised. Supportive working environments would usually have systems in place whereby personal work needs, objectives and skills are reviewed and reflected upon. Appraisal systems and peer review activities are a useful means to explore all these areas. Managers and employees alike would do well to explore mechanisms for broadening and deepening understanding of work-related activities and relating them to career needs and opportunities.

It is suggested that the factors highlighted in Box 6.6 are ones which may help you to develop reflective aspects of your portfolio.

Sources of career-related information

As well as developing insight and understanding of personal and professional needs as they impact on

---

Box 6.6 Factors influencing job satisfaction in a clinical post

- Factors relating to care and the client/patient group
- The clinical specialty
- The pace of work, e.g. patient turnover, day care
- Organisational factors relating to care delivery, the dynamics of the health care team
- Opportunities to develop the nurse–patient relationship
- Support for learning, team support, staff support network
- Style of leadership by managers
- Morale of staff
- Team membership
- Opportunities for teaching, learning, professional development and promotion

---

your career, gaining access to up-to-date factual information about career options, job availability, courses and programmes of study is an essential prerequisite to informed career decision-making. The main sources of career-related information may be accessed from:

- the local university or college of higher education
- managers, ward sisters, team leaders, etc. in the trusts
- the national boards' career services.

The local university or college of higher education

Now that colleges of nursing, midwifery and health studies have merged with a university, you will find lecturers with special interest in career guidance; they may be ENB network members, which ensures that they receive the latest information relating to professional requirements, for example for teacher preparation, and listings for courses of study for practice in clinical settings.

In addition, universities and colleges update their prospectuses annually. It is useful to request full-time and part-time course prospectuses to identify the full range of courses available. Then, follow up this request with course-specific requests to the faculty or department to view a more detailed course outline. As well as nursing degrees and diplomas there are a range of full- and part-time courses under the title of, for example, Diploma or Degree in Health Studies, Community Studies, Health Service Management, which may contain a significant proportion of nursing input. For degree courses at Master or Bachelor level, opportunities on these courses to undertake a clinically oriented dissertation may exist and therefore give students a good opportunity to study aspects of their own specialist area.

Managers, ward sisters, team leaders, etc. in the trusts

Many senior members of staff in the trusts have a good working knowledge of career options available to nurses. You may find senior nurses with specific responsibility for professional development of staff and who have particularly good knowledge of the local opportunities.

If you need information about, for example, surgical posts in a particular trust, then it is not unreasonable to write to the nursing manager of the surgical directorate or unit for information about opportunities and options. Enclose a curriculum vitae if you are serious about wishing to work there. You could also approach the trust's personnel department for information about forthcoming posts.

The national boards' careers services

All the national boards have information relating to careers in their respective country (see Useful addresses, p. 128). This tends to take the form of factsheets and details relating to professional requirements and available courses and their location.

MANAGING YOUR CAREER OPPORTUNITIES AND WORK-RELATED APPLICATIONS

Making the decision to apply for a new post is a significant step in anyone's life. It is tempting to assume that the grass is greener elsewhere but this is not always the case. It is sometimes difficult to assess and evaluate whether one is in the 'best' place which will result in growth, development and opportunity.

The RCN (1995) suggests that the following features are those that will enhance and support the individual at work:

- Nursing and nurses are valued
- An investment is made in education and training
- Individuals are provided with tailor-made development programmes
- Innovation and the development of practice is encouraged
- The success of individuals and teams is celebrated
- Team working and supportive relationships are in evidence throughout
- Mistakes are used as an opportunity for learning
- Those with ability are regarded as an asset and not a threat
(RCN 1995, p. 5)

If you find that your working environment is unable to satisfy these criteria it may be time for you to move on.

Making decisions and plans relating to short- and long-term needs and opportunities is dependent, as we have seen, on a range of complex and interrelated factors which have personal, professional and social implications. Despite these factors, when faced with the necessity to apply for a post, it is essential that everything is covered to ensure that you know as much as possible about the post and the process of application. So, before you apply you need a range of information about the post.

Information needed prior to application

Pre-application information about a post may be gleaned from:

- the advertisement
- the role specification
- staff already in post
- previous personal experience of working there, e.g. as a student
- an informal visit.

  Aim to seek information about:

- the purpose and grade of post
- the requirements of the post, e.g. responsibilities, qualifications, previous experience
- details of the contract and opportunities for renewal and upgrading, e.g. from grade E to F
- the system of staff support
- teaching and learning opportunities
- the appraisal system
- the style of management on the ward/unit
- how care is managed
- the closing date for applications.

The application form

Ensure that this is completed to the highest standard and that all information requested is given. If your profile is requested, ensure that this is also up to date. Often information requested on the application form is duplicated on your curriculum vitae (CV) (see Box 6.7 for a suggested layout). Remember application forms are copied and distributed to all members of an interview panel so it is helpful to have the form completed in full, and typed in black ink, with a handwritten covering letter unless you are requested to do otherwise.

Your referees

Select your referees wisely – remember they are your backers. For initial posts following registration a reference will be requested from your university, usually through the course leader. Referees are asked for a range of details relating to your character, personality,

---

Box 6.7 A suggested layout for a curriculum vitae

Name
Address   Date of birth   Age
General education
Professional qualifications
Professional education
Present appointment
Previous appointments
Research
Publications
Professional interests/membership of professional organisations
Referees

(If one or more headings are not applicable, simply omit them.)

---

previous experience, professionalism, suitability for the post, and sickness and absence records, which are read after an interview. It is important that your referees know you well. Keep in touch with them – use them as mentors and guides as your career develops and inform them of your plans and the posts you are applying for. This is an important relationship to nurture. The more your referees know of your plans, the more appropriate and supportive the references are likely to be. Then when you are offered a post – let them know!

Curriculum vitae (CV)

A CV is a clear summary of personal and professional profile details which should be adapted to support and complement your application form. Use the job specification to help you adapt your CV as you may be able to give details of, for example, previous experience which is particularly relevant to the post being applied for. You may find that a CV is requested at the time of application and your portfolio is required at interview. There will be some repetition between these two records.

Informal visit

If you are applying for a post in a new area or one unfamiliar to you, aim to book an informal visit through the ward/unit manager or personnel department. Some posts detail that opportunities for tours etc. are available on the day of interview. However, you need to judge whether this is going to be enough for you to be confident about what you are applying for. It is in your interest to undertake a visit to meet staff, view the workplace and to ask questions to clarify your knowledge of the post. An informal visit is vital for you to develop insight, knowledge and understanding of the local culture, staff relationships, values about nursing and the management ethos.

The interview process

There are many styles of interviewing used in the health services. They will depend on the seniority of the post and the role specifications. The more senior the post the greater the range of techniques employed.

The panel interview

This is the most common approach used for clinical nursing posts. Panel members are usually two to four in number. The ward sister and senior nurse manager for the unit may be accompanied by a member of the personnel department and an external member from another trust. If the post involves other organisations, e.g. the local university department of nursing, senior lecturing staff may be represented. Panel members will usually decide on the area of questioning and ask a range of open questions each in turn which usually relate to the following topics.

Background issues:
- Reasons for applying
- Previous experiences – clinical and educational
- Aspects of previous job satisfaction
- Features described in the application form, CV or portfolio
- Aspects of previous academic and/or professional education
- The person specifications.

Clinical and practice-related issues:
- Why you have applied for this post
- What skills you are bringing to the post
- What you hope to learn
- What you need to learn
- Knowledge of current research relevant to the post
- What would you do if ... – clinical issues/incidents to check and assess your potential actions
- Sources of job satisfaction
- Opinions about current clinical issues, e.g. advanced practice, care pathways, expanded role developments for nurses.

Professional issues:
- Nursing values, commitment and insight into nursing-related issues
- How you keep up to date, professional awareness.

Particularly for E grade and above:
- Working as a team
- Leadership potential
- Your teaching needs and experience
- Your management needs and experience
- Research interests
- Plans for future development/study.

Open questioning. These are opportunities for you to ask questions – have some prepared, e.g. in relation to preceptorship, orientation to the post, the contract and clinical developments in the unit.

Interviewers adopt a range of skills to build up pictures of candidates to judge their suitability for a post. Applicants' papers are scrutinised in advance – some, if not all, interviewers will have been involved in short listing. Questions are prepared to ensure that the role specification is covered, to test candidates' understanding and suitability for the post and how their personal and professional skills will contribute to the area of practice. Interviewers will aim to establish a rapport and inform candidates of how the interview will be conducted. They ask probing questions to deliberate and explore important issues in depth and will often take notes during the process.

In addition to informal and formal interview activities, some selection processes will include other demands, particularly those which will reveal a candidate's skills and insights relating to the post.

The presentation

Being requested to prepare a topic for presentation is a more common strategy for those applying for senior posts. Usually a topic is identified by the interview panel which is pertinent to the post. The same topic is given to all candidates who are advised about the criteria for the process, e.g. the length of the presentation, who will be in attendance, the location and time and whether questions will be asked by the 'audience'.

Presentations allow members of staff associated with the potential new staff members to meet, witness and provide informal feedback about candidates. They also provide opportunities for candidates to communicate their insight, professional awareness and understanding of topical issues. The use of and reference to research is an advantage, and candidates being able to analyse, relate and evaluate items will reveal how 'up to date' they are and how adaptable they are to the experience of those in attendance. It is usual for candidates to prepare visual aids, to be prepared to use an overhead projector and to provide a short but clear summary of the content of the presentation for distribution to each member of the audience.

Social activities

For senior positions, the selection process may extend over a number of days. If a range of selection activities is being utilised, then social activities may also become part of the process. Gathering staff and candidates over a lunch to encourage as many staff as possible to meet and discuss issues is commonplace. Though it may seem as though this style of activity is more revealing for staff, candidates can benefit from social discourse with staff and members of the interview panel, particularly when this type of activity is prior to the formal interview. Candidates should take full advantage of meeting a range of staff to communicate their values, commitment and potential suitability for the post.

After the interview and selection activities

Offering a post

Following any selection interview, decisions are usually reached which result in a candidate being matched to a post. Panel members reserve the right to decide a time limit for this activity. It is not unusual for candidates to be asked to wait for the decision, which is reached after all the candidates have been interviewed. Increasingly, particularly for senior posts (F grade and above), candidates are advised that they will be informed by a member of the panel later that day or the following day. There are occasions when decisions are delayed further, for example if references are not available, or if other interview dates have been organised for another group of applicants. Also, verification for a post sometimes needs to be made by the head of an organisation, so the panel do not have the power to recommend that a post is offered until all details have been scrutinised appropriately.

The panel have the responsibility to ensure that there is evidence that the candidate most suitable for the post meets the criteria set for the post. Obtaining optimum evidence depends on thorough preparation by the panel, the scrutiny of all relevant data from candidates, the preparation and asking of questions which probe, explore, search and direct the candidate to reveal information from which fair judgements may be made.

Feedback

Offering feedback to candidates whether they have been successful or not, is a perspective often requested by candidates. Giving formal or informal feedback to candidates is the responsibility of the interview panel but they are under no obligation to provide it. However, most candidates appreciate explanation of reasons why a post has been offered or not. When informing candidates of the outcome of the selection process, interviewers should be prepared to offer feedback either verbally or in written form. It is useful for a panel to decide how this is to be managed as it gives employers the opportunity to advise and perhaps encourage candidates not successful with the post to consider an alternative post in the future, hence maintaining contact with the potential employers.

CONCLUSION

Career opportunities for surgical nurses are many but so are the demands both for clinical development and the acquisition of the necessary educational and managerial skills. This chapter has revealed ways of assessing and focusing on necessary activities to make the process of career development as positive as possible. To underestimate career opportunities is to underestimate your potential as a surgical nurse, so make use of the information, resources, your peers, mentors and colleagues to make this aspect of your life an enjoyable yet fruitful one.

USEFUL ADDRESSES

Careers information for nurses, midwives and health visitors and information regarding continuing education

NHS Careers
PO Box 376
Bristol BS99 3EY
0845 6060655

The National Board for Nursing, Midwifery and Health Visiting, Northern Ireland
RAC House
79 Chichester Street
Belfast BT1 4JE
01232 238152

National Board of Nursing, Midwifery and Health Visiting for Scotland
Careers Information Service
22 Queen Street
Edinburgh EH2 1NT
0131 226 7371

The Welsh National Board for Nursing, Midwifery and Health Visiting
Floor 2
Golate House
101 St Mary's Street
Cardiff CF1 1DX
01222 261 400

Open and Distance Learning providers for Nurses, Midwives and Health Visitors

Distance Learning Centre
South Bank University
Southwark Campus
103 Borough Road
London SE1 0AA
0171 815 8297

Macmillan Open Learning (MOL)
EMAP Health Care Ltd
Portess South
4–6 Crinan Street
London N1 9X4
0171 843 4850

National Extension College
18 Brooklands Avenue
Cambridge CV2 2HN
01223 316644

Nursing Standard Open Learning
Nursing Standard House
17–19 Peterborough House
Harrow
Middlesex HA1 2AX
0181 423 1066

Nursing Times Open Learning
4 Little Essex Street
London WC2R 3LF
The Open University
Walton Hall
Milton Keynes MK7 6AA
01908 274066

Ms M Kirwan
Regional Development Officer
The Open University
10 Drumsheugh Gardens
Edinburgh EH3 7QJ
0131 226 3851

School of Health Care (ENB 998 & 934 courses only)
Liverpool John Moores University
Whiston Hospital Site
Prescot
Merseyside LE35 5DR
0151 231 2121

Open Learning Unit
Northumberland College of Arts and Technology
College Road
Ashington
Northumberland NE63 9RG
01670 841200

RCN Institute
Royal College of Nursing
20 Cavendish Square
London W1M 0AB
0171 409 3333

Statutory and advisory bodies

Department of Health
Quarry House
Quarry Hill
Leeds
Yorkshire LS2 7UD

Department of Health, Northern Ireland
Dundonald House
Upper Newtownards Road
Belfast BT4 3SB

The King's Fund
11–13 Cavendish Square
London W1M 0AB

Nurses Central Clearing House
PO Box 346
Bristol BS99 7FB

Royal College of Nursing of the United Kingdom
20 Cavendish Square
London W1M 0AB

Royal College of Nursing
17 Windsor Avenue
Belfast
Northern Ireland
Royal College of Nursing
Ty Maeth
King George V Drive East
Cardiff CF4 4XZ

Royal College of Nursing
Glenbourne House
42 South Oswald Road
Edinburgh EH9 2HH

Scottish Home and Health Department
St Andrew's House
Regent Road
Edinburgh EH1 3DE

The English National Board for Nursing, Midwifery and
Health Visiting
Victory House
170 Tottenham Court Road
London W1P 0HA

The National Board for Nursing, Midwifery and Health
Visiting in Scotland
22 Queen Street
Edinburgh EH2 1JX

The National Board for Nursing, Midwifery and Health
Visiting, Northern Ireland
RAC House
79 Chichester Street
Belfast BT1 4JR

The Welsh National Board for Nursing, Midwifery and
Health Visiting
13th Floor
Pearl Assurance House
Greyfriars Street
Cardiff CF1 3AG

United Kingdom Central Council for Nursing, Midwifery
and Health Visiting (UKCC)
23 Portland Place
London W1N 4JT

Other useful organisations for career support

Association of Paediatric Nurses
c/o Central Nursing Office
Hospital for Sick Children
Great Ormond Street
London WC1N 3HN

District Nurses Association
57 Lower Belgrave Street
London SW1 0LR

Health Visitors Association
50 Southwark Street
London SE1 1UN

Occupational Health Nurses Association
c/o Royal College of Nursing
20 Cavendish Square
London W1M 0AB

QARNNS, Matron in Chief
First Avenue House
High Holborn
London WC1 6HE

QARANC, Liaison Officer
Ministry of Defence, Army
Empress State Building
Lillie Road
London SW6 1TR

RAF, Director of Nursing Services
Ministry of Defence
First Avenue House
High Holborn
London WC1 6HE

Scottish Office Home and Health Department
Prison Service Recruitment (Nursing)
Calton House
5 Redheughs Rigg
Edinburgh EH12 9HW

H M Prison Service Headquarters
Cleland House
Page Street
London SW1P 4LN

REFERENCES

Brown R A 1992 Portfolio development and profiling for nurses. Quay Publishing, Lancaster

Castledine G 1996 Clarifying and defining nursing role developments. British Journal of Nursing 5(21): 1338

Castledine G 1998 The role of the clinical nurse consultant. British Journal of Nursing 7(17): 1054

Department of Health (DoH) 1996 The development of nursing and health visiting roles in clinical practice. (Letter 4.7.96.) DoH, London

Department of Health (DoH) 1999 Making a difference: strengthening the nursing, midwifery and health visiting contribution to health and healthcare. The Stationery Office, London

Department of Health and Social Security (DHSS) 1977 The extending role of the clinical nurse: legal implications and training requirements. HC (77) 22. HMSO, London

English National Board (ENB) 1991a A framework for continuing professional education and the Higher Award for nurses, midwives and health visitors. ENB, London

English National Board (ENB) 1991b The professional portfolio. ENB, London

Goodman J 1998 Evaluation and evolution: the contribution of the advanced practitioner to cancer care. In: Rolfe G, Fulbrook P (eds) Advanced nursing practice. Butterworth-Heinemann, Oxford

Handy C 1985 The future of work. Blackwell, Oxford

Manley K 1997 A conceptual framework for advanced practice: operationalising the advanced practitioner/consultant nurse role. Journal of Clinical Nursing 6:(3): 179–190

Manley K, Cruse S, Keogh S 1996 Job satisfaction of intensive care nurses practising primary nursing. Nursing in Critical Care 1: 31–41

NHS Executive 1998 Nurse consultants. (HSC 1998/161, 22 September) DoH, London

Nurses, Midwives and Health Visitors Act 1979 HMSO, London

Nurses, Midwives and Health Visitors Act 1992 HMSO, London

Pedler M, Burgoyne J, Boydell T 1986 A manager's guide to self development. McGraw Hill, Berkshire

Royal College of Nursing (RCN) 1995 A guide to planning your career (RCN nurses in leadership project). RCN, London

Royal College of Nursing (RCN) 1996 Nursing workforce. RCN Factsheet. RCN, London

Sanderson J 1993 Career development for nurses. Opportunities and options. Scutari Press, London

Schober J 1988 The career guidance experiences of registered nurses (Cardiff University). Unpublished thesis available in the Steinberg collection, The Library, Royal College of Nursing, London

Schober J E 1990 Your career – making the choices. In: Tschudin V, with Schober J Managing yourself.

Macmillan, London

Seccombe I, Ball J 1992 Motivation, morale and mobility. A profile of qualified nurses in the 1990s. Institute of Manpower Studies, Brighton

Seccombe I, Ball J, Patch A 1993 The price of commitment: nurses' pay, careers and prospects 1993. Institute of Manpower Studies, Brighton

Smith G, Seccombe I 1998 Changing times: a survey of registered nurses in 1998. Report 351. Institute for Employment Studies, Brighton

Stechmiller J, Yarandi H 1992 Job satisfaction among critical care nurses. American Journal of Critical Care 1(3): 37–44

United Kingdom Central Council for Nursing, Midwifery and Health Visiting (UKCC) 1985 Advertising for nurses, midwives and health visitors. UKCC, London

United Kingdom Central Council for Nursing, Midwifery and Health Visiting (UKCC) 1987 Confidentiality. UKCC, London

United Kingdom Central Council for Nursing, Midwifery and Health Visiting (UKCC) 1989 Accountability. UKCC, London

United Kingdom Central Council for Nursing, Midwifery and Health Visiting (UKCC) 1991 Post registration education and practice proposals. UKCC, London

United Kingdom Central Council for Nursing, Midwifery and Health Visiting (UKCC) 1992a The scope of professional practice. UKCC, London

United Kingdom Central Council for Nursing, Midwifery and Health Visiting (UKCC) 1992b The code of professional conduct for the nurse, midwife and health visitor, 3rd edn. UKCC, London

United Kingdom Central Council for Nursing, Midwifery and Health Visiting (UKCC) 1994 The future of professional practice – the council's standards for education and practice following registration. UKCC, London

United Kingdom Central Council for Nursing, Midwifery and Health Visiting (UKCC) 1995 PREP and you. Factsheets 1–8. UKCC, London

United Kingdom Central Council for Nursing, Midwifery and Health Visiting (UKCC) 1996a Guidelines for professional practice. UKCC, London

United Kingdom Central Council for Nursing, Midwifery and Health Visiting (UKCC) 1996b Register No 17. UKCC, London

United Kingdom Central Council for Nursing, Midwifery and Health Visiting (UKCC) 1997 PREP and you. UKCC, London

United Kingdom Central Council for Nursing, Midwifery and Health Visiting (UKCC) 1998 A higher level of practice: consultation document. UKCC, London

Welsh Language Act 1992. HMSO, London

FURTHER READING

Department of Health (DoH) 1996 Nursing: The leading edge of health care. A focus on developing nursing leadership. Nursing Standard Publication, RCN, London

English National Board for Nursing, Midwifery and Health Visiting Resource and Careers Department 1994 Post registration courses – opportunities for continuing education. ENB, London

Hull C, Redfern L 1996 Profiles and portfolios: a guide for nurses and midwives. Macmillan, Basingstoke

Royal College of Nursing (RCN) 1995 A guide to planning your career (RCN nurses in leadership project). RCN, London

United Kingdom Central Council for Nursing, Midwifery and Health Visiting (UKCC) 1996 Guidelines for professional practice. UKCC, London

United Kingdom Central Council for Nursing, Midwifery and Health Visiting (UKCC) 1997 PREP and you. UKCC, London

United Kingdom Central Council for Nursing, Midwifery and Health Visiting (UKCC) 1998 A higher level of practice: consultation document. UKCC, London

The person undergoing surgery

7

The person as a holistic being

Sharon L. Edwards

AIMS

The aims of this chapter are:

- to explore the history and meaning of holism
- to clarify the concept of holism, identify related concepts and propose a model for holism
- to highlight the debate surrounding holism
- to review holism in relation to nurse education, in an attempt to increase its understanding among surgical nurse practitioners.

INTRODUCTION

Holism has a long history dating back as far as Hippocrates in the 5th century, who viewed the mind and body as closely linked. This belief remained popular in the 17th century, when it began its demise. The practice of viewing the body as separate from the mind became known as dualism and this notion became more popular as medical discoveries continued to increase in the late 18th century. It is suggested that holism is overlooked by medicine as it is against the ideology of scientific enquiry, which attempts to view the individual as a set of parts to be broken down and studied. Holism is opposed to this form of reductionism. During the early 20th century medical science continued to grow and dominate society. Holism became overall ignored by medicine and other health care practitioners, who were also dominated and controlled by medical science.

The concept of holism only regained gradual importance during the 1960s and has since become a central tenet of nursing in both the UK and the USA. A review of holism in the British and American literature and research studies indicates that holism is a complex and multidimensional concept, which is widely accepted as a pivotal concept in the provision of high-quality nursing care. This acknowledgement of holism is long overdue.

The literature on holism today appears to reveal a plethora of articles written on the subject, but there seems to be no clear consensus on what constitutes holism. A number of terms are used to describe the concept of holism, such as complementary therapies, biopsychosocial, 'whole' as well as 'parts', nursing models, nursing process, nursing diagnosis and caring. Others consider totality; whole person; body, mind, emotion and spirit acting together; multiple interacting subsystems. There seems to be confusion over the definitions of the concepts involved. The terms are often used interchangeably and indiscriminately in the literature. This lack of agreement regarding holism is suggested to be due to a lack of a clear definition of what the concept holism is. Holism as a concept needs to be further clarified so that it may be used more effectively, its strengths and limitations evaluated, and variations introduced that enhance the contribution that the concept makes to the development of nursing knowledge for practice.

The most quoted understanding in the literature of the concept of holism is that it is a philosophy (Allen 1991a). This view of holism lends itself to interpretation and can therefore be a belief about nursing held by surgical nurses and how they wish to practise. Through understanding the concept of holism as a philosophy, and its many varied facets, the understanding of this important concept may develop, and its application into practice may be encouraged.

HISTORICAL PERSPECTIVE

Holism and holistic practices are steeped in history, from both sociological and nursing perspectives. In this section both of these viewpoints will be discussed.

Early origins

Early beliefs emphasised links between the mind and body. For instance, Hippocrates in the 5th century advocated environmental causes and treatment of illness, the importance of emotional factors, nutrition in health and disease and the healing power of nature (Griffin 1993). Chinese and Indian healing included the need for harmony between the individual, society, natural world, diet, exercise, meditation, and self-regulation as a whole (Griffin 1993). In addition, the ancient Greeks certainly believed that human beings were complete wholes rather than reducible mechanisms (Taylor 1988).

The mind and body link theory began its demise with the emergence of the science of medicine in the 17th century (Owen & Holmes 1993). The practice of viewing the body as separate from the mind became known as dualism, and separation of the two

increased as a result of the medical discoveries of the late 18th century. The arguments for dualism were further supported by Descartes in the late 19th century (Owen & Holmes 1993). Hegal attempted to heal the rift between the mind and body in the early 19th century (Owen & Holmes 1993), but it was not until the South African scientist, philosopher and politician, Jan Smuts (1926), that the concept of holism began to be associated with a systematic set of ideas. He postulated a philosophy in which the interdependent and interrelated parts were treated not within the dominant positivistic scientific paradigm, but from a new perspective for which he coined the term 'holism' (Smuts 1926).

1890–1930

Dualism between the mind and body continued to grow in popularity as a belief in the late 19th and early 20th centuries, possibly owing to further medical discoveries around this time. The acceptance of medical science, and the augmentation of new technology grew in importance (Boschma 1993). With the growth of clinical research, hospital medicine became the dominant medical practice by the end of the 1930s (Boschma 1993). Hospital medicine saw disease as a specific entity with a diagnosis and specific treatment, rather than as an imbalance between the body and its environment. Rather than attending to the patients in their social and family context, clinical medicine sought to improve the diagnosis and treatment of the diseased body. The efforts of the advocates of preventive and social medicine to advance living conditions in large urban centres were disregarded, and the major focus of medicine turned towards inpatient hospital care and clinical pathology (Rosenberg 1987).

Care of the hospital patient became increasingly complex and technical during the first three decades of the 20th century. This development had a powerful effect on nursing and other health care professionals. The community perspective of care disappeared, the need to improve the unhygienic living conditions and poor housing, rife during this period, were ignored, and hospital practice became the primary focus of nursing study and thought (Boschma 1993). This was despite Florence Nightingale and Lillian Wald who promoted holistic principles (Allen 1991a Boschma 1993, Shealy 1985, Wilson-Barnett 1988), for they challenged nurses to identify the influences of the social setting on patients, focus attention on prevention, extend nursing care beyond the purely physical, consider the natural responses to disease, show concern about the whole person in mind, body and spirit

(Owen & Holmes 1993). They recognised the patient's family, friends, and neighbours, as well as the environment, and recommended that they be included in care if health was to be restored and disease prevented (Allen 1991a).

1930–1985

By the First and Second World Wars and through the setting up of the power base of medicine by the National Health Service (NHS) in the 1940s, more surgery was performed, and the number of acutely ill patients treated in hospitals expanded (Boschma 1993). Society became dominated by the medical model, characterised by scientific rationality, emphasis on objective, numerical measurements, biochemical data, mind and body dualism, disease seen as an entity, individuals seen as complex machines, the whole as the 'sum of its parts'. The domination of science and technology, despite achieving spectacular advances, had not led to definitive cures for stress-related conditions such as hypertension, depression, alcoholism and insomnia (Gordon 1988). Trying to explain all phenomena, including human beings, in terms of only their most basic biological processes was not logical (Griffin 1993).

This brief history of the medical viewpoint reflects nursing's struggle to gain status as a profession, as nursing knowledge was not deemed to be scientific since it often tended to reflect only aesthetic and personal knowing (Carper 1978). It also serves to explain the complicated relationship of nursing with medicine. Medicine viewed patients as the sum of their parts and nursing was struggling to maintain individualised holistic care in a hostile environment, through viewing patients as more than the sum of their parts. Therefore, within this climate of differing viewpoints, individualised care became fragmented and difficult to achieve (Boschma 1993).

By the 1960s nurses became dissatisfied with the medical view of the person, as it omitted the influence of family, friends, significant others, the community, and social and environmental factors on the individual. It failed to identify the broad scope of needs required by the individual, but more importantly did not acknowledge health as an integral concept of nursing. As a reaction, nursing leaders attempted to formulate the profession's rationale for certain practices in holistic terms, which cast the focus of care on to the individual as a whole (Allen 1991b).

In America, the nursing process was introduced as a method of problem-solving and hospital nursing care began to be redefined. The integrity of the totality of the life of the individual patient was emphasised and became an accepted instrument for improving patient care. The nursing process was defined as a psychodynamic interpersonal relationship (Orlando 1961, Peplau 1966). It resulted in the individualised nursing care plan and a model to define nursing as a professional process or method which was comprehensive and patient-centred (Allen 1991b). The nursing process became incorporated into the new definitions of nursing. It identified the needs and problems of the patient, and the role of the nurse was to assist patients in meeting their needs and resolving the subsequent problems. Central to the nursing process was the nurse–patient relationship, considered instrumental to resolving patients' problems (Boschma 1993).

With the growth of the nursing process, the use of the medical model began to diminish. Nurses began to develop questions, possible concepts to study, and hypotheses that demanded research to test them. Nurses began to question nursing practices, develop research, form the pattern of empirical knowing identified by Carper (1978), and began to understand their practice. Through this understanding of practice, nursing theories and models began to develop.

Yet, it was becoming clear that nurses lacked the formal education necessary to provide the foundation for holistic practice. In America at this time, nurse curricula began to focus more on preventive health concepts as well as viewing the person as a holistic being. By incorporating a model, these two aims could be achieved and many of the nursing models seen in this country today grew out of the need to develop a curriculum that reflected this changing view of nursing. The integrated curriculum in Britain, therefore, began to provide the student with the opportunities to develop knowledge and skills imperative to holistic practice (Allen 1991b).

The increasing interest is illustrated by a growing literature, for between the years 1870–1960 holism was almost completely ignored in the nursing literature. This began to change between the years 1966–1970 when there were 18 articles mentioning holism, a number which increased to 220 between 1980 and 1985 (Kobert & Folan 1990). The increase in the number of articles on holism is evidence of an emerging set of values, beliefs and professional interest in holism (Johnson 1990, Sarkis & Skoner 1987). Among nurses, the holistic movement has continued to spread, with innovators in holistic nursing establishing professional nursing organisations such as the Nurse Healer – Professional Associates Inc. in 1979 and the American Holistic Nursing Association (AHNA) in 1980 (Johnson 1990).

In describing the focus of nursing as holistic, nursing's independent professional responsibility to use personal interaction to contribute to the recovery of the patient has become evident. The nurse is no longer perceived as 'hand maiden to the physician' (Peplau 1966). The term 'holism' attained a different meaning and was now used to identify the unique role of the nurse, while medicine was presented as reductionistic (Levine 1971, Rogers 1970). Within this context, nursing saw itself as being the patient's advocate and the holistic caretaker of patients. Holistic patient care legitimised nursing's unique, independent identity within hospital and community systems.

1986–present day

Nursing thought became dominated by the effort to identify a unique theoretical nursing perspective of study and work. New theories and models, such as Watson's Theory of Human Caring (Watson 1989), have resulted, emphasising the importance of the holistic approach. Additionally, modern, more holistic friendly qualitative research paradigms have emerged, which generate valuable nursing knowledge and provide a more holistic understanding of the whole. These include naturalistic enquiry, phenomenology, ethnography, action research, narrative research and grounded theory, all of which are committed to the naturalistic, interpretive approach and to capturing the individual's point of view, examining the constraints of everyday life and securing rich descriptions (Denzin & Lincoln 1994).

Yet, there still remains resistance to qualitative research studies, mainly from the positivist sciences (physics, chemistry, economics and psychology), which often consider such work as unscientific, or only exploratory, or entirely personal and full of bias (Denzin & Lincoln 1994). The opposition of positivist science to the qualitative research paradigm is the continued attempt to legitimise one version of truth over another, and it fails to encourage reason and truth (Reason & Rowan 1993). This discourse in the development of nursing knowledge threatens the future of holism. If nursing is to accept holism, it needs to forget the criticisms from positivist science in relation to qualitative research, and observe the prominent principle of the holistic philosophy – 'the whole'. In this sense, all ways of generating knowledge and undertaking research must be valued in holistic practice, now, and in the future.

THE CONCEPT OF HOLISM

There remains very little explanation of the concept of holism, and holism is generally used in the context of biological, psychological and sociological (biopsychosocial) processes. It appears that there is some discord between what is written about holism and what actually occurs in practice. The criticisms of holism are those generally steeped in scientific principles. The mechanistic systems are still followed and, as such, nursing often fails to recognise the complexity of holism.

Reflective point

Reflect upon what holism actually means to you when caring for a surgical patient and how you would recognise a holistic stance in the practice of other surgical nurses.

Rather then just provide a linguistically based analysis of the term holism, it is more important to understand the actual phenomenon and its underlying values, beliefs and assumptions (Rodgers 1989). Therefore to explain and understand the concept of holism is not to base it upon positivist philosophy or to reduce the essence of the concept, but to focus on the interrelationships that exist within it.

Analysis of the term

According to Sarkis & Skoner (1987) the origin of the word 'holism' is attributed to Jan Christiaan Smuts who wrote a treatise entitled *Holism and Evolution* (Smuts 1926). This work described holism as 'the principle which makes for the origin and progress of wholes in the universe'. However, the word holism was traced by Blattner (1981), who suggested that it is derived from the Anglo-Saxon word *hal*, which means 'whole', 'to heal', 'sound', or 'happy'.

In Middle English it can also be spelled 'wholism', which is equivalent to holism (Blattner 1981). The words holism and holistic are originally derived from the Greek word *holos*, meaning whole (*Oxford English Dictionary* 1993). Gordon (1988) suggests that there is no tangible difference between the words 'holistic' and 'wholistic', nor do there appear to be any distinctions between the words 'holism' and 'holistic'.

In *Roget's Thesaurus* (1982) a number of synonyms of the word holistic are identified, e.g. comprehensive, total, all, exhaustive and entire. Thus, both the words 'holism' and 'holistic' suggest completeness or wholeness and will be used synonymously in this chapter.

Related concepts used to explain holism

Despite the increasing popularity of the use of the term holism within the context of nursing, it cannot be assumed that all users share a common definition and understanding of the concept. Rodgers (1989, p. 330) asserted that when a definition, or attributes, of a concept are not clear, the ability of the concept to assist in fundamental tasks is greatly impaired.

The purpose of this section of the chapter is to clarify holism, the use and meaning of the word within the context of surgical nursing, and to explore the various interpretations of the concept.

Complementary therapies

Complementary therapy is often considered as a related concept to holism, because a number of complementary therapies are based on the concept of 'holism' (McGourty & Hotchkiss 1993). Complementary therapies include aromatherapy (Buckle 1993), massage and osteopathy (Trevelyan 1993a), therapeutic touch and yuleopathy (Booth 1993a,b), aromatherapy (Trevelyan 1993b), hypnotherapy (Booth 1993c) and reflexology (Booth 1994). Often nurses are ridiculed by colleagues and questioned by nursing union representatives for incorporating complementary therapies (Passant 1990), but hold fast that this is holistic care. Gordon (1988) described holistic medicine as the inclusion of complementary medical practices as well as treatment without medication, which included self-regulation strategies, relaxation therapies, biofeedback, hypnosis, guided imagery and meditation.

This suggests that holism can be defined as incorporating complementary therapies into nursing care. This definition is a mistake. It is not wrong to suppose that through the use of complementary therapies, nurses are becoming sensitive to the individual needs of their patients as well as being creative in meeting those needs. In complementary therapies nursing has found a new dimension to care, and the nursing profession is in a privileged position to be able to learn and offer this care to help their patients. Yet, incorporating complementary therapies into practice does not necessarily mean holistic care (Newbeck 1986), and medical and nursing practitioners may propose to deliver holistic care but not utilise complementary therapies. Therefore, you can incorporate the concept of holism into practice but not offer complementary therapies. Equally, you can be a complementary practitioner but not be holistic. Consequently, it is suggested that complementary therapies enhance the holistic approach, but alone do not constitute holistic care or demonstrate the concept of holism in its entirety.

Biopsychosocial

Holism is viewed by some as an explanation for those clinical practitioners who include biopsychosocial aspects of the human being into their care (Owen & Holmes 1993, Sarkis & Skoner 1987). Shaver (1985) proposed that nursing is concerned with human responses to a compromised or potentially compromised health status, and that a model of care is needed that takes into account a host of factors that impinge on the health status of an individual. Shaver suggests that the holistic model to achieve this is the physical and psychosocial model, and states: 'So rather than cause/disease/health problem/cure model, nursing uses a vulnerability/risk/human response/ care model, such a model describes integrated functioning of the whole individual from a bio-psycho-social view and explains the interaction among environment, mind, and body as it affects health status.' (Shaver 1985, p. 188).

This suggests that holism is represented by the biopsychosocial model. Engal's work is also based on the use of the term biopsychosocial, as he preferred it to 'holism' (Sarkis & Skoner 1987).

The biopsychosocial view of holism is criticised for omitting integrated aspects of the whole person, such as culture, religion, spirituality (Buckle 1993) and sexuality (Fugate-Woods 1987, Lewis & Bor 1994, Weston 1993). Buckle (1993) proposed that for nurses to truly practise holistic nursing they need to become in touch with their own spiritual self as 'whole' people; then they can become comfortable about meeting the spiritual needs of their patients. Meerabeau (1991) suggests that nurses are rarely approached by patients on a spiritual level as they are often either embarrassed or afraid. Spirituality is often not mentioned in pre-registration nursing courses and when it is, it is only to say that nurses cannot lay out Orthodox Jews, and that Moslems must be turned to the East within an hour of death (Buckle 1993). Interestingly, Gordon (1988) used terms such as biochemical, physiological, emotional, mental and spiritual to explain holistic medicine. However, many nurse theorists view the person as a biopsychosocial being and have made no explicit reference to the person's spiritual nature (Ham-Ying 1993).

Fugate-Woods (1987) and McHaffe (1993) expressed the importance that sexuality has to our image of ourselves, and our social relationships, and thus it requires to be included in the holistic perspective. Webb (1987) highlighted the need for greater consideration of the sexuality of the individual within the context of viewing the person as a biopsychosocial being. She also contended that holistic care cannot be provided if sexuality is ignored. In addition, Leininger (1978) stressed the influence of culture on the total being of the person, which is generally ignored by viewing the person as a biopsychosocial being.

Therefore, are those nurses who include biopsychosocial aspects in the care of their patients practising holism, and as such can this approach be designated as holistic? There is evidence to suggest that the majority of nurses and medical practitioners view holism in this way (Sarkis & Stoner 1987), and both Fuller (1987) and Shaver (1985) appear to confirm this by emphasising: 'the whole person is multidimensional, having biological, psychological, and sociological dimensions.' (p. 188).

'Whole' as well as 'parts'

Modern medicine considers the body to be a machine which is made up of separate parts. These parts can be studied and explained through rigorous scientific enquiry (Kottow 1992). The total sum of all the parts therefore, makes up the whole. This view tends to be reductionist and attempts to explain human beings in terms of only their most basic biological parts. This is reflected in systems theory, used in many nursing models, which may be perceived by some as reductionist, as it is concerned with achieving a balance between body systems (homeostasis), be they physical or psychosocial (Walsh 1991). This method of explaining all phenomena, including human beings, does not work (Griffin 1993). On the other hand, holism is the opposite, in that all the parts combine to make up the whole (Griffin 1993). This means that the whole is greater than and different from the sum of its parts.

Therefore, can a science that views a person as only a set of parts, e.g. modern medicine, or through a systems model, be practising holism, or can only those who view the whole person as one, be classed as practising holism? Is it those who see people, not as a whole, but as a set of parts who are practising holism? Whatever the outcome, an individual is a whole as well as made up of parts (Owen & Holmes 1993). The parts are all interdependent and interrelate to each other, which determines the nature of the entire person, who, as such, cannot be understood by isolated examination of the distinctive parts. As a result, holism cannot be explained as 'whole' or 'parts', owing to the complex interrelationships between parts. No part, however small, functions in isolation; no part of us works or fails to work without affecting the whole. So to use this explanation to understand holism is ambiguous, unreliable and poses more questions than it answers.

Nursing models and theories

Nurse theorists have used the term holism to refer to the patient in different ways: as a biopsychosocial adaptive system (Roy 1980); as a behavioural system (Johnson 1974); as a physiological, psychological, sociocultural, developmental being (Neuman 1974); as a unity functioning biologically, symbolically, and socially (Orem 1985). However, it is argued that the definitions used by these theorists perpetuate the reductionistic male view of human beings as a collection of parts, and dilute the meaning of the concept of holism as originally conceived. Often nurses applying reductionistic theories, such as Roy, Orem, Neuman and Johnson, have believed that they are functioning under a holistic philosophy simply because the theory uses the term holism (Kobert & Folan 1990).

Other theorists such as Parse (1981), Watson (1989), and Newman (1987) define nursing and person in terms that are more closely related to feminine ideas and values that are in opposition to the mechanistic male world view of logical empiricism (Agan 1987). They demonstrate a concern for the person within a contextual whole, they interrelate the mind and body, and they rely on research techniques that do not depend on empirical measurement. Yet, whichever model is used in clinical practice, none solely necessarily explains or demonstrates holism.

The nursing process

The nursing process refers to a framework for organising and providing care through a prescribed sequence of unalterable steps. Most commonly, these steps involve patient assessment, planning care, implementation of interventions, and evaluation of the process or patient status (Barnum 1987). It is argued that the nursing process and holism originate from two different world views. The nursing process originated from a reductionist scientific background and, as such, is not representative of holism, as it divides the patient into a predetermined list of processes. These two world views have been described in non-nursing literature as representing masculine and feminine approaches to the world (Belenky et al 1986, Gilligan 1982), suggesting, therefore, that the nursing process and holism are inconsistent with each other and cannot exist simultaneously in the same practice.

However, it is not suggested that by using the nursing process surgical nurses are not using holism, even though some authors would disagree (Caper & Kelly 1987, Kobert & Folan 1990). At clinical level, to reconcile the philosophical and practical disharmony from thinking holism while writing the nursing process, nurses need to be aware that their written record reflects nursing's values within the health care system, and thus provides an opportunity to demonstrate their value as nurses, and promote holistic nursing. Barnum (1987) brings both views together by suggesting that, while holism represents the philosophical context within which nursing is viewed and delivered, the nursing process refers to a distinct method by which nursing care is documented.

Nursing diagnosis

Nursing diagnosis was initially introduced as a step to the care-planning process. It was recognised explicitly by several nurse theorists as a stage of the nursing process (King 1981, Roy 1980). However, it has since been promoted as something different from, and more than just a part of, problem identification within the boundary of the nursing process (Booth 1992).

However, certain questions have been raised by Mills et al (1997) and Mason & Webb (1993) with regard to nursing diagnosis and holism, only one of which is relevant here: is nursing diagnosis congruent with seeing the patient as a whole or is it mechanistic and reductionist? (Mills et al 1997). Humanistic approaches are enhanced through a thorough psychological and social assessment. It is often these aspects of care which are missed out in surgical ward care plans, mainly because it can be hard for surgical nurses to articulate the information in a written format. It is suggested that, by using nursing diagnosis and developing knowledge and skills in this area, a more holistic approach to care could ultimately result. Therefore, nursing diagnosis is not in conflict with holism, but works in collaboration with the holistic paradigm to enrich holistic practice (See also Ch. 19).

Caring

Holism includes the preconditions of caring (Blattner 1981, Griffin 1993). It has long been considered that caring is the essence of nursing (Boykin & Schoenhofer 1990, Dunlop 1986, Forsyth et al 1989, Morrison 1989). Nevertheless, the term 'care/caring' is frequently and inconsistently used by the discipline of nursing (Kyle 1995). Leininger (1981, p. 3) defines care/caring as: 'Those assistive, supportive, or facilitative acts toward or for another individual or group with evident or anticipated needs to ameliorate or improve a human condition or lifeway.'

Watson (1979) views caring in nursing practice as a therapeutic interpersonal process, making the assumption that caring can only be demonstrated on an individual basis. Watson lists 10 'carative' factors that constitute caring (Box 7.1). These caring activities present nursing care as a deeply human activity.

The majority of caring models such as that of Watson (1979) focus on caring behaviours. This view of caring is shared by McFarlane (1976), who considers caring as a series of 'helping' activities, as do Griffin (1980, 1983), Orem (1985) and Weiss (1988). To view caring as a set of caring behaviours and activities has been criticised within the literature. Benner (1984) warns that when caring is separated into individual behavioural parts we do it violence. Dunlop (1986) also believes that by operationalising caring as a finite set of caring behaviours 'we are likely to end up with something different to what we now recognise as caring' (p. 667).

Duke & Copp (1992) expanded this argument and described caring as the hidden ingredient of nursing, the common thread running through all we do as nurses: 'Like a string in a necklace, it holds all the beads together. However, in the same way that a string is often hidden, so is caring in nursing' (p. 40).

This indicates that there is more to caring than what one can see (Kyle 1995). Consequently, a number of authors have described caring as an ethic (Carper 1979, Fry 1988, Harrison 1990, Kelly 1988, Kurtz & Wang 1991), indicating that there is a moral component to caring. Griffin (1983) emphasises the need for a moral component in caring. Several authors view the principle of respect for persons as the basis for all caring relationships (Gaut 1986, Kitson 1987). According to Fry (1988), for caring to have a moral value, it must be viewed as 'good' or 'right' for the specific reasons outlined in Box 7.2, and it is when caring has these

---

Box 7.1 The 10 carative factors (Watson 1979)

1. The formation of a humanistic–altruistic system of values.
2. The instillation of faith–hope.
3. The cultivation of sensitivity to oneself and others.
4. The development of a helping–trusting relationship.
5. The promotion and acceptance of the expression of positive and negative feelings.
6. The systematic use of the scientific problem-solving method of decision-making.
7. The promotion of interpersonal teaching–learning.
8. The provision for a supportive, protective, and (or) corrective mental, physical, sociocultural, and spiritual environment.
9. Assistance with the gratification of human needs.
10. The allowance for existential–phenomenological focus.

> **Box 7.2** Characteristics that give caring its moral value (Fry 1988)
>
> 1. Caring must be viewed as an ultimate or overriding value to guide one's actions.
> 2. Caring must be considered a universal value.
> 3. Caring must be considered prescriptive in that certain behaviours (empathy, support, compassion, protection, etc.) are preferred.
> 4. Caring must be other-regarding, it must consider the human flourishing of others and not one's own welfare.

characteristics that it can be regarded as a moral value. Therefore, in order for nursing to be caring it involves more than a set of activities; it encompasses the manner in which these activities are carried out, which should reflect the moral value of respect for persons (Kyle 1995).

Despite the discussions in relation to caring, it appears to be more of a hidden practice in nursing which has a moral element attached to it and, as such, the term does not define the concept of holism. However, caring can obviously play an integral role in practising holism, which can help to expand surgical nurses' comprehension of holism and assist them in acquiring a set of inner values compatible with holistic nursing. Yet what are these inner values that surgical nurses require?

HOLISM AS A PHILOSOPHY

In the previous section holism is represented as incorporating a wide range of interests. It is suggested to include complementary therapies as a new dimension of care which serves to enhance the holistic approach. It can also include biopsychosocial aspects of the human being, the view taken by the majority of nurses and medical practitioners. In addition, it confirms that holism cannot be explained as 'whole' or 'parts' because no part of a person works, or fails to work, without affecting the whole. Holism encompasses caring which emphasises moral values in the delivery of patient care. Yet it is not solely explained by incorporating a nursing model, the nursing process or nursing diagnosis. So what is holism and why is it so important to surgical nursing?

It is emerging in the literature that holism is an attitude or belief, an approach to living and dying, life and health, not to disease. It recognises the individual's ability to heal.

The holistic approach accepts scientific methods and knowledge but does not exclude other areas of maintaining and restoring health. It is a unified view (Kolcaba 1997), a way in which both the male and female world views, mentioned throughout this chapter, can unite. Ruskin (1865) stated that:

We are foolish, and without excuse foolish, in speaking of the superiority of one sex to the other, as if they could be compared to similar things. Each has what the other has not: each completes the other and is completed by the other; they are nothing alike, and the happiness and perfection of both depends on each asking and receiving from the other what the other only can give.

This suggests, if idealistically, that by being together a man and a woman constitute a whole, as each imparts something which the other does not have. Hence, holism is not complete without theories, conceptions, ideas, insights and views on the world. In this way, holism offers more scope for progression, action, creation, decision, discovery, self-development, speculation, invention, and enthusiasm in defence and support of nursing actions in surgical patient care. Consequently, holism offers more than interdependence of mind, body and soul within the environment. It could contribute to other health sciences, instead of being something for nursing alone. Overall, holism is a philosophy, a vast construct with many facets and various descriptions, and before nurses state that they are practising holism they first need to understand the basic principles of what it encompasses.

Allen (1991b) proposed that because nursing exhibits a continuing acceptance of holistic ideas, the understanding of the philosophical concept of holism is important mainly because of the fact that it underlies both theory and practice in nursing. Holism appears in virtually all nursing theories and as a justification for specialty areas of practice such as surgical nursing, and also for the introduction of innovations in nursing care, as in the case of primary nursing. Therefore, a critical evaluation of statements, conclusions, predictions, or explanations of the sciences regarding holism is important in nursing (Allen 1991b), as it contributes heavily to the essential knowledge base in nursing curricula (Forbes & Fitzsimons 1993). Some researchers propose that to determine if holism works it should be vigorously exposed to scientific empirical research. Others suggest that it transcends this type of testing. Allen (1991b) highlighted the methodological dilemma in applying holism as a theoretical concept to the traditional empirical research model.

Nurses must temporarily abandon questions of whether holism works in the context of clinical practice or research and look instead at what contributions can be made to holism from both surgical nurses and the supporting sciences, and consequently accept those that are necessary and reject those which are unsuitable. It is essential that if nursing is to subscribe to holism as its philosophical stance, then all the facets surrounding it are regarded as what is good and valuable in nursing. Many facets of holism are outlined in the literature and these are listed in Box 7.3. All facets of holism are vast topics in themselves and it is not within the confines of this chapter to discuss them all. But by identifying them it is hoped to help nurses to formulate a precise and coherent position on which to

---

Box 7.3 The facets of holism identified in the literature so far

Adaptation to change
Biopsychosocial (cultural, religious, sexual)
Caring
Collaborative practice
Communication
Complementary therapies
Counselling skills
Decision-making
Education/teaching
Empathy
Empowerment
Environment
Ethical principles
Evidenced-based practice
Freedom
Health promotion
Knowledge – all types
Knowledge from other disciplines/professions
Learning
Listening
Management skills
Medical practices
Negotiation
Nursing diagnosis
Nursing models
Nursing process
Nutrition
Practice development
Primary nursing
Professional organisations
Reflection on and in practice
Relatives and significant others
Research (all paradigms)
Resource management
Self-awareness
Self-esteem
Self-healing
Sleep
Standard setting
Supporting each other
Therapeutic relationships
Transitions in life
Valuing individuals

---

base the philosophy of holism and add an element of reality that will prevent holism from becoming so abstract and idealistic that it is rendered useless to the profession (Allen 1991b).

A study by Johnson (1990) attempted to identify through three phases the key words used to explain holism (Table 7.1). The purpose of the research was to identify the important concepts and activities that represent the holistic paradigm of health in nursing. It does not, however, explain the concept of holism but represents a list of concepts that are viewed to be synonymous with holism.

In identifying the many facets and synonymous terms that encompass the philosophy of holism, a problem arises as to how they should be put together to form a model for holistic practitioners. Ham-Ying (1993) identified two common usages for holism: as a view of the person and as an approach to the delivery of nursing care. By merging these aspects with those listed in Box 7.3, a practical model to guide the philosophy of holism is proposed (Box 7.4).

It is these differing facets of holism that make it important to surgical nurses, as it serves to:

- encourage practice development in the form of research and education
- formulate effective leadership within the surgical practice setting
- nurture change
- improve the quality of care.

Boxes 7.5 and 7.6 demonstrate how the model of holism can be put to effective use in surgical wards.

As knowledge and application of the model expand and develop, more insight will be gained into the nature of the person as a total entity. As a result, aspects of the philosophy may be rejected, new ones accepted or the two usages of holism may be continually refined. In this way, holism is addressed in the form of related concepts, which recognises the likelihood of change, rather than attempting to determine holism as static or constant with rigid lines of division. For, through this definition of holism, nursing is nearer to understanding the whole person, and attempts to care for and value individuals as a whole.

Moreover, some consideration needs to be given to the areas which encompass holism. For can individual nurses include all of the elements proposed in the philosophy of holism outlined in Box 7.4, and if they do not are they therefore not practising holism? This may be compounded by other factors such as stress levels and the lack of clinical resources. It is suggested that an individual may not be able to deliver all of those elements of holism mentioned. Yet every nurse generally

Table 7.1 Key words used to identify holism (Johnson M B 1990 The holistic paradigm in nursing: the diffusion of an innovation. Research in Nursing and Health 13 (2). Copyright © 1990 Wiley-Liss, Inc. Reprinted by permission of Wiley-Liss, Inc., a subsidiary of John Wiley & Sons, Inc.)

Category	Words	
Beliefs, values and philosophy	Body/mind/spirit	Interconnected
	Community	Lifestyle
	Consciousness	Parapsychology
	Environment	Preventive medicine
	Expanding consciousness	Process
	Holistic health	Psychosomatic
	Humanism	Spirituality
	Humanistic	Wellness
	Integration	Wholeness
Role of client	Awareness	Partnership
	Balance	Self-care
	Harmony	Self-concept
	Healing/healer	Self-healing
	Health promotion	Well-being
	Interrelationship	Whole person
Role of the nurse	Caring	Health counselling
	Education	Health promotion
	Energy	Partnership
	Energy field	Self-actualisation
	Empowerment	Self-awareness
	Guide	Whole person
	Healing/healer	
Activities and modalities	Acupressure	Music therapy
	Acupuncture	Relaxation
	Art therapy	Stress management
	Biofeedback	Therapeutic touch
	Hypnosis	Touch
	Imagery	Visualisation
	Massage	Yoga
	Meditation	

has a special or a variety of special interests. These may include counselling relatives or patients, ethics, wound care, communication, diabetes, stoma care, research, primary nursing, etc. Therefore could holistic practice as a philosophy perhaps be better delivered as a ward team?

Three questions still remain. First, can all those areas of holism be incorporated into practice, even by a team? If surgical nurses are not including all the areas, then are they practising holism? Third, how many facets or concepts do nurses need to embody before a surgical ward team can be certain that they are putting into practice a holistic philosophy? The answers to these three questions are not for academics or theorists to explore, but for clinical practitioners themselves to consider. Holism is a philosophy and, as such, the basic principles of what it encompasses need first to be understood by nurses; then they can move on to decide which elements they believe will enhance

the care delivery to their patients. The holistic philosophy is an attitude towards a patient, and it is about having a set of moral and philosophical values whether individual or as a ward team, which strives to deliver the highest quality of care to the patient.

Reflective point

Consider the three questions highlighted above for yourself.

The third question is, can an individual facet within holism (e.g. sexuality, wound care, nutrition, reflective practice, caring, pain) be treated holistically? This question can be answered: 'Yes'. This is because some of the facets described within holism (Box 7.3) can be applied to an individual topic area or concept, for

---

Box 7.4   A practical guide to the philosophy of holism

As a view of the person	**As an approach to the delivery of nursing care**
Adaptation	Adaptation to change
Attitudes	All paradigms of research
Biopsychosocial (cultural, religious, sexual)	All types of knowledge valued
Communication	Caring
Community	Clinical supervision
Education/teaching	Collaborative practice
Empathy	Complementary therapies
Empowerment	Duty to care
Environment	Education/teaching/learning
Experiences	Ethics
Family	Evidenced-based practice
Health promotion	Health promotion
Individual	Include relatives, friends, patient, significant others in the
Involved in decision-making	delivery of care
Lifestyle	Knowing self
Listening	Management skills
Medical practices	Multidisciplinary team
Membership of groups	Negotiation
Partnership	Non-judgmental counselling skills
Personality	Nursing diagnosis
Rights of the individual	Nursing model
Role in society/family	Nursing process
Self-care	Practice development
Self-concept	Primary/team nursing
Self-esteem	Professional organisations
Stress management	Reflection on and in practice
The patient's rights	Resource management
The whole is more than the sum of its parts	Self-awareness
Touch	Standard setting/audit
Transitions in life	Supporting each other
Trust	Therapeutic relationships
Values and beliefs	

---

example, pain. Research will be imperative if one is to explore pain: the treatment or method chosen may have ethical implications, there may be an advantage to using complementary therapies, developing a relationship with patients, using the nursing process, demonstrating empathy, all of which are included in the philosophy of holism, and as such can be applied to pain or any other concept(s) that surgical nurses wish to evaluate in a holistic manner.

However, surgical nurses need to be constantly mindful of a personal functional definition of holism, and should be careful to promote the philosophy of holism and not just the word.

THE OBJECTIONS TO HOLISM

There are objections to holism identified in the literature and warnings to its shaping nursing care (Griffin 1993). So what are the objections to holism? The fact that not all patients may need this broad intervention in every situation, that it may be introduced to cut costs, and the power base outside of nursing may not endorse its application. These factors could hinder the implementation of holism in surgical wards.

The overuse of holism principles

Holism can undermine the precise focusing on a clinical condition. Yet it is not every condition that requires the use of holistic practices, e.g. a broken finger may not require the nurse to consider any additional problem except that of the broken finger (Griffin 1993), although, depending on circumstances, this may be debatable. Yet, what this attempts to show is that the practice of holism has a broad remit, but there may be times when nurses are not required to function within this broad arena. Nurses need to recognise that occasionally a single problem or need is just that and nothing else. Griffin (1993) warns that: 'Working on a broad canvas can facilitate a dangerous superficiality if one is not trained and willing first to recognise what may be single and special' (p. 312).

Box 7.5 A model case for holism in surgical nursing practice

A surgical ward develops a new philosophy in collaboration with all the staff. The ward philosophy focuses on holism. The designated staff search the literature to help guide them toward achieving their pledge for holistic care, decide upon this model, and set about choosing which aspects they wish to add or include in their holistic approach.

1. The approach to the delivery of nursing care may include areas such as:
   a. Staff require to gain self-awareness; this can be facilitated through clinical supervision and/or reflection.
   b. Primary nursing may be accepted and incorporated into the organisation of delivering care.
   c. Education on the ward is valued, and a needs assessment is undertaken amongst staff to determine educational needs, and thus arrange ways in which these needs can be met.
   d. All ways of knowing are valued, and designated staff set about investigating more effective use of knowledge on the surgical ward.
   e. Research may be chosen, and staff set about incorporating research meetings whereby staff analyse a particular piece or a collection of research on the same topic relevant to surgical nursing each week, or on a fortnightly or monthly basis, to determine the research for use in clinical practice.

   f. (c), (d) and (e) incorporate practice development and enhancing clinical skills.
   g. Some of the above issues will require negotiation and leadership skills, collaborative practice, supporting each other, adaptation to change, all of which assist in the application of the holistic model.
   h. Many of the above may lead to further developments, such as standard-setting and audit, including complementary therapies; all serve to build on the holistic approach to surgical patients.
2. The view of the person may include:
   a. Incorporating a model which truly reflects the holistic philosophy, such as Watson (1979).
   b. The chosen model reflects the view of the person, and values patients as individuals with their own attitudes, values and beliefs, personality, family, roles, lifestyle, self-concept, and experiences which will at all times be considered.
   c. Patients have a right to be informed about their illness, and take part in the decision-making process.

These areas are just a suggestion. The transition to these and other holistic principles may not be easy. They require vigorous investigation by individuals or groups of staff, motivation, and most of all belief in the value of holism and holistic practice(s).

However, by discouraging an unjustifiable broad intervention it could be argued that the nurse demonstrates respect for that person. Respect has been demonstrated by many writers as an element of caring (Kyle 1995), which plays an integral role in the practice of holism. Thus, holistic principles can be embraced to a lesser or a greater degree, depending on the circumstances required.

Holism used to cut costs

The new 'holistic medical' model underscores the uniqueness and unity of the individual and emphasises the potential for self-actualisation (Boschma 1993). It has a major emphasis on self-help and self-awareness; people have responsibility for their own health and well-being. They are responsible for their own promotion of health, their habits in the areas of nutrition, exercise, stress reduction, and lifestyle patterns to increase wellness.

However, emphasising self-responsibility has negative aspects, which were identified in the late 1970s (Crawford 1977) and were subsequently raised again by Lowenberg (1989). As long as illness is attributed to external factors, as in the biomedical model, the only moral responsibility the patient has is to comply with the treatment. The holistic emphasis on self-responsibility and personal choice, however, makes people responsible for unhealthy behaviours that are considered risk factors for disease. Consequently, blame and guilt may be laid on patients, and they may be subjected to moral condemnation (see Ch. 4).

Therefore, self-responsibility might be a welcome argument to withdraw money and resources because of apparent irresponsible behaviours, especially in the light of rising costs of health care and political controversy about health care policy (Griffin 1993). Consequently, cultural factors that influence lifestyle and the social production of disease might be ignored (Crawford 1977, Lowenberg 1989). There is uncertainty about any long-term effects of holistic thought, if these ideas are popularised and diffused through the media in a simplistic way.

Box 7.6   A model case for holism in surgical nursing practice

Medical practices may be continually undervaluing nursing practice, and as such the emphasis on holism is not currently focused on the surgical ward. Efforts of the staff are to make this more clear, and set about using the model in the following way:

1. The approach to the delivery of nursing care may include areas such as:
    a. Through collaborative practice it could be made clear to doctors that their current medical practices are valuable but focus mainly on just one area of knowledge, e.g. scientific, reductionist, which has been identified as being narrow and as such unable to explain all aspects of the patient.
    b. Surgical nurses want to focus on a more multidisciplinary approach to delivering care to their patients, using primary nursing.
    c. It is decided that to focus more on the nursing role, nursing diagnosis should be included, to

facilitate the development of new knowledge and skills in interpreting psychological and psychosocial care. This will require education of staff together with adaptation to change and resource management.
    d. Many of the above may lead to further practice developments, such as multidisciplinary care planning, standard setting or complementary therapies, or improved therapeutic relationships, all of which serve to build on the holistic approach to surgical patients.

This is all that may be required to enhance the holistic view on a surgical ward, but still may not be easy. The necessity to implement the above will continue to require vigorous investigation by individuals or groups of staff, motivation, and most of all belief in the values of holism and holistic practice(s).

Management

The nursing profession may decline in status as it faces a variety of problems in which holism may be partially implicated. Continuing government and local government cutbacks in funding have threatened the scope and even the existence of many nursing programmes in many areas (Allen 1991b). The position of 'nursing manager' continues to be abolished and business managers are placed in control of the profession in many areas, with the power to influence nursing care decisions significantly (Ralph 1989). In this way the holistic practice of nursing may have become constricted.

A contributing factor to these problems may well be the generalised, global nature of the holistic goals that are valued in nursing. A long-standing problem has been how to translate such goals into measurable outcomes, as they do not lend themselves readily to evaluational research methodologies. This has led to the inability of nursing to demonstrate that the holistic care it purports to give makes any real difference. This is a critical failure in such financially insecure times.

If nurses are to provide holistic care, this ideal has to be shared by the business managers who make the policies, and by resource budget holders. Business managers need to understand that holistic principles cannot be researched using traditional scientific approaches. It needs to be stated that holism works because of the facets it encompasses, not because of

the philosophy itself. Without acceptance of the nature of holism, the concept of holism may not be fully brought into operation within the context of nursing.

Reflective point

Begin to consider how you would explain to a non-nurse business manager the benefits of a holistic approach.

THE CONFLICTING VIEWS REGARDING HOLISM

There are some contradictory views within holism, which mainly arise between the specialist nurse and the generic nurse, and the duty to care and holism.

The specialist and the generic nurse

Specialist nurses are currently advocated in clinical practice and a number of them are already in post performing such roles as nutrition nurse, stoma nurse, research nurse, wound care nurse, diabetic nurse. In addition, there are specialist nurses who work with a particular client group, rather than have a specific role, for example surgical nurses themselves. However, it is argued that the integration of specialist nurses is a move away from the holistic approach and a return to empiricism which embraces the linear, reductionistic and mechanistic masculine world view, which provides a great measure of power, tradition and acceptance for science, particularly medicine (Kobert & Folan 1990). Medicine follows the tradition of specialists, e.g. nephrologist, orthopaedics, gynaecologist, neurologist and neurosurgeon, cardiologist or cardiac surgeon, which is congruent with a reductionist approach. Similarly, the stoma nurse, the research nurse, diabetic nurse, nutritionist are all part of the same fragmentation of nursing, identical to medicine, as it breaks the person down into parts. If just the specialist nurse were to emerge in nursing, who would be looking after the patient? The specialist nurse will be looking after individual areas or groups of clients, as observed in medicine.

Therefore, there is a strong argument for a more generic nurse rather than a specialist nurse. This would serve to ensure that nurses lead care through the holistic approach they have to offer. However, the role of the generic nurse is criticised, for how can a nurse be 'an all singing and all dancing nurse' and be expected to do everything for patients. Similarly, there is the problem of the generic nurse 'knowing something about everything', implying that the generic nurse might be unable to have the depth of knowledge and experience of the specialist nurse in every area. In addition, to maintain the generic role of the nurse and to maintain their holistic approach, nurses may be expected to transfer from ward to ward.

These contrasting points of view suggest that nursing is so diverse and expansive that we need all types of nurses. Thus it appears that there is room for both a specialist nurse and the generic nurse. Generic nurses will be holistic in focus, will coordinate the care of the patient, recognise when it is necessary to bring in a specialist, be educated to a high level to be able to cope with this role, and have the holistic approach to care as their philosophy. Specialist nurses, in contrast, would maintain their holistic focus and have the same high level of education, but only be called upon when the knowledge or experience of the generic nurse is insufficient.

Thus the 'generic nurse would remain on top, but the specialist nurse will be on tap'.

This view suggests that holistic nurses do not necessarily know everything about all the problems associated with their patients. Therefore, the generic nurse will not be 'an all singing and all dancing nurse', a view the majority of nurses have of the generic nurse. In this way, holism on surgical wards may be conveyed through the generic and specialist nurses working together to deliver holistic care as part of a team.

Some of these principles were highlighted by Manley (1997), who proposed practice development as an eclectic mechanism for integrating all nursing

professional functions, e.g. generic and specialist nurse, for the benefit of patients. Manley (1997) went on to state that practice development: 'is a prerequisite for clinical effectiveness, quality improvement and the development of a culture which facilitates the responsive and proactive action necessary to lead and influence today's health care provision' (p. 5).

The duty to care and holism

The duty to care means that health care must be administered to patients without any personal regard to any individual qualities, faults and idiosyncrasies (Pratt 1996), implying perhaps that during the delivery of care these specific peculiarities should be ignored. Yet holism advocates paying special attention to an individual's unique and distinct characteristics, such as marks or particular features, sexual habits, personal beliefs or attitudes, diagnosis, weight, as these are what constitute, and helps the nurse to understand, the whole person. Griffin (1993) suggests that to take on board all the patient's imperfections and peculiarities is invasive and presumptuous. Indeed, some people hate being understood for fear of being controlled.

This suggests that the duty to care strongly conflicts with holism. Yet it is obvious that what is required to solve this argument, is for nurses to consider in their care the patients' faults, qualities and idiosyncrasies, as this will help them to deliver holistic care. But as nothing should influence how a surgical nurse delivers care to a patient, the duty of care will always be adhered to. It is suggested that a duty to care is within the realms of holism and not in conflict with it.

These objections and conflicts within the concept of holism need to be taken very seriously, for so doing will assist in a deeper and more precise understanding of the meaning of holism and continue to map out the ideal processes for practice.

HOLISM AND NURSE EDUCATION

The principles of holism are generally the same for all nurses whatever area they practice in, be it surgical, medical or community nursing, but it is the education of the surgical nurses of the future which is important if the philosophy of holism is to survive and shape future health practices. As a surgical nurse you may be a future member of curriculum planning groups.

The holistic curriculum

Educators are in a particularly advantageous position to introduce and promote the practice of holistic nursing.

From curriculum development to role-modelling behaviour, teachers and advanced practitioners involved in curriculum planning, can have a profound impact on pre- and post-registration nurses. If holism is taught as a philosophy, then both pre- and post-registration nurses may gain a solid foundation from which to practice (Forbes & Fitzsimons 1993).

Nurse education prepares nurses to be leaders and prepares individuals to be autonomous practitioners (Forbes & Fitzsimons 1993). It is ultimately the nursing curricula which should be designed to educate nurses to have a holistic view. This will ultimately prepare a pre- and post registration nurse to be aware of the need for a comprehensive approach greater than solely nursing. Introducing holism to nurses at all levels allows them to have an understanding of the attitudes, values, and methods of not only their own profession, but other professions as well (White 1989). With this knowledge base, pre- and post-registration students of nursing are empowered to employ effective strategies to promote holistic care. This effort entails far more than merely 'doing' nursing. It has an objective to communicate the essentials of nursing so that they are understood by health team professionals, patients and their families.

Curriculum content and methods must teach group activities grounded in the humanistic view of learning (Forbes & Fitzsimons 1993, Rodgers 1983). Therefore, surgical nurse practitioners involved in curriculum planning must insist on a humanistic approach to unfold the experiential and interconnected nature of nursing with no possibility of separating emotions, rationality, or development; encourage nurses to explore their feelings and engage in varying forms of self-expression; move students towards exploring their positive contributions to patient care in an enthusiastic way; and help to develop self-esteem and self-assurance. Embracing humanistic thinking in curriculum planing will ensure that surgical nurses of the future become fully aware of their healing contributions to their patients (White 1989). This level of holism must be developed and achieved through the curriculum, and will hopefully go some way towards providing the relevant knowledge that will equip surgical nurses with sufficient knowledge and skills to give holistic care.

The holistic teacher

The holistic (surgical) nurse teacher is concerned with human growth, individual fulfilment and self-actualisation of staff/students, and prefers to emphasise the importance of the cognitive and psychomotor elements in the student (Quinn 1992). Rodgers (1983) identified two main principles that apply to the holistic approach to teaching, namely teacher–student relationships, and the clinical learning environment. Embracing these two principles can be someone who shares feelings as well as knowledge with the learners; has awareness of self and concentrates on being him- or herself; has acceptance, trust of the learners, understanding and empathy. Jacono & Jacono (1994a,b) suggest that teachers demonstrate holism by relating to a student as they truly are, which will help illuminate the meaning of situations (identified as the therapeutic use of self) and increase the value of learning.

Jacono & Jacono (1994b) defined holistic teachers by their characteristics and by their chosen teaching methods. Mynaugh (1991) noted that the characteristics of a teacher were important. Rice (1992) mentioned the particular characteristics as warmth, flexibility, ability to negotiate and compromise. Halldorsdotter (1990), Miller et al (1990), Nehms (1990) attributed these characteristics to the success of the holistic teacher.

The influences on holism in nurse education

There are two areas that may influence holism in the education of nurses: the modular system being imposed on pre- and post-registration nurse curricula, and the power base of management and the allocation of resources within higher education.

Higher education and the modular system

With the move into higher education, the majority of nurse curricula are embracing the higher education ethos of modular courses (Akinsanya 1990). This form of curriculum separates a nursing course into parts, therefore suggesting that the whole is the sum of its parts, e.g. the total of all the modules makes up a diploma or degree in nursing. It fails to recognise that the whole is more than and different from the sum of its parts, which forms the basis of the holistic philosophy. It could be argued that by moving into higher education nursing is moving away from holistic principles, as higher education can be considered to be very traditional, exerts a great measure of power, and unequivocally accepts the majority of its knowledge from the quantitative paradigm of pure science. This could mean a move away from the holistic focus in nurse education and a return to empiricism which embraces the reductionistic and mechanistic masculine world view.

Rodgers (1983) would suggest that with this predominate set of values and this type of system, holistic nurse teachers could become repressed by administration. In addition, they might be in danger of becoming specialists in a specific module area or of being absorbed into a particular subject which they teach. This way of delivering nurse education through a collection of teachers with specialist knowledge or interest, in areas such as biosciences, research, psychology, ethics, pharmacology, who also have a high level of education and experience in these areas, emphasises the potential for nurse education to become fragmented and distant from the importance of holistic principles in the delivery of nursing care.

For, if it is just the specialist teacher who emerges in nurse education as in clinical practice, who would be able to bring all the knowledge gained from all of the modules together, to ensure that the curriculum maintains and adheres to the holistic philosophy? This is not to propose that the specialist teacher does not have a holistic focus, as this is also necessary, but to suggest that it is imperative that some teachers are able to bring to the forefront the holistic principles so valued in nursing, e.g. that nursing is more than and different from the sum of all the different and relevant modules. The holistic teacher must remain educated to a high level, preferably with a graduate or higher degree in nursing.

The bringing together of a modular curriculum may only be essential for pre-registration nursing students, because in many post-registration nurse courses students have already acquired a great deal of clinical experience and knowledge in the field of nursing. Therefore they should be able to digest all the modules and then relate them to the holistic philosophy. This serves to enhance the postgraduate surgical nurses' knowledge and to achieve a greater understanding of the extent and limits of holistic nursing practice. However, the pre-registration nurse generally has little experience of clinical practice and the theory that underpins it, and as such might require more emphasis on bringing all of the modules together as an integrated whole.

Management

In higher education, as in clinical practice, there are continuous government and local government cutbacks in funding, and educational managers are placed in control of nurse education budgets which have the power to significantly influence nurse education decisions. In this way the education of holistic practices in nurse education could become impeded.

This could be because higher education has a tradition that accepts and values empiricism as a way of generating knowledge, which embraces the reductionistic and mechanistic masculine world view. This could mean that nurse educationalists have to work hard to translate their holistic goals, which do not lend themselves readily to the quantitative numerical paradigm of cause/effect or correlation research methodologies, to gain acceptance of a way of delivering education that views people and the world they live in differently. If nurse educationalists cannot do this in such financially insecure times, then holism may not survive within the context of higher education.

CONCLUSION

If nurses are to provide holistic care, surgical nurses must temporarily abandon questions of whether holism works in the context of clinical practice or research and look instead at what contributions can be made to holism from both nursing and the supporting disciplines. This has been attempted by the model of holism suggested by this chapter. Once this has been achieved, surgical nurses need to accept those that are necessary and reject those which are unsuitable. Through the concepts identified by this model, surgical nurses may be able to identify the broad scope and range of their holistic practices and determine how holism may be effective in clinical practice. When continually applied to practice, the identified model may be continually refined, and variations and innovations introduced to enhance surgical nurses' understanding of the person as a whole.

It is essential if nursing is to understand and subscribe to holism as its philosophical stance, that all the facets surrounding it are identified and regarded as what is good and valuable in nursing. This ideal then has to be shared by clinical practitioners, those who educate them, by health care policy makers, by business managers and by resource allocators. Without all this, the concept of holism may not be fully brought into operation within the context of nursing.

Nursing must continue to develop, evaluate, and maintain the full scope of its holistic practices. The professional must be proactive when holistic ideals are threatened; this may involve strategies that articulate to policy makers, the public and managers, the value of incorporating the philosophy of holism into clinical and educational practices. This has to be done early enough to influence nursing services which are vital in areas where such services are being cut. In addition, holistic ideas must continue to become influential in the practice philosophy of nursing care.

REFERENCES

Agan R D 1987 Intuitive knowing as a dimension of nursing. Advances in Nursing Science 10(1): 63–70

Akinsanya J A 1990 Nursing links with higher education: a prescription for change in the 21st century. Journal of Advanced Nursing 15(9): 744–754

Allen C E 1991a Holistic concepts and the professionalisation of public health nursing. Public Health Nursing 8(2): 74–80

Allen C E 1991b An analysis of the pragmatic consequences of holism for nursing. Western Journal of Nursing Research 13(2): 256–272

Barnum B J 1987 Holistic nursing and the nursing process. Holistic Nursing Practice 1(3): 27–35

Belenky M F, Clinchy B M, Goldberger N R, Tarule J M 1986 Women's ways of knowing: the development of self voice and mind. Basic Books, New York

Benner P 1984 From novice to expert: excellence and power in clinical nursing practice. Addison-Wesley, Menlo Park

Blattner B 1981 Holistic nursing. Prentice Hall, Englewood Cliffs

Booth B 1992 Nursing diagnosis: one step forward. Nursing Times 88(7): 33–34

Booth B 1993a Therapeutic touch. Nursing Times 89(31): 48–50

Booth B 1993b Yuleopathy. Nursing Times 89(50): 48–49

Booth B 1993c Hypnotherapy. Nursing Times 89(40): 42–45

Booth B 1994 Reflexology. Nursing Times 90(1): 38–40

Boschma G 1993 The meaning of holism in nursing: historical shifts in holistic nursing ideas. Public Health Nursing 11(5): 324–330

Boykin A, Schoenhofer S 1990 Caring in nursing: analysis of extant theory. Nursing Science Quarterly 3(4): 149–155

Buckle J 1993 When holism is not complementary? British Journal of Nursing 2(15): 744–745

Caper C F, Kelly R 1987 Neuman nursing process: a model of holistic care. Holistic Nursing Practice 1(3): 19–26

Carper B 1978 Fundamental patterns of knowing in nursing. Advances in Nursing Science 1: 33–44

Carper B A 1979 The ethics of caring. Advances in Nursing Science 1(3): 11–19

Crawford R 1977 You are dangerous to your health: the ideology and politics of victim blaming. International Journal of Health Services 7(4): 663–680

Denzin N K, Lincoln Y S 1994 Handbook of qualitative research. Sage Publications, Thousand Oaks

Duke S, Copp G 1992 Hidden nursing. Nursing Times 88(17): 40–42

Dunlop M J 1986 Is a science of caring possible? Journal of Advanced Nursing 11(6): 661–670

Forbes E J, Fitzsimons V 1993 Education: the key for holistic interdisciplinary collaboration. Holistic Nursing Practice 7(4): 1–10

Forsyth D, Delaney C, Maloney N, Kubesh D, Story D 1989 Can caring behaviour be taught? Nursing Outlook 37(4): 164–166

Fry S T 1988 The ethic of caring: can it survive in nursing? Nursing Outlook 36(1): 48

Fugate-Woods N 1987 Toward a holistic perspective of human sexuality: alterations in sexual health and nursing diagnosis. Holistic Nursing Practice 1(4): 1–11

Fuller S S 1987 Holistic man and the science and practice of nursing. Nursing Outlook 26: 700–704

Gaut D A 1986 Evaluating caring competencies in nursing practice. Topics of Clinical Nursing 8(2): 77–83

Gilligan C 1982 In a different voice: psychological theory and women's development. Harvard University Press, Massachusetts

Gordon J S 1988 Holistic medicine. Chelsea House Publishers, New York

Griffin A P 1980 Philosophy and nursing. Journal of Advanced Nursing 5(3): 261–272

Griffin A P 1983 A philosophical analysis of caring in nursing. Journal of Advanced Nursing 8(4): 289–295

Griffin A 1993 Holism in nursing: its meaning and value. British Journal of Nursing 2(6): 310–312

Halldorsdotter S 1990 The essential structure of a caring and uncaring perspective of the nursing student. In: Leininger M, Watson J (eds) The caring imperative in education. National League for Nursing, USA

Ham-Ying S 1993 Analysis of the concept of holism within the context of nursing. British Journal of Nursing 2(15): 771–775

Harrison L L 1990 Maintaining the ethic of caring in nursing. Journal of Advanced Nursing 15(2): 125–127

Jacono B J, Jacono J J 1994a How should holism guide the setting of educational standards? Journal of Advanced Nursing 19(2): 342–340

Jacono B J, Jacono J J 1994b Holism: the teacher is the method. Nurse Education Today 14(4): 287–291

Johnson D E 1974 The behavioral systems model for nursing. In: Riehl J P, Roy C (eds) Conceptual models for nursing practice. Appleton-Century-Crofts, New York

Johnson M B 1990 The holistic paradigm in nursing: the diffusion of an innovation. Research in Nursing and Health 13(2): 129–139

Kelly L S 1988 The ethic of caring: has it been discarded? Nursing Outlook 36(1): 17

King I 1981 A theory for nursing: systems, concepts and processes. John Wiley, New York

Kitson A L 1987 A comparative analysis of lay-caring and professional (nursing) caring relationships. International Journal of Nursing Studies 24: 155–165

Kobert L, Folan M 1990 Coming of age in nursing: rethinking the philosophies behind holism and nursing process. Nursing and Health Care 11(6): 308–312

Kolcaba R 1997 The primary holisms in nursing. Journal of Advanced Nursing 25(2): 290–296

Kottow M H 1992 Classical medicine v alternative medical practices. Journal of Medical Ethics 18(1): 18–22

Kurtz R J, Wang J 1991 The caring ethic: more than kindness, the core of nursing science. Nursing Forum 26(1): 4–8

Kyle R V 1995 The concept of caring: a review of the literature. Journal of Advanced Nursing 21(6): 506–514

Leininger M 1978 Transcultural nursing: concepts, theories, and practices. John Wiley, New York

Leininger M M 1981 The phenomenon of caring: importance, research questions and theoretical considerations. In: Leininger M M (ed) Caring an essential human need. Wayne State University Press, Detroit

Levine M A 1971 Holistic nursing. Nursing Clinics of North America 6(2): 253–264

Lewis S, Bor R 1994 Nurses' knowledge of and attitudes towards sexuality and the relationship of these with nursing practice. Journal of Advanced Nursing 20(1): 251–259

Lowenberg J S 1989 Caring and responsibility: the crossroads between holistic practice and traditional medicine. University of Pennsylvania Press, Philadelphia

McFarlane J 1976 A charter for caring. Journal of Advanced Nursing 1(3): 187–196

McGourty H, Hotchkiss J 1993 Study rules. Nursing Times 89(36): 42–45

McHaffe H 1993 Improving awareness. Nursing Times 89(18): 29–31

Manley K 1997 Practice development: a growing and significant movement. Nursing in Critical Care 2(1): 5

Mason G, Webb C 1993 Nursing diagnosis: a review of the literature. Journal of Clinical Nursing 2: 67–74

Meerabeau L 1991 The presentation of competence in health care. Journal of Advanced Nursing 16(1): 63–67

Miller B, Haber B, Byrne M 1990 The experience of caring in the teaching–learning process. In: Leninger M, Watson J (eds) The caring imperative in education. National League of Nursing, USA

Mills C, Howie A, Mone F 1997 Nursing diagnosis: use and potential in critical care. Nursing in Critical Care 2(1): 11–16

Morrison P 1989 Nursing and caring: a personal construct theory study of some nurses' self-perceptions. Journal of Advanced Nursing 14(5): 421–426

Mynaugh P 1991 A randomised study of two methods of teaching perineal massage: effects on practice rates, episiotomy rates, and lacerations. Birth 18(3): 153–159

Nehms T 1990 The lived experience of nursing education: a phenomenological study. In: Leninger M, Watson J (eds) The caring imperative in education. National League for Nursing, USA

Neuman B M 1974 The Betty Neuman health care systems model: a total person approach to patient problems. In: Riehl J P, Roy C (eds) Conceptual models for nursing practice. Appleton-Century-Croft, New York

Newbeck I 1986 The whole works. Nursing Times 82(30): 48–49

Newman M A 1987 Theory development in nursing. F A Davis, Philadelphia

Orem D E 1985 Nursing: concepts of practice. McGraw-Hill, New York

Orlando I J 1961 The dynamic nurse–patient relationship. Putnam, New York

Owen M J, Holmes C A 1993 'Holism' in the discourse of nursing. Journal of Advanced Nursing 18(11): 1688–1695

Parse R 1981 Man living health: a theory of nursing. John Wiley, New York

Passant H 1990 A holistic approach in the ward. Nursing Times 86(4): 26–28

Peplau H E 1966 Nurse–doctor relationships. Nursing Forum 5: 61–75

Pratt R 1996 HIV & AIDS: a strategy for nursing care. Arnold, London

Quinn F M 1992 The principles and practice of nurse education, 2nd edn. Chapman and Hall, London

Ralph C 1989 Nursing management and leadership – the challenge. In: Jolley M, Allan P (eds) Current issues in nursing. Chapman and Hall, London

Reason P, Rowan J (eds) 1993 Human inquiry: a sourcebook of new paradigm research. John Wiley, Chichester

Rice C 1992 Strategies and faculty roles for teaching RN students. Nurse Educator 17(1): 33–37

Rodgers B L 1989 Concepts, analysis and the development of nursing knowledge: the evolutionary cycle. Journal of Advanced Nursing 14(4): 330–335

Rodgers C 1983 Freedom to learn for the 80s. Macmillan, New York

Rogers M E 1970 An introduction to the theoretical basis of nursing. F A Davis, Philadelphia

Rosenberg C E 1987 The care of strangers: the rise of America's hospital system. Basic Books, New York

Roy C 1980 The Roy adaptation model. In: Riehl J P, Roy C (eds) Conceptual models for nursing practice. Appleton-Century-Croft, New York

Ruskin J 1865 Sesame and lilies. Oxford University Press, Oxford

Sarkis J M, Skoner M M 1987 An analysis of the concept of holism in nursing literature. Holistic Nursing Practice 2(1): 61–69

Shaver J F 1985 A biopsychosocial view of human health. Nursing Outlook 33(2): 188

Shealy M C 1985 Florence Nightingale 1820–1910: an evolutionary mind in the context of holism. Journal of Holistic Nursing Practice 3(1): 4–6

Smuts J C 1926 Holism and evolution. Macmillan, New York

Taylor E J (ed) 1988 Dorland's illustrated medical dictionary, 27th edn. W B Saunders, Philadelphia

Trevelyan J 1993a Osteopathy. Nursing Times 89(34): 46–48

Trevelyan J 1993b Aromatherapy. Nursing Times 89(25): 38–40

Walsh M 1991 Models in clinical nursing: the way forward. Baillière Tindall, London

Watson J 1979 Nursing: the philosophy and science of caring. Little Brown, Boston

Watson J 1989 Nursing: human science and human care. Appleton-Century-Croft, Norwalk

Webb C 1987 Sexual healing. Nursing Times 86(4): 29–30

Weiss C J 1988 Model to discover, validate, and use care in nursing. In: Leininger M M (ed) Care, discovery and uses in clinical and community nursing. Wayne State University Press, Detroit

Weston A 1993 Challenging assumptions. Nursing Times 89(18): 26–29

White A K 1989 Bringing out the best in all of us. Heart and Lung 18: 27A–30A

Wilson-Barnett I 1988 Nursing values: exploring the clichés. Journal of Advanced Nursing 13(6): 790–796

8

Stress in surgical patients: a physiological perspective

Agnes Hibbert

AIMS

The aims of the chapter are:

- to examine the various approaches to studying aspects of stress in surgical patients
- to describe different methods of measuring stress with emphasis on physiological assessment using levels of hormones as indicators of stress
- to discuss the role of the 'stress' hormone cortisol and the implications of elevated levels for the surgical patient
- to outline the proposed links between stress and health or illness outcomes for the surgical patient
- to analyse critically three studies which set out to study stress by measuring anxiety in patients undergoing surgery.

INTRODUCTION

For patients undergoing surgery, stress may appear to be an inevitable feature of the whole event. Yet it may be useful to consider whether certain practices, such as preoperative procedures or the behaviour of carers, may lead to higher levels of stress. Stress as a concept is difficult to define, but as a response both psychologically and physiologically, it is believed to be experienced with varying degrees of severity. Interactions with the patient may therefore aim at altering the severity of stress or associated emotions such as anxiety or fatigue.

This chapter begins with a description of the various approaches to studying stress, including a discussion of Selye's (1956) work which helped popularise the modern use of the word stress. Selye's theory of stress and adaptation underpins many studies of surgical patients referred to in the literature. His work underpins Roy's (1976) Adaptation Model for nursing practice, which is discussed in Chapter 20. Moving on to physiological and psychological measures of stress, the chapter focuses on endocrine and immune responses, with an outline of the concept of homeostasis which explains changes to a challenging situation such as surgery. As the hypothalamus is the integrating centre of homeostatic mechanisms involving endocrine and immune responses, the hypothalamus and the pathway by which its actions are instigated are further explored. A distinction is made in the chapter between the various hormones which have been associated with stressful situations, namely the catecholamines, adrenaline and noradrenaline, and cortisol. Historically, the catecholamines have become synonymous with stress as a result of the work of Cannon and De La Paz (1911) who described the 'flight or fight' response. This led to many nursing texts describing the patient who, for example, may be facing a surgical procedure as having symptoms such as a rapid heart rate, high blood pressure, dry mouth and dilated pupils. Such responses, however, are more likely to be seen on admission to the ward, rather than during the whole period prior to surgery. This does not necessarily mean that surgical patients are not feeling anxious or that their adrenaline level is not raised. It simply highlights the way responses obtained from animal studies under extreme circumstances, or laboratory studies far removed from normal circumstances, are misinterpreted by suggesting that they resemble the experiences of patients. The chapter will therefore discuss the studies which have tried to establish the significance of elevated levels of hormones. The functions of cortisol, whose levels are shown to be elevated at times of reported anxiety, are considered in more detail and an attempt is made to draw a link between stress and immune responses. This leads on to a suggestion of what the implications of elevated cortisol levels might be for the surgical patient.

An important aspect of traditional scientific research is concerned with generalising about a certain population of people from studies using a sample. The purpose of such research is to assist in understanding the way in which the majority of individuals respond and may therefore be helpful in predicting outcomes following various treatments. It is clear, however, that whilst generalisations can be useful, the importance of individual differences should not be overlooked. Various personal characteristics such as age, sex, state of health, nutritional status, presence of disease, personality, coping styles, as well as the nature of the operation itself, can all influence the patient's response to surgery and recovery back to health. Individuals may therefore differ in their response to the same surgical operation. Highlighting individual differences can pose a challenge to current thinking regarding variables, thus helping to improve experimental measures and the testing of scientific generalisations and hypotheses (Lykken 1976). Several researchers have set out to establish the most appropriate preoperative nursing interventions for bringing about a speedy postoperative recovery. As we shall see from the studies discussed in this chapter, it is difficult to identify a procedure or action which is best for all patients, for such a conclusion is dependent on carefully conducted experiments. The studies, all of which are about surgical patients' responses to stress, illustrate emphatically that the findings of any study are constrained by its design and the literature relied upon for interpreting the results.

MODELS OF STRESS

Three types of model have been used to describe the process underlying stress. The first is known as the Stimulus Model, which describes anxiety-eliciting events (Stokes & Kite 1994). This model has been used to identify factors which are associated with reported feelings of stress by an individual or group of individuals. The disadvantage of this model is that it makes generalised statements about a particular identified factor, or stimulus, whereas what is stressful for one individual may not, in fact, be stressful for another (Montague 1987). Many biological studies approach stress by measuring the response to a stimulus or a 'stressor'. This second approach has been labelled the Response Model and in the main looks at physiological responses to a threat or challenge. For example, the experiments carried out by Selye in the 1930s on rats used the Response Model to evaluate physiological changes to stressors (Selye 1956). A third model called the Transactional Model of stress (Cox & Mackay 1976) is based on individuals' perceptions of the 'stressful' situation and their perceived capabilities of coping with it (Lazarus 1966). In this model, stress is designated to occur only when there is a mismatch between perceived demand and the perceived ability to cope with the demand (Lazarus 1966). The Transactional Model therefore considers that individuals evaluate a situation in the light of their beliefs, experience and their ability to respond. The model encompasses the influence that the individual and the environment have on each other, and takes into account the psychological state of the person more than the Stimulus Model and the Response Model. The definition of stress according to the Transactional Model is similar to that adopted by Lazarus (1971) in that it is the mismatch between individuals' perception of demands and their perception of their resources to cope with it (Stokes & Kite 1994).

Establishing the approach to studying stress is important as it determines the dimension of the findings. For example, studies which set out to identify factors which may influence a person's perception of stress will be able to suggest changes in the behaviour of that person's carers. Similarly, the Transactional Model will enable the researcher to see the person as an individual and approach the study from a truly holistic stance (see also Ch. 7). More specific models related to surgery have been proposed, for example to investigate the possible link between preoperative anxiety and postoperative recovery (Johnston 1988). The models can be described as cognitive–behavioural, communication and psychophysiological. The cognitive–behavioural model provides a framework within which to investigate the way patients think about surgery and the care they receive. It therefore examines motivation, coping strategies and emotions. The communication model incorporates the interpretation of patients' behaviour by medical staff and the consequences of this. For example, the communication model could be used to examine the relationship between anxiety perceived by others or communicated to nursing staff from patients and the postoperative recovery following the subsequent nursing interventions. The psychophysiological model of stress and surgery adopts a holistic perspective. A holistic stance is to see the 'nature of the body as a whole' as entreated by Hippocrates (cited in Cooper 1996). The Transactional Model assesses patients' perceptions of emotions (such as anxiety) and measures physiological changes simultaneously.

Several texts in nursing refer to Selye's work which used the Response Model approach to measure outcomes of stressful stimuli (Selye 1956). As a medical student in the 1920s, Selye was interested in the common symptoms presented by patients rather than the specific ones which aided diagnosis. He named the characteristic signs of illness 'the general sickness syndrome' which included fatigue, general aches and pains and coated tongue (Selye 1976). Selye first published a 'brief note' in 1936, where he categorised stages of the reaction in rats to various chemicals or noxious stimuli, and referred to the responses as a 'general syndrome' (Selye 1976). Selye's work, in turn, was greatly influenced by the findings of Cannon earlier in the century. For example, Selye (1936) described an initial 'alarm reaction' to a noxious stimulus which was similar to the 'flight or fight' response reported by Cannon and De La Paz (1911) where activation of the sympathetic–adrenal–medullary system increased levels of adrenaline and noradrenaline from the adrenal medulla, although in Selye's case he observed changes in the adrenal gland as a whole (Selye 1956). Selye further developed the Response Model, which is underpinned by the concept of homeostasis, whereby the body tries to return the internal environment to normal, by investigating the key processes involved in the reaction to stressors. Montague (1987) gives a concise account of the work by Selye and the possible relevance to clinical practice. In short, the reactions to noxious stimuli in rats were categorised into:

- The *general alarm reaction* where the animal suffered weight loss and the adrenal cortex was depleted of cortisol. If stressful stimuli continued the animal died.
- The first phase was followed by the *stage of resistance* if the animal survived the alarm stage without further noxious stimuli. Selye (1936) suggested that this was the opposite of the first stage as the adrenal cortex hormone had replenished itself, which he concluded after seeing enlarged adrenal glands following dissection at this stage. However, Selye was unaware at the time that cortisol, a steroid, is not stored and therefore this could not possibly be the adaptation phase suggested.
- If the noxious stimuli continued, the animal entered into the *stage of exhaustion* which was similar in signs to the alarm stage.

The three stages were called the general adaptation syndrome, which describes the several effects on the body of non-specific stimuli. The animal was, according to Selye, showing adaptation to the stressors and these responses may be coordinated. From a clinical point of view, Selye (1976) suggested that patients undergoing stress such as surgery can develop the adaptive defensive mechanisms necessary to overcome the stressor.

Issues raised by Selye's work

1. The adaptive responses to stress must include behavioural and psychological responses in an attempt to re-establish homeostasis (Johnson et al 1992). Therefore omission of psychological measurement in stress research is outmoded (Baum et al 1982). Selye (1956), for example, included no psychological measure of stress, which was later shown to be important in physiological responses in other animals (Mason 1968b).

2. It is difficult to extrapolate findings from one animal model to another, and especially to humans, and although Selye's (1956) findings have not been reported using other animals, Mason (1959, cited in Mason 1968b) found monkeys habituated, that is,

became used to a stimulus such as a continuous stressor; this was not the case with rats. It was postulated by Manyande et al (1995) that preoperative preparation to reduce anxiety may sensitise cortisol and adrenaline responses to surgery. However, whether humans habituate to stressful stimuli or can be sensitised to them is still a matter of speculation.

3. Selye (1956) used high doses of biochemical agents foreign to the animal and this could nowadays be considered 'unphysiological' and therefore not comparable to real-life concentrations of hormones. The experiments were also laboratory studies under controlled conditions, whereas field studies carried out in the normal environment for human subjects move closer towards reflecting real responses (Vingerhoets & Marcelissen 1988). Field studies on humans have already begun to show markedly different levels of hormone responses to stress compared to those measured in laboratory controlled experiments (Pollard et al 1992).

Nevertheless, Selye paved the way for discussing the possible effects of stress on health and illness outcomes. Selye (1976) also suggested that adaptation is a normal response and inappropriate responses may result in 'diseases of adaptation'. The link between the endocrine and immune systems was postulated by Selye (1976) referring to chronic conditions associated with the inflammatory response, such as rheumatoid arthritis. This link between the endocrine and immune systems through the central nervous system has gained popularity and continues to be investigated to this day, particularly in relation to stress (Steptoe 1991).

> **Reflective point**
>
> How do you think the points raised by Selye's work apply to other studies on stress?

MEASURING STRESS

Psychological assessment tools

Psychological assessment tools for measuring stress fall into two main categories: those that rely on self-reporting of subjective feelings, and those which measure performance. Performance measures assess the effects of stress on some ability or skill, e.g. problem-solving (Meijman & O'Hanlon 1984). The limitation of using mental tasks in performance measures is the lack of an agreed typology of mental workload,

that is, the degree of taxing the mind (Meijman & O'Hanlon 1984).

In addition to assessing emotions or affective states, self-report measures can be used to determine life events associated with stress. For example, negative life events, such as death of a loved one or divorce, can be assessed in relation to health outcomes (Holmes & Rahe 1967). The Social Readjustment Rating Scale (SRRS) was designed to measure major life events (Holmes & Rahe 1967). Daily life events, on the other hand, have different instruments which can measure activities during the day that may be stress inducing (Sarasen et al 1978). For example, the Daily Hassles Scale (Kanner et al 1981) claims to be predictive of stress, as physical symptoms are correlated with reports of hassles (Lazarus et al 1985, cited in Pennebaker & Watson 1988). The SRRS and the Daily Hassles Scale identify stressors which are related to stress or ill health. A similar tool was developed to identify specific events which were stressful to patients and ranked them according to severity (Volicer & Bohannon 1975). Examples of specific events which were ranked as most stressful included 'thinking you may lose your sight', 'thinking you may lose a kidney or some other organ' and 'not having your questions answered by staff'. Examples of the least stressful events included 'having strangers sleep in the same room' and 'having to wear a hospital gown'.

Psychological measures of stress and well-being

Psychological measures of stress can include the assessment of emotions such as anxiety, fatigue and depression, which are associated with perceived stress (Pennebaker 1982). Pennebaker & Watson (1988) found that self-reports of physical symptoms related to stress, such as headaches, general aches and pains, dizziness and difficulty in concentrating, correlated highly with perceived stress. The degree of emotions or symptoms could be used to determine the amount of stress (Baum et al 1982). In other words, a self-report of emotions or physical symptoms such as headaches and aches and pains can provide a direct access to subjective experiences associated with stress and can be used to assess well-being (Morrison & Peck 1990).

Physiological assessment

Both the Response Model and the Transactional Model consider stress to be initiated by increased demand or challenge. Such demand is detected by the body and results in imbalance of the internal environment. Homeostasis refers to the mechanisms involved in bringing about a state of equilibrium following changes in the internal or external environment, so restoring the body to an optimal functioning level.

HOMEOSTASIS

Homeostasis was described by Cannon and Britton in 1927 as the processes involved in maintaining a stable internal environment. This requires integration and coordination of all the organs and systems of the body. The coordinated homeostatic mechanisms depend upon good communication between an integrating centre and the various actions or responses of the systems. Figure 8.1 shows that homeostatic mechanisms consist of a receptor to detect any changes internally or externally to the body. This information is relayed to an integrating centre where a coordinated response is communicated via nervous and endocrine pathways to an effector, for example increasing activity of an endocrine gland. Regulating the response relies on a feedback mechanism to the integrating centre which is essential for coordination.

The hypothalamus is an integrating centre which controls homeostatic mechanisms. The hypothalamus receives information about changes in the internal and external environment and initiates processes which maintain a balance between input and output. Figure 8.1 shows a schematic view of the integrating centre which receives information, e.g. neural information via afferent nerves, or in the case of the endocrine system, chemicals in the blood. The appropriate response is relayed by efferent pathways, that is, messages are sent via the nervous system to the effector, e.g. an

organ, muscle or gland. An endocrine response involves releasing-hormones from the hypothalamus which stimulate the anterior pituitary to release hormones directed at specific tissue types. A neuroendocrine response involving the hypothalamus and posterior pituitary is an example of the close relationship between the nervous system and the endocrine system. This relationship, together with the integration of the immune system, is described concisely by Griffen & Ojeda (1996). The hypothalamus plays a particularly important role in regulating homeostatic mechanisms associated with stress (Dallman et al 1992). Box 8.1 lists some of the many functions of the hypothalamus.

An example of the role of the hypothalamus in regulating homeostatic mechanisms is temperature control. Alterations in environmental temperature will result in effector responses such as changes in behaviour (e.g. curling up if cold or removing clothing if hot), stimulation or inhibition of mechanisms concerned with sweating, skeletal muscle contraction, dilatation or constriction of blood vessels near the skin surface influencing the amount of radiated heat loss. The hypothalamus regulates these effector responses in order to maintain the constant body temperature necessary for optimal cellular functioning.

In addition to being an example of maintaining a constant internal environment, temperature regulation also demonstrates that homeostasis is about maintaining a balance between input and output even if the equilibrium point is at a higher absolute value. If the hypothalamus has a new 'set point' at a temperature level that is higher than usual, homeostatic mechanisms will bring about changes to raise the body temperature and maintain this temperature at the new level. A temporary increase in temperature may be seen, for example, in patients following surgery. This is brought about by release of cytokines (chemicals released from cells, principally immune cells) or microorganisms. It is not entirely clear why the

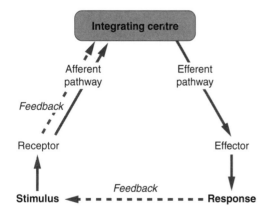

Figure 8.1 Schematic view of homeostasis (adapted from Hinwood 1993).

Box 8.1 Functions of the hypothalamus

- Produces hormones which are stored in the posterior pituitary
- Influences the activity of the anterior pituitary by producing releasing factors which stimulate production of hormones
- Regulates body temperature
- Controls eating (appetite) and drinking (thirst) behaviour
- Is involved in emotional and motivational behaviour

cytokines influence a new higher set point but it is now considered to be an adaptive response. Although careful monitoring of the body temperature postoperatively is important to detect any changes from the body's normal range of 36.1–37.8°C, efforts are no longer made to reduce the temporary slight pyrexia.

PRINCIPAL PATHWAY ACTIVATED DURING STRESS

The principal pathway activated in response to stressful events is the hypothalamic–pituitary–adrenal (HPA) axis, illustrated in Figure 8.2, which incorporates both the nervous and endocrine systems. The HPA axis is activated by stimuli to the hypothalamus, the categories of which are also shown in Figure 8.2. Two distinct components make up the HPA axis: first, the sympathetic–adrenal medullary (SAM) system involving release of catecholamines, principally adrenaline and noradrenaline, and second, the pituitary–adrenal cortical (PAC) system, which alters levels of corticosteroids such as cortisol (Mason 1968a,b).

Cannon and De La Paz (1911) reported an increase in the catecholamines, adrenaline and noradrenaline, in response to emotional stimuli as well as preparedness by the organism to perceived threat, which they termed the 'fight or flight' response. The activation of the SAM system was accompanied by many physiological changes, such as increased pulse rate, increased blood pressure, dilatation of pupils, inhibition of gastrointestinal function and increased sweating. These physiological changes are often quoted in the literature as signs and symptoms of stress; however, some of the changes are related to other factors, for example pulse rate increases with physical exertion, while blood pressure elevation may be associated with disease. Such arousal is seen at times of immediate threat and has become synonymous with acute challenge.

Catecholamines as markers of stress

Adrenaline and noradrenaline have frequently been used as markers of stress (Baum et al 1982). For example, increased catecholamine levels were seen in patients on the first day of hospital admission but these declined once individuals were accustomed to the new environment (Tolsen et al 1965). In addition to measuring hormones, however, other signs and symptoms can be quantified, for example from self-reports of physical symptoms or the objective measure of the palmar sweat test. Although palmar sweating has been associated with stress, Johnston (1975, unpublished work, cited in Johnston 1988) reported that differences in palmar sweating in surgical patients did not correlate with 'fear' or anxiety but with arousal. Surgical patients who were trained in relaxation techniques had greater adrenaline levels, measured increased activity and made a quicker recovery (Wilson 1981). These findings are consistent with a series of experiments by a Swedish team led by Frankenhauser in the late 1970s and early 1980s, who demonstrated that adrenaline secretion equated with effort whereas cortisol secreted from the adrenal cortex was associated with distress and reported feelings of anxiety (Lundberg & Frankenhauser 1980). Increases in adrenaline and noradrenaline and their effects are often quoted as a response to stress. However, several workers now believe that elevated levels are indications of effort or arousal in a new situation rather than necessarily always being associated with negative events (Shulkin et al 1994).

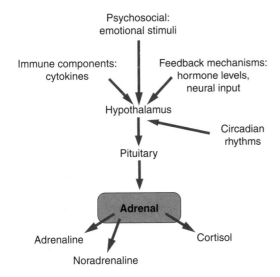

Figure 8.2 The hypothalamic–pituitary–adrenal axis.

Reflective point

How would you assess patients' feelings over time during their stay in hospital? If the majority of patients are anxious on admission to hospital, what may help to reduce this anxiety?

Glucocorticoids as markers of stress

The second component of the HPA axis is the pituitary–adrenal cortical system where activity was particularly demonstrated to be related to stress (Selye 1936). Frankenhauser (1980) demonstrated that distress without effort, that is, raised cortisol, and unchanged adrenaline and noradrenaline levels, results in stress. Raised circulatory cortisol levels are therefore interpreted as an indication of stress (Baum et al 1982). Cortisol levels are therefore a useful indicator of stress and steroid hormone concentrations have been measured both in blood and in urine (Wild 1994). However, more sensitive experiments have enabled cortisol to be quantified using saliva. The non-invasive method of collecting a sample makes this an ideal technique for field studies and it may be a valuable tool for studying stress in patients in the future. Levels of cortisol have been shown to be raised during severe exercise but psychological variables such as emotions are the most potent stimuli for cortisol release (Mason 1968b).

ACTIONS OF CORTISOL

At times of stress new demands are placed on the body to maintain changes such as increased heart rate, respiratory efficiency and the provision of energy substrates. Regulatory mechanisms are activated which play a role in the synthesis of complex substances (anabolism), for example new tissue growth in a surgical wound, or enzymes concerned with driving the metabolic pathways to provide energy needed for other processes. All cellular processes require energy and the demand increases at times of trauma or surgery. Complex substances such as proteins and fats are broken down (catabolism) in many tissues in order to provide molecules which are usable for energy production. For instance, the fasted state of the surgical patient preoperatively will result in mobilisation of amino acids from proteins, providing substrates for the synthesis of glucose. This process is referred to as gluconeogenesis, where production of glucose is from non-carbohydrate sources such as amino acids and fatty acids. Gluconeogenesis predominantly occurs in the liver and results in maintaining blood glucose levels. The regulatory mechanisms ensure that glucose is made available for the brain whilst simultaneously maintaining stores in other tissues. These mechanisms are influenced by glucocorticoids such as cortisol, which alter carbohydrate, protein and fat metabolism.

Cortisol has several functions: it plays a key role in metabolic processes particularly in response to stress; it is involved in the immune response in resistance to noxious stimuli; it affects mineralocorticoid activity and excretion of water load; and it influences cardiovascular tone. The ability of cortisol to be so versatile is due to direct activity on the cells concerned as well as facilitating permissive and suppressive actions of other hormones (Greenspan & Baxter 1994). Anabolic and catabolic actions are insulin-dependent, demonstrating how cortisol interacts with other hormones in order to exert its effects. Cortisol may have a stimulatory effect, stimulating enzymes concerned with gluconeogenesis, increasing hepatic glucose production from products of anaerobic respiration and protein and fat breakdown. Cortisol may also have a permissive effect as it increases hepatic responsiveness to hormones such as glucagon and catecholamines, stimulating gluconeogenesis. In other tissues, such as adipose tissue, cortisol stimulates lipolysis, mobilising fatty acids, perhaps by potentiating the effects of catecholamines (Berne & Levy 1997).

Elevated levels of cortisol will therefore maintain circulatory glucose levels, which ensure that vital areas of the body, such as the brain, are protected against sudden increased demands for energy. These mechanisms conserve carbohydrate resources and stores, for example by synthesising glycogen whilst simultaneously inhibiting its breakdown. Physiologically, then, elevated cortisol levels may be a useful adaptive response. On the other hand, cortisol is associated with negative affective states, for example anxiety (Frankenhauser 1980). From an evolutionary perspective, such emotions may have been an important signal to protect the organism in some way by ensuring withdrawal from the situation where possible. This may suggest that although elevated cortisol levels are adaptive, prolonged exposure is not. Surgical patients are exposed to elevated levels of cortisol and depending on the type of surgery this may be for a considerable time (Slade et al 1975). What is difficult to determine is whether elevated cortisol levels place surgical patients at greater risk of tissue harm or increase patients' susceptibility to infection.

Implications of elevated cortisol levels

The initial metabolic response to trauma such as surgery is dominated by direct effects of adrenaline and noradrenaline as well as cortisol and its effects on insulin and glucagon. Peripherally, glucocorticoids antagonise effects of insulin on glucose uptake in muscle and adipose tissue (Laycock & Wise 1996). Insulin secretion is increased if there is chronic glucocorticoid excess. The increase in levels of insulin may be interpreted as a change in the resistance to a hormone. Insulin resistance at the peripheral tissues occurs so glucose is destined for brain and cardiac tissue (Halpin 1988). The time period for such changes is longer term than the effects of, say, catecholamines. The insulin increase may take more than 1 week to peak and may be accompanied by insulin resistance. However, insulin resistance is seen in patients who have been 'nil by mouth' prior to surgery (Halpin 1988). Elevated cortisol levels would therefore not only increase blood glucose levels, but also result in insulin resistance, particularly in peripheral tissues. Although surgery may result in only a temporarily elevated plasma cortisol level, some individuals with particular disorders display a type of exaggerated response (hyperreactivity); that is, they have 'vulnerable' systems (Steptoe 1991). Examples of disorders which may cause some individuals to display disturbances to elevated hormone levels are diabetes mellitus, hypertension and myocardial ischaemia. It therefore suggests that elevated cortisol levels in surgical patients with underlying conditions may not be adaptive but potentially harmful.

Cortisol is particularly active in the fasted state where glucocorticoids maintain plasma glucose levels and glycogen disposition (Laycock & Wise 1996), although glucocorticoids increase glycogen in the liver in both the fed and fasted states (Felig et al 1987). There may be several reasons why starvation of patients occurs. The underlying condition may reduce the appetite prior to admission to hospital. The surgical patient may not have eaten for some time because of being nil by mouth prior to surgery and before diagnostic tests as well as immediately postoperatively. The surgical patient might have a wound or injury and may possibly have an infection, and these demands increase catabolism (Kispert 1992). The surgical patient therefore has increased breakdown of large molecules such as proteins in order to provide the necessary glucose needed to drive metabolic and chemical processes. Cortisol ensures that circulatory glucose levels are maintained, and insulin resistance at peripheral tissues results in reduced uptake of glucose from the blood. High blood glucose levels can have detrimental effects on wound healing (MacSween & Whaley 1992).

The increased rate of metabolism and protein breakdown following trauma and surgery was first suggested over 100 years ago by Malcolm (Kispert 1992). In the 1930s the measurement of nitrogen (excreted) after trauma demonstrated changes in the balance of protein. Cuthbertson (1932) named responses following trauma to muscle 'ebb' and 'flow' phases after recognising that the components excreted

were similar to those of skeletal muscle. Cuthbertson suggested that the 'ebb' phase decreases metabolism at a period during cardiovascular shock following injury. The 'flow' phase saw an increased metabolism, raised temperature, elevated blood sugar and increased pulse and respiratory rate, and increased excretion of nitrogen, sulphur and potassium in the urine, indicating protein breakdown. The similarities between these symptoms and those seen postoperatively led to the belief that the nitrogen excreted was due to stress, and that surgery results in large skeletal muscle losses. However, improved techniques allowed the isolation of an amino acid which reflects skeletal muscle breakdown. By measuring the amino acid from the muscle and that excreted in urine before and after surgery, Rennie et al (1984) showed the nitrogen loss could not be solely from skeletal muscle.

The relationship between protein breakdown as a whole and the various tissues is a complex one. Although it appears that there is an overall catabolism which must involve the skeletal muscle mass, the amount of involvement seems to be dependent on several other factors, such as the illness itself. Changes in protein stores and metabolism therefore occur in surgery where glucocorticoids such as cortisol are likely to play a major role. These responses could be adaptive responses; however, it is clear that undernourished patients prior to surgery will be placed in a more vulnerable position (Windsor 1993). This emphasises the importance of objective measurements of nutritional status, which in some cases may include hepatic secretions of proteins in addition to anthropometric evaluation to ascertain whether protein–calorie malnutrition is present prior to surgery (Baker et al 1982).

Other effects of glucocorticoids are seen in more extreme circumstances where levels may be excessive or deficient. However, these effects are findings from either animal studies or in vitro assays (test-tube experiments) which are not always reflected in vivo, where tests are completed on reactions which have occurred in the body. The significance to the surgical patient therefore remains questionable. Nevertheless, there is an increased speculation as to whether it is these pathways and processes which account for why some patients make a poor postoperative recovery. Box 8.2 lists suggestions of the possible links between elevated cortisol levels and a poor outcome postoperatively for the surgical patient.

In addition to the association between psychophysiological pathways and stress, recent work has turned its attention to psychoneuroimmunology (Ader et al 1991). There is evidence that psychological factors influence immune function (Ader et al 1991, Jemmott & Locke 1984).

Box 8.2 Possible links between elevated cortisol levels and poor postoperative outcome

1. Glucocorticoids such as cortisol regulate glucose metabolism, albeit secondary to insulin, which influences blood glucose levels and protects against glucose deprivation. Elevated cortisol levels therefore have a protective role in stressed states, e.g. hypoglycaemia seen in undernourished patients or in times of increased demands such as surgery. The increased hepatic glycogen and glucose production from excess glucocorticoids and decrease in glucose uptake and utilisation in peripheral tissues results in a tendency for hyperglycaemia and decreased carbohydrate tolerance. Increased levels of blood glucose may increase the risk of poor wound healing postoperatively as seen in diabetic patients (Young 1988). The effects of insulin resistance may increase susceptibility to diabetes mellitus in some individuals who respond in a hyperactive manner to elevated levels of cortisol (Steptoe 1991).

2. Cortisol excess is involved in regulation of salt metabolism by binding to aldosterone receptors on renal tubular target cells. Glucocorticoids may increase the glomerular plasma flow rate by acting on the vasculature, thereby increasing the glomerular filtration rate, resulting in water loss and dehydration of tissues. So far there is yet to be established a strong or well-defined relationship between cortisol secretion and water excretion seen in humans (Pollard 1993).

3. Glucocorticoids have also been associated with increased systemic vascular tone, resulting in high blood pressure possibly through potentiating vasoconstrictor effects of catecholamines and antidiuretic hormone (ADH). Elevated adrenocorticotrophic hormone (ACTH) levels and subsequent increase in glucocorticoids seen in chronic stress suggest a possible relationship between the development of hypertension and HPA axis stimulation (Gamallo et al 1988). These findings were derived from studies on rats and, to date, transient elevated levels of cortisol have not been shown to be associated with hypertension in humans. However, individuals with underlying disorders such as myocardial ischaemia have been shown to react differently to raised hormone levels (Steptoe 1991).

In a series of studies on stress and social deprivation, immune responses were seen to differ in individuals who reported less support and more stress (Kiecolt-Glaser & Glaser 1988, cited in O'Leary 1990). The link between stress and illness which concerns psychological influences has been extensively studied. Immunological changes in healthy individuals undergoing surgery have been reported, demonstrating that it was surgery itself rather than the presence of disease which altered immune functioning (Bradley & Calman 1988). Surgery will therefore bring about immunological changes, the significance of which is not entirely clear (Ballieux 1994). Indirectly determined factors related to personality type, perception of the event and coping style play a significant role in the stress-induced changes in immune responses (Ballieux 1994). Certain immune changes are measured alongside psychological measures, for example changes in numbers of total lymphocytes or subsets. The activity of immune cells such as natural killer (NK) cells to allergens, or macrophage function, may be measured in induced stress states, or one parameter of behaviour is compared to several immune responses (Kusnecov & Rabin 1994). Surgical stress has been shown to alter a variety of immune parameters, which include alteration in natural killer cell activity, macrophage function and cytokine production (Kusnecov & Rabin 1994).

However, the link between stress and immune response may be explained through the actions of cortisol. Cortisol has been shown to alter immune responses when pharmacological levels such as steroid treatments are used. The mechanisms through which cortisol exerts its effects on the immune system may be active when cortisol is elevated during times of stress as seen in surgical patients. The question is whether these effects significantly affect the patients' susceptibility to infection, and if so, whether they can be altered if psychological factors are such potent stimuli.

Effects of cortisol on immune responses

Increased illness was reported after stressful life events (Holmes & Rahe 1967). This finding led to further work on quantifying stress and its association with increased susceptibility to illness and infection (Khansari et al 1990). Several hormones are altered at times of stress but the pituitary–adrenal cortical (PAC) system and glucocorticoids have been the most extensively studied (Mason 1968b). Figure 8.3 shows a schematic view of the possible links between the three systems.

The action of hormones is mediated by components of the immune system and, in turn, hormones such as cortisol influence the immune response. In pharmacological concentrations, cortisol is inhibitory rather than permissive, preventing the stages of the inflammatory response which are shown in Box 8.3.

High concentrations of cortisol inhibit the stages of the inflammatory process (Box 8.3) and also decrease the number of lymphocytes which are involved in both humoral (e.g. antibody-producing) and cell-mediated immune responses. Basophils and eosinophils are also reduced in number. The actions of these two types of cells help regulate the inflammatory

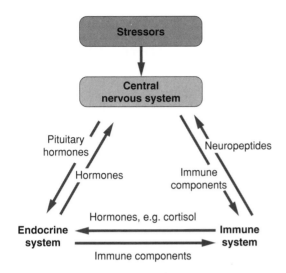

Figure 8.3   Influence of stressors on endocrine and immune systems (adapted from Immunology Today 11(5) Khansari et al, Effects of stress on the immune system, 170–175 (1990) with permission from Elsevier Science).

Box 8.3   Stages of the inflammatory response

- Increased permeability of capillaries.
- Diffusion of plasma-like fluid.
- Migration of white blood cells (WBCs) into the area.
- Lysosomal membranes in WBC rupture releasing enzymes.
- Proteolytic enzymes destroy damaged cells.

---

response by regulating the release of substances such as heparin, histamine and bradykinin, which influence blood clotting and blood vessel permeability. However, cortisol increases neutrophils which play a role in phagocytosis ('cell eating'), for example where foreign microorganisms are engulfed, as well as red blood cells (RBC) and platelets. Cortisol also inhibits synthesis and release of histamine from tissue mast cells, which originate from the basophils in the blood and are responsible for alleviating the effects of an allergic response. A protein synthesised in response to cortisol action on immune cells is known to inhibit the enzyme responsible for the production of the precursor molecule of prostaglandins and leukotrienes.

Prostaglandins and leukotrienes are both synthesised from arachidonic acid, which is a molecule found in cells in almost every organ of the body (Colbert 1993). Prostaglandins are biologically active lipids which are important intracellular mediators acting as local hormones. In addition to playing an important role in the immune response, prostaglandins are involved in a vast number of biological reactions which include: haemostasis, fever, control of blood vessel diameter, bronchial diameter, uterine contraction and cervical dilatation, and electrolyte and water absorption in kidneys and the gastrointestinal tract (Colbert 1993). Leukotrienes are involved in the inflammatory response and activation of platelets in blood clotting (Griffen & Ojeda 1996). Chemicals released from lymphocytes in an immune response, such as interleukin 1 (IL-1), interleukin 2 (IL-2) and gamma interferon (IFNγ) are influenced by glucocorticoids (Besedorsky et al 1986). In turn, receptors for IL-1, IL-2 and IFNγ have been found on tissue other than immune cells including endocrine glands (Abraham 1991). Cortisol, therefore, modulates the immune response by directly influencing synthesis of prostaglandins and cytokine production, and affects the action of other hormones. In turn, the products of the immune responses may regulate the hypothalamic–pituitary–adrenal cortical axis (Munck & Guyre 1991).

Activation of the above components is, however, reported from studies using pharmacological levels of cortisol. Munck et al (1984) suggested a move away from seeing cortisol as an anti-inflammatory agent unless used in such doses. They postulated that glucocorticoids actually protect the body from damage by various actions on the immune and endocrine systems, thereby preventing mechanisms from overshooting. They describe the effects of glucocorticoids as demonstrating a homeostatic mechanism which is permissive at low concentrations and suppressive at high ones. In a study measuring postoperative circadian rhythms and cortisol stress response in two types of cardiac surgery, Lanuza (1995) discusses prolonged elevation of plasma cortisol adversely affecting health because of its anti-inflammatory actions and antipyrogenic properties. However, this is clearly referring to actions of cortisol at pharmacological levels. Whilst the levels reported by Lanuza (1995) were elevated, they were not equivalent to pharmacological doses. What may have been of significance, however, is the relatively long period of time for which these elevated levels were sustained. Similar arguments were put forward by Boore (1976) to account for increased infection in patients who reported more stress. However, only animal studies were referred to in support of such claims. Further work is needed to investigate everyday levels of cortisol and their relationship to immune responses in patients undergoing surgery.

The effects of stress on the nervous, endocrine and immune responses are important for surgical patients if susceptibility to illness and infection is increased. Sepsis, for example, is a major problem in critical illness (Schkichtig & Ayres 1988). Immune responses must be intact to promote recovery. The cells of the immune system must work optimally. For example, a rapid response from macrophages is needed, as these cells are responsible for integrating responses between the B cells and T cells. T cells also need to be efficient as they are necessary for recognising invading antigens or infectious agents, generating lymphokines, and are involved in the synthesis and activation of B cells (antibody production). Other organs must also be functioning at an optimum level, as they may be concerned with providing the materials necessary for immune responses. For example, the liver manufactures proteins such as the coagulation factors involved in blood clotting. Complement components which play a major role in opsonisation, a process which aids phagocytosis, as well as escalating and integrating the immune response, are synthesised in the liver.

Increase in protein synthesis, necessary for the above functions, has been reported in surgical patients (Schkichtig & Ayres 1988). Stores of proteins are therefore in constant flux with a resultant metabolic cost for this turnover. The primary source for increased protein synthesis is from endogenously derived amino acids which appear to be from skeletal muscle (40% of total body protein) and 60% from dietary protein. During periods of starvation, such as prior to surgery in some patients, all synthesis comes from endogenous sources. This would place these particular patients at risk of not being able to maintain protein synthesis necessary for immune functioning and hence may increase their susceptibility to infection postoperatively.

STUDIES OF STRESS IN SURGICAL PATIENTS

A stimulus approach to identifying stressors

Using the Hospital Stress Rating Scale (HSRS), Volicer et al (1977) reported that surgical patients were more stressed than medical patients. The instrument was used to pinpoint the experiences which were stressful for surgical patients, for example not getting relief from pain medication was ranked 10th out of 49 events. However, comparing responses to stress between surgical and medical patients presents great difficulties, as there are several factors, including age and genetic make-up of the individual, which may account for any changes measured (Steptoe 1991).

Surgery could be considered a stressful event because of the major changes to the physical and psychological well-being of the person. Various methods are used to assess the amount of stress a person may perceive and, further, to identify specific stressors for surgical patients. Volicer & Bohannon (1975) devised a Hospital Stress Rating Scale (HSRS). The HSRS was proposed as a tool to identify the specific events or items which both medical and surgical patients found most stressful. The tool was developed using the Holmes and Rahe (1967) Social Readjustment Rating Scale (SRRS) as a basis. Similarly to the SRRS, the HSRS listed a number of events which the patients were asked to score in terms of most to least stressful. However, the tool was developed using American patients' responses, which may be different from what UK patients would identify and rank. For example, a major worry for patients in the US using the HSRS was 'not having enough insurance to pay for your hospitalisation'. This may not apply to UK patients using the National Health Service, although UK patients may still have financial concerns due to hospitalisation.

A response-based approach using a cognitive–behavioural perspective to study anxiety

In a study of nurses' perceptions of stress in preoperative surgical patients, Biley (1989) found that nurses were not accurate in perceiving stress in their patients. Nurses consistently overestimated the anxieties of patients. These findings were consistent with research by Johnston (1982, cited in Johnston 1988) with the exception of major worries where nurses were fairly accurate in predicting those which were important to the patient. In addition to the results from this study being drawn from a small sample, there are other limitations. Suggesting questions to patients may result in 'false positives' where the patients and the nurses respond to questions which they may not have considered. Patients may even under-report their anxieties and they may not wish to admit to anxiety (Johnston 1988). Furthermore, it would be important to consider individual differences. Nevertheless, Biley (1989) suggests that general stress reduction could be beneficial, rather than attempting to identify specific responses to stress. In other words, individual differences are not taken into account.

Biley's (1989) study highlights that patients' actual worries may not coincide with nurses' perceptions of their worries. Although tools are available for nurses to assess anxiety and worry, they appear to make little use of them (Johnston 1988). Nurses may, however, assess a patient's anxiety levels in an overall assessment and not treat it as a separate entity. However, the findings by Biley (1989) of the principal stressors for surgical patients do not match those identified in an earlier study conducted by Carr & Powers (1986). This may suggest that different studies might identify different 'priorities' of stressors, demonstrating that the findings are dependent on the right questions. For instance, Johnston (1988) reported that factor analysis demonstrated that surgical patients did feel more stressed than medical patients and that the loss of independence was the major stressor for the majority of surgical patients, but that this needed to be asked.

There have been a number of studies which measure self-reports of anxiety and compare these with outcome or recovery. For example, a comparison of patients' anxiety levels showed that those patients with higher anxiety levels required more anaesthesia (Williams et al 1975). Hayward (1975) suggested that more analgesia was requested postoperatively by patients who were anxious prior to surgery. These are two fairly typical studies which use the request for analgesia as an indicator of poor recovery. It is questionable, however, whether such a request is a sign of poor recovery. It would be interesting to carry out similar experiments in which there is patient-controlled analgesia and a shift in the locus of control to the patient. Recovery may not be linked so much to the need for analgesia but more to coping strategies and the need to feel in control of one's condition (see also Ch. 2). Patients taken through imagery experienced less pain, were less distressed, requested less analgesia and felt that they coped better (Manyande et al 1995).

The Transactional Model – a psychophysiological perspective to study anxiety

Immune responses may alter susceptibility to infections, which may be directly related to elevated cortisol levels. Boore (1976) set out to examine preoperative interventions which reduce anxiety in surgical patients. Although there were limitations in the method, the study warrants further discussion. Its aim was to test whether interventions prior to surgery, such as giving information, influenced postoperative recovery. Boore (1976) measured physiological parameters associated with stress, which in this case was a derivative of cortisol, 17-hydroxycorticosteroid (17-OHCS), in the urine of surgical patients. One group of patients who received guidance regarding postoperative leg exercises, deep breathing and what to expect were compared with another group who received none of this information. Boore (1976) reported results where elevated levels of 17-OHCS in patients who received no information also coincided with a greater incidence of complications after surgery, such as respiratory infections, deep vein thrombosis and wound infections.

However, the study has a number of limitations. First, the effect of urine flow rates on urinary hormone concentrations is not entirely clear (Pollard 1993) and the approach used by Boore (1976) gives no indication of the reliability or validity of the method. Second, it is assumed that giving information to patients prior to surgery is the same for all recipients. However, patient reports show that receiving information about the surgery was not as important as the outcome of the operation and concerns about family and home (Johnston 1988). In other words, it was the practical or psychosocial consequences of operation that were most worrying for patients. Thirdly, the main aim of giving information prior to surgery is to reduce anxiety and aid recovery. However, there has been variable success with giving information preoperatively to patients. Johnston (1988) gives a comprehensive account of studies which investigate different personality types and coping styles with the variable responses to giving information as an intervention. Only one out of nine studies measuring the effects of giving information on reducing anxiety showed a positive relationship (Johnston 1988). Finally, nurses were the ones who gave information to surgical patients in Boore's (1976) study when research assistants could not be obtained. The nurses were asked to give information dispassionately in order that only the act of giving information intervention could be tested. The study was therefore not about nurses giving information but rather the intervention itself.

Reflective point

How appropriate is it to provide care in a dispassionate way? Do you think nurses give information in a different way from other carers? How would you go about identifying what it is that nurses do differently from others?

From a physiological perspective the interpretation of levels of hormones requires careful consideration. For instance, Boore (1976) interpreted higher levels of urinary 17-OHCS as an indication of increased anxiety and a worse outcome postoperatively. By contrast, Udelsman et al (1986) suggested that high levels of corticosteroids in primates after surgery did not result in a worse outcome such as inhibiting wound healing, whereas lowering levels resulted in a clear disadvantage. Boore (1976) assumed that elevated levels of 17-OHCS accounted for increased infections because of its inhibitory effects on the immune system. However, Mason (1968b) had already challenged this view, suggesting that only pharmacological doses of cortisol inhibited the immune system and real-life levels of cortisol played more of a permissive role. The lack of detail of the type, severity and time of infections of the patients with higher levels of 17-OHCS mentioned in Boore's (1976) study, as well as the circumstances surrounding these infections, makes it difficult to comment further. However, Jenner & Richards (1985) suggested that increased cortisol levels, which are associated with infection, would be maladaptive if they inhibited the immune response but may play a role in regulating the response to an invading antigen. A study by Slade et al (1975) showed depression of the immune response after major surgery in normal patients; clinically, however, significant problems such as increased infection rate did not arise. Poor correlation was seen between cellular immunity activity and postoperative infection (Slade et al 1975). There are, however, many factors which influence infection and the true complexity of the physiological mechanisms involved may be more difficult to grasp (Munck et al 1984); for instance, not all immune responses are regulated by glucocorticoids.

Another study involving physiological measurement and information-giving was designed to assess the effects of music treatment on salivary cortisol in patients exposed to pre-surgical stress (Miluk-Kolasa et al 1994). Salivary cortisol was measured in patients receiving information about the surgery about to be performed the following day. The 34 patients were split into two groups. One group listened to a selected music programme after being given information and the other group did not listen to music. The information received resulted in a 50% rise in salivary cortisol within 15 minutes. The cortisol levels of the group not listening to music gradually decreased but remained higher than the original level 1 hour later. The group listening to music showed a marked reduction in salivary cortisol which after 1 hour was similar to non-surgical patients. What is interesting about this study is that it suggests that music may have a positive effect on patients by reducing cortisol levels more quickly.

CONCLUSION

For the nurse caring for the surgical patient, a thorough assessment of the patient's needs is of paramount importance. Nursing models may offer a framework within which to carry out an assessment from a holistic perspective, but there is a need for development of tools specifically for assessing anxiety in surgical patients to which nurses can gain access. A critical analysis of studies which purport to identify the most appropriate nursing interventions for reducing stress and improving patient care serve only to highlight the complexity of the phenomenon. Such studies reveal problems associated with experimental design, limitations of available research tools, and difficulties in trying to establish a relationship between findings associated with stress and the nursing care given. Perhaps the best example of a study requiring careful methodology and interpretation of data is provided by Boore (1976). The study demonstrated among other things difficulties in isolating the different variables impinging on the surgical patient's situation, as well as the need for reliable and valid instruments and appropriate literature for interpreting the results.

Similar problems are encountered by researchers who use physiological measures to try to demonstrate the links between stress and illness. From a physiological perspective, the recent discovery of receptors on cells which play a part in the immune response and endocrine activity suggests it may only be a matter of time before establishing the links between stress and susceptibility to illness. Improved experimental design within traditional scientific methodology may provide one approach to determining what constitutes appropriate nursing interventions for surgical patients in the future. As nurses are faced with an increasing demand to provide evidence-based care, it may be opportune to take a closer look at what scientific research can offer. Furthermore, there is a need to identify precisely what it is that nurses do before any attempt can be made to quantify how well they do it in terms of measuring patient outcome. Nevertheless, the tools needed for the psychological and physiological assessment of the patient awaiting surgery currently lack sophistication and are in need of further refining. This opens the way for surgical nurses to consider how to develop tools of assessment and to investigate the procedures and interventions which will enhance patient care.

REFERENCES

Abraham E 1991 Effects of stress on cytokine production. Methods and Achievements in Experimental Pathology 14: 45–62

Ader R, Felton D L, Cohen N 1991 Psychoneuroimmunology, 2nd edn. Academic Press, London

Baker J P, Detsky S, Wesson D E et al 1982 Nutritional assessment: a comparison of clinical judgement and objective measurements. New England Journal of Medicine 306: 969–974

Ballieux R E 1994 The mind and the immune system. Theoretical Medicine. An International Journal for the Philosophy and Methodology of Medical Research and Practice 15(4): 387–395

Baum A, Grunberg N, Singer J E 1982 The use of psychological and neuroendocrinological measurement in the study of stress. Health Psychology 1: 217–236

Berne R M, Levy M N 1997 Cardiovascular physiology, 7th edn. CV Mosby, St Louis

Besedorsky H, del Rey A E, Sorkin E, Dinarello C A 1986 Immunoregulatory feedback between interleukin-1 and glucocorticoid hormones. Science 233: 652–654

Biley F C 1989 Nurses' perception of stress in preoperative surgical patients. Journal of Advanced Nursing 14(7): 575–581

Boore J R P 1976 An investigation into the effects of some aspects of pre-operative preparation of patients on post-operative stress and recovery. Thesis, RCN Steinbeck Collection, London

Bradley A J, Calman K C 1988 Immunology and surgery. In: Ledingham I McA, MacKay C (eds) Jamieson and Kay's textbook of surgical physiology, 4th edn. Churchill Livingstone, London

Cannon W B, Britton S W 1927 Studies on the conditions of activity in endocrine and emotion on medulliadrenal secretion. American Journal of Physiology 79: 433–465

Cannon W B, De La Paz D 1911 Emotional stimulation of adrenal secretion. American Journal of Physiology 27: 64–70

Carr J A, Powers M J 1986 Stressors associated with coronary bypass. Nursing Research 35(4): 243–246

Colbert D 1993 Fundamentals of clinical physiology. Prentice Hall International, London

Cooper C 1996 Handbook of stress, medicine, and health. CRC Press, London

Cox T, Mackay C J 1976 A psychological model of occupational stress. A paper presented to the Medical Research Council meeting Mental Health in Industry, November, London

Cuthbertson D P 1932 Observations on the disturbance of metabolism produced by injury to the limbs. Quarterly Journal of Medicine 1: 233–246

Dallman M F, Akano S F, Scribner K A, Bradbury M J, Walker C D, Strack A M, Cascio C S 1992 Stress, feedback and facilitation in the hypothalamo-pituitary–adrenal axis. Journal of Neuroendocrinology 4(5): 517–526

Felig P, Baxter J D, Broadus A E, Frohman L A 1987 Endocrinology and metabolism. Prentice Hall International, London

Frankenhauser M 1980 Psychoendocrine approaches to the study of stressful person–environment interactions. In: Selye H (ed) Selye's guide to stress research. Van Nostrand Reinhold, New York, pp 46–70

Gamallo A, Alario P, Villanua M A, Nava M P 1988 Effect of chronic stress in the blood pressure in the rat: ACTH administration. Hormone and Metabolic Research 20: 336–338

Greenspan F S, Baxter J D 1994 Basic and clinical endocrinology. 4th edn. Prentice Hall International, London

Griffen J E, Ojeda S R 1996 Textbook of endocrinology. Oxford University Press, Oxford

Halpin 1988 Glucose homeostasis. In: Fisher R, Reason J (eds) Handbook of life stress cognition and health. John Wiley, Chichester

Hayward J 1975 Information: a prescription against pain. RCN, London

Hinwood B 1993 A textbook of science for the health professions, 2nd edn. Chapman and Hall, London

Holmes T H, Rahe R 1967 The social readjustment rating scale. Journal of Psychosomatic Research 11: 213–218

Jemmott L B III, Locke S E 1984 Psychosocial factors, immunological mediation, and human susceptibility to infectious diseases: how much do we know? Psychological Bulletin 95: 78–108

Jenner D A, Richards J 1985 Determination of cortisol and cortisone in urine using high performance liquid chromatography with UV detection. Journal of Pharmaceutical Biomedical Analysis 3(3): 251–258

Johnson E O, Kamilaris T C, Chousos G P, Gold P W 1992 Mechanisms of stress: a dynamic overview of hormonal and behavioural homeostasis. Neuroscience and Behavioural Reviews 16(2): 115–130

Johnston M 1982 Recognition of patients' worries by nurses and by other patients. Journal of Clinical Psychology 21: 255–261

Johnston M 1988 Impending surgery. In: Fisher R, Reason J (eds) Handbook of life stress cognition and health. John Wiley, Chichester

Kanner A D, Coyne J C, Schaefer C, Lazarus R S 1981 Comparison of two modes of stress measurement: daily hassles and uplifts versus major life events. Journal of Behavioral Medicine 4: 1–39

Khansari D N, Murgo A J, Faith R E 1990 Effects of stress on the immune system. Immunology Today 11(5): 170–175

Kiecolt-Glaser J, Glaser R 1988 Methodological issues in behavioural immunology research with humans. Brain, Behaviour and Immunity 2: 67–78

Kispert P H 1992 Metabolic response to stress. In: Simmons R L, Steed D L (eds) Basic science review for surgeons. W B Saunders, London, ch 7

Kusnecov A, Rabin B S 1994 Stressor-induced alterations of immune function: mechanisms and issues. International Archives of Allergy and Immunology 105: 107–121

Lanuza D 1995 Postoperative circadian rhythms and cortisol stress response to two types of cardiac surgery. American Journal of Critical Care 4(3): 212–220

Laycock J, Wise P 1996 Essential endocrinology, 3rd edn. Oxford University Press, Oxford

Lazarus R S 1966 Psychological stress and the coping process. McGraw-Hill, New York

Lazarus R S 1971 The concepts of stress and disease. In: Levi L (ed) Society, stress and disease. Oxford University Press, London, vol 1

Lazarus R S, Delongis A, Folkman S, Green R 1985 Stress and adaptational outcomes: the problem of confounded measures. American Psychologist 40: 770–779

Lundberg U, Frankenhauser M 1980 Pituitary–adrenal and sympathetic–adrenal correlates of distress and effort. Journal of Psychosomatic Research 24: 125–130

Lykken T 1976 The role of individual differences in psychophysiological research. In: Venables P H, Christie M J (eds) Research in psychophysiology. Academic Press, New York, ch 1

MacSween R N M, Whaley K (eds) 1992 Muir's textbook of pathology, 13th edn. Edward Arnold, London

Manyande A, Berg S, Gettins D, Stanford S C, Mazhero S, Marks D F, Salmon P 1995 Pre-operative rehearsal of active coping imagery influences subjective and hormonal responses to abdominal surgery. Psychosomatic Medicine 57(2): 177–182

Mason J W 1959 Psychological influences on the pituitary–adrenal cortical system. Recent Progress in Hormone Research 15: 345

Mason J W 1968a A review of psychoendocrine research on the sympathetic-adrenal medullary system. Psychosomatic Medicine XXX(5: part II): 631–653

Mason J W 1968b A review of psychoendocrine research on the pituitary–adrenal cortical system. Psychosomatic Medicine XXX(5: part II): 576–607

Meijman T F, O'Hanlon J F 1984 Workload: an introduction to psychological theories and measurement methods. In: Drenth P J D, Thierry H, Willems P J, de Wolff C J (eds) Handbook of work and organizational psychology. John Wiley, Chichester, vol 1

Miluk-Kolasa B, Obminski Z, Stupnicki R, Golec L 1994 Effects of music treatment on salivary cortisol to pre-surgical stress. Experimental Clinical Endocrinology 102(2): 118–120

Montague S E 1987 Nursing the physically-ill adult. In: Boore J R P, Champion R, Ferguson M C (eds). A textbook of medical–surgical nursing. Churchill-Livingstone, London, ch 8

Morrison D P, Peck D F 1990 Do self-report measures of affect agree? A longitudinal study. British Journal of Clinical Psychology 29: 395–400

Munck A, Guyre P 1991 Glucocorticoids and immune function. Psychoneuroimmunology, 2nd edn. Academic Press, New York

Munck A, Guyre P, Holbrook N 1984 Physiological functions of glucocorticoids in stress and their relation to pharmacological actions. Endocrine Reviews 5: 25–44

O'Leary A 1990 Stress, emotion, and human immune function. Psychological Bulletin 108(3): 363–382

Pennebaker J W 1982 The psychology of physical symptoms. Springer-Verlag, New York

Pennebaker J W, Watson D 1988 Self-reports and physiological measures in the workplace. In: Hurrell J J, Murphy L R, Sauter S L, Cooper C L (eds) Occupational stress: issues and developments in research. Taylor & Francis, London, pp 184–199

Pollard T 1993 Variation in mood and adrenal 'stress' hormone levels and blood pressure associated with everyday working experience in a British population. DPhil Thesis, Department of Anthropology, University of Oxford

Pollard T, Ungpakorn G, Harrison G A 1992 Some determinants of population variation in cortisol levels in a British urban community. Journal of Biosocial Science 24: 477–485

Rennie M F, Bennegard E, Eden E et al 1984 Urinary excretion and efflux from the leg of 3-methylhistidine before and after major surgical operation. Metabolism 33: 250–256

Roy C 1976 Introduction to nursing: an adaptation model. Prentice Hall, Englewood Cliffs

Sarasen I G, Johnson J H, Siegel J M 1978 Assessing the impact of life changes: Development of life experiences survey. Journal of Consulting and Clinical Psychology 46: 932–946

Schkichtig R, Ayres S M 1988 Nutritional support of the critically ill. Year Book Medical Publishers, London

Selye H 1936 A syndrome produced by diverse noxious agents. Nature 138: 72–75

Selye H 1956 The stress of life. McGraw-Hill, New York

Selye H 1976 The stress of life, 2nd edn. McGraw-Hill. New York

Shannon I, Prigmore J, Brooks R, Feller R 1959 The 17-hydroxycorticosteroids of parotid fluid, serum and urine, following intramuscular injection of repository corticotropin. Journal of Clinical Endocrinology 19: 1477–1480

Shulkin J, McEwen B S, Gold P W 1994 Allostasis, amygdala, and anticipatory angst. Neuroscience and Biobehavioural Reviews 18(3): 385–396

Slade M, Simmons R L, Yunis E, Greenberg L J 1975 Immunodepression after major surgery in normal patients. Surgery 78(3): 363–372

Steptoe A 1991 The links between stress and illness. Journal of Psychosomatic Research 35(6): 633–644

Stokes A, Kite K 1994 Flight stress: stress, fatigue and performance in aviation. Avebury Aviation, Hants

Tolsen W W, Mason J W, Sachar E J, Hamburg D A, Handlon J H, Fishman J R 1965 Urinary catecholamines response associated with hospital admission in normal subjects. Journal of Psychosomatic Research 8: 365–372

Udelsman R, Ramp J, Gallucci W T, Gordan A, Lipford E, Norton J A, Loriaux D L, Chrousos G P 1986 Adaptation during surgical stress: a reevaluation of the role of glucocorticoids. Journal of Clinical Investigation 77(4): 1377–1381

Vingerhoets A J J M, Marcelissen F H G 1988 Stress research: its present status and issues for future developments. Social Science and Medicine 26(3): 279–291

Volicer B J, Bohannon M W 1975 A hospital stress rating scale. Nursing Research 24(5): 352–359

Volicer B J, Isenberg M A, Burns M W 1977 Medical–surgical differences in hospital stress factors. Journal of Human Stress 3: 62–77

Wild D (ed) 1994 The immunoassay handbook. The Macmillan Press, Hants

Williams J G J, Jones J R, Workhoven M N, Williams B 1975 The psychological control of pre-operative anxiety. Psychophysiology 12: 50–54

Wilson J F 1981 Behavioural preparation for surgery: benefit or harm? Journal of Behavioural Medicine 4: 79–102

Windsor J A 1993 Underweight patients and the risks of major surgery. World Journal of Surgery 17: 165–172

Young M E 1988 Malnutrition and wound healing. Heart and Lung 17(1): 60–67

FURTHER READING

Ballieux R E 1994 The mind and the immune system. Theoretical Medicine. An International Journal for the Philosophy and Methodology of Medical Research and Practice 15(4): 387–395

Brook C, Marshall N 1996 Essential endocrinology, 3rd edn. Blackwell Science, Oxford, Oxford

Cerrato P L 1991 Surgery, stress, and metabolism. Registered Nurse 54(8): 63–65

Fisher S, Reason J 1988 Handbook of life stress cognition and health. John Wiley, Chichester

Garvey A, Hibbert A, Manley K 1992 Nutrition and nursing. A resource for teachers. Royal College of Nursing and National Dairy Council, London

Greenstein B 1994 Endocrinology at a glance. Blackwell Science, Oxford

Hadley M E 1992 Endocrinology, 3rd edn. Prentice Hall International, London

Hill G L, Blackett R L, Pickford I et al 1977 Malnutrition in surgical patients: an unrecognized problem. Lancet 1: 689–692

Hobsley M, Imms F J 1992 Physiology in surgical practice. Edward Arnold, London

Ledingham I McA, MacKay C (eds) (1988) Jamieson and Kay's textbook of surgical physiology, 4th edn. Churchill Livingstone, London

Peterson P K, Chao C C, Molitor T, Murtaugh M, Strgar F, Sharp B M 1991 Stress and pathogenesis of infectious disease. Reviews of Infectious Diseases 13: 710–720

Porterfield S P 1997 Endocrine physiology. Mosby-Year Book, New York

Rivier C 1991 Role of interleukins in the stress response. Methods and Achievements in Experimental Pathology 14: 63–79

Scheuch K 1986 Theoretical and empirical considerations in the theory of stress from a psychophysiological point of view. In: Appley M H, Trumbull R (eds) Dynamics of stress. Physiological, psychological and social perspectives. Plenum Press, New York, ch 7

Simmons R L, Steed D L 1992 Basic science review for surgeons. W B Saunders, London

Young V R 1990 Protein and amino acid metabolism with reference to ageing and the elderly. In: Prinsley D M, Sandstead H H (eds) Nutrition and ageing. Progress in Clinical and Biological Research 326: 279–300

9

Psychological, existential and spiritual aspects of surgery

Ruth Davies

AIMS

This chapter aims to:

- explore the meaning of surgery for the individual from psychological, existential and spiritual perspectives
- identify a framework for holistic assessment.

INTRODUCTION – WHY YOU SHOULD READ THIS CHAPTER

There is no such thing as a routine operation or surgical procedure. If this is all you remember from this chapter, I will be satisfied. Of course we knowledgeable and experienced nurses know that we care each week for several people having various types and forms of surgery, and the care of these people may be 'routine' to us as we work to well-proven care plans and familiar procedures. For the person undergoing surgery, it is likely to be a unique experience, and as no two people are alike, we must not generalise about the experience of surgery for people.

Any of us may ourselves undergo surgery. It may not be until that happens that some of the material I include in this chapter makes sense to you or becomes real, but I hope you will continue to read and perhaps reflect on some of the thoughts and information which follow. Surgical nurses must include psychology and spirituality in their assessment of patients and their families in order to provide holistic care.

It is almost impossible to separate out psychological, existential and spiritual issues as they are so closely related to each other. I will, however, try to identify what I mean by each for the purposes of this chapter, but would ask you to remain aware that addressing need in one area will impact on the others, and on the physiological status of the body too. The deep experience of peace and acceptance as a result of meditation or prayer, for example, will have an effect on vital signs, and may influence a patient's choices and behaviours with regard to accepting or rejecting treatments or prognosis.

WHY SHOULD SURGICAL NURSES KNOW ABOUT PSYCHOLOGY?

This is a necessary question, as nurses must not unquestioningly accept contributions from other academic disciplines. It is important that nurses are helped to assess theory, to question its value, to consider the issues of validity and reliability, and formulate their own applications where appropriate. Psychology is hugely relevant to surgical nurses as I hope I will demonstrate in this chapter. Definitions of some terms will be found in the glossary. Psychology is the scientific study of human behaviour and experience (Caws 1975) and although this is an old definition, and simple, it is comprehensive.

SCHOOLS OF PSYCHOLOGICAL THOUGHT

There are four major schools of psychological thought: the psychoanalytic, the behaviourist, the humanistic and the transpersonal. These all complement and extend each other, although at times it is for us, the users, to integrate these approaches. The psychoanalytic approach was originated by Freud (1856–1939), who proposed a model of the unconscious, a model of personality development and a treatment method (psychoanalysis). This has been much refined since his original work, but credit must be given for the insights into the unconscious world and its role in behaviour. It provides a useful framework for analysing what is going on intra- and interpersonally and helps us to explore blocks to action or understanding. The second is the behavioural approach, pioneered by Skinner (1904–1990) and Watson (1878–1958), which concentrates on that which is directly measurable and observable, i.e. behaviour. Originally, consciousness and introspection were omitted but increasingly these are being included in a behaviourist approach. A major contribution to nursing here is in helping us to understand and teach skills and to identify the effect of tissue damage on cognition, for example. The third approach is humanistic psychology, with which many nurses will be familiar, through the client-centred approach which it advocates. Rogers (1902–1987) and Maslow (1908–1970) are key authors here and Maslow, along with Assagioli (1888–1974), is also considered to be central in 'fourth force' or transpersonal psychology. This latter is relatively recently becoming addressed and includes the spiritual nature of being.

With any one patient we might draw on theory from any of these approaches to assess need, to plan and implement care and to define outcomes.

It is noteworthy that all the psychological approaches, particularly when applied to the helping arena, stress that the nature of the relationship between client and helper is paramount, and in therapeutic terms may be more important than the actual practice orientation. In other words, it is the qualities of the helper which are essential in whether patients feel cared for and helped, rather than the psychological treatment techniques. In this vein, Jacobs (1993, p. 43) writes, 'It is clear from much of the research that has been undertaken on the effectiveness of therapists and counsellors that, despite there being differences of method, of theoretical understanding, and also various levels of experience, a consistent and key factor in the felt success of therapy is the relationship between the helper and the client'. Peplau (1988) writes of the relationship itself being a nursing aim, not something to be taken for granted. The importance of the relationship cannot be overemphasised.

INDIVIDUAL DIFFERENCES

This area is frequently discussed within psychology and is often posed as: why does one person feel/think/behave like this and another like that? This is of course, fascinating to explore and hypothesise about but what matters on a practical, surgical nursing level, is that people are different. This is immediately apparent when we begin to explore the meaning of surgery and the various forms which it may take.

For any individual, surgery may be planned or unplanned, the result of an emergency, accident, chronic disease or sudden diagnosis; the person may anticipate surgery with fear, with hope, with eagerness. Surgery may be performed in order to confirm a diagnosis; there will certainly be a prognosis to be given. A person may be clearly ambivalent about the outcome of surgery – whilst accepting the need for surgery, the loss of a limb or body part may not itself be welcomed. Add to this the uncertainty and anxiety that accompanies admission to hospital (Pitts 1991), whether for a short or long stay, perhaps in a regional or specialist unit, the absence or presence of the patients' own support networks, their understanding, comprehension and acceptance of what is happening to them, their ability to talk freely about fear or their tendency to close down, their fear of illness, their resistance to accepting a traditional patient role, and we can begin to see why we cannot generalise. We must also not forget the individual's response to pain and other physiological processes such as tissue healing, tiredness or hunger, which can affect attention, perception and memory, and we must therefore consider when is the best time, physiologically, as well as psychologically, to talk to someone.

If we are able to use an individual client-centred approach, we will be able to identify not only what an individual needs to know, for example, but also any of the age-related, spiritual or cultural beliefs or activities which may be in operation. A child may need simple language, which he can understand in line with his cognitive development, whereas an adolescent may be intrigued by the workings of the body and want as much detail as possible. Another person may, owing to cultural or spiritual beliefs, or personal preference, not wish to know anything. For people to say 'I trust in God' is not to be dismissed, rather to be accepted as their way of coping with the current trauma and perhaps included in making necessary decisions, for example about consent to treatment.

It may seem that if individual differences are so great that few generalisations can be made about behaviour, cognition and emotion, then psychology has little to contribute to nursing. On the contrary, it is because psychology has demonstrated such a wide range of human experience that we can begin to understand that many responses are normal rather than abnormal. Psychology therefore provides the base for individualised rather than routinised care. Psychology can also inform us about principles, for example that information is best delivered in both verbal and written format in order to enhance perception and memory.

With reference to the definition of psychology as the scientific study of human behaviour and experience, we can explore what psychologists have discovered about responses to surgery and how their findings can be related to practice.

Responses to surgery begin, for most people, before the actual operation, when surgery first enters their awareness as a possibility. This may be at the GP's surgery, the outpatient clinic or as a result of individual reflection. There may be a time of acute anxiety and worry while appointments and results are waited for, a different set of anxieties related to admission to hospital and still more regarding the anaesthetic and the surgical procedure. To this can be added concerns about the outcome of the surgery and the losses which will result.

Johnston (1987) is a psychologist who has researched widely about the concerns of surgical patients. She found, when exploring anxiety in 135 female preoperative patients undergoing a range of gynaecological procedures, that their most common worries were concerned with absence from home, for example how husbands and children would cope. However, their major (most important) worry was about the outcome of the operation, specifically whether it would be a success and the time required to return to normal. It seemed that this was the same, regardless of procedure, which ranged from dilatation and curettage to total hysterectomy. She does not, unfortunately, specify what was meant by a 'success', whether this meant a cure, or whether it was without complications, but the work overall is of significance to us and merits further study, perhaps along the lines of whether men and women worry about different issues. It is noteworthy that to define 'success' is difficult and is often not attempted, and is itself worthy of further study.

Reflective point

Identify two different patients. What would be a successful outcome for each of them? What would you, the patients and members of their families call a success? How far does your own idea of success influence the care you give and your relationship with the patient and family?

Many nurses will be familiar with the work of Hayward (1975) who suggested that providing information preoperatively reduced the levels of pain experienced postoperatively. Johnston (1987) challenges this and similar work, claiming that only one of nine experiments and studies involving information-giving showed any significant benefits to the patients. This is not to say that we should not provide information, but it must make us more aware of the need to find out what the patient actually wants to know and to what level. What is clear is that where we make assumptions about people's needs we may not have much success in reducing anxiety. In earlier work, Johnston identified that nurses were generally mistaken or wrong in assessing patients' anxieties (Johnston 1976) and that patients did better than nurses in identifying other patients' concerns (Johnston 1982). This might indicate that the relationship is central to such disclosures – patients in adjacent beds may talk much more to each other than to 'busy' nurses. Does this mean that we should ask one patient about the concerns of another? No, but it must indicate that attention should be paid to the time needed to form a therapeutic relationship.

Although Johnston's work is now 10–20 years old, the findings are important for education and practice development. It could for example indicate a training need which enables nurses to develop awareness of and then address the worries of people about outcome, which often seem to be ignored. Heaven & Maguire (1996) found, however, that simple skills training is insufficient in helping nurses to elicit patient concerns, and much more research and practice development is needed in this area, with regard to attitudinal and behavioural change, and clinical support and supervision. In an earlier chapter (Ch. 5) I wrote about supervision for the emotional aspects of our roles, which will be challenged and stretched if we begin to talk with our patients about major worries, outcome and survival. We need support in order to do this.

Suls & Wan (1989) conducted a meta-analysis of the effects of sensory and procedural information on coping with stressful medical procedures and pain. They concluded that combined sensory–procedural information was the most useful. Sensory information is about how the procedure feels – uncomfortable, temperature changes, localised pain, etc. – and procedural information is about what actually happens in a technical sense (this would include getting results). It can be very useful to tell patients, particularly in today's day care settings, that the effect of an invasive technique and the sedation for it may last several days. It may not be appropriate to return to work the following day and it may be normal to feel more tired than usual for a week or so (this will of course depend on the actual procedure and chemicals used). A risk of short admission is that the impact of the procedure on the patient may be minimised (Parry 1995) and patients may worry about feeling unwell or unusually tired a few days later when they only went into hospital for a morning. Equally after major surgery, many patients may not know how long it may take for them to recover and heal, and think they have problems when their experiences are within normal ranges.

More recently, Teasdale (1993) has challenged the information-giving strategies, commenting on the lack of replication of earlier studies. He makes the point that no information is ever complete or impartial, that there is always a motive in giving information. He writes: 'to ask whether "information" relieves anxiety is conceptually flawed. Relief of anxiety will depend not on the words uttered or written, but upon meanings which nurses intend to convey and upon the inferences drawn by patients' (Teasdale 1993, p. 1128). He continues to identify that some studies which have helped patients have control over aspects of their admission and treatment show promising results (e.g. the use of relaxation) but notes also that opportunities for patients to have meaningful control over events are limited.

Further work is also indicated on cognitive reframing strategies, where patients are helped to identify the meaning of an event, recognise that original fears, thoughts and expectations may not be accurate and then consider other possible, positive outcomes. These must then be tested. An example may be of a previously fit woman of 65 who has no experience of being an inpatient before. She develops arthritis of the knee and rapidly becomes immobile. The GP and consultant recommend a joint replacement but she is unhappy about this and agrees only reluctantly to go to hospital for the replacement. On talking to the nurse, she expresses her fears more fully. She has previously been able to do everything for herself but is now dependent on her family for help. Her self-esteem is low and she is sure that many others need the operation more than she does. She is immobile and in considerable constant pain and does not know how the new joint will help her. She is afraid of the general anaesthetic and thinks she may die on the operating table. The nurse can help by gaining an understanding of the patient's meanings and attributions about the event (surgery) and acknowledging the reality and the fantasy of the situation. She may provide information about the anaesthetic, she may be able to introduce other patients who have had the operation and are now pain-free. She may also validate that constant pain and immobility are very sound reasons for surgery and she (the patient) does merit such intervention. The patient can then test her new thoughts and attributions and will hopefully be less anxious as she realises that there are positive reasons for having the surgery. In terms of control, she may also be able to make requests which will help ease her admission. This would be an example of how the relationship underpins a particular style of intervention (in this case cognitive–behavioural) as referred to at the beginning of the chapter. All this, of course, requires time to get to know the patient and training for the nurse in reframing techniques. A considerable amount of time for training and supervision may be required in order that these techniques are used in a collaborative rather than an authoritative (and possibly degenerate) manner.

Reflective point

How do you elicit patients' concerns? What information do you provide and how? Is this appropriate given some of the issues raised above?

SURGERY AND LOSS

Murray Parkes & Napier (1975), two psychiatrists who explored the psychiatric after-effects of amputation, relate loss of a limb to grief and depression similar in process to that following the death of a loved one. They suggest that there are two reactions to the loss event, one of alarm due to stress and danger and a second of grief related specifically to the expected or sustained loss. Although their focus was amputation and their work is now old, their findings can inform all surgery. Not all patients will require psychiatric intervention, but early, sensitive care might prevent this.

All surgery involves loss, in all sorts of ways, and I will spend some time looking at this. I would not suggest that all these areas are or can be addressed during an acute surgical admission, but it may help to understand the psychological experiences which may account for immobility, lack of interest, restlessness, withdrawal, anger, or resentment in surgical patients. Sleeplessness may be due to inadequate pain control, or unfamiliar position but may also be due to psychological pain, worry and challenge. Medication may not be the best choice for the patient.

What is lost (actually or potentially) when someone requires surgery?

The most obvious loss is of life. When we are well, we imagine that we will live forever, that illness is for other people, we feel inviolate. On one level we know that we will die sometime, but we do not believe that time is now. Having a condition which requires surgery confronts us with our own morbidity and mortality and sometimes that of others, as for example when an emergency caesarean section saves or ensures the life of mother and baby. We fear and deny death, whether this be fast or slow. We know as well that many people work through this and approach death with a sense of peace and completeness, but the initial reaction is always likely to be one of shock and grief.

With a feared loss of life, our whole world is challenged, both in its current form and in the form of dreams and aspirations for the future. We all have our own dreams for the future, whether they be of living to a ripe old age, seeing children grow up, or reaching the moon. What matters is that these dreams are not judged but are accepted as important potential losses.

One result of a diagnosis, for example cancer, is that as well as a fear of loss of life, support may disappear, at the time it is most needed. Family and friends may be unable to support the patient as they have their own grief to deal with, and perhaps relief that it has not happened to them. It is not just the bereaved who are avoided by people who do not know what to say: it is those whose life is threatened. Some friends and relatives will deal with this by denial, by focusing on tasks, just as nurses do, ignoring or not seeing or hearing the emotional needs, but concentrating instead on the physical ones. Look around next visiting time and see how much actual conversation is occurring – visitors will be tidying lockers, sorting out laundry, showing photographs, talking to each other, perhaps saying 'we'll talk when we get home'. How often as well do relatives not want each other to know a diagnosis, for fear of upsetting one another. As nurses we might know that everyone does know that the patient has cancer or is dying, but somehow they keep it secret from each other. It is often a relief when talking can start, but it may take time for people to feel ready. The nurse does, I believe, have a responsibility to point out that talking to each other is a possibility and could support the family in this. Not all families have time on their side, and as nurses we should not assume that families are aware how close to death a patient may be. One family I know were devastated when the mother died soon after discharge home – they had not understood that 'there's nothing more we can do' meant that she was so close to death. Later they were very angry that they had not had more clear information.

Secondary to loss of life and security are other losses which relate more specifically to the body part affected. Each body part, whether it be a limb or an organ, has a practical function, an expressive function and a symbolic function. For example, a hand holds, grips, feels, touches, and also expresses emotion in the form of gestures. Furthermore it is symbolic of power, agreement, strength, dexterity, completeness, normality and much more. A uterus, likewise, is where a foetus matures until birth, expresses menstrual flow (often experienced as cleansing) and symbolises femininity, reproduction and sexuality. For a woman undergoing hysterectomy, the latter loss may be of much greater concern than the actual surgery. Once again, patients know their needs best and these should be explored. Using Johnston's (1987) themes of common and major worry, it behoves us to find out and not judge the patient's specific concerns regarding the surgery.

Reflective point

Think of a patient and how your own and the patient's views have differed. How did this influence the care and relationship between you?

Another loss is of an intact body boundary. Surgery probes, cuts, removes parts of, inserts, stitches, our bodies. Prior to surgery we will have had an intact skin (cuts and grazes excepted) and no one will have violated this. Now, however rational the reasons for the surgery, people will have had access to our bodies in a totally new and bizarre way. They will see and touch our bodies in a way which we and our most loved ones never will. This requires a huge amount of trust on the part of patients, not just in the skill of the surgeons but in their ability to show respect for someone else's body. Further, the scar is always there to be seen, even if it is as small as the site of insertion of the endoscope. This feeling of violation may not cause long-term difficulties for patients, but is often thought to be abnormal. It is not so. All surgery is invasive – whether it is perceived as such or not depends on the individual.

For the patient who is confined to bed, the body boundary may extend to include the bed itself, the catheter tubing and bag, the drainage tubing and bottles, the infusion set, the nasogastric tube, the leads to ECG machines, etc. A movement of any of these may cause anxiety as they pull on a tender body. The discomfort and lack of mobility associated with infusions is not to be underrated either. It is difficult to lift yourself up the bed with a painful abdomen and only one workable arm, for example.

Body image is often changed as a result of surgery, whether this be due to loss of a limb or visible body part or a scar which, as mentioned above, changes the previously intact nature of our skin. Sundeen and colleagues (1994) define body image as: 'the sum of the conscious and unconscious attitudes the individual has toward his body. It includes present and past perceptions as well as feelings about size, function, appearance, and potential. Body image is a dynamic entity, because it is continually being modified by new perceptions and experiences' (Sundeen et al 1994, p. 64). From this definition, we can see that surgery will change a person's body image and may bring to the surface unconscious attitudes or feelings towards our bodies. Individuals may never have thought about the value they put on a body part until they are threatened with its loss or alteration. Some people have a distorted body image, feeling that they are heavier or lighter, taller or shorter than they actually are, and others will be more accurate. Body image is associated with how attractive we feel and our self-esteem and there will be individual variation here. Some people will feel that they are loved because they have a 'perfect' body and to have a stoma or a mastectomy may result in loss of a partner who is essential to their self-esteem. Others may feel that survival matters more than the intact, complete body and will not be concerned to the same extent about the stoma or mastectomy. I use these as examples because both can have a profound effect on sexuality and sexual behaviour and will influence the degree to which surgery is judged successful by the patient.

Where people feel that they are loved on condition that they have a perfect body, the threat of surgery is great. Rogers (1951), a humanistic psychologist, writes of unconditional positive regard and this is one example where nurses can demonstrate unconditional acceptance of a patient. The theory supports our practice in not showing distaste for a wound, or for changing a colostomy bag. If we can show acceptance, we may help towards rebuilding a patient's self-esteem. We are also modelling this response to family and friends. Equally, Kaufman (1985) writes about shame and the sense of being a disappointment to others (initially parents), and this may be a feature of mutilating surgery, that the person feels ashamed at not living up to a particular standard. As nurses, we might also be guilty of shaming patients who we feel are not making progress, or who seem to need more analgesia than we think they should. 'This is Mrs Davies, she needs a *lot* of pain relief' was the content of an end-of-bed handover in my recent experience. I was asking for my regular, prescribed, postoperative analgesia, assertively attempting to ensure that it was given prior to acute pain setting in. This experience made me very wary of further surgery, but sharing my concerns about postoperative pain relief did have good effect the second time. I certainly felt shamed by the first nurses though, whose judgement of me clearly influenced their comments and my care.

A related concept is of stigma, where people often feel shame. Goffman (1964) writes of hidden and visible stigmas, the latter being obvious to see, such as paralysis or facial scarring. Hidden stigmas can be 'covered' in that very few people will be aware that the person next to them has a colostomy or one breast. Some amputations can be hidden while people are sitting but are evident on movement. What matters, though, is how people feel about themselves. Goffman makes the point that on one level every person has reason to feel stigmatised, but most are 'covered'. This is similar to Kaufman (1985) with his work on shame. If we feel shame, we cannot be free to be ourselves.

It is also possible that judgements that we as nurses make arise from ignorance or lack of awareness. I remember how having seen a person undergo an emergency appendicectomy in theatre, it suddenly made sense that he needed substantial analgesia postoperatively and that paralytic ileus was only to be expected, so much of the gut had, necessarily and respectfully, been explored. I was able to tell my colleagues on the ward what I had seen and to educate them too. It is possible that because surgery and many investigative procedures do happen away from the ward, we find it difficult to appreciate the patient's experience. Perhaps an annual trip to the diagnostic suite and theatre would keep this fresh.

In summary, Pitts (1991) suggests that there are three reasons why surgery is stressful: the anaesthetic and related fears of losing consciousness and control; the degree of pain anticipated postoperatively; and the nature of surgery, the fact that the body is incised and the use of instruments on the body. She writes: 'It may be that each of these separate elements is stressful, but that their unique combination in surgery is particularly difficult to anticipate and cope with' (Pitts 1991, p. 67). She does make reference to the fear of not waking up from the anaesthetic, but it is worthy of note that there is no other mention of the issues of life and death, survival and the critical nature of surgery to the individual. Often surgery occurs as the result of an emergency, perhaps an accident; equally often it is planned but is concerned with a life-threatening situation. It is also commonly reported that surgery is psychologically as well as physically invasive; the idea that someone has been inside one's skin, incised and manipulated organs, is bizarre and can raise questions and feelings regarding the violation of being, the sanctity of the body and one's vulnerability and lack of control over life. These issues will be addressed in the next section.

How then, can surgical nurses begin to meet the psychological needs of patients? I have already identified that individual differences are great and present considerable methodological challenges to research which can form a basis for practice recommendations. We can only conclude that patients must be treated as individuals, with time spent finding out how much and in what manner to help each patient psychologically. This means that we must be willing and able to explore those issues which arise as a result of a person requiring surgery. Given, also, that the relationship is paramount, we must spend time attending to and reflecting on our behaviour and attitudes in this respect. Clinical supervision has an important part to play here (see also Ch. 5).

WHY SHOULD SURGICAL NURSES KNOW ABOUT EXISTENTIAL ISSUES?

I will now proceed to the area of existential issues and challenges in more detail. The realisation that surgery is required is confronting – suddenly the individual has to deal with issues of morbidity, mortality, life and death. Heron (1990) tells us that confronting is 'about waking people up to what it is they are not aware of in themselves that is critical for their own well-being and the well-being of others' (Heron 1990, p. 44). Arguably, when surgery is required, we are confronted with a challenge to our existence, about which Yalom (1985) writes:

The existential approach posits that the human being's struggle is with the givens, the ultimate concerns, of existence: death, isolation, freedom, and meaninglessness. Anxiety issues from basic conflicts in each of these realms: we wish to continue to be and yet are aware of inevitable death; we crave ground and structure and yet must confront groundlessness; each of us desires contact, protection, to be part of a larger whole yet experiences the unbridgeable gap between self and others; we are meaning-seeking creatures thrown into a world that has no meaning.

(Yalom 1985, pp. 95–96)

The cry of 'why me' stems from this search for meaning, and the lack of meaning is itself painful. There are no answers to such a question. Likewise, Bullock et al (1988) write, 'Existential psychology … emphasises that each individual is constantly making choices, great and small, which cumulatively determine the kind of person he becomes … it is concerned with the individual's attempts to discover a satisfying sense of his personal identity and to give meaning to his life' (Bullock et al 1988, p. 296). In some ways, cognitive reframing (see above) is about making choices to think differently. One challenge is that for most of the time most of us are unaware of the multitude of choices we make each day – when to get up, what to wear, which teeth we brush first and, suddenly, when confronted with the threat of illness and surgery, these choices are both highlighted and meaningless.

Surgery (or indeed any severe illness) requires us to live with and come to terms with uncertainty, pain, grief, isolation. In Yalom's (1985) research, he asked patients who had been in group psychotherapy what had helped them and in one category of responses, which he called 'existential factors', the following were identified:

- 'recognising that at times life is unfair and unjust'
- 'recognising that ultimately there is no escape from some of life's pain and from death'
- 'recognising that no matter how close I get to other people I must still face life alone'
- 'facing the basic issues of my life and death, and thus living my life more honestly and being less caught up in trivialities'

- 'learning that I must take ultimate responsibility for the way I live my life no matter how much support and guidance I get from others' (Yalom 1985, p. 92).

You may be reading this and thinking, 'but most of my patients seem all right in themselves. I don't see or hear people asking why me, what's the point in going on? I don't see people who are desperately struggling with these issues.' There are at least three possible explanations for this, the first being that perhaps much of this work will be done in the non-ward environment. Nurses in surgical outpatients will often be involved in breaking bad news and later follow-up, the practice nurse may be visited in the period after diagnosis but before admission to hospital, and community staff will be involved postoperatively. These people may be more likely to be participants in such discussions, particularly where a relationship is built up over the course of wound dressing or chemotherapy for example. It is also possible that the patient addresses many of these questions in the time between diagnosis and admission and has had the opportunity to work through some of the shock. Janis (1969) refers to the work of worrying as a necessary part of preoperative preparation on the part of the patient, and although his work has not been replicated, the concept would seem reasonable. Many patients may not speak at all to health care professionals, preferring instead to use their own support networks of family and friends. It is probably worth remembering, though, that family and friends may not always be able to speak freely and will have their own grief to deal with. In terms of assertive care, taking the initiative and broaching these areas yourself will require courage but may also be well worthwhile.

The second explanation concerns the role of denial, which is increasingly considered worthy of respect for its psychological protective features. Freud, with his theorising about the unconscious, used the term 'mental defence mechanisms', of which denial is probably the most important. This is not to say that denial is not to be challenged and explored, more that it is to be respected and worked with appropriately. This move is echoed within the psychotherapy arena. However, Parkes writes, 'if it is necessary for the bereaved person to go through the pain of grief in order to get the grief work done, then anything that continually allows the person to avoid or suppress this pain can be expected to prolong the course of mourning' (Parkes 1972, p. 173). Although he is writing about death and bereavement, the response to loss as identified earlier will follow a similar path. At some stage, people will need to grieve for the actual and potential losses brought about by surgery.

The third reason is more concerning and it is of whether you, as a surgical nurse, are open to seeing and hearing these cries of existential pain. Is the person who is withdrawn seen as an 'easy patient' who does not make demands, or is he someone to sit with and get to know? Is the patient who denies any emotion similar? Are you willing and able to talk with a patient about death or loss of meaning in life, or do you prefer to deny this to yourself and avoid such encounters? Worden (1983) suggests that it is difficult to talk to the bereaved for several reasons, and again these can be transferred to the patient experiencing grief in other situations. He suggests that it is simply uncomfortable to witness pain in another person, and relationships may be cut short as a result. Further, we can be made more aware of our own losses, our own feared losses and our own death. Parkes (1972) writes, 'Pain is inevitable in such a case [death] and cannot be avoided. It stems from the awareness of both parties that neither can give the other what he wants. The helper cannot bring back the person who is dead, and the bereaved person cannot gratify the helper by seeming helped' (Parkes 1972, p. 163). Polishuk (1991) begins a poem with:

They tell us it's an acceptable risk,
Only three per million.
All I know is
I have cancer

(Polishuk 1991, p. 65)

Reflective point

Let this evoke in you a memory of when you were helpless to do anything for a patient, perhaps regarding a terminal prognosis, and the patient could not be made better nor pretend to you that she felt better for talking. Later you might realise that you helped by being present with the patient.

A key point to remember is that the person asking 'why me?' or 'why my loved one' (in whatever form this takes) or who feels no sense of purpose in life, is struggling with deep personal issues. This does not mean the person is in imminent need of referral to psychiatric services, rather that he or she is in crisis. Stone (1993) writes, 'For a crisis to occur people must view the precipitator as a profound threat to their well-being or to the well-being of their family. They see it as a very dangerous situation, one that most likely will adversely affect their lives' (Stone 1993, p. 19). He continues to tell us that a crisis is a normal human reaction to an emotionally hazardous situation and reminds us that conflict and unhappiness are not synonymous with mental illness. He is clear that intervention is necessary – 'although persons in crisis are not necessarily mentally ill, they may experience remarkably strong emotional reactions such as anxiety, depression, tension, panic, a personal and social sense of confusion and chaos, feelings of loss, helplessness, hopelessness and disorganisation. The emotional pain can lead to more serious distress if it is not resolved adequately' (Stone 1993, p. 23). He argues that positive interpersonal relationships will aid the successful resolution of a crisis. Being with someone in emotional distress is difficult but it is through being present (Ersser 1991) that we can help, without apparent action. Being present is seen as an expression of the transpersonal (the fourth school of psychological thought) by the fourth force psychologists.

Reflective point

Identify a time when you have asked 'why me?' or 'why that patient?' Remember how you felt and notice how you feel now. What did you learn from that episode? How has this influenced you in your personal and professional life?

Returning to Yalom's existential factors, we can see that there is little we can do to answer these 'why me' questions for anyone other than ourselves. Talking may help us to explore ideas and reach conclusions, as may techniques such as guided imagery and emotional expression. It may be that we can help people with their existential struggles about life and death, isolation, meaninglessness and purpose only when we have confronted these ourselves and this is where spirituality might be relevant.

WHY DO SURGICAL NURSES NEED TO KNOW ABOUT SPIRITUALITY?

The simple and short answer to this is that if you do not include spirituality in your nursing care, then you are not practising holistic nursing. The biopsychosocial model is incomplete without spirituality (see also Ch. 7). Oldnall (1996) in a review of nursing theorists identified only two who wrote with any clarity about spirituality (Neumann and Watson) and cites Carson (1989) who calls for spirituality to become the fourth recognised domain of nursing and an integral part of theory development. He also suggests that nurse education fails to meet the needs of students in preparing for working with patients in this domain.

The term 'spirituality' is very difficult to define and the tendency in the literature is to characterise it, to tell us its purpose, its forms. The only clarity in current definitions is that it is not synonymous with religion, and reference is usually made to a higher or deeper dimension in life, the desire and ability to transcend the material realm (O'Brien 1982) and that meaning and purpose are integral concepts.

It is possible that a spiritual domain in us enables us to find ways of dealing with the 'why me' type of question and, for example, Oldnall (1996) tells us that 'Highfield and Cason (1983) argue that the spiritual dimension of a human being encompasses the inherent need to find satisfactory answers to the ultimate questions concerning the meaning of life, illness and death. The individual's deepest relationships with others, himself and God (or other influential focus) are the centre of the individual's spiritual dimension' (Oldnall 1996, pp. 21–22). In a different but related vein, Labun (1988) introduces the concept of spiritual health or integrity, writing: 'Spiritual integrity is present when the person experiences wholeness within the self, with other human beings, and in transcendence with another realm. Spiritual integrity is demonstrated through acts that show qualities such as love, hope, trust and forgiveness' (Labun 1988, p. 315). In one sense, we show love when we care fully for a patient and this would come from our own spiritual integrity. This relates also to transpersonal psychology, as mentioned at the start of this chapter. Whitmore (1991) explains that the transpersonal dimension:

is that area of the human psyche which is qualitatively higher than, and which transcends, personal existence. It is the home of greater aspirations, the source of higher feelings like compassion and altruism, and forms the roots of intuition and creative intelligence .... Transpersonal experiences have a reality which many feel to be more profound than normal everyday existence ... they leave the individual with a deepened sense of value and meaning.

(Whitmore 1991, pp. 9–10)

Here, compassion is a quality which is often demonstrated by the nurse. A transpersonal experience is similar to Maslow's (1970) concept of a peak experience which might include a sense of peace, stillness, acute presence in the world and awareness of how small a part one plays in the universe. Key themes related to spirituality then, are of meaning, relationship, the source of some qualities, of transcendence. Is surgical nursing ready to address these?

How can we meet the spiritual needs of our patients? Oldnall (1996) writes of spiritual needs without providing examples of these, which is unfortunate. Without stating a need it is difficult to begin to identify ways to meet it. Perhaps a spiritual need is to search for meaning or purpose. This would fit with the existential tradition. It might also include the need for time for ourselves, for reflection, meditation or prayer, or religious or devotional acts. A spiritual need might also be for someone to be present or absent during these times, to participate or not. A location might be an essential part of this – how many of you actually take patients to a site of beauty – a lake, a park, the hospital chapel, for example? Hospital chapels are often places of richness, sanctuary and peace from the busyness and drab decor of the main hospital, but are still an artefact. Contact with the natural, living world is sometimes most refreshing and renewing – do not discount the value of flowers as representing this.

Reflective point

Are you willing to ask patients what they might need and then provide it, or know who might if you are not able to?

Some nurses have trained in massage, deep relaxation, guided imagery for example, and might use these skills at such times, but most will not have these in their repertoire. We can, however, use those qualities and skills which are within us as part of our own spirit.

Heron (1990) defines helping as 'supporting and enabling the well-being of another person' and writes: 'People who help people move by the grace within the human spirit. This grace is the primary source of effective helping behaviour' (Heron 1990, p. 11). He describes five key attributes in this helping grace: warmth and acceptance; openness and being in tune with the other's experience; a grasp of what the other needs; the ability to help meet those needs appropriately; authenticity. He summarises this as: 'This combination of concern, empathy, prescience, facilitation and genuineness is, I believe, the spiritual heritage of humankind' (Heron 1990, p. 11). The effective helper, according to Heron (1990), comprises the interaction of inner grace, character and cultural influence. 'Inner grace is a spiritual endowment and potential which everyone has. Character is what persons make of themselves in response to their culture. The way in which these three factors influence each other will determine whether or how the capacity for helping emerges' (Heron 1990, p. 12). This point is important – the culture of a ward will interact with our own inner grace and character to influence our own being and

nursing behaviour. (We may not always be consciously aware of this interaction.) Some of you may have worked on one ward where you experienced the culture as oppressive and moved to another where you were more able to express your inner grace, for example, and felt more 'at home'. Some people choose to work in the community where the environment and culture is more suited to their character and grace. Returning to the culture of a ward, it may be that the culture influences you in such a way that you are not open to seeing or hearing patients' existential or spiritual needs. The ward exists within its own culture, the hospital and the State, all of which may be concerned with economic rather than spiritual issues.

Reflective point

When does your heart sing? Does this happen in your work environment? Could you make it happen for you? How?

Wright (1991) calls for environments in which nurses can nurse and refers to 'high touch' and 'high tech' skills. Without the former, the patient may be treated but is not healed. In an environment which emphasises the latter, there may be little you can do to build relationships with patients in which existential and spiritual issues can be broached at length or in depth. This is not to say that you should not try. Rather that it is even more important to use effectively the short time available. A central part of holistic care and working with grace is being able to use the moment. A word of kindness, attention to physical comfort, being silent with, are all expressions of grace.

In summary then, spirituality involves a search for meaning and purpose, a sense of wholeness, an ability to transcend the everyday realm, and it is in the individual's spirit (or soul) that love, compassion, joy, creativity, courage, sensitivity, grace are located. An individual who has this sense of wholeness may be able to practise surgical nursing in its most holistic fashion. Oldnall (1996), however, questions whether this is possible, as it would seem that the biopsychosocial needs of patients are not fully met and to add a further dimension is unrealistic when nurses are already fully stretched. If we are to meet the spiritual needs of patients, our own spiritual needs must also be met (we must first identify that they exist in us). One result of living a spiritual life is that one aims to become free of attachments (e.g. to perfection, money, ambition) and far more realistic and able to make choices about what can and should be done. It also opens us to working with and through grace. A note of caution, though – the journey is never complete – it requires consistent reflection and openness, introspection and change as our lives continue.

HOLISM AND REDUCTIONISM

Surgery can easily be approached on a reductionist model, in fact it is sometimes jokingly referred to as 'spare part', 'plumbing', relatively straightforward procedures. I'm getting my hip done, someone might say, without reference to the rest of her body and the impact a hip replacement will have on her whole being. Equally we all know of the old days when people were identified by their condition, e.g. the appendix in bed 8. I am not sure that we have completely moved on from this reductionism, although bed 8 is more likely to have a named person in occupation now. The current culture within which we work may also mean that the practicalities of holistic care are very difficult to implement. With reduced length of admission, it is very difficult to get to know a patient in a whole sense, and much easier to concentrate solely on the reason for admission (the disease, rather than the dis-ease).

One holistic assessment framework, see Fig. 9.1, is to consider someone's life in terms of occupation, leisure, relationships and spiritual aspects. Freud originally wrote of the healthy individual who has pleasure or satisfaction in work, play and relationships, and the spiritual dimension has been added by the transpersonal psychologists such as Assagioli (1991). This framework is often used in counselling assessments and a balance in these four areas may be seen as healthy. For example, some individuals may have too much work, too much leisure, no meaning in their life, unhappy relationships. This same framework can be used to assess the impact of surgery on the individual as I will demonstrate. I would add that this has yet to be tested in practice – perhaps the time is ripe. As a surgical nurse, you might like to reconsider your approach to assessment.

Occupation does not refer simply to employment, but to how people fill their lives with purposeful activity. It is also important to acknowledge that not everyone who has work is happy with it or derives satisfaction from it; some work solely to earn money. Many patients will not have formal work, which may have an impact on how much money is available for the family to visit. Surgery will affect people in their occupations, either through absence from work, or the inability (perhaps temporarily, perhaps permanently)

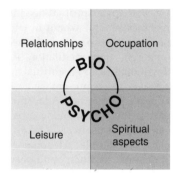

Figure 9.1 A framework for holistic assessment.

to do their chosen tasks. Alternatively, they may be more mobile as a result of surgery and work opportunities result. Asking about occupation in such a way will provide valuable information with which to plan care. It may also be a relatively 'safe' place to start, in terms of levels of disclosure.

Likewise with leisure, individuals undergoing surgery may find they have to cope with more leisure, or change the way they use this time. Leisure may be enforced, resulting in boredom, perhaps through lack of mobility pre- or postoperatively, or may be welcomed as an opportunity to slow down in order to gather strength before surgery. The link between isolation and depression is worth exploring where mobility or social life changes as a result of surgical intervention and it may be worth exploring how contact with others can be maintained. Asking people how they use their leisure time may lead in to specific foci such as taking an alcohol history, or noting that a regular runner has a normally slow pulse rate, all of which information is essential to the overall care of the patient.

Surgery may have a profound effect on relationships, when we consider the anxiety which is often associated with not knowing what will happen, the separation and isolation which occurs during hospitalisation and the effects of the actual operation on the individual's body image and function (and perhaps partners' ideals too). As well as partners, other significant relationships can be addressed, for example with children, colleagues and friends, and parents. Many people will have surgery for cancer and will find that people do not know what to say to them, as the close ties and the tragedy of a situation cause anxiety, sadness and fear. Also surgery can affect mobility and body function and appearance. Psychosexual issues are rarely addressed, even where there is an established risk to sexual functioning as in abdominoperineal resection, or hysterectomy, and this is your opportunity to discuss these areas.

Finally, undergoing surgery may challenge our beliefs about life. It is one thing to know that we are mortal, it is quite different to be confronted with that fact not only through diagnosis of disease but also through having to trust someone to be sufficiently skilful and caring to help us and, hopefully, ameliorate our condition. It is no surprise then that individuals undergoing surgery may choose consciously or unconsciously to deny the challenge to current self-knowledge and themselves remain reductionist in their thoughts and conversation. This is to be respected and if we remain aware of the need for psychological defence we can be client-led in our care and serve the patient well. The question, 'how are you in yourself' often gives us valuable information about how a person is dealing with existential issues. An answer such as 'Deep down, I'm all right, and I feel really sad' is quite different from 'I can't see any point in going on'. A recent study asking people to subjectively rate their emotional health with the question, 'How would you rate your current emotional health – good, fair, poor or very poor?' identified that this was a robust predictor for clinical depression in the following year, those patients who said 'very poor' being at much greater risk (Hoff et al 1997). If we ask people about their spiritual needs, they may not know what we mean (neither may we) but if we inquire about regular behaviours or rituals, time alone, religion and how they are in themselves, we will probably get a better response.

The depth of exploration in any of the above four areas will lead to relevant information, and will require skilful observation, listening and questioning on the part of the nurse. Sleep patterns, diet, medication have to be addressed when there is an appropriate opening. It is useful to know how people cope with stress, sadness, bereavement, whether they have a history of depression or mental illness, and rather than taking a task-focused history, the nurse can explore the lack of relationships, the changing job history, the people who are friends, etc. This sometimes takes courage, and it certainly takes time, much more than a quick check about 'alcohol use – social?' or 'expressing sexuality – wears make-up' on the assessment sheet. One great advantage of this form of assessment is that it is holistic and will enable relationships to develop as more time is taken getting to know the patient. This is also perhaps its greatest challenge.

CONCLUSION

The aims of this chapter were to explore the meaning of surgery for the individual from psychological, existential and spiritual perspectives and secondly to provide a framework for holistic assessment. In terms of meeting the needs of patients with regard to psychological, existential and spiritual issues, you will, by now, have realised that there are no easy answers to this or quick-fix skills to be acquired, but that key features can be identified, for example:

- a willingness to care, to love, to be authentic, to feel and express emotions yourself
- a willingness to explore your own psychological, existential and spiritual aspects of being
- an openness to meeting patients' needs without judgement
- the willingness and courage to be with as well as to do for patients
- a commitment to reflection, meditation and transcendence
- an openness to your own creativity, beauty and joy and that of others.

When these features underpin our practice, we are willing and able to really hear what patients need – we can assess them fully, and work with them throughout our time with them to meet shared objectives and promote health and independence throughout. However, this is not easy as the demands on ourselves are great. Few of us wish to address our own issues, waiting instead for this to be forced upon us by our own life events. Few of us find it easy to seek help, or to go to awareness or growth workshops where some of this exploration can be undertaken. However, the attitude of openness to experience and willingness to reflect is essential, wherever you learn, whether this be classroom or forest. I wrote earlier of support and supervision (Ch. 5) and I believe that it is through this process that we can begin to use, examine and apply knowledge, technical skills, presence and grace in order to help patients with their psychological, existential and spiritual issues. There is no way that a recipe book approach can be used as no two patients are the same.

At the beginning of this chapter I wrote that I will be satisfied if you remember that there is no such thing as a routine operation or surgical procedure. I will be more satisfied if through reading this chapter you have been able to reflect and perhaps change your practice for the better. I hope that through reading this chapter you have gained a greater understanding of the human being, from psychological, existential and spiritual perspectives. I would ask you to remember that they are all interwoven and that if we are to practise true holistic care, we must include these domains. I wish you and your patients well.

If nursing is to be healing, we work with grace.

REFERENCES

Assagioli R 1991 Transpersonal development: the dimension beyond psychosynthesis. Crucible, London

British Association of Counselling Guidelines 1992. BAC, Rugby

Bullock A, Stallybrass O, Trombley S 1988 Fontana dictionary of modern thought, 2nd edn. Fontana, London

Caws A G 1975 Introduction/preface. In: Altschul A 1975 Psychology for nurses. Baillière Tindall, London

Ersser S 1991 A search for the therapeutic dimensions of nurse–patient interaction. In: McMahon R, Pearson A 1991 (eds) Nursing as therapy. Chapman and Hall, London

Goffman 1964 Stigma: notes on the management of spoiled identity. Penguin, London

Hayward J 1975 Information – a prescription against pain. Royal College of Nursing, London

Heaven C N, Maguire P 1996 Training hospice nurses to elicit patient concerns. Journal of Advanced Nursing 23: 280–286

Heron J 1990 Helping the client. Sage, London

Hoff R A, Bruce M L, Kasl, S V, Jacobs S C 1997 Subjective ratings of emotional health as a risk factor for major depression in a community sample. British Journal of Psychiatry 170: 167–172

Jacobs M 1993 Still small voice: an introduction to pastoral counselling, 2nd edn. SPCK, London

Janis I L 1969 Stress and frustration. Harcourt Brace & Jovanovich, New York

Johnston M 1976 Communication of patients' feelings in hospital. In: Bennett A E (ed) Communication between doctors and patients. Oxford University Press, Oxford, pp 30–43

Johnston M 1982 Recognition of patients' worries by nurses and by other patients. British Journal of Clinical Psychology 21: 255–261

Johnston M 1987 Emotional and cognitive aspects of anxiety in surgical patients. Communication and Cognition 20(2/3): 245–260

Kaufman G 1985 The psychology of shame. Routledge, London

Labun E 1988 Spiritual care: an element in nursing care planning. Journal of Advanced Nursing 13: 314–320

Maslow A H 1970 Motivation and personality, 2nd edn. Harper and Row, New York

Murray Parkes C, Napier M M 1975 Psychiatric sequelae of amputation. In: Silverstone T, Barraclough B 1975 Contemporary psychiatry: selected reviews from the British Journal of Medicine. Royal College of Psychiatrists, London

O'Brien M E 1982 The need for spiritual integrity. In: Yura H, Walsh M B (eds) Human needs and the nursing process. Appleton-Century-Crofts, Norwalk, Connecticut, pp 85–95

Oldnall A 1996 A critical analysis of nursing: meeting the spiritual needs of patients. Journal of Advanced Nursing 23: 138–144

Parkes C M 1972 Bereavement: studies of grief in adult life. International Universities Press, New York

Parry A 1995 The lived experience of day surgery. MSc Thesis, Royal College of Nursing, London

Peplau H 1988 Interpersonal relations in nursing. Macmillan, London

Pitts M 1991 The experience of treatment. In: Pitts M, Phillips K (eds) The psychology of health. Routledge, London

Polishuk S 1991 All I know. In: Brady J (ed) 1 in 3 women with cancer confront an epidemic. Cleis Press, Pittsburgh

Rogers C R 1951 Client centred therapy. Constable, London

Stone H 1993 Crisis counselling: caring for people in emotional shock. SPCK, London

Suls J, Wan C K 1989 Effects of sensory and procedural information on coping with stressful medical procedures and pain: a meta-analysis. Journal of Consulting and Clinical Psychology 57(3): 372–379

Sundeen S, Stuart G, Rankin E, Cohen S 1994 Nurse client interaction: implementing the nursing process, 5th edn. CV Mosby, London

Teasdale K 1993 Information and anxiety: a critical reappraisal. Journal of Advanced Nursing 18: 1125–1132

Whitmore D 1991 Psychosynthesis counselling in action. Sage, London

Worden J W 1983 Grief counselling and grief therapy. Tavistock, London

Wright S 1991 Facilitating therapeutic nursing and independent practice. In: McMahon R, Pearson A 1991 Nursing as therapy. Chapman and Hall, London

Yalom I D 1985 The theory and practice of group psychotherapy, 3rd edn. Basic Books, New York

FURTHER READING

Goddard 1995 Spirituality as integrative energy: a philosophical analysis as requisite precursor to holistic nursing practice. Journal of Advanced Nursing 22: 808–815

Johnston M, Vogele C 1993 Benefits of psychological preparation for surgery: a meta-analysis. Annals of Behavioural Medicine 15(4): 245–256

Salmon P 1992 Psychological factors in surgical stress – implications for management. Clinical Psychology Review 12: 681–704

10

Culture: the social context of surgery

Helen Allan

AIMS

The aims of this chapter are:

- to introduce the surgical nurse to the concept of *culture* and how it frames the social context of surgery
- to present an overview of current social and cultural issues which affect surgical nursing
- to suggest areas for practice development in surgical nursing in the context of a *multicultural society*
- to develop the surgical nurse's awareness of the need for *culturally sensitive care*.

INTRODUCTION

Surgical nurses care for patients from different cultural backgrounds and need to provide care in a culturally sensitive way. This chapter will provide knowledge to enable them to do so. It will avoid an approach which specifies cultural differences based on ethnicity. Culture is broader than *race* or *ethnicity* and the surgical nurse needs to be sensitive to different aspects of a patient's cultural background, such as religion, age, gender, sexuality and social class as well as ethnic background. Instead, the discussion will look at the nurse's options while working within the surgical patient's cultural frame of reference.

Why should surgical nurses find this chapter essential for their practice? There are basically five reasons: first, it will assist them in meeting the demands of the Patient's Charter (DoH 1991, 1995) in a meaningful and respectful way. Second, it will assist them to explore their own self-awareness about their own culture and translate those insights into caring.

Third, there are current debates within academia and politics generally on cultural issues within a multicultural society which nursing needs to be part of:

• Initiatives from government on meeting ethnic minorities' health needs (DoH 1993) and from professional organisations (RCN Race and Ethnicity

Committee 1993) have also stimulated discussion among nurses regarding their practice.

- Studies of culture, stigma and deviancy within sociology have been introduced to nursing with the increased input of sociological theory to nursing curricula.
- Debates within anthropology about an anthropology of nursing (largely carried out by anthropologists on nurses) or an anthropology for nurses (carried out by nurses with nurses) are currently taking place, while at the same time there is interest in the nursing press in clinically applied anthropology (Allan & Wiseman 1995, Littlewood 1989).
- Debates within the science of knowledge have influenced nursing theory, e.g. Watson's (1988) phenomenological philosophy of nursing. Inter-subjectivity (a key feature of the nurse–patient relationship for Watson) acknowledges what both the nurse and the patient bring to the relationship and the effect this has on the care delivered; it is a development of the ideas of phenomenologists who look at the 'here and now' experience (Rose 1990, p. 59). Watson suggests that intersubjectivity includes the acknowledgement of culture as a feature of the nurse–patient interaction.
- Leininger (1978, 1991) has focused on culture as a key concept within her *transcultural* theory of care since the 1960s, but nursing within the UK has been slow to develop her concepts and apply them to British society.

The remaining two reasons why the surgical nurse needs to study this chapter are reflected in two themes within the medical sociology and critical medical anthropology literature which are relevant when considering the implications that sociocultural factors have for surgical nursing.

The first theme is the clinical application of sociological and anthropological findings. Nurses have studied these in relation to patients' beliefs about health and illness and related behaviours. However, although relevant to surgical nursing, the applications of these findings are few (Baxter 1988, Henley 1987, 1988). Surgical nurses should ask themselves: how have the patient's beliefs about health contributed to this admission for surgery? How will these beliefs affect the patient's recovery? How will my *sociocultural* background affect our relationship and how can I facilitate meaningful communication?

This self-awareness on the part of nurses will allow them to address how they, the experts, define the surgical situation, how the patient defines it and how this potential difference impinges on care. Are there negotiated or common meanings between nurse and patient? Fox (1992) argues that the surgical experience

is shaped by the power of the expert because of the history of surgery as a discipline. What effects does this power of the expert to shape the social meanings of surgery have on patients in their sociocultural contexts?

The second theme is the discussion of the effects of wider political and economic forces on surgery. These forces 'pattern human relationships, shape human behaviour and condition collective experience, including forces of institutional, national and global scale' (Singer 1986, p. 128, cited in Chrisman & Johnson 1990). What are the wider political issues which affect surgery and surgical nursing? A key political and economic force has been the pressure to reduce waiting lists and increase throughput of surgical patients (Fox 1992).The development of day care surgery is a result of these forces which has led to developments in surgical nursing. The social construction of surgery as a medical specialty, the meaning of surgery in western medicine and the differences in surgical rates cross-culturally as a reflection of these differences in meaning are exactly those issues that surgical nurses ought to examine if they wish to develop nursing practice in this area of specialty.

The meanings attached to surgery for individual patients will depend on the sociocultural and historical contexts of their lives. These meanings may be more or less shared by those caring for them (the nurses and other members of the multidisciplinary team). The goal of nursing in this respect is to care for patients in a culturally sensitive way (McGee 1994, p. 789). Nurses need to develop awareness of their own culture, to identify what is important to them, in order for them to care for their patients holistically and to meet their patients' specific cultural needs.

Nursing theory, Leininger's theory of cultural care diversity and universality (1978, 1991), Littlewood's generalised nursing model (1989), Geissler's work on culture and the nurse–patient dyad (1995) and Denny & McCrea's work on human sociocultural needs (1991), will be used to explore ways in which culturally sensitive care can be delivered. These theories have been applied to practice, and the nurse's options in caring for surgical patients in a culturally sensitive way will be discussed. Also, suggestions will be made within the chapter on how surgical nurses might look at their own practice to develop culturally sensitive care and initiate change to set quality standards in line with policy.

Culturally sensitive care

Culturally sensitive care is a term which describes how care might be delivered to ethnically, linguistically and culturally diverse groups of patients (Fee 1994). Fee suggests that there are five issues which are relevant:

1. developing greater sensitivity and respect for individual differences among clients of a specific cultural group
2. separating the effects of culture from the effects of *socioeconomic status*
3. exercising caution in interpreting and generalising research findings
4. exercising caution in the use of standardised tests
5. obtaining the best written and spoken language translation.

Leininger (1985) has developed the concept of culturally sensitive care in nursing in her theory of cultural care diversity and universality. She describes this theory as the development of a knowledge base which incorporates an awareness of the nurse's own culture, preferences and prejudices alongside specific information about local ethnic groups. She argues that to provide culturally sensitive care (Leininger 1991), the nurse needs to understand the concept of culture and how culture is communicated within and between groups. The following questions need to be asked and understood by the surgical nurse:

• What is culture?
• How is it transmitted?
• How does it affect health?
• How does it affect health care provision?

What is culture?

What is culture? Culture is a slippery concept – one which appears self-evident yet is difficult to define. Nurses use the terms cultural, sociocultural and social to describe attributes of patients' behaviour which may or may not affect their health. It helps the nurse build up a holistic picture of a patient's life. But what exactly is culture? Does it differ from society? Can the two terms be used interchangeably?

Culture as behaviour

Culture refers to the ways we live and the meanings that we apply to those behaviours. Keesing (1982) cites Goodenough (1961) to explain that there are two aspects to culture which are important to establish. Firstly, culture refers to 'the pattern of life within a community – the regularly recurring activities and material and social arrangements' which are characteristic of a human group (Goodenough 1961, p. 521). This means that culture concerns the behaviours an outsider would observe about the ways we live.

In the same way, in nursing, a patient's cultural behaviours would be the observable ways of living which affected the patient's health and with which we, as nurses, would concern ourselves. Observable ways of living include household living arrangements, eating arrangements, kinship systems, marriage, divorce, education and socialisation of children, sexual behaviours, economic systems, communication networks, language, play. As Herskovits (1955) suggested, culture is 'all the man-made part of the environment' which we observe and has been created by humans. This form of culture Keesing (1982) calls the sociocultural system. This view of culture is also described as the *functionalist* or *structural–functionalist* tradition (Jenks 1993) as it concerns itself with observable social structures and how these interrelate to form society, to make society function. From this perspective, cultural behaviours are understood in terms of society as a whole. It is how individuals' behaviour may affect their roles in society and may threaten or enhance society's cohesiveness and functioning which becomes important. An example might be a young man who sustains a head injury and multiple fractures through competing in a dangerous sport without the recommended equipment or protective clothing. His behaviour endangers his life and will have social and economic consequences for his personal well-being. But his injuries are costly to the NHS in terms of immediate and long-term care. His absence from work will also have an added cost for his employer and the State. Seen from this perspective, the young man's behaviour has individual and social consequences.

Culture as beliefs

Secondly, culture refers to the meanings of the observed behaviours – the 'organised system of knowledge and belief whereby a people structure their experience and perceptions, formulate acts and choose between alternatives' (Keesing 1982, p. 68) – the reasons why we, as individuals, do things and how we understand our own actions. As nurses we would want to understand, as far as we could and in as much as the patient is able to tell us, why patients behave in certain ways. We can then, perhaps, through that familiarity with the patient, care empathically (Malek 1989).

Cultural knowledge and beliefs are shared by a social group and are based on assumptions about reality: 'the nature of the social and physical environment and one's place within it' (Marshall 1990). A student nurse quickly becomes knowledgeable about the kind of behaviour acceptable on a new ward. This cultural knowledge is shared by all the nurses who work on a particular ward. Further, Geertz (1966) argued that culture is understood and transmitted through meanings in the forms of symbols which act as a framework for understanding experience. An example of a symbol in health assessment is the meaning attached to smoking. It is just a behaviour but it has become filled with meaning outside of the simple act of inhaling cigarette smoke. It 'means' (among other things) risk, enjoyment, rebellion, fashion, death, cancer. Therefore, the symbol of a cigarette is a potent message understood by many groups of people in different ways. Culture is 'an historically transmitted pattern of meanings embodied in symbols, a system of inherited conceptions expressed in symbolic form by means of which men communicate, perpetuate and develop their knowledge about and attitudes towards life' (Geertz 1966). This way of looking at culture places great importance on ideas and thoughts rather than observed behaviours (Keesing 1982). Jenks (1993, p. 48) states that culture, in this tradition, is 'the practice of humankind, as is its understanding'.

Why is it important to clarify the difference between these two aspects of culture? Weber, a 19th century sociologist, identified the concept of 'verstehen' to explain that to understand how society works we need to understand two meanings about any behaviour: what the outside observer understands about the behaviour and what the actor, the insider, understands about the behaviour. He argued that we can observe and understand through empathy but that the observer then needs to explain and generalise the behaviour to other situations (Swingewood 1984, p. 145). He described explanation and generalisation in terms of ideal-types which exist to enable humans to communicate meanings about culture. Empathy allows us to understand through another's eyes and explanation allows us to generalise from these understandings and observation and to compare cultures.

Anthropologists have described these two types of understanding as the *etic* (outsider) and *emic* (insider) views. Therefore, to understand culture, social scientists have argued that both views are needed. Culture does not exist as an entity on its own, 'out there', but only through the meaning that humans attach to it.

A nursing example to demonstrate this is provided in Case studies 10.1 and 10.2.

Case study 10.1 shows the nurse applying her own meaning to the woman's smoking behaviour as an outsider (*etic*), i.e. smoking damages health and may

---

Case study 10.1   Patient A

A woman arrives for her outpatient appointment in the gynaecology department. She is suffering from menorrhagia and the consultant suggests an investigative hysteroscopy under general anaesthetic which the woman consents to. The named nurse begins to inform the woman about the operation and assess her anaesthetic risk status. The woman smokes 30 cigarettes a day. The nurse points out that this is harmful, gives her a leaflet on giving up smoking and advises her to do this before she is admitted for her operation.

Case study 10.2   Patient A: an alternative approach

A woman arrives for her outpatient appointment in the gynaecology department. She is suffering from menorrhagia and the consultant suggests an investigative hysteroscopy under general anaesthetic which the woman consents to. The named nurse begins to inform the woman about the operation and assess her anaesthetic risk status. The woman smokes 30 cigarettes a day. The nurse starts to explore with this woman the reason why she smokes, what pleasure it gives her, what her level of knowledge is about the health risks of smoking heavily and what positive and negative feelings giving up smoking have for her.

---

be an anaesthetic risk. Case study 10.2 shows the nurse exploring the woman's behaviour by trying to understand the meaning that smoking and giving up smoking have for her. The nurse tries to understand the insider (*emic*) view. Which nursing action would be the more effective? Current evidence in health promotion research suggests that Case study 10.2 would be, because the nurse empowers the woman by empathising and trying to understand her reasons for smoking. She also empowers the woman to articulate her concerns in a meaningful way to her (see Ch. 3).Wilson-Barnett & Macleod Clark (1993) suggest that nurses have to incorporate empowerment into their health education and promotion work if health promotion is to be successful (for further discussion, see also Calnan 1987).

Case study 10.2 also shows that Keesing's definition of culture is relevant to nursing. The nurse in Case study 10.2 is facilitating the woman to articulate her knowledge and beliefs whereby she forms her perceptions and makes sense of her experiences, plans actions and chooses between alternatives (Keesing 1982, p. 68).

Society and ethnicity

How does culture differ from society? Society is the group of people who share a common culture and by whom it is understood. The terms *ethnicity* and *race* or racial group are important characteristics of groups which are often used interchangeably with cultural or social. They are very different. Ethnicity derives from the concept of belonging to a people or tribe (Senior & Bhopal 1994). Senior & Bhopal argue that it implies one or more of the following: a shared origin or social background; shared culture and traditions that are distinctive, maintained between generations and lead to a sense of identity and group; and a common language or religious tradition. Ethnicity is not nationality (which has been imposed on most ethnic groups since the emergence of the nation state). It is affected by migrant status but the migrant group remains ethnically distinct from the host community. Ethnicity is also distinct from race. Race is a term used to describe the divisions of humankind by physical characteristics. (For further discussion, see Giddens 1993, Miles 1989, Baxter 1988.) Senior & Bhopal (1994) point out that a group of people may be racially similar but culturally distinct; for example Serbian Muslims, Serbian Orthodox and Croatian Roman Catholics.

Nurses may, therefore, refer to patients' cultural beliefs and behaviours, and their social and ethnic group/background when communicating their care to others. But can we refer to all members of social groups with shared cultures and ethnic backgrounds as being essentially the same, that is, *homogeneous*? Leach (1982) points out that all cultures have different subcultures which divide the larger culture. This means that societies are divided by social class, caste, ranks, wealth, gender, religion and ethnicity into subcultures whose members have different behaviours and understandings of their behaviour. But he goes on to say that no subcultures are homogeneous. This is because culture changes and individuals within cultures and subcultures interpret and change culture which is then passed on to the next generation. There are also differences between the rules or guidelines that should govern behaviour and how members of the culture actually behave (Helman 1990, p. 6).

Scaffa & Davis (1990), in their study on the effects of culture on patients with acquired immune deficiency syndrome (AIDS), argue that not all descriptions of a culture are applicable to all members in all situations, which means that nurses have to approach patients as individuals, with an awareness of their differing subcultures and the effects these might have on the way patients interpret their illness and any interaction with a nurse. However, they also state that the differences between cultures and subgroups of those cultures are greater than the differences within the subgroups. Therefore, if there are sufficient similarities identified by group members within the group compared to another culture, then it makes sense to speak about a cultural identity and to plan care accordingly, while remaining aware that not all members will wish to behave in the same way all the time in different situations.

Transmission of culture

How is culture transmitted? Helman (1990, p. 5) argues that culture provides a set of guidelines (explicit and implicit) which are inherited by members of groups or societies. These guidelines inform the members of the group how to view the world, how to experience it emotionally and how to behave in relation to other people, to supernatural forces or gods and to the natural environment. *Enculturation* is the process by which one learns to become a member of a cultural group. This socialisation process takes place within the context of personal relationships, often within kinship networks, and community networks (Marshall 1990). It means that children become socially and culturally competent in their environment. Ways of transmitting culture are symbols, language, art and ritual. There are debates about how much of culture is learnt by an individual and how much is acquired (Keesing 1982, pp. 91–107).

The migration status of groups is important when considering culture and ethnicity (DoH 1993). The homogeneity of subcultures is affected by *acculturation* which is how an outsider, immigrant or subordinate group, assimilates and adapts to the dominant group or culture to become culturally and socially indistinguishable (*Concise Oxford Dictionary of Sociology* 1994). A dominant culture is one which, through economic or political power, is able to impose its culture on subordinate groups so that the latter's culture becomes devalued. This affects the transmission of the subculture's beliefs and behaviours which results in acculturation. Nurses can impose their nursing culture (the occupational culture which they learn as students and junior staff nurses) on patients when they come within their influence. This can be benign, for example when the patient learns to be on the ward for meal times. It can also be damaging, for example when visitors are restricted to certain numbers, which devalues, through lack of awareness, the need in some cultures for all family members to visit the sick person. Nurses may also be aware of how the process of enculturation in nursing works for them personally when they enter a new ward environment.

Reflective point

Can you think of a positive example of how acculturation may work for students working within a surgical area?

How does culture affect health?

In this section the effects of culture on health will be discussed. There are five issues which are relevant for nurses in this discussion:

- lay beliefs about health and illness
- the symbolic nature of surgery
- health behaviours
- the effect of stress
- the effect of individual or collective approaches to health.

Lay beliefs about health and illness

One way that nurses attempt to understand the effect of cultural background on health is through learning about their patients' lay beliefs about health and illness (Leininger 1985, Littlewood 1989). Acknowledging that there are lay beliefs which may be different from professional ones was first discussed by Kleinman (1978), who argued that culture affected health in one major way unrecognised by western biomedicine: the doctor thinks of disease and the patient of illness. The medical perspective is expressed in terms of disease, diagnosis and treatment. The lay perspective is expressed in illnesses, experiences of changes in states of being and social function – the human experience of sickness. Illness and disease do not stand in a one-to-one relation to each other (Kleinman 1978) but exist as two clinical realities. The professional clinical reality is based on 'scientific logic' grounded in biomedical explanations of disease. The lay clinical reality is idiosyncratic and changeable, heavily influenced by personality and cultural factors (Kleinman 1980). The lay belief about health and illness will also be influenced by past responses to illness episodes; Case study 10.3 illustrates this point.

Patients' understanding of illness and their experiences are described as health and illness beliefs (Calnan 1987) and have been utilised by nurses in developing nursing models (Leininger 1985, Littlewood 1989, Scaffa & Davis 1990), although more extensively in the USA than in the UK. Patients' health and illness beliefs are important in understanding the

Case study 10.3   Patient B

A patient with a diagnosis of peripheral vascular disease refuses to give up smoking after the removal of his foot. The 'rotten' part of his body which has been treated is now no longer there and he cannot 'see' the damage smoking may be doing to the rest of his body. He does not feel ill but much better now that his pain has gone. He looks forward to returning to work. The nurse caring for him understands his disease in biomedical terms and realises that smoking is causing hidden damage which will, in all likelihood, progressively affect his peripheral circulation and mean further amputations in the future. The lay perspective in this case is expressed in terms of lack of pain and the regaining of social function; it is not understood in pathophysiological terms.

totality of a patient's illness experience (Helman 1990, p. 86). However, the application of this knowledge to surgical nursing appears to be slow. There are few articles discussing this aspect of care in the surgical environment although nursing initiatives such as information sheets in different languages, improving equal access and policies on interpreters are evidence of cultural sensitivity in practice.

Kleinman argued that the doctor and nurse presume that health care takes place within a professional framework and are ignorant of the popular and folk sectors where the majority of illness is treated. The popular sector includes complementary therapists who may treat cancers, fertility problems and eating disorders (Helman 1990). The folk sector includes self-treatment, self-help groups, family care, religious practitioners, spiritual healing. The extent of these health sectors is important for pre-admission clinics and discharge planning. As Kleinman suggested, 'changes in the interaction between professional and popular care have the potential for far greater effects on cost, access and satisfaction than changes in professional care alone' (1978, p. 251).

These two differing versions of *clinical reality* (i.e. an etic and emic perspective), what symptoms mean to the nurse and patient in a clinical context and where health care is thought to take place by the professional, have resulted in patient dissatisfaction, inequality of access to care and spiralling costs of health care. Konner (1993) argues that there is now dissatisfaction from both patients and doctors who realise the inadequacy and inefficacy of biomedicine. The Community Care Act 1990 and Patient's Charter (DoH 1991, 1995) may be seen, partly, as political moves to recognise the importance of the non-professional health care sectors.

Malin (1994, p. 27) argues that the participation of users and carers is central to the success of the Community Care Act reforms and is a direct challenge to the biomedical orthodoxy. The inclusion of users and carers at the level of planning and provision of services was stimulated by criticism of the lack of involvement of users in assessment; the inadequacy of data on user needs; and the need for collaboration among professional groups in designing care packages.

Reflective point

Reflect on how patients' understanding of health may influence interactions with doctors and nurses.

The symbolic nature of surgery

In a later article (Csordas & Kleinman 1990), these ideas about lay and professional clinical realities were developed and are important for explaining how culture affects health and surgical care. Even if there are two clinical realities in a medical consultation (a lay and a professional one), therapy, treatment and healing are an active response to disease and illness understood by both patient and doctor. Surgery is part of this active response and may be a continuation of therapy started in the folk and popular sectors. Just as patients have understandings of illness, their experiences of changes in their state of being, so they have beliefs about treatments and the potential of the doctor or nurse to heal. Csordas & Kleinman argue that any healing system (western biomedicine, Ayurvedic medicine, Chinese medicine, psychotherapy) includes symbolic and non-symbolic components. They mean that the treatments may work of themselves but they may work because the patient and doctor or nurse believes they will. Moerman (1979) found that the effectiveness of surgery relied, in part, not on the specific surgical procedure but on its generalised placebo effect. He observed that the surgical 'laying on of steel' may be parallel to the ritual laying on of hands. Other symbols in the surgical relationship between doctor and patient may be starving for theatre, shaving and skin preparation, bowel preparation, signing the consent form, the surgeon's visit after the operation and the surgeon's 'ward round'. Fox (1992) found that practices dealing with sterile technique, particularly the wearing of surgical masks in theatre, were grounded in beliefs not facts. Nurses and doctors realised that surgical masks were an inefficient means of preventing infection and wore them incorrectly but resisted abolishing their use because they served some symbolic function.

Csordas & Kleinman (1990) are clear that all medical and healing systems have a therapeutic process, including procedure and outcome, which are culturally defined. The symbolic value of western surgery is based on distinctions between diagnosis and treatment, between medical and non-medical healing, between technological and non-technological treatments and between religious and non-religious healing. Culturally, western surgery has separated itself from medicine as a specialty and from the folk and popular health sectors. Surgical patients, however, bring to the surgical therapeutic process their experiences of the illness leading up to surgery, including all the carers who make up their therapy management group. These include their families and other practitioners as well as the surgical team. Recognising this, therapy management group is vital to effective discharge planning (Community Care Act 1990).

Health behaviours

Health is affected by cultural factors in other ways. Brown & Inhorn (1990) argue that culture determines patterns of disease and death in a population for two reasons: first, culture shapes important behaviours which predispose people to disease, such as smoking and diet leading to coronary heart disease and peripheral vascular disease where surgical treatments have become widely accepted; second, through culture, people change their environment, i.e. agriculture, which affects their health through the type of diet they eat and the diseases that they suffer as a result. For example, bowel surgery for cancer and Crohn's disease is directly affected by the diet that is available for us to eat. Brown & Inhorn (1990) classify cultural risk factors which predispose to disease into two categories: endogenous and exogenous.

Endogenous risk factors:
- genetic (inherited predisposition), e.g. haemoglobinopathies
- congenital (effect of intrauterine environment), e.g. club foot.

Exogenous risk factors:
- biotic (microorganisms)
- non-biotic (workplace, environment, war, political, economic, ideological), e.g.: dietary deficiency/overconsumption responsible for diabetes, coronary heart disease, hypertension, cancer (Brown & Inhorn 1990).

Culture, health and stress

One particular field of research that has looked at culture and disease is the literature on stress. Early work, focusing on cultural factors, showed how essential hypertension and related health problems were associated with cultural change or *modernisation* (Cassel et al 1960, Henry & Cassel 1969). Cultural change was taken to be stressful. Other work in this field included the relationship between social class and disease (Dressler 1990). However, these models of cultural stress and disease have been criticised because they give little or no attention to how or why behaviours are embedded in cultural contexts (Young 1980). So doctors, nurses and psychologists may use a model of life-crises to explain the social stress experienced by an individual which may result in disease. But the life-crises are not understood in the larger cultural contexts of particular communities. Dressler (1990) suggests that there are cross-cultural similarities between stressors (both acute and chronic) which can be clinically applied (general stressors). There are also particular stressors which need to be understood in a cultural context (racism for example). He argues that general stressors, which do not vary cross-culturally, may have more impact on disease risk than particular stressors. However, Dressler does not suggest that cultural variability can be ignored.

Stressful life events result in the same risk of disease but not the same disease, which varies cross-culturally. This may be affected by the resistance resources that are available in different communities. The most important resistance resource is social support (Dressler 1990). Significantly, the meaning of support is more risk-reducing than actual support. Other resistance resources are the timing of support and the effect of migration and personal coping resources (Dressler 1990).

Individualism or collectivism?

The issue of how cultural factors affect health at an individual or collective level is important and appears to influence whether the nurse ignores culture or attempts to identify cultural differences. An individual approach to care which is culturally sensitive should include an awareness of the collective culture while acknowledging that individuals interpret their culture in their own way. Backett & Davidson (1995) in their study into the effects of life-course on health promotion found that cultural factors are both unique to any individual and, at the same time, influenced by patterns of accepted cultural behaviour. Individual factors may include family history, past illness experiences,

personally valued health advice, individual social circumstances and personal interpretations of health promotion knowledge. Wider patterns of cultural factors are age, marriage and responsibilities, which they discuss as life-course. These personal and collective cultural factors influence how an individual behaves in relation to drinking alcohol, smoking tobacco and exercise.

In this section we have looked at how culture directly affects health and illness at the level of population risk factors to disease, the effect of general and specific cultural stressors on health, the influence of lay and professional health and illness beliefs and, at the individual level, how culture affects the patient's contact with doctors and nurses. The last question Leininger (1985) asks is: how does culture affect how we nurse?

How does culture affect nursing care in the surgical environment?

There are several important ways in which the culture of the surgical environment affects the nursing care of the surgical patient. Nurses may be unaware of these effects, as they form part of the world with which they are familiar. Some of these effects can arise out of the potentially different backgrounds of both staff and patients. This may lead to misunderstandings and, in the extreme, labelling of patients. It is the nurse's duty to be aware of potential cultural differences which may affect the patient's experience of hospital and the surgical ward.

Attitudes of nurses and doctors

Culture has a direct bearing on the provision of nursing care for the surgical patient. Fisher & Peterson (1993) and Fox (1992, 1994) both argue that surgeons strongly influence how surgical personnel (including nurses in operating theatres and in the surgical ward) treat patients. In operating theatres the surgeon's ultimate control and unquestioned authority in surgical technique, combined with the depersonalisation of the patient, compromise quality of care for the surgical patient (Fisher & Peterson 1993). Fox (1994), in an English study, found that surgeons' and anaesthetists' images of surgical patients were grounded in their understandings of surgery: the 'good' that the operation would do; the power of surgery to heal; the superiority of medical knowledge over lay knowledge. However, surgical personnel were unaware of the effects that these images had on the care they delivered. Fox argues that nurses and doctors saw the surgical experience from their professional perspective based on biomedicine or ignorance of others' viewpoints ('biomedical centrism'). The doctors and nurses believed that their actions were for the good of the patients and the side-effects a necessary evil. They failed to see outside of their own viewpoint because they were ignorant of alternatives. Fox argues that the alternative viewpoint was that of the patient who experienced the surgical admission and procedure from his or her own cultural background. What the nurses and doctors failed to understand was that the surgical admission is not simply a biomedical episode but a cultural experience for the patient. A cultural experience occurs whenever and wherever the patient enters the health care system. Patients interpret events from their 'lay' world view which may or may not include an understanding of the medical and nursing worlds and the power of surgery to heal.

Ethnocentrism

Weidman (1979) argues that an understanding of 'health culture' is important for health care professionals because of the emergence of multi-ethnic populations with traditional beliefs from the folk and popular sectors which affect how the western medical system of health care is viewed. There are competing systems of medical care which health care professionals need to be aware of if they are to deliver effective health care. Health cultures are 'the phenomena associated with the maintenance of well-being and the problems of sickness with which people cope in traditional ways within their own social networks' (Weidman 1979, p. 85). In fact, the dominance of the western medical world view leads to ignorance of other systems. Encounters between medicine (nursing) and patients which ignore cultural differences, result in 'unintended but real intolerance and possibly contempt for the patient's cognitive system' (Weidman 1979, p. 86). This inability to see others' world views is called *ethnocentrism*. Ethnocentrism within the doctor–patient or nurse–patient interaction occurs when the patient's belief system is invalidated and the patient is asked to accept unquestioningly the western (dominant) medical world view, its efficacy, assumptions and understandings.

Reflective point

Can you think of situations where you have experienced ethnocentrism as a patient or as a nurse? Discuss this experience with a colleague.

Outcomes of surgery

The process of the surgery, the attitudes of the medical and nursing staff encountered by the patient and the way these attitudes shape the care given are one way that cultural issues affect surgery. Cay et al (1975) argued that the outcomes of surgery are also affected by culture. The success of surgery is traditionally measured in biomedical terms by medical and nursing staff. This is because the dominant culture within western health care is biomedical. However, patients measure success in terms of psychosocial rather than physical factors, not necessarily the absence of symptoms. This suggests that patient criteria, which are influenced by non-biomedical cultures (Csordas & Kleinman 1990, Kleinman 1978), are subordinate to the dominant biomedical culture and ignored. Cay et al argue that if surgery is to be adequately evaluated, patients' criteria need to be included in evaluation. The use of patient narratives may be one approach to achieving such an evaluation.

Cultural brokerage

Fitzgerald (1992) suggests that it is the culture of the clinical interaction which also directly affects the provision of care. It does this through the presence of multiple cultures and medical systems which are involved in every clinical interaction. These are:

- the personal or familial culture of the care provider
- the culture of the client or patient
- the culture of the dominant medical (or nursing) system
- the culture of the traditional medical culture.

Difficulties arise when there is little shared knowledge between patients and doctors/nurses about these multiple cultures. The knowledge that the nurse or doctors have about the different cultures depends on their level of self-awareness about their own culture and other cultures. Fee (1994), in a study on the rehabilitation of patients with spinal cord injury after surgery, proposed a framework of cultural brokerage based on increasing the self-awareness of the psychologist, doctor or nurse about the multiple cultures described by Fitzgerald. He suggested that rehabilitation for these patients has limited effectiveness if the culture of the clinical interaction is not recognised. *Cultural brokerage* describes how the cultural awareness of both professional and patient can be increased by sharing cultural knowledge and meanings (Weidman 1979, p. 211). Increasing cultural sensitivity establishes new meanings for both patient and carer.

But Fitzgerald (1992) points out that a cookbook approach to cultural brokerage, where the beliefs, attitudes and behaviours of a society are compiled and used as a formula, achieves the opposite effect and may lead to stereotyping and increased stigma, as beliefs and behaviours are not understood and the distance between the cultures is increased.

An example of the multiple cultures that patients may bring to the surgical encounter is Bendelow's (1993) study on pain perceptions, emotions and gender. She found that lay perceptions of pain were influenced by the gender of the person experiencing pain. Men and women perceived women to be stronger in coping with pain both in physical terms, as a preparation for and an experience of childbirth, and through cultural expectations as a result of their socialisation as girls and mothers. Women's ability to tolerate pain was also seen to be affected by the inner-city, multiracial community they came from. Cultural brokerage in this case, women's tolerance of pain, would need to understand three aspects of gender to fully understand the culture of the client or patient.

Surgical practice

Lastly, culture at a global level affects the practice of surgery: the techniques developed, the technologies used, the types of diagnostic procedures and operations carried out for particular disorders and diagnoses. The differences in surgical rates internationally and nationally have been long been recognised (Ham 1988, McPherson 1990, OECD 1993). What are the cultural influences which may affect these differences? The number of surgeons per head of population, and age and gender distribution of population were found to influence differences in surgical rates, but, interestingly, not disease of population (Ham 1988, p. 10). McPherson et al (1982) suggested that the degree of variation was more heavily influenced by controversy and uncertainty among professionals than by the system of health care.

Some variation within the UK is thought to occur because of differences in rates of morbidity and age and sex distribution (McPherson 1990). Variations in surgical rates between regions in the UK are increasingly explained by variations between individual surgeons and by GP referral preferences (Ham 1988, p. 13). Reasons for these cultural variations appear to be clinical judgement, prevailing custom and the supply and availability of resources (McPherson 1990, p. 21). Operations such as appendicectomy and cholycystectomy have low variation within the UK but high variation internationally. Tonsillectomy, hysterectomy and prostatectomy have high variation between areas in the UK and hysterectomy has a high international variation. McPherson (1990) states that so far:

In health care, there is a diversity of accepted opinion on the need for and value of alternative treatments. In many situations, equally qualified physicians might disagree on which treatment is optimal. There is often no scientifically correct way to practice much of medicine. Many accepted theories concerning the treatment of illness have not been adequately assessed, and consensus based on knowledge of treatment outcomes is the exception rather than the rule.

(McPherson 1990, p. 17)

Health policy research suggests that cultural influences, such as those quoted above, which affect the practice of medicine need to be acknowledged and medical procedures evaluated critically (for further discussion, see Cochrane 1971).

CRITICAL THINKING ABOUT NURSING THE SURGICAL PATIENT

Understanding culture, how it affects the care we give and the immediate environment we care in, is not sufficient to realise the full impact culture has on surgical nursing. Surgery, as part of the medical establishment, developed into a profession over a period of 100 years, from an unregulated world of barbers, healers and quacks (Stacey 1988) whose competence and judgement were variable and whose power depended on the patronage extended to them from their rich, elite clients. (See Waddington 1973 and Jewson 1976 for further discussion.) The medical profession in the 20th century has evolved into a professional body with authority, status and power whose members work within the NHS and the private sector (Gabe et al 1994), thus adapting to societal changes but also retaining a body of rich patrons. Initially the history of medicine was documented as the logical progression from ignorance to expertise by an emerging expert group using its knowledge and skills for the benefit of society. This cultural history is important to understand when considering how culture affects nursing the surgical patient, as Fox (1992), Britten (1991), Bendelow (1993) and Fisher & Peterson (1993) have found.

This view of medicine as essentially beneficent was challenged in the 1970s and 1980s by a more critical view – one which analysed the medical profession as an elite occupational group whose claim to power, authority and status rested on the exploitation of the knowledge gap between doctors and patients. The medical profession was seen to be responsible for creating demand for its services by medicalising everyday life (Illich 1975, Gabe et al 1994). Medicine's claims to therapeutic effectiveness were also challenged at this time by historical research (McKeown 1979).

Fox's (1992) study into surgery is the first of its kind to critically examine how surgeons and surgery function to maintain this power, authority and status, to analyse the challenges to surgeons' power from nursing and management and to evaluate surgery's claim to heal through its specific skills. Fox argues that surgery in the UK has evolved for over a century into a specialty within medicine which can claim 'to stand for all that medicine as a whole claims for itself in terms of expertise and heroism' (Fox 1992, p. 1). The prestige associated with surgery has long been part of television programmes, both documentaries and fictionalised accounts (Karpf 1988).

Human aspects of surgery

Fox argues that surgery is not 'just' surgery, not just a technical intervention, but a human activity which is embedded in the social importance of the activity to the surgeons, the nurses, the anaesthetists and the patients. Surgery is about the power of the surgeon to be an expert. This power has cultural meaning and operates through the culture of the surgical environment.

Fox has looked at surgery and surgeons with a critical eye and suggested ways in which surgery has been socially constructed by surgeons to benefit the profession rather than the patient. There are four key areas where the culture of surgery works to enhance surgeons' control over patients and other professional groups involved in surgery (nurses, operating department assistants and anaesthetists):

- asepsis
- dominance over surgery
- patient as expert
- challenges to medicine.

Asepsis

Fox found that surgeons and surgical procedures maintain that asepsis and the demarcation of the aseptic area in the operating theatres is essential to prevent infection. However, Fox observed that asepsis was continually disregarded, particularly by medical staff. Asepsis, rather than a scientific fact on which rested the healing power of surgery, had a more symbolic role in identifying surgery as different and better than other medical specialties. Nurses in this situation tried to enforce asepsis but were ignored. Fox concluded that the wearing of surgical masks depended on the status of the person wearing it.

Dominance over surgery

Fox observed that there was a struggle for control of the surgical procedure, from the operating theatre to the discharge of the surgical patient, between surgeons and anaesthetists primarily, but also in the surgical ward between surgeon and nurses. Fox found that surgeons shaped the behaviour of surgical nurses. The nurses either submitted passively or developed ways of manipulating the surgeon sometimes to their advantage without a confrontation. In this quotation from his fieldwork, the nurse is discussing aseptic technique in the operating theatre:

> Nurse C: X is always reaching over and taking instruments. I slapped him on the hand. I feel like saying, 'Stop it, that's my domain.' But I'll say that I'm learning, and I can't learn if he takes the instruments.
>
> (Fox 1992, p. 36)

Patient as expert

Fox found that surgical patients, in terms of their knowledge about their bodies and their illnesses, were ignored by surgeons. Surgeons, whose power over the patient was almost complete in the operating theatre, continued to view themselves as experts in the ward where the patients were now recovering and beginning to see themselves as capable of making decisions about their progress. Nurses tried to use this situation as a means of challenging the surgeons' control over the ward stay. In particular, he observed nurses acting as advocates for patients and contesting surgeons' control over wound healing and discharge. Fox concluded that surgeons appeared at their most authoritative on the postoperative ward round, where their authority could, of course, be challenged by patients and nurses. He observed only one patient who managed to set an agenda for the interaction and she had to write her questions down to ensure that they were answered.

Challenges to medicine

Lastly, Fox found that surgeons' authority which has become part of their professional culture was being challenged by the political and economic changes within the NHS. Day care surgery, in particular, reduced the surgeon to a 'cog in the technical machine' where the mystique and aura surrounding surgical techniques are reduced to measuring outcomes in economic terms, for example throughput of patients. Managers challenge the occupational power of surgeons as the following quotation shows: 'Surgeons will only change the way they work if they are forced to by re-organization' (Fox 1994, p. 16).

The culture of gender

The last environmental and cultural factor which affects the delivery of nursing is that of gender. Witz (1994) suggests that biomedical values and beliefs are culturally reinforced through gender. The majority of nurses are female and women are cross-culturally inferior to men, especially in the world of work. Nursing as an occupational group has emerged out of Victorian ideals about womanhood and these are still culturally important (for further reading on this topic, see Ehrenreich & English 1979). Armstrong (1983) argues that the cultural devaluing of caring skills and women's position as carers adversely affects women working in professional caring and the status of nursing work. The wider cultural issues which affect surgery and surgical nursing turn out to be political and economic but also shaped by gender. Witz argues that the 'problem for nursing has been and continues to be the problem of gender' (1994, p. 23). In Fox's study (1992) he observed nurses challenging surgeons' power sometimes effectively and at other times ineffectively (the majority of nurses being female and the surgeons male). Witz (1994) maintains that nurses need to recognise that culturally gender is the fact which prevents the development of professional autonomy through practitioner status.

Reflective point

Are you aware of how gender roles influence your interactions with your colleagues? Discuss these thoughts with someone you work with.

Marriage, family life and immigration

The sociocultural implications for caring for the surgical patient are affected by two factors: (1) sociocultural changes in the UK, in particular in relation to the family; (2) the changing demographic and ethnic profile of local populations. Social changes in the UK have affected cultural behaviours and beliefs. These changes have been the result of global movements such as feminism, information technology and international markets and trade as well as local movements of peoples or immigration. These changes means that British culture is no longer homogeneous (it may have only been so in ideal terms) and to care for surgical patients the nurse has to be aware of and understand the cultural shifts that have taken place and place them in their historical context.

Marriage and family life

There have been changing family patterns cross-culturally over the 20th century which are the result of immigration, economic developments, increased communication and mass culture (Giddens 1993, p. 397). These are very broadly:

- a declining influence of kin groups (including extended families)
- an increased trend for individuals to choose their own spouses
- an increased attention to and action for the rights of women
- changing attitudes to sexual activity, which include both sexual freedom and restriction in sexual activity
- an increased concern with the human rights of children.

These movements have been reflected in family life in the UK. Although monogamy remains the only form of legal marriage, the most common marriage pattern may be called 'serial monogamy' where individuals are married to one person at a time but have more than one marriage. Sexual relations outside of marriage are common. Marriage is based on the ideal of romantic love and couples are expected to find self-fulfilment through partnership with each other (Giddens 1993). Sexuality has become a human rights issue and a political movement. Choice of sexual expression has moved on to the political agenda and become a concept nurses have had to deal with in caring for surgical patients (Corless 1992; for further reading see Lawler 1992, Webb 1994).

Families are patrilineal, that is, they follow the male line for inheritance and the woman more commonly takes the man's name on marriage. Families are nuclear and have ties with extended families but tend not to live local to their kin (for further discussion see Young & Wilmott 1973, Rapaport et al 1982, Allan 1985). Divorce remains at a higher level than at any other period since its legalisation (Clark & Haldane 1990); 40% of children born in the UK will live in a one-parent family and, as remarriage is also increasing, they will become members of 'reconstituted' families (Giddens 1993, p. 404, Haskey 1994a,b). Three-quarters of those divorced remarry. Concern about the effects of divorce on children has been well documented and changes in attitudes to divorce have been reflected in the Children Act 1989 and changes to the adversarial divorce proceedings. Divorce has an economic impact as well as an emotional one (Bohannon 1970, Vaughan 1986). Women suffer economic effects more than men after divorce, particularly if they remain as lone parents. There are 1.3 million lone-parent families and they comprise 1 in 5 of all households with dependent children (Haskey 1994b). The number of single and separated lone-parent families compared with widowed lone-parent families has increased. The nuclear family as a household is declining and accounts for 24% of all households compared with 37% of households with cohabiting or married couples with no dependent children and 26% households with single people (Pearce & White 1994). (See Social Trends 24: OPCS 1994) for further discussion of the types of family life in the UK.) The surgical nurse needs to be aware of the patient's family history and set-up in order to plan for discharge and to arrange visiting of significant others whilst the patient is in hospital. The nurse can no longer rely on the presence of a carer, who will be at home and not working, to care for the patient on discharge. One way of mapping these family relationships is to draw genograms with the patient and to highlight the patient's significant relationships. One example of this approach to mapping important relationships is a 'friendship' circle discussed by Allan & Harding (1994).

One major change in family set-ups since the Second World War has been in the role of women. The position of women has changed within the family owing to paid work outside the home, which tends to be part time, increased unemployment of men from the manufacturing industries, and the women's movement, which has challenged and changed cultural beliefs and values about women's roles in society. Women working full time are 36% and part time are 89% of the workforce (Pearce & White 1994) and 59% of married women work (Graham 1993). This poses an extra burden on many women: the dual burden of work within the household, including child care, and paid employment (Gittins 1985, Graham 1993).

Another cultural shift has been the increase in the population over 65 years old and the increase in the elderly infirm (DoH 1990). This has an impact on the family, work, health and social care, and differences in life-courses between the elderly and the young in society. An example of the effects these demographic changes might have on surgical nursing is the increasing popularity of day care surgery. There are specific criteria used to select appropriate day care surgical patients which specify among others that the patient will be accompanied home and will have a companion for 24 hours. For the elderly this may be a problem if they are widowed or have a dependent relative to care for. But it also poses problems for younger adults who have dependent relatives or children.

Table 10.1 The ethnic composition of the population of England and Wales

Ethnic group	Number (000s)	Percentage
White	46 938	94.1
Black Caribbean	499	1.0
Black African	210	0.4
Black other	176	0.4
Indian	830	1.7
Pakistani	455	0.9
Bangladeshi	162	0.3
Chinese	146	0.3
Other Asian	193	0.6
Other	281	0.6
England and Wales	49 890	100

Source: 1991 Census (DoH 1993)

Immigration

Immigration into the UK has also altered family life in ways that affect nursing (Chan 1994, Doolin 1994, Lea 1994). Immigration of ethnic minorities to the UK refers to those peoples who immigrated in the late 19th and early 20th centuries from Europe for political and religious reasons and those who have immigrated since the early 20th century largely from the New Commonwealth (which includes the Indian subcontinent, the African Commonwealth, and the Caribbean Commonwealth) for largely economic reasons (DoH 1993). The British government differentiates between political and economic immigration, regarding the former as valid and the latter invalid. This decision is a political one and open to interpretation at different times in history (Giddens 1993). The ethnic minority population distribution is given in Table 10.1. (See Owen (1994) and Heath & Dale (1994) for further discussion of ethnic minorities within the UK.)

There is a wealth of data on country of origin for British residents but until the 1991 census no data were collected on ethnic origin. This means that figures of ethnic minorities are underestimated in official statistics. It highlights the blurred distinctions between ethnicity, nationality and race which affect the family lives of immigrants and their children (Giddens 1993, p. 401). For surgical nurses who wish to increase their knowledge of the local population profile, local government surveys collect data on ethnic origin. The 1991 census records ethnic origin by County District and this is used to plan care for local populations. The Chinese and Irish populations have little epidemiological data and there has been criticism that their health needs are rarely discussed in relation to health care provision (DoH 1993, Doolin 1994).

Graham (1993) discusses the differences between ethnic minority and white family life in the UK in respect of women's lives. There is a youthful age structure of black families compared to the ageing structure of the white population. There are also a greater proportion of households with dependent children among ethnic minority families: 46% Afro-Caribbean households have dependent children (a child under 16 years of age), 60% of Indian households and 78% of Pakistani–Bangladeshi households compared to 29% of white households (General Household Survey 1989).

Reflective point

What implications do these statistics have for the surgical nurse caring for women from ethnic minority families?

Graham (1993) points out that ethnic minority communities are also changing as a result of migration in respect of marriage and kin networks, and cites two challenges to cultural stereotypes which have been researched recently among UK ethnic communities. Brah (1992) and Bhachu (1991) both looked at changes to traditional, cultural gender roles expressed by young Asian girls and the effects of these on their attitudes to family and marriage.

The Health of the Nation strategy (DoH 1993) includes specific policy statements which apply to surgical nursing and the sociocultural needs of patients. Firstly, some ethnic groups are at higher risk of illness in the five key areas. This needs specific action in screening and health promotion, particularly as the ethnic minorities have a younger age structure and are potentially at risk of developing those illnesses for which surgery is a palliative treatment, for example heart disease, peripheral vascular disease, diabetes, cancers. Secondly, ethnic minorities have poorer access to care, including surgery. Thirdly, specific illnesses which are no longer prevalent in the white community, are still problems for the ethnic communities.

NURSING THE SURGICAL PATIENT IN A CULTURALLY SENSITIVE WAY

These cultural changes have meant that surgical nursing, pre-admission clinics, arrangements for day case surgery, hospital care, discharge planning and community follow-up, can no longer rely on the presence of carers in the community who will be members of a family group living in the same household. There is discussion of issues related to caring for ethnic minority patients in the nursing literature; however, very little of this literature has focused on surgical patients. How does the surgical nurse care in a culturally sensitive way?

Culturally sensitive care is respectful of differences between groups and individuals within groups (Fee 1994). Nurses have to be aware of their own prejudices and have specific information to enable them to provide care that is based on a knowledge of culture, the transmission of culture, and how culture affects health and health care provision. Four nursing models will now be discussed. Leininger's theory of cultural care diversity and universality (1985) is the most developed in its theoretical thinking. It remains the only theory of cultural care. The other three are frameworks which will introduce the reader to the current thinking in the field.

Cultural interactionist nursing model

Denny & McCrea (1991), in a qualitative study of the needs of patients undergoing stoma formation, identified three groups of needs: sociocultural, psychological and biophysical. They found that patients felt that individual psychological and biophysical needs were met but did not feel that their sociocultural needs were met. Denny & McCrea suggested that human needs are in constant interaction with the environment, which includes the family and society. In hospital this interaction focuses on the surgeons and the nursing staff as well as on the family and significant others. Nurses and surgeons become the stimuli and satisfiers of needs. Psychological and biophysical needs were identified by the staff and responded to but cultural needs were not identified. Denny & McCrea argued that sociocultural needs were difficult to identify because they did not impinge on hospital care and remained the province of the family and the individual. However, this did not remove nursing responsibility for identifying and responding to sociocultural needs. An example of a sociocultural need which was not identified was the need for information about stoma care. Patients felt that they were not informed about stoma care before they left hospital; only one patient was given the ward booklet on stoma care. This patient was asked if the nurses came back to discuss the booklet: 'No, they didn't come back. I suppose they left it up to my own intelligence. I am sure if I had asked them they would have' (Denny & McCrea 1991, p. 42).

What this demonstrates is that the nurses may have assumed that the patient's understanding was the same as their own and that he had no need of explanation. This is an example of ethnocentrism (Weidman 1979) where professionals are largely unable to see outside their world view, their clinical reality. The remaining patients received information from their health centres but this was not planned as part of their discharge. The nurses focused on the physical needs of changing the stoma bag and dealing with the odour, and teaching patients to do this for themselves. They remained ignorant of wider sociocultural needs that might have been the concern for patients, such as sexual intercourse, and did not discuss the non-professional sectors of health care and the networks of support that patients might use on discharge. Denny & McCrea (1991) discuss the application of a cultural interactionist model of nursing which plans care around the needs identified by patients (see Fig. 10.1).

The key to this model of nursing is the assessment stage. Needs can only be identified if they are expressed, and the nurse, as both stimulus and satisfier of needs during surgical care, is responsible for this in planning care.

Leininger's theory of cultural care diversity and universality

Health and illness beliefs are culturally diverse but all cultures interpret illness in culturally meaningful ways and respond to illness in different ways. Leininger (1985) argues that care, which she sees as central to nursing, is universal but that different cultures care in different, culturally meaningful ways.

Her theory attempts to identify the differences and similarities of care between cultures which will provide the basis for nursing knowledge which will guide nursing actions (1985, p. 210). She has focused on universalities and diversities of human care. Cultural care diversity is the variability of assistive, supportive or facilitative acts towards or for an individual or group which nursing carries out. Cultural care universality is the uniform phenomena found in specific cultures through which care is expressed. She argues that there are more care diversities than universalities because of the variability of human life, but that this may change as acculturation progresses with the mix of people from different cultures and ethnic backgrounds, principally through information technology.

The aim of her theory is to establish meaningful congruent and holistic care for the patient. Her theory explains and predicts human care patterns of cultures and nursing care practices. Transcultural nursing uses the discussion of culture, health and illness beliefs, and the effect of culture on caring, to formulate three culturally based nursing care activities which enable the nurse to work within the patient's cultural frame of reference (see Fig. 10.2). Again, care given is based on an assessment of the social world of patients, their position and beliefs as individuals and within families and social groups, and their beliefs about health care. This assessment is called the Sunrise Model (Leininger 1985, p. 210).

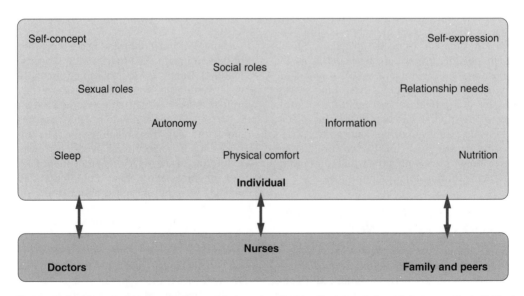

Figure 10.1 The cultural interactionist model of nursing showing the interrelationship between the individual and the health care professional (adapted from Denny & McCrea 1991).

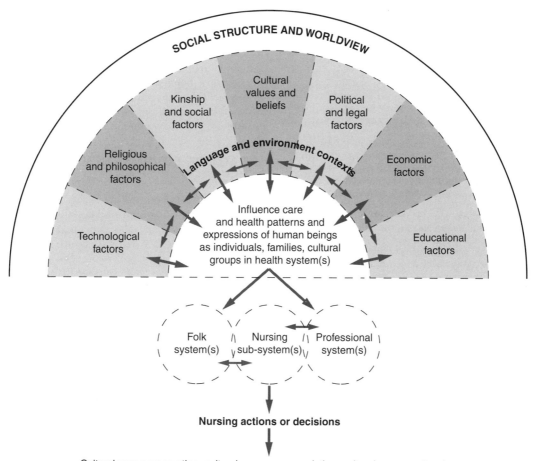

Figure 10.2   Sunrise theoretical and conceptual model of transcultural care diversity and universality (adapted from Leininger 1985).[1]

Box 10.1 shows how this model assists the surgical nurse in caring for a patient undergoing stoma formation in the three cultural care activities.

Leininger predicts that culturally congruent and sensitive care will reduce stresses and conflicts which arise from differences in cultural backgrounds of carers and patients.

Intercultural communication model

'Intercultural communication' is the study of 'concepts and skills of face-to-face interaction between people who are culturally different' but also emphasises the need to understand the impact of the nurse's cultural

patterns as well as those of the patient (Geissler 1995, p. 69). The nurse has to understand the function of communication and the unspoken understandings which are presumed by people engaged in communication. Therefore, intercultural communication acknowledges that there are differences and seeks to explore these to give culturally sensitive care. An intercultural communication model for nursing is based on the reality of the clinical dyad: a nurse from one culture and a patient from a different culture. The skills needed in this model are communication skills and a degree of self-awareness. As Geissler argues, cultural variations:

illustrate the need to understand self as a basis for understanding the culturally diverse patient. Because culture equals communication, nurses must recognise and address much more than language barriers and the need for interpreters … To work effectively with culturally diverse

---

[1]From: *Nursing & Health Care* 6 (4). Reprinted with permission. Copyright 1985 National League for Nursing.

Box 10.1 An example of culturally sensitive care using Leininger's nursing actions (adapted from McGee 1994)

- *Cultural care preservation* which is essentially helping patients to preserve their existing lifestyle by drawing on culturally based knowledge and skills, e.g. acknowledging the preference for and facilitating the presence of a relative during clinical examination. This may be a spouse who had concerns centred on their sexual relationship.
- *Cultural care accommodation* which involves helping patients to adapt to change in a manner which is culturally acceptable to them, e.g. a change in diet after surgical bowel resection. This may mean translation of information leaflets or appointment with a dietitian with an interpreter or the presence of whoever will be cooking the new diet for the patient.
- *Cultural care repatterning* in which the nurse helps the patient to adapt to major changes, e.g. managing a stoma in a culturally acceptable way. This may involve adapting health education about handwashing to incorporate beliefs about cleanliness.

---

patients, their families and with culturally diverse colleagues, nurses must first examine their own culturally learned values and behaviours.

(Geissler 1995, p. 72)

Geissler (1995) uses three examples of cultural variations – thinking patterns, cleanliness and perceptions of time – to discuss how communication about cultural differences needs to be explored to deliver culturally sensitive care. Geissler does not provide a framework for using this approach to nursing. However, in discussing cultural variations in thinking patterns, she suggests the use of mind-maps to illustrate how the nurse might chart the patient's cultural values associated with pain. Although this is not a concrete framework for the nurse to implement, it does provide a way of thinking about culture and how the nurse might focus on communication to develop culturally sensitive care.

Generalised nursing model

Littlewood's generalised nursing model is based on Kleinman's insight that the biomedical model does not acknowledge the difference between disease and sickness (Kleinman 1978). Patients' beliefs about sickness are grounded in their own lives and patients ascribe meanings to their symptoms (Littlewood 1989, p. 225). She argues that nurses are ideally situated to give culturally sensitive care because they are with patients and deal with patients' understandings about their illness (sickness). Nurses mediate between the worlds of

patients (sickness) and doctors (disease). The generalised nursing model uses an assessment to find out patients' beliefs about their admission, illness or surgical procedure. It is an ethnoscientific model – that is, it attempts to obtain, systematically, an accurate account of people's behaviour and how they perceive and interpret their environment. Box 10.2 gives some examples of questions which nurses might ask to complete their assessment in this model.

PRACTICE DEVELOPMENT: ASSESSMENT

The four models outlined above are developments in the fields of transcultural nursing and anthropology applied to nursing. The key features of these approaches are understanding culture and its effects on health and illness; self-awareness and the effect the nurse has on the nurse–patient interaction; cultural relativism – the need to accept 'other'; and the importance of assessment.

Fee (1994) argues that a structured assessment guide is a useful first step in delivering culturally sensitive care. He suggests that such a guide would need to include:

- sociological data, including economic status, educational status, social networks, valued social institutions
- psychological data, including self-concept, family, significant others and peers, external environment and response to stress
- biophysiological data.

In particular, nurses should be specific in asking questions that reflect their awareness of other healing systems: Does the patient consult with any other health practitioners? What cultural beliefs does the patient have about the cause(s) of illness and health? Would the patient like any other health practitioner to be included in the surgical care? Fee argues that an assessment based on data outlined above would allow patients to express their explanatory model about their admission for surgery. Case studies 10.4 and 10.5 will illustrate this in relation to sexuality. Sexuality has been deliberately selected as an important aspect of surgical nursing and one which has implications for all three areas outlined in Fees' assessment guide

Savage (1987) makes clear that surgery can affect patients by its direct surgical intervention on the physiological sexual response and by its effect on body image. In Case study 10.4 there is direct physiological damage and an altered body image.

Box 10.2   The nursing process using the generalised nursing model (adapted from International Journal of Nursing Studies 26(93) Littlewood J A model for nursing using the anthropological literature, 221–229 (1989) with kind permission from Elsevier Science Ltd)

Assessment
- Why has the patient used this particular healing system, i.e. agreed to hospitalisation?
- What does the patient see as the cause of his or her presenting problem?
- What does the patient feel are the consequences of the problems?
- What does the patient feel are the cures – what can help?
- What does the patient feel are the causes for disturbances in terms of the basic physiological needs?
- What metaphors are used to describe the person's experiences?
- How would the treatment of the disturbance be effected within the patient's peer group and family?
- Are there any rituals surrounding this problem?
- When will the patient feel that he or she is better/has a better quality of life?
- How well does what the person says about causes/cures concord with significant others and/or peers?

Planning
- Care is planned with the patient and discussions as to who else might be brought in to help determine needs/care/cures.
- Mediation by the nurse takes place, doctor–patient interaction, patient–ward interaction, or patient–environment interaction.

Nursing intervention
- Involvement of agreed agencies and recognised healers.
- Nursing treatments carried out as negotiated with patient.

Evaluation
- Does the person feel healed?
- Is the person able to fulfil all the basic needs?
- Has the cause of the disorder been understood and discussed?
- What does the person feel the consequences of the intervention might be?

Case study 10.4   Patient C

A woman has undergone radical vulvectomy for cancer. She is married and her partner visits every day and has been involved in her care. She has two children and works part time as a teacher in a primary school. She has been visited and supported by relatives and friends during her stay in hospital. She has consulted a reflexologist during recent years for general health problems. She is anxious over the possible recurrence of her cancer and feels 'dirty' around her operation site. She has said that she has enjoyed sex before the operation and is worried that her sexual fulfilment may now be impeded.

Her partner has asked the nurses about sexual intercourse in the future. He is anxious not to appear undesiring of his wife because of her altered body image but not over keen, which may make her feel under pressure to have sexual intercourse with him.

One of the nurses explains to him, and later to the couple together, about the physiological and psychological effects of the surgery. She explores the meanings that different expressions of sexual activity have for them both and they are referred to a sex therapist. The couple also decide to consult the patient's reflexologist about complementary therapy in the rehabilitation stage.

Grossman (1982) gives examples of different surgical procedures which commonly affect a patient's sexuality. She suggests that there are five problem areas relating to sexuality when nursing the surgical patient:

1. impaired body image

2. loss of self-esteem owing to dependency on others
3. differences in gender identity and gender role
4. difficulties in decision-making and responsibility for sexual functioning
5. possibility for becoming a victim of sexual exploitation by others including health care staff.

Grossman (1982) suggests that seemingly non-sexual areas of the body may be affected by surgery and cause sexual difficulties (Case study 10.5).

Savage (1987) suggests that nurses have to imagine the effect any surgical procedure might have on their patients' expression and experience of sexuality to empathise with and consequently care for them. By assessing the whole experience of the patient's surgical experience, the nurse may care in a culturally sensitive way.

Reflective point

Reflect on a critical incident where you have cared for a patient's sexual needs. What did you find difficult? Why? Discuss these feelings with a colleague.

CONCLUSION

This chapter has set out to introduce the surgical nurse to the concept of culture and how it frames the social context of surgery by presenting an overview of

---

Case study 10.5   Patient D

A young woman has maxillofacial surgery and finds, postoperatively, that her scars affect how she feels about being kissed and kissing her partner. Kissing has played an important part in their previous sexual relationship and this situation has upset both partners involved.

---

current social and cultural issues which affect surgical nursing. It has been suggested that central to practice development in surgical nursing is the need for the surgical nurse to develop awareness of the need for culturally sensitive care. Building on self-awareness about ethnocentricity and social change, the nurse may develop practice in the context of a multicultural society; to do this, a cultural nursing model needs to be developed, and assessment of the surgical patient's cultural background needs to be undertaken.

A cultural nursing model for surgical nursing

There is no one nursing model which enables the surgical nurse to implement sociocultural care in the surgical environment, as developing culturally sensitive care is dependent on self-awareness about one's own culture (Chrisman & Johnson 1990, Geissler 1995, Leininger 1985).

At the heart of caring for patients in a culturally sensitive way is the ability of the nurse to tolerate ambiguity and to share and value cultural difference and similarity. Chrisman & Johnson (1990) argue that this anthropological approach, which values cultural relativity, is inherently at odds with the biological and reductionist way of thinking that characterises the biomedical model of health care and much nursing care. It may be that nursing the surgical patient in a culturally sensitive way begins with that insight to change and develop practice.

However, Chrisman & Johnson (1990) acknowledge that health care practitioners need 'prescriptive theory' – a rationale for using this approach to enable them to work in the biomedical world. They point out that practitioners use indicators to help them give cultural care, such as the patient is identified as ethnically 'other' and the disease is associated with 'other'. This has given rise to many excellent books on ethnic and religious differences. Chrisman & Johnson (1990) suggest that a prescriptive theory for an anthropological health model needs to concern itself primarily with culture. The basics of this theory would include how culture is learnt; how culture is shared; what customs are evident in different groups; how value is assigned

to behaviours and beliefs; ethnocentrism and cultural relativity; and the illness/disease distinction. These are all incorporated in Leininger's theory of cultural care diversity and universality (1991) which is the most developed model available.

However, Chrisman & Johnson (1990) argue that medical anthropology needs to become more critical of medical practice and to examine the power relationships involved in the therapeutic encounter. Fox's (1994) study showed how nurses were involved in a subordinate position in many surgical encounters. Leininger's (1985) theory has not developed this critical thinking, and any model applied to surgical nursing needs to incorporate critical thinking to care in a culturally sensitive way. Littlewood's generalised nursing model is based on this critical insight.

Assessment

This self-awareness might start with the surgical nurse asking herself:

- How have the patient's beliefs affected and possibly contributed to this admission for surgery?
- How will these beliefs affect the patient's recovery from surgery?
- How will my sociocultural background affect our relationship?
- How does the culture of the ward/outpatients' department affect our relationship?
- How can I facilitate meaningful communication?

Developing practice

To develop practice, surgical nurses need to decide on the standards they want to set for quality care in meeting the sociocultural needs of patients. These might involve a ward philosophy, assessment tools which reflect the understandings about culture discussed in this chapter, language which is non-discriminatory and relevant to the ethnic minority needs of the local community, information sheets which are culturally relevant and sensitive, and initiatives which seek to develop equal access to surgical services for the local community.

Surgical nurses need to develop evaluation strategies to measure the care they are delivering in terms of these standards, and to liaise with the local community to meet local needs.

The sociocultural implications of caring for the surgical patient are broad. They require the surgical nurse to be reflective, ethically aware and self-motivated because it is easier and much more comfortable to be unaware of another's culture. A multicultural society calls for a multicultural nurse and nursing culture.

USEFUL ADDRESSES

Council on Nursing and Anthropology
Jody Glittenberg
President CONAA
School of Nursing
University of Arizona
Tucson AZ 85721
USA

Anthropology in Action
Dean Powley
Administrator
CCS, Arts B
University of Sussex,
Falmer
Brighton BN1 9QN

REFERENCES

Allan G 1985 Family life. Basil Blackwell, Oxford
Allan H T, Harding I G 1994 Happy families. Nursing Standard 8(43): 36–37
Allan H T, Wiseman T W 1995 Establishing an anthropology for nurses within Project 2000 common foundation programme. Anthropology in Action, Journal for Applied Anthropology in Policy and Practice 2(3): 2–7
Armstrong D 1983 Medicine as a profession: time of change. British Medical Journal 301: 691–693
Backett K C, Davidson C 1995 Life-course and life-style: the social and cultural location of health behaviours. Social Science and Medicine 40(5: 629-638
Baxter C 1988 Ethnic minorities. Culture shock. Nursing Times 84(2): 36–38
Bendelow G 1993 Pain perceptions, emotions and gender. Sociology of Health and Illness 15(3): 273–294
Bhachu P 1991 Culture, ethnicity and class among Punjabi Sikh women in 1990's Britain. New Community 17(3): 401–412
Bohannon P 1970 The six stations of divorce. In: Bohannon P (ed) Divorce and after. Doubleday, New York
Brah A 1992 Women of South Asian origin in Britain – issues and concerns. In: Braham P, Rattansi A, Skellington R (eds) Racism and antiracism: inequalities, opportunities and policies. Sage Publications, London
Britten N 1991 Hospital consultants' views of their patients. Sociology of Health and Illness 13(1): 83–97
Brown P J, Inhorn M C 1990 Disease, ecology and human behaviour. In: Johnson T M, Sargent C F (eds) Medical anthropology: contemporary theory and method. Praeger, New York, ch 11
Calnan M 1987 Health and illness: the lay perspective. Tavistock, London
Cassel J C, Patrick R, Jenkins D 1960 Epidemiological analysis of the health implications of culture change. Annals of the New York Academy of Sciences 84: 938–949
Cay E L, Philip A E, Small W P, Neilson J, Henderson M A 1975 Patient's assessment of the result of surgery for peptic ulcer. Lancet 1(7897): 29–31
Chan T T L 1994 Black and ethnic minority clients: meeting needs. Nursing Standard 9(11): 3–13
Children Act 1989 HMSO, London
Chrisman N J, Johnson T M 1990 Clinically applied anthropology. In: Johnson T M, Sargent C F (eds) Medical anthropology: contemporary theory and method. Praeger, New York, ch 5
Clark D, Haldane D 1990 Wedlocked? Intervention and Research in Marriage. Polity Press, Cambridge

Cochrane A L 1971 Effectiveness and efficiency: random reflections on health services. Nuffield Provincial Hospital Trust, London
Community Care Act 1990 HMSO, London
Corless R 1992 Caring for a homosexual man undergoing a colostomy formation. British Journal of Nursing 1(10): 502–506
Csordas T J, Kleinman A 1990 The therapeutic process. In: Johnson T M, Sargent C F (eds) Medical anthropology: contemporary theory and method. Praeger, New York, ch 1
Denny P, McCrea H 1991 Stoma care: the patient's perspective. Journal of Advanced Nursing 16(1): 39–46
Department of Health (DoH) 1990 Health of the nation. HMSO, London
Department of Health (DoH) 1991 The patient's charter. HMSO, London
Department of Health (DoH) 1993 Health of the nation ethnicity and health, a guide for the NHS. HMSO, London
Department of Health (DoH) 1995 The patient's charter and you. HMSO, London
Doolin N 1994 The luck of the Irish?… Nursing Standard 8(46): 155–165
Dressler W W 1990 Culture, stress and disease. In: Johnson T M, Sargent C F (eds) Medical anthropology: contemporary theory and method. Praeger, New York, ch 14
Ehrenreich B, English D 1979 For her own good: 150 years of advice to women. Pluto Press, London
Fee F A 1994 An introduction to multicultural issues in spinal cord injury rehabilitation. SCI Psychosocial Process 7(3): 104–108
Fisher B J, Peterson C 1993 She won't be dancing much anyway: a study of surgeons, surgical nurses and elderly patients. Qualitative Health Research 3(2): 165–183
Fitzgerald M H 1992 Multicultural clinical interactions. Journal of Rehabilitation 58(2): 38–42
Fox N J 1992 The social meaning of surgery. Open University Press, Buckingham
Fox N J 1994 Anaesthetists, the discourse on patient fitness and the organisation of surgery. Sociology of Health and Illness 16(1): 3–18
Gabe J, Kelleher D, Williams G (eds) 1994 Challenging medicine. Routledge, London
Geertz C 1966 The impact of the concept of culture on the concept of man. In: Platt J R (ed) New views on the nature of man. Reprinted 1973, University of Chicago Press, Chicago

Geissler E M 1995 Culture and the nurse–patient dyad. Medisurg Nursing 4(1): 69–72

General Household Survey 1989 HMSO, London

Giddens A 1993 Sociology, 2nd edn. Polity Press, Cambridge

Gittins D 1985 The family in question. Macmillan, Oxford

Goodenough W H 1961 Comment on cultural evolution. Daedalus 90: 521–528

Graham H 1993 Hardship and health in women's lives. Harvester Wheatsheaf, Hemel Hempstead

Grossman S 1982 Surgical conditions. In: Weinberg J (ed) Sexuality: human needs and nursing practice. W B Saunders, Philadelphia

Ham C 1988 Health care variations: assessing the evidence. King's Fund Institute, London

Haskey J 1994a Stepfamilies and stepchildren in Great Britain. In: Population trends. OPCS: Government Statistical Services, London, Summer no 76, pp 17–28

Haskey J 1994b Estimated numbers of one parent families and their prevalence in Great Britain in 1991. In: Population trends. OPCS: Government Statistical Services, London, Winter no 78, pp 5–19

Heath S, Dale A 1994 Household and family formation in Great Britain – the ethnic dimension. In: Population trends. OPCS: Government Statistical Services, London, Autumn no 77, pp 5–13

Helman C 1990 Culture, health and illness. Butterworth-Heinemann, Oxford

Henley A 1987 Supplement on racism, nursing and the health service. Nursing Times 83(24): 24–31

Henley A 1988 Caring in a multi racial society. Bloomsbury and Islington Southside Public Health Department, London

Henry J P, Cassel J C 1969 Psychosocial factors in essential hypertension. American Journal of Epidemiology 90: 171–200

Herskovits M J 1955 Culture anthropology. Alfred A Knopf, New York

Illich I 1975 Limits to medicine. Marion Boyars, London

Jenks C 1993 Culture. Routledge, London

Jewson N 1976 The disappearance of the sick man from medical cosmology. Sociology 10(2): 225–244

Karpf A 1988 Doctoring the media: the reporting of health and medicine. Routledge, London

Keesing R M 1982 Cultural anthropology, 2nd edn. Holt-Saunders, New York

Kleinman A 1978 Culture, illness and care, cultural lessons from anthropologic and cross-cultural research. Annals of Internal Medicine 88: 251–258

Kleinman A 1980 Patients and healers in the context of culture. University of California Press, Berkeley

Konner M 1993 The trouble with medicine. BBC Books, London .

Lawler J 1992 Behind the screens, nursing somology and the problem of the body. Churchill Livingstone, Melbourne

Lea A 1994 Nursing in today's multicultural society: a transcultural perspective. Journal of Advanced Nursing 20(2): 307–313

Leach E 1982 Social anthropology. Fontana, Glasgow

Leininger M M 1978 Transcultural nursing: concepts, theories and practices. John Wiley, New York

Leininger M M 1985 Transcultural care diversity and universality: a theory of nursing. Nursing and Health Care 6(4): 209–212

Leininger M M (ed) 1991 Cultural care diversity and universality: a theory of nursing. National League for Nursing, New York

Littlewood J 1989 A model for nursing using the anthropological literature. International Journal of Nursing Studies 26(93): 221–229

McGee P 1994 Culturally sensitive and culturally comprehensive care. British Journal of Nursing 3(15): 789–792

McKeown T 1979 The role of medicine, 2nd edn. Oxford University Press, Oxford

McPherson K 1990 International differences in medical care practices. In: Health care systems in transition: the search for efficiency. OECD, Paris

McPherson K, Wennberg J W, Hovind O et al 1982 Small area variations in the use of common surgical procedures: an international comparison of New England, England and Norway. New England Journal of Medicine 307: 1310–1314

Malek C 1989 The socialisation of empathy. PhD Thesis, University of Boston

Malin N 1994 Development of community care. In: Malin N (ed) Implementing community care. Open University Press, Buckingham

Marshall P P A 1990 Cultural influences on perceived quality of life. Seminars in Oncology Nursing 6(4): 278-284

Miles R 1989 Racism. Routledge, London

Moerman D E 1979 Anthropology of symbolic healing. Current Anthropology 20: 59–80

Office of Population Censuses and Surveys (OPCS) 1994 Social trends 24. Government Statistical Office, London

Organization for Economic Cooperation and Development (OECD) 1993 Variations in common medical practices of large areas. In: Health policy studies no 3: OECD health systems facts and trends 1960–1991. OECD, Paris

Owen D 1994 Spatial variations in ethnic minority group populations in Great Britain. In: Population trends. OPCS: Government Statistical Services, London, Winter no 78, pp 23–33

Pearce D, White I 1994 1991 census of great Britain: summary of results. In: Population trends. OPCS: Government Statistical Services, London, Winter no 78, pp 34–43

Rapaport R N, Fogarty M P, Rapaport R 1982 Families in Britain. Routledge and Kegan Paul, London

Rose J F 1990 Psychologic health of women: a phenomenologic study of women's inner strength. Advances in Nursing Sciences 12(2): 56–70

Royal College of Nursing Ethnicity Committee 1993 Action on race and health. RCN, London

Savage J 1987 Nursing, gender and sexuality. Heinemann Medical Books, London

Scaffa M E, Davis A D 1990 Cultural considerations in the treatment of persons with AIDS. Occupational Therapy in Health Care 7(2/3/4): 69–85

Senior P A, Bhopal R 1994 Ethnicity as a variable in epidemiological research. British Medical Journal 309(July): 327–330

Singer M 1986 Developing a critical perspective in medical anthropology. Medical Anthropology Quarterly 17(5): 128–129

Stacey M 1988 The sociology of health and healing. Routledge, London

Swingewood A 1984 A short history of sociological thought. Macmillan Educational, London

Vaughan D 1986 Uncoupling: turning patients in intimate relationships. Oxford University Press, Oxford

Waddington I 1973 Role of the hospital in the development of modern medicine. Sociology 7(2): 211–224

Watson J 1988 Nursing: human science and care. National League for Nursing, New York

Webb C 1994 Living sexuality: issues for nursing and health. Scutari Press, London

Weidman H H 1979 The transcultural view: prerequisite to interethnic intercultural communication in medicine. Social Science and Medicine 13b: 85–87

Wilson-Barnett J, Macleod Clark J 1993 Research in health promotion and nursing. Macmillan, London

Witz A 1994 The challenge of nursing. In: Gabe J, Kelleher D, Williams G (eds) Challenging medicine. Routledge, London, ch 2

Young A 1980 The discourse on stress and the reproduction of conventional knowledge. Social Science and Medicine 14b: 133–146

Young M, Wilmott P 1973 The symmetrical family. Routledge and Kegan Paul, London

11

Surgery and the older person

Rhona Meek

AIMS

This chapter aims to:

- consider the effects of demographic trends on surgical health care demand
- examine the changes associated with normal ageing and analyse the implications of these changes for the specialist nursing care required by older people undergoing surgery
- critically analyse the relationship between age and surgical risk
- critically appraise the theories underpinning the care of older surgical patients.

INTRODUCTION

Caring for older people is possibly the most complex and challenging area of nursing. As a result of an increasing number of older people in the UK, there has been a rapid demand for health care; people are falling ill with age-related conditions who, not many years ago, simply would not have lived long enough for these to develop. Surgery is seen as an important means to improve function and quality of life. However, older people are at a higher risk for postoperative complications than younger patients and as a result, there is a growing need for nurses skilled in the care of older people, whatever the surgical setting.

When nurses are cognisant of the changes associated with the processes of ageing, implementation of preventive actions intraoperatively have the potential to positively alter the surgical course. By developing an increasing body of knowledge about the nursing needs of older people undergoing surgical procedures, nurses can provide care that not only will prolong lives, but will help to give those lives meaning, comfort and dignity (Jackson 1988).

Current perspectives

During the 20th century, Britain, in common with other industrialised countries, underwent a major demographic transformation. As a result of decreased mortality among all ages (but especially in the first year of life) and reduced fertility there has been a change in the nature of the population age distribution. Women aged 60 years and over and men aged 65 years and over, the ages usually taken as indicating the start of the later phases of the life course, now represent about 18% of the population compared with just 5% at the turn of the century (CSO 1990).

In 1991, the population of the UK was 57.6 million of which 10.5 million people were over pensionable age (Age Concern 1993). If the current demographic trends continue, then the early decades of the 21st century will see a further numerical increase in this age group. Current forecasts predict that the population of the UK will increase to approximately 61 million by the year 2025 (CSO 1990) including 11.3 million over pensionable age.

As the number of elderly people continues to rise, there has been a simultaneous increase in demand for health care services for older people, as well as an increase in treatment options (Lusis 1994). Operative and anaesthetic risks of many surgical procedures have changed. As a result of improved intraoperative techniques, there is now more rigorous and accurate preoperative evaluation and closer perioperative monitoring. Increasingly, older clients and their doctors are more likely to choose a surgical course, where indicated, in spite of old age (Dodson & Seymour 1992).

Individuals are no longer being denied the benefit of surgery because of age alone and consequently nurses are now confronted with a changing profile of patients undergoing surgery. However, surgical interventions, despite their advances, do present greater problems in later life. Changes associated with normal ageing and the presence of underlying disease contribute to higher morbidity and mortality in the older surgical patient. To combine the principles and practice of surgical nursing with the unique characteristics of the elderly patient is an immense challenge to the nurse, demanding perceptive assessment, careful identification of actual and potential problems and meticulous care planning and implementation (Garrett 1991). Consequently, essential knowledge for the surgical nurse includes an understanding of the processes of ageing and their effects on daily living activities, postoperative progress, the likely speed of rehabilitation and discharge needs.

THEORETICAL FOUNDATIONS AND IMPLICATIONS

Ageing and the older adult

Age is not a simple concept and has many meanings. Traditionally, the transition to retirement at age 60 for women or 65 for men heralds the onset of old age. But of course, nobody grows old overnight; the process of ageing is something in which everyone is involved from the moment of birth. It is a complex process and although it does not occur in the same way, at the same rate or to the same extent in all individuals, there are some commonalities of ageing.

It is not the intention of this chapter to discuss theories of biopsychosocial ageing in depth. It is rather to analyse the implications of the normal ageing processes for older adults who are in need of surgery, and the nurses who care for them. The theories of biopsychosocial ageing are well covered in texts by Kimmel (1990) and Bond et al (1993), included in the list of further reading at the end of the chapter.

Beginning in early adulthood, there are a number of internal biological and physiological changes taking place which eventually show up as external physical changes. During young adulthood, most biological and physiological functions are at their peak, or most efficient level. However, changes are indeed taking place but are internal and therefore not generally experienced or observed directly by the individual. Thus, they have little impact on behaviour.

For most people, it is when they reach their 40s and 50s that they take note of these changes. During middle to late adulthood the physical changes begin to affect individuals functionally, influencing behaviour and adaptation to the everyday environment (Hayslip & Panek 1993).

Despite the commonalities, not all individuals of a given age will share the same attitudes or have similar performance levels, since normal ageing processes proceed at different rates for different people. For example, some older men lose hair during their late 20s or have grey hair by 40, while others have a full head of hair in their 60s. Since all body systems do not age at the same rate, there is great variability among individuals.

According to Keene (1991) the major physical changes related to ageing are tissue deterioration, slowed cell division and atrophy, impaired homeostasis, decreased efficiency of the immune system and decreased neuromuscular response. These changes result in a decreased ability to respond quickly to stress and trauma, an increased need for intensive monitoring for complications, a longer postoperative recovery and rehabilitation period and an urgent need for a thorough assessment to prevent intra- and postoperative complications.

The major changes that occur as a result of normal ageing processes have been identified within Table 11.1, grouped together within the body systems, and their significance for the older person and the health care team demonstrated. It must be reiterated that ageing is a complex, unique process and, although these changes cannot be prevented, older people will not all experience them at the same rate or to the same extent. Different parts of the body age at different rates and an elderly person may therefore exhibit the features to a greater or lesser degree – or not at all.

Table 11.1 Changes related to the normal ageing process

Changes	Significance
Integumentary system	
Thinning of subcutaneous fatty layers; loss of collagen and elastin fibres; atrophy of the epidermis; sebaceous glands become less productive	Skin becomes dry and inelastic; patient increasingly susceptible to cold environmental temperatures; decreased resilience and bruises easily
Epithelial cells thin; sharper body contours; perception of pain reduced by 5%	Increased risk of pressure sores
Reduction in number of sweat glands	Increased susceptibility to heat exhaustion
Cell mitosis is slower; increased fragility of blood vessels leads to compromised peripheral circulation	Delayed wound healing; increased risk of superficial haemorrhage with minor trauma
Special senses	
Decreased lens transparency and elasticity; diminished eye muscle tone and narrowed blood vessels	Decreased visual acuity; reduced adaptation to changes in light (light to dark and vice versa)
Degeneration of the hair cells and the cochlea; cerumen is drier and often results in impaction	Progressive hearing loss; diminished ability to hear high-pitched sounds
Respiratory	
Respiratory muscles weaken; sensitivity to stimuli decreases	Cough reflex may be less sensitive and coughing less effective
Epithelium atrophies	Cilia decrease in number and mechanism less efficient
Alveolar membrane thickens as collagen increases; air spaces dilate; lung tissue loses elasticity; decreased functional alveolar surface	Vital capacity of lung decreased by 25%; reduction in alveoli leading to inadequate elimination of carbon dioxide; blood oxygen levels decrease
Thoracic cavity increases in the anteroposterior diameter; ribs become less mobile; postural changes occur; degeneration of intervertebral discs	Limitation of lung expansion; respirations shallower; reduction in vital capacity
Cardiovascular	
Decrease in elastic fibres in the heart, resulting in rigidity; thickening of the cardiac wall and endocardium; mitral and aortic valves become rigid	Cardiac output and stroke volume decrease; contractility of the heart muscle and heart rate decrease; dysrhythmias more common
Nervous supply to the heart (sympathetic and parasympathetic) decreases	Maximum heart rate decreases; reduced ability to increase cardiac output
Arteries less elastic as concentration of collagen increases; calcium and cholesterol and calcium accumulate in the vascular walls	Reduction in peripheral circulation; peripheral resistance increases; blood pressure increases

Table 11.1 (Contd.)

Changes	Significance
Gastrointestinal system	
Loss of teeth; poor dentition; atrophy of taste buds and muscles used in mastication	Loss of taste acuity, potential poor appetite and inability to eat
Decrease in production of saliva and oesophageal peristalsis	Excessively dry mouth and difficulty in swallowing
Decreased production of hydrochloric acid and digestive enzymes	Anaemia due to impaired absorption of iron and vitamin B12
Intestinal motility decreases; loss of muscle tone	Constipation occurs
Genitourinary system	
Narrowing and loss of blood vessels; vasoconstriction is persistent	Renal blood flow is reduced by 53%
Reduction of 40% in the number of functional glomeruli by age 75; decrease in connective tissue within kidney; effectiveness of antidiuretic hormone is diminished	Glomerular filtration rate decreases by up to 50%; renal plasma flow and reabsorption time increases affecting the diluting, concentrating and excreting ability of the kidney
Anatomical changes – loss of muscle tone and weakening pelvic floor muscles – lead to retention and stasis of urine	Decreased bladder strength, capacity and incomplete emptying; decreased awareness of the need to void; residual volume increases; risk of urinary infection: risk of incontinence
Prostate gland enlarges	Obstruction of normal urinary flow
Neurological system	
Neurons decrease in number	Losses occur in sensory functions: tactile sensation blunted, pain tolerance increases; intellectual ability remains stable
Nerve fibres degenerate with loss of conduction velocity in nerve fibres; fibres decrease in number	Reaction time is slower; prone to acute confusional states while in hospital
Degenerative thermoregulating mechanism	Slower to respond to environmental temperature change
Musculoskeletal system	
Gradual decrease in bone mass: 25% in women and 12% in men	Bone weakness and a predisposition to fractures
Thinning of cartilage around joints	Loss of height and postural change; varying degrees of joint stiffness
Decline in muscle mass as cellular loss and atrophy occur, large muscle groups more than small	Muscle strength, endurance and agility decrease

The nursing implications of these normal changes of ageing are numerous. It is not so much that there are major differences in the planning and implementation of nursing care, but rather differences in the emphasis and attention to various aspects of care (Keene 1991). Successful surgical management of older people's health problems is dependent upon the nurse's understanding of age-related factors and consequent adaptation of surgical nursing practice.

Reflective point

As you consider the changes identified within Table 11.1, how might their effects increase the risk of intraoperative problems? How do (or will) you assess, plan and evaluate care to ensure that older patients proceed through their surgical stay with a minimum of complications?

Much confusion exists about what differentiates the normal changes of biological ageing from age-related disease. Latz & Wyble (1987) stress that changes due to normal biological ageing must be universal, intrinsic, progressive and deleterious. This means that all members of the species must experience the change (universal), the change must occur regardless of the environment (intrinsic), the change will continue to occur in one direction (progressive) and the change will eventually lead to death (deleterious).

Age-related diseases are health conditions that occur almost exclusively in older age groups, for example osteoarthritis or emphysema. The distinction is that the occurrence is not universal, the causation is not necessarily intrinsic, the course may be arrested and the pathology managed.

SURGICAL INTERVENTIONS

Though the largest percentage of hospitalisations of older people are for medically related conditions, 35% of inpatient admissions are for surgical services (Palmer 1990) and more elderly people are undergoing surgery than ever before. Indeed, surgical operations are more frequent in older adults (Nolan 1992, Thomas & Richie 1995). Surgical rates are 55% higher in those aged over 65 years – 215 operations per 1000 compared to 120 per 1000 in people under 65 – with those individuals over 75 years of age requiring one-third more surgery than all other groups.

The aim of any surgery is for older people to enjoy at least as good and preferably greatly enhanced quality of life after surgery. Indeed, surgical intervention has provided many older people not only with more years to live their lives but also with more functional years. New surgical procedures and techniques have transformed the lives of many older people (Garrett 1991). Replacement of arthritic hip joints, for example, has meant a new lease of life for older people previously seriously immobilised and in pain, and ophthalmic procedures have restored useful sight to many.

Box 11.1 lists the 10 most frequent surgical procedures for older people. However, gender influences the type of surgical interventions performed. Palmer (1990) demonstrates that the most common surgical procedures for older women are lens extraction, reduction of fractures, cholecystectomy and hip replacements. For elderly men, prostatectomy, inguinal hernia repair and lens extraction are the most frequently performed surgery.

Is age a risk factor for surgery?

The short answer to this question is a definite yes, and no, depending on how you view the data. If raw

---

Box 11.1 The 10 most frequent surgical procedures in older people (Palmer 1990)

- Operations on the prostate gland
- Total hip replacement
- Coronary artery bypass graft
- Partial excision of large intestine
- Operations on the eye
- Pacemaker insertion or replacement
- Open reduction of fracture with internal fixation
- Removal of coronary obstruction
- Operations on the central nervous system
- Cholecystectomy

---

statistics are examined, a definite and significant increase in mortality with increasing age is evident (Lubin 1993): older people are at higher risk than younger people and mortality rates for surgery increase with each decade.

According to Arron et al (1992) the overall surgical mortality in older people has been shown to be:

- less than 65 years old: 1%
- 65–80 years old: 5–10%
- more than 80 years old: 10%.

Over time, improved surgical and anaesthetic techniques, advanced monitoring systems and more thorough preoperative assessment of risk factors have contributed to significant decreases in surgical mortality rates for older adults. Before 1960, when surgical mortality was 18% in the older age group and greater than 30% for older adults undergoing emergency surgery, avoiding surgery was a reasonable approach. The decline in overall surgical mortality in later years has influenced a change in attitude toward estimation of surgical risk in older people (Thomas & Richie 1995), so that age is no longer considered as a contraindication for most surgical procedures and age alone should not deter anyone from having a necessary operation.

Indeed, Catlic (1985) reported the cases of six patients between the ages of 100 and 104 who underwent anaesthesia and surgery. Three patients had major orthopaedic surgery and one a cholecystectomy. All patients survived and lived 1 or 2 years following their procedures. Catlic stated that 'elective surgery should not be deferred nor emergency surgery denied even for centenarians on the basis of chronological age'. This is a far cry from a 1907 report (Smith 1907) that described 167 operations performed on patients older than 50 and described this 'advanced age' as a contraindication to surgery.

So, if age alone cannot be regarded as a contraindication for surgical treatment, consideration of, and adjustments for, other factors must be made. These factors include physiological changes that occur with the ageing process, the presence of underlying diseases, the surgical procedure being performed and the timing of diagnoses and surgical intervention. Although Thomas & Richie (1995) argue that older patients are to be considered at higher risk, Lubin (1993) stresses that age alone should not be used as the sole criterion to deny older patients indicated for surgical procedures, pointing to the importance of assessing all risk factors in determining outcome.

As has been demonstrated (Table 11.1), physiological changes occur in many organ systems with ageing and may result in decreases in physiological reserve. The precise implications of these changes for surgical mortality are unknown but decreases in cardiac, respiratory and renal function are known to have adverse effects on surgical outcome (Lubin 1993). Physiological changes affect all patients to some degree. However, there are important factors that are patient-specific. One of the most important is the degree of underlying illness in the patient who is to undergo surgery.

Vaz & Seymour (1989) studied underlying diseases in 288 patients between the ages of 65 and 97 undergoing a general surgical procedure. Almost one-third of the patients had at least three different medical diagnoses: 18% had a history of respiratory disease and 37% a history of cardiovascular disease; 14% had suffered heart failure, and 9% had a history of angina. Neurological disease, including Parkinson's disease and cerebrovascular disease, accounted for 7% of the patients and a further 7% had diabetes mellitus. Significantly, only 28% of the patients were taking no medications, while 30% were on three or more daily.

Mohr (1983) argues that most of the excess morbidity in the aged surgical patient has its foundation in these pre-existing medical problems, not simply the patient's chronological age. Furthermore, increased mortality for both elective and emergency surgery is related to factors other than age, particularly pneumonia, cardiac compromise and malignancy. Older people with diabetes (Mohr 1983) and dementia (Bernstein & Offenbartl 1991) are at greater risk.

A category to be considered in determining surgical risk is the type of surgery to be performed. Common surgical procedures are easily divided into two types: relatively safe and relatively risky (Thomas & Richie 1995). Relatively safe procedures include prostatectomy and operations on the eye, where the likelihood of postoperative complications is small. Relatively risky procedures are cholecystectomy, coronary artery bypass, appendicectomy and hip surgery. When emergency surgery is undertaken in older people for whatever reason, the mortality rate is more than double that for elective surgery (Arron et al 1992).

The timing of diagnosis and surgical intervention is an important factor in determining surgical risk. Older people may be at greater risk for serious, life-threatening illness. When surgical disease occurs in older people the onset may be more sudden or the illness may be more difficult to diagnose, and hence treat accordingly, because of the lack of classical signs. For example, older people with appendicitis exhibit atypical symptoms, perforate more often and evolve the illness at a faster rate (Burns et al 1985). As a result, mortality from appendicitis for elderly patients is four times that of the general population.

Because emergency surgery has a higher risk than an elective operation, surgical intervention should not be delayed if there is a good chance that the disorder might become significantly worse. Judicious timing of elective surgery in early old age, for example the repair of an inguinal hernia, will pre-empt the need for emergency surgery at a later, and perhaps less robust, stage.

Seymour & Pringle (1981), in studying specifically abdominal surgery, found that the age-specific rates for emergency abdominal surgery rose with age, but the rates actually decreased with age for elective surgery. From these data they argued that elderly patients were having emergency surgery in greater numbers because they were not receiving medical or surgical care that might have prevented these emergencies. For women there was a large increase in the rate of emergency surgery for femoral hernias; in men there was an increase in the rate of emergency surgery for inguinal hernias. They believe that it is likely that at least some of these hernias could, and should, have been repaired electively, thereby reducing the risk of individual patient mortality.

The treatment of choice?

Although surgery is an option in the treatment of many of the conditions older people experience, it is not always the treatment of choice as far as the surgeon or the patient is concerned. In addition to addressing the patient's chance of surviving the operation, the surgeon, together with the whole care team, including the patient and the patient's family, must consider many factors in the decision to operate.

Vowles (1979) has identified questions that every surgeon should consider with older clients:

- Which is likely to be longer, the natural course of the disease or the patient's expectation of life?
- Without surgery, what will be the patient's quality of life?
- What chance has the patient of surviving surgery?
- Should the operation be elective and soon or is it better to leave well alone and risk surgery later?
- Should the operation be radical and heroic or modified and palliative?

In addition to a decline in surgical risk, there has been a move in the benefit side of the equation. The current life expectancy of a man aged 65 is on average another 13.2 years and for a female of the same age another 17.2 years (Victor 1991). This increase in survival has had a profound impact on evaluating the benefit of surgery. If the patient is only expected to survive 1–2 years, the patient and physician may be reluctant to pursue potentially life-threatening surgery to correct an elective problem. If the patient is expected to survive 8–10 years, Thomas & Richie (1995) suggest that the proposal for potentially life-threatening surgery to correct an elective problem may be viewed more enthusiastically.

There has been a shift from the tradition of paternalism to a primary focus on respecting patients' self-determination in choosing the treatment that will provide the most benefit and do the least harm. The surgeon should discuss all the surgical options and the alternatives to surgery with the patient and should help the patient make the final decision. If the patient makes an informed choice and rejects surgery, provided the patient is judged competent to make that decision, then it should be respected.

I clearly remember an elderly patient who after long and frank discussions with the surgeons, but against the wishes of her children, refused to consent to surgery for the amputation of her gangrenous leg. In her late 80s, she was not prepared to take the risk of surgical intervention and truly believed that her quality of life would not be improved with the amputation of her leg. The medical and nursing team supported the patient in her decision and cared for her until her death some weeks later. However, it was not an easy time; the family required much support during the difficult weeks and each one of the team questioned what we might experience in similar circumstances.

PREOPERATIVE NURSING CONSIDERATIONS

On admission to hospital, elderly people have on average nine separate diagnoses (Garrett 1991) so nursing assessment is often more complicated than with younger people. Obtaining a clear picture of the patient's medical, functional, social and psychological situation requires a multi-professional approach and collation of community and hospital-acquired information. Nurses play a key role in preoperative assessment of older people and the data utilised will include the objective information contributed by other members of the health care team.

Changes as the result of normal ageing vary considerably within and between individual older people. These may be further influenced by the presence of both acute and chronic health problems, perhaps unrelated to the surgery being performed, which themselves can have a tremendous impact on the outcome of surgery. Each client is unique and requires an in-depth nursing assessment, focusing on physiological, psychological, sociocultural, developmental and spiritual aspects of the client.

Functional assessment

Setting the environment for the assessment of older patients includes minimising distractions, providing privacy and explaining that sharing the information is important to ensure a safe and speedy recovery. If a hearing deficit is noted, the nurse needs to face the light to facilitate lip-reading and use short, direct questions which focus on important data. Shouting is to be avoided as it alters pronunciation and makes speech perception difficult.

Functional assessment is an integral part of the nursing assessment of the older surgical patient and addresses those physical and 'instrumental' activities of living which are required in order to live independently (Lusis 1994). The assessment should focus on a nursing model whose goal is returning patients to their optimum level of functioning. For some older patients, this may not be a state of total independence, because of limitations arising from ageing or chronic disease processes. It is therefore imperative that the assessment establishes the 'baseline' for each patient and determines the balance between what the patient needs to manage in daily living and what resources are available to help in this (Squires & Taylor 1988). If assistance to meet daily living activities is required, both the type of assistance and what is acceptable to the patient are documented. Knowledge of the patient's physical limitations before surgery facilitates the planning of appropriate interventions to maintain abilities in the preoperative period and the restoration of optimum independence postoperatively.

It is not unusual for patients to hesitate about giving information; Lusis (1994) suggests that older people may be reluctant to give functional information or may overstate their abilities, interpreting questions as concern about their ability to live independently. If there is any doubt about the patient's accuracy, the nurse must, within the boundaries of patient confidentiality, tactfully verify information with a family member or seek additional information from other members of the multiprofessional team.

Psychosocial assessment

Assessment of the patient's social situation is crucial in determining the availability and ability of the spouse or family members who may be needed, at least temporarily, to provide competent care following the older patient's discharge. Similarly, questions regarding the patient's home environment are relevant since certain characteristics of the home could become problematic after surgery, demanding adaptations or the supply of aids.

Addressing these issues during the nursing assessment is vital since worries concerning social and family life may be of more concern to the patient than the need for surgery and add to stress levels. Often, through collaboration with the patient and family, these problems can be anticipated and managed. However, circumstances could demand the patient's referral for health and social care, either temporarily or on a permanent basis, once discharged.

Adaptations that will be necessary as a result of the surgery and the postoperative quality of life may have an important impact on the patient's willingness to undergo surgery and ultimately postoperative recovery. Jackson (1988) demonstrates that elderly patients who have high levels of motivation, a will to live, positive expectations of the surgery and a proven ability to cope successfully with stress have significantly lower rates of postoperative complications and disabilities than those who see little value in their lives and have high levels of preoperative anxiety.

During the nursing assessment, the nurse must consider the patient's emotional status and 'readiness' for surgery. Many old people fear hospitalisation and surgical intervention with its potential of forced dependency on others. Fear of the unknown, pain, mutilation, destruction of the already altered body image are experienced to varying degrees and may contribute to a confusional state in the pre- and postoperative periods.

Emotional support in the preoperative period is an extremely important nursing intervention. Any apprehension must be recognised and allayed by attending to the patient's specific concerns, before giving balanced and often much needed repeated explanations of what to expect both before and after surgery (see also Chs 9 and 10).

Cognitive and mental status assessment

An assessment of the patient's cognition and mental status, including memory and problem-solving, is vital and can readily occur in the context of the nursing assessment. Asking the patient to describe events leading up to the need for surgery, how the activities of living are managed and what plans have been made for post-discharge care will give a fairly good indication of the patient's cognitive processes.

Whilst stress and anxiety contribute to a temporary confusional state, a more permanent cognitive impairment is not a part of the normal ageing process and the patient's usual cognitive status may be verified with family members and validated by the physician through mental status screening (Goldfarb 1960, Hamilton 1960).

Since the patient will need to be taught about the surgical procedure and his role in managing care afterwards, deficits in any of these functions will affect his ability to participate in and cooperate with the planned treatment.

Skin assessment

Skin assessment is most important prior to surgery to provide a baseline for colour, oedema or presence of breakdown. All older patients should be evaluated for risk of skin breakdown on admission, using a recognised tool (Gosnell 1987, Pritchard 1986, Waterlow 1988) and, for those shown to be at risk, a regimen of mobilisation, pressure-relieving mattresses and nutritional support should be commenced. The nurse must maintain patients' mobility during the preoperative phase or, if they are immobile, teach passive and active exercises and encourage frequent changes of position.

Medication

Despite the fact that older people comprise only 18% of the population, they receive between 30–40% of prescribed drugs (Woodhouse 1994). Potentially dangerous adverse drug reactions are due to multiple prescribing and age-related changes in pharmacodynamics and pharmacokinetics. Changes in drug absorption, metabolism and elimination may result in drugs still being effective hours, and even days, after the patient has taken them, and they may potentially interact with the anaesthetic agents during surgery.

It is therefore crucial for the surgical nurse to take an accurate medication history of all prescribed drugs, over-the-counter drugs and home remedies, which many elderly people do not consider as medication because they were not prescribed by their doctor.

Lusis (1994) stresses that the nurse should collaborate with the surgeon to determine how the patient's drug regimen will be maintained in the immediate postoperative period when the patient is not allowed oral intake and how soon drugs can be restarted. The regimen may be altered by the need for postoperative pain control; adding even one medicine to an already complex regimen must be considered carefully in view of potential drug interactions or adverse effects.

Nutritional assessment

The importance of a thorough preoperative nutritional assessment for elderly patients cannot be overemphasised. Older people are known to be commonly deficient in protein, vitamins A, C, D and E, thiamine, folic acid and iron (Latz & Wyble 1987) and studies have found evidence of protein–calorie malnutrition in as high as 50% of hospitalised elderly patients. Poor dentition, decrease in thirst and taste, poor eating habits and social and financial considerations may all result in poor nutritional status (Webb & Copeman 1996).

Nutritional status is further depleted post-admission by the withholding of oral intake for diagnostic tests, prolonged intravenous fluid use and delay in implementing nutritional support, often until the patient is severely depleted. McWhirter & Pennington (1994) found a 43% prevalence of undernutrition in their study of elderly patients, and furthermore, Klipstein-Grosbuch et al (1995) noted that the nutritional status of elderly people declined during hospital admission, especially in the most undernourished, unless nutritional support was provided.

Malnutrition is a risk factor for postoperative morbidity and mortality, since the older person may be less able to successfully manage the stresses associated with surgery and is at risk for postoperative skin breakdown, impaired wound healing, wound dehiscence, evisceration and infection. Barstow et al (1983) report that 18% of severely malnourished patients with fractured neck of femur died following surgery, compared with 4% of well-nourished patients, a difference not due to associated illness or age.

Nurses should structure their assessment of a patient's nutritional status on determining the presence of risk factors and indicators (shown in Box 11.2) and confer with the dietitian to ensure improved nutrition for elderly clients in both the pre- and postoperative periods. Surgical patients have varying nutritional needs, dependent on their age, type of operation, preoperative nutritional status and the expected extent of postoperative losses. However, patients with moderate or severe malnutrition will require preoperative nutritional support, which reduces the risk of surgical morbidity and mortality.

Box 11.2   Malnutrition risk factors and indicators

Risk factors
- Ignorance of basic facts of nutrition
- Inadequate housing, poor storage and/or cooking conditions
- Social isolation: living and/or eating alone
- Low social class: IV and V
- Reduced income
- Inappropriate food intake: inadequate or poorly balanced
- Prolonged adherence to poorly designed therapeutic diet
- Inadequate dentition, dentures, periodontal disease, dental caries
- Malabsorption
- Physical disability affecting mobility and dexterity
- Mental disability: anxiety, depression, confusion, dementia
- Multiple medicines
- Cultural or religious factors
- Alcohol abuse
- Increased nutritional needs: prolonged bedrest, pressure sore, chronic ulcer

Indicators
- Unintentional weight loss of over 5% over preceding 3 months
- Under/overweight: body mass index under 20 or over 25
- Muscle wasting and lack of subcutaneous fat
- Dehydration
- Oedema
- Anthropometric measures, e.g. triceps skin fold 80–85% of standard
- Biochemical assessment, e.g. serum albumin below 3 g/dL, Hb under 10 g/dL
- Vitamin B12 deficiency
- Listlessness, apathy, low mental test score
- Anorexia, nausea, dysphagia
- Change in bowel habit
- Delayed wound healing and bruises easily
- Nutrition-related disorders: osteoporosis, osteomalacia, anaemia
- Angular stomatitis, glossitis, bleeding gums

Nutritional supplements are important to improve nutritional status of elderly patients and Lusis (1994) argues that nasogastric feeding may be required for those who cannot take enough calories orally. When identifying nutrition preoperatively as difficult, perhaps because of persistent vomiting or oesophageal obstruction, parenteral feeding should be considered to improve the patient's condition before surgery. Mullen et al (1980) highlight several small studies where improvement in postoperative outcome has been achieved with the administration of preoperative total parenteral nutrition (TPN).

Teaching and learning

Surgical nurses must ensure that when older people return home following surgery they are able to act as autonomously and independently as possible. Preoperative teaching is a priority. Unless patients have a serious mental impairment, ageing does not mean that they cannot learn; but it often means that they learn differently than younger patients. Fromm & Metzler (1993) suggest strategies to maximise teaching and learning.

Learning cannot proceed if the elderly patient has unmet needs. If patients have anxieties, fears or worries, memory deficits become more pronounced and it is more difficult to attend to information that may be vital to their welfare. It is important for the nurse to dispel any unfounded fears regarding surgery or its effects with accurate and balanced information.

The speed of information processing does slow with age so nurses must allow extra time for each teaching session, dividing complex material into short sections to enable patients to assimilate new material with knowledge they have already acquired. Sensory defects are minimised by patients wearing their aids and glasses and providing a quiet area where distracting background noise will be at a minimum. Using more than one sense helps, such as following up spoken instruction with written material printed with sharp contrasts, preferably black on white.

Preoperative pulmonary exercises

Degrees of pulmonary insufficiency are common in older people; decreased vital capacity, increased residual volume, impaired gas exchange and reduced bronchopulmonary movement are normal ageing changes. Coughing is less efficient and the depressant effects of medications and anaesthesia further increase the older surgical patient's risk for pneumonia and respiratory complications. According to Thomas &

Richie (1995) the most lethal postoperative infection is pneumonia, with an attributable mortality of 27%. For older people with a chronic obstructive airway disease the risk of pulmonary complications is even greater.

As well as ensuring a detailed baseline preoperative respiratory assessment for later comparisons, preoperative teaching regarding deep breathing and coughing is essential to avoid postoperative complications. Nurses need to assist and support older patients to perform exercises correctly. Coughing exercises traditionally taught to younger patients preoperatively may be contraindicated for older clients, particularly if undergoing abdominal surgery, since vigorous coughing can interfere with wound healing and rupture wounds.

Luckman & Sorenson (1980) suggest that the following judicious coughing exercises be taught and supervised:

- Lie on back or side or sitting position.
- Splint abdomen by lacing hands across abdomen over a folded towel or pillow.
- Inhale through the nose.
- Exhale through the mouth, giving two short coughs with tongue extended.

This will assist in loosening and removing secretions from the base of the lung.

Fluid balance

Decreased renal perfusion and changes in the concentrating ability of the kidney, long-term diuretic use and decreased thirst sensation predispose many older people to dehydration. Hoot Martin & Larsen (1994) demonstrate that dehydration is associated with increased mortality and morbidity among older people, particularly infections (pneumonia and urinary tract infections), renal failure, increased skin breakdown, confusion and increased incidence of falls and injuries.

Assessment of an older person's hydration status will note possible physical findings associated with dehydration (Box 11.3). Alert nurses must intervene to prevent or lessen the impact of dehydration. Interventions preventing dehydration are preferable since the process of fluid replacement is not without complications (Hoot Martin & Larsen 1994). Owing to decreased efficiency of renal excretion and reabsorption, older patients have less ability to compensate for large shifts in fluid and electrolyte balance, and further imbalances may contribute to cardiac or mental status complications. Input and output recordings, especially

---

Box 11.3 Physical findings associated with dehydration

- Deep tongue furrows
- Low oral intake
- Dry tongue and mucous membranes
- Low urine output
- Warm, dry skin
- Raised urea and electrolytes
- Tachycardia, thready pulse
- Confusion, disorientation, changes in mood and disposition

---

in emergency situations, should therefore begin on admission and be regularly documented throughout every shift.

It is important for the nurse to determine with the anaesthetist the specific length of 'nil by mouth'(NBM) status needed for each patient by scrutinising the specific type of surgical procedure to be performed and reviewing the patient's history and physical assessment. An individual length of NBM (rather than the standard 6–8 hours) and the possibility of drinking clear fluids a few hours prior to the procedure can often prevent dehydration in the elderly patient (Hoot Martin & Larsen 1994). However, Dodson & Seymour (1992) suggest for the mildly dehydrated patient, at risk of hypotension at induction of anaesthesia, it is wise to have an intravenous infusion in place before theatre.

Consent

The decision to proceed with surgery must truly be an informed one: the nature of the surgery, the risks involved, the discomfort and restrictions before, during and after the procedure, and ultimate quality of life to be expected must all be clearly presented by the surgeon. The British Medical Association and the Royal College of Nursing (1995) explore ethical issues surrounding the complex concepts of consent, treatment and confidentiality, recommending guidelines and suggestions for good practice (see also Ch. 4).

While family members and patient may disagree on whether the surgery be performed, the decision ultimately rests with the older patient unless competence is an issue. The decision for surgery can be a difficult one for patients. They need the nurse's support for their right to make their decision and to do so without feelings of guilt. Explanations are necessary and the nurse can encourage questions and clarify misunderstandings, feeding back information to the surgeon. The nurse must contact the surgical team if he or she

believes that the patient does not understand the procedure and needs more information.

I clearly remember an incident when an independent and alert 80-year-old lady, with carcinoma of the bowel, had been referred to the surgeon. This recent diagnosis was deeply distressing to the patient; she was experiencing difficulty coming to terms with it and at times became quiet and withdrawn. The surgeon came to see her one afternoon to discuss surgery and when he had left, the patient had a beaming smile. She explained that a doctor had been to see her and was taking her to the theatre in the next few days and that she would come back with a bag. Her interpretation of the prospect of an abdominoperineal resection and formation of colostomy was a trip to the local theatre to see a show and the purchase of a new handbag before the return to the ward.

INTRAOPERATIVE NURSING CONSIDERATIONS

Communication

Regardless of age, the strange environment of an operating department can be intimidating and threatening to security and self-esteem. It can be especially frightening for older people with hearing or visual deficits and is compounded when glasses and hearing aids have been removed (Jackson 1988). Whenever possible, communication aids should be left in place and the nurse and other members of the surgical team should directly face older patients when communicating with them, without wearing a mask. This allows patients to use lip-reading and to see facial expressions, mechanisms compensating for hearing loss (Latz & Wyble 1987). Female nurses could wear bright lipstick to make their lips more visible.

Since elderly people may have difficulty processing more than one stimulus, only one member of the care team should talk to the patient at a time and use touch to communicate support and reassurance (Moore & Proffitt 1993). Time must be allowed for older patients' vision to adapt when moved from one light level to another, and the nurse should attempt to reduce glare by leaving the overhead lights off until needed.

Anaesthesia choice

Few studies have specifically examined the effects of various anaesthetic agents in older people. The decision to use general anaesthetic or regional anaesthetic is determined by the patient's age, medical conditions, site of operation and type of surgery being performed. Dodson & Seymour (1992) argue that regional anaesthesia has advantages over general since it causes less confusion, reduces bleeding and stress response, extends pain relief and reduces the risk of postoperative circulatory and respiratory problems. However, there are difficulties in performing the procedure because of arthritic changes and calcium deposits along the vertebral column.

Palmer (1990) argues that general anaesthesia may have an advantage when used for confused, disoriented and agitated patients who are uncooperative. Certainly for tense, anxious patients the use of general anaesthesia will produce better relaxation, prevent pain and lessen fear, since the patient will not worry about being awake in the operating theatre. Older people are more prone to hypotension, hypothermia and hypoxaemia after general anaesthetic, but complications are reduced when the patient's overall medical condition has been stabilised and short-acting agents are used (see also Ch. 23).

Hypothermia

Impaired thermoregulatory mechanisms and loss of subcutaneous tissue result in a significant threat of hypothermia for older people during surgery. A cool operating room environment, topical applications of cold solutions and intravenous fluids can cause shivering which, Palmer (1990) asserts, may increase oxygen demand by as much as 300–500%. An increased oxygen demand leads to increased cardiac output and ventilation, causing tissue ischaemia in the heart and brain.

Hypothermia impedes elimination of anaesthetic agents and delays wakening and return of reflexes, so other drugs must be reduced to avoid overdosage. Furthermore, it may result in apathy, disorientation, listlessness and slurring of speech in the conscious patient, signs often misinterpreted as a transient ischaemic attack or a stroke.

Close monitoring of body temperature (Garrett 1991), preferably with a rectal probe while the patient is unconscious, and cardiac function during operative procedures and in the recovery room is crucial. Jackson (1989) suggests the use of warmed blankets under and over the body, warmed gowns and caps, covers on unaffected extremities, prewarmed intravenous fluids and blood products, and warm, humidified oxygen as preventive measures.

Joint and skin care

Positioning of the older patient for procedures may be challenging to the surgical nurse because of structural changes, such as kyphosis, limited joint movement or paralysis and concern over fragile skin. Dellasega & Burgunder (1991) claim that malpositioning of joints and limbs may lead to increased postoperative stiffness, discomfort and pain, not necessarily related to the operative site. Joints that are not positioned in neutral alignment are subject to stress and possible bone injury. Where possible, nurses should assist patients to place themselves in the position of greatest comfort, particularly if they have arthritic joints. Support for the head with at least one pillow when patients are in a supine position is especially important so as not to hyperextend the neck or compress neck vessels, compromising blood flow to the brain.

Prolonged immobility, loss of adipose tissue and decreased peripheral circulation combine to put older patients at high risk for pressure sores. The time of immobility is longer than the actual time in the operating room: prolonged pressure may begin with preoperative sedation and continue through postoperative recovery (Scott et al 1992). Skin integrity must be protected while positioning and transferring the patient on and off the operating table to avoid shearing, and all areas subject to pressure should be well supported and padded. Slight position changes, when possible, relieve pressure areas and improve circulation to compressed tissues.

The use of tape to secure limbs, tubes or dressings should be avoided (Latz & Wyble 1987) since it can tear fragile skin, and the nurse should provide alternative methods of securing dressings, including the application of protective skin barriers and tubular stockinet.

Recovery

Elderly patients are at increased risk for hypoxia during the recovery room stay as a result of the sedative effects of tranquillisers administered prior to surgery, residual anaesthesia, narcotics and muscle relaxants. Careful observation of the older patient following surgery is essential. The nurse must watch for signs of hypotension and depression of the cardiovascular, respiratory or central nervous systems. The monitoring of oxygen saturation with a pulse oximeter will help rational decision-making regarding the need for supplemental oxygen.

POSTOPERATIVE NURSING CONSIDERATIONS

Surgical nurses are in a key position to assist older people in achieving maximum benefit from surgery. The most sophisticated surgical procedures in the world, performed by the most skilled surgeon, are of little value if poor rehabilitative care causes disability or death from avoidable complications.

The goals in postoperative care for older people are, as in any age group, the prevention of complications, or early detection and management should they occur, and returning patients to their optimum level of independence as soon as possible.

Postoperative recovery may take longer in the older patient because body systems have more difficulty in coping with the stress of anaesthesia and surgery, and because of the effects of chronic disease and changes associated with ageing. These factors also make the development of complications more likely.

As older people often do not manifest typical symptoms, early identification of complications can be challenging, demanding an informed awareness and particular vigilance from nursing staff (Garrett 1991). Adverse reactions to surgery are rarely due to one factor (Jackson 1989) and are often not as dramatic and marked as in younger patients: silent infarcts may occur with little or no pain, and fever may present as acute confusion in the absence of a pyrexia (Jackson 1988). Careful, constant monitoring by the nurse, combined with knowledge of the individual patient's baseline, are crucial in detecting a change in status (Lusis 1994).

Restoring body temperature

Since elderly people have a lowered ability to combat hypothermia and take longer for the body temperature to return to normal, temperature monitoring is a high priority. Rewarming patients must be done slowly, since if it is done too quickly, many complications are possible including hypoxia, acid–base disturbances, pulmonary oedema, pneumonia, dehydration, hyperglycaemia and acute tubular necrosis.

Maintenance of adequate cardiovascular function and tissue perfusion

Myocardial depression, arrhythmias and hypotension are the most significant complications during the immediate postoperative period and are the result of the cumulative effects of anaesthesia, overdose of preoperative medicines, blood and fluid loss and peripheral pooling of blood. Elderly patients with preexisting heart disease are most prone to myocardial infarction postoperatively (Thomas & Richie 1995).

Careful monitoring of vital signs is important: changes in rate, rhythm and quality of radial/apical pulses and systolic blood pressure reductions should

be promptly recognised and reported. Palmer (1990) suggests that a systolic blood pressure drop greater than 20 mmHg, drops with each reading of 5–10 mmHg or a pressure falling below 80 mmHg are indicators of problems. In high-risk patients, monitoring of cardiac status by electrocardiogram (ECG), central venous pressure (CVP) lines and arterial blood gases may be indicated for several days.

Immobility, arteriosclerosis and intraoperative trauma to veins contribute to an increased risk of thrombophlebitis (Dodson & Seymour 1992). Early ambulation is the best preventive measure in addition to passive and active movements and antiembolic stockings. For patients forced to undertake prolonged bed rest, low-dose (5000 units/12 hours) subcutaneous heparin may be considered (see also Ch. 25).

Fluid and electrolyte balance

Fluid replacement during surgery is necessary to replace blood and fluid loss and to maintain electrolyte balance. However, because elderly people's fluid and electrolyte margins of safety are so narrow, complications of circulatory overload or hypovolaemia tend to advance quickly in older patients to life-threatening proportions (Menyhert 1988).

Nurses must be cognisant of the risk of fluid imbalance and patients should be monitored for signs of overload or dehydration. Skin turgor is best assessed by pinching the skin over the sternum or forehead. Early recognition and correction of fluid and electrolyte imbalance can prevent serious complications in the postoperative period.

Hypovolaemia, caused by blood and fluid loss during surgery, may impair the older patient's renal function, already reduced by 50% as a result of ageing, and lead to necrosis. Approximately 20% of the perioperative deaths of elderly surgical patients are directly attributable to acute renal failure (Kelly 1995). Recognition of acute renal insufficiency should trigger a rapid, aggressive evaluation of the cause. Reduced urinary output can indicate this, so hourly documentation of a patient's immediate postoperative intake and output, including non-measured fluid losses such as in diaphoresis, is essential.

Intravenous fluids, administered to prevent or correct hypovolaemia, must be carefully administered, as circulatory overload readily occurs giving rise to pulmonary congestion and heart failure. Central venous pressure readings may be necessary to monitor the situation.

In addition to careful fluid management, serum electrolyte levels must also be monitored. Hyponatraemia, resulting from over-administration of intravenous fluids or too much water orally, is a common postoperative occurrence, which can contribute to acute confusion and drastically influence patient outcomes (see also Ch. 26).

Respiratory function

Decreased vital capacity, reduction in total alveolar surface and diminished cough reflex, together with the effects of surgery, influence the incidence of pulmonary complications in older patients in the postoperative period, particularly in the first 48 hours. Patients with an underlying disease such as chronic obstructive airway disease (COAD) or asthma are especially at risk. Furthermore, the anatomic location of the surgical site has a direct effect on the rate of complications (Nolan 1992). Risk is highest in upper abdominal surgery, lower in lower abdominal surgery and lower still in vaginal or extremity surgery.

Respiratory complications are the most common cause of death in elderly surgical patients, the most lethal being pneumonia, with an attributable mortality of 27% (Thomas & Richie 1995).

In older patients, small and seemingly insignificant changes in vital signs or behaviour may be early signs of impending problems, so skilled observation is essential. While not being fully conscious from surgery, the elderly patient may demonstrate combativeness (Lusis 1994) or restlessness as the first symptom of hypoxia. It is crucial that restlessness is not mistaken for pain since the administration of a narcotic could deplete the body's oxygen supply even more. A mild loss of energy or intermittent confusion may be the primary symptoms of pulmonary complications and must be investigated.

Hypoxia in the postoperative period may contribute to acute confusion. Rosenberg & Kehlit (1993) found a significant correlation between mental function and oxygen saturation in older patients undergoing both minor and major surgical procedures. Nurse monitoring and correction of oxygenation should continue throughout the postoperative period; pulse oximetry monitoring of oxygen saturation should be routine in all patients and oxygen administered as indicated. Oxygen administration helps prevent respiratory distress and promotes optimal mental function. Replacing dentures as soon as possible restores functional position of the oral tissues to improve respiratory efforts.

Hypoxaemia has been documented up to 10 days postoperatively in elderly patients and may be a factor in nocturnal confusion (Jackson 1988). Early ambulation is the most important preventive measure. Because of its stimulation of deep breathing, ambulation can increase the patient's lung capacity by 15–20% and can assist in the prevention of deep vein thrombi. This may be difficult, especially if the patient is fearful of falling or believes that bed rest and healing are synonymous. However, if the importance of early ambulation is understood by patients, most will try to comply with the need to be mobile as soon as possible (see also Chs 23 and 24).

Cognitive function

An older patient's mental status is easily compromised during hospitalisation and surgery (Keene 1991). Acute confusion, one of the most common and serious postoperative complications in elderly patients, may be the result of numerous reversible, organic causes (Box 11.4) and affects between 10 and 15% of patients (Dellasega & Burgunder 1991). If confusion does develop, the patient will exhibit fluctuating level of consciousness, sleep disturbances, orientation and memory deficits and changes in psychomotor behaviour.

A postoperative acute confusional state may be a common occurrence in elderly patients but it is not normal and demands a thorough and immediate investigation to identify a cause or causes. This involves comparing current mental status with preoperative baseline data, and reviewing vital observations, drugs and anaesthesia used during surgery, and

---

Box 11.4 Causes of postoperative acute confusional states

- Electrolyte and metabolic imbalance
- Reduced oxygen supply:
  – increased CO_2
  – anaemia
  – infection
  – fever
  – hypotension
  – cardiac failure
  – compromised pulmonary function
- Urinary tract infection or retention
- Impaired renal and hepatic function
- Constipation
- Multiple medicines
- Adverse drug effects, especially tranquillisers and sedatives
- Surgery lasting more than 4 hours
- Postoperative haemorrhage
- Alcohol or drug withdrawal
- Anxiety
- Frequent environment change
- Sensory deprivation or overload

current and preoperative medications. If treatment is not given, or is unsuccessful, the patient may die or be left with permanent brain damage.

I recollect one incident when an elderly lady became confused and agitated following surgery to repair a fractured neck of femur. Although a provisional diagnosis of an acute exacerbation of dementia was made by the doctor and no treatment was prescribed, consultation with the named nurse confirmed that the patient had previously been alert and independent. Blood analysis demonstrated that the patient was severely uraemic. Intravenous fluids were commenced and within 24 hours, the patient had become alert, oriented and eager to commence mobilisation. The careful assessment by the surgical nurse had enabled prompt interventions and prevented further complications for the patient.

Lusis (1994) argues that, with knowledge of the patient's history and a thorough preoperative assessment, the nurse should be able to identify those patients at risk of developing acute confusion in the postoperative period and plan interventions to reduce the incidence or decrease the length of a patient's transient cognitive impairment.

Reflective point

When admitting patients to the surgical environment, what information must you gain to assess their risk of developing a postoperative acute confusional state? How would you use that information to plan strategies to reduce the risk of confusion developing in individual patients?

Time and space are associated with confusion. Time is relational in that successive events are related with one another and give constancy to an environment. Jackson (1989) states that when periods of time are lost, for example when events immediately following surgery cannot be remembered, time sequences are lost and confusion and fear may result. Frequent explanations, reassurance and reorientation will assist the patient regain time sequence. The sooner older patients are able to keep track of time and regain a sense of control over their own environment and activities, the sooner they become reoriented to time, place and person.

Orientational devices, such as calendars, clocks and familiar objects from home, will assist patients regain a sense of control, and increasing their level of activity will ensure that they move around the ward area

obtaining different sensory inputs. Ensuring that patients wear their glasses or hearing aid will help them relate more clearly to the environment.

The nurse should focus on supportive care and preventing secondary complications such as falls, dehydration and poor nutritional intake, which may worsen confusion and contribute to the increased morbidity and mortality.

Early ambulation and movement

The importance of early and consistent mobilisation for the older patient cannot be overemphasised. The benefits of surgery will be diminished if the patient becomes debilitated from the complications of loss of muscle tone and strength, endurance and circulatory tone which arise from immobility. These occur rapidly in elderly patients and may result in permanent loss of function. The ability to walk without lightheadedness or the ability to stand long enough to prepare a meal may be compromised by just a few days confined to bed (Lusis 1994). Early ambulation is therapeutic in the prevention of many complications, facilitates the resumption of previous activity levels and provides another parameter for evaluating recovery from surgery.

Postural hypotension is a common postoperative complication for elderly patients and results from prolonged bed rest, analgesia/anaesthetic effects, hypovolaemia, chronic venous insufficiency, hypertension and antihypertensive drugs (Palmer 1990). Measuring blood pressures and pulse rate in the postoperative period gives an indication of the patient's vascular tone and ability to tolerate ambulation.

Early mobilisation should include active and passive leg exercises and movement of hip and ankle joints through their full range of motion in the hours after surgery (Palmer 1990). The nurse assists patients to change position slowly, especially from a lying position to sitting upright, dangling their feet over the side of the bed and eventually ambulating (Keene 1991). Patients should have hearing aids and glasses in place, to ensure comprehension of instructions and awareness of the environment. Footwear with non-skid soles should be worn and the mobility aids normally used should be available (Lusis 1994).

Early ambulation may not be easy to achieve with arthritic or debilitated patients and must always be gentle and slowly progressive. Garrett (1991) stresses that patients' capabilities must not be overtaxed in the early postoperative period as fatigue may lead to frustration, loss of confidence and subsequent lowering of motivation. Patients should have early evaluation and follow-up by the physiotherapist and occupational therapist.

Pain relief

Relief of pain is essential. Studies have demonstrated that older people do not experience less pain than younger patients (Harkins & Chapman 1976, 1977), but they may be less able to distinguish between different intensities of pain (Dodson & Seymour 1992) and are less willing to label a sensation as painful.

Furthermore, Herr & Mobily (1991) suggest that older people may also hold myths and misunderstandings about pain, which interfere with the frequency and accuracy of reporting. They may believe that pain indicates serious illness or impending death, that they must live with the pain or that it is unacceptable to show pain. Thus, older people's reactions may at times seem inappropriate or inconsistent and demand perceptive assessment of verbal and nonverbal pain by the surgical nurse.

In the immediate postoperative period, analgesia is important as severe pain may inhibit deep breathing, raise or lower the blood pressure, precipitate dysrhythmias and induce confusion. A cautious approach to the intramuscular administration of narcotics in the hypothermic patient must be taken because of delayed absorption by cold muscles. If several doses are given because of apparent lack of response, an overdose can occur when the muscles warm and the blood vessels dilate. Dodson & Seymour (1992) argue that narcotics should be administered intravenously until the patient is warm, while Wild & Coyne (1992) suggest that epidural analgesia affords improved pain relief with less sedation.

In succeeding postoperative days, analgesic drugs should be administered freely in a reduced dosage that is titrated for relief and monitored carefully, as there is a narrow margin between effective pain control and the onset of complications such as confusion, incontinence, hypotension and loss of balance. Slowed circulation in older patients predisposes them to drug overdose from delayed distribution, detoxification and excretion. Doses of analgesics may need to be reduced as much as one-quarter to one-third, and sufficient time must be allowed for a drug bolus to act before a second dose is administered. Non-steroidal anti-inflammatory drugs are effective for mild to moderate pain and should be employed as soon as pain severity allows.

Nurses also have available to them, depending on the patient's physical and mental status, an extensive repertoire of non-invasive nursing measures, including comfort and relaxation techniques, imagery and cutaneous stimulation. Breathing exercises and active progressive relaxation exercises are detailed by McFarland & Thomas (1991). Such measures are low risk, can be used in conjunction with or to supplement analgesia and can be easily adjusted without undesirable side-effects. Equally important is the presence and reassurance of the nurse and supportive visits from the family and friends, which do much to relieve the anxiety and tension that contribute to the perception of pain (see also Ch. 24).

Wound healing

A variety of ageing processes, such as decreased peripheral circulation, diminished immune and inflammatory responses, decreased production of neutrophils and lymphocytes and a slowed rate of cell proliferation, can delay all stages of wound healing. Surgical experience shows that even the very old can effectively repair extensive wounds, but on the whole, the wounds do take longer to heal; re-epithelialisation takes twice as long for a 75-year-old as is does for a 25-year-old (Orentreich & Selmanowitz 1969). Latz & Wyble (1987) point out that older people are at increased risk of dehiscence, evisceration and formation of fistulous tracts.

Age is not an independent risk factor in the incidence of surgical infection. However, the prevalence of medical conditions such as diabetes, heart disease, pneumonia and urinary tract infection predisposes older people to a higher risk of wound infection. Nosocomial infections account for 24% of wound infections and remain a major source of postoperative morbidity (Nichols 1991). Because an older patient's susceptibility to infection is greater than that of a younger patient, strict adherence to aseptic principles and the implementation of practices to reduce the risk of infection are essential (see also Ch. 13).

Even in the absence of pyrexia or fever in the patient, any incision that is inflamed and tender indicates the presence of infection and must be treated accordingly (see also Ch. 28).

DISCHARGE PLANNING

Older people are heavily dependent on their period in hospital being as restorative as possible and enabling them to maintain or regain confidence in their ability to manage at home. However, changes in the organisation of health care services (King's Fund 1994) in recent years have led to earlier discharge of patients from hospital into the community; the average length of stay in acute hospitals has fallen from 20 days in 1948 to just 5 days in 1991 (Age Concern 1995). As a result, older people are being discharged more quickly and in frailer health than ever before with carers, both informal and professional, assuming greater responsibility for older clients' continuing rehabilitation and longer-term needs.

Recent reports from the King's Fund (1994) and Age Concern (1995) found that elderly people were discharged from hospital without suitable preparation or arrangements in place in the community. Older people in acute wards were not routinely asked about their home circumstances or how they would cope after discharge, and information on discharge procedures was not widely available in wards. There were delays and inadequacies in the provision of community services and evidence of poor communication between professionals in hospital and the community health and social services.

The reports highlight the importance of the need for a comprehensive nursing assessment at the time of the patient's admission and an awareness of family and social support. Liaison between hospital and community staff, both on the patient's admission to hospital and before discharge, is essential to ensure continuity of care for older surgical patients. Designated liaison workers or hospital aftercare schemes (Age Concern 1995) assist in a smooth transition from hospital to home and can make a significant contribution to an older person's recovery.

Discharge plans made preoperatively are only tentative and must be reviewed in the light of postoperative progress and evaluation of the patient's progress in self-care abilities. One area of major concern is patients' activity tolerance in relation to their home environment. When it is determined that the patient's functional needs for assistance are greater than can be met by the present support systems, additional planning is necessary. Some patients may be able to return home with extra support from family or an outside agency, and hospital discharge may need to be delayed until this can be arranged. Others, however, may need referral to residential or nursing home placements.

The more comprehensive existing discharge policies are, and the more closely they are followed, the more likely it is that the necessary aftercare will be in place. This may only be necessary in the short term but it is nevertheless important to ensure the patient's full recovery.

Surgical nurses are challenged to provide safe and effective care for older patients undergoing surgical interventions. Careful assessment throughout the perioperative period enables the nurse to anticipate older patients' needs and intervene appropriately to yield the best possible outcome. By strengthening older adults' physical and psychological status prior to surgery, recognising and minimising risks, and facilitating a prompt return or improvement of function postoperatively, nurses can ensure that maximum benefit from surgery will be achieved.

FUTURE PERSPECTIVES

The trend in the UK, as throughout industrialised countries, for the ageing of the population looks set to continue into the early decades of the next millennium. Victor (1995) argues that it is not yet possible to predict with any certainty what proportion of the population the older age groups will represent. That depends upon the birth rate and this, if past experience is anything to go on, shifts unpredictably with transient social circumstances and attitudes to child bearing. Demographic forecasts for the numbers of older people are much more reliable as these people are already born. Unless there are radical changes in migration to and from the UK, or in mortality rates in middle age, or an unprecedented natural disaster, the numbers can confidently be predicted. By the year 2025, the population over 65 years old will be 11.3 million (CSO 1990).

While it needs to be emphasised that old age does not automatically mean ill health and dependency, there are clear associations between advancing years and increasing levels of ill health and disability (Victor 1991). As people age, they encounter a higher incidence of disease processes that require surgical intervention as a result. Elderly people will continue to take advantage of surgical techniques that can not only add years to their lives but also improve their functioning in their remaining years. Kelly (1995) predicts that approximately 50% of those currently over the age of 65 will undergo an operative procedure in their remaining lifetime.

It must be remembered that the cohorts of people now past retirement age had the experience of childhood during the interwar depression years and then young adulthood in the war, when they were encouraged rather than discouraged from smoking. The legacy of those eras, which fortunately have not been repeated since, is with them today.

According to Jefferys & Thane (1989), there is evidence that those people aged 60–74 today are generally both more affluent and in better physical and mental shape than were their counterparts a generation ago at the same age. It is therefore likely that, as they age and become the 'older' (75–84) and 'oldest old' (85 and over), their health will be better than that experienced by the present cohort of over 80-year-olds.

Reflective point

Will older people in future cohorts experience the same health problems as their predecessors? How might current medical advances and behaviour patterns associated with healthy lifestyles and fitness influence health at a later stage for the cohorts which adopt them? Look back at the 10 most frequent surgical procedures in older people (Box 11.1). How different do you think the list might look in 10, 20 or even 50 years time?

The growing population of older individuals is providing many challenges and opportunities for innovation in health care. Recognising that ageing is a process beginning at birth, the surgical nurse, in caring for individuals of all ages, has the opportunity to promote clients' healthy futures. Through patient and family education the nurse can help patients appreciate how environmental conditions and healthy lifestyles influence the changes that occur with age.

Greater attention must be paid both to alleviating existing chronic conditions among older people through tertiary health promotion, and to preventive strategies throughout the life cycle. The aim must be to maintain the highest possible level of physical and cognitive functioning throughout life.

Information about prevention, early diagnosis and appropriate treatment can reduce the incidence of disease and disability and enable individuals of all ages to enjoy healthier lives.

With the rapid advance in technology and the onset of minimally invasive surgery, Harvey (1987) estimates that up to 80% of surgical procedures may be provided on an outpatient basis within the next decade. What is now a trend towards less invasive, less radical surgery whenever possible will be a way of life in the 21st century. Whilst not every older patient will be suitable for minimally invasive surgery, it has the potential to reduce the risk of patient exposure to hospital pathogens, decrease patient anxiety and allow family and friends to be present during the pre- and postoperative periods.

Dellasega & Burgunder (1991) assert that the principle that all individuals are of equal moral worth should mean equity of access to services and equal quality of treatments and care for all individuals. However, in the climate of finance reform, where care costs are increasingly closely scrutinised and challenged, resources are finite and choices will have to be made between competing priorities and needs. If older people are not to be disadvantaged or, solely on the basis of chronological age, treated as a separate class, Henwood (1990) argues that it is vital that the debate about rationing care is a public one where principles of equity and individual value are considered alongside economic imperatives.

REFERENCES

Age Concern 1993 Older people in the United Kingdom. Age Concern England, Mitcham, Surrey

Age Concern 1995 Hospital afterthought. Age Concern London, London

Arron M, Martin G, Webster J 1992 Perioperative care of the elderly. Comprehensive Therapy 18: 4–10

Barstow M D, Rawlings J, Allison S P 1983 Undernutrition, hypothermia and injury in elderly women with fractured femur: an injury response to altered metabolism? Lancet 1: 143–146

Bernstein G M, Offenbartl S K 1991 Adverse surgical outcomes among patients with cognitive impairments. American Surgeon 57: 682–690

British Medical Association and Royal College of Nursing 1995 The older person: consent and care. BMA, London

Burns R P, Cochran J L, Russell W L, Bard R M 1985 Appendicitis in mature patients. American Surgeon 201: 695–703

Catlic M R 1985 Surgery in centenarians. Journal of the American Medical Association 253: 3139

Central Statistical Office (CSO) 1990 Social trends 20. HMSO, London

Dellasega C, Burgunder C 1991 Perioperative nursing care for the elderly surgical patient. Today's Operating Room Nurse 13(6): 12–17

Dodson M E, Seymour G 1992 Surgery and anaesthesia in old age. In: Brocklehurst J C, Tallis H M, Fillit P (eds) Textbook of geriatric medicine and gerontology, 4th edn. Churchill Livingstone, Edinburgh

Fromm C G, Metzler D J 1993 Preparing your older patient for surgery. Registered Nurse (Jan): 38–41

Garrett G 1991 Surgery in old age. In: Garrett G (ed) Healthy ageing: some nursing perspectives. Wolfe, London

Goldfarb A I 1960 Psychiatric disorders of the aged: symptomology, diagnosis and treatment. Journal of the American Geriatrics Society 8: 698–707

Gosnell D J 1987 Assessment and evaluation of pressure sores. Nursing Clinics of North America 22(2): 399–416

Hamilton M 1960 A rating scale for depression. Journal of Neurology, Neurosurgery and Psychiatry 23: 56–62

Harkins S W, Chapman C R 1976 Detection and decision factors in pain perception in young and elderly men. Pain 2: 253–264

Harkins S W, Chapman C R 1977 The perception of induced dental pain in young and elderly women. Journal of Gerontology 32: 428–435

Harvey C K 1987 Future trends in perioperative nursing and technology. Nursing Administration Quarterly (Winter): 39

Hayslip B, Panek P E 1993 Adult development and ageing. HarperCollins, New York

Henwood M 1990 No sense of urgency. In: McEwen E (ed) Age: the unrecognised discrimination. Age Concern, London

Herr K A, Mobily P R 1991 Pain assessment in the elderly. Journal of Gerontological Nursing 17(4): 12–19

Hoot Martin J, Larsen P D 1994 Dehydration in the elderly surgical patient. Association of Operating Room Nurses Journal 60(4): 666–671

Jackson M F 1988 High risk surgical patients. Today's Operating Room Nurse 10(2): 26–33

Jackson M F 1989 Implications of surgery in very elderly patients. Association of Operating Room Nurses Journal 50: 859–869

Jefferys M, Thane P 1989 Introduction: an ageing society and ageing people. In: Jefferys M (ed) Growing old in the twentieth century. Routledge, London

Keene A 1991 Perioperative assessment and nursing: implications for the elderly. Plastic Surgical Nursing 11(4): 143–150

Kelly M 1995 Surgery, anaesthesia and the geriatric patient. Geriatric Nursing 16(5): 213–216

King's Fund 1994 Seamless care or patchwork quilt? King's Fund, London

Klipstein-Grosbuch K, Reilly J J, Potter J, Edwards C A, Roberts M A 1995 Energy intake and expenditure in elderly patients admitted to hospital with acute illness. British Journal of Nutrition 73: 323–334

Latz P A, Wyble S J 1987 Elderly patients: preoperative nursing implications. Association of Operating Room Nurses Journal 46(2): 238–253

Lubin M F 1993 Is age a risk factor for surgery? Medical Clinics of North America 77(2): 327–333

Luckman J, Sorenson K C 1980 Medical–surgical nursing: a psychophysiologic approach. W B Saunders, Philadelphia

Lusis S A 1994 Nursing management of the elderly surgical patient. Plastic Surgical Nursing 14(3): 139–146

McFarland G K, Thomas M D 1991 Psychiatric mental health nursing. J B Lippincott, Philadelphia

McWhirter J P, Pennington C 1994 Incidence and recognition of malnutrition in hospital. British Medical Journal 308: 945–948

Menyhert L R 1988 Special considerations in geriatric care: an overview. Journal of Post Anaesthesia Nursing 3(3): 162–164

Mohr D N 1983 Estimation of surgical risk in the elderly: a correlative review. Journal of the American Geriatrics Society 31(2): 99–102

Moore L W, Proffitt C 1993 Communicating effectively with elderly surgical patients. Association of Operating Room Nurses Journal 58(2): 345–351

Mullen J L, Busby G P, Matthews D C 1980 Reduction of operative morbidity and mortality by combined preoperative and postoperative nutrition support. Annals of Surgery 192: 604–613

Nichols R 1991 Surgical wound infections. American Journal of Medicine 91: 54S–64S

Nolan T 1992 Surgery in the elderly: lowering risks by understanding special needs. Postgraduate Medicine 91(2): 199–208

Orentreich N, Selmanowitz V J 1969 Levels of biological functions with ageing. Trans Academic Science Series B 31: 992–1012

Palmer M A 1990 Care of the older surgical patient. In: Eliopoulos C (ed) Caring for the elderly in diverse settings. Lippincott, Philadelphia

Pritchard V 1986 Calculating the risk. Nursing Times 82(48): 40–55

Rosenberg J, Kehlit H 1993 Postoperative mental confusion: association with postoperative hypoxia. Surgery 114(1): 76–81

Scott S M, Mayhew P A, Harris E A 1992 Pressure ulcer development in the operating room. Association of Operating Room Nurses Journal 56(2): 242–250

Seymour D G, Pringle R 1981 Surgical emergencies in the elderly: can they be prevented? Health Bulletin 41: 112–131

Smith O C 1907 Advanced age as a contraindication to operation. Medical Researcher 72: 6240

Squires A J, Taylor M 1988 Assessment of the older patient. In: Squires A J (ed) Rehabilitation of the older patient: a handbook for the multidisciplinary team. Chapman and Hall, London

Thomas D R, Richie C S 1995 Preoperative assessment of older adults. Journal of the American Geriatrics Society 43: 811–821

Vaz F G, Seymour D G 1989 A prospective study of elderly general surgery patients: pre-operative medical problems. Age Ageing 18: 309–315

Victor C R 1991 Health and health care in later life. Open University Press, Buckingham

Victor C R 1995 Old age in modern society, 2nd edn. Chapman and Hall, London

Vowles K D J 1979 Surgery for the aged. In: Vowles K D J (ed) Surgical problems in the aged. Wright, Bristol

Waterlow J 1988 The Waterlow card for the prevention and management of pressure sores: towards a pocket policy. Care: Science and Practice 6(1): 8–12

Webb G P, Copeman J 1996 The nutrition of older adults. Edward Arnold, London

Wild L, Coyne C 1992 Epidural analgesia: the basics and beyond. American Journal of Nursing 92(4): 26–30, 32–34

Woodhouse K W 1994 Pharmacokinetics of drugs in the elderly. In: Crome P, Flanagan R J (ed) Drugs and the ageing population: current issues. Journal of the Royal Society of Medicine Supplement 23(87): 2–4

FURTHER READING

Bond J, Coleman P, Peace S (eds) 1993 Ageing in society, 2nd edn. Sage, London

British Medical Association and Royal College of Nursing 1995 The older person: consent and care. BMA, London

Crome P, Flanagan R J (eds) Drugs and the ageing population: current issues. Journal of the Royal Society of Medicine 87(suppl 23): 1–30

Keller S M, Markovitz L J, Wilder J R 1987 Emergency and elective surgery in patients over age 70. American Surgeon 53: 636–640

Kimmel D C 1990 Adulthood and ageing, 3rd edn. Wiley, New York

Redfern S J (ed) 1991 Nursing elderly people, 2nd edn. Churchill Livingstone, Edinburgh

Squires A J (ed) 1988 Rehabilitation of the older adult: a handbook for the multidisciplinary team. Chapman and Hall, London

Victor C R 1991 Health and health care in later life. Open University Press, Bucks

Victor C R 1995 Old age in modern society, 2nd edn. Chapman and Hall, London

Webb G P, Copeman J 1996 The nutrition of older adults. Edward Arnold, London

PART 3

The environment for surgery

PART CONTENTS

12

The changing policy context of surgical nursing

Abigail Masterson   Ailsa Cameron

AIMS

The aims of this chapter are:

- to stimulate an awareness amongst surgical nurses of the fundamental importance of an understanding of health and social policy to their everyday practice
- illustrate the relationship between health and social policy and the work of the surgical nurse
- identify ways that surgical nurses can influence the policy agenda.

INTRODUCTION

Nursing in the United Kingdom (UK) has continually been influenced by the directions, goals and principles of government and dominant groups in the policy-making process (Robinson et al 1992). For too long nurses have failed to acknowledge that their work exists within a wider context which controls and rations the resources that support the health care system, ultimately affecting what nursing is and the way in which nursing care is delivered. This chapter aims to stimulate an interest in social policy and awareness amongst surgical nurses of the fundamental importance and relevance of an understanding of social policy to their everyday practice with patients.

WHAT IS SOCIAL POLICY?

Social policy in its broadest sense encompasses Acts of Parliament, and central government and local government directives as well as the operationalisation of decisions at grass roots level. It may not appear to be relevant to everyday surgical nursing practice, yet it is our contention that changes in social policy can and do have a direct impact on nursing.

Social policy has been defined as the rationale underlying the development and use of social institutions which affect the distribution of resources, status, and power between different individuals and groups in society (Bulmer et al 1989). Social policy is concerned with the values and principles which govern such distribution as well as their outcomes. It develops from and responds to ideas about how society ought to be and involves action or inaction on the part of central government and/or other interest groups such as professionals (Gough et al 1994). Policy making and implementation involve negotiation and bargaining between competing demands, in what has been called the policy community (Kingdom 1991). Historically the medical profession has always maintained a powerful position in the policy-making process (Ham 1992), whereas nursing has been characterised by its weak voice and relative invisibility (Robinson et al 1992). Nursing's participation in the development and advancement of surgical care has of course been crucial but surgical nurses have a potentially even more important role to play in the formulation of policy to affect the way in which care is given in the future.

Social policy in its broadest sense can be seen as comprising legislation, government initiatives and social trends. To illustrate the impact of social policy on the profession in general, and surgical nursing in particular, we will look at examples of how one Act of Parliament – the NHS and Community Care Act 1990 – has had a major impact on the way that nursing services are provided. We will outline the impact of two government initiatives – the reduction of waiting lists and the reduction in junior doctors' hours – on the roles of surgical nurses. We will consider the interaction between changes in health technology and the development of health policy, and the effect of changes in demography on the role of the profession and the composition of the nursing workforce. Studying social policy in this way, we believe, can enable nurses to gain a greater understanding of the processes by which policies are developed and implemented and the consequences of such policies for society and nursing. Through such study, nurses may be able to predict many future policy changes, and influence rather than react to the course of events, as advocated in the recent White Paper (DoH 1997a).

Why is social policy important to nursing?

There is no doubt that British health care has changed markedly over the last two decades (Ham 1992) but nursing has not always been ready for the changes that have taken place, particularly in the organisation and delivery of services. As a result, the profession often appears to react too late. For example much of the

debate about the desirability, preparation and evaluation of nurse practitioners came after their introduction into the acute and primary care services. Consequently, the profession was in a much weaker position to plan, manage and control the development (UKCC 1997). At the same time health care assistant roles are developing in all care areas in response to changes in pre-registration nursing education, and skill mix and reprofiling projects to meet the cost-effectiveness agenda. In some areas it can now be seen that the work of nurses has increasingly become that of supervisors rather than hands-on carers. Yet both the RCN membership and the UKCC (unlike the Chartered Society of Physiotherapists, for example) have refused to allow membership of their organisations to health care assistants and health care support workers. Although this exclusion has been argued on the basis of their being *professional* organisations, clearly the existence of a large number of support workers who remain outside of professional control has implications for safety, standards of care and ultimately the viability of the profession.

Indeed, at a time when the composition of health services is being radically altered, for example as a result of the move from acute to primary care, serious doubts are being raised about the contribution of various professional groups. The future of health visiting and school nursing in particular has been questioned. In 1997 the Lifespan Trust in Cambridgeshire fought a highly publicised battle to introduce the role of generic community health nurse at the expense of specialist health visiting and school nursing services (Hancock 1997). At first glance, this policy development may not appear to be particularly relevant to surgical nurses, but coupled with other debates, such as the 1996 report from the University of Manchester Health Services Management Unit on the future of the health care workforce, it highlights the pressure for change in the structure of the nursing profession. Of greater concern is that both initiatives can be seen as evidence of an undervaluing of the traditional nursing role by policy makers and policy analysts generally. The 'Manchester Report' argued for the creation of a generic health worker from which specialisms such as physiotherapy could emerge. Many of the duties expected of this generic health care worker appeared to closely resemble traditional conceptualisations of nursing.

Despite the well-publicised shortage of nurses, the Government has professed an interest in the development of the nurse anaesthetist role to compensate for the shortage of anaesthetists (Audit Commission 1997). Nurses' voices need to be heard in health and social policy debates, otherwise decisions about the way health care is provided and the composition of the health care workforce will be taken without consideration of professional nursing issues (Gough et al 1994). The development of a cadre of nurses who can competently and effectively analyse and influence the formulation of health policies to support nursing objectives is therefore crucial. At the time of writing, the new White Paper on the NHS identifies a stronger role for 'expert' nurses in all areas of care delivery and health policy-making (DoH 1997a).

The experiences of nurses in the USA may provide a useful model, as they have recently adopted a much more proactive stance in terms of their interaction with the development of health and social policy. American nurses have developed strong political affiliations; they view lobbying as part of their normal role and actively encourage practitioners to go into politics at all levels (Girouard 1989). The endorsement of Clinton and the Democrats by the American Nurses' Association is perceived to have been important in securing their re-election (Rafferty 1997). In return for this support there have been attempts to reform many aspects of health and welfare services, for example enabling nurses to claim reimbursement privileges as independent practitioners. It has been argued that if nurses in the UK could follow this model we might be able to challenge successfully the negative effects of many policies for us and our patients, and empower nurses and nursing to achieve their fullest health promotion potential. However, the situation is much more complex. Despite American nurses' move towards politicisation and their active involvement in supporting Clinton in his first presidential election, they now find themselves facing multiskilling and down-sizing, and nursing jobs being threatened by unlicensed personnel. Having already established a role for themselves within the policy-making process, they may find it easier to challenge these developments from within rather than arguing from outside.

In the UK, however, nursing has not demonstrated such political activity. The RCN has steadfastly refused to align itself with any particular political party, believing its members' interests are better served by providing a source of objective advice on political issues to all political parties. May 1 1997 was an historic moment for nurses and nursing in the UK when Anne Keene, the former general secretary of the Community Practitioner and Health Visitor's Association, was one of the first nurses ever to be elected to parliament. Her maiden speech and personal manifesto was to ensure that nursing is represented in Parliament. If nursing is to have a significant voice in the formation of health and social policy, other nurses most follow this lead.

Reflective point

Consider how surgical nurses can adopt a proactive stance to influence the policy agenda. By taking an active role in a trade union or professional organisation you can begin to set the agenda for change.

THE NATIONAL HEALTH SERVICE

The majority of nurses in the UK work within the NHS. In order to understand how social policy shapes the profession and the work that nurses do, it is necessary to briefly review the history of the NHS and its development to the present day.

The NHS was formally established on 5 July 1948 but its final shape was the result of a trend that started in the late 19th century of progressive state involvement in health care. The two world wars highlighted the marked disparity in service provision across the UK and the feasibility of centralising the organisation and management of health care. Advances in medical science and effective utilisation of the policy process ensured that medicine had a significant influence on the final shape of the service. Consequently, the model of health and health care which has had the greatest influence on the NHS is the 'medical model'. Indeed, health has usually been seen as synonymous with the elimination of medically defined disease and, as a result, acute and curative services such as surgery have been a priority for funding, although this is currently under review (Ham 1992).

Since its inception the NHS has constantly been scrutinised on grounds of cost and efficiency. As early as 1953 a commission was set up in response to the perceived spiralling of health costs (Guillebaud Committee 1956). Successive reorganisations of the service, coupled with initiatives such as the resource allocation working party in 1976, have been motivated at least in part by a desire to cut costs, even though the percentage of gross national product (GDP) spent on health care in the UK is much lower than that in comparable countries. Possibly the most radical of these reviews resulted in the NHS and Community Care Act 1990 which led to the introduction of the concept of the internal market to health care services in Britain.

The impact of legislation on the way in which health care is provided

The importance of government legislation in the shaping of health care is beyond doubt. In order to illustrate this relationship we will consider the impact of the 1990 NHS and Community Care Act on the provision of health services.

As we have said the 1990 Act led to the introduction of what has become known as the internal market. The Act aimed to foster some of the qualities of competition and choice which are found in private enterprise (Ham 1992). In essence the Act led to a split between the purchasing and providing functions of the NHS. Individual hospitals or groups of hospitals could apply for trust status which gave them the independence to determine:

- what services they would supply
- the terms and conditions of staff they employed
- the opportunity to generate income.

In other words, trusts were encouraged to provide responsive, market-driven services. They no longer had to provide a full range of services, which has led some commentators (Robinson & Le Grand 1994) to suggest that hospitals have developed services focusing on the needs of patients with acute, self-limiting illness which is more profitable than providing long-term rehabilitation services.

These reforms precipitated changes in referral patterns which highlighted the vulnerability of some hospitals (Glasman 1994). Purchasers attracted by lower costs and better quality were able to place contracts with different providers making some hospitals unviable. Reducing length of stay and expanding day surgery has been crucial to providers' survival although these initiatives also involve bed reductions, thus leading to increased overheads which in turn can make hospitals uncompetitive (Tomlinson 1992). The internal market actively encouraged individual trusts to compete against one another for business. Anglia Harbour Trust was one of the first casualties of this policy when it was forced out of business in 1996. Other trusts have had to respond to these new challenges by drastically reconfiguring the services that they provided; for example setting up their own chemotherapy service or hiring consultants on a sessional basis to provide specialist services rather than losing their cancer patients to specialist centres.

The 1990 Act also allowed general practitioner (GP) practices to apply to become fundholders. By becoming fundholders, GPs were given a budget that was judged to reflect the health needs of their local population.

The formula used to calculate the budget was weighted, to reflect factors such as age and social deprivation within the locality. In turn, GPs used their allocation to purchase or rather contract with health care providers to supply particular services, for example elective orthopaedic surgery. Many questions have been raised about how these financial allocations were derived. For example were the allocations responsive to the changing needs of the population? Was there flexibility in the allocation to cope with unexpected health needs such as an outbreak of *E. coli*? Were the allocations weighted appropriately to meet the age structure of the local population?

Some commentators (Robinson & Le Grand 1994) suggested that fundholding was seized upon by those practices in relatively affluent areas where there was a greater chance of making a profit. Concerns were also expressed that so-called 'expensive patients', i.e. those who require complex long-term support, had problems registering with such practices. Poorer inner city areas continued to be served mainly by non-fundholding practices and their health care continued to be purchased by health authorities (Appleby et al 1994). Some commentators suggested that fundholders received priority from trusts and that patients from fundholding practices were able to jump the queue in accessing hospital beds, particularly for elective surgery (Glennester et al 1994). In other words, a two-tier system was emerging despite the original philosophy of the NHS that all sections of the population would have equal access to services.

Clearly this fundamental change in the way services were purchased and provided had implications for the delivery of surgical services. The introduction of trusts as independent financial units forced a re-examination of the most cost-effective means of providing services and this led to initiatives such as re-engineering of the workforce, skill mix reviews and in many instances the development of new professional roles. Some trusts have introduced nurse-led preoperative clinics and rapid discharge programmes in an attempt to make services more efficient (Ong 1997). In addition, new clinical roles such as nurse anaesthetists (Audit Commission 1997), nurse endoscopists (UKCC 1997) and surgeons' assistants (Tuthill 1995) have been established. These developments deserve greater consideration, since they have implications for the future of the nursing profession, and we will return to the issue of new roles later in the chapter. Another consequence of the increased number of purchasers has been the lack of a purchasing consensus and fragmentation of service planning and development. Ultimately this fragmentation may cause uncertainty to educational planners and providers about the nature and size of the workforce needed to support the service.

The 1990 Act and the mixed economy of care – the legitimisation of independent hospitals

The split between the purchaser and provider function and the rhetoric of the private sector economy has also allowed and even encouraged purchasers of health care to look actively for new health care providers outside of traditional models.

A common assumption is that before the 1990 NHS and Community Care Act there was no mixed economy of health care, but in reality a buoyant private health sector existed. The Conservative governments of 1979–1997 had given tax breaks and other financial incentives to encourage sectors of the population to invest in private health care insurance. Such benefits were often seen as a desirable employment perk and recruitment incentive. This led to an increase in the range of private sector provision and many new private hospitals were built which offered care ranging from cosmetic surgery to cardiac bypass surgery. This expansion of the private sector also allowed some patients to make choices about phases of care. For example, a patient might have cardiac surgery within the NHS but choose to convalesce in a private hospital. In addition, the 1990 Act explicitly sanctioned the acceptability of multiple providers of health care to meet a range of different needs. So the Act enabled purchasers of health care, be they GPs, health authorities or insurance companies, to choose providers from any sector that best met their requirements (Ham 1994).

The 1990 legislation also encouraged wider discussions of the appropriateness of state funding for certain surgical interventions. As a result, surgical procedures like breast reduction and the removal of varicose veins were increasingly only provided within the private sector. Consequently, the patient group that surgical nurses work with depends on whether the nurses are employed by the NHS or the private sector. The patient group in private hospitals is generally likely to be younger, fitter, wealthier and undergoing less radical surgery. Such patients consequently will have less need for extensive postoperative support. Inevitably this will affect the type of nursing required and therefore the composition and preparation of the nursing workforce in surgical services.

As a result of these changes, private hospitals have become significant employers of surgical nurses. This has implications for the education, professional support and development of nursing. The profession needs to ensure that nurses employed in the private sector enjoy the same opportunities as nurses in the NHS. Private hospitals have always been able to set their own rates of pay and remuneration packages, which have often been less beneficial than the employment conditions in the state sector. In addition, the education needs of nurses in the independent sector are not covered by the education purchasing consortia, which only purchase education for the state sector (DoH 1997b). Therefore nurses working in the independent sector may have more difficulty accessing post-registration courses and continuing professional development of all kinds. Professional associations used to working with the institutions of the NHS have been criticised by nurses from the private and independent sectors for not promoting their interests. Nurse leaders need to have a broader understanding of the changing pattern of services and the context in which they are delivered if they are to lead the whole profession in the next century.

'The New NHS – Modern. Dependable'

In December 1997 the new Labour Government outlined its proposals for reforming the NHS (DoH 1997a). The White Paper 'The New NHS – Modern. Dependable' stated that from April 1999 GPs and community nurses would have the opportunity to work together in Primary Care Groups (PCGs) to improve the health of the population they serve. PCGs will serve a population of approximately 100 000 patients and will commission services to meet the population's health care needs from a cash-limited budget. PCGs will commission services from the appropriate NHS trusts and will work in partnership with local authorities to ensure that primary and community health and social care services are better integrated.

In other words, despite the rhetoric of partnership, health services will continue to be configured around a division between those who commission services and those who provide them. This raises several important issues that need to be considered by the nursing profession. First, the trend towards involving primary health care workers, particularly nurses, in the commissioning of services is set to continue. In order to maximise the potential for health gain, the profession needs to ensure that it supports individual nurses to make an effective contribution to the commissioning process. For example, PCGs may herald the emergence of a new managerial role for nurses or the rise of a public health nurse who is a specialist in epidemiology. Indeed the White Paper (DoH 1997a, p. 46) explicitly stated that the Government wishes to encourage and 'extend the recent developments in the roles of nurses working in acute and community services. The Government is committed to encouraging and supporting the development of nursing practice in these ways.'

Clinical effectiveness and service quality are major strands of the Government's drive to develop and modernise the NHS (DoH 1997a). In the White Paper 'A First Class Service: Quality in the New NHS' (NHSE 1998) the government sets out a framework for quality improvement based on the concept of clinical governance. The new National Institute for Clinical Excellence will provide clinicians with clear authoritative guidance on clinical and cost effectiveness. In addition, the ongoing development of evidence-based service frameworks will set national standards and define models for specific services and care groups. Surgical nurses need therefore to acknowledge that the continued move towards evidence-based commissioning and clinical governance will require all professional groups to audit their practice. Nursing specialties will need to articulate and justify their contribution to health gain or will risk being omitted from the list of commissioned services. The new professional roles that surgical nurses have developed over the past decade will not be exempt from this trend. Indeed, it could be argued that this trend will be of particular importance to those nursing roles that transcend professional boundaries, whether they are at the nursing/medicine interface or the nursing/therapist interface. Similarly, research evidence will be important to support developments within the nursing profession, for example practice nurses assisting GPs to carry out minor surgical procedures, thereby taking over some of the traditional activities of surgical nurses. Thus the integration of research evidence into the management and practice of surgical nursing is fundamental to the profession's future (DoH 1997a).

Reflective point

Acquire a copy of the White Paper (DoH 1997a) and consider the impact it has had or may have on your professional development and service delivery in your area.

POLICY INITIATIVES

As we discussed in the introduction to this chapter, the shape of health services owes as much to the operationalisation of particular government initiatives as it does to Acts of Parliament. To illustrate this point we will consider two highly publicised government initiatives that in our belief have dramatically affected the way in which health care services have been provided and specifically the role of surgical nurses.

Waiting list initiatives

Although waiting lists had long been a cause for concern, they had reached the top of the health policy agenda in the early 1990s. The Conservative Government saw the reduction of waiting lists as a way of cosmetically improving services without dealing with the issues of chronic under-funding. Central government issued guidance to health authorities indicating that no patient should wait more than 2 years for admission to hospital. One hundred new consultant posts were created to help achieve this and £33 million was made available during 1990/91 to tackle this issue (Ham 1992). The Patient's Charter (DoH 1991a) consolidated the initiative and gave patients the right to be seen within 2 years.

Individual trusts have developed their own strategies to reduce waiting lists. Some used the extra funding to open operating theatres and day surgery units at the weekend in an effort to increase levels of activity; others circumvented the directives by delaying outpatient assessment appointments so that they appeared to have reduced waiting times. Other trusts employed locum doctors and GPs on short contracts to run minor operation lists and some purchased a full range of services from private hospitals.

Waiting list initiatives also had a direct impact on the health professions. Nursing and therapy roles in outpatient clinics were expanded in many trusts in order to free surgeons to spend more time in theatre. For example, orthopaedic physiotherapy practitioner posts were created to take those patients directly off a consultant's waiting list who were unlikely to require surgical intervention. Preoperative assessment roles, which include a full medical clerking and presurgical work-up, have become popular in some trusts. New ways of managing certain health problems which avoided the need for surgery were also encouraged. Indeed nurses have set up complete services for the conservative management of patients with intermittent claudication (Binnie 1997). The skill mix in theatres has also been reviewed with the result that nurses have become more involved in the process of surgery as the emergence of nurse anaesthetist and first assistant roles demonstrates.

Clearly, the waiting list initiative has had and will continue to have major implications for nursing but it appears that rather than being involved in the planning and implementation of the initiative, nursing has had to reactively manage the consequences. It is interesting to note that despite these highly publicised attempts to reduce waiting lists, the Department of Health revealed in 1997 (press release on DoH website, 97/351) that the number of patients waiting for treatment in England had risen to a record high of 1.2 million and 818 patients had waited more than the revised Patient's Charter (DoH 1995) guarantee of 18 months. This represented a 14% increase on 1996. Health Minister, Frank Dobson, reacted by appointing Stephen Day, NHS Regional Director in the West Midlands, to head an action team to tackle the problem (Batty 1997). We are not suggesting that greater nursing involvement in the waiting list initiative would have altered the course of events but it may have led to more sensitive role development and a more coherent approach to the management of theatre time and waiting lists.

Junior doctors' hours

Another government initiative which appears to have had a major impact on the way in which health services are delivered has been their 1991 plans to reduce the hours worked by junior doctors to keep them in line with European directives and to reduce progressively the contribution of doctors in training to service provision in the NHS (Calman 1993, NHSME 1991). The media had long been campaigning about juniors working too many hours, leading to mistakes, stress and even death amongst the profession and worries that many students were leaving the profession. The Government directed that employers should ensure that as soon as practicable no doctor in training should have to work longer than 83 hours a week. The maximum was to fall to 72 hours a week by the end of 1994 for those doctors working in posts that were described as 'hard pressed'. No junior doctor should be working in excess of 72 hours a week by the end of 1996 (DoH 1991b). As part of the mechanisms used to achieve these targets the Government urged employers to make best use of the skills of nurses and other allied staff to help reduce the junior doctors' workloads and ultimately their hours of work.

To enable this reduction, the Government allocated money to each region to fund new developments. Some trusts invested their 'taskforce' money in the development of new clinical roles, often nursing, to facilitate the reduction in junior doctors' hours of work. For example Trent Region used £500 000 of taskforce money to pump-prime a raft of new nursing roles to fill the gaps left by the junior doctors (SCHARR 1997). Many of these new roles were developed within surgical specialities and involved the establishment of nurse-led services such as preoperative clinics in ENT and gynaecology. Unfortunately much of the literature around such new roles is anecdotal or descriptive and there is very little outcome research. As a result, it is difficult to say whether these developments have been beneficial for patients and staff.

Much has been written about the negative and positive implications of this initiative for nursing. For example, the negative view implies that nurses have had to pick up the tasks that junior doctors no longer had the time, or inclination, to do, whilst the positive view identifies this as an opportunity for nursing to achieve its full potential by developing into new areas. Whatever one's view about such developments it appears that nursing had to react to the reduction in junior doctors' hours rather than being welcomed as an equal partner in proactive discussions about the future shape of the health care workforce and significant changes in the form of medical training. It would surely have been of more benefit to the profession and therefore the patient if the view of nurses had been sought at the inception of such initiatives. Full discussion would have enabled a coherent and systematic approach to the education and assessment of competence needed to underpin such new roles, rather than the development of posts in an ad hoc and incremental manner. Unfortunately, discussions around policy-making and funding for education and training of health professionals are dealt with separately, which makes coherent strategic planning across the professions difficult (DoH 1997b). The UKCC and RCN now meet on a regular basis with the General Medical Council and the medical Royal Colleges. However, it is still rare that such meetings are used as an opportunity for joint planning (Dowling et al 1996). At local levels, devolvement of budgetary responsibility to directorates has also worked against strategic multidisciplinary approaches to the development of health care roles.

THE RELATIONSHIP BETWEEN TECHNOLOGICAL ADVANCES, SOCIAL POLICY AND NURSING

As we argued in our opening section, the way nursing is delivered and the policies that are developed to support this is often driven by external factors, that is, factors outside of government health policy. In this section we would like to consider the impact of changes in technology on the way health care is delivered.

Technology has always had a significant influence on health and social policy and nursing practice. Before the development of safer anaesthesia and antibiotic therapy the surgical procedures possible were extremely limited. Surgery was only contemplated if the risk to life of not proceeding with an intervention was greater than the risk to life posed by the surgery itself.

Day surgery

One of the most profound changes in modern times to have affected surgical nursing and acute care in general has been the growing number of patients undergoing day surgery (Audit Commission 1990). Many conditions which used to require hospital admission can now successfully be treated as day cases – for example, cholecystectomy, hernia repair and removal of varicose veins. Technological and pharmacological advances have supported this expansion in day surgery and non-invasive therapies. It is likely that the types of conditions deemed to be appropriate for day surgery will grow as these advances continue and trusts are pressured to keep waiting lists short. However, these developments have implications for the way in which health services are provided. As Miller (1997) points out, the expansion in day case surgery has profound effects on community health services such as GPs and community nurses, who increasingly have to deal with postoperative conditions as well as their traditional caseloads, and it is unclear whether or not they have the appropriate skills for this changing caseload.

In an effort to respond to these changes, some trusts have developed new types of services that will support patients postoperatively in the community. For example, hospital at home schemes have been established to support patients following day surgery. There is some debate as to whether these services are economically viable (Coast 1993) but for those trusts who want to increase throughput and thereby reduce waiting lists they may appear an attractive option.

Wickham (1993) suggests that the development of day surgery has fundamentally changed the nature of the professions involved in surgical care and will continue to do so. For example, a number of specialists, such as the interventional radiologists and the physician gastroenterologists, are already assuming a therapeutic role which was until recently restricted to surgeons. Wickham restricted his analysis to medicine but clearly these developments have implications for nursing too. The ENRiP database (SCHARR 1997) identifies that nurses are taking on new technical procedures such as intravenous cannulation, epidural management and top-up, and the recording and interpretation of electrocardiograms, which has resulted in a shifting of the boundaries between medicine and nursing (Murray et al 1995). Nurses are also delivering traditional medical interventions within a nursing paradigm, for example curettage, cryosurgery and endoscopy. These developments will no doubt lead to further changes in speciality and professional boundaries and necessitate changes in training/education. Some techniques which in the past required inpatient surgical stays – the removal of moles and benign cysts – are being performed in GP surgeries. Surgical interventions now regularly take place in areas outside of the traditional surgical departments such as obstetric units, radiology units, cardiac catheter laboratories, endoscopy suites and accident and emergency departments (Vincent 1997). Consequently, the work that would traditionally have been carried out by surgical nurses is now being undertaken by X-ray department nurses, practice nurses and radiographers. Such developments will arguably reduce the total number of nurses required in the acute sector (Jones 1985, King's Fund Commission 1992). It is likely, however, that the rising number of older patients will result in increasing activity on surgical wards, high dependency units and intensive therapy units. To meet future health needs, many nurses who are presently working in acute hospital services may need to be redeployed in the community or will be increasingly confined to high-dependency and intensive-care services.

The growth in day surgery, although apparently welcomed by patients and professionals alike, has to be critically evaluated to ensure that only appropriate patients and interventions are selected for this changing mode of service delivery. Gelijns & Fendrick (1993) argue that the rapid increase in the professional and patient demand for some techniques, for example the removal of gallstones, precluded the use of controlled trials to establish efficacy, safety, and probably economic performance for laparoscopic cholecystectomy. Although the early pilots in day surgery had strict selection protocols restricting such services to young, essentially fit patients with good support at home, there is some evidence that older, frailer patients are frequently being steered towards this option, with severe consequences for their carers and the community nursing services. It seems surprising that the full range of emotional and psychological support associated with traditional services can be managed through the day surgery system. Searching questions need to be asked by nurses, such as in whose interests are these innovations being promoted or developed, the patients or the service? Day surgery may be wholly appropriate and desirable in some instances but in others it may not (Thatcher 1996) (see also Ch. 15).

Similarly, the growth in minimally invasive surgery has great financial costs in terms of equipment, training, theatre and hospital design. Wickham (1993, p. 12) claims that in the future, health care delivered in 'single story stand alone production line units in areas with good car parking and rapid transport facilities will and should replace the old type of 355–500 bed mega institutions'. Within these centres, operating room design will also change radically from the simple concept of the operating table and scalpel to the purpose-built interventional suite containing radiological, ultrasonic and endoscopic facilities, multiple monitor displays and other ancillary instrumentation. A total reappraisal of the mechanisms of achieving asepsis during operation will have to be undertaken. For many procedures it would seem totally unnecessary for the operator to wear a gown and mask. Changes in the design of buildings will also affect the working environment and social relationships between health professionals and the public. Surely nursing should be involved in such discussions about how surgical care is to be provided in the future.

Reflective point

You might like to consider whether or not Wickam's view of the future health care environment seems appropriate to the needs and requirements of an ageing population (See also Ch. 11.)

Reduced length of stay

Dramatic reductions in the length of stay for all surgical interventions have occurred over the last decade. In part the pressure has been economic, a need to increase through-put, thereby increasing efficiency. However, developments in surgical techniques, advances in the scientific knowledge base and changes

in philosophies regarding rehabilitation and normalisation have also contributed to these reductions. This has had significant impact on the model of care underpinning surgical nursing. No longer is the role one of doing for dependent patients but rather one of nurturing independence postoperatively.

One example of this change in philosophy has been the care of patients undergoing joint replacement, which has changed from a focus on bed rest and passive recuperation to aggressive rehabilitation in the immediate postoperative period. Many trusts have invested in preoperative assessment clinics run by nurses, or home visits by an outreach nurse, at which the presurgical work-up is completed, discharge arrangements are begun and rehabilitation regimes are taught (UKCC 1997). A similar model has been developed for cardiac patients. Those patients undergoing cardiac surgery who are believed to have appropriate levels of support are sometimes fast-tracked through the process and discharged on day 5 postoperatively. These services are normally backed up with outreach cardiac home care nurses who visit and monitor the patients daily. In some instances, the nurses have laptop computers which enable them to transmit an ECG via a modem to the patient's consultant who can then order changes in prescriptions which can be transmitted back to the nurse in the patient's home. Once again, the examples above illustrate how developments in surgical techniques and technology have radically altered the function of surgical nurses and the knowledge base required to underpin their practice. Nurses need to be able to evaluate these changes within a professional framework and also within a health policy context in order that appropriate resources can be accessed and the professional view inform the policy debates.

DEMOGRAPHIC TRENDS

Surgery and surgical nurses are also affected by changes in the structure of the population. The average life span is increasing by an average of 2 years every decade (Central Statistical Office 1995). OPCS data (1993) suggest that by 2001 16% of the total population will be aged 65 or more and 2% will be aged at least 85. Older people have a high usage of all health services; consequently, surgical nurses need to expand their knowledge of multiple pathology associated with ageing and the increased need for active rehabilitation in the older patient group. However, as we have suggested, it is unclear whether surgical and rehabilitation services will continue to be provided by the NHS; a few trusts and purchasers of services already have explicit age-related criteria for accessing particular types of surgical procedures. Other trusts have significantly reduced rehabilitation and convalescence facilities. Either the population will choose increasingly to purchase services from the private sector if they have the means or they may go without. The efficacy and impact of such developments needs wider public debate.

The age structure of the nursing profession itself has also changed markedly over the last 20 years. A recent analysis by the UKCC of the professional register showed that the percentage of nurses under the age of 29 has plunged to an all-time low, whilst the percentage of nurses in the older age categories is increasing steadily and the number of new admissions to the register is dropping (Nursing Times 1997). Recent figures from the English National Board's Annual Report highlighted that there are currently more training places available than candidates wanting to fill them – only 15 362 people applied for 16 126 training places last year (Waters 1997). The NHS Executive *Education and Planning Guidance* (1997) notes that national workforce modelling indicated that commissioning levels were insufficient to meet the future demand for qualified nurses predicted by employers. A survey by the Association of Healthcare Human Resource Managers found that 60% of employers were experiencing significant problems recruiting registered staff (Stock 1997). In many areas of the country, trusts are carrying vacancies even in traditionally popular specialisms such as surgical nursing. Increasing attention to cost-effectiveness and value for money in association with difficulties in recruiting and retaining qualified nursing staff have resulted in changes in the role and function of the nurse in surgical areas. Health care assistants supported by NVQ training are undertaking many traditional nursing tasks such as the monitoring of vital signs and dressing uncomplicated wounds. The profession needs to consider seriously why so many nurses continue to leave and why school leavers decide against joining the nursing profession, and how we can change their minds (see Ch. 5).

Reflective point

What might encourage nurses to stay in your clinical area? How would you recommend attracting more school leavers and mature entrants into the profession?

NEW ROLE DEVELOPMENT

The chapter, so far, has attempted to illustrate how social policy interacts with and shapes nursing. One of the underlying themes of our discussions has been the impact on the profession of key pieces of legislation and policy changes which have resulted in the emergence of a new role for surgical nurses. Any cursory review of the professional literature demonstrates a proliferation of new roles in nursing. We now examine these developments in more detail and investigate the implications for the profession.

The nursing development movement was established in the 1980s on the back of initiatives such as the nursing process, which was intended to be not only a system of documentation but also a way of illustrating the unique contribution of nursing to health care. The nursing literature in the mid-1980s was characterised by pleas to regain the fundamental value of nursing. Arguments were constructed to illuminate nursing's therapeutic contribution in its own right. Jane Salvage, author of the seminal text *The Politics of Nursing* in 1985, and long-time member of the radical nurses' group, was appointed Head of Nursing Developments at the King's Fund. In the late 1980s the nursing development movement grew rapidly and appeared to have a significant influence on the policy and professional agenda. For example the Department of Health supported the establishment of 30 nursing development units as a means of encouraging excellence in practice. The self-confidence of the profession was manifest in the empowering rhetoric of primary nursing and the legislative support for educational change (UKCC 1986, Salvage & Wright 1995).

Some commentators saw *The Scope of Professional Practice* (UKCC 1992) as the culmination of a decade of nursing emancipation (Land et al 1996, Paniagua 1995). The document enabled individual nurses to take responsibility for the expansion of the service they provided. It emphasised professional accountability and placed decisions about the boundaries of practice in the hands of practitioners (Redfern 1997).

However, the UKCC document could equally be seen as enabling the resubordination of nursing. It was launched at the same time as the drive towards a reduction of junior doctors' hours and arguably has been used to justify and promote the development of new roles that supported the needs of medicine and management rather than the needs of patients and nursing development (Denner 1995, Dimond 1995). Many of the service developments discussed earlier would not have been possible without a flexible adaptable workforce, eager to develop their professional practice in the light of 'Scope'. As we have argued, waiting lists could not have been reduced without nurses being prepared to take on the physical assessment skills traditionally performed by junior doctors. Similarly, the complex needs of patients on surgical wards at night required an expanded repertoire of skills and the transformation of the night sister role into that of the night nurse practitioner. In addition, the changes in service delivery, such as day surgery and hospital at home schemes, rely on nurses being comfortable to work across the primary–secondary care interface and reclassify themselves as educators for self-care rather than providers of care. At the same time, technological developments have enabled nurses to perform, rather than support, many diagnostic procedures such as endoscopy and Doppler ultrasound.

Whether or not the reader believes that these developments are a positive move for nursing, attention needs to be paid to the very real professional issues they raise. For example issues of clinical competence, the availability of appropriate training, potential conflict with regard to accountability and how these posts fit into a coherent personal and organisational career development strategy. Once again, we would argue that nursing needs to engage actively in both the formation of policy and the critiquing of that same policy in order that appropriate responses are developed to meet the challenges that face the profession.

HOW YOU CAN SHAPE THE POLICY AGENDA

When you have read this chapter, we hope that you will feel inspired to take a more active part in the decisions that affect your profession and service. There are many ways nurses can become involved in health policy debates. Below are a few examples of strategies you may wish to employ:

- Why not join and take an active role in your professional association or trade union. For example, all members of the RCN have the right to attend Congress and speak during the debates where the future direction of RCN activity is determined. Regular attendance at your local trade union meetings will keep you up to date with current debates in the union locally and nationally – you may even learn more about what is going on in your trust.
- By joining a special interest group you may be asked to give evidence to select committees and to comment on proposed government policy. For example, the Nurse Practitioner Association within the RCN contributed to debates around the supply and administration of medication.

- Letter writing campaigns have been used successfully by many groups, for example breast cancer campaigners. You should write to your Member of Parliament, health authorities and trust boards about any issue you feel strongly about.
- You could also attend your local community health council (CHC) meetings in your capacity as patient or health professional to make sure that your voice is heard. CHCs have recently raised the profile of waiting times in accident and emergency departments by unofficially auditing their local services.
- By joining a political party, you could become involved in determining internal policy and commenting on the strategic direction of the parliamentary party. You could even follow in the footsteps of Anne Keene and Laura Moffat who in 1997 became the first nurses ever to be elected to parliament.
- Finally, if there is a particular issue affecting your service, why not form your own campaign group? There are numerous examples of local action groups formed to deal with specific issues such as the Save Barts Campaign which have successfully attracted media coverage to their cause, which may have contributed to securing the hospital's future.

CONCLUSION: WHY AN UNDERSTANDING OF SOCIAL POLICY CAN HELP

As we have demonstrated, nurses and the patients that nurses care for are all affected in many ways by health and social policies. However, little attention has been paid by most nurses to health policy formulation and implementation. Nevertheless, health policy affects surgical nurses' daily work: it controls what nurses can and cannot do; dictates who receives nursing care and where that nursing care takes place. Increasing technological developments and advances in therapeutics have implications for the ways in which surgical nurses will work in the future, and the changing demographic structure of our society will affect not only the patient population but the composition of the nursing workforce.

Nursing is a valuable resource which must be actively utilised in health care policy and planning. If nurses are restricted to implementing the decisions made by others and working under conditions established by others, they may feel disempowered, realising that they have little impact on health care policy and provision. This in turn promotes a cycle of frustration, detachment and powerlessness (Tierney 1990). An understanding of the policy process and the underlying reasons for changes in the provision of health care can enable nurses to influence that process. If nurses are to gain and maintain autonomous control over the practice of nursing, they must be involved in defining the scope of that practice. And if nurses want to have an impact on access, quality, allocation and delivery of health care they must make that impact through the policy-making process.

Policy analysis enables a look into the future and offers an attempt to predict the challenges that will face nursing in the next century. A full discussion of all of the policy trends is beyond the scope of this chapter but the following issues seem likely to need discussion and resolution:

- The changing demographic structure of the nursing and medical workforce and recruitment problems which will lead to more new-role development and changes in functions of the multidisciplinary team in health care.
- The change in the age profile of the population and patterns of morbidity which will affect the demand for different types of health care, particularly surgical care.
- Further developments in laser treatment, keyhole and minimally invasive surgery which will continue to both reduce the incidence of major surgical intervention and fundamentally alter traditional patterns of care.

- Assessment of competence will become a key issue for all health personnel in a climate of rapidly changing health care techniques and an increasingly litigious society.
- Public expenditure on health care will continue to be reduced and rationing will become explicit rather than implicit.
- More nurses will be employed outside of the NHS than within it as privately funded health care grows.
- State-funded health care will be provided increasingly through an insurance-based system rather than being funded from general taxation.
- Long term, the distinction between medical and surgical nursing may be increasingly seen as of little importance and as having more to do with the historical development of medicine than patient and nursing needs.

The policy gaze, as we have demonstrated, encourages a refreshing analysis of the macro sociopolitical context within which nursing takes place. The tools of policy analysis, if harnessed by nurses, can encourage proactive professional and personal development. In order to control the future of the profession, surgical nurses must participate actively in policy making at all levels.

REFERENCES

Appleby J, Smith P, Ranade W, Little V, Robinson R 1994 Monitoring managed competition. In: Le Grand J, Robinson R (eds) Privatisation and the welfare state. Allen and Unwin, London

Audit Commission 1990 A short cut to better services: day surgery in England and Wales. HMSO, London

Audit Commission 1997 Anaesthesia under examination. HMSO, London

Batty D 1997 Waiting list buster. Nursing Standard 12(10): 14

Binnie A 1997 Nursing therapy for patients with chronic vascular disease. Paper given at the RCN Critical Care Forum Conference – Developing your practice through research: ideas and innovations in critical care, Birmingham

Bulmer M, Lewis J, Pichaud D (eds) 1989 The goals of social policy. Unwin Hyman, London

Calman K (Chair) 1993 Hospital doctors: training for the future. The report of the working group on specialist medical training. DoH, London

Central Statistical Office 1995 Social trends. HMSO, London

Coast J 1993 The role of economic evaluation in setting priorities for elective surgery. Health Policy 24: 243–257

Denner S 1995 Extending professional practice: benefits and pitfalls. Nursing Times 91(14): 27–29

Department of Health (DoH) 1991a The patient's charter. HMSO, London

Department of Health (DoH) 1991b Hours of work of doctors in training: the new deal. (Executive Letter: EL(91)82) NHSE, Leeds

Department of Health (DoH) 1995 The patient's charter and you. HMSO, London

Department of Health (DoH) 1997a The new NHS – Modern. Dependable. The Stationery Office, London

Department of Health (DoH) 1997b Devolution of responsibilities to education consortium. (Executive Letter: EL(97)30) NHSE, Leeds

Dimond B 1995 UKCC's standards for incorporation into contracts. British Journal of Nursing 4(18): 1045–1046

Dowling S, Martin R, Skidmore P, Doyal L, Cameron A, Lloyd S 1996 Nurses taking on junior doctors' work: a confusion of accountability. British Medical Journal 312: 1211–1214

Gelijns A C, Fendrick A M 1993 The dynamics of innovation in minimally invasive therapy. Health Policy 23: 153–166

Girouard S A 1989 Health policy: implications for the CNS. In: Hamric A B, Spross J A (eds) The clinical nurse specialist in theory and practice, 2nd edn. J B Lippincott, Philadelphia

Glasman D 1994 Ulster fundholders send patients to Scotland to ease long waiting lists. Health Service Journal 104(5407): 8

Glennester H, Mataganis M, Owens P, Hancock S 1994 GP funding: wild card or winning hand? In: Le Grand J, Robinson R (eds) Privatisation and the welfare state. Allen and Unwin, London

Gough P, Maslin-Prothero S, Masterson A 1994 Nursing and social policy: care in context. Butterworth Heinemann, Oxford

Guillebaud Committee 1956 Report of the Committee of Enquiry into the cost of the National Health Service. Cmnd 966 3. HMSO, London

Ham C 1992 Health policy in Britain: the politics and organisation of the National Health Service, 3rd edn. Macmillan, Basingstoke

Ham C 1994 Reforming health services: learning from the UK experience. Social Policy and Administration 17: 87–101

Hancock C 1997 Selling out school nurses. Nursing Standard 26(12): 19

Jones C 1985 Patterns of social policy: an introduction to comparative analysis. Tavistock, London

Kingdom J 1991 Government and politics in Britain. Policy Press, Cambridge

King's Fund Commission 1992 London health care 2010: changing the future of health services in the capital. King's Fund, London

Land L, Mhaolrunaigh M A, Castledine G 1996 Extent and effectiveness of The Scope of Professional Practice. Nursing Times 96(35): 32–35

Miller B 1997 Home economics. Nursing Times 93(38): 32–33

Murray C, Read S, McCabe C 1995 Reduction in junior doctors' hours: the nursing contribution. SCHARR, Sheffield

NHS and Community Care Act 1990 HMSO, London

National Health Service Executive (NHSE) 1997 Education and planning guidance. DoH, Leeds

National Health Service Executive (NHSE) 1998 A first class service: quality in the new NHS. NHSE, Leeds

NHS Management Executive (NHSME) 1991 Junior doctors: the new deal. NHSME, London

Nursing Times 1997 UKCC figures warn of nursing's lost youth. Nursing Times 19(93): 6

Office of Population Censuses and Surveys and General Register Office for Scotland (1993) 1991 census: persons aged 60 and over. HMSO, London

Ong B N 1997 Patients approve of pre-operative assessments. Nursing Times 93(40): 57–59

Paniagua H 1995 The scope of advanced practice: action potential for practice nurses. British Journal of Nursing 4(5): 269–274

Rafferty A 1997 If the past was tense, can the future be perfect? Nursing Times 93(5): 28–31

Redfern S 1997 Reactions to nurses expanding practice. Nursing Times 93(32): 45–47

Robinson J, Gray A, Elkan R (eds) 1992 Policy issues in nursing. Open University Press, Milton Keynes

Robinson R, Le Grand J 1994 Evaluating the NHS reforms. King's Fund Institute, London

Salvage J 1985 The politics of nursing. Heinemann, London

Salvage J, Wright S 1995 Nursing development units: a force for change. Scutari, London

SCHARR 1997 The ENRiP data base. SCHARR, Sheffield

Stock J 1997 Vital statistics. Nursing Standard 26(12): 16

Thatcher J 1996 Follow-up after day surgery: how well do patients cope? Nursing Times 92(37): 30–32

Tierney R 1990 Strategies for empowerment. Nursing Standard 4(47): 32–34

Tomlinson B 1992 Report of the inquiry into London's health service, medical education and research. HMSO, London

Tuthill V 1995 The training of nurse surgical assistants. Surgical Nurse 4(21): 1240–1245

United Kingdom Central Council for Nursing, Midwifery and Health Visiting (UKCC) 1986 Project 2000: a new preparation for practice. UKCC, London

United Kingdom Central Council for Nursing, Midwifery and Health Visiting (UKCC) 1992 The scope of professional practice. UKCC, London

United Kingdom Central Council for Nursing, Midwifery and Health Visiting (UKCC) 1997 Scope in practice. UKCC, London

University of Manchester Health Services Management Unit 1996 The future healthcare workforce. University of Manchester, Manchester

Vincent S 1997 The changing role of peri-operative nursing. Nursing Times 93(40): 56–57

Waters A 1997 Worrying decline in student applicants. Nursing Standard 12(9): 5

Wickham J 1993 An introduction to minimally invasive therapy. Health Policy 23: 7–15

FURTHER READING

Ackers L, Abbott P 1996 Social policy for nurses and the caring professions. Open University Press, Buckingham. *An introductory text aimed at students of the caring professions. The book offers a step-by-step guide to the policy process and a useful overview of policy issues that cross the health and social care divide.*

Gough P, Maslin-Prothero S, Masterson A 1994 Nursing and social policy: care in context. Butterworth Heinemann, Oxford. *An innovative book that focuses on concepts rather than the policy process. Accessible for both pre- and post-registration nurses and other health care professionals.*

Ham C 1992 Health policy in Britain: the politics and organisation of the National Health Service, 3rd edn. Macmillan, Basingstoke. *An invaluable introduction to health policy in Britain. The book provides an insight into the substance of health policy, the process of policy making and the implementation of policy.*

Robinson J, Gray A, Elkan R (eds) 1992 Policy issues in nursing. Open University Press, Milton Keynes. *A seminal text that examines a range of issues facing nursing from a variety of different perspectives.*

13

Infection control: maintaining a safe environment

Rozila Horton

AIMS

The aim of this chapter is to enable the nurse to man-age infection risks in surgical patients by gaining an insight into:

- intrinsic and extrinsic factors which increase patient susceptibility
- microorganisms of clinical significance
- practical issues relating to surgical practice
- environmental and health and safety issues affecting both patients and staff
- the contribution of the infection control nurse/department in developing a programme of safe and informed infection control practice.

INTRODUCTION

Infections in a hospitalised patient remain, by far, the most serious cause of morbidity and mortality. Postoperative patients risk acquiring more than just surgical wound infection. Chest, urinary tract, intra-venous related bacteraemia/septicaemia, skin, mouth, eye, and gastrointestinal infections are some of the complications encountered by these patients. Additional problems include adverse effects of antibi-otics such as multiresistant microorganisms and diar-rhoea, which can spread with sufficient ease to become an outbreak requiring rigorous management.

Humans live in a symbiotic relationship with mil-lions of bacteria. The constant presence of bacteria and some fungi which cover the skin and populate the gut limits the action of so-called invasive, pathogenic microorganisms. However, even these commensal microorganisms take on a sinister role of colonisers and/or invaders when the body's epithelial barrier is broken or bypassed and the host is physiologically and immunologically compromised. In surgery the transgression of the first line of defence, the skin, is the first step in a cycle of wound infection in patients who may be already compromised. Patients' intrinsic risk factors may be beyond the control of health professionals but it is possible to influence many external agents. The steps taken by health care workers to identify hazards and prevent or minimise infection risks to patients remain crucial to safe and informed care. This will help nurses to define the infection control quality elements in nursing practice. Since the development of the purchaser/provider fundholding system (DoH 1989a), the surgical patient throughput has remained an important measurement of performance. There is now, however, an increasing shift of attention from purchasing activity to purchasing evidence-based protocols. The protocols suggest to the commissioners of care that the most effective set of actions will be taken (Sheldon & Borowitz 1993). It is therefore paramount that nurses have sufficient knowledge and insight into the factors which contribute to the development of infections in surgical patients in order to determine and define the most effective set of actions to safeguard their patients. Furthermore, there is an increasing demand for providers to produce data on infection rates, in particular in surgical patients. Whilst it is recognised that a number of wound infections, especially in clean surgery, can be reduced, there is little evidence to indicate that nurses have much control over the primary infections of these wounds. Health service provider managers may, however, be asked to produce evidence of all possible preventive measures employed in both unavoidable and preventable infections. It is hoped that the text of this chapter will aid nurses in developing an effective infection-control protocol for patients undergoing surgery.

CURRENT PERSPECTIVES

The separation of provider and purchaser services and the creation of an internal market as a result of the introduction of the previous Government's White Paper 'Working for Patients' (DoH 1989a) produced a 'quality'-conscious health service. The internal market introduced an element of competition, and trusts were expected to provide efficient and quality care in return for payment. Provision of quality care and effective use of resources became and continue to be the driving force on the health care agenda. The importance of hospital-acquired infection (HAI) as one of the criteria for judging the quality of patient care is increasingly being recognised. It is the aim of all health professionals to provide patients with the best possible care; care which reduces the discomfort and distress associated with illness and which maximises the chances of full recovery. Features of a service which fulfil these requirements are described as quality. Any complication in a patient episode becomes a marker of quality. Hospital-acquired or nosocomial infections are a complication of hospital stay and remain an important indicator of quality care.

A hospital-acquired infection causes discomfort, reduces quality of life and creates anxiety for patients and their relatives. All infections carry with them a degree of morbidity by interfering with the recovery process. Infections are also an important cause of mortality. The level of mortality associated with hospital-acquired infections in the UK is difficult to assess because of the absence of accurate data. The Hospital Infection Working Group (DoH/PHLS 1995) has made a crude comparison with the data available in the USA and concluded that 5000 deaths (1% of all deaths) might be primarily attributable to hospital-acquired infections, and in a further 15 000 cases (3% of all deaths) hospital-acquired infections might be a substantial contributor. According to the Group, hospital-acquired infections could be more common than traffic accidents or suicides as a primary cause of death.

Resource implications of hospital-acquired infections

The first national prevalence survey in 1980 (Meers et al 1981) showed that around half of the 19.1% infections in hospital were hospital acquired. The second survey was carried out in 1993/4 and would suggest similar figures (Emmerson et al 1996). Currie & Maynard (1989) estimated the cost to the National Health Service of the extra treatment and delayed discharge of patients with hospital-acquired infections in England to be about £115 million and 950 000 lost bed days per annum. A third of these infections are said to be preventable by good infection control, resulting in a saving of around £36 million for the NHS. The cost to the hospital relates to the increased use of drugs, especially antibiotics, dressings, medical, nursing and therapy staff time and of prolonged bed occupancy (Ayliffe et al 1990).

The Patient's Charter (DoH 1991) is concerned with raising the standards of care for patients in hospitals and the community. Amongst other things, the Charter focuses attention on the length of time a patient needing surgery has to wait before admission to hospital because of lack of beds. One of the recognised reasons for the extended length of stay of patients in hospital is hospital-acquired infections. The length of stay varies from between 3 and 30 days with an average of 7 days.

INFECTION RISKS AND SURGICAL PATIENTS – THEORETICAL BACKGROUND

SURGICAL WOUND INFECTIONS

Stakeholders of health care are likely to be influenced by the best possible outcome of in-hospital treatment. In a postoperative patient, the ideal operation results in the cure of the condition, primary healing and uneventful recovery. Surgical wound complications result in human suffering and extended hospital stay and treatment, which consume scarce resources and lead to patients' loss of income and productivity (Cruse 1992). Surgical wound infections accounted for 18.9% of hospital-acquired infections in the 1980 prevalence survey (Meers et al 1981) and 10.7% in 1993/4 (Emmerson et al 1996). The move to early discharge and the increase in day surgery provision may account for the lower figure in the latter survey.

The length of inpatient stay increases significantly in patients with surgical wound infections: the average length of stay is said to range from 5–20.5 days (Bremmelgaard et al 1989). Mishriki and colleagues (1992) identified an extra 480 bed days in a surgical wound survey of 1242 consecutive patients where 83 became infected. The budget holder, therefore, has a vested interest in requesting an audit of wound infections and whenever possible demanding a reduction in the rate of wound infections which are known to be preventable. Although the promotion of a safe environment and prevention of cross-infection constitute good practice, most factors associated with the development of surgical wound infections are outside the control of nurses.

INTRINSIC AND EXTRINSIC FACTORS INFLUENCING WOUND INFECTIONS

The risk of infection in surgical wounds is dependent upon the contamination that occurs at the time of surgery and the ability of the body to resist that contamination. An insight into how wounds are classified and what factors, both intrinsic and extrinsic, increase the patient's susceptibility to infection is desirable.

Classification of surgical wounds

Wounds may be classified at the time of surgery into clean, clean-contaminated, contaminated and dirty.

- *Clean wounds* – operations in which a viscus is not opened. This category also includes non-traumatic, uninfected wounds where no inflammation is encountered and where no break in technique has occurred.
- *Clean-contaminated* – a viscus is entered but without spillage of contents. Also included in this category are non-traumatic wounds where a minor break of technique has occurred.
- *Contaminated* – gross spillage has occurred or a fresh traumatic wound from a relatively clean source. Acute non-purulent inflammation may also be encountered.
- *Dirty* – old traumatic wounds from a dirty source, with delayed treatment, devitalised tissue, clinical infection, faecal contamination or a foreign body (Altmeier 1979, Ayliffe & Lowbury 1982, NAS 1964).

Risk factors which increase patient susceptibility to infection

A number of factors which increase the host susceptibility to infection are identified in Box 13.1.

Infection risks are identified as host related (intrinsic) or resulting from prescribed therapeutic treatment procedures related to medical and nursing care (extrinsic).

Some of these components are considered here.

Intrinsic risk factors

Extremes of age

'Extremes of age' are defined as children aged 1 year and under, and people aged 65 years and over.

The newborn infant of normal weight relies on maternal antibodies for protection against infection for a period of 3–6 months until its immune system is fully developed. Premature delivery and low birth weight add significantly to the infant's susceptibility.

Older people suffer changes in their cell-mediated and humoral immunity which can lead to poor healing

---

Box 13.1 Risk factors which increase the patient's susceptibility to infection (Donowitz 1987)

- An underlying disease such as diabetes, blood and respiratory disorders.
- The therapy for disease, e.g. chemotherapy used to suppress the bone marrow in patients with leukaemia, lymphoma and those undergoing bone marrow or organ transplant.
- The use of steroids and cancer cell-suppressing (cytotoxic) drugs may result in interference with the host defences and in depression of immunity. Medications such as steroids are known to increase the risk of infection
- Treatments and procedures carried out whilst in hospital, especially invasive techniques such as surgery, urinary catheterisation and intravenous therapy.

---

ability. The elderly population also tend to suffer from many underlying diseases which render them prone to infection (see also Ch. 11).

All studies have shown not only an increase in wound infection rate with advancing age but that age influences infection rate independently of other factors (Cruse & Foord 1980, Davidson et al 1971, Farber & Wenzel 1980, Leigh 1981, Mishriki et al 1990, Mishriki et al 1992, NAS 1964).

Underlying conditions/disorders

Diabetes. Cardiovascular disorders are more common in people with diabetes than in the general population. There may also be accompanying degenerative changes in blood vessels and decreased nutrition to cells which can affect the natural healing process (Jarrett 1985).

Respiratory disorders. A disorder which interferes with respiratory airflow is likely to result in complications. Conditions likely to obstruct the smooth passage of air through the lungs are chronic bronchitis, emphysema, asthma, bronchiectasis and cystic fibrosis. Impaired coughing mechanism, increased secretions, ischaemia, and susceptibility to colonisation of the lower respiratory tract with Gram-negative microorganisms are some of the problems encountered in people with chronic obstructive airways disease. These invariably increase the host's susceptibility to infection.

Blood disorders. Blood disorders range from anaemia to leukaemia, lymphoma, myeloma, agranulocytosis and thrombocytopenia.

In most instances of blood disorder, there is a degree of anaemia. Anaemic patients may have poor nutrition as well as poor skin condition, predisposing them to pressure sores and infection. Leukaemia is characterised by an abnormal proliferation of immature white cells which tend to interfere with bone marrow function leading to the production of fewer normal blood cells. The resulting anaemia, leukopenia or thrombocytopenia increases the patient's vulnerability to infections from agents which are normally considered to be of low pathogenicity.

Lymphoma is characterised by an abnormal structure of cells in lymph nodes. Many symptoms associated with lymphoma create a favourable medium for infection development.

A partial or complete absence of neutrophils in agranulocytosis makes the patient extremely susceptible to serious infection.

When platelet disorders occur, there is an interference in the number or the function of platelets which affects the coagulation process. The tendency to bleed easily leads to anaemia and associated complications.

Smoking

Tobacco-related complications such as coronary heart disease, chronic obstructive airways disease, and atherosclerotic peripheral vascular disease increase the smoker's risk of infection.

Nutrition and build

Both obese and emaciated individuals are susceptible to complications (NAS 1964). Obese people may be lacking in many elements required for healing. The blood supply to fatty tissue is poor, so the tissue heals more slowly. There is also an increased risk of contamination of a wound during surgery for people with surplus fat, since the procedure may take longer. Obese people may not follow a balanced diet with essential nutrients, hence they may be as malnourished as underweight and emaciated individuals. Possibilities of postoperative chest infections are high in obese people because of their poor mobility.

Reduction in infections, including surgical wound infections, have been shown to be commensurate with improved nutrition (Hamilton 1982). Malnutrition impairs host defences by weakening immune response. The metabolic reserves are decreased and the integrity of the epithelial surfaces are affected in emaciated and malnourished people (see also Ch. 27).

Extrinsic risk factors

Drug therapy as a risk factor

Conditions such as leukaemia and lymphoma are treated with radiotherapy and/or chemotherapy to suppress abnormal cell production. Unfortunately, the cytotoxic nature of the treatment results in the destruction of normal cells as well, thus leaving the patient highly susceptible to infectious agents. Patients suffering from malignant tumours are exposed to similar treatments with subsequent immunosuppression.

Steroid therapy, the use of an anti-inflammatory drug used to treat many conditions, will interfere with the important inflammatory phase of the healing process.

Breach in the integrity of skin

Trauma, surgical wounds, venous and pressure ulcers, and stab wounds such as cannulae through the skin are examples of transgression of the first line of defence. Apart from creating a portal of entry for microorganisms, lesions and wounds are susceptible to colonisation with pathogenic microbials, including antibiotic resistant microorganisms of significant concern.

Traumatised surfaces are open to contamination with microbes which bypass the first line of defences. The devitalised or ischaemic soft tissue provides an ideal environment for pathogens to multiply; and invasive procedures such as those involving respiratory tubes, urinary or vascular catheters, and wound drains create a portal of entry for these microorganisms. Multiple trauma cases are nursed in intensive care units where further colonisation of injured surfaces and devices with hospital flora is inevitable. The host defence mechanism is unable to clear this microbial colonisation of wound, drains and catheters. Tracheostomy, so often a feature in intensive care patients, becomes an added focus of colonisation, leading to infections of the lower respiratory tract. Long-term immobility and bedsores create further colonisation and infection problems. The critically injured patient loses the protection provided by normal gut flora because injury, ischaemia, impaired motility, pH changes, fasting and antibiotics disrupt the normal environment. The hypermetabolic state, often produced by traumatic injury, results in a relative nutritional deficiency which compromises wound healing and immunity.

Items as foreign bodies

Any foreign material in the wound reduces local host defences. Factors associated with sutures and wound drains are discussed later (p. 249).

Microorganisms may be introduced during the placing of any invasive device such as intravascular and urinary catheters, respiratory therapy appliances and nasogastric feeding tubes. These devices also carry an added risk of becoming a focus for many microorganisms, which may result in infection. The reservoir created by this focus can become a potential threat of transmission of infection to other patients.

Bypass of defence mechanism through devices

Procedures such as intubation or tracheostomy bypass the normal array of defences. Apart from any interference with the normal filtration through the nose and clearance by cilia, the inhaled air may lack warmth and humidification. The process of insertion can be accompanied by trauma and subsequent colonisation of the mucous membrane of the system by Gram-negative microorganisms. The device can also become contaminated during manipulation and suctioning. Masks, nasal cannulae, suction catheters, humidifiers and breathing tubings are all potential sources and routes for infectious microorganisms. Contamination may be present on the hands of health care personnel or may originate from microorganisms which colonise the critically ill patient. The device may continue to be a source of infection if not adequately and appropriately decontaminated between each use.

Aerosol-producing respiratory therapy equipment such as nebulisers may become contaminated if not washed and dried thoroughly between each use.

As with endotracheal procedures, nasogastric tubes can be accompanied by trauma to the mucosal surface, or, through prolonged use, by erosion. Colonisation of the damaged tissue with Gram-negative microorganisms can be a precursor to infections such as pneumonia.

Any body system can thus be compromised because of inherent factors or as a result of treatment and care practices.

Reflective point

Based on the information provided, examine risk factors, both intrinsic and extrinsic, of two patients, and consider how these may increase their susceptibility to infection.

MICROORGANISMS OF CLINICAL SIGNIFICANCE

Infection is defined as invasion and multiplication of microorganisms in body tissues, which may be clinically unapparent or result in local cellular injury because of competitive metabolism, toxins, intracellular replication, or antigen–antibody response (Hentges 1995).

A detailed discussion on microorganisms and microbiology is beyond the scope of this chapter; two comprehensive text books are cited in the Further Reading section (Greenwood et al 1999 and Mims et al 1993). A brief overview of microorganisms which have particular significance in surgical clinical situations is provided here.

Microorganisms commonly encountered in surgical practice

Any microorganism may be encountered in surgical practice. A patient infected with one of the blood-borne viruses such as human immune deficiency virus (HIV) or hepatitis virus may require surgical intervention. Alternatively, a viral infection such as herpes varicella (chickenpox) or herpes zoster (shingles) may manifest following admission. Viral gastroenteritis is frequently encountered in all clinical practices including surgery.

The microorganisms predominantly affecting wounds are bacteria and fungi. As stated earlier, many bacteria and fungi live on the human skin and in the gut in a commensal relationship but become invaders when the barrier is broken and the human body is compromised. More harmful and pathogenic microorganisms are also given free access to a vulnerable site in a susceptible host. Most pathogenic bacteria release a chemical toxin or enzyme that injures cells or disrupts their function. Some bacteria can form spores in order to survive an unfriendly environment. These hard shells (spores) provide an armour for bacteria to resist destruction by disinfection and temperatures lower than 121°C. This has an implication for rendering items safe after use and will be discussed later.

Bacteria

Recognition. Bacteria are classified by their shape (into rods, cocci and spirochaetes), their preference for oxygen (aerobic) or not (anaerobic). Bacteria appear as clear bodies under a microscope and require identification by staining. The bacterial cell wall structure and permeability allow bacteria to absorb and retain stain. However, not all bacteria are able to hold on to the same stain on decolorisation with acetone and

require counter-staining. Gram-positive bacteria retain the initial blue dye and Gram-negative bacteria are recognised by their ability to retain the red counter-stain. The purpose of such staining in clinical practice is to allow the microbiologist to proceed with further testing of the culture and/or to advise medical colleagues on the appropriate therapy and intervention.

Characteristics of bacteria which make them of clinical significance:

- *Invasiveness* – relates to the ability of bacteria to enter the body and spread throughout the tissue.
- *Pathogenicity* – some bacteria produce toxins and therefore have a greater ability to cause disease than others.
- *Virulence* – refers to the degree of pathogenicity or ability of the organism to cause disease.
- *Infectious dose* – the more pathogenic the organism, the lower the dose required to produce an infectious reaction.

Fungi

Fungi are plants which feed on dead plant and animal matter. They are opportunistic in nature and cause diseases in humans whose immune status is compromised. Although normal body flora are destroyed by antibiotics, fungi remain relatively unaffected by these antimicrobials and can proliferate. Candida infections are the common fungal infections encountered in clinical situations.

Table 13.1 demonstrates the nature of microorganisms commonly encountered in surgical practice.

SURGICAL PATIENTS – PRACTICAL ISSUES

Patients in virtually any speciality can be vulnerable to infection and will require safe and informed care. Safe and informed infection control care would suggest that factors relating to the development of infection in a given situation have been recognised and understood and appropriate actions taken to prevent or minimise these risks.

The following section considers the components of safe and effective infection control care of surgical patients, taking into account each of the factors identified in Figure 13.1.

Table 13.1   The nature of organisms commonly encountered in surgical practice

Microorganism	Characteristics	Habitat/transmission	Diseases	Prevention	Resistance
Bacteria *Staphylococcus aureus*	Gram-positive cocci in grape-like clusters	Skin, nose and perineum (carriage rate high in hospital staff and patients). Spread by contact and airborne route	Postoperative wound infection; boils; skin sepsis; catheter-related infection; septicaemia; food-borne infection; pneumonia, etc.	Hand hygiene	Methicillin-resistant strains (MRSA) may require isolation and follow an MRSA regime
Staphylococcus epidermidis	Gram-positive cocci in grape-like clusters	100% skin carriage rate. Spread by direct and indirect contact. Almost always a hospital-acquired infection although may be endogenous	Opportunistic pathogen responsible for infections related to invasive devices, artificial prosthesis, urinary tract infections	Strict hand hygiene; aseptic device care	Often multi-resistance problems associated with this microorganism
Beta-haemolytic streptococci *Streptococcus pyogenes* (group A streptococci)	Gram-positive cocci in chains	Human respiratory tract and skin. Spread by airborne droplets and contact	Tonsillitis, erysipelas, impetigo, cellulitis, scarlet fever, puerperal fever	Strict contact precautions; isolation for 24–48 h after the start of antibiotic therapy	
Streptococcus agalactiae (group B streptococci)		Gut and vagina. Infants acquire organisms from mothers at birth. Also by contact spread between infants in nursery	Neonatal meningitis and septicaemia, gynaecological sepsis	Strict hand hygiene	
Alpha-haemolytic streptococci *Streptococcus pneumoniae*	Gram-positive cocci in pairs (diplococci)	Human respiratory tract (4% population). Transmission by droplet spread	Septicaemia, pneumonia, meningitis	Hand hygiene	Some penicillin resistance
Enterococcus faecalis (faecal streptococci)	Gram-positive cocci	Gut of humans and animals. Infections mainly endogenous but can be cross-transmitted	Severe septicaemia in the immunocompromised and sometimes after surgery, urinary tract infection	Strict hand hygiene	Resistance to cephalosporins
Clostridium perfringens (*welchii*)	Anaerobic Gram-positive rods, spore forming	Widespread in soil and normal flora of man and animals. Infection can be endogenous from own faecal flora or exogenous from external contamination ingestion of contaminated food	Gas gangrene; food poisoning from food contaminated with enterotoxin-producing strain	Thorough cleaning of traumatic wounds	

Table 13.1 (Contd.)

Microorganism	Characteristics	Habitat/transmission	Diseases	Prevention	Resistance
Clostridium difficile	Anaerobic spore-forming Gram-positive rods	Normal gut flora in some humans, growth encouraged by antibiotics. Spread from person to person by faecal–oral route	Antibiotic-associated diarrhoea (pseudomembranous colitis). Can be rapidly fatal in immunocompromised hosts	Isolation and strict enteric precautions until diarrhoea subsides	Metronidazole not always effective
Escherichia coli	Gram-negative rods	Normal habitat in gut of humans and animals, can colonise lower end of urethra and vagina. Spread by contact, faecal–oral route, can be food-associated, can be endogenous	Urinary tract infection, diarrhoeal disease (associated with haemolytic–uraemic syndrome), neonatal meningitis, septicaemia	Strict hand hygiene	Resistance to a number of antibiotics
Proteus spp.	Gram-negative rods (fishy odour)	Found in human gut, soil and water. Infection can be endogenous but also spread by contact	Hospital-acquired wound infection, septicaemia, pneumonia; urinary tract infection	Hand hygiene; good aseptic technique	Resistance to a number of antibiotics
Klebsiella spp.	Gram-negative rods	Habitat: gut of humans and animals; moist inanimate environments. Endogenous but infection can be spread by contact	Opportunist infections – urinary and respiratory tract	Scrupulous hand hygiene and aseptic technique	Multiple antibiotic resistance
Pseudomonas aeruginosa	Aerobic Gram-negative rods	Found in gut in a small percentage of healthy humans and in a large number of hospital patients. Direct and indirect spread but can be endogenous – mainly opportunistic	Urinary tract, respiratory tract (a major problem in cystic fibrosis), septicaemia, infections of skin and burns	Strict hand hygiene, aseptic technique, appropriate processing of patient care items	Resistance to many antibiotics
Bacteroides fragilis	Gram-negative anaerobic rod	Habitat: gut of humans. Mainly endogenous	Wound infections; abscesses of liver, brain, intra-abdominal, aspiration pneumonia	Good surgical technique; hand hygiene	Resistance to a number of antibiotics
Fungi *Candida albicans*	Occurring as yeast	Part of normal flora in mouth and intestine. Opportunist infections in immunosuppressed and antibiotic-treated people. Contact spread	Candidiasis, thrush	Strict hand hygiene	

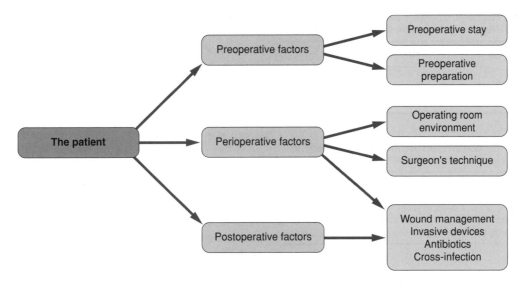

Figure 13.1   External factors known to be responsible for surgical wound and other infections.

PREOPERATIVE FACTORS

Length of preoperative stay

A direct link between the length of preoperative stay and succeeding wound infections has been well established. Table 13.2 shows the relation between the number of preoperative days' stay and likelihood of infection determined by Cruse (1992).

There are two possible explanations for this: patients requiring extended preoperative stay are likely to be debilitated or present with a coexisting illness; or preoperative stay results in lowered patient resistance or increased pathogenic skin contamination (Mishriki et al 1992).

Preoperative preparation

There is a strong association between preoperative shaving and wound infection (see Table 13.3). Other studies have shown a wound infection rate of 5.6% in shaved patients as opposed to 1% in those not shaved or using depilatory cream (Seropian & Reynolds 1971).

Dry, and sometimes clumsy, razor shaving, damages the deeper layers of skin causing bleeding or wound exudate which acts as a medium for bacterial growth. Abrasions and damage to the dermal layer from shaving are also open to bacteria liberated during contaminated and dirty operations.

Preoperative shaving remains a tradition despite this knowledge. The reasons for shaving may be purely aesthetic and/or to allow easy changes of postoperative wound dressings. If hair removal is unavoidable, shaving should be effected *immediately* before surgery to prevent bacterial multiplication in the serum oozing from the damaged skin (Mishriki et al 1992). A depilatory cream is less damaging but is associated with skin sensitivity in some patients (see also Ch. 20).

> **Reflective point**
>
> Are patients in your clinical area shaved as a routine? If so, what evidence is there to support this practice? What preoperative general skin hygiene measures are advocated in your practice area to minimise the risk of infection?

PERIOPERATIVE FACTORS

Operating room environment

The majority of postoperative infections in wounds other than clean wounds, appear to be from endogenous sources, i.e. from the patient's own flora. The operating room environment can influence some surgical wound infections, which suggests that a degree of environmental control is necessary.

Ventilation

The operating room ventilation serves a dual purpose: to prevent infection of the patient's wound and provide a comfortable atmosphere for the surgical team.

Table 13.2   Relationship between percentage of wound infections and length of preoperative stay (Cruse 1992)

Number of days	Wound infections (%)
1	1.1
7	2.1
14 or more	3.4

Table 13.3   Relationship between preparation method and infection rate in clean surgery (Cruse 1992)

Method of preparation	Wound infections (%)
Razor shaving (2 hours preoperative)	2.3
Hair only clipped	1.7
Neither shaving nor clipping	0.9

Microbial contamination in the form of skin scales is generated within the operating room through the physical activities of staff members. Although most people disperse bacteria of low pathogenicity, around 10% of males and 1% of females also disperse *Staphylococcus aureus*, the microorganism commonly associated with wound infection from exogenous sources. It is generally accepted that microorganisms in the air of operating rooms are associated with infections. Airborne contamination in prosthetic joint surgery has been highlighted by Lidwell et al (1983). Thus the air movement in operating rooms is designed to curtail the transfer of bacteria from less clean to clean areas and to reduce the airborne bacterial contamination.

Only a small number of bacteria are required to produce deep infection in orthopaedic surgery. Here an ultra-clean air system which allows a further reduction of airborne contamination is generally used.

Operating room clothing

There is a constant shedding of microorganisms from exposed skin and from mucous membranes, and use of barrier clothing in operating rooms is needed to minimise the contamination of the air as well of the wound.

Gowns. Shedding from the skin is increased by friction from clothes during activity. Dispersal of *Staphylococcus aureus* amongst theatre personnel can be profuse, especially from the perineal area (Polakoff et al 1967). Clothing made of non-woven fabric rather than loose-weave cotton is generally considered appropriate (Whyte et al 1983). Total body exhaust suits are recommended for the scrub team during elective joint replacement surgery.

Headwear. Human hair is known to be a potential carrier of *Staphylococcus aureus*, especially where skin or scalp diseases such as eczema and psoriasis are present. Keeping hair clean and tidy should be a prerequisite for all operating room personnel. The helmet total exhaust system is well established for elective joint replacement surgery but traditional headgear is considered necessary only for the scrub team. Effective ventilation is thought to counteract any bacterial shedding and wearing of traditional headgear by non-scrub staff is considered unnecessary (Humphreys et al 1991).

Masks. The use of masks to reduce postoperative wound infection remains controversial. Few microorganisms are dispersed from mouth and nose during normal breathing and talking but they are expelled with forced ventilation. Masks for general surgery are considered unnecessary (Orr 1981), but if worn, should be changed after each operation. Careful manipulation of worn masks is essential to prevent contamination of hands.

Nowadays, masks are increasingly worn to protect the wearer from blood and body fluid splashes from patients during procedures (Advisory Committee on Dangerous Pathogens 1990a).

Gloves. Gloves protect the surgeon from contamination by blood and exudate from the patient and protect the patient from transfer of microorganisms from the surgeon's hands. Damage to gloves, in the form of minute holes, during surgery is well known. This may place both the patient and surgeon at risk of acquiring infection. Fresh gloves should be worn for each new procedure.

Footwear. The floor of the operating room is thought to play little part in the spread of infection and routine mopping with detergent and water will help keep the level of contamination low. The use of disposable overshoes by visitors is unnecessary and even hazardous; putting on overshoes may lead to contamination of hands. Theatre shoes should be worn for their antistatic, antislip properties rather than as an infection control measure.

Cotton drapes

Drapes are used to create a barrier between wound site and the patient's own skin bacteria. A 'bacterial strike-through' has been shown to occur with cotton drapes when these become soaked with wet instruments. Cruse (1992) suggests a layer of sterile plastic on the thigh under cotton drapes. This inexpensive draping has been shown to be as effective as expensive disposable drapes.

Plastic adhesive sheets. Cruse (1992) quotes 1.5% infection rate in clean surgery when using cotton drapes, which increased to 2.3% when plastic adhesive drapes were used in addition. However, French et al (1976) have shown a reduction in the level of bacterial contamination when plastic drapes were used. The use of a wound-adhesive drape is generally thought *not* to add significantly to the wound infection outcome.

Operating room practice

Sterility of instruments

Sterilising is a process which kills or removes all microorganisms. A sterilisation process is necessary if the instrument penetrates intact skin or mucous membranes, enters sterile body cavities or is in contact with a breach in the skin or mucous membrane. Most operating rooms are served by an efficient sterile services department. However, it falls to all staff to check the integrity of sterile packages.

Processing of some heat-labile items (high-level disinfection) is often carried out by theatre personnel and it is imperative that they are appropriately trained before taking on such an important responsibility.

Surgical handwash

During surgery, the first line of defence, the skin, is normally breached, allowing microorganisms direct and easy access to internal tissues and organs. Lengthy duration of many surgical procedures and the fact that a large proportion of gloves may be perforated at the end of the operation demand antisepsis that provides both immediate as well as prolonged antibacterial activity. Aqueous 4% chlorhexidine or 7.5% (w/v) povidone–iodine is generally used (Paulssen et al 1988).

Nail brushes, if used, should be limited to nails only. Brushing damages the skin, with the attendant risk of the emergence of microorganisms from the deeper layers of skin (Ojajarvi et al 1977).

Duration of surgery

A report on the incidence of wound infection in England and Wales (PHLS 1960) identified a direct link between the length of the operation and the infection rate. Cruse (1992) identified a similar link and has provided the following explanation:

- Bacterial contamination increases with time.
- The tissues in the operative area are damaged by drying and retractors.

- A longer operation is usually associated with increased use of sutures and electrocoagulation which reduces the local resistance of the wound.
- Longer procedures are more likely to be associated with blood loss and shock, thereby reducing the general resistance of the patient.

Use of sutures and drains

The number of microorganisms required to produce infection is lowered substantially in the presence of sutures, clips and staples (Edlich et al 1973).

Wound drains are useful in reducing dead space and prevent collection of blood, exudate or other body fluid (haematoma) which may act as a culture medium. Drains can, however, afford an entry point for bacteria at the tip of an open drain or, in cases of closed drains, introduce a foreign body reaction and increase the risk of infection (Magee et al 1976).

Skill of the surgeon

A very significant association has been identified between the skill of the operator and the wound infection rate (Mishriki et al 1992). Wounds are said to heal without complication when there is gentle handling of tissue, careful haemostasis, adequate blood supply, removal of devitalised tissue, absolute reduction of dead space and wound closure without tension.

POSTOPERATIVE FACTORS

As mentioned earlier, infections in a surgical patient are not limited to wound infections: virtually any body system may be affected. Consideration of postoperative factors should include practices and treatments which may result in an adverse outcome.

Wound management

Wound dressing material

Wounds can readily acquire bacteria and need to be covered. The protection provided by the traditional dressings such as dry gauze and Gamgee is limited in the presence of wound exudate. Modern dressings, such as hydrogels and hydrocolloids, afford the moist environment required to improve wound epithelialisation and granulation. They are impermeable to bacteria but allow moisture vapour to escape and retain heat and the antimicrobial effect of wound exudate (see Ch. 28).

Polymer films, used as primary adhesive transparent dressings, also maintain the moist environment and wound exudates and are equally effective.

Principles of asepsis

The term asepsis is familiar to nurses who are involved with the management of surgical wounds and in the insertion and manipulation of invasive devices. Principles of asepsis suggest that every effort has been made to:

- guarantee the safety of the equipment used (cleaning/disinfection/sterilisation)
- reduce the level of microbial contamination of the site requiring manipulation (antisepsis)
- ensure that no microorganisms are introduced (asepsis).

Cleaning is the removal of dirt, debris and organic material. Such decontamination is easily achieved by washing with detergent and running warm water. *Cleaning is an important first stage in the processing of items for disinfection or sterilisation.*

Disinfection removes or destroys harmful microorganisms but not bacterial spores or slow viruses.

Sterilisation is the complete destruction or removal of all living microorganisms including bacterial spores.

For the purpose of rendering an item safe for patient use it should be either clean, disinfected or sterilised. The process used depends on the risk involved in the use of items (see Table 13.4).

Antisepsis is the reduction of the number of microorganisms already present on the body site prior to a procedure. An alcohol-based antiseptic such as chlorhexidine or povidone–iodine is generally used to reduce the skin flora prior to surgery. Overzealous wound cleansing during a wound dressing procedure is not recommended and a gentle lotion such as sterile water or normal saline is considered adequate.

Asepsis suggests a procedure designed to prevent any introduction of microorganisms to the site and is achieved by a non-touch technique and use of sterile gloves.

Wound dressing procedure

Almost all clinical areas will boast their own individual wound dressing technique. There is little scientific basis for these procedures. The intention of the dresser is to keep the bacterial contamination down. The level of airborne bacterial contamination of the immediate surrounding during wound dressing is considerably lower with hydrocolloid dressings compared to conventional absorbent cotton wool or gauze (Lawrence 1994). Irrespective of the type of dressing used, the question that should always be asked is: does the wound require dressing at this time?

Reflective point

In some clinical areas nurses remove flowers from bed areas before dressing a wound. Does this occur in your practice area? The water in the vase will yield Gram-negative bacteria but there is no evidence to suggest that wounds have acquired microorganisms from flowers or flower water. Removing flowers from bed areas before dressing wounds adds little to the principles of asepsis.

Antibiotics

The role of antibiotics as both prophylaxis and therapy in surgical patients in minimising infection-related morbidity and mortality is well established. Unfortunately, the development of resistance by many bacteria has generated different and sometimes very serious problems both for patients and the clinical environment in which they are treated. These are summarised by Mehtar (1992) as follows:

1. The antibiotics required to treat multiple-resistant bacteria are usually more potent, costly and require a parenteral route of administration.

2. The morbidity, and occasionally mortality, is increased with multiple-resistant bacteria, particularly those involved in nosocomial (hospital-acquired) infections.

3. The hospital environment becomes colonised with resistant bacteria and the spread of these bacteria is further increased via clinical and non-clinical equipment.

4. Hospital stay is prolonged and, occasionally, further surgical intervention is required.

Antimicrobials are also known to be associated with increased risk of infection, especially pneumonia. Other complications include antibiotic-associated diarrhoea.

Invasive devices

Intravascular therapy

Intravascular (i.v.) therapy carries a high risk of the introduction of microorganisms at the time of insertion,

Table 13.4 Classification of items and surfaces in relation to risk (Babb J In: Taylor E W (ed) Infection in surgical practice (1992) by permission of Oxford University Press)

Risk category	Method of decontamination	Process options	Examples of items/surfaces
High risk In contact with a break in the skin or mucous membrane or introduced into a sterile body area (if sterilisation is not practicable, high-level disinfection may be adequate)	Cleaning and sterilisation	**Heat tolerant** Autoclave Hot air oven **Heat sensitive** Single use Ethylene oxide Low-temperature steam and formaldehyde Sporicidal disinfectants, e.g. glutaraldehyde	Surgical instruments, laparoscopes arthroscopes, cardiac catheters, implants, infusions, injections, needles, syringes, swabs, surgical dressings, sutures
Intermediate risk In contact with intact mucous membranes, body fluids, or contaminated with particularly virulent or readily transmissible organisms, or if the item is to be used on highly susceptible patients or sites	Cleaning and disinfection (or sterilisation)	All the above and **Heat tolerant** Boiling Pasteurisation Low-temperature steam washer disinfectors **Heat sensitive** Disinfectants, e.g. glutaraldehyde, chlorine-releasing agents, alcohol, clear soluble phenolics	Respiratory and anaesthetic equipment. GI endoscopes, bronchoscopes, thermometers, vaginal speculae, body fluid spillage, dirty instruments prior to reprocessing, bed pans
Low risk In contact with normal and intact skin	Cleaning usually adequate Disinfection if known infection risk	Manual cleaning with detergent Automated cleaning/ disinfection Disinfectants	Trolley tops, operating table, wash-bowls, lavatory seats, baths, wash hand basins, bedding, patient supports
Minimal risk Remote, not in direct contact with patients or immediate surroundings Unlikely to be contaminated with a significant number of pathogens or be transferred to a susceptible site	Cleaning alone	Manual or automated cleaning, damp dusting, wet mopping, dust-attractant mops, vacuum cleaners	Floors, walls, furniture, ceilings, drains

or from subsequent contamination of the device or its insertion site. As stated earlier, intravascular devices known to be associated with infections are peripheral lines, central intravenous lines, total parenteral nutrition (TPN) catheters, arterial lines, and catheters used to provide long-term central venous access, amongst many. Infections of the vascular system range from local cellulitis, abscess formation, septic thrombophlebitis to bacteraemia. Between 0.2% and 8% of patients receiving i.v. infusion develop septicaemia (Shanson 1989). Many primary infections that are related to intravascular devices are known to originate from the patient's own flora or from microorganisms transmitted from the hands of the person inserting the

device. These devices also provide a direct pathway for microorganisms between the person's external environment and the bloodstream.

Certain *basic* precautions are considered here.

Setting up an intravenous infusion: the use of aseptic technique. The aim of aseptic technique is to prevent the contamination and subsequent spread of microorganisms to susceptible patient sites. The use of this principle is paramount when siting an intravascular infusion because the infusion site affords a *direct* entry point for bacteria. This is achieved by:

• *Handwashing by the operator.* Bacteria carried on the hands of the operator will enter the bloodstream through the insertion site.

- *Cleaning of the insertion site.* An alcoholic chlorhexidine solution or an iodophor in alcohol should be used to clean the site, allowing 30 seconds for application and further 30 seconds to dry (Maki et al 1991).
- *Choosing the insertion site.* Catheters placed in the lower part of the body, especially femoral veins, are more likely to result in complications and infection than those placed in the upper limbs. Lower extremities are frequently colonised with bowel microorganisms (Shanson 1989)
- *Anchoring of the cannula.* The cannula needs to be stable to prevent inward migration of microorganisms due to movement of the cannula. The insertion site should be secured with a *sterile* tape and dressing but enabling observation.
- *Recording date and time of insertion.* Leaving the cannula in place for longer than 72 hours significantly increases the risk of infection (Elliot 1993, Henderson 1995, Shanson 1989). The cannula should be changed and resited every 48–72 hours (Shanson 1989). If blood has been transfused, the entire giving set, down to the cannula, should be changed every 48–72 hours or sooner.

Maintenance of the intravenous device: inspection of the site. This should be done daily and at each use. Signs of erythema, oedema, phlebitis or pus are the first indications of complications. This may be accompanied by pain, tenderness and possible pyrexia. Early identification of problems may prevent subsequent morbidity or mortality in the patient. At the first sign of symptoms, the entire i.v. equipment should be withdrawn immediately and the cannula sent for culture and sensitivity testing. The resiting should take place using an aseptic technique and a new set of equipment, including the cannula. In some circumstances, prompt removal of the cannula may be impracticable and this remains the responsibility of the clinician in charge of the patient.

Maintenance of asepsis during manipulation of the device. *Handwashing is paramount.* Contamination of the system during repositioning, changing the solution, obtaining samples, handling the catheter hub, etc., have all been associated with bacteraemia. Many microorganisms, including coagulase-negative staphylococci, e.g. *Staphylococcus epidermidis*, are known to colonise the hub–tube junction (Duggan et al 1985). Swabbing with an alcohol-based antiseptic prior to manipulation is considered to be effective in reducing the number of these microorganisms (Duggan et al 1985).

Total parenteral nutrition (TPN)

The delivery of total parenteral nutrition is commonly used in critically ill and severely compromised patients whose susceptibility to bacteraemia is vastly increased. Complications such as septicaemia have been associated with TPN (Henderson 1995). The management of TPN should include:

- maintenance of asepsis
- strict protocol with regard to using the TPN line for the delivery of TPN fluids *only*
- prompt discontinuation if any signs of complications appear.
(See also Ch. 27.)

Dialysis, either peritoneal or haemodialysis, provides a direct entry point for microorganisms and requires a similarly strict code of practice.

Reflective point

Based on the hazards associated with intravenous devices as discussed here, consider how these risks are managed in your clinical area.

Urinary catheterisation

The genitourinary tract is the most common site of infection both in hospitals and nursing homes (Ouslander 1987, Roe & Brocklehurst 1987) 86% of urinary tract infections (UTI) are said to associated with instrumentation, usually catheterisation (Roe et al 1986, Slade & Gillespie 1985). The 1994 Prevalence Survey (Emmerson et al 1996) found 23.2% of hospital-acquired infections to be those of the urinary tract. Catheters bypass the normal clearing mechanism of the urinary system and carry the bacteria colonising the distal portion of the urethra. The presence of bacteria in urine (bacteriuria) is associated with catheterisation in 1 in 5 patients (Mulhall et al 1988, Murphy et al 1983). The consequences of bacteriuria may be urinary tract infection or bacteraemia and septicaemia with significant patient morbidity. There is also a potential for creating a reservoir for multiple-resistant microorganisms which has implications for both the patient and the organisation. Highly toxic and expensive antibiotic therapies have to be used, as the choice is reduced by the resistance of the microorganisms.

A number of factors have been identified as contributing to urinary infections (Garibaldi 1993). These are listed as points to ponder:

- *The indiscriminate use of catheters.* Millions of patients are catheterised in hospital settings and nursing homes. There may be alternatives to catheterisation.

- *Preparation of the genital region.* The distal urethra and the area surrounding the genitalia are normally colonised by skin and faecal flora. Thorough cleaning with an antiseptic solution is necessary.
- *A strict code of asepsis.* A break in the aseptic technique can lead to the introduction of microorganisms into the urinary system and can also contaminate the drainage system.
- *Trauma.* A lack of expertise or a large-bore catheter can result in meatal and urethral damage leading to further colonisation with hospital flora.
- *Inadequate light.* An absence of adequate lighting, especially when catheterising females, can result in the catheter inadvertently touching the surrounding area or being placed in the vagina (the catheter must be discarded and gloves changed).
- Maintenance of the integrity of the drainage system:
  - Continuous movement of an unanchored catheter can cause irritation of the urethra and also introduce microorganisms from the external meatus into the urinary system.
  - Other components include frequent breaks in the drainage system and lack of unobstructed urine flow.
  - Urine specimens should be obtained from the sampling port and not by opening the catheter–drainage tube connection.
- The emptying procedure:
  - The bag should be emptied when it contains 500 ml or every 8 hours unless the patient's condition demands otherwise.
  - Strict observance of handwashing before and after the procedure and appropriate decontamination and storage of collecting jugs must be maintained.
- Meatal care: faeces, exudate or encrustation may collect round the meatal–catheter junction and become a focus for microorganisms; the site should be washed with soap and water and dried.
- Duration of catheterisation: there is a direct link between the duration of catheterisation and increased risk of infection. Catheters should be removed as soon as possible.

The risk of infection in suprapubic and intermittent catheterisation is lower than in urethral catheterisation.

Respiratory therapy devices

Both upper and lower respiratory tract infections (RTI) are encountered in surgical settings. Infections of the lower respiratory tract, especially pneumonia, carry a high mortality rate. Lower respiratory tract infections accounted for 22.9% of hospital-acquired infections in the 1994 Prevalence Survey (Emmerson et al 1996). Nosocomial chest infections can be encountered in any area of patient care but are more commonly associated with intensive care, neonatal care units, and postsurgery patients.

Many factors interfere with a person's impressive array of respiratory defences. Some are host related such as age, chronic lung disease, immunosuppression. Many infections are, however, the result of hospital procedures and treatment (Pennington 1995).

Intubation of the respiratory tract, either for surgery or long-term respiratory assistance, is associated with a high incidence of pneumonia. Tracheostomy further increases this risk (Cross et al 1981). Respiratory therapy equipments serve as a source of bacterial contamination. Pulmonary function test apparatus has been associated with cross-infection with tuberculosis (Hazaleus et al 1981). Even nasogastric tubes have been associated with nosocomial pneumonia (Veazey 1981).

A number of preventive measures are considered here:

- Strict hand hygiene both before and after contact with susceptible patients and equipment.
- Prevention of contamination of respiratory therapy equipment. This includes face masks, nasal cannulae, tubes such as oral, endotracheal, anaesthetic and ventilator, humidifiers, rebreathing bags, oxygen tents and equipment producing aerosols such as nebulisers.
- Employment of single-use items wherever possible. Sterilisation or high-level disinfection of reusable articles after use and/or every 24–48 hours.
- Use of high-efficiency bacterial filters to prevent contamination of the spirometer and machinery.
- Filling of humidifiers with sterile fluids only. Do not 'top-up' the solution; discard the remnant of fluids before replenishing.
- Thorough washing of mini-nebulisers, drying and wiping with an alcohol-impregnated swab after each use.
- Use of a plastic apron and gloves when dealing with secretions from infected patients.
- Use of masks and protective eyewear is recommended if contamination of the face is likely during cough-inducing procedures.

Gastrointestinal infections and other complications

Many infection-related gastrointestinal symptoms mimic conditions which require surgical intervention. This can present a genuine dilemma to the surgical team. The nursing staff must view all cases of diarrhoea and/or vomiting or nausea with suspicion and take enteric precautions. Ideally, isolation should be considered until the diagnosis is confirmed; in this way cross-transmission and possible outbreaks of infection may be prevented.

Another well-established cause of diarrhoeal disease in care settings is antibiotics. Antibiotics disrupt the normal gut flora leading to recolonisation of the gut. The usual anaerobes are replaced with microorganisms such as *Staphylococcus aureus* or *Candida*. Many broad-spectrum antibiotics inhibit the normal flora, allowing the microorganism *Clostridium difficile* to multiply. The toxin produced by *Clostridium difficile* causes severe diarrhoea requiring treatment. Cross-infection amongst patients receiving antibiotic therapy is common.

Outbreaks of gastrointestinal infections affecting patients and staff in care settings are well recognised. The main aim during such outbreaks is to identify the pattern of the disease and curtail its spread. The movement of staff and patients between wards and within the affected area creates an ideal environment for the spread of infection.

Methicillin-resistant Staphylococcus aureus (MRSA)

Infections caused by staphylococci are an important cause of morbidity and mortality. Staphylococcal infections, especially those associated with methicillin-resistant *Staphylococcus aureus* (MRSA), are costly in terms of treatment as well as the disruption of hospital routine by outbreaks. MRSA are said to vary in their 'virulence and epidemic potential' (Cox et al 1995). Some strains, known as epidemic methicillin-resistant *Staphylococcus aureus* (EMRSA), cause severe and life-threatening infections and require aggressive and costly measures to curtail their spread. Outbreaks of MRSA infections are very difficult to control and require rigorous measures entailing considerable expense. MRSA outbreaks are difficult to control because:

- Asymptomatic carriage may often occur for long periods.
- Current methods to detect colonisation of patients are slow and insensitive and an outbreak may be underway for some time before it is recognised.
- Carriage may be at a variety of sites, any one of which may be the dominant reservoir for spread.
- The need for scrupulous handwashing is often underestimated.

- There is a need to provide isolation facilities, which may be insufficient in numbers (Keane et al 1991).

Both patients and carers are affected by these rigorous measures. Keane et al (1991) have issued guidelines on MRSA which form the basis of local protocols in most health care settings. The community control of MRSA is, however, less well defined. There is a constant movement of patients between community and hospitals. Patients colonised with MRSA in hospital have been known to carry the microorganism for months or years afterwards. Nursing homes have also been affected by MRSA with risks of infection higher in nursing home patients colonised with MRSA compared to those colonised with methicillin-sensitive *Staphylococcus aureus* (MSSA). The constant movement of patients between nursing homes and hospitals creates a potential for outbreaks in both institutions. Health professionals caring for MRSA-positive patients are also at risk of becoming colonised with the organism and subsequently transmitting it to other patients. It is, therefore, considered necessary to attempt to eradicate the organism wherever possible.

Precautionary measures have to be instituted when the microorganism is first isolated. The rigorous measures can be modified if the microorganism is of a less aggressive strain and/or if the carriage sites are found to be negative at screening.

Policies and procedures relating to MRSA are now based on the revised guidelines released in August 1998 by the Working Party of the British Society for Antimicrobial Chemotherapy, the Hospital Infection Society and the Infection Control Nurses Association (Ayliffe et al 1998). The condition generates anxiety and confusion in patients and their relatives and they may find a simple information or advice sheet helpful. For example see Figure 13.2, the Royal College of Nursing (1992) MRSA Patient Information Leaflet.

CROSS-INFECTION

Cross-infection occurs because microorganisms have been afforded an opportunity to travel from an infected or contaminated source to a vulnerable site in another patient. Any patient care item can become contaminated and require appropriate processing. This is covered earlier (see Table 13.4). Another well-recognised means of cross-transmission of microorganisms between patients is the hands of health care workers. Since handwashing remains the most fundamental principle in controlling infection, the issues surrounding this practice are explored in detail.

METHICILLIN-RESISTANT STAPHYLOCOCCUS AUREUS

(M.R.S.A.)
PATIENT INFORMATION LEAFLET

ROYAL COLLEGE OF NURSING

1 **What is this bug?**
It is a bacterium which is not easily killed by the more commonly used antibiotics.

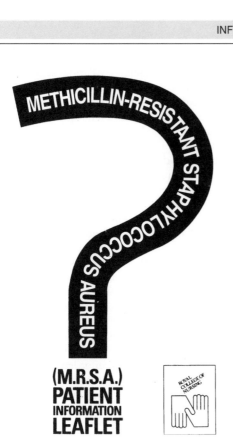

2 **How does it affect me?**
Nothing is visible but it may delay the healing process.

3 **How did I catch MRSA?**
It is one of the bacteria found in the environment from time to time and will do little or no harm unless it invades the body. The spread is usually by human contact.

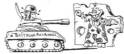

4 **How is MRSA identified?**
By taking a specimen and sending it to the laboratory to be examined.

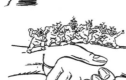

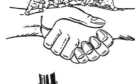

5 **Can it be treated?**
Yes, very successfully, by prescribed ointment, washes or antibiotics.

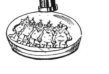

6 **How do I know when the bug has gone?**
Only when repeated specimens show no growth of the bacterium.

7 **Can it come back?**
Yes. Be careful with personal hygiene and handwashing. Be especially careful not to touch areas of broken skin and keep damaged skin covered.

8 **Why are patients with MRSA nursed in an isolation ward or room?**
To prevent the spread of the bacterium to other patients, who may be more vulnerable.

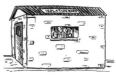

9 **How can the spread of the MRSA be minimised?**
By the thorough washing and drying of hands of everyone involved.

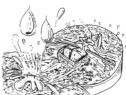

10 **Can visitors to the ward catch MRSA?**
Healthy people are at very little risk of catching MRSA. They should keep cuts covered with a waterproof dressing and ensure they wash their hands thoroughly on leaving the ward. All visitors should see the nurse in charge before visiting. The nurse will give guidance and instruction on the prevention of spread of infection.

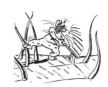

11 **Can visitors infect other people?**
Not if they wash and dry their hands before and after visiting.

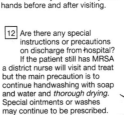

12 **Are there any special instructions or precautions on discharge from hospital?**
If the patient still has MRSA a district nurse will visit and treat but the main precaution is to continue handwashing with soap and water and *thorough drying*. Special ointments or washes may continue to be prescribed for a while after discharge.

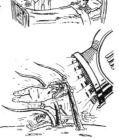

13 **Will my marital and sexual life be affected?**
No.

If you have any other questions or would like more information, please contact: The Ward Sister/District Nurse or your own G.P.

MRSA/js *Drawings produced by Colin Charlton, graphic worker.*

Figure 13.2 Methicillin-resistant *Staphylococcus aureus*: patient information leaflet (reproduced by kind permission from RCN 1992).

Handwashing

A strong relationship has been established, since the middle of the 19th century, between the hands of health care workers and cross-transmission and spread of microorganisms between patients. This route remains, by far, the most hazardous, since large numbers and more virulent microorganisms can be transferred to a susceptible person at one time. Hospitals are admitting more severely ill patients who require frequent invasive procedures and devices with an increasing risk of transmission of pathogenic microorganisms between patients. A simple but effective means of protecting patients from nosocomial infections is handwashing.

Handwashing agents and types of handwashing

The purpose of handwashing is to remove dirt and/or to reduce the level of microorganisms present on the hands. The microorganisms likely to cause problems are those picked up during care activities that use the hands of the health care workers as a means to travel to susceptible patients. The vulnerability resulting from the illness which necessitated hospital admission and from the interventions prescribed increases the patient's susceptibility to infection from transient microorganisms. *The majority of these microorganisms are removed by the mechanical action of handwashing or chemical action of hand disinfection.*

The choice of handwashing agent, the duration of the wash and the technique used will depend on the nature of the procedure to be undertaken and the susceptibility of the patient. Three methods of rendering hands safe are commonly used: social, antiseptic and surgical handwash.

Social handwash. This is by far the most common form of handwashing practised in both home and care situations. The aim is to remove all transient microorganisms. Blowing the nose, visiting the lavatory, handling soiled nappies and cleaning toilets at home are some of the personal actions which result in significant hand contamination. Practices which involve direct contact with patients and used equipment often produce high levels of contamination. These microorganisms are easily removed by washing for 10–15 seconds with plain soap and running water and mechanical friction, friction being the most important element in effective handwashing (Ayliffe et al 1978).

It is important to note that short nails are desirable since the majority of microorganisms are found under or around the fingernails. The bacteria counts are also higher under and around rings but the microorganisms can be removed effectively by manipulating rings during handwashing. Wearing of jewellery in clinical settings should be limited to a wedding ring.

Antiseptic/disinfectant handwash. In an antiseptic or disinfectant handwash, chemical substances possessing antimicrobial activity are applied to the skin. Antisepsis is paramount in cases where patients' high vulnerability predisposes them to infection from resident microorganisms. Newborn infants, severely immunosuppressed patients and patients receiving intensive care fall into this category.

Surgical handwash. The conditions during surgery (see p. 249) demand a handwash which is effective in removing the transient microorganisms as well as in reducing resident microorganisms to a safe level. Although soap, water and friction are effective in removing transient microbes, there is a possibility of an increase in the level of resident microorganisms following a social handwash. This is thought to be a result of increased shedding of desquamating epithelium which contains microorganisms. These resident bacteria can be pathogenic if afforded an opportunity to invade a site in a vulnerable patient. An antimicrobial wash is needed to kill or inhibit the resident microorganisms and reduce the number still further. A further advantage of using an antiseptic agent is the persistent antibacterial activity of the residue on the skin following the handwash. Such antibacterial action is desirable when frequent handwashing is impossible, such as during prolonged surgical procedures. Box 13.2 provides information about when hands should be washed.

Reflective point

Since handwashing is key to the prevention of cross-infection, how do you ensure good practice amongst all health care professionals in your practice area?

CROSS-INFECTION – ISSUES TO ADDRESS

Cross-infections are confirmed by carrying out certain identification tests on the microorganisms. In many cases the likelihood of the same infection is based on more than one patient presenting similar or the same clinical symptoms. Whether cross-infection is suspected or confirmed, it is useful to establish a method of evaluation which can help identify gaps in the knowledge and practice of all practitioners.

The framework in Figure 13.3 suggests a systematic and reflective investigation of any untoward

---

> **Box 13.2**   When hands should be washed
>
> **Before:**
> * performing invasive procedures
> * caring for susceptible patients
> * preparing or handling food
> * any other activity where a risk of transmitting infection is anticipated
> * leaving work areas (e.g. before going to the lavatory, visiting the canteen or going home).
>
> **Before and after:**
> * touching wounds and dressings of any type.
>
> **Between:**
> * significant or prolonged contact with different patients, particularly in high-risk areas such as intensive therapy units.
>
> **After:**
> * situations likely to cause microbial contamination such as contact with blood and body fluids, secretions or excretions
> * touching sources likely to be contaminated with medically significant microorganisms (such as urine measuring devices, suction bottles, sputum collection pots)
> * caring for patients infected or colonised with important bacteria, e.g. methicillin-resistant *Staphylococcus aureus* and gentamicin-resistant *Klebsiella pneumoniae*, where there is a risk of serious cross-infection
> * personal contamination such as using the toilet, blowing or touching one's nose.

occurrence, especially cross-infection in a patient, by identifying:

* the knowledge base of all care workers
* breaks in practices
* the approach taken to patient care in different clinical areas
* the level and effectiveness of communication
* the quality element in the care provided
* practices which merit audit.

Health and safety issues

The aim of the care organisation is to manage risks to patients, staff and visitors. Staff should develop sufficient expertise to identify and analyse the infection hazards posed to patients, staff and visitors and take appropriate action to prevent or minimise the risks.

Hazards are associated with practices as well as with health care settings. Patients and staff are at risk from practices and from each other. It is almost impossible to

legislate for all eventualities when an exposure to infection may occur. By far the biggest reminder was the transmission of acquired immune deficiency syndrome (AIDS) to health care workers as a result of occupational exposures (Communicable Diseases Report 1993). A case of primary cutaneous tuberculosis was reported in a nurse following a needlestick injury from a patient with AIDS and undiagnosed tuberculosis (Kramer et al 1994). Such unfortunate episodes remind the health professionals that many disease-producing microorganisms may be present in the blood, body fluids, secretions and excretions of an otherwise healthy and undiagnosed person. The accepted advice is that some basic precautionary steps need to be taken at all times when dealing with body excretions and secretions.

Universal precautions

The concept of *universal precautions* was introduced in the USA in the late 1980s in order to minimise the occupational risk of blood-borne viral infections in health care workers (Center for Disease Control 1987) and is generally recommended in this country (Advisory Committee on Dangerous Pathogens 1990b). The following recommendations by the Advisory Group on Hepatitis (UK Health Departments 1993) can be described as the basis of universal precautions (see Box 13.3).

Figure 13.4, the safety aspect of employee health, also relates to further health and safety components of health care. Further reading regarding employee health can be found in Bamford (1995) and ROSPA (1986).

The principles of a safe environment (Fig. 13.5) include adherence to the Control of Substances Hazardous to Health (COSHH) Regulations 1993 (HSE 1993). The COSHH Regulations require employers to evaluate the control of the risk to health for all their employees from exposure to hazardous substances at work. These include microbiological agents, dusts of any kind in substantial quantities and all chemicals hazardous to health except lead and asbestos, the control of exposure to which is covered by other regulations. Radiation is also excluded. COSHH applies to everyone who is exposed to risks to health, immediate or delayed, which arise from hazardous substances in a work activity. These regulations lay down the essential requirements both for a sensible step-by-step approach to the control of hazardous substances and for the protection of the people exposed to them. Further reading regarding the principles of health and safety may be found in publications by the Health and Safety Commission (1999) and the Department of Health (1989b).

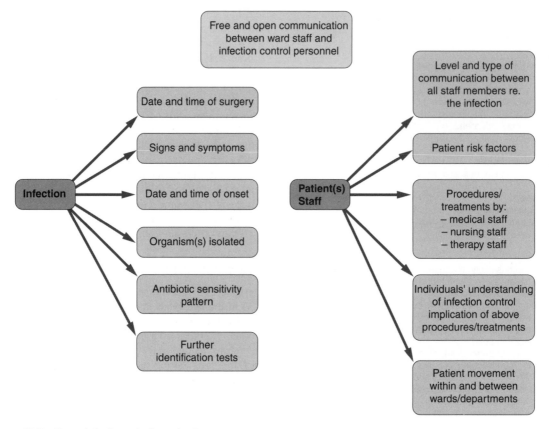

Figure 13.3 Cross-infection – the investigation.

- Apply good basic hygiene practices with regular handwashing.
- Cover existing wounds or skin lesions with waterproof dressings.
- Avoid invasive procedures if suffering from chronic skin lesions on hands.
- Avoid contamination of person by use of appropriate protective clothing.
- Protect mucous membranes of eyes, mouth and nose from blood splashes and bloodstained body fluids.
- Prevent puncture wounds, cuts and abrasions in the presence of blood/bloodstained body fluids.
- Avoid sharps usage wherever possible.
- Institute safe procedures for handling and disposal of needles and other sharps.
- Institute approved procedures for sterilisation and disinfection of instruments and equipment.
- Clear up spillages of blood and other body fluids promptly and disinfect surfaces.
- Institute a procedure for safe disposal of contaminated waste.

Specific practical issues

Patients requiring surgical interventions may present with underlying infectious conditions which necessitate specific actions and precautions to protect health professionals and/or other patients. The measures taken should reflect the following:

- the infectious agent
- the reservoir or the site in the body where the microorganism resides
- portal of exit of the microorganism
- means of transmission of the microorganism
- route by which the microorganism enters the vulnerable patient
- the susceptible patient.

For example, in a patient presenting with hepatitis B infection, the 'chain' components shown in Figure 13.6 have to link to enable a non-immune staff member to contract the virus.

The chain can be interrupted at any point to prevent or curtail the spread of any microorganism or infection.

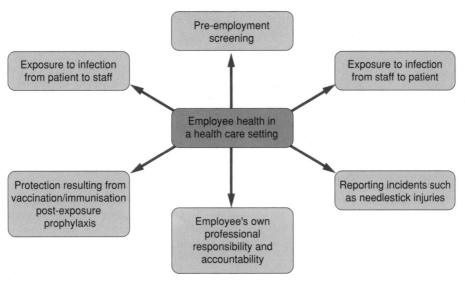

Figure 13.4 Safety aspects of employee health.

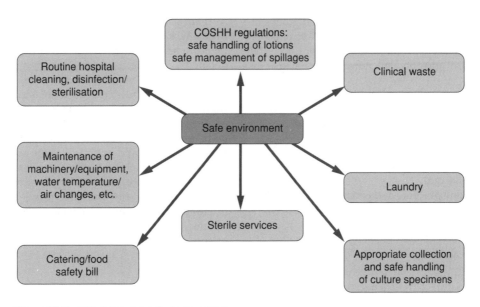

Figure 13.5 Principles of a safe environment.

In the majority of cases, the link can be readily broken by using some basic precautions such as sensible handwashing and environmental hygiene (Fig. 13.7), whereas isolation and specific measures may be required in some instances (Fig. 13.8). The chain can also become a useful tool for evaluating care as well as assessing individual staff member's knowledge and understanding of the microorganism, disease and the relevant practice.

THE INFECTION CONTROL NURSE

Infection control is one aspect of good practice amongst many. Much of infection control is based on 'common sense' derived from an in-depth understanding of the reasons for each action or inaction. The person with a level of 'expertise' who can help, guide and support the bedside and community nurses is the

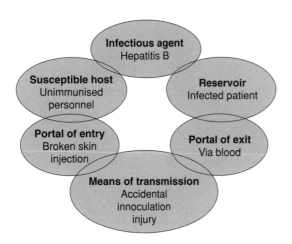

Figure 13.6 The chain of infection: hepatitis B.

infection control nurse, a clinical nurse specialist. Increasingly, the concept of 'link or liaison' nurses (Horton 1988) is used by infection control nurses to impart the necessary knowledge to identified groups of bedside nurses, making them the ambassadors of good, safe and research-based infection control practice. The infection control nurse and link nurses work together to:

- identify the infection control educational requirement for staff in an individual workplace
- implement safe measures on recognition of infection
- investigate infections to establish the avoidable and non-preventable elements in this outcome, and evaluate care
- identify good practices and commend colleagues
- recognise aspects of care which could have been tackled differently, for future reference
- carry out surveillance of infection, investigation of outbreaks and audit of knowledge and practice.

The link nurses are pivotal in providing safe and informed care and work collaboratively with all staff to achieve these aims.

CONCLUSION

All stakeholders are increasingly being influenced by parameters of outcome of in-hospital treatment in choosing the 'best' option for their patients. Health professionals are required to ensure that patients under their care are at no time placed at risk of being harmed. There is an increasing expectation that there are regular reviews of practice to ensure and assure safety, appropriateness and effectiveness of treatments and procedures. Additionally, this includes defining standards, measuring achievements and identifying mechanisms to improve performance.

Infection rates in clean operations are expected to be the best measure of effective infection control programmes in surgery. This chapter has explored all the relevant components which contribute to the development of a wound infection. In many cases the patient's own inherent factors will have played a major part in this outcome, whereas in others the skills and expertise of the operator may have been the deciding factor.

If surgical wound infection rates are to become a benchmark for successful infection control practice, then nurses need to be involved in the effectiveness debate by making a positive and 'informed' contribution. Surgical wound infections may be outside nurses' control but they need to argue this point from an informed basis. Furthermore, infections in surgical patients are not limited to wounds; other body systems are equally vulnerable. The assessment of patients and appraisal of the outcome needs to encompass each and every variable. Audit and evaluation of care surrounding infected and non-infected patients can provide nurses with a solid foundation from which to develop a proactive programme of care which can be presented as an example of good practice.

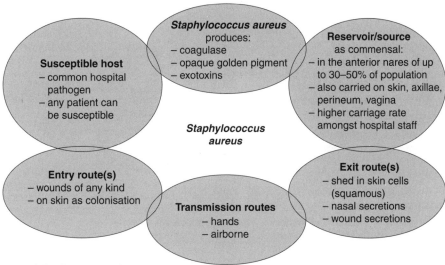

Symptoms – infections caused
SUPERFICIAL
– affects skin and surface structures, e.g. boils, sticky eyes in babies, breast abscess in breast-feeding mothers, wounds and burns (found in 5% of clean surgical wounds)
SYSTEMIC
– osteomyelitis, septicaemia (often relates to vascular access sites or surgical wounds), endocarditis (following cardiac surgery; in drug addicts), etc.
TOXIN RELATED
– food poisoning following ingestion of preformed enterotoxin
– toxic shock syndrome (mainly women using vaginal tampons)
– scalded skin syndrome

Principles of management
– hands remain the main method of transferring *Staphylococcus aureus* from a source to a susceptible patient
– contaminated used equipment can transmit organism if not decontaminated between uses
– handwashing is the fundamental infection control measure
– environmental hygiene of clinical areas should be of a high standard

Figure 13.7   The chain of infection: *Staphylococcus aureus*.

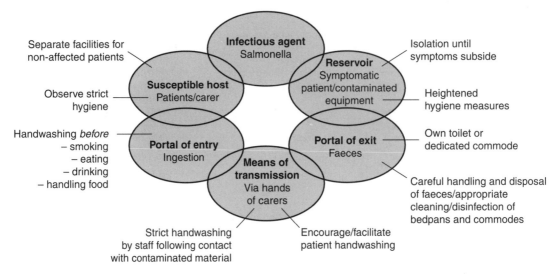

Figure 13.8 Steps required in source isolation of a salmonella infection (reproduced by kind permission from Horton & Parker 1997).

REFERENCES

Advisory Committee on Dangerous Pathogens (ACDP) 1990a HIV – the causative agent of AIDS and related conditions, 2nd revision of guidelines. HMSO, London

Advisory Committee on Dangerous Pathogens (ACDP) 1990b Categorisation of pathogens according to hazard and categories of containment, 2nd edn. HMSO, London

Altmeier W A 1979 Surgical infections; incisional infections. Little Brown, Boston, pp 287–306

Ayliffe G A J, Lowbury E J L 1982 Hospital-acquired infection: principles and prevention. Wright, Bristol

Ayliffe G A J, Babb J R, Quoraishi A H 1978 A test for hygienic hand disinfection. Journal of Clinical Pathology 31: 923–928

Ayliffe G A J, Collins B, Taylor L J 1990 Hospital acquired infection. Principles and practice, 2nd edn. Butterworth, London

Ayliffe G A J, Buckles A, Casewell M W et al 1998 Revised guidelines for the control of methicillin-resistant Staphylococcus aureus infection in hospitals. Journal of Hospital Infection 39(4): 253–285

Babb J 1992 Action of disinfectants and antiseptics and their role in surgical practice. In: Taylor E W (ed) Infection in surgical practice. Oxford University Press, Oxford

Bremmelgaard A, Raahave D, Beier-Holgersen R, Pedersen J V, Andersen S, Sorensen A I 1989 Computer-aided surveillance of surgical infections and identification of risk factors. Journal of Hospital Infection 13: 1–3

Center for Disease Control 1987 Recommendations for prevention of HIV transmission in health-care settings. Morbidity and Mortality Weekly Report 36(suppl 2S): 1S–18S

Communicable Diseases Report 1993 Health care workers and HIV: surveillance of occupationally acquired infection in the United Kingdom. Public Health Laboratory Service (PHLS), London

Cox R A, Conquest C, Mallaghan C, Marples R R 1995 A major outbreak of methicillin resistant Staphylococcus aureus caused by new phage type (EMRSA-16). Journal of Hospital Infection 29: 87–106

Cross A S, Roup B 1981 Role of respiratory assistance devices in endemic nosocomial pneumonia. American Journal of Medicine 70: 681

Cruse P J E 1992 Classification of operations and audit of infection In: Taylor E W (ed) Infection in surgical practice. Oxford University Press, Oxford

Cruse P J E, Foord R 1980 The epidemiology of wound infection: a 10 year prospective study of 62939 wounds. Surgical Clinics of North America 60: 1

Currie E, Maynard A 1989 The economics of hospital-acquired infection. Discussion Paper 56. Centre of Health Economics, University of York, York

Davidson A I G, Clark C, Smith G 1971 Postoperative wound infection: a computer analysis. British Journal of Surgery 58: 333–337

Department of Health (DoH) 1989a Working for patients. HMSO, London

Department of Health (DoH) 1989b The control of substances hazardous to health – guidance for the initial assessments in hospitals. HMSO, London

Department of Health (DoH) 1991 The patient's charter. HMSO, London

Department of Health and Public Health Laboratory Service 1995 Hospital infection control. DoH, London

Donowitz G R 1987 The immunosuppressed patient. In: Farber B F (ed) Infection control in intensive care. Churchill Livingstone, Edinburgh

Duggan J M, Oldfield G S, Ghosh H K 1985 Septicaemia as a hospital hazard. Journal of Hospital Infection 6: 406–412

Edlich R F, Panek P H, Rodehaever G T et al 1973 Physical and chemical configuration of sutures in the development of surgical infection. Annals of Surgery 117: 679

Elliot T S 1993 Line-associated bacteraemias. Communicable Diseases Report. Public Health Laboratory Service (PHLS), London

Emmerson A M, Enstone J E, Griffin M, Kelsey M C, Smyth E T M 1996 The second prevalence survey of infection in hospitals – overview of the results. Journal of Hospital Infection 32 (3): 175–190

Farber B F, Wenzel R W P 1980 Postoperative wound infection rates: results of prospective statewide surveillance. American Journal of Surgery 140: 343–346

French M L V, Eitzen H E, Ritter M A 1976 The plastic adhesive drape: an evaluation of its efficiency as a microbial barrier. Annals of Surgery 184: 46–50

Garibaldi R A 1993 Hospital acquired urinary tract infections. In: Wenzel R P (ed) Prevention and control of nosocomial infections, 2nd edn. Williams & Wilkins, Baltimore, pp 600–613

Hamilton D 1982 The nineteenth century surgical revolution – antisepsis or better nutrition. Bulletin of History of Medicine 56: 30

Hazaleus R E, Cole J, Berdichewsky M 1981 Tuberculin skin test conversion from exposure to contaminated pulmonary function test apparatus. Respiratory Care 26: 53–55

Health and Safety Commission 1999 General COSHH ACOP (control of substances hazardous to health) carcinogens ACOP (control of carcinogen substances) and biological agents (control of biological agents) ACOP. Stationery Office, London

Health and Safety Executive (HSE) 1991 Successful health and safety management. HSE, London

Health and Safety Executive (HSE) 1993 Control of substances hazardous to health and control of carcinogenic substances: control of Substances Hazardous to Health Regulations 1988. HSE Books, Sudbury

Henderson D K 1995 Bacteraemia due to percutaneous intravascular devices. In: Mandell G L, Dolin R, Bennett J E (eds) Principles and practice of infectious diseases. Churchill Livingstone, New York

Hentges D J 1995 Medical microbiology and immunology. Little Brown, Boston

Horton R 1988 Linking the chain. Nursing Times 84(26): 44–46

Horton R, Parker L 1997 Informed infection control practice. Churchill Livingstone, Edinburgh

Humphreys H, Russell A J, Marshall R J, Ricketts V E, Reeves D S 1991 The effect of surgical theatre head-gear on air bacterial counts. Journal of Hospital Infection 19: 180

Jarrett J 1985 The natural history and prognosis of diabetes. Medicine International 2(13): 1311–1312

Keane C T, Coleman D C, Cafferkey M T 1991 Methicillin resistant *Staphylococcus aureus* – a reappraisal. Journal of Hospital Infection 19(3): 147–152

Kramer F, Sasse S A, Simms J C, Leedom J M 1994 Primary cutaneous tuberculosis after a needlestick injury from a patient with AIDS and undiagnosed tuberculosis. American Journal of Infection Control 3: 341–344

Law D J W, Mishriki S F, Jeffery P J 1990 The importance of surveillance after discharge from hospital in the diagnosis of postoperative wound infection. Annals of the Royal College of Surgeons, England 72: 207–209

Lawrence J C 1994 Dressings and wound infection. American Journal of Wound Infection 167(1A)(suppl): 21S–24S

Leigh D A 1981 An eight-year study of postoperative wound infection in two district general hospitals. Journal of Hospital Infection 2: 207–217

Lidwell O M, Lowbury E J L, Whyte W, Blowers R, Stanley S J, Lowe D 1983 Airborne contamination of wounds in joint replacement operations: the relationship to sepsis rates. Journal of Hospital Infection 4: 111–113

Magee C, Rodehaever G T, Golden G T 1976 Potentiation of wound infection by surgical drains. American Journal of Surgery 131: 547–549

Maki D G, Ringer M, Alvardo C J 1991 Prospective randomized trial of povidone iodine, alcohol and chlorhexidine for prevention of infection associated with central venous and arterial catheters. Lancet 338: 339–343

Meers P, Ayliffe G A J, Emmerson A, Leigh D, Mayon-White R, Mackintosh C, Strong J 1981 Report on the national survey of infections in hospitals. Journal of Hospital Infection 2(suppl): 1–51

Mehtar S 1992 Action of antibiotics and the development of antibiotic resistance. In: Taylor E W (ed) Infection in surgical practice. Oxford University Press, Oxford

Mishriki S F, Law D J W, Jeffery P J 1990 Factors affecting the incidence of postoperative wound infection. Journal of Hospital Infection 16: 223–230

Mishriki S F, Jeffery P J, Law D J W 1992 Wound infection: the surgeon's responsibility. Journal of Wound Care 1(2): 32–36

Mulhall A B, Chapman R G, Crow R 1988 Bacteriuria during indwelling urethral catheterization. Journal of Infection 11: 253–262

Murphy D M, Faulkner F R, Cafferkey M T, Gillespie W A 1983 Septicaemia after transurethral prostatectomy. Journal of Urology xxii: 133–135

National Academy of Sciences 1964 Ad hoc committee of the Committee on Trauma: post operative wound infections: the influence of ultraviolet irradiation of the operating room and of various other factors. Annals of Surgery 160(suppl 2): 1–92

Ojajarvi J, Makela P, Rantasalo I 1977 Failure of hand disinfection with frequent handwashing: a need for prolonged field studies. Journal of Hygiene 79: 107–119

Orr N 1981 Is a mask necessary in the operating theatre? Annals of the Royal College of Surgeons of England 63: 390–392

Ouslander J G 1987 Complications of chronic indwelling urinary catheters among male nursing home patients: a prospective study. Journal of Urology 138: 1191–1195

Paulssen J, Eidem T, Kristiansen R 1988 Perforations in surgeons' gloves. Journal of Hospital Infection 11: 82–85

Pennington J E 1995 Nosocomial respiratory infections. In: Mandell G L, Dolin R, Bennett J E (eds) Principles and practice of infectious diseases. Churchill Livingstone, New York

Polakoff S, Richards I D G, Parker M T, Lidwell O M 1967 Nasal and skin carriage of *Staphylococcus aureus* by patients undergoing surgical operation. Journal of Hygiene, Cambridge 65: 559–566

Public Health Laboratory Service (PHLS) 1960 Incidence of surgical wound infection in England and Wales: a report of the Public Health Laboratory Service, Great Britain. Lancet 2: 659–663

Roe B, Brocklehurst J C 1987 Study of patients with indwelling catheters. Journal of Advanced Nursing 12(6): 713–718

Roe B, Chapman R G, Crow R 1986 A study of the procedures for catheter care recommended by district health authorities and schools of nursing. Nursing Practice Research Unit, University of Surrey

Royal College of Nursing (RCN) 1992 Introduction to methicillin resistant *Staphyloccocus aureus*. RCN, London

Royal Society for the Prevention of Accidents (ROSPA) 1986 Health and safety practice. Pitman, London

Seropian R, Reynolds B M 1971 Wound infection after preoperative depilatory versus razor preparation. American Journal of Surgery 121: 251–254

Shanson D 1989 Microbiology in clinical practice, 2nd edn. Wright, London

Sheldon T A, Borowitz M 1993 Changing the measure of quality in the NHS: from purchasing activity to purchasing protocols. Quality in Health Care 2: 149–150

Slade N, Gillespie W A 1985 Urinary tract and the catheter. Infection and other problems. Wiley, Chichester

UK Health Departments 1993 Protecting health care workers and patients from hepatitis B. HMSO, London

Veazey J M Jr 1981 Hospital-acquired pneumonia. In: Wenzel R P (ed) Handbook of hospital-acquired infections. CRC Press, Florida

Whyte W, Bailey P V, Hamblen D L, Fisher W D, Kelly I G 1983 A bacteriologically occlusive clothing system for use in the operating room. Journal of Bone and Joint Surgery 65B: 502–506

FURTHER READING

Bamford M 1995 Work and health. Chapman and Hall, London

Greenwood D, Slack R, Pentherer J 1999 Medical microbiology, 15th edn. Churchill Livingstone, Edinburgh

Mims C A, Playfair J H L, Roitt I M, Wakelin D, Williams R, Anderson R M 1993 Medical microbiology. Mosby, London

14

The hospital surgical unit, the operating theatre and recovery unit

Deena Graham

AIMS

This chapter aims to provide the reader with an opportunity to:

- explore the changing surgical environment within the operating theatre and recovery room in relation to the nature of the surgical unit and future clientele
- identify the important role of communication within the surgical environment
- consider how the physical environment impinges on patient care
- explore the changing role of nursing in providing an environment to meet the needs of patients.

INTRODUCTION

The focus of this chapter will be an investigation into the nature of the environment in which surgical care takes place. The first part of the chapter will address the care environment generally and the second part will focus on components of the surgical environment.

It is important that nurses working in the surgical environment have an overall understanding of the perioperative experience of patients, in order to be able to apply this to patient care and nursing practice.

Alterations in the economic, social and political agendas of the health care system in the 1990s have influenced and modified the nature of care provided in the surgical setting. The technological developments of the last few years have been numerous and varied. Endoscopy, angioplasty and lasers have changed the profile of the surgical patient. Diagnostic tools such as ultrasound and X-ray procedures allow for more precise localisation of problems and have reduced the need for surgical exploration of tissues. Accordingly, the need for extensive invasive surgery is now declining and this has impacted on the practice of surgical nursing. Technological and medical advances have altered the time span of patients' stay in the surgical unit and the process of care provision. There is no doubt that surgical technology will continue to expand and make operative procedures quicker and safer. The nurse's role in the health care matrix is constantly adapting to meet and provide a service which suits a changing society, and scientific and medical advancement. As a result, it can be argued that no one type of nurse provides care for patients during their stay in the surgical unit.

Application to nursing

The chapter aims to explore how the physical environment impinges on patient care and how open lines of communication are important in the surgical environment so that all nurses are well informed about events that take place during the perioperative phase and their effects on patient care. Consideration will also be given to how stimuli from the external environment may cause the patient to encounter problems of adaptation and alienation within what may be unfamiliar surroundings.

There is a need for interaction between all areas of care provision to help promote continuity of care. This chapter aims to bridge the gap between areas so that nurses who work on surgical units have a knowledge of the changes in nursing in the operating department and how this may bring them closer together in collaboration in care.

The chapter is written in four distinct sections which all interlink. This is an attempt to draw together the individual perspectives on the surgical care environment and produce an overall holistic picture of surgical nursing which is greater than the sum of the parts. The four sections are:

- The changing surgical environment
- The effect of the physical environment of care
- The changing role of nursing in the environment of the operating department
- The role of nursing in providing an environment to meet the needs of patients.

THE CHANGING SURGICAL ENVIRONMENT

The changing surgical environment is conceptualised in Figure 14.1 and will be explored from the perspective of the nature of the surgical unit and the future clientele.

The surgical unit

In order to provide continuity, the issues involved in providing care require a holistic perspective (Moss Jones 1994). Consequently, the provision of patient care is an important issue that needs to be examined in a wider perspective.

General systems theory (Bertalanffy 1968) provides a conceptual framework for studying the development of integrated health care systems and is a useful model to use in an attempt to examine the physical, social and psychological aspects of care provision. Most

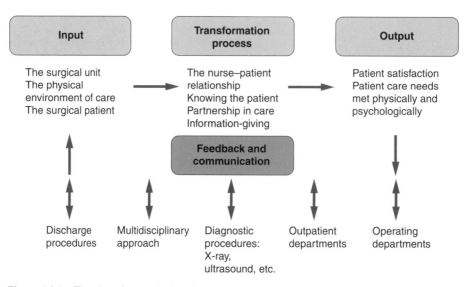

Figure 14.1 The changing surgical environment.

theorists describe a system as a set of elements in inter-action or relationship with one another (Fig. 14.1). Interactions occur in the system and between the system and its environment (Handy 1984). This is particularly pertinent to the relationship between the surgical ward and interrelated units such as outpatients, anaesthetics and the operating department.

A system is more than the sum of its parts because there is interaction among the parts. This produces an outcome that is greater than the sum of the outcomes of the individual parts. When the systems approach is applied to organisations, it highlights the point that if any part of the system is altered it is likely to have repercussions for the system as a whole (Stichler 1994). Therefore, feedback and communication is a vital aspect of systems theory. It is also recognised that the needs of an organisation often change with time, and systems must respond to changing needs. Feedback and communication are central ideas in systems thinking. Having the clearest possible understanding of the 'current reality' of the whole situation in which the unit is embedded is essential for effectiveness. Information and evaluation are essential for the system to be responsive and react to the dynamic changes in the external environment (Moss Jones 1994)

The surgical unit is a component of a much larger unit such as an NHS trust or private hospital. As such, the unit also needs to be able to interact effectively with other systems within the organisation. Using general systems theory, the surgical unit can be viewed as part of an interacting and interdependent group of health care units that have their own separate identity and organisational structure. These health care units work interdependently to respond to external forces and achieve outcomes that could not be accomplished if they worked separately. They work together, serve a common purpose, the provision of quality care, and communicate with exterior forces in the external environment. The units within this system need to be adaptive to responses and to changes in the market forces within the health care industry (Stichler 1994). Within the system, adaptation is a necessary response to a changing environment. The system must either change itself to adapt, change the surrounding environment or adjust both in order to survive. According to Rea (1995), most hospital units are managed as clinical directorates. A clinical directorate is a small unit of management within a hospital or trust which is largely organised around patient groups or medical specialties. These directorates are responsible for their own day-to-day affairs and doctors usually play a major role in their management. The clinical directorate management approach is intended to involve clinicians in a patient-focused approach to management which also has an overall view of the business aspect of providing care. It is argued by Rea (1995) that there is a danger that directorates will become the new power bases of trusts and that this could be detrimental to the system, in that they are focusing on the needs of a small part of the organisation rather than taking a view of the needs of the whole organisation. Accordingly, the feedback and communication aspects of the systems theory model become almost redundant. Consequently, coordination and integration across directorates could become arduous and there could be inefficiencies associated with the provision of services to and the support for several small management teams. Therefore, it is also increasingly important that each directorate provides an input to strategic decision-making policies as well as day-to-day management responsibilities.

Subsequently, effective communication is essential between clinical directorates. It is vital that organisational and strategic management decisions about care provisions are made in view of the whole picture. This enables the organisation to respond rapidly and effectively and to adapt to the ever changing environment of health care provision.

It is therefore important to view the surgical unit as part of an interacting and interdependent group of health care units. Feedback and communication are essential between units to allow a rapid response and adaptation to the changing environment of health care provision.

Reflective point

Consider the ease of communication between directorates in your organisation.

The future clientele for hospital surgery

We are now experiencing a dramatic shift in the delivery of surgical care, as economic incentives drive surgical care out of hospitals and back into the community. Consequently, the lengths of inpatient hospital stays are dramatically decreasing as patients are discharged increasingly earlier following surgery. Improved anaesthetic agents and techniques have also played a part in the changing face of the surgical unit. New anaesthetic agents such as midazolam hydrochloride are metabolised rapidly and allow patients to return to a conscious state more quickly than traditional agents. This facilitates earlier discharge after surgery.

Pain management is also more adequately controlled with many patients experiencing more effective control of acute pain which enables them to return home more quickly (Llewellyn 1991, Partridge et al 1991) (see Ch. 24).

A government report by Partridge et al (1991) 'Day Surgery – Making it Happen' acknowledged that day surgery was an economical, practical and highly successful method of providing quality treatment for a wide range of elective surgical procedures. Surgeons now perform many surgical techniques as day surgery which were previously considered to be the remit of intermediate surgery (see Ch. 15).

The surgical unit no longer just includes the traditional surgical ward. There is an increasing use of high-turnover 5-day wards, open from Monday to Friday and providing care for patients who are having minor/intermediate procedures but are not suitable candidates for a day surgery unit. Usually these units close on Fridays and if patients cannot be discharged by then they are transferred to another unit that can meet their needs. The advantages of these units are that they are cost-effective (Llewellyn 1991) and can be tailored to meet the specific needs of short-stay patients. Such units usually have admission guidelines to prevent them from becoming overflow admission units.

Admission criteria for 5-day wards

Admission criteria for 5-day wards tend to focus on the following factors (adapted from Llewellyn 1991):

• The anticipated length of stay for the patient should be no longer than 72 hours.
• There is a reasonable expectation that pain control can be achieved within 72 hours.
• The patient has the ability to meet basic self-care needs.
• The patient has the cognitive and psychomotor capabilities for learning any new self-care demands.

As technological advances move surgery forward, there will still be the need for more specialised major surgery, and so routine inpatients will by definition need more specialised and highly skilled nursing care because of the types of surgery being performed. Therefore nursing roles within the health care matrix will need to constantly adapt to society's expectations, scientific and medical advancement, and social change.

Nursing has changed and surgical patients' needs can no longer be met by the generalist nurse from the surgical unit alone. Nurses who work on surgical units

may have a limited knowledge of what occurs in the outpatient department, radiology department or the operating room and the effects of these intraoperative occurrences on patients. No one nurse provides care in all areas during the patient's stay in the surgical unit and there needs to be interaction between all areas of care provision to help promote true continuity of care.

Reflective point

You may want to consider the following:

1. how case management (see Ch. 2) as a strategy could overcome some of the continuity problems identified above
2. how case management could work in your area, and from whom you might expect resistance and support for such a change
3. the impact of shorter hospital stays on turnover
4. the changing nature of surgical inpatients as a result of demographic changes and the growth in day surgery.

THE EFFECT OF THE PHYSICAL ENVIRONMENT OF CARE

According to Wilson Barnet (1988) it is all too easy for a nurse to forget the strangeness of a hospital ward for first-time patients and their significant others. It is maintained that feelings of helplessness and fear are experienced by most patients at some time during their stay and may affect their rate of recovery. Hospitals provide a strange and threatening environment which imposes various demands on the patient. This stress should be seen as an interaction between the environment and the individual.

When the National Health Service was established in 1948 it inherited around 3000 hospitals and clinics of enormously varied standards. Development or conversion of these Crown services was slow and underfunded; therefore even today there are many hospitals which still occupy outdated buildings that are located on crowded sites with little space for expansion (Rogers & Salvage 1988).

In many hospitals change is continuous. Something is always in the process of being added, remodelled or moved. Very little of this kind of change occurs within the frame of any sort of long-range plan. The result is that the functions of departments are split and fragmented and spaces are unsuited to their function (Allen et al 1976). It can be argued that the age of the buildings need not itself be a problem, but regular renovation is necessary in order to keep pace with modern needs. Regular maintenance and repairs are also matters of good housekeeping in keeping the environment fit for up-to-date practice.

The Department of Health and the Welsh Office (1990) maintains that adult acute care wards are the largest single element in a hospital. Therefore their design, grouping and relationships with diagnostic treatment and service departments are major influences on the form of the whole hospital. It is also suggested that surgical wards should have easy access to the operating theatres and the intensive care unit. It is argued that there are advantages in grouping wards together according to specialty as they can share accommodation and equipment, and management can be easier and more responsive to changing needs.

In a 'patient-focused environment' staff and services are organised around the care needs of the client group. The main concept behind this approach is the decentralisation of the delivery of care to the specific team or teams looking after the client group. However, one of the major disadvantages of this approach to designing the environment of care is that the cost of capital equipment, e.g. X-ray, ultrasound, etc., may not be affordable and may not prove to be cost-effective when measured against the growing and dynamic changes made in technology and medical science (Partridge et al 1991, RCN 1994).

Lighting

Aspect, view and sunlight are matter of first importance to the sick

(Nightingale 1859)

Modern building design sometimes favours environments with little or no natural light, while old buildings are often dark and obscured from daylight by other building near by (Rogers & Salvage 1988). Rooms that are likely to be occupied for any length of time by patients need to have neutral light. Subsequently, although internal rooms may contribute to economy in the planning stages of a new unit, because they require artificial lighting and mechanical ventilation, capital and running costs are increased. Lighting should be sufficient and suitable, whether natural or artificial. Many lighting problems can be solved through good design and better equipment (DoH and the Welsh Office 1990). It can be argued that natural light is more soothing than artificial light and everyone likes to see out of a window, which provides a visual link with the outside world.

The decor should be light and pleasant with natural lighting being essential to the well-being of the patients. Sunlight enhances colour and shape and helps to make a room bright and cheerful.

In general, a mixture of artificial and natural light is best for staff and patients. The design of windows in a unit must meet the various demands of the rooms they are required for. In addition to the diverse statutory requirements, the following aspects also demand consideration:

- illumination and ventilation
- insulation against noise
- thermal insulation
- the prevention of glare
- the provision of a visual link with the outside world (DoH and the Welsh Office 1990).

Surroundings are attractive to people if they appeal to their senses; that is, if they enjoy looking at them, if they touch them with pleasure and if the atmosphere is fragrant or free from disagreeable odours and free from attention-getting noise.

Whether people are conscious of it or not, the design or arrangement of a room contributes to its harmony. Balance or symmetry should be a guiding principle and is sometimes achieved through the use of contrasting colours in curtains, screens and furniture. Colour can influence the morale of patients and staff and can be used to help patients to orient themselves and to recognise particular rooms more quickly. Biley (1993) contends that colour may influence the promotion of relaxation or activity. However, it is also important to take into account that accurate assessment of the colour of a patient's skin is of clinical importance, therefore surface colours should not distort the colour rendering of light sources.

Good illumination is indispensable to good nursing and to the safety of both nurses and patients. The goal should be to get enough light at the right location to perform the tasks necessary without subjecting the patient to uncomfortable brightness. Provision should be made to prevent glare, as contrasts in brightness are uncomfortable. Glare can be reduced by attention to the detail of window design and can be controlled by curtains or blinds.

Adequate lighting is essential for efficient sight. Sufficient lighting should be provided for all activities performed in the area. Poor lighting leads not only to mistakes and lower efficiency but also to poor health for patients and staff. Consideration needs to be made of safety and accident prevention (Rogers & Salvage 1988).

Noise

Unnecessary noise or noise that creates an expectation in the mind, is that which hurts a patient

(Nightingale 1859)

According to Synder-Halpern (1985) noise is defined simply as unwanted sound that can cause stress fatigue or loss of concentration. Almost unconsciously the nurse may become used to a noisy ward or department. However, with some thought much of the disruption could easily be prevented, reduced or confined to specific times.

Topf (1992) states that the psychological annoyance of noise arises from various factors such as intensity and frequency. Since one person's reaction to sounds may be negative and another's positive, noise-induced subjective stress has been defined not as the objective decibel level, but as individually different annoyance due to sound. The inability to control stress resulting from noise creates a sense of helplessness and hopelessness. Unpredictable and uncontrollable sound levels have been described as being more stressful compared to those under control (Topf 1992).

Voice levels, working with and using equipment, environmental noises caused by telephones, patient call systems, etc., visitors and the heightened sensitivity of the hospitalised patient are noise stressors that may be potentially detrimental to health and sufficient to extend illness (Topf 1992).

Careful consideration should be given to ensuring a quiet environment for patients. Sounds from utility rooms should be isolated and absorbed at source where possible with acoustic materials. Noise should be reflected and reduced by the use of soft floor coverings, curtains and other materials. Nurses can introduce practical measures; for example they should wear quieter footwear, place the telephone on a gentler tone and encourage the use by other patients of headphones with television and radio sets (DoH and the Welsh Office 1990).

On the other hand, a ward can be too quiet. Quiet, like other therapeutic activity, may be frightening or depressing and must therefore be used with discretion and consideration for the individual's needs. Indeed a low level of background sound can assist in maintaining some degree of privacy (Topf 1992).

Noise and sleep disturbance

Individuals may have difficulty achieving and maintaining a sleep state in a noisy unfamiliar environmental setting. In such a setting, noise will arouse an individual sufficiently to prevent relaxation and sleep. It is important that patients in hospital obtain good quality and length of sleep especially after surgery. Sleep is thought to conserve energy and restore the body and brain after the day's wear and tear (Haddock 1994).

Patients may suffer sleep disturbances due to changes in the environment, temperature and diet. Other factors affecting sleep include anxiety, depression, respiratory difficulties, pain and noise (Closs 1988). Patients who have had surgery may suffer a more specific sleep deprivation due to the effects of anaesthesia, narcotics, postsurgical stress and postoperative nursing interventions (Irwin 1992). If sleeplessness is a common problem for hospital patients which nurses fail to take seriously, then there is some cause for concern. The nurse is in a unique position to facilitate and enable adequate rest and sleep, not only because of high levels of contact with patients at night, but also because the nurse is often the culprit when it comes to high levels of noise and activity at night (Duxbury 1994). Activity that may sometimes be unnecessary could, with a little forethought and sensitive nursing care, be either reduced or not undertaken at all (Duxbury 1994).

Reflective point

Consider strategies you could introduce to further reduce noise for the patients in your area from both staff and the environment generally.

Time

Time plays a very important part in the psychological aspect of the environment of care. An individual's perception of time is affected by many variables. It varies for each individual from one situation to another, depending on age, level of anxiety and the role in a given situation (Henderson & Nite 1978). It is important to remember that the measurement of time is not the same for the patient, the nurses, visitors or other members of the multidisciplinary team, but nevertheless it is equally as important for each.

Time and the passage of time may be disturbed by any illness, especially when patients are forced to give up their usual routine and activities. Consequently, when hospitalisation is necessary, the artificiality of the hospital routine accentuates and distorts time. For patients this timeless quality is emphasised by rising early in the morning, the absence of clocks, calendars and current literature, and by their isolation from the daily routines of the outside world (Henderson & Nite 1978).

However, the passage of time can be helped with new and sophisticated nurse call and communication systems now available. Some of these systems have a dual function in allowing communication between nurse and patient but also incorporate such aspects as cable television and nationwide access to radio stations. The units are provided as a console on a swing arm which can be rotated around the bed space. Communication is via a telephone line which allows the patient to telephone the nurses' console. Outside calls can also be made and incoming calls received. These systems may have a charge for such aspects as the cable television and telephone calls but they do enable patients to keep in contact with relatives and significant others even when confined to bed. Patients therefore have some control over the use of equipment and how they maintain contact with their outside world.

According to Peplau (1955) loneliness (or lonesomeness) is a common experience. It implies being without the company of others but recognising a wish to be with others. Loneliness can occur when an individual is isolated or it can be felt despite proximity to others in a group. It is an individual psychological state, but remains a social phenomenon because it is related to the interactions of human beings. Stated simply, it is the result of being separated from loved persons and things. It is an unwelcome feeling of a lack of companionship and a wish for interaction different from that being experienced. It takes on individual characteristics and can manifest itself differently in different persons (Francis 1980).

This concept of loneliness (or lonesomeness) is particularly important for ill patients who need to remain in hospital for some time after the surgical procedure. It could be argued that the less acutely ill patients are, the more lonely they become as there is a risk that the nurse–patient contact time could decrease. At this stage patients may begin to feel alienated and powerless within the acute care setting. The ward routine may accentuate the loss of control and contact with the outside world.

Personal space and the culture of mixed wards

Each person has a way of finding some kind of space for his or her own use and everyone tries to create a space no-one else invades. Henderson & Nite (1978) describe the distances that human beings keep between themselves and others as 'body buffer zones'. These zones vary with each individual and may be affected by circumstances such as mood and social setting. They may also be culturally determined. Body buffer zones are also related to the need to interact with each other as well as the need for privacy. The way in which space is arranged and organised largely determines and controls the kinds of activities and behaviour that take place within it. Certain activities are unlikely when the arrangement of space is not optimum (Henderson & Nite 1978).

The issues surrounding the use of mixed beds units are pertinent in the present climate of the Health Service. It can be argued that the philosophy of the introduction of mixed-sex wards was born from the need to increase economic productivity and produce a faster turnover of bed usage (RCN 1993). At the onset it was usual for the ward to be split into two halves, male and female; as time progressed, this became male and female bays. In Nightingale-style wards without a partition, men may be placed on one side of the ward and women on the other. Eventually the situation deteriorated into mixed bays and patients being placed wherever a bed was available (Nursing Standard 1994). The needs of the individual were never taken into account, and patients, some of whom had waited years for elective surgery, did not feel strong enough to complain about such a situation or understand the procedure by which they might choose to do so. All intentions of respecting the patient's right to privacy and dignity seem to have been forgotten in the rush for economic viability.

On the other hand, with the high profile of the Patient's Charter (DoH 1991a) and consumer organisations, the issue of mixed-patient wards has again been highlighted as an area of concern by a growing number of complaints made to Patients Associations (Nursing Standard 1994). However, according to Burgess (1994), who undertook a review of the literature and research studies looking at the issue of mixed-sex wards, this concept appears to be acceptable to the majority of patients. Despite adverse publicity, mixed bays, especially those of a bay design and those with separate bathroom and toilet facilities were not a matter of high priority for patients. According to the Nursing Standard (1994) there is an argument for mixed-sex wards in that they aim to provide an environment which presents a 'normal lifestyle' for patients. However, this can be disputed because it can be maintained that being in an environment where the patient has had or is about to experience a surgical intervention does not lend itself to a 'normal lifestyle'.

The research shows that admission to an unfamiliar hospital environment is a time of anxiety for most patients (Wilson Barnett 1988). Consequently, it could be argued that clients finding themselves in the environment of a mixed ward could have increased stress and anxiety levels. Subsequently during a period of illness and vulnerability it can be more restful and supportive to be in a single-sex environment (RCN 1993).

Accordingly, it is suggested that patients should not be pressured to accept a mixed-sex ward on the grounds that single-sex facilities are not available and admission will otherwise be delayed. Mixed-sex wards should be modified to provide privacy for washing, sleeping and toilet facilities and alternatives should be available for anybody unhappy within a mixed-setting environment (See also Ch. 20).

Technology and patient care

Surgery generally has an intensive psychological impact on patients and, whatever the reason for surgery, when patients come to the surgical unit they have a need for emotional support (Kneedler & Parsons 1987). Evolving technology enables frequent and accurate monitoring of a patient's condition but, it is argued by Mann (1992), may distract attention from the patient's needs. It is maintained that the increased use of technical equipment may cause conflict between the 'art of nursing' and the 'science of technology'.

However, with the increased use of technology in providing surgical care many more patients in the surgical unit have now to compete with bedside technology for personal space and emotional support. The use of electronic monitoring (e.g. oxygen saturation, parenteral feeding, syringe pump drivers) leads to a perception of immobilisation and confines patients to their bed space, potentially heightening their feelings of anxiety, loneliness and powerlessness. Halm & Alpen (1993) consider that this increase in technology may evoke further fear and anxiety in patients and significant others. In an area where there is much technology it is claimed that this may also lead to depersonalisation. It is further argued that technology does have the potential to dehumanise the nurse–patient relationship, but it is the nurse's responsibility not to see the patient as just a collection of medical information.

The physical impact of bedside technology brings together all the aspects of the environment of care so far discussed. Consequently, the patient perceives that the lights are constantly on as the nurse needs lighting in order to undertake a physiological assessment. There may be constant disruption in the bay or in a specific area because of the sound of alarms or the high noise levels attributed to machinery. Patients' sleep patterns are disturbed and patients' personal space is invaded by machinery, intravenous lines and monitoring wires. It is important that the nurse educates the patient and family members as to the need for the technology, its purpose and its function. This may help to address concerns and also decrease feelings of anxiety and helplessness. Nurses need to acknowledge that the more technological the environment becomes the more important it is to respond to individual human needs (Curtin 1984).

Transportation

For many surgical patients, trips for investigative procedures and the journey to the operating room are events that may cause them to confront the reality of their illness. This has been described by one patient as 'going to the gallows' (Parry 1995) (see Ch. 15). It is therefore not surprising that patients at these times feel vulnerable and helpless.

Corridors in hospitals are not part of a controlled environment and have a tendency to be chaotic. Patients are aware of the frenzied activity around them and subjected to loud and frightening noises. In such situations it is imperative for the nurses to support patients.

According to Phippen (cited in Kneedler & Dodge 1987), an important goal of transportation is patient safety, particularly if the patient has had premedication and may be suffering from altered physiological conditions, for example weakness, confusion and sedation. Ideally, a nurse should accompany each patient who leaves the department in a chair or on a trolley, especially if the patient is about to undergo an invasive procedure. This provides for continuous monitoring by the nurse and assures continuity of care and communication between departments.

Communicating with the patient is an important transportation goal. Often, however, the porter and the nurse may get caught up in the technical details of the task and the more human elements of this patient care activity can be ignored. Appropriate use of therapeutic touch and nonverbal communication can convey a feeling of being in a safe environment.

However, the process of transporting the patient to and from the surgical unit is often viewed as trivial and a chore by nursing staff, particularly if the workload and skill mix are uneven. More and more often, the ideal of the nurse accompanying the patient is becoming impracticable to achieve, and the role of patient escort is therefore delegated to the least skilled worker; and yet this is at a time when the patient requires skilful nursing attention.

From the perspective of equipment, patient trolleys must be equipped with working brakes and side rails that can easily be elevated or lowered. There also need to be attachments for placing intravenous stands, and for transporting the patient having oxygen therapy, a device that will secure the cylinder is essential. Another requirement for a trolley is the capability of placing the patient in Trendelenburg's and sitting positions with controls that are easy to operate and within quick reach (Phippen, cited in Kneedler & Dodge 1987).

The patient's bed is another possible means of transportation, especially if the patient is unable to be transferred easily. When using a bed for transportation, manoeuvrability is an important consideration. Unfortunately hospital beds are notorious for having small wheels that become locked in crevices. The brakes often do not work and the mechanism for adjusting the height is sometimes fixed in the lowest position which makes lifting and handling very hazardous. In units where patients' beds are used as the main mode of transportation to and from operating departments, routine preventive maintenance is essential.

When transferring a patient from one department to another it is important to ensure that all connections for intravenous infusions, catheters and chest drains are secure and tight. It is also important to check that the patient is not lying on tubing and that it is not kinked. Intravenous infusions containers need to be elevated to prevent a backflow of venous blood into the tubing (Phippen, cited in Kneedler & Dodge 1987).

Often while transferring patients, catheter bags are placed on the trolley and covered with a blanket to prevent embarrassment for the patient. However, this is a poor technique which may lead to reflux of urine into the tubing. This will become a source of potential urinary tract infection. All catheters and drainage tubes must be free from kinks and the drainage bag hung on the side of the trolley during transportation (Winn 1996).

Patients with chest drains should always be accompanied by a nurse who is competent in the management of chest drains. The basic principle is to keep the chest bottle below the level of the chest and the tubes connected at all times (Campbell 1993). If the bottle is elevated above the level of the chest fluid, the fluid may reflux into the pleural space eventually leading to a mediastinal shift (Campbell 1993). Two chest drain clamps must be readily available in case of tube disconnection or accidental breakage of the chest drain bottle, thereby allowing the pleural tube to be clamped off quickly and prevent a renewed pneumothorax and subsequent collapse of the lung. However, these clamps should not be left on for long periods as a tension pneumothorax can develop (Campbell 1993).

The operating suite

The operating department should be isolated from the main stream of corridor traffic in the hospital. The

Reflective point

Consider the ways that patients are transferred between departments in your unit. Are there specific reasons for the methods used or is it that no-one has questioned this aspect before?

How do you implement your lifting and handling policy when transferring patients onto trolleys or into chairs?

How do you protect your patients' dignity when transferring them between beds, trolleys and chairs?

suite should be adjacent to the recovery rooms and in an area easily accessible to central supply, pathology, radiology, blood bank and critical care areas. The flow of traffic should be such that contamination from outside the area is excluded and within the area the separation of clean and contaminated areas should exist. The three main areas of the operating department are the anaesthetic room, the operating theatre and the recovery unit (Aitkenhead & Smith 1990).

Anaesthetic room

Anaesthetic rooms are the norm in the UK but not in many other countries. An anaesthetic room allows for a quiet area for induction of the patient. It is a more appropriate environment for the patient who is usually already vulnerable and anxious. It is also a less terrifying experience for the patient than lying on the operating table and having to listen to and observe preparations which may be still occurring (Yentis et al 1995).

The anaesthetic room is designed to support the patient awaiting surgery. Consequently the area should be quiet and restful. It should be away from the mainstream traffic in the department and should provide privacy and seclusion. It should not be used as a short cut into the operating theatre when patients are present, and talk and noise should be kept to a minimum (Groah 1990).

Having an anaesthetic room also allows for an increased throughput in the operating department, as one anaesthetist can be beginning the anaesthetic while another is taking the previous patient off the table.

Although generally speaking the use of a separate anaesthetic room is advisable, there are times when high-risk patients may be induced on the operating theatre table to keep the delay between the onset of unconsciousness and the start of the operative procedure to a minimum. It also prevents the discontinuation of monitoring equipment during transfer.

According to Aitkenhead & Smith (1990), the design of the anaesthetic room should allow for easy access all around the patient trolley and should provide space for anaesthetic and monitoring equipment. It is suggested that a floor space of 21 m² is appropriate. There should also be adequate storage space in cupboards and shelves so that the equipment being used during induction of anaesthesia may be stored in a readily accessible manner. The work top must be of sufficient size to allow for preparation of the anaesthetic.

Piped gases and suction and electrical sockets should be available near the head of the patient trolley. An anaesthetic machine, mechanical ventilator and appropriate breathing system and invasive monitoring systems are also necessary. It is also vital to have available a selection of suction tubes, bronchial catheters and connection tubing. Other vital equipment includes:

- intubation equipment, laryngoscopes with a standard and long blade, a selection of endotracheal and nasopharyngeal tubes of various sizes
- laryngeal masks
- anaesthetic face masks
- a selection of anaesthetic drugs
- emergency resuscitation equipment and drugs
- facilities for the administration of intravenous fluids (Yentis et al 1995).

The operating theatre

Aitkenhead & Smith (1990) maintain that a modern theatre should incorporate the following features:

- measures to ensure the safety of patients and staff
- services for anaesthetic and surgical equipment
- environmental controls to reduce the risk of airborne infection
- artificial lighting appropriate for the requirements of both the surgeon and anaesthetist.

In addition, provision should also be made for preparing instrument trolleys, cleaning dirty instruments and scrubbing up.

The standard operating room is rectangular or square in shape and should provide floor space of approximately 45 m². Rooms designed for cardiac surgery and neurosurgery which require additional equipment will require more floor area. Those designed for day surgery and endoscopy will require less.

The finish for floors, walls and ceilings should be fire resistant, hard, smooth and non-porous so that these surfaces are easy to clean and do not readily permit adherence of bacterial particles. If possible, the surfaces should be as free as possible of seams, joints and crevices, for the above reasons. Traditionally, cool pastel colours have been used to paint the walls. There is no special requirement of colour, except that it be free from glare, and recently a wide variety of warmer colours have been introduced (Groah 1990).

Daylight per se is not necessary in the operating theatre although it is more pleasant for staff if windows are present. The level of illumination of general lighting in theatre is vital to both the anaesthetist and the surgeon, as an appreciation of the skin colour is affected by the spectrum of the source of illumination. As a high level of illumination is required over the operating table, specific ceiling-mounted lamps are standard.

It is important that the temperature in the theatre and anaesthetic room is high enough to reduce the chances of the patient developing hypothermia; this is particularly important in paediatric surgery and operations on the elderly. However, the temperature also needs to be comfortable for the theatre staff. Temperatures of 22–24°C are normally acceptable in the operating room with a relative humidity of 50% (± 10%).

There has been considerable controversy regarding the risk to theatre staff from atmospheric pollution by anaesthetic gases and vapour. However, according to Aitkenhead & Smith (1990), none of these problems have been substantiated by randomised trials. Nevertheless, government guidelines recommend the use of a scavenging system and it is deemed sensible to minimise the level of atmospheric pollution in the operating department.

When designing new departments, the storage facilities should exceed the current requirements and be located throughout the suite. The need for storage space is frequently underestimated and therefore large pieces of equipment, for example image intensifiers and laser machines, occupy the corridors. It is important to take into account that rapidly changing technology will ultimately produce new equipment requiring additional space.

A reliable communication system is also an essential prerequisite in the operating theatre. Dependable communication links with the reception area and the recovery unit are important. As well as the telephone link, an auxiliary intercom system can also provide links between the theatres, recovery rooms, reception and other areas.

The recovery unit

According to Dodge et al (1987), it is important in the recovery period that each patient has an optimal physical and psychological environment. This includes proper emergency and monitoring equipment and provisions for continuous physical safety and emotional comfort.

The early 1940s saw the development of the recovery unit. Before recovery areas became common, postoperative patients were returned to an annex of the ward where a trainee nurse would observe the patient and help to forestall any complications (Pipkin 1991). This procedure could often last for days. Moreover, the policy of isolating these patients was often not to facilitate their recovery but to prevent other patients having to witness the trauma of pain, vomiting and death (Pipkin 1991).

The recovery unit developed because the types of anaesthetic agents developed during the war years allowed operative procedures to become more complex (Pipkin 1991).

The first recovery unit was opened in 1942 in the USA by the eminent anaesthetist Dr Lunday at the Mayo Clinic. The first recovery unit to be opened in the UK was in Birmingham by Dr Flemming in 1955.

The ideal site for a recovery unit is within the operating department and close to the theatres themselves. This enables the anaesthetists to have ready access to the patients in the recovery room and for the recovery staff to have medical help immediately available. It also reduces to a minimum the risks involved in transporting unconscious patients long distances.

The ideal number of recovery bays depends on the number of operating rooms being served and the type of surgery undertaken (Eltringham et al 1985). In general, an average of 1.5 bays per theatre is recommended, but this may be increased where the turnover of operations is faster.

The immediate post-anaesthetic phase presents multifaceted challenges that require special clinical expertise to assure the return of patients to physiological homeostasis equivalent to or improved over their preoperative state. It is important that patients have continuous individual care in this unit until they are able to maintain their own airway.

Each trolley space needs to have the following basic equipment:

- a suction unit with a variety of suction catheters including a Yankeur suction catheter and disposable bronchial suction catheters in varying sizes
- an oxygen outlet with a working flow meter and humidifier – disposable oxygen face masks with

tubing for attachment to the oxygen supply should also be available
- external monitoring for vital signs and oxygen saturation levels
- adequate lighting
- an emergency call system easily activated from each bed space.

Other important accessories are tissues, vomit bowl, gauze and non-allergenic tape. There also has to be appropriate space for nursing documentation to take place. Furniture that takes up minimum floor space allows for easier cleaning and better access to the patients. It is also important that attention is given to each patient's privacy and dignity in large open areas of care.

Scavenging systems are now widely used in operating departments but their introduction to the recovery area has been slow (Eltringham et al 1989). It is possible that high concentrations of anaesthetic gases are being exhaled by the patient during the early stages of recovery when the recovery staff must, of necessity, remain in close proximity to the patient's airway. It is suggested that further research is needed to determine the requirement for active scavenging in the recovery unit. However, atmospheric pollution can be reduced and working conditions improved by the provision of good ventilation and possibly air conditioning.

Recovery care centres

As technology changes the face of surgical procedures, the concept of postsurgical recovery care centres may be developed further in this country as the need for fast turn-over surgery continues to grow. This innovation is developing in the USA where day surgery is very popular (Carr & Webster 1991).

The postsurgical recovery centre is a special health care facility designed for generally healthy patients who require nursing care and pain control in an overnight environment. The concept is to provide an integrated facility of surgery and overnight care in a non-hospital environment. The recovery care centre is designed to provide a friendly environment that is sensitive in meeting the needs of clients and their families. The design reflects a calm and friendly atmosphere and there are facilities for relatives to stay overnight with patients and participate as 'care partners'. It is argued that these centres provide an excellent opportunity to maintain a more personal, private, comfortable and non-institutional environment.

THE CHANGING ROLE OF NURSING IN THE ENVIRONMENT OF THE OPERATING DEPARTMENT

Figure 14.2 illustrates a number of interacting factors impinging on the role of the nurse within the operating theatre.

There are many changes under way in the health care delivery system which have guided nurses to inspect and closely define their nursing role, using nursing concepts and theories. Consequently, as the fundamental ideas about nursing care are changing, so it is time to question the attitudes, beliefs and values of the role of the nurse in the operating department.

In the past, nursing in the operating department was viewed as an isolated aspect of nursing practice. The perception has developed that the nurse is subject to the surgeon's/anaesthetist's wishes and is a technician, who is interested in the handling of 'high-tech' instruments and equipment but has very little to do with 'hands-on' patient care. This picture presents an image of nursing practice that is highly technical and committed to task allocation rather than responsive to patient care (Fennell 1989).

Many practising nurses in the operating department were educated before the developments in nursing theory and accordingly may feel devalued by a definition of professional nursing, which seems foreign to them (Smith 1990). It is also possible that there is a discrepancy between what theatre nurses see as the 'ideal and academic' world of contemporary nursing practice, as portrayed by nursing education, and what they perceive as the 'real' world of the day-to-day care they provide.

Changes in practice

Innovation implies that there has been a change in the status quo as a result of creativity. This change may be a new product or service, or a way of doing something (Manion 1993). Specialist and advanced practice as a nursing innovation in the operating department are new ways of defining the developments in skills and levels of nursing expertise needed to practise in this area in the present health care environment. Before such innovations can become a reality in nursing practice there needs to be a culture which supports and values the innovation (Manion 1993).

Nursing practice should no longer consist of ritualistic actions, the nurse carrying out tasks without thinking them through in a problem-solving, logical and critical way. All nurses in the operating department need to do more than just understand and describe care, they need to be able to analyse and evaluate that care and make changes as and when appropriate. There needs to be a theory of why and how nursing is carried out in order to make predictions of what is good nursing practice for each

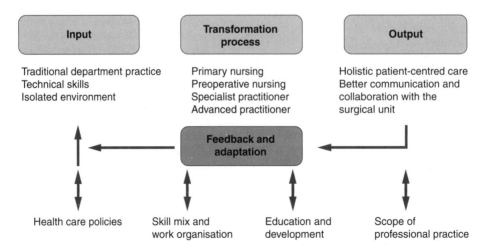

Figure 14.2 The changing role of the theatre nurse.

patient (Binnie 1990). Hunt & Evans (1994) suggest that as the amount of knowledge becomes too complex for a profession, so it will divide into new sub-disciplines, and new occupations may emerge as sub-disciplines. It is therefore unwise to consider any profession as a static entity with closed boundaries as this may impinge on innovation, change and development.

As regions look at skill mix and the development of the role of multidisciplinary practitioners, nurses in the operating department need to define what they believe nursing to be. Nurses do not have the monopoly on skills and caring, and there are many other members of the multidisciplinary team who also care. Therefore, if caring is to be seen as something specific to nursing, professional caring needs to be demonstrated, described and analysed (Dunlop 1986).

The introduction of the economic market into the health service has been accompanied by greater emphasis on unit labour costs and the need to determine skill mix. In order to examine the potential for reducing nursing budgets, managers are looking to replace highly qualified nursing staff with operating department practitioners, less-qualified nurses and health care assistants. The purpose of skill mix seems to relate the effectiveness of assorted skills from a range of grades to delivering either quality or cost-efficient care or both. Operating department nursing finds itself in the position of facing the critical choice of promoting innovation and change in relating skill- and grade-mix issues to the practice of professional nursing while demonstrating nursing worth, or being replaced, albeit slowly and insidiously, by another more cost-effective occupational group. Manion (1993) describes this type of position as a choice between chaos and transformation.

There have been several attempts in both the British and American literature to try to transform and prescribe a role for nursing in the changing environment in which surgery takes place. Even so, within this aspect of the speciality of surgical nursing, a common role and definition of the changing role of nursing seems to be elusive.

Fennell (1989) asserts that initially nurses gained status from working with the surgeon and anaesthetist, who came to rely on a highly technically trained nurse. This, coupled with an increased knowledge of asepsis, which created a secluded and isolated environment, led to nurses in the operating department becoming isolated from other aspects of patient care and other nursing colleagues.

The technical role

During the 1940s there was a severe shortage of staff in the operating department. In order to overcome this shortage, the grade of operating department assistant was introduced. It was intended that this grade would relieve nurses of the technical aspects of work in the department and allow them to concentrate on patient care. However, McGee (1991) maintains that nursing in the operating department still appears to be firmly committed to task allocation and policies and procedure, with the emphasis being operation centred, not patient centred. Baxter (1987) argues that there is a definite role for the nurse in the operating department but also claims areas of interchangeability in the assistant to the surgeon/anaesthetist role and the circulating role. Carrington (1991) describes the function of the theatre nurse as a person with complex technical knowledge which is required in the care and maintenance of instruments and procedures to preserve a safe environment for the patient. It is indicated that the nurse has advanced technical expertise which is necessary for the rotation of stocks and supplies and the selection of appropriate instruments and sutures. Carrington also contends that part of the nurse's role is to maintain a calm and mature attitude when the surgeon encounters periods of stress. It is also important that the nurse is able to concentrate and anticipate during long operations.

The Bevan Report (NHSME 1989) examined the role of the nurse in the operating department as part of a larger study concentrating on the utilisation of operating departments in general. The results of this descriptive survey study were that all nurses, in the anaesthetic room and operating theatre, and operating departments assistants, were interchangeable and should be trained together and become known as operating department practitioners. The inability to make competencies explicit to nursing practice is also demonstrated by other authors (Holden 1992, Wicker 1987) and in reality there is still no real clarification of the role.

Holden (1992), working with the recommendations of the Bevan Report (NHSME 1989), asserts that there is no specific role for the theatre nurse, and claims that all grades of staff should agree on a core educational series. Developing the role of the operating department practitioner is seen as a practical answer to the staffing needs in this environment. Taking the technical role further, Curry & Poole (1991) and Wicker (1991) argue that the next logical step for nurses working in the operating department is to perform surgery as a surgeon's assistant. This would be seen as a progression of the nurse's role towards advanced practitioner and has now been taken as the way forward for nursing in anaesthetics with discussions, at present, on the role of the nurse anaesthetist. However, nurses need to examine this development in the light of the 'Scope of Professional Practice' (UKCC 1992).

The perioperative role

Caring can be seen to be central to effective nursing practice (Leininger 1988). The operating department is an environment that values technology and thus skilful and compassionate caring may be overlooked (see Ch. 7). As a result the nurse may be carrying out procedures on the patient rather than with the patient (Dunlop 1986). Raatikainen (1989) contends that nurses in a technical environment may view the patient as an object and, as such, regard the individual as lacking the ability to feel pain, fear and distress. Often nursing in this context is determined by the medical model of care, and lack of time can reduce nursing practice to the delivery of technical tasks. Care in this environment tends to be limited by the assumption that the nurse knows exactly what the outcomes should be and is only concerned with the most efficient ways of achieving these aims (Benner & Wrubel 1989).

According to Meleis (1991), the domain of nursing has both theoretical and practical boundaries, and encompasses knowledge of practice which is based on philosophy, common sense and research findings. Marks-Maran (1992) considers nursing to be a dynamic process where nurses know why they have made nursing care decisions and can account for their action. Nursing practice is seen as sensitive, relevant and responsive to the needs of individual patients (UKCC 1992). The concept of perioperative nursing was developed in the late 1970s by the American theatre nurses as nursing philosophy was being developed and the medical model was beginning to be abandoned (Dodge 1987). In the past, perioperative nursing was defined as the nursing activities performed by the professional operating room nurse during the preoperative, intraoperative and postoperative phases. It is maintained that the contemporary role of the perioperative nurse is patient-oriented, not environment- or surgeon-oriented.

There is an assertion (Dodge 1987) that the perioperative nurse should realise that the patient may need personal contact, information to help cope with fears and anxieties, and explanations other than those provided by medical colleagues. This combines caring and compassion with a professional knowledge base which encompasses the nursing process and a philosophy which increases responsibility to the patient. The perioperative role, according to Kneedler & Dodge (1987), is not for nurses who prefer technical to professional activities (See also Ch. 20).

Towards primary nursing

The National Association of Theatre Nurses (1991) put forward the perspective that nurses should set standards of care, ensure a systematic approach to care and maintain continuity of that care. Accordingly, it is asserted that part of the nurse's role is to coordinate patient care and lead and supervise nursing practice.

Baxter (1987) attributes the provision of physical care, psychological support and a safe environment as specific to operating department practice. The role has also been defined as assessing, planning and evaluating patient care. To assess the patient and plan appropriate care, it is necessary for theatre nurses to observe and collect data with the patient, thereby assessing the patient's psychological as well as physical needs. Wicker (1987) claims that patients' care needs are often not assessed and the nursing care received in the operating department rotates around operations and work routines, not individualised patient care. Accordingly, in order to undertake an assessment, it has been argued that operating department nurses need to leave the theatre environment and learn about patients through pre- and postoperative visits (Dodds 1991, Shaw 1983).

Tudor (1992) portrays the function of the nurse as a primary nurse who accepts a workload, plans care for the individuals in that case group and supervises others, including associate carers, in providing and evaluating that care. The role of the operating department nurse is, therefore, to provide care with the support of others which meets the individual's care needs. It is recognised that to implement such a structure, departments need to consider carefully skill mix and rethink the role of nursing in the department. This concept would fit well with multidisciplinary or nurse-led assessment clinics (see also Ch. 2).

Specialist and advanced practice in the operating department

The role of the specialist practitioner is considered to be broader than that of a nurse working within a general specialty. The professional model of practice underlying the specialist role is concerned with promoting nursing functions which will be of benefit to the patient and family and significant others

(UKCC 1994). This concept of specialisation gives nurses the opportunity to focus on a specific field of nursing, thereby applying a broad range of theories to that field of practice. Specialist practitioners will be developing a clinical nursing role, not a role which is predominantly an expansion of technical skill in favour of the assumption of medical tasks. Specialist practitioners in the operating department will be able to exercise a higher level of clinical judgement and discretion in providing clinical care (Davies & Burnard 1992, Ellis 1992).

Advanced nursing practice is developed by experts who are analytical in their thinking about nursing practice and can use this skill to motivate and improve patient care. They are also able to articulate and describe this way of thinking to others. Therefore, practitioners at this level provide excellence in nursing practice and give a clear sense of direction for other nurses to follow (Calkin 1984, Kappeli 1993).

There has been a great deal of discussion about the role of advanced practice in the UK and especially regarding the role of surgeon's assistant and the development of nurse anaesthetists in the operating department. It has been claimed that nurses seek to increase their status and expertise by emphasising and developing the highly specialised knowledge and skills of science and technology, rather than caring knowledge. It is recognised that technical expertise is necessary and the range of technical expertise will change over time, but the role of the nurse is centrally one which emphasises certain personal skills and qualities of patient care (Ashworth & Morrison 1994, Ford & Walsh 1994).

McKee & Lessof (cited in Robinson et al 1992) argue that if the long hours worked by junior doctors are to be reduced, leading to fewer mistakes and safer treatment for patients, it may be necessary for nurses to assume responsibility for many of the junior doctors' technical tasks. This they claim would provide a safer service for the client and continue to provide holistic care. However, there is no discussion or debate on how handing down medical tasks to nurses could improve and provide holistic care. There is an assumption that competence to practice as a nurse is only concerned with undertaking tasks and that the nurse being able to undertake tasks of a technical nature equals quality care (see Ch. 12).

Advanced practice in the operating department can be viewed in terms of the knowledge, skills and competence needed to perform highly technical tasks. It has already been acknowledged that elements of the nurse's role that were considered areas of nursing care can now be broken down and allocated to a person with the appropriate skills and knowledge (NHSME 1989). Nevertheless, this argument can be seen to be flawed, as it raises concerns that specifically focus only on the technical aspect of the nurse's role. It reduces the special caring quality of nursing and the nurse's ability to blend knowledge, skills, experience and empathy into seemingly effortless clinical practice (Ashworth & Morrison 1994, RCN 1992). Brykczynska (1992) insists that before a nurse can demonstrate professional care, the nurse must be a competent practitioner of nursing. This involves understanding, articulating, and demonstrating care and caring attitudes as a professional nurse. It implies that nursing work involves more than just performing skills and tasks.

As technical roles develop and nurses' and junior doctors' roles merge, it can be argued that nurses should take delegated tasks from medicine in order to advance their own practice (Grimaldi 1990, Holmes 1992). Subsequently, it could be argued that it does not matter who performs the task, provided that the person has been trained for it, is assessed as competent, is acceptable to the patient and achieves the same standards (Ellis 1992).

Advanced practice in operating departments is not about advancing technical roles, however, but about being able to define humanistic and caring ways of providing care for the patients who need a surgical procedure. In order to achieve such nurse-led innovations in practice, nurses need to feel supported and empowered to begin to make the change. If such philosophies are not encouraged within the organisation and nursing work is not seen as being valid and important, then nurses will lack the decision-making powers to enable them to change their practice. To become true advanced practitioners, nurses working in operating departments need to have a united and clear identity. They also need to value the humanistic nature of nursing and develop role models who can demonstrate through theory and research the value of nurse-led advanced practice to operating departments (see Ch. 1).

THE ROLE OF NURSING IN PROVIDING AN ENVIRONMENT TO MEET THE NEEDS OF PATIENTS

The nurse–patient relationship and knowing the patient

Caring in nursing is often viewed as a humanistic process which allows the nurse to respond to the needs of the patient (Leininger 1988). It can be seen to be central to effective nursing practice and can be understood as the human expression of respect and value for the person. Therefore inherent in the notion of caring is the commitment that all individuals have the right to be treated with integrity and dignity (Boykin & Schoenhoffer 1990).

It could be argued that the patient who arrives at hospital for treatment in the surgical unit has no expectation of the nurse apart from a skills-based competence approach to care, which means that the nurse provides the care that is necessary, quickly, efficiently and in a professional manner. This task-oriented pattern of providing care allows for minimal and superficial interaction between the nurse and patient with little space for negotiation and is all that is necessary within this clinical environment (Morse 1991, Ramos 1992).

However, it can also be maintained that one of the characteristics of professional nursing is allowing the patient to be the focus of care. Therefore, the nurse needs to be aware of the concerns of the patient, notice the behaviour of the patient, both verbal and nonverbal, and be mindful of the messages that may be present (Morse 1991).

All that patients want to know to a greater or lesser extent is what is going to happen to them during their stay in the department. It is now generally accepted in nursing that giving patients information relieves anxiety, reduces the patient's need for analgesia and enhances a more rapid recovery (Wilson Barnet 1988). Information-giving is an essential concept in nursing and should be a very important aspect of care for all patients entering the surgical unit either as inpatients or as day surgery clients.

The aim of giving information is to give patients an awareness of what is unfamiliar, making it recognisable and thus less frightening for them (Benner 1984). Therefore, an explanation of the procedures that take place when the patient is admitted for a surgical procedure is a key part of the nurse's role. Information-giving increases patients' understanding about their environment of care, treatment and rehabilitation by giving specific information in a planned and structured way.

There are limits to the amount of information that can be assimilated on one occasion (Goods Reis & Pieper 1990). The nurse also needs to take into consideration the fact that anxiety surrounding admission and surgery may decrease the amount of information that is assimilated by the patient. Benner (1984) contends that if patient teaching is to be effective it must meet the needs expressed by patients themselves. It is valuable to see how patients perceive the problems they may have and to recognise that the nurse's perception may not equal that of the patient. It is also necessary to assess patients' level of understanding and correct any possible misconceptions they may have.

In order for the process to be effective, the nurse needs to use good counselling and interpersonal skills so that the process becomes a two-way exchange of information in which the person feels comfortable to ask questions and does not feel threatened in the environment. Patients need to feel that nurses have time for them and so it is important that nurses sit down with patients, maintain eye contact and actually listen to what patients have to say (Fox 1986) (see also Chs 9 and 10).

Range of approaches available for giving patients information

By understanding what is happening to them, patients have some form of control over their fears and anxieties. However, patients admitted on the day that surgery is performed have a greatly reduced amount of time in which important information can be given to them. The strategies used for giving information and the timing need to be given detailed consideration if information-giving is to be maximally effective for the patient (Haines 1992, Oberle et al 1994).

There are several methods of giving patients information, but the research suggests that whatever method is used the information given should be presented in such a format that it is not haphazard, inconsistent or vague (Rothrock 1989).

Structured versus unstructured

According to Fortin & Kirouac (1976), structured information-giving has been planned and is given in a systematic way. Unstructured information is presented informally to individual patients, there is no format and the level of information given may not be consistent between nurses. Felton et al (1976) suggest that patients who receive information in a structured way assimilate the information better and are able to recall it better.

Group versus individual

King & Tarsitano (1982) imply that people who are taught in groups learn more quickly. Group instruction for patients who are having similar types of surgery has the benefit of providing peer support and encouraging relatives and significant others to take part. However, Hathaway (1986) argues that the concept of individualised patient care does not run congruent with teaching groups of patients. Consequently, it is important to identify each patient's needs and provide information aimed at meeting those needs.

Preadmission booklets/information leaflets

These could be sent to patients with their admission information. It is important that these booklets contain only the type of information that is essential for the patient. They should be clearly set out, easy to read and available in a variety of languages. Written information can be referred to by patients in the days prior to surgery and they can ring the unit if they have questions about the admission (Wallace 1985) (see also Ch. 3).

While planning how to give information to patients it is important for nurses to appreciate that patients need to be treated as individuals who have previous experiences in life that they may be able to bring to the situation (Fox 1986). The nurse needs to provide an environment in which the patient feels at ease, from a physical and psychological point of view. Nurses need to use good counselling and interpersonal skills so that the process becomes a two-way exchange of information. They also need to provide an environment which encourages friendliness, trust and reassurance and allows for two-way communication. This provides a psychological climate which allows patients to feel respected and supported and enables them to ask questions as appropriate (Cupples 1991) (see also Ch. 9).

Collaborative multidisciplinary preadmission clinics

In line with the systems approach to care management discussed earlier, it can be argued that if groups of practitioners work together, the effects of their combined efforts will produce a better outcome than that which would be produced from the mere sum of the individual efforts (Gilbert 1995).

Consequently, a multidisciplinary approach to providing care involves a team with varied skills and specialist knowledge working together to coordinate and provide a comprehensive assessment and information-giving service for all patients undergoing surgery (Fountain 1993).

In order to conserve time and to prevent an overlap of information being given, preadmission education clinics have an important role. Such clinics can involve staff working collaboratively in presenting different aspects of surgical care, e.g. a ward nurse and a nurse from the operating department and a member of the medical team. The benefits are twofold: the time spent providing information would be reduced, and patients would be given the correct information once, instead of having variations of the same theme repeated in several different inconsistent forums. This would also allow lines of communication and feedback to be maintained between the different units providing care, and enable the sharing of information and better continuity of patient care.

Patients attending outpatients appointments can be seen in multidisciplinary preadmission clinics where they would be assessed by medical and nursing staff (Dixon 1994).

It is suggested that the staff in these departments have a shared philosophy of mutual respect, understanding and acceptance of each other's disciplines in order that patients are assessed effectively. Fountain (1993) maintains that there are four important considerations in developing a multidisciplinary team. These are:

- The team needs to have a purpose and develop team goals.
- There need to be agreed standards for excellence in care.
- The goals of the team need to be guided by the needs of the client.
- The whole team needs to be 100% responsible and accountable for success.

According to Øvretveit (1990), the main function of working in a multidisciplinary team is to ensure that the patients get a better service than they would otherwise from one individual perspective. There may be overlap in some of the roles in a multidisciplinary team and consequently efforts must be made to coordinate how team members will function and organise themselves in a collaborative manner. It is important to also remember that each member of the team brings a new and individual perspective about the needs and care provision of the clientele. Fountain (1993) further argues that for a multidisciplinary team to be effective no one person in the team should be seen to be more important than the others in the care being delivered. This may be difficult in a health care system which has a very traditional hierarchical system built on control and routine duties (Engstrom 1986). Each role within the multidisciplinary team has its special and important qualities. Therefore, a multidisciplinary team working together can provide a comprehensive assessment and information-giving service which would utilise the skills of all members of the surgical multidisciplinary team. Figure 14.3 illustrates the members of the surgical multidisciplinary team (see also Ch. 2).

Communication is one of the most important issues relating to collaboration in multidisciplinary work. There should be positive communication and teamwork between disciplines and, if a multidisciplinary care plan is used, information should be collected once

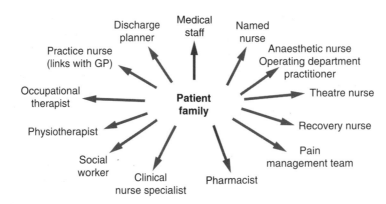

Figure 14.3 Members of the surgical multidisciplinary team (adapted from Fountain 1993).

and not duplicated. Therefore all the information collected about the patient is stored in one specific area (Swann 1994). The medical staff take a patient history and perform a physical examination. They would also check that routine X-ray examinations, blood tests and other investigations have been undertaken. If results are not available, the relevant tests are ordered (Dixon 1994).

On the other hand, nurses assess gaps in areas of care, such as the psychological and social support that the patient may need (Llewellyn 1991). Nurse assessment is concerned with identifying over-anxious patients, the information these patients may need and family support and discharge needs. The nurse also examines the physical assessment of the patient in order to make special note of any circumstances that may be appropriate to perioperative management during the patient's stay in the unit (Swann 1994).

This joint approach to managing the preadmission environment provides a quality, efficient patient- and family-centred service which should, through teaching and planning, reduce the anxiety of patients and their relatives. This process would create an opportunity to begin the planning of the most appropriate perioperative management, including discharge planning and the required follow-up care, if appropriate. The patients could then be given written information to reinforce important points imparted during the session, and which could be referred to by patients in the days prior to surgery (Wallace 1985). During these sessions patients need to be informed of the role of the named nurse in providing any further information they perceive themselves to need as well as providing information about the perioperative period when they come into hospital. This information will also need to be reinforced in any written information given to patients.

Øvretveit (1990) maintains that given the time and skills available, difficult decisions may have to be made about priorities in effectively resourcing multidisciplinary teams, particularly in new ventures. Consequently, setting up preadmission clinics may be difficult in terms of human resources, time, skills and equipment. Teams should be planned, funded, nurtured and regularly reviewed. There needs to be recognition from management, that time must be set aside for staff education and possible training for new competencies. There also needs to be recognition that resources will be necessary for the development of care plans, providing information and contacting patients to attend the clinics. However, Llewellyn (1991) maintains that developing this type of service can be exciting and challenging and help to develop effective working relationships with the ward staff, staff from the operating department and the anaesthetic department (see also Ch. 15).

Reflective point

You could perhaps think about what it means to work collaboratively. How would you recognise it? How is it similar to or different from cooperation? It would be worth brainstorming your own list of indicators of collaboration, then using your list to analyse your own multidisciplinary team for evidence of collaboration.

Additionally, consider the factors which hinder collaboration and those which enhance it within your own team. (See also Ch. 2.)

The Community Care Act (DoH 1991b) is about providing services and support which enable people to live as independently as possible in their community. The arrangements under this Act require local government, the Health Service and the independent sector to work in partnership to assess health needs and provide care, taking account of the views of those for whom they are providing care.

The objective is to provide a service in which the boundaries between primary health care, secondary health care and social care do not form barriers as seen from the perspective of the service user, i.e. the client. In the changing environment of surgical care and with the decrease in the length of stay in the surgical ward, assessment of need and the provision of care in the community are paramount in order to provide continuity of quality care for these patients. Surgical units need to develop greater links with community nurses and general practitioner units in order to break down the barriers of the primary–secondary care interface and provide continuity of care for patients who are being discharged back into the community earlier than ever with little or no social back-up.

The need for collaboration between the acute service provision and the primary health care provision is now greater than ever. The frequency of clinics, the number of hours for which they are held and the type of written information, all need to be evaluated on a regular basis for effectiveness and efficiency. It is suggested that a strategy for evaluation should be developed and the evaluation results should be produced both as qualitative and quantitative data on a regular basis (Rankin & Duffy 1983).

CONCLUSION

By considering the environment of care from a general systems theory perspective it has been possible to examine the physical, social and psychological aspects of care provision for patients during their stay in the surgical unit.

There is no doubt that surgical technology is continuing to develop, making operative procedures quicker and safer, and patient discharge times are constantly being reduced. Consequently, the impact on the role of the surgical nurse is the need to be aware of both the physical and psychological aspects of patient care. This does not just involve aspects of the surgical procedure but also the impact that the physical environment of care has on the patient's psychological and social well-being. One of the aims of the chapter was to explore how open lines of communication could inform nurses about events that take place during the perioperative phase. The concept of collaborative multidisciplinary preadmission clinics is not new, but it is hoped that by discussing them in this forum it can be seen how groups of practitioners could work together to improve communications and produce better outcomes for the patient. This could also be a forum for health care workers to develop an informal networking system, share information and learn from each other.

Although the chapter has been written in separate sections, it is hoped that it has drawn together the individual perspectives on the impact that the physical environment may have on surgical care, and produced an overall picture of surgical nursing related to the environment of care which is greater that the sum of the individual parts.

REFERENCES

Aitkenhead A R, Smith G (eds) 1990 Textbook of anaesthesia, 2nd edn. Churchill Livingstone, Edinburgh

Allen R, Von Karolyi I 1976 Hospital planning handbook. John Wiley, London

Ashworth P, Morrison P 1994 The notion of competence in nursing In: Hunt G, Wainwright G (eds) Expanding the role of the nurse. Blackwell Scientific, London

Baxter B 1987 Staffing of operating theatres – the role of the nurse ATN News (Oct.): 21–24

Benner P 1984 From novice to expert. Addison-Wesley, California

Benner P, Wrubel J 1989 The primacy of caring. Addison–Wesley, California

Bertalanffy L von 1968 General systems theory: foundation, development, applications, revised edn. George Braziller, New York.

Biley F 1993 Creating a healing patient environment. Nursing Standard 8(5): 31–35

Binnie A 1990 The potential of professional practice. Nursing Standard 4(2): 34–37

Boykin A, Schoenhoffer S 1990 Caring in nursing, analysis of extant theory. Nursing Science Quarterly 3(4): 149–155

Brykczynska G 1992 Caring a dying art? In: Jolley M, Brykczynska G (eds) Nursing care : the challenge to change. Edward Arnold, London

Burgess L 1994 Mixed responses. Nursing Times 90(2): 30–34

Calkin J D 1984 A model for advanced nursing practice. Journal of Nursing Administration 1: 24–30

Campbell J 1993 Making sense of underwater sealed drainage. Nursing Times 89(9): 34–36

Carr T, Webster C S 1991 Recovery care centres – an innovative approach to caring for healthy surgical patients. Association of Operating Room Nurses Journal 53(4): 986–995

Carrington A 1991 Theatre nursing as a profession. British Journal of Theatre Nursing 1(1): 5–7

Closs J 1988 Patient's sleep–wake rhythms in hospital. Nursing Times 84(1): 48–50

Cupples S 1991 Effects of timing and reinforcement. Heart and Lung 6(1): 654–660

Curry I, Poole D 1991 The question of the operating department. British Journal of Theatre Nursing 1(7): 4–9

Curtin L 1984 Nursing: high-touch in a high tech world. Nursing Management 15: 7–8

Davies D B, Burnard P 1992 Academic levels in nursing. Journal of Advanced Nursing 17: 1395–1400

Department of Health (DoH) 1991a The patient's charter. HMSO, London

Department of Health (DoH) 1991b Community care in the next decade and beyond. HMSO, London

Department of Health and the Welsh Office 1990 Adult acute wards (4). Health Building Note. HMSO, London

Dixon L 1994 Preadmission clinic in an ENT unit. Nursing Standard 23: 23–26

Dodds F 1991 First class nurses or second class doctors? British Journal of Theatre Nursing 1(9): 6–8

Dodge G 1987 A philosophical approach to perioperative nursing. In: Kneedler J, Dodge G (eds) Perioperative patient care, 2nd edn. Blackwell Scientific Publications, London

Dodge G, Jensen A, Rice H 1987 Immediate post operative care. In: Kneedler J, Dodge G (eds) Perioperative patient care, 2nd edn. Blackwell Scientific Publications, London

Dunlop M J 1986 Is a science of caring possible? Journal of Advanced Nursing 11: 661–670

Duxbury J 1994 Avoiding disturbed sleep in hospitals. Nursing Standard 9(Nov 30): 31–33

Ellis H 1992 Conceptions of care. In: Soothill K, Henry C, Kendrick K (eds) Themes and perspectives in nursing. Chapman and Hall, London

Eltringham R et al 1985 Post anaesthetic room facilities. Association of Anaesthetists of Great Britain and Ireland, London

Eltringham R, Durkin M et al 1989 Post anaesthesia recovery, 2nd edn. Springer-Verlag, London

Engstrom B 1986 Communication and decision-making in a study of multidisciplinary team conference with the registered nurse as conference chairman. International Journal of Nursing Studies 23(4): 299–314

Felton G et al 1976 Pre-operative nursing interventions with patients for surgery: outcome of three alternative approaches. International Journal of Nursing Studies 13: 83–96

Fennell L 1989 But is it nursing? British Journal of Theatre Nursing (Feb): 13–17

Ford P, Walsh M 1994 New rituals for old: nursing through the looking glass. Butterworth Heinemann, London

Fortin F, Kirouac S 1976 A randomized controlled trial of preoperative patient education. International Journal of Nursing 13: 11–24

Fountain M J 1993 Key roles and issues of the multidisciplinary team. Seminars in Oncology Nursing 9(1): 25–31

Fox V 1986 Patient teaching: understanding the needs of the adult learner. Association of Operating Room Nurses Journal 44(2): 234–240

Francis G M 1980 Loneliness: measuring the abstract – II. International Journal of Nursing Studies 17: 127–130

Gilbert T 1995 Nursing: empowerment and the problem of power. Journal of Advanced Nursing 21: 865–871

Goods Reis D, Pieper B 1990 Structured versus unstructured teaching – a research study. Association of Operating Room Nurses Journal 51(3): 1334–1339

Grimaldi C 1990 The nursing science: a need for specialists. In: Lindeman C A, McAthie M (eds) Nursing trends and issues. Springhouse, Pennsylvania

Groah L K 1990 Operating room nursing, 2nd edn. Appleton Lange, Connecticut

Haddock J 1994 Reducing the effects of noise in hospital. Nursing Standard 8(43): 25–28

Haines N 1992 Same day surgery: co-ordinating the education process. Association of Operating Room Nurses Journal 55(2): 573–579

Halm H A, Alpen M A 1993 The impact of technology on patients and families. Nursing Clinics of North America 28(2): 443–455

Handy C 1984 Understanding organisations. Penguin, London

Hathaway D 1986 Effects of pre-operative instructions on post operative outcomes. Nursing Research 35(5): 269–275

Henderson V, Nite G 1978 Principles and practice of nursing, 6th edn. Collier Macmillan Publications, London

Holden J 1992 Theatre opportunities. Nursing Times 88(22): 34, 35

Holmes S 1992 Pioneering assistants. Nursing Times 88(40): 16, 17

Hunt G, Evans W 1994 Health care assistants and accountability. In: Hunt G, Wainwright G (eds) Expanding the role of the nurse. Blackwell Scientific, London

Irwin P 1992 The physiology of sleep. In: McMahon R (ed) Nursing at night. Scutari Press, Harrow

Kappeli S 1993 Advanced clinical practice – how do we promote it? Journal of Clinical Nursing 2: 205–210

King I, Tarsitano B 1982 The effect of structured and unstructured preoperative teaching: a replication. Nursing Research 36(6): 324–329

Kneedler J, Dodge G (eds) 1987 Perioperative patient care, 2nd edn. Blackwell Scientific Publications, London

Kneedler J A, Parsons A 1987 Psychological support. In: Kneedler J, Dodge G (eds) Perioperative patient care, 2nd edn. Blackwell Scientific Publications, London

Leininger M M 1988 Care: the essence of nursing and health. Wayne State University Press, Detroit

Llewellyn J G 1991 Short stay surgery. Association of Operating Room Nurses Journal 53(35): 1179–1191

McGee P 1991 Perioperative nursing: a review of the literature. British Journal of Theatre Nursing (Oct): 12–17

Manion J 1993 Chaos or transformation: managing innovation. Journal of Nursing Administration 23(5): 41–48

Mann R 1992 Preserving humanity in an age of technology. Intensive and Critical Care Nursing 8(4): 240–244

Marks-Maran D 1992 Rethinking the nursing process. In: Jolley M, Brykczynska G (eds) Nursing care – the challenge to change. Edward Arnold, London

Meleis A I 1991 Theoretical nursing: developmental and progress, 2nd edn. J B Lippincott, London

Morse J M 1991 Negotiating commitment and involvement in the nurse patient relationship. Journal of Advanced Nursing 16: 455–468

Moss Jones J 1994 Learning organisations concepts, practices and relevance. NHS Training Directorate Unit, Bristol

National Association of Theatre Nurses (NATN) 1991 A strategy for nursing in the operating theatre. NATN, Harrogate

NHS Management Executive (NHSME) 1989 The management and utilisation of operating departments. (The Bevan Report) HMSO, London

Nightingale F 1859 Notes on nursing … what it is and what it is not. Republished 1980, Churchill Livingstone, London

Nursing Standard 1994 Mixed sex wards: the choice of patients? Nursing Standard 8(33): 32–33

Oberle K, Allen M, Lynkowski P 1994 Follow up of same day patients. Association of Operating Room Nurses Journal 59(5): 1016–1025

Øvretveit J 1990 Making the team work! Professional Nurse 5(10): 284–288

Parry A 1995 The lived experience of day surgery. Unpublished MSc dissertation. Royal College of Nursing, London

Partridge A, Brennan M, Gray N H 1991 Day surgery – making it happen. HMSO, NHS Management Executive, London

Peplau H E 1955 Loneliness. American Journal of Nursing 55(12)

Pipkin I 1991 Evolution of post anaesthesia care. Cited in: Allen A (ed) Core curriculum for post anaesthesia nursing practice. W B Saunders, London

Raatikainen R 1989 Values and ethical principles in nursing. Journal of Advanced Nursing 14: 92–96

Ramos M C 1992 The nurse patient relationship – themes and variations. Journal of Advanced Nursing 17: 46–56

Rankin S, Duffy K 1983 Patient education: issues, principles and guidelines. Lippincott, Philadelphia

Rea C 1995 Clinical directorates. British Journal of Health Care Management 1(4): 213–214

Robinson J, Gray A, Elkan R (eds) 1992 Policy issues in nursing. Open University Press, Milton Keynes

Rogers R, Salvage J 1988 Nurses at risk – a guide to health and safety at work. Heinemann Professional Publishing, London

Rothrock J 1989 Perioperative nursing research: preoperative psychoeducational intervention. Association of Operating Room Nurses Journal 49(2): 597–602

Royal College Of Nursing (RCN) 1992 The value of nursing. RCN, London

Royal College of Nursing (RCN) 1993 Mixed sex wards. Issues in nursing and health (No. 23). RCN, London

Royal College of Nursing (RCN) 1994 Guidance on patient-focused care. Issues in nursing and health. RCN, London

Shaw H 1983 What aspects of the nursing process are applicable in theatre nursing and how can they be implemented? ATN News, May 11–13

Smith M 1990 Nursing practice: guided by or generating theory. Nursing Science Quarterly 34: 147–148

Stichler J 1994 System development and integration in healthcare. Journal of Nursing Administration 24(Oct 10): 48–52

Swann B A 1994 A collaborative ambulatory preoperative evaluation model. Association of Operating Room Nurses Journal 59(Feb 2): 430–437

Synder-Halpern R 1985 The effect of critical care unit noise on patient sleep cycles. Critical Care Quarterly 7(4): 41–51

Topf M 1992 Effects of personal control over hospital noise on sleep. Research in Nursing and Health 15: 19–28

Tudor M 1992 The endangered species. Nursing 5(7): 24–26

United Kingdom Central Council for Nursing, Midwifery and Health Visiting (UKCC) 1992 Scope of professional practice. UKCC, London

United Kingdom Central Council for Nursing, Midwifery and Health Visiting (UKCC) 1994 The future of professional practice – the Council's standards for education and practice following registration. Position statement on policy and implementation. UKCC, London

Wallace L 1985 Surgical patients' preferences for pre-operative information. Patient Education and Counselling 7(4): 377–387

Wicker P 1987 The role of the nurse in theatre. Senior Nurse 7(4): 19–21

Wicker P 1991 Back to the future. Nursing Standard 6(2): 52–53

Wilson Barnett J 1988 Patient teaching – recent advances in nursing. Churchill Livingstone, London

Winn C 1996 Basing catheter care on research principles. Nursing Standard 10(18): 38–40

Yentis S, Hirsch N P, Smith G B 1995 Anaesthesia A to Z. Butterworth Heinemann, Oxford

15

Day surgery

Michèle Malster   Angela Parry

AIMS

The aims of this chapter are:

- to clarify the concept of day surgery
- to increase the surgical nurse's awareness of day surgery
- to highlight the importance of patient selection
- to consider the patient's and carer's perspectives of the day surgery experience.

INTRODUCTION

In recent years there has been a great increase in day surgery in this country and, indeed, internationally. The reader might be forgiven for thinking that the concept of day surgery is new, but the history of day surgery in this country dates from the beginning of this century. Its origin is attributed to James Nicholl, who operated on nearly 9000 children between 1900–1909 in Glasgow, on an outpatient basis. However, it was not until the 1980s that day surgery was 'rediscovered' and began to proliferate into a recognised surgical specialty. This chapter will consider the current state of day surgery, within its history, and the possibilities for the future.

THE CONCEPT OF DAY SURGERY

'A surgical day case is a patient who is admitted for investigation or operation on a planned non-resident basis and who nonetheless requires facilities for recovery. The whole procedure should not require an overnight stay in hospital' (Commission on the Provision of Surgical Services 1992). The term 'day surgery' is commonly used in this country to describe surgery that is performed on a day-care basis, i.e. on average between the hours of 8 a.m. and 6 p.m., following which the patient is discharged home. However, the term 'ambulatory surgery' is also used, particularly in the USA where the 'day' represents

23 hours 59 minutes. This refers to any patient who has had surgery and is discharged within 24 hours. The terms are often used interchangeably.

Day surgery in well-established centres probably accounts for 50% of elective surgery, depending on specialty; for example, the figure is nearer 80% for cataract surgery. The advantages of day surgery are presented in Box 15.1.

The success of day surgery depends on ensuring that the patient is 'street fit' following surgery. There are a number of factors which contribute to this, particularly: the type of surgery, the type of anaesthesia and patient selection.

Type of surgery

Examples of routine operations being performed on a day-care basis are presented in Box 15.2, which also shows the original 'basket' of day surgery procedures deemed suitable by the Audit Commission (1990a). In general, the type of surgery performed on a day-care basis in this country falls within the categories of minor and intermediate. However, increasingly more complex procedures are being undertaken as technological advances in surgery are being made and the scope now far exceeds the Audit Commission's original list. Arguably the main criteria for day surgery are that procedures should:

- not last longer than 60 minutes, although this time is increasing
- not cause excessive blood loss
- not cause excessive postoperative nausea and vomiting (PONV).

Currently, many minor surgical procedures which originally were performed in day surgery centres are being performed in outpatients departments and in GPs' surgeries, e.g. excision of sebaceous cyst, skin tags, small lipoma, etc. This has made way for an expansion in day surgery.

Box 15.1 Advantages of day surgery

- Minimal disruption to normal lifestyle
- Rapid return to familiar surroundings
- Patients like it
- Reduced risk of cross-infection
- Decreased waiting time
- Not dependent upon availability of a hospital bed
- Fixed date for surgery
- Increased numbers of patients treated

Box 15.2 Examples of commonly performed operations in day surgery

General surgery
- Varicose vein stripping and ligation*
- Excision of anal fissure, skin tags, etc.*
- Haemorrhoidectomy
- Excision of pilonidal sinus
- Breast lump excision*
- Excision of lipoma
- Wedge resection of toenail
- Excision of sebaceous cysts
- Hernia repair
  - inguinal*
  - femoral
  - umbilical

Orthopaedics
- Carpal tunnel decompression*
- Excision of ganglion*
- Release of trigger finger
- Bunion surgery
- Excision of exostosis
- Excision of bursa
- Release of Dupuytren's contracture*
- Removal of metalwork:
  - pins
  - plates
  - screws

Gynaecology
- Termination of pregnancy*
- Dilatation and curettage*
- Colposcopy
- Diagnostic and operative laparoscopy*
- Cervical polypectomy
- Excision of Bartholin cyst
- Hysteroscopy
- Intrauterine contraceptive device:
  - insertion
  - removal

Genitourinary
- Circumcision
- Orchidopexy
- Varicocele excision
- Ureteric stent insertion
- Excision of epididymal cyst
- Urethral dilatation
- Vasectomy/reversal
- Cystoscopy*
- Testicular biopsy
- Urodynamic studies
- Excision of hydrocele
- Resection of bladder tumour

Ophthalmic
- Cataract excision and lens implant*
- Correction of strabismus*

ENT
- Submucous resection*
- Adenoidectomy

Box 15.2 (Contd.)

ENT
- Insertion of grommets*
- Myringotomy*
- Tonsillectomy
- Microlaryngoscopy
- Nasal fracture reduction*
- Antral washout

Plastic surgery
- Revision of scar
- Excision of skin lesion

Dental
- Extraction of teeth
- Conservation treatment under general anaesthetic
- Removal of wisdom teeth
- Osseo-integration

Endoscopic procedures
(See Box 15.3)

Day treatment centres may include other non-surgical procedures:

- gastrointestinal endoscopy and procedures
- cytotoxic therapy
- pain management procedures
- haematological treatments

*Included in the Audit Commission's original 'basket' of procedures for day surgery (1990a)

Technological advances in surgery have also enhanced day surgery. These include improved surgical techniques, new suturing materials and endoscopic techniques. New techniques, such as phacoemulsification for cataract removal, have reduced the operating time and enabled greater numbers of patients to be treated using local anaesthesia. Phacoemulsification is a means of chemically dissolving the lens, prior to insertion of an artificial lens, during cataract surgery. New suturing materials such as Vicryl Rapide are absorbable and therefore do not require a visit to the GP's surgery for removal. Surgical techniques via endoscopy are increasing and examples of endoscopic procedures performed as day surgery are presented in

---

Reflective point

Why might the term minimal access surgery be considered more appropriate?
Do you know someone who has had an endoscopic procedure? How did he or she feel afterwards?

Box 15.3. Originally described as 'minimal invasive techniques', endoscopic procedures are now often referred to as 'minimal access surgery' (Johnson 1997).

Originally it was felt that the endoscopic technique, resulting in a smaller incision, would cause less pain and therefore the patient would be able to return to work sooner. However, there is evidence to suggest that this is not so (Johnson 1997). One needs to consider the body's physiological response to surgery and anaesthesia. A patient who has a hernia repaired endoscopically, still requires anaesthesia, has the same operation performed, and undergoes the same physiological stress response – only the size of the wound has changed. It is worth noting that some operations, such as inguinal hernia repair, are reverting back to 'open' surgery, because there is arguably little cost-effective benefit to the patient or the day surgery centre (Lawrence et al 1995, Rudkin & Maddern 1995).

Type of anaesthesia

New anaesthetic agents have made an impact on day surgery; these include the volatile agents desflurane and sevoflurane, which give a faster recovery time (Jones 1990, Nathanson et al 1995). New induction agents for general anaesthesia, such as propofol, promote quicker recovery and reduce the incidence of postoperative nausea and vomiting (PONV) (Carroll & Ogg 1996). PONV is a common problem following day surgery and has been described as 'the big, "little" problem' (Kapur 1991, p. 244). It is distressing for the

---

Box 15.3 Examples of endoscopic procedures undertaken in day surgery

Diagnostic/operative arthroscopy
- Shoulder
- Elbow
- Wrist
- Knee
- Ankle

Laparoscopy
- Diagnostic
- Sterilisation
- Cholecystectomy
- Hernia repairs

Hysteroscopy

Urethroscopy
- Ureteroscopy (± stent insertion)
- Prostatectomy (laser)

patient and failure to manage the problem effectively may well influence the patient's willingness to have further day surgery, if it were necessary. Measures which can be instituted to minimise the risk include:

- avoiding the use of nitrous oxide
- total intravenous anaesthesia (TIVA) thereby avoiding inhalational agents which might precipitate PONV
- pre-emptive anti-emetics
- use of local and regional anaesthetic techniques.

Local and regional anaesthetic techniques are a common alternative to general anaesthesia in day surgery and regional techniques are also useful for providing postoperative analgesia (Raeder 1997). However, discharge criteria may have to be adapted to accommodate the use of regional anaesthesia. For example, patients need to be warned about the lack of sensation, so that they are able to protect the area from any trauma. Patients who have had spinal anaesthesia will need to be warned about the risk of headache, while the ability to pass urine is particularly important following epidural or spinal anaesthesia (Peng et al 1997).

The development and introduction of the laryngeal mask airway (LMA) for airway management has also advanced general anaesthesia for day surgery (Brain 1983). It provides better airway management than the Guedel airway and mask, without the risks associated with endotracheal intubation (Alexander et al 1988), and this will be discussed later.

The most important impact on the success of day surgery is good patient selection. The process of 'pre-assessment' is now widely accepted as essential in promoting patient safety, minimising cancellations on the day of surgery and reducing postoperative hospital admissions.

PRE-ASSESSMENT

The pre-assessment process takes place usually 2–4 weeks prior to surgery and has several functions:

- to assess patient's suitability for day surgery
- to provide the patient and, where possible, the carer with information
- to prepare for discharge
- to identify individual needs.

Who should perform the pre-assessment? The initial decision to refer the patient for day surgery will be made by the patient's clinician. In some areas this may be the general practitioner, but more often it is the clinician in the outpatients department. If the patient is

to have surgery within 4 weeks, and resources permit it, there is no reason why the pre-assessment could not be performed by the patient's clinician. However, it is generally recognised that the nursing staff in the day surgery centre are more ideally suited to assess patients, particularly when the patient may have to wait several months for surgery.

Patient selection aims to ensure that the patient, following day surgery, is 'street fit' prior to discharge. The original criteria for suitability for day surgery suggested by the British Association of Day Surgery (1991) are presented in Box 15.4. However, most established day surgery units are now using these criteria more flexibly in order to optimise patient care.

Originally only ASA Grade 1 patients were deemed suitable for day surgery (see Box 15.5), while at present ASA Grade 3 may be considered suitable. It is more important to consider the welfare of the patient than to adhere rigidly to the set criteria. For example, it may be safer for an immunosuppressed patient to have surgery on a day-care basis, rather than as an inpatient exposed to the risk of nosocomial infection. Flexible use of patient selection criteria may optimise patient safety by causing least disruption to the patient's normal lifestyle.

Reflective point

Which other client groups might benefit from having surgery as a day case, rather than as an inpatient?

You have probably considered well-controlled insulin-dependent diabetic patients as one of your groups, but what about those patients who might well become extremely stressed by a change from their normal environment, such as patients with learning disabilities or the elderly (Davies & Ogg 1993)? Day surgery allows a quick return to normal surroundings and social contacts, as it aids continuity of autonomy and emotional state (Rowe & Kahn 1987).

Box 15.4 Original criteria for suitability for day surgery (British Association of Day Surgery 1991)

- Below age limit of 70 years.
- Fit and healthy patients, ASA grades 1 and 2.
- Exclude procedures where severe postoperative pain and haemorrhage may arise.
- Exclude patients who are obese, diabetic or with chronic respiratory or cardiovascular disease.
- Operations which take longer than 60 minutes should be excluded.
- Food or oral fluids have not been taken for 6 hours prior to anaesthesia.
- Patients must live within a 20-mile radius.
- Patients must be accompanied home.

Box 15.5 The American Society of Anesthesiologists' physical status classification (ASA status) (ASA 1963)

ASA 1	A healthy patient
ASA 2	Mild systemic disease, no functional limitation
ASA 3	Severe systemic disease, some functional limitation
ASA 4	Severe systemic disease, incapacitating and a constant threat to life
ASA 5	Moribund patient not expected to survive for 24 hours with or without operation

It is important that there is a clear framework for the pre-assessment process. In general, the areas of assessment include:

- medical history
- psychological preparation
- socio-domestic situation.

A suggested framework for a patient medical screening questionnaire is provided in Box 15.6. However, this needs to be evaluated in conjunction with the socio-domestic assessment, which will be discussed later. It is important that the selection process is a collaborative process. Consultation with the anaesthetist will assist the nurse in risk assessment for individual patients and optimising safety, together with minimising the risk of cancellation on the day of surgery. The inclusion of lay carers in the pre-assessment interview can:

- enhance the carer's preparation for the role
- allow assessment of the carer's suitability
- clarify the socio-domestic situation
- enhance patient communication
- reinforce patient information.

If the carer is not present at the pre-assessment interview, the nurse is reliant upon the patient giving the carer the relevant information for postoperative care in the form of written information. There is no guarantee that the patient will remember to do this. However, there is another opportunity to ensure that this information is communicated to the carer, albeit rather late, when the patient is discharged following surgery.

The situation described in Case study 15.1 is unusual, but a similar concern for the nurse might be the postoperative care of an elderly patient, by a frail elderly spouse, following cataract surgery (see also Ch. 11). To minimise this problem following day

Reflective point

In general, lay carers are not specifically assessed for their suitability to care for the patient following day surgery. Consider the scenario outlined in Case study 15.1 and see if you can suggest how the situation might be managed and how it might be avoided in the future.

surgery, the patient should be cared for by a 'robust' person.

Criteria for patient selection

There are recognised criteria used for selecting patients for day surgery. However, as previously stated, these are being used more flexibly in order to allow more patients access to day surgery. There is anecdotal evidence to suggest that patients who were deemed unsuitable for day surgery and who were treated as inpatients often did not need to stay in overnight. It has been suggested by Hitchcock (1998) that, before judging a patient unsuitable for day surgery, one should consider what would be done differently if the patient were treated as an inpatient.

Age

In the early 1990s when day surgery was being promoted, age was a factor which assumed some importance when selecting patients. At that time, the recommended upper age limit was 70 years and very few children were considered for day surgery (Commission on the Provision of Surgical Services 1992). At the present time, there is no upper age limit and generally no lower age limit although some centres are reluctant to treat babies; this is probably due to the specialised resources and staff required. In health care, physiological age is more important than chronological age. As you may recall, when you reflected about specific client groups who might benefit from day surgery, it was suggested that patients with learning disabilities and the elderly might benefit from day surgery, because it could minimise the risk of anxiety and disorientation (Briggs et al 1995, Davies & Ogg 1993, Farquharson 1993). However, the elderly do need careful assessment as they may be suffering systemic disorders which require polypharmacy for their management and which could compromise their safety for general anaesthesia. Nevertheless, exclusion from day surgery on grounds of age per se cannot be justified (see also Ch. 11).

Box 15.6   Framework for patient selection

Day surgery medical screening questionnaire (reproduced by kind permission from Whitwam 1994)

1.	Have you had an operation before?	Yes/No
2.	Have you had any problems with anaesthetics?	Yes/No
3.	Have any of your relations had problems with anaesthetics?	Yes/No
4.	Are you taking any medicines (tablets, patches, inhalers, injections)?	Yes/No
5.	Are you taking steroid tablets currently/recently?	Yes/No
6.	Have you any allergies (drugs, plasters, etc.)?	Yes/No
7.	Have you had serious illnesses in the past?	Yes/No
8.	Do you have high blood pressure?	Yes/No
9.	Do you get chest pains. indigestion or heartburn?	Yes/No
10.	Do you have blackouts or faint easily?	Yes/No
11.	Do you get breathless easily?	Yes/No
12.	Do you have asthma or bronchitis?	Yes/No
13.	Do you smoke?	Yes/No
14.	Have you ever had a convulsion or a fit?	Yes/No
15.	Do you have arthritis?	Yes/No
16.	Do you have muscle disease?	Yes/No
17.	Do you have anaemia or other blood disorder?	Yes/No
18.	Do you know your sickle status (if relevant)?	Yes/No
19.	Do you bleed badly or bruise without cause?	Yes/No
20.	Have you been jaundiced (turned yellow)?	Yes/No
21.	Do you drink alcohol?	Yes/No
22.	Do you have kidney disease?	Yes/No
23.	Do you have diabetes (sugar in the urine)?	Yes/No
24.	Do you have a hiatus hernia?	Yes/No
25.	Do you get heartburn or tummy acid in the throat?	Yes/No
26.	Do you have crowns, loose or artificial teeth?	Yes/No
27.	Do you have contact lenses or hearing aid?	Yes/No
28.	If female, are you/could you be pregnant?	Yes/No
29.	If female, are you taking an oral contraceptive pill?	Yes/No

---

Case study 15.1   Patient A

A 48-year-old lady has arrived in the day surgery centre for stripping of varicose veins in her legs. She has not brought her husband with her, because 'he is not an early riser'. Following her surgery, she makes a satisfactory recovery and her husband is notified that she is ready for collection. Her husband arrives by taxi to collect her. The nurse caring for the patient is concerned to note that he is obviously suffering from Parkinson's disease, has difficulty in walking and is unsteady on his feet.

Obesity

One of the most controversial criteria relates to the assessment of obesity. The common measurement used is the body mass index (BMI) or weight : height ratio (calculated as weight (kg) divided by height $(m)^2$). Generally the acceptable BMI is increasing and 30 is often regarded as within safe limits, although 35 is now becoming the accepted norm. The concomitant disease processes of obesity, such as cardiac disease, hypertension, hiatus hernia, diabetes mellitus and sleep apnoea, might well preclude the patient from day surgery, rather than obesity itself. For day surgery the most common problems relate to:

- intraoperative positioning
- airway management during and following general anaesthesia or sedation
- risk of aspiration of gastric contents during anaesthesia or sedation
- drug metabolism
- surgical access
- mobilisation following surgery.

The distribution of fat is recognised as an important factor in assessing the risk associated with obesity. The well-recognised 'pear-shaped' figure is associated with less risk to health, than the 'apple-shaped' figure where the fat is distributed around the waist. For this reason, waist measurement (> 88 cm for women and > 102 cm for men) might be more accurate in risk assessment (Bray & Gray 1988, Jointhorp 1990, cited in Bullock & Rosendahl 1992).

Respiratory disease

In assessing a patient with chronic obstructive airways disease, exercise tolerance may be a good indicator of the patient's suitability for day surgery. Patients with obvious restricted pulmonary function and/or a productive cough should be referred to the anaesthetist for assessment.

In this country, particularly in urban areas, there has been a significant increase in asthma in recent years. If patients are well controlled there should be no contraindication to day surgery. Episodes of hospitalisation to manage the problem would indicate the need for referral to an anaesthetist for risk assessment. Measurement of the peak expiratory flow rate (PEFR) may be helpful. Enquiring about triggers for asthmatic attacks is useful and it is essential to establish whether or not the patient is able to tolerate non-steroidal anti-inflammatory drugs (NSAIDs). These drugs are widely used for the management of postoperative pain, but are known to trigger bronchospasm in susceptible patients (see Ch. 24). All asthmatic patients should be encouraged to bring their inhalers with them on the day of surgery (see also Ch. 23).

Cardiac disease

Exercise tolerance is a useful guide in assessing a patient's suitability. Patients with asymptomatic valvular disease will be suitable, but will require antibiotic cover. Patients who are on warfarin therapy will need to be discussed with the surgeon. Otherwise, the main contraindications for day surgery are:

- myocardial infarction or cerebrovascular accident < 6 months ago
- poor exercise tolerance (cannot climb two flights of stairs without chest pain)
- second or third degree heart block
- sick sinus syndrome
- rhythm disturbances, e.g. atrial fibrillation, ventricular dysrhythmias
- antidysrhythmic therapy or digoxin.

Hypertension

Hypertension is a common reason for postponing a patient's day surgery, but should not ultimately preclude the patient. The recognised definition of hypertension is systolic pressure > 140 mmHg and diastolic pressure > 90 mmHg. It is important to remember that the patient may be very anxious and this can influence the blood pressure measurement. Other factors which might adversely influence the accuracy of the recording should be eliminated (British Hypertension Society Working Party 1997) and the measurement repeated after several minutes. If the diastolic pressure is still higher than 100 mmHg, the patient's surgery will have to be postponed. It is common practice to refer patients back to their general practitioner for blood pressure monitoring and possible treatment. Following three successive blood pressure recordings within recognised norms, the patient can be referred back to the day surgery centre.

Diabetes mellitus

Patients who are non-insulin-dependent diabetics and well controlled with hypoglycaemic tablets are suitable for day surgery, but should omit their tablet on the day of surgery. Well-controlled insulin-dependent diabetics are suitable for day surgery, in the absence of any concomitant disease. Ideally, these patients should be first on the morning operating list and advised to omit the morning dose of insulin. Monitoring of blood glucose levels for both groups should include pre- and postoperative recordings. It is important that both groups should resume their normal regime as soon as possible.

It is important that patients are assessed on an individual basis with referral to the anaesthetist, as necessary. The risk of postoperative nausea and vomiting needs to be minimised for these patients, which for some individual patients will mean considering alternatives to general anaesthesia. Local or regional anaesthesia with or without sedation may be preferable.

Drug history

Identification of drug therapies is sometimes difficult, because patients cannot remember the names of the drugs they are taking. In some cases, they may not be sure why they are taking them and this can hinder the assessment process. To minimise the risk to patients, it is useful to ask patients to bring their medication with them on the day of surgery and/or during the pre-assessment process.

Individual assessments will be required for those patients regularly taking any of the following drugs:

- steroids
- anticoagulants
- antidysrhythmics
- digoxin
- monoamine oxidase inhibitors.

Patients taking the combined oral contraceptive pill should be managed according to local policy, in order to minimise the risk of deep vein thrombosis. The literature suggests that the pill should be stopped 4 weeks prior to surgery on the lower limbs, especially if a pneumatic tourniquet is required intraoperatively (British Medical Association and Royal Pharmaceutical Society of Great Britain 1999).

Recreational drugs. It is important that patients are encouraged to disclose information about their use of recreational drugs without fear of censure, so that an accurate assessment can be made. While the use of cannabis is generally accepted as not being a contraindication for a patient's suitability for day surgery, the use of heroin may be more controversial. Ecstasy is known to interact with some anaesthetic agents to produce a reaction similar to malignant hyperthermia (Aitkenhead & Smith 1996). Patients who use Ecstasy or cocaine should be advised to abstain for 2 weeks prior to surgery (see also Ch. 4).

Social history

The selection criteria for day surgery patients having general anaesthesia or sedation include:

- responsible adult to escort home and stay 24 hours
- lives no more than 1 hour's drive away
- must travel home in car or taxi, not public transport
- access to a telephone
- registered with a general practitioner.

It is important to remember that if the patient were having surgery as an inpatient, a qualified nurse would be providing the postoperative care. Following surgery, the patient will rely on informal carers, i.e. family or friends. In other words, one might say that the nurse is delegating this duty to a total stranger.

Reflective point

Imagine you are going to care for a relative following day surgery. What information would you need? How long will you take off work? What would you be expected to do for your relative? Whom would you contact in an emergency? (This reflection will be followed up shortly.)

The social criteria for day surgery provide a basis for ensuring the safety of the patient. Travelling home by car with an escort, for not more than 1 hour, should minimise the risk to the patient of injury and postoperative nausea and vomiting (PONV), although there is some disagreement about a link between prolonged travelling time and the incidence of PONV (Boulton et al 1994, Fogg & Saunders 1995).

Other factors to be assessed

Other factors which might contribute to improving the patient's experience of day surgery need to be assessed. These include, for example:

- willingness to be a day surgery patient
- level of anxiety
- risk of PONV
- risk of morbidity
- allergies
- previous experience of day surgery
- occupation and return to work.

The original criteria for suitability for day surgery produced by the British Association of Day Surgery (BADS 1991), included the statement 'the patient must be willing' (to have day surgery). It is probably fair to say that, on the whole, patients are not specifically asked if they would prefer to have day surgery or be an inpatient. However, if the patient expressed an objection, this would be respected. Likewise, it is not routine to offer day surgery patients premedication, but if the patient obviously required it, it could be given. There appears to be an assumption that day surgery may be less stressful for the patient, so premedication can be avoided. In Chapter 20 the use of premedication is mentioned and there is the suggestion that this may delay discharge. In fact, there is evidence to suggest that day case patients do experience significant levels of anxiety (MacKenzie 1989, Young & Munro 1995) and that premedication in day surgery may have several benefits, without delaying discharge (Shafer et al 1989). There is also the concern that anxious patients may express dissatisfaction with the information they are given, and may also experience more postoperative symptoms (Linden & Engberg 1996).

Risk of postoperative nausea and vomiting

PONV is distressing for the patient and its optimal management remains a problem. The incidence of PONV is increased in:

- females (Cookson 1986)

- obese patients (Lerman 1992)
- individuals susceptible to travel sickness (Kamath et al 1990)
- particular types of surgery (Beattie et al 1991, Cookson 1986)
- patients with a history of PONV (Muir et al 1987)
- anxious patients (Sleight & Henderson 1995)
- patients with delayed gastric emptying (Palazzo & Strunin 1984)
- the phase of the menstrual cycle (Honkavaara et al 1991)
- the use of opioids for analgesia (Forrest et al 1990).

Early studies of ondansetron indicated that it could provide optimal relief for PONV if given pre-operatively (Alon & Himmelseher 1992, Wechtler et al 1990), but more recent studies provide evidence which does not support this (Pueyo et al 1996, Rowe et al 1994, Tramer et al 1997). Management might be improved by better risk assessment which could identify the need for pre-emptive anti-emetic therapy in susceptible individuals. For example, anecdotally, there is evidence to suggest that the smell of toast (a common source of nutrition given prior to discharge) is nauseating to some patients. For this reason, some centres offer sandwiches or fruit buns instead. This example highlights the multifaceted nature of PONV.

Risk of morbidity

Information from the pre-assessment interview needs to be communicated to the other members of the health care team. For example, there is little point in carefully documenting that the patient has arthritis in the spine or hips if this is not taken into account when positioning the patient in the operating theatre. Likewise information about a patient's previous experience of day surgery may identify an individual risk. One also needs to consider what one regards as morbidity.

Case study 15.2   Patient B

A 43-year-old female patient has surgery for the varicose veins on her left leg. Her surgery was in the morning and she has made a routine recovery, but she is complaining of a slight headache. When she gets home the headache is worse and she then begins to feel nauseated. She spends the rest of the day in bed and most of the next day. She rings up the day surgery centre, nearly 36 hours after her discharge, seeking help.

When does a patient problem become morbidity? Headache is a common problem following day surgery (Chung et al 1996), but is usually relieved by drinking fluid and taking a mild analgesic. However, if the patient is unable to return to normal activity within 12 hours of surgery, as in Case study 15.2, one would arguably regard this problem as morbidity.

Investigations

Preoperative investigations are required to ensure patient safety during anaesthesia and surgery. If there are no recent blood results on record from outpatient clinic visits, it may be necessary to organise the relevant tests during the pre-assessment process. Many day surgery centres are able to offer a 'one-stop' service, as their staff have the requisite skills to perform venepuncture and electrocardiograph (ECG) recording.

The indications for various blood tests, ECG and chest X-ray examinations are suggested in Figure 15.1. As well as these commonly accepted investigations, a cervical spine X-ray may be indicated in patients with a history of rheumatoid arthritis in order to identify potential problems associated with mobilisation of the neck for airway maintenance during general anaesthesia.

Patient information

Providing patient information is always a source of concern for staff working in the day surgery setting. There is a limited time available, both at pre-assessment and also during the day surgery episode to provide and reinforce information. Much has been written about patient information in general in this book (See Ch. 3), and about pre-operative information, in particular, in Chapters 20 and 23. Factors affecting the retention of information include:

- amount of information
- timing of information
- relevance
- method of communication
- barriers to communication, e.g. anxiety, stress, hearing loss, etc.
- language.

Reflective point

Consider the scenario in Case study 15.2. The patient is experiencing a recognised postoperative problem. What might be the possible cause of her headache? What advice would you give to her? At what stage would this be considered morbidity?

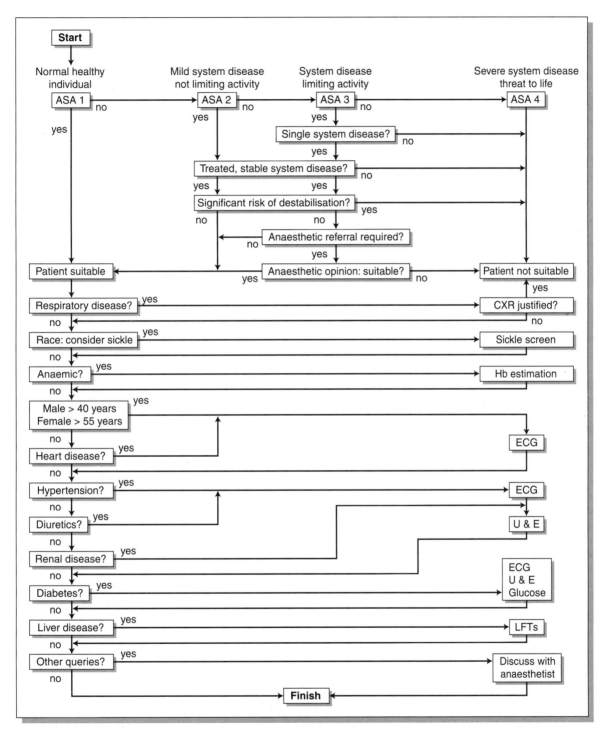

Figure 15.1   Medical selection and investigation algorithm: CXR – chest X-ray; Hb – haemoglobin; ECG – electrocardiography; U & E – urea and electrolytes; LFTs – liver function tests (reproduced by kind permission from Whitwam 1994).

Several audits of the day surgery patient's experience have identified dissatisfaction with information about the day surgery episode (Willis et al 1997). To try to relieve anxiety about day surgery, there is a lot of information to give the patient. However, one needs to have a realistic approach to communicating this information.

Reflective point

Imagine that you have been referred to the outpatients department at your local hospital, which you have never visited before. The surgeon tells you that you need to have an operation and sends you to see a nurse in the day surgery centre. What would you want to know?

The timing of the information is important, as stated in Chapter 20. Optimal timing is suggested as 10–14 days preoperatively and this is the general aim in day surgery. As mentioned, there needs to be a compromise between all the information that the patient may require and the essential information to safeguard the patient. One also needs to consider the information that will require reinforcing. For this reason the common methods of communication are oral and written information.

The essential information is given orally (and reinforced in written form) and includes:

- date and time of admission
- fasting instructions
- instructions about medication, if appropriate
- transport and escort arrangements
- return to work
- contact telephone numbers for day surgery.

Fasting instructions

In day surgery, the fasting times have radically changed over the past few years. In 1990, the standard fast from midnight for patients having morning surgery was relatively common (Strunin 1993). More recently, the norm has become 6 hours for food and up to 2 hours preoperatively for clear fluids (Pandit 1998). To reinforce this, some centres are actively encouraging patients, last on the operating list, to have a drink while they are waiting. This should minimise the dehydration which can occur preoperatively and which may contribute to vasovagal incidents postoperatively.

Instructions about medication

In terms of preoperative instructions, these need to be individualised according to the patient's needs, or in accordance with local protocols. The pre-assessment interview also provides the opportunity to discuss the means of analgesia relevant to individual patients, both intraoperatively (e.g. rectal diclofenac) and postoperatively. At this stage oral consent for use of diclofenac (Voltarol) per rectum may be gained and reinforced by written consent when the consent form is signed.

Transport and escort instructions

As previously mentioned, travel home via public transport is not recommended following day surgery. Indeed, in most day surgery centres, when signing the consent form, patients also agree to the terms agreed for day surgery.

Return to work

The term 'day surgery' often seems to mean different things to different people. To staff caring for patients having day surgery it means that the patient will be treated on a day care basis, but otherwise postoperative recovery will probably be the same as that for an inpatient. However, patients may expect to return to work within 1–3 days. Employers often expect the patient to return to work the next day. Somehow this situation needs to be resolved. At pre-assessment, patients should be advised to negotiate a return to work with their employer and given individual recommendations about the recovery time required. This may involve further questioning about the patient's occupation.

Reflective point

Mr Jones, aged 34 years, is scheduled to have a right inguinal hernia repair in 2 weeks' time. He is a long distance lorry driver and needs to return to work as soon as possible.

Mr. Jones asks you how soon he can return to work. What advice would you give him?

The issues you need to consider relate to Mr Jones' job. It is probably physically demanding. Physical activities may include climbing on and off the back of the lorry, assisting with securing the load, climbing in and out of the driver's cab. All of these activities are challenging after surgery, particularly surgery in the groin area. However, from personal experience, I know that some patients following hernia repair do feel particularly well, ignore the advice they are given and return to work earlier than expected. These are the patients who ring up the day surgery centre 2 weeks postoperatively complaining that they are in agony and feel exhausted.

A further word of caution related to the scenario involving Mr Jones: what about the other aspect of his work – the driving? When is it safe to drive following general anaesthesia and surgery? Postoperative advice often relates to 'not operating machinery for 24–48 hours'. Research studies indicate that the advice given about driving following general anaesthesia varies greatly (Goodwin, cited by Davenport 1998, Kortilla 1982). Of course, not all patients have a general anaesthetic for their hernia repair. Once the local anaesthesia has worn off, patients will probably manage their pain with non-steroidal anti-inflammatory drugs (NSAIDs). These drugs can also affect a patient's judgement (APBI 1997). Whilst driving, it may be necessary to perform an emergency stop – would the patient hesitate, anticipating the pain this may cause? Your advice would need to highlight this point. Finally, what does the patient's driving insurance policy state about cover following surgery?

Contact numbers for the day surgery centre

Both patients and carers do find contact numbers reassuring (Malster et al 1998). Patients should be encouraged to telephone the centre prior to, or following, surgery if they have any queries. Some centres provide an 'on-call' telephone service, so that patients can contact day surgery staff in an emergency at night. There have been various studies evaluating the efficacy of this service (Heseltine & Edlington 1998, Jackson et al 1997, Knowles & King 1995).

This section has highlighted the amount of information which needs to be communicated to the day surgery patient during the pre-assessment interview. As previously stated, essential information can be reinforced by written information in the form of patient information leaflets. Entering the patient's individual information (e.g. date and time of admission, fasting times, etc.) at the time of pre-assessment, may draw the patient's attention to reading other information also included. Other written information given to the patient may include details about the day surgery centre, an explanation of the proposed procedure together with postoperative instructions and carer's information.

Reflective point

Earlier you were asked to reflect on what information you would need if you were going to care for a relative following day surgery. How might you obtain this information?

You could check whether or not carers can attend the pre-assessment interview. Most day surgery centres invite carers to attend for all or part of the process, according to the patient's preference. If you were unable to attend, for personal reasons for example, you could advise your relative of any questions you would like answered. Bear in mind, that your relative might be preoccupied with his or her own concerns, so that it might be useful to write down your questions, as a reminder.

If the pre-assessment process has already taken place, check whether your relative has been given information which relates to his or her aftercare. Day surgery staff often give the carer's information sheet to the patient to give to the carer. If you still have concerns, you could ring up the day surgery centre for advice.

ORGANISATION OF CARE

Preoperative care

On the day of admission, patients are oriented to the day surgery environment and prepared for their surgery. This preparation includes undressing and undergoing the usual preoperative checks carried out by the nurse as described in Chapter 20. The patient is also seen by the surgeon to discuss any concerns the patient may have about the surgery, gain consent, and mark the operation site, if applicable. The anaesthetist, too, visits the patient to verify suitability for day surgery anaesthesia and to assess the need for premedication or preoperative monitoring, e.g. blood glucose level.

This may be a stressful time for patients: being anxious about the forthcoming surgery and possible sequelae; trying to get used to unfamiliar surroundings; and wondering what time they will go to the operating theatre. This waiting time has been identified as a major cause for concern among patients (Cripps & Bevan 1996, Malster et al 1998) and it is important that staff recognise this and try to minimise the patients' anxiety by keeping them informed of progress or delay in the operating list. For some surgical specialities, it is possible to give each patient an individual appointment time in order to minimise the waiting time.

Intraoperative care

The principles of safe intraoperative care are the same as those for inpatients (see Ch. 21); however, day surgery does have significant implications in terms of ensuring that the patient is 'street fit' following surgery and anaesthesia.

Anaesthesia

In contrast to inpatient anaesthesia, most of the drugs used for anaesthesia for day surgery patients are short-acting. For example, total intravenous anaesthesia (TIVA) is common in day surgery, the most usual drugs being propofol and alfentanil, supplemented by nitrous oxide and oxygen via a laryngeal mask airway (LMA). Propofol is a short-acting intravenous induction agent, which can also be given by incremental doses or infusion to maintain general anaesthesia, and

which has a short recovery time. It works synergistically with the commonly used opioids, fentanyl, alfentanil and remifentanil, which provide good analgesia and quick recovery. As previously mentioned, the LMA has had a great impact on day surgery because it allows safe management of the patient's airway without the risks associated with endotracheal intubation: tachycardia (Wilson et al 1992); hypertension (Wilson et al 1992), dysrhythmias (Fujii et al 1995) and raised intraocular pressure (Myint et al 1995). These risks are due in part to the type of muscle relaxant used, but also to stimulation of the upper airway during endotracheal intubation. Following insertion, the LMA rests in the hypopharynx. As can be seen in Figure 15.2, it is possible for the LMA to provide a conduit between the oesophagus and the trachea. For this reason, patients at risk of regurgitation of gastric contents would still require endotracheal intubation. Likewise, as the cuff of the LMA is confined by soft tissue structures (unlike the rigid structure of the trachea in which an endotracheal tube would be situated), inflation pressures during intermittent positive pressure ventilation should

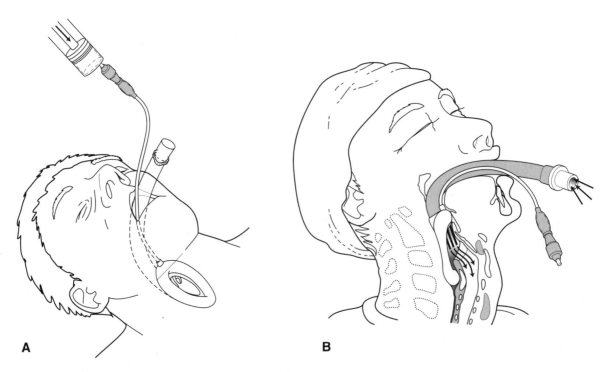

A **B**

Figure 15.2 (**A**) The laryngeal mask airway. When in situ in the hypopharynx (**B**), the LMA rests at the junction of the gastrointestinal and respiratory tracts and, with its cuff inflated, forms a seal with the glottis. ((**A**) from McCrirrick et al 1991 by kind permission; (**B**) from Davies et al 1990 Laryngeal mask airway and tracheal tube insertion by unskilled personnel. 336: 977–979. With permission.)

not exceed 1.7 kPa, as this could result in air escaping around the cuff, or being forced into the oesophagus (Broderick et al 1989). As a result, the latter could increase the risk of regurgitation.

Analgesia

The use of intraoperative wound infiltration is common in day surgery, even if the operation is being performed under general anaesthesia. The efficacy of various techniques has been studied, e.g. intra-articular infiltration (Cook et al 1997, Elhakim et al 1996), and topical application to, or infiltration of, the fallopian tubes during laparoscopy (Alexander 1997, Fiddes et al 1996). Another significant development is the use of diclofenac per rectum. Ideally this should be inserted intraoperatively to provide immediate postoperative analgesia. It is important to gain the patient's consent preoperatively; failure to do so could constitute assault.

Positioning

As with any patient undergoing surgery, safe optimal positioning must be achieved. Care must be taken to ensure that there is no risk of nerve damage. However, day surgery patients are usually at minimal risk of developing pressure sores or deep vein thrombosis, because of the relatively shorter duration of surgery and early ambulation. Day surgery patients are probably more at risk of morbidity from pre-existing pathology (e.g. osteoarthritis in the hips or knees which could impede optimal positioning), if caution is not exercised. This reinforces the importance of the pre-assessment process in identifying potential risks to the individual.

Blood loss

Unlike inpatient surgery, operations performed on a day surgery basis are selected so that the risk of significant blood loss is kept to a minimum. However, the future of day surgery may well include surgery which is associated with significant blood loss, but this should not exceed 10% of the total blood volume. Methods of blood loss estimation are described in Chapter 25 and while, at present, one would not expect a day surgery patient to have a significant loss of blood, untoward incidents do occur (Biswas & Leary 1992, Linares-Gil et al 1997, Twersky et al 1995). In such circumstances, immediate i.v. fluid replacement is essential, prior to admission as an inpatient for further management.

Recovery

First stage

The immediate post-anaesthetic recovery phase is variously described as 'first stage' or 'early' recovery and refers to care of the patient in the recovery room. The principles of post-anaesthetic recovery are described in Chapter 22. Although a high proportion of day surgery patients may already be awake on transfer to the recovery area, particularly if they have had TIVA, others may be unconscious with the LMA still in situ. During the past 10 years, there has been considerable discussion regarding who should remove the LMA (Brimacombe & Berry 1993), but it is now generally regarded as the role of the recovery staff (Brain 1991, Dingley et al 1994). Originally, it was suggested that the LMA should be removed while the patient was still anaesthetised to avoid the risk of laryngospasm and airway irritation (Pollard & Cooper 1995). Currently, it is more common to leave the LMA in situ until the patient is awake and/or removes it (Brain 1991, Milligan 1994).

Recovery times vary and it is therefore unusual to have fixed times for patients to stay in the recovery area. Before discharge from the post-anaesthetic recovery area, the patient should be awake and oriented to person, time and place, have stable vital signs within own norms and be able to respond to commands. There are scoring systems available which may be useful for auditing this process. These include the Aldrete post-anaesthesia score (Table 15.1) and the Steward score (Box 15.7). Each of these has its own merits according to the parameters which are measured.

Second stage

Following discharge from the post-anaesthetic recovery area, the patient's recovery is referred to as 'second stage' or 'intermediate' recovery and this takes place in the ward or second stage recovery area. During this phase, the patient is prepared for discharge by gradually gaining return to normal function and therefore 'street fitness'. Initially the main concerns relate to patient comfort and safety: ensuring the patient's observations remain stable and that the patient is pain-free, with no nausea and vomiting.

Analgesia is achieved by various means, including intraoperative analgesia using local anaesthesia and the use of diclofenac per rectum. Postoperatively, many centres have introduced protocols or guidelines for the management of postoperative pain, using a combination of NSAIDs such as ibuprofen, ketoprofen, diclofenac, ketorolac, codeine phosphate and

Table 15.1 Aldrete post-anaesthesia scoring system (reproduced by kind permission from Aldrete JA, Kroulik D 1970 A post-anaesthetic recovery score. Anaesthesia and Analgesia 49: 924–934)

Post-anaesthesia recovery score	In	15	30	45	Hours	Out
Activity						
Able to move voluntarily or on command						
4 extremities	2	2	2	2	2	2
2 extremities	1	1	1	1	1	1
0 extremities	0	0	0	0	0	0
Respiration						
Able to deep breathe and cough freely	2	2	2	2	2	2
Dyspnoea, shallow or limited breathing	1	1	1	1	1	1
Apnoeic	0	0	0	0	0	0
Circulation						
Preoperative blood pressure in torr						
BP 20 mm of pre-anaesthesia level	2	2	2	2	2	2
BP 20–50 mm of pre-anaesthesia level	1	1	1	1	1	1
BP 50 mm of pre-anaesthesia level	0	0	0	0	0	0
Consciousness						
Fully awake	2	2	2	2	2	2
Arousable on calling	1	1	1	1	1	1
Not responsive	0	0	0	0	0	0
Colour						
Normal	2	2	2	2	2	2
Pale, dusky, blotchy, jaundiced	1	1	1	1	1	1
Cyanotic	0	0	0	0	0	0
Total						

Dismissal criteria: total score of 10, plus stable vital signs

---

Box 15.7 Steward simplified post-anaesthesia score (reproduced by kind permission from Steward 1975)

Consciousness
Awake	2
Responding to stimuli	1
Not responding	0

Airway
Coughing on command or crying	2
Maintaining a good airway	1
Airway requires maintenance	0

Movement
Moving limbs purposefully	2
Non-purposeful movements	1
Not moving	0

---

paracetamol. At pre-assessment, as mentioned, it is important to identify those patients in whom NSAIDs cannot be used. While these drugs are the most common means of providing analgesia, opioids are still used for 'rescue' analgesia if, at any stage, the patient's pain management requires them (Vijay & King 1995).

Nausea and vomiting

This problem has already been highlighted, but it is a major concern for day surgery patients. Not only is it distressing for the patient, but it can also delay discharge. Studies have shown that the incidence of PONV ranges from 30–68%, depending on the type of surgery (Watson, cited in Millar et al 1997). Another consideration is that, as part of the discharge criteria following day surgery, there is the recommendation that patients are able to tolerate fluids and food. However, this may actually increase the risk of PONV. In many centres, this criterion has changed to fluids only and there is the suggestion that this should not be mandatory. The problem is: how does one ensure that the patient returns to normal hydration and nutrition after discharge?

Case study 15.3 Patient C

A 28-year-old female has had a laparoscopic sterilisation. Following surgery, her postoperative observations are normal and she has passed urine. On the whole she feels comfortable, but feels slightly nauseated and is reluctant to drink more than a few sips of water. She is due to be discharged and is becoming anxious because she is afraid of being sick, but she also wants to go home as soon as possible.

Reflective point

How would you manage the patient described in Case study 15.3? Remember that you need to justify your actions.

The problem of PONV needs to be managed on an individual basis. If the unit policy states that patients must tolerate fluids before discharge, discharge must be delayed until this can be achieved. Giving a patient fluids may provoke vomiting and this may then require the administration of an anti-emetic drug. Alternatively, if allowed, the patient could be discharged, but there would need to be arrangements for follow-up communication to ensure that the patient does return to normal oral hydration within a few hours following discharge.

Mobilisation

Mobilisation following day surgery will start as soon as the patient feels able to get up. Careful supervision is required in case the patient has a vasovagal response. This response may not occur immediately, but may be precipitated by ambulation or going to the toilet and for this reason the patient is escorted by a member of the health care team. Patients recover at different rates, so it is not possible to anticipate how much discharge will be delayed, but generally patients do not require overnight admission.

DISCHARGE

To try to ensure the safety of the day surgery patient, the need for criteria to assess a patient's readiness for discharge has been identified by Stephenson (1990). The generally recognised criteria for discharge are those presented in Box 15.8. More recently, with the advances that are being made in day surgery and

---

Box 15.8 Criteria for discharge

- Vital signs stable
- Oriented to person, time and place
- Has passed urine
- Tolerates oral fluids
- Minimal nausea
- No evidence of haemorrhage
- Pain adequately controlled
- Able to walk without difficulty
- Has been given written postoperative instructions
- Suitable transport available
- Companion for 24 hours postoperatively
- Has postoperative medication, if required

---

anaesthesia, these criteria are being modified to provide more flexibility and will reflect the changes in day surgery care and management. A post-anaesthetic discharge scoring system for ambulatory surgery has been devised by Chung et al (1991) and is presented in Table 15.2.

Case study 15.4 **Patient D**

A 50-year-old man has come to day surgery for repair of his inguinal hernia. He had his operation at 8.30 a.m. and it is now 12.30 p.m. He is ready for discharge, but is unable to pass urine. The discharge criteria state 'The patient must be able to void'.

Reflective point

Why might the patient in Case study 15.4 be unable to pass urine? Would you allow him to go home?

Factors you might consider in relation to the patient described in Case study 15.4 include:

- anxiety about passing urine on demand
- postoperative discomfort
- type of intraoperative analgesia
- fasting time.

The first two factors are arguably not going to improve by delaying discharge. The type of intraoperative analgesia might be significant. If the patient has had an ilioinguinal block for intraoperative analgesia, it is important to ensure that he is able to void. The fasting time may be of particular relevance. If the patient has had nothing to eat or drink since midnight,

Table 15.2 Post-anaesthetic discharge scoring system (adapted from Chung et al 1991)

	Score		
	2	1	0
A: Vital signs	Within 20% of preoperative value	20–40% of preoperative value	Greater than 40% of preoperative value
B: Activity and mental state	Oriented × 3 (to person, time and place) with steady gait	Oriented × 3 with unsteady gait	Not oriented × 3 with unsteady gait
C: Pain, nausea and/or vomiting	Minimal	Moderate needing treatment	Severe needing treatment
D: Surgical bleeding	Minimal	Moderate	Severe
E: Intake and output	Has had oral fluid and voided	Has had oral fluid and not voided	Has neither had oral fluid nor voided

A total score of greater than or equal to 8 indicates street-worthiness.

it may be unrealistic to expect him to void; on the other hand, if he has had clear fluids in the early morning prior to admission, one would expect him to be able to pass urine.

Most of the discharge planning will have taken place at pre-assessment. However, much of the information about postoperative care will need to be reinforced, and possibly modified, during the discharge process. When the patient has met the required criteria for discharge, specific postoperative instructions can be given. These will include care related to the surgery, activity level, follow-up arrangements and analgesia. This information is usually given orally and reinforced with written information. Follow-up arrangements may include visiting the practice nurse for suture removal, postoperative check at the hospital and future outpatients appointment. The presence of the carer at this time is invaluable in reinforcing this information. It is also the carer's opportunity to gain further information about caring for the patient at home, and gaining reassurance from obtaining contact numbers in case of emergency or query (Malster et al 1998).

Some day surgery centres provide a follow-up service, by telephoning the patient on the day after surgery. This service has been positively evaluated (Knowles & King 1995, Heseltine & Edlington 1998) and its provision is recognised as desirable by day surgery staff. However, it is very time-consuming to provide this service and requires extra resources to maintain.

NEEDS OF SPECIFIC CLIENT GROUPS

It is not possible, in this text, to consider the needs of all the adult client groups in the day surgery setting. Indeed, the needs of some client groups have already been mentioned in this chapter. However, in view of the changing patterns of health care, it would be a major omission not to consider the needs of the increasing population of elderly patients. Chapter 11 discusses this client group in detail, so this section will only highlight special considerations associated with the day surgery environment. There is evidence to suggest that elderly patients prefer day surgery (Audit Commission 1991). It has already been stated that there is no upper age limit when assessing patient suitability, but it is important to consider the implications for performing surgery on a day-case basis.

Factors which need to be taken into consideration include:

- physiological fitness
- communication barriers
- preparation for surgery
- type of anaesthesia
- lay carers

Physiological fitness

While many adults stay fit and healthy until late in life, a significant proportion do develop some form of dysfunction or systemic disease associated with the ageing process. This means that the pre-assessment process must ensure that any risk factors are identified. Pathology may affect more than one system resulting in the need for polypharmacy for its management. This might increase the risk of interaction with anaesthetic drugs. Other drug therapy which might be particularly associated with the elderly is the use of low-dose aspirin to reduce platelet aggregation.

Communication

The ageing process is often associated with some degree of sensory loss which could impede communication.

Elderly patients may be reluctant to admit that they have a problem and may mask the deficit well and develop coping strategies. Throughout the day surgery episode, patients should be encouraged and assisted to continue using any aids, as appropriate.

Reflective point

What strategies might an individual employ to cope with a hearing deficit? How might you identify these? How could you check that the patient has received information that you have given him or her?

Particularly at the pre-assessment interview, any sensory loss should be identified. Failure to communicate effectively can place the patient at risk, may cause the patient to arrive ill-prepared for surgery or may result in the patient not arriving on the day of surgery. Hearing loss can result in misunderstanding or misinformation. The presence of the lay carer can greatly assist in the communication process. If the patient is unaccompanied, it is essential to assess the patient's understanding of the procedure and the preparation required. This may be achieved by a variety of methods, but one way might be to ask the patient to repeat any preoperative instructions that have been given.

For patients with defective eyesight, patient information leaflets in large-size print may be helpful. This may be particularly indicated for instructions about self-instillation of postoperative eye drops following ophthalmic procedures.

Memory loss presents a serious problem for managing patients during the whole day surgery episode and recovery. These patients may become easily distressed by the change in their surroundings and become reassured by returning to their normal environment. The attendance of the carer is essential to gaining patient cooperation and ensuring patient safety and continuity of care.

Preparation for surgery

Elderly patients often have a routine to their lives; if this is disrupted, they may become anxious and/or confused. For this reason, it is important to check that any arrangements for the day of surgery are negotiated with the patient. While some individuals do not require much sleep and like to get up early in the morning, other less mobile patients may have to get up more slowly and would become distressed by having to interrupt their routine. The risks of preoperative

anxiety have been highlighted in Chapters 9 and 20. It should be noted, however, that elderly patients have their own coping strategies. This may be observed by checking arrival times of elderly patients, who often come early for their appointments so that they can familiarise themselves with their surroundings, or in the, often erroneous, belief that they will be seen or treated sooner. This fact was corroborated by a recent local audit (Malster et al 1998).

Type of anaesthesia

If general anaesthesia is not possible or appropriate, local anaesthesia with or without sedation might be an alternative. Local anaesthesia is particularly useful for ophthalmic procedures such as cataract removal. However, when considering local anaesthesia, the patient's ability to cooperate needs to be assessed. Some elderly patients may have difficulty keeping still for the duration of the surgery. This may occur in individuals with little subcutaneous fat who could feel pressure pain, while lying on the operating table, or movement may occur because the patient forgets to keep still.

Davies & Ogg (1993, p. 17) have identified that altered pharmacokinetics which present in the elderly are related to:

- reduced absorption
- altered distribution
- increased end-organ sensitivity
- reduced metabolism
- reduced renal clearance.

In terms of general anaesthesia they suggest that elderly patients require smaller doses of anaesthetic agents and that anaesthesia takes longer to wear off (Davies & Ogg 1993). Disorientation following surgery may occur, possibly owing to hypoxaemia or hypotension, but may be minimised by using some of the more recently developed anaesthetic agents such as desflurane (Bennett et al 1992).

Lay carers

The role of the lay carer for elderly patients is crucial in optimising the day surgery experience. The need to assess the suitability of the carer has already been highlighted. The pre-assessment nurse is arguably best placed for this role. An elderly spouse may not realise his or her limitations in being able to care for the patient postoperatively at home. If the carer is not present, the nurse may need to use gentle probing questions to obtain the necessary information.

PERCEPTIONS OF DAY SURGERY

The patient's perspective

Given the prevailing conditions in today's NHS, day surgery is seen as the way ahead for an efficient, cost effective patient-oriented service (Audit Commission 1990a). However, the importance of considering the patient's perspective cannot be overemphasised, if the day surgery service is to provide meaningful patient care (Harju 1991, James 1993, Tinkle & Beaton 1983).

In the early 1990s, the Audit Commission stressed the importance of gaining the consumer's perspective of day surgery. The response to their commissioned patient perception questionnaire (Audit Commission 1990a,b, 1991) indicated that 80% of those who responded were satisfied with the day surgery experience. This positive response has also been borne out by several single-centre surveys which, using a retrospective quantitative design, have highlighted overall patient satisfaction in conjunction with minimal postoperative complications (Fenton-Lee et al 1993, Ghosh 1994, Hawkshaw 1994, Ramachandra 1994). Yet, whilst the demand for users' views about the service offered by day surgery centres has never been so great, the limits of this approach to data collection are well documented (Brant 1992). Authors have concerns about the validity and reliability of patient satisfaction questionnaires because these are often completed by the patient prior to discharge (Meredith & Wood 1994). However, it is possible for patients to be satisfied but also identify aspects of care that require improvement, as studies have shown (Hawkshaw 1994, James 1993, Rhodes 1991). Parry (1995) demonstrated that, in some cases, patient satisfaction, reported after the day surgery episode, may be influenced by having survived the ordeal and this highlights that major concerns on the day appear insignificant once the surgery is over. One patient in her study illustrated this by saying: 'I would suggest, all the points that I made at the beginning, I realise now are not important. They are minor things – you forget about them – that is not so important. But now the recovery, that is important'. Another patient identified a particular source of distress to him was being expected to walk to the operating theatre – a common expectation in many day surgery centres. He likened it to Alcatraz and 'walking to the gallows'.

Two studies, in particular, have taken as their starting point the patient's experience of day surgery from a qualitative perspective and, whilst identifying overall satisfaction with the day surgery experience, have identified areas of concern. These include the need for more information, misunderstanding of the term 'day surgery', and care following discharge (Parry 1995, Otte 1996).

The need for more information

One of the major causes of patient dissatisfaction with health care is inadequate preparation (Malin & Teasdale 1991). Meredith & Wood (1994) suggested that staff need to be more explicit when describing the day surgery episode so that, when patients encounter the process, they are better prepared. This is particularly necessary when the contact with health professionals is brief and intense (Neve 1995).

Reflective point

Imagine that you are describing the day surgery episode to a patient, during the pre-assessment interview. How might you make this more meaningful for the patient?

You might, for example, compare or contrast the day surgery episode to a previous experience of hospital treatment. Other strategies might include incorporating the patient's previous life experiences. An obvious example might be to describe the pain that a patient might experience following specific gynaecological operations as similar to 'period pains', which the patient might have experienced previously.

What other examples can you give?

It is important to remember that entering a hospital can be seen as a source of threat and anxiety and that the amount of stress experienced is independent of the size of the operation being performed (Long & Phipps 1985). People in good physical health are more anxious on admission to hospital than those who are unwell (Cochran 1984, cited in Bailey & Clarke 1989).

A small study by Neve (1995), focusing on patients' and nurses' perceptions of caring in a day surgery unit, used a Q sort technique to identify 'most caring' and 'least caring' behaviours. While patients focused upon the need for honest information about their treatment and condition, nurses, in contrast, emphasised the need for physical care – 'caring for' – at the expense of 'caring about' behaviours. The nurses' perspective may be partly explained by the day surgery environment and the sudden change in dependency of the client, whilst also focusing on the need for patients to gain 'street fitness' in a short space of time. This study serves to emphasise that information-giving is an essential component of caring from the patients' perspective.

Parry (1995) in a phenomenological study with eight patients sought to portray their experience of contemplating, undergoing and recovering from day surgery for hernia repair. Patients felt that they lacked knowledge concerning day surgery and had a need for more information. As one patient stated: 'Although I fully agree with day surgery I would like to know a bit more. For people who have not experienced hospital or surgery before, the need for information is important'. It would appear, however, that, for some, the uncertainty holds no fears, with another patient stating: 'It's a bit of an adventure, not actually knowing what will happen on the day' – not a situation to be encouraged. We must never lose sight of the enormous trust patients place in us or their belief that we will always act in their best interests.

It is important to realise that the need for information is highly individual and this is particularly relevant, as nurses in the day surgery setting are required to work with a wide range of clients. Day surgery does pose a challenge for providing adequate education and, as studies have indicated (Otte 1996, Parry 1995), there is no room for complacency.

Misunderstanding the term 'day surgery'

Parry's study in 1995 highlighted that there was a misunderstanding of the term 'day surgery' from two perspectives: firstly, that the stay in hospital is shorter than a 'day'; and, secondly, that the recovery time is longer than a 'day'. In this study patients' comments included: 'The fact that he said to me, "Oh yes, you'll be in and out in a day" meant that I'd be fit to go to work the following day'.

As practitioners working in the day surgery setting, we need to ensure that patients gain a better understanding of the concept of day surgery. It would appear that patients can find the day surgery experience similar to a conveyor belt feeling (Parry 1995). As one patient remarked: 'and it seemed a bit of a factory job, rather than care ... sort of in and out'. Indeed, one patient likened the experience to going to the local supermarket.

Given the compact time frame, it is understandable how this impression could be gained. Clearly, day surgery is often seen, by staff, as a way of minimising disruption to the patient's normal pattern of living. However, whilst it is only natural that many patients want to get home as quickly as possible (Buckley 1993), others may prefer a more leisurely approach to their care. Treatment on a day-surgery basis should remain a choice for the patient, as highlighted

by one patient in Parry's study (1995) who stated: 'I remember saying before the operation that I'd prefer to be in overnight, but now it seems simple to come home on the day'. In this study, some patients were clearly expecting to remain in hospital for longer than they did and consequently were concerned at being discharged so early, and about the burden this placed on their carers. As one patient remarked: 'It was my daughter who pointed it out. She said it's quite a big responsibility having you home straight away'.

Reflective point

How do we prepare carers for their continuing responsibility?
  You may wish to refer to your reflections earlier in this chapter.

As previously mentioned, the other misunderstanding about day surgery relates to the recovery time. In essence, because the patient is discharged so soon after surgery, the postoperative recovery which would previously have taken place in hospital (as an inpatient) now occurs at home. Patients need to be made aware of this (Robinson 1994). The author naively assumed that having an arthroscopy as a day case would be like having a tooth out, and confidently arranged his work and family commitments on that assumption. Fortunately, he revised his plans following pre-assessment.

Continuity of care

In Parry's study (1995), patients were concerned as to 'who was in charge' of them, following discharge. They felt that the hospital stay was so short and the discharge was too swift. Once they got home, the patients felt someone should be 'looking after' them, but were not sure who that 'someone' should be. This bewilderment was expressed by one patient, after he had visited his general practitioner to hand over his discharge letter: 'Well, I'm left with not knowing. Should I go back? Does he need to know?'.

The importance of discharge planning cannot be overemphasised. There is concern that patients may not be adequately prepared for discharge because of the reduced amount of patient contact (Markanday & Platzer 1994). As one patient in Parry's study (1995) remarked: 'There's no chatting anymore. I mean, in a week, you would talk to people and you would go away with a lot more information', and this was reinforced by another who stated: 'I thought somebody might just have come along and said, 'Do you feel all right to go?'. These views are supported by Otte (1996) who, using grounded theory, interviewed eight ENT patients approximately 3 weeks after day surgery. She identified the need for a more coordinated follow-up procedure on an individual basis, because patients were not prepared for the increase in independence and felt that they were being left to their own devices. Upon reflection, could it be that staff are failing to recognise the patient's need for a more formalised discharge procedure, as noted by Moran & Kent (1995), in their desire to provide 'seamless care'? Bailey & Clarke (1989) highlighted that discharge home requires a period of adjustment and coping, which will, in part, depend on support available, but also on the preparation that has been given. The amount of preparation that is required will vary for each individual, but it is important that patients are encouraged to assist in coordinating their own care.

Several of the studies mentioned here have used small sample groups, but this has arguably provided more in-depth insights than might have been gained by larger studies. However, it is important to remember that the experiences highlighted here may not be representative of the majority of day surgery patients. From the literature, it appears that, in many day surgery centres, auditing the service that they provide is a high priority. As part of this, patients' perspectives during and following the day surgery experience can be used to reshape and develop health services.

Commonly, patients express a high level of satisfaction with day surgery, but there are also common concerns about car parking space, inadequate information, length of wait in the day surgery centre prior to surgery and untimely discharge (Cripps & Bevan 1996, Malster et al 1998). It has been suggested that patients who are dissatisfied with the level of information provided may experience more postoperative symptoms (Linden & Engberg 1996).

The carer's perspective

Lay carers make a significant contribution to the success of day surgery. This sometimes occurs at the personal expense of the individual, as demonstrated by Willis et al (1997) who found that 13% of carers took time off work, with 7% indicating a loss of earnings, and a 1-week survey by Malster et al (1998) revealed that 35% of carers took unpaid leave to care for patients. In our opinion, this may represent one of the hidden costs of day surgery. In the latter survey, 89%

of carers felt confident about caring for the patient. Factors which influenced their confidence included: the 'excellent written information', 'the patient recovered well', attending the pre-assessment process and because one carer had experienced the same operation. Carers were asked what advice they would offer other carers. In relation to the day of surgery, they suggested 'leave plenty of time to park' and 'be prepared to spend most of the day at the hospital'. Following surgery, the advice was to 'make sure they get a lot of rest', 'help out where necessary' and 'stay by the patient – they may need you most of the time'. Other studies have identified the need for lay carers to be educated for their role (Rush et al 1995).

The impact of day surgery on the workload of community health care staff

Throughout the past decade, concern has been expressed regarding the impact of day surgery on the community health care staff. Several audits have been carried out to assess how an increase in day surgery impinges on their workload. The main reasons for patients contacting the primary health care team are presented in Box 15.9.

It has been suggested that providing medical certificates, before patients are discharged from the day surgery centre, could reduce the number of visits to general practitioners' surgeries (Woodhouse et al 1998). Better pain control and information about what to expect after surgery may also help (Willis et al 1997). It is difficult to produce an overall estimate of the impact of day surgery. One study indicated that as many as 50% of patients contacted primary or community health care staff within 21 days following surgery, but the postoperative visit rate was remarkably low (Lewis & Bryson 1998). Another study suggested that only 4.3% of patients consulted their general practitioner,

---

Box 15.9 Common reasons for patients contacting the primary health care team

- Analgesia
- Nausea and vomiting
- Wound infection
- Bleeding
- Headache
- Dizziness
- Sore throat
- Suture removal
- Sickness certificates

with 1.4% contacting the district nurse (Ghosh & Sallam 1994), and other studies have indicated similarly low figures (Elwood et al 1995). This wide variation indicates the difficulty in predicting how an increase in day surgery might affect individual community health care teams. However, one might anticipate that performing more complex surgical procedures on a day-care basis could well have a more pronounced effect.

Some day surgery units have identified the need for better liaison with their local general practitioners and practice nurses. This has sometimes been achieved by the introduction of 'open evenings' at day surgery centres, so that staff from the community can meet staff in the day surgery centre to discuss concerns about the continuity of care delivery. In other centres, nursing staff have taken on a liaison role with local general practitioners. In 1995, Cavill surveyed 60 local general practitioners: 16 responded, and the results revealed that one-quarter of respondents were not in favour of a liaison nurse. Personal experience suggests that this liaison role is of limited value.

THE FUTURE OF DAY SURGERY

The recent expansion of day surgery over the last 10 years has given rise to many well-established centres, some of which have already reached the millennium targets proposed by the NHS Executive's day surgery task force (NHS Executive 1994), while others have reached their individual capacity. There is a need to continue the impetus in day surgery and individual centres may well have to decide their own initiatives. The options include improvement in quality, extended day surgery units or the movement into day treatment centres.

The need to monitor quality has been debated at several day surgery conferences and various criteria have been suggested. In terms of new initiatives, the extended day surgery unit is an option preferred by some units who feel that, by extending the operating hours, they can achieve more throughput. Several examples of this have been presented and there is evidence that day surgery in this country may progress to the 23 hour 59 minute day favoured by the USA (Healy et al, unpublished work, 1998). However, there is a limit to the amount of day surgery which can be performed without increasing the complexity of surgery. So, it is likely that a greater amount of day surgery will be of an intermediate to major nature, as increasing numbers of minor surgical procedures are performed on an outpatient basis. The third option of incorporating day surgery within day treatment centres is arguably an attractive option for centres which are just being developed or which are in the process of being relocated to newly designed centres. Incorporating day surgery with other day treatments such as haematological, oncological and other therapies, suitable on a day-care basis, may make economic sense and could possibly be accommodated within stand-alone or free-standing units.

When considering the future of day surgery, it is important not to discount government initiatives which may or may not be counterproductive. Over the recent years we have seen ebbs and flows in the quantity of day surgery performed, related to the frailties of the contracting systems in health authorities. When the Government's latest initiative of creating primary care groups has been established, it will be interesting to note its influence on the quantity and quality of day surgery.

REFERENCES

Aitkenhead A R, Smith G (eds) 1996 Textbook of anaesthesia. Churchill Livingstone, Edinburgh

Aldrete J A, Kroulik D 1970 A post-anaesthetic recovery score. Anesthesia and Analgesia 49: 924–934

Alexander C A, Leach A B, Thompson S R et al 1988 Use your brain! Anaesthesia 43: 893–894

Alexander J I 1997 Pain after laparoscopy. British Journal of Anaesthesia 79: 369–378

Alon E, Himmelseher S 1992 Ondansetron in the treatment of post-operative vomiting: a randomised double-blind comparison with droperidol and metoclopramide. Anesthesia and Analgesia 75: 561–565

American Society of Anaesthesiologists (ASA) 1963. Anesthesiology 24(11)

Association of the British Pharmaceutical Industry (ABPI) 1997 Compendium of data sheets and summaries of product characteristics. Datapharm Publications, London

Audit Commission 1990a A short cut to better services. Day Surgery in England and Wales (October). HMSO, London

Audit Commission 1990b Day surgery audit guide and data collection. Internal Publication, Audit Commission, London

Audit Commission 1991 Measuring quality: the patient's view of day surgery. Occasional Paper. HMSO, London

Bailey R, Clarke M 1989 Stress and coping in nursing, Chapman and Hall, London

Beattie W S, Linblad T, Buckley D N et al 1991 The incidence of postoperative nausea and vomiting in women undergoing laparoscopy is influenced by the day of the menstrual cycle. Canadian Journal of Anaesthesia 38: 298–302

Bennett J A, Lingaraju N, Horrow J C et al 1992 Elderly patients recover more quickly from desflurane than isoflurane anaesthesia. Journal of Clinical Anaesthesia 4: 378–381

Biswas J K, Leary C 1992 Post-operative hospital admission from a day surgery unit: a 7 years retrospective survey. Anaesthesia and Intensive Care 20: 147–150

Boulton B B, Wood S, Mackenzie S I P 1994 Does distance travelled affect day surgery morbidity? Journal of One Day Surgery (Summer): 10–12

Brain A I J 1983 The laryngeal mask: a new concept in airway management. British Journal of Anaesthesia 55: 801

Brain A I J 1991 Studies of the laryngeal mask – first learn the art. Anaesthesia 46: 417–418

Brant R, Clarke M 1992 Hearing the patient's story. International Journal of Health Care Quality Assurance 5(6): 5–7

Bray G A, Gray D S 1988 Obesity part 1: pathogenesis. Western Journal of Medicine (149): 429

Briggs T P, Anson K M, Jones A Coker B J, Miller R A 1995 Urological day case surgery in elderly and medically unfit patients using sedoanalgesia: what are the limits? British Journal of Urology 75: 708–711

Brimacombe J, Berry A 1993 The laryngeal mask airway – the first ten years. Anaesthesia and Intensive Care 21: 115–116

British Association of Day Surgery 1991 Day surgery. (Companion notes to teleconference) Medical Television Network, London

British Hypertension Society Working Party 1997 Blood pressure measurement. British Medical Journal Publishing Group, London

British Medical Association and Royal Pharmaceutical Society of Great Britain 1999 British national formulary. BMA and RPS, London

Broderick P M, Webster N R, Nunn J F 1989 The laryngeal mask airway: a study of 100 patients during spontaneous ventilation. Anaesthesia 44: 238–241

Buckley P 1993 Utilisation of day surgery. Journal of One Day Surgery 2(3): 21–24

Bullock B L, Rosendahl P P 1992 Pathophysiology, 3rd edn. Lippincott, Philadelphia

Carroll P H, Ogg T W 1996 Recovery after day surgery with intravenous anaesthetic agents. Ambulatory Surgery 4: 19–23

Cavill K M 1995 Thoughts on liaison nurses in a day case unit. Journal of One Day Surgery (Winter): 13

Chung F, Un V, Su J 1996 Postoperative symptoms 24 hours after ambulatory surgery. Canadian Journal of Anaesthesia 43: 1121–1127

Chung F et al 1991 A new post-anaesthetic discharge scoring system for ambulatory surgery. Anesthesia and Analgesia 72: S42

Commission on the Provision of Surgical Services 1992 Guidelines for day case surgery. Royal College of Surgeons, London

Cook T M, Tuckey J P, Noland J P 1997 Analgesia after day case knee arthroscopy: double blind study of intra-articular tenoxicam, intra-articular bupivacaine and placebo. British Journal of Anaesthesia 78: 163–168

Cookson R F 1986 Nausea and vomiting: mechanisms and treatment. Springer-Verlag, Berlin, pp 130–150

Cripps M, Bevan L 1996 A report of patients' experiences after day surgery. Journal of One Day Surgery (Spring): 7–8

Davenport H T 1998 Anaesthesia for day surgery: fings aint wot they used to be. Journal of One Day Surgery (Summer): 24–25

Davies P R F, Ogg T W 1993 Managing anaesthesia for geriatric day surgery. Journal of One Day Surgery (Spring): 16–18

Davies P R F, Tighe S Q M, Greenslade G L, Evans G H 1990 Laryngeal mask insertion by unskilled personnel. Lancet 336: 977–979

Dingley J, Whitehead M J, Wareham K 1994 A comparative study of the incidence of sore throat with the laryngeal mask airway. Anaesthesia 49: 251–254

Elhakim et al 1996 Intra-articular tenoxicam relieves post arthroscopy pain. Acta Anaesthesiologica Scandinavica 40: 1223–1226

Elwood J H, Godden S, Barlow J 1995 General practitioners and community staff contacts after day care. Journal of One Day Surgery (Autumn): 17–18

Farquharson M 1993 Day surgery for patients over 70 years old. Journal of One Day Surgery (Summer): 20–21

Fenton-Lee D, Riach E, Cooke T 1993 Outcome in day surgery. Journal of One Day Surgery 3(3): 13–14

Fiddes T M, Williams H W, Herbision G P 1996 Evaluation of postoperative analgesia following laparoscopic application of Filshie clips. British Journal of Obstetrics and Gynaecology 103: 1143–1147

Fogg K J, Saunders P R I 1995 Folly! The long distance day surgery patient. Ambulatory Surgery 4(3): 209–210

Forrest J B, Cahalan M K, Rehder K 1990 Multicentre study of general anaesthesia. Anesthesiology 72: 262–268

Fujii Y, Tanaka H, Toyooka H 1995 Circulatory responses to laryngeal mask airway insertion or tracheal intubation in normotensive and hypertensive patients. Canadian Journal of Anaesthesia 42(1): 32–36

Ghosh S 1994 Are the Audit Commission's targets realistic? Journal of One Day Surgery 4(2): 19–21

Ghosh S, Sallam S 1994 Patient satisfaction and post-operative demands on hospital and community services after day surgery. British Journal of Surgery 81(11): 1714–1715

Harju E 1991 Patient satisfaction among day surgery patients in a central hospital. Quality Assurance in Health Care 3(2): 83–88

Hawkshaw D 1994 A day surgery follow-up survey. British Journal of Nursing 3(7): 348–351

Heseltine K, Edlington F 1998 A day surgery post-operative telephone call line. Nursing Standard 13(9): 39–43

Hitchcock M 1998 Unpublished paper. 4th National Conference on Managerial and Professional Issues in Day Surgery. London

Honkavaara P, Lehtinen A M, Horvorka J et al 1991 Nausea and vomiting after gynaecological laparoscopy depends upon the phase of the menstrual cycle. Canadian Journal of Anaesthesia 38: 876–879

Jackson I J B, Paton R H, Hawkshaw D 1997 Telephone follow-up the day after day surgery. Journal of One Day Surgery (Spring): 5–7

James R 1993 Night and day. Health Service Journal 103: 22–24

Johnson A 1997 Laparoscopic surgery. Lancet 349: 631–635

Jones R M 1990 Desflurane and sevoflurane: inhalation anaesthetics for this decade? British Journal of Anaesthesia 65: 527–536

Kamath B, Curran J, Hawkey C et al 1990 Anaesthesia, movement and emesis. British Journal of Anaesthesia 64: 728–730

Kapur P A 1991 The big 'little' problem. Anesthesia and Analgesia 73: 243–245

Knowles I, King T A 1995 A note on a day care postoperative telephone helpline. Journal of One Day Surgery (Autumn): 20

Kortilla K 1982 Recovery and driving after brief anaesthesia. Anaesthetist 30: 377–382

Lawrence K, McWhinnie D, Goodwin A L et al 1995 Randomised controlled trial of laparoscopic and open repair of inguinal hernia: early results. British Medical Journal 311: 981–985

Lerman J 1992 Surgical and patient factors involved in postoperative nausea and vomiting. British Journal of Anaesthesia 69 (suppl 1): 24S–32S

Lewis C, Bryson J 1998 Does day case surgery generate extra workload for primary and community health service staff? Annals of the Royal College of Surgeons of England 80: 200–202

Linares-Gil M J, Pelegri-Asanta M D, Pi-Siques F et al 1997 Unanticipated admissions following ambulatory surgery. Ambulatory Surgery 5: 183–188

Linden I, Engberg I B 1996 Patients' opinions of information given and post-operative problems experienced in conjunction with ambulatory surgery. Ambulatory Surgery 4: 85–91

Long B, Phipps W J 1985 Essentials of medical/surgical nursing. C V Mosby, St Louis

McCrirrick A, Ramage D T O, Pracilio J A, Hickman J A 1991 Experience with the laryngeal mask airway in two hundred patients. Anaesthesia and Intensive Care 19(2): 256–260

MacKenzie J W 1989 Day case anaesthesia and anxiety. A study of anxiety profiles amongst patients attending a day bed unit. Anaesthesia 44: 437–440

Malin N, Teasdale K 1991 Caring versus empowerment: consideration for nursing practice. Journal of Advanced Nursing 16: 657–662

Malster R M J, Solly J, Schofield S et al 1998 From beginning to end: an audit of the patient's experience of the day surgery. Journal of One Day Surgery (Spring): 18–21

Markanday L, Platzer H 1994 Brief encounters. Nursing Times 90(7): 38–42

Meredith P, Wood C 1994 The introduction of an audit programme to measure patient satisfaction with surgical care. Journal of One Day Surgery 4(2): 15–16

Millar J M, Rudkin G E, Hitchcock M 1997 Practical anaesthesia and analgesia for day surgery. Bios Scientific, Oxford

Milligan K A 1994 Laryngeal mask in the prone position. Anaesthesia 49: 449

Moran S, Kent G 1995 Quality indicators for patient information in short stay units. Nursing Times 91(4): 37–40

Muir J J, Warner M A, Offord K P 1987 Role of nitrous oxide and other factors in postoperative nausea and vomiting: a randomised and blinded prospective study. Anesthesiology 66: 513–518

Myint Y, Singh A K, Peacock J E et al 1995 Changes in intra-ocular pressure during G.A. Anaesthesia 50: 126–129

Nathanson M H, Fredman B, Smith I et al 1995 Sevoflurane versus desflurane for outpatient anaesthesia: a comparison of maintenance and recovery profiles. Anesthesia and Analgesia 81: 1186–1190

Neve C 1995 Patients' and nurses' perceptions of caring in a day surgery unit. Unpublished MSc dissertation, City University, London

NHS Executive 1994 Day surgery task force report and tool kit upgrade. EL(94) 76. October

Otte D 1996 Patients' perspectives and experiences of day surgery. Journal of Advanced Nursing 23: 1228–1237

Palazzo M G A, Strunin L 1984 Anaesthesia and emesis 1: aetiology. Canadian Journal of Anaesthesia 31: 178–187

Pandit S K 1998 Current issues in ambulatory surgery. Ambulatory Surgery 6: 5–11

Parry A 1995 The lived experience of day surgery. Unpublished MSc dissertation. Royal College of Nursing, London

Peng P W H, Chan V W S, Chung F F T 1997 Regional anaesthesia in ambulatory surgery. Ambulatory Surgery 5: 133–143

Pollard R C, Cooper G M 1995 The laryngeal mask in day surgery: a survey of current practice and usage. Ambulatory Surgery 3(1): 37–42

Pueyo F J, Carrascosa F, Lopez L, Iribarren M J, Garcia-Pedrajas F, Saez A 1996 Combination of ondansetron and droperidol in the prophylaxis of postoperative nausea and vomiting. Anesthesia and Analgesia 83: 117–122

Raeder J C 1997 Epidural and spinal anaesthesia have no place in a busy day unit? Ambulatory Surgery 5: 113–116

Ramachandra V 1994 Day surgery pain. Journal of One Day Surgery 3(4): 14–15

Rhodes S 1991 A follow-up of patients following day care cataract operations. Journal of One Day Surgery 1(2): 16–19

Robinson H 1994 An unorchestrated encounter – a user's account of day surgery. Surgical Nurse 7(4): 28–30

Rowe J W, Kahn R L 1987 Human ageing: Usual and successful. Science 237: 143

Rowe L, de Boer F, Crocker S 1994 Nausea and vomiting following gynaecological surgery: a comparison of ondansetron and droperidol as prophylaxis. Journal of One Day Surgery (Winter): 9–10

Rudkin G E, Maddern G J 1995 Perioperative outcome for day case laparoscopic and open hernia repair. Anaesthesia 50: 586–589

Rush J D, Harris K, McLouglin A P et al 1995 Consideration for the escort's role underestimated. Journal of One Day Surgery (Winter): 6–7

Shafer A, White P F, Urquhart M L 1989 Outpatient pre-medication: use of midazolam and opioid analgesics. Anesthesiology 71: 495–501

Sleight J W, Henderson J D 1995 Heart rate variability and pre-operative anxiety. Acta Anaesthesiologica Scandinavica 39: 1059–1061

Stephenson M E 1990 Discharge criteria for day surgery. Journal of Advanced Nursing 15: 601–613

Steward D J 1975 A simplified scoring system for the post-operative recovery room. Canadian Anaesthetic Society Journal 22: 111–113

Strunin L 1993 How long should patients fast before surgery? Time for a new guideline. Editorial. British Journal of Anaesthesia 70: 1–3

Tinkle M, Beaton J 1983 Toward a new view of science: implications for nursing research. Advances in Nursing Science (January): 27–36

Tramer M R et al 1997 A quantitative systematic review of ondansetron in treatment of established postoperative nausea and vomiting. British Medical Journal 314: 1088–1092

Twersky R S, Abiona M, Thorne A C et al 1995 Admissions following ambulatory surgery: outcome in seven urban hospitals. Ambulatory Surgery 3(3): 141–146

Vijay V, King T A 1995 Postoperative intramuscular opiates in day surgery. Journal of One Day Surgery (Summer): 6–7

Wechtler B V, Sung Y F, Duncalf D, Josylin A F 1990 Ondansetron decreases emetic symptoms following outpatient laparoscopy. Anesthesiology 73: A36

Whitwam J G (ed) 1994 Day-case anaesthesia and sedation. Blackwell Scientific Publications, London

Willis C E, Watson J D, Harper C V et al 1997 Does day surgery embarrass the primary health care team? An audit of complications and consultations. Ambulatory Surgery 5: 71–75

Wilson I G, Fell D, Robinson S L et al 1992 Cardiovascular responses to insertion of the laryngeal mask. Anaesthesia 49: 733–734

Woodhouse M, King T A, Challiner A 1998 Impact of day surgery on community services . Journal of One Day Surgery (Summer): 3–4

Young S J, Munro F J 1995 Some patient pre-operative anxieties about day surgery. Journal of One Day Surgery (Autumn): 21

16

The high dependency unit

Carolyn Mills

AIMS

This chapter aims to provide the reader with an opportunity to:

- explore the history of the high dependency unit (HDU) and its relationship with intensive care
- consider the purpose of the HDU
- identify key issues to consider in setting up an HDU
- consider the nature of nursing in high dependency settings
- explore nurse–patient issues
- review the advantages and disadvantages of high dependency units.

INTRODUCTION

The upsurgance and role of the high dependency unit (HDU) are related to issues concerning the care of the critically ill, and the nature and role of intensive care. In the last 30 years the care of critically ill patients has developed rapidly. Intensive care units (ICU) now epitomise the challenge of high technology care and, with increasingly complex therapeutic techniques, advances in technology and new practices, have the ability to care for increasingly sick and challenging patients. As a consequence intensive care units make heavy demands in terms of staff, equipment and other resources.

Within the UK, the overall availability of intensive care beds is substantially less than in mainland Europe (Singer et al 1994). Therefore, compared with Europe, a higher proportion of intensive care patients in British ICUs are likely to require mechanical ventilation (Rennie 1995), leaving many acutely ill, but non-ventilated patients to be managed in non-intensive care areas. For this type of patient, treatment in an ICU may potentially represent overtreatment, and treatment in a general ward may potentially represent undertreatment; care in an intermediate care area such as a high dependency unit would be more appropriate. A recent report commissioned by the Department of Health investigated the demand for intensive care beds with respect to supply. During a 3-month audit of six intensive care units, 712 patients were admitted of which 75 were seen to be inappropriate admissions. Clinicians identified that 49 of these patients could have been more appropriately admitted to a high dependency unit (DoH 1995, p. 40). Specifically relating to surgical patients, the National Confidential Enquiry into Perioperative Deaths (Campling et al 1992) stated that inadequate provision of high dependency units in hospitals continues to put patients at risk in the vital days following an operation. The report recommended that any hospital admitting complex elective patients for surgery should review its provision of intensive and/or high dependency care to ensure adequate provision is made.

In today's health care climate the appropriateness of caring for patients in an ICU or an HDU will inevitably be translated into monetary terms, relating to issues such as patient mix, admission patterns, outcome and the relative cost of ICUs and HDUs. The financial advantage of caring for patients in the HDU rather than the ICU is persuasive; Singer et al (1994) cited the comparative costs in 1991 as being £437 versus £1149 per day.

Currently less than 10% of hospitals in the UK have high dependency units (Thompson & Singer 1995). However, with an increasing amount of evidence that appears to support the case for HDUs (Crosby & Rees 1983, Crosby et al 1990, Kilpatrick et al 1994, Ridley et al 1991) their number looks set to rise in the next decade. The Association of Anaesthetists in a report published in 1990 stated that the provision of a high dependency unit in every acute hospital would allow rationalization of patient care … improve the care of many patients currently nursed on general wards … and decrease the pressure on scarce intensive care facilities.

Application to nursing

The above factors combined with the predicted changes in nursing and health care provision in the next decade (DoH 1994); increasing technology and the ability to keep people alive for longer; the shift from acute to primary care and the associated increase in the acuteness of illness in hospital inpatients, combined with the probable change in the traditional role of the nurse working in hospitals, reinforces further the need for all nurses to have knowledge about the purpose and functioning of HDUs. As the majority of

patients admitted to HDUs have undergone surgery, either being admitted to the HDU electively postoperatively or as a postoperative emergency (Thompson & Singer 1995), there is a particular need for surgical nurses to have an awareness of the purpose and functioning of HDUs to enable them to be responsive to the changing needs of patients and their families and to provide a high-quality service.

Quality is an abstract concept which is difficult to define, but relates to attainment of the highest degree of excellence in patient care (Van Maanen 1981). Donabedian (1989) considers that quality has three key components: the quality of technical care, the goodness of the interpersonal relationship and the goodness of the amenities of care. Today clients know more about health services; consequently, they have greater expectations, and at the same time are more critical in their attitudes. This represents a challenge for all health care professionals.

For nurses to meet the challenges resulting from the changing environment of health care, as previously highlighted, and to ensure provision of a high-quality service, all nurses, but particularly surgical nurses, need to have knowledge and skills in caring for critically ill patients requiring high dependency care.

HISTORICAL PERSPECTIVE

What is an HDU?

An HDU is defined by the Association of Anaesthetists of Great Britain and Ireland (1990) as 'an area for patients who require more intensive observation, treatment and nursing care than can be provided on a general ward.' It would not normally accept patients requiring mechanical ventilation, but could manage those receiving invasive monitoring. It is viewed by the Intensive Care Society (ICS 1990a) as an area offering a standard of intermediate care between the general ward and full intensive care.

A high dependency unit therefore provides a level of care intermediate between that on a general ward and that on an ICU. It can act as a 'step up' or a 'step down' between the levels of care delivered on a general ward and on an ICU. A high dependency unit does not provide a full range of support services for patients requiring very high levels of care such as in an intensive care unit; it monitors and supports patients with or likely to develop acute (or acute on chronic) single organ failure. The types of patients for whom HDU care may be most appropriate are outlined in Box 16.1.

Box 16.1 Appropriate patients for high dependency care

- Patients requiring support for single organ failure (excluding those requiring advanced respiratory support)
- Patients who would benefit from more detailed monitoring and supervision than can be provided on a general ward
- Patients who no longer require intensive care, but are not well enough to return to a general ward
- Postoperative patients needing close monitoring
- Patients not undergoing specific medical or surgical intervention but who require close monitoring

---

However, Box 16.1 can only be a guide to the type of patients who would benefit from being cared for in an HDU as there appears to be no common agreement as to what services an HDU would specifically offer. There is bound to be variation at local level, as there is also with intensive care provision. Generally, however, a high dependency unit would not care for patients requiring mechanical intervention or patients requiring multiple organ support.

The history of critical care

Historically the term critical care has been associated with intensive care. There is a paucity of literature focusing on what constitutes critical care nursing practice, and those studies that are available focus on intensive care areas for their data (Breu & Dracup 1982, RCN 1969). Hudak et al (1990) see that the 'essence of critical care nursing lies not in special environments, nor amid special equipment, but in the nurses' decision making process and willingness to act on decisions made'.

The arena of critical care nursing in the 1990s is considerably different from the 1970s and 1980s. With advances in biotechnology and medical progress there has been an expansion in hi-tech areas, providing a high level of care and specialist nursing knowledge and skills. The Institute of Manpower Studies (1992), in a recent study on nurses and technicians, terms such areas 'high technology areas'. They do not offer a definition as to what constitutes a high technology area but the areas considered in the study include intensive care, coronary care and renal units. Although not included in this study, high dependency units could also be considered as offering a similar service.

Critical care nursing is a specialty that has become established in the last decade. Florence Nightingale in her *Notes on Nursing* (1859) alluded to the need for critical care by recognising the value of having one place where postoperative and other patients needing close attention could be watched.

During the Second World War the concept of intensive care was seen in the specialised teams which were formed to provide pre- and postoperative intensive care to men at the battle front, with seemingly positive results (Lenihan 1979).

In the 1950s medical specialties began to develop rapidly. At this time the first units for assisted ventilation were set up initially in response to the polio epidemic that was affecting most of western Europe at that time.

The 1960s and 1970s saw the development of intensive care units on a relatively rapid scale, accompanied by advances in technology and new practices. Today almost every hospital in the UK has an intensive care unit, with many larger hospitals in fact having several specialist intensive care units, e.g. cardiothoracic, neurosciences. The origin of HDUs is unclear in the literature, but the development of ICUs and then CCUs in the 1960s can be seen as a precursor.

Today continued advances and developments in medicine have resulted in the ability to care for sicker and sicker patients, patients that a few years ago would have had little or no chance of surviving. This in itself raises the issue of the ethics of concentrating a lot of resources on a relatively small number of patients (see Ch. 4). But the main consequence has been an increasing pressure on intensive care resources. In 1990 the Intensive Care Society recommended that the number of ICU beds needed to rise from 1% to 2% of acute hospital beds to cope with the increasing pressure on ICU resources. Today the situation appears unchanged with several recent reports highlighting the problems of providing sufficient ICU beds to meet demand (DoH 1995, Mitchell et al 1995).

One of the key issues emerging from such reports is the issue of appropriateness of referrals to the ICU. The increasing pressure on ICU resources led both the Intensive Care Society (1990b) and the Association of Anaesthetists (1988, 1989) to look closely at the patients in ICUs. They recognised the existence of a patient group who, although critically ill and requiring monitoring and close supervision, had a relatively low risk of dying and could be cared for in an area providing acute care, somewhere between the general ward and the ICU. The Association of Anaesthetists (1990) stated that the provision of a high dependency unit in every acute hospital would allow rationalization of patient care … improve the standards of care of many patients currently on general wards and … ease the pressure on scarce ICU facilities. It seems, however, that the problem remains, as it continues to be identified and highlighted in more recent reports (DoH 1995).

Currently in the UK there are over 300 designated intensive care units; however, less than 15% of these hospitals have an HDU (Donnelly et al 1995). The future for health care implies a substantial shift in the balance of health care provision from acute care to community care, with only the very sick requiring hospital care (DoH 1993a). Combined with the increasing financial evidence to support the development of HDUs (Singer et al 1994); and the potential for improved quality of care that can be offered to patients who would be appropriately admitted to a high dependency unit (DoH 1995); and an ageing population who will potentially require high dependency nursing if they undergo major surgical intervention,, the interest in high dependency care is growing.

To date, no formal evaluation of the cost benefits of HDU care has been conducted. But the provision of a high dependency service will increasingly be on the agenda of most acute hospitals as an intermediate facility requiring less capital expenditure and lower staffing levels than an ICU. It is somewhere that can potentially ensure that patients receive care appropriate to their needs, while retaining the more expensive and increasingly scarce intensive care beds for the critically ill patients.

However, it is vital that the role of such units is clarified and past work reflected on and learnt from before more resources are committed.

PURPOSE AND STRATEGY
Provision of facilities in HDUs

Within the UK there is variation in relation to the provision of facilities and monitoring procedures offered in a high dependency unit. However, all HDUs should be able to provide the following:

- a clear operational policy based on a background of multidisciplinary care and effective communication
- a nurse–patient ratio of 1 : 2 (ICS 1990a)
- a designated consultant as a director, with continuous support from an ICU or admitting consultant
- administrative, technical and secretarial support
- continuing education and training of all staff
- evidence of audit of the service
- a sufficient caseload to maintain expertise and skills of all staff.

The technical capability of HDUs will also vary from unit to unit. Most HDUs would provide a broad range of monitoring and support facilities very similar

to those offered in the ICU environment but with no mechanical respiratory support. Box 16.2 identifies a range of monitoring and support facilities most commonly found within HDUs

Admission to and discharge from an HDU

Admission and discharge policies are key to ensuring the most effective use of high dependency beds. The purpose of such policies is to ensure that patients admitted are appropriate for an HDU, to reduce and prevent cancellation of elective patients, and to ensure availability of beds for emergency admission requests. In order to achieve realistic and workable policies on admission and discharge, there needs to be collaboration between medical and nursing staff within and external to the HDU and also with the bed manager.

Box 16.2   Monitoring and support facilities commonly offered by HDUs

Monitoring
- Intra-arterial pressure
- Pulmonary artery catheter
- Central venous pressure
- Pulse oximetry
- Continuous ECG

Respiratory support
- Facial/nasal continuous positive pressure ventilation (CPAP)
- Tracheostomy
- Arterial blood gas monitoring
- Oxygen therapy
- Airway management

Cardiovascular support
- Inotropes
- Vasodilators
- Intra-aortic balloon pumps
- Pacing
- Cardioversion
- Thrombolytic therapy
- Autotransfusion

Renal support
- Haemofiltration
- Heamodialysis
- Plasma exchange
- Peritoneal dialysis

Analgesia and sedation
- Epidural analgesia
- Heminevrin infusions
- Patient-controlled analgesia
- Continuous intravenous sedation

To date, there are no national recommendations concerning admission and discharge policy for HDUs, as there are for ICUs, although some HDUs have locally developed policies to fit their individual needs. If the number of HDUs is set to increase, there will certainly be a need for these policies in the future.

Reflective point

How would you begin to go about introducing admission and discharge guidelines for an HDU in your own locality? Who would you need to liaise with; who would you get involved; who would support you; and from whom would there be resistance and why?

Admission

The purpose of high dependency units is to offer a standard of care intermediate between the general ward and ICU. Patients admitted to a high dependency unit usually require one or more of the following:

- Continuous monitoring (can be invasive) and close supervision. As previously stated, this could be a step up from the general ward for a patient whose condition gives concern and may prevent the need for admission to ICU. It could be a step down from intensive care for patients who no longer require intensive care but are not well enough to go to a general ward. It could be for a patient who is admitted specifically for close supervision who does not require mechanical ventilation, e.g. a patient for whom there were problems with cardiac rhythm during surgery and who experienced dysrhythmias.
- Rapid and effective intervention for a known complication, e.g. cardioversion, insertion of pacing wires.
- Optimisation preoperatively, to reduce the potential for complications and possible ICU admission postoperatively, e.g. a patient undergoing elective surgery for repair of an aneurysm.

Specific admission criteria may need to be developed to define for stakeholders of the HDU service, either internal or external, what type of patients are considered suitable for admission to such areas. Although there are some general criteria which appear to be common in relation to admission to an HDU, e.g. that HDUs do not accept patients requiring mechanical ventilation, each HDU will vary in the level and type of facilities that they are able and prepared to offer. This in turn will affect their specific admission criteria. This variation is demonstrated by the examples that follow.

Admission criteria could be developed around areas such as the status of the potential patient's respiratory system, cardiovascular system, central nervous system, renal system, temperature and analgesia. For example, a patient who was in need of ventilation or intubation would be admitted to an ICU area, while a patient who required 60% oxygen with adequate oxygen saturation (over 90%) would be considered suitable for an HDU area. A patient who required 60% oxygen with inadequate oxygen saturations (under 90%) may go to either area depending on the patient's general condition, past medical history and local needs in relation to bed availability. The following example relates to the provision of analgesia. In some hospitals, patients receiving analgesia through an epidural infusion would be considered appropriate to be cared for in an HDU; elsewhere patients with epidural infusions are commonly cared for in ward areas.

At the present time the majority of HDU beds are used for postoperative care (Thompson & Singer 1995). However, with the change in the balance of health care provision between community setting and acute care settings, and acute hospitals becoming more like 'high technology centres offering intensive, and specialized care' (DoH 1993a) this may be set to change in the coming decade.

Discharge

General criteria for discharge from the HDU would be when patients no longer require close observation and any threat to them has been alleviated. Again, criteria for discharge will vary between individual units, and to some extent will reflect their admission criteria.

Both admission to the HDU and discharge of patients from it will be influenced by one overriding factor, that is, demand on beds. This potentially has a twofold effect: that of premature discharge from the HDU to the ward to make way for a patient whose need is judged to be greater; and also, the placing of patients who would ideally be nursed in a high dependency environment in a ward area. This reinforces the point made earlier about the need for all nurses to have some knowledge of high dependency nursing to ensure that such patients and their families receive safe and appropriate standards of care regardless of the setting.

Nursing considerations in admitting and discharging patients

There is little literature available on the experiences of patients and their families, either on admission to or discharge from an HDU. However, one small study focusing on the experience of family members having a relative transferred from an ICU to a general ward (Mills 1995) provides some insight. It found that the experience was isolating for families who had previously felt secure within the ICU environment. Overall, relatives felt positive about the transfer, seeing it as indicating progress towards health. These positive feelings, however, were easily changed to negative feelings as a result of undergoing the actual experience of transfer.

Key reasons for families feeling like this seemed to relate to noticeable differences experienced within the high technology area compared with the general ward, notably in the level of technology and intervention, the nurse–patient ratio and, specifically, in this study, the organisational approach. As the ICU practised primary nursing, particularly supportive and therapeutic relationships with families had resulted, whereas the ward did not practise primary nursing and so a lack of continuity became more obvious to the relatives when directly experienced and compared (Mills 1995).

Although this study was based on families in an ICU, there are parallels that can be drawn with patients and families being discharged from an HDU. The importance of the family in the discharge process from ICU has been recognised through other studies and has been linked to patients' outcomes (Carr 1988, Saarmann 1993).

For nurses admitting patients to HDU areas there is a need to have an understanding of how an HDU runs and the reasons for admission, to allow them to prepare the patient (and family) to be admitted to the HDU. Key issues which would need to be explored with all patients would relate to the technology that patients would expect to find, and that this is 'normal', the increased number of nurses available to care for each patient, and the size of the area. Specific information will also need to be given pertaining to each individual patient's reason for admission.

With regard to discharge from the HDU, this potentially could be a less traumatic experience for patients and relatives than discharge directly from an ICU, as the patients and their families may have already experienced changes in the transition from ICU to HDU. Or, if patients had been admitted to the HDU directly from a ward, they would have already experienced being cared for in a ward area. But for patients who are admitted directly rather than via a ward or ITU to an HDU, and then discharged from it, this may not be the case. Again, patients and their families need to be made aware of the differences between an HDU and the ward as identified above so that they do not come as unexpected.

Overall, communication between ward areas and the HDU is the key to making transfer to and from the HDU as seamless as possible and the least stressful for patients and their families as well as nursing and medical staff.

Interface with the hospital

Within the UK, high dependency units currently are sited in a variety of settings: as part of a general ward, usually surgical; as a discrete unit; or combined with an ICU. Most HDUs in the UK are geographically separate from the intensive care unit, with almost 50% of these being part of a general ward (Thompson & Singer 1995). This is a situation which will potentially change in the future, as the acuteness of illness in hospital patients rises and the number of HDU beds increases. Issues concerning HDU beds and their best position within the hospital will undoubtedly arise.

Centralisation of high dependency care in a hospital (disregarding its actual physical position) has the potential to ensure a high level of nursing and medical expertise in an 'appropriate' area, and to reduce costs through rationalising ICU resources and potentially sparing some ICU resources (Donnelly et al 1995, Rennie 1995, Singer et al 1994). The interface a high dependency unit has with the rest of the hospital will vary considerably depending on the positioning of the unit.

There is a paucity of literature about the advantages and disadvantages of different geographical positions for the HDU within a hospital. South East Thames Regional Health Authority recommended in 1994 that by December 1998 all hospitals with a high dependency unit in their area should have it placed adjacent to the intensive care unit. The rationale cited for this recommendation was that high dependency care was a service closely relating to intensive care. As one of the arguments supporting the need for more HDUs concerns more effective use of resources, it is essential that staff and other resources are managed carefully, as identified resource utilisation will be influenced by the positioning of an HDU. Choice will probably be dependent on local circumstances, predicted clinical course and on the facilities already available. Regarding the actual geographical positioning of HDUs, there appear to be advantages and disadvantages for each of the main options.

Some of the more generic advantages and disadvantages are now briefly explored.

The HDU as part of a general ward

Advantages.   Patients do not have to move to a new area when their condition starts to improve or deteriorate; this allows patients to become used to an area. They would probably not be exposed to the potential stressors associated with transfer from a completely separate unit. There is potential for better continuity of nursing care between the HDU area and the ward area. In fact it may be possible for the patients' named nurses to continue to care for them. Staff also increase their skills in HDU nursing because of the increased exposure.

Disadvantages.   Expertise in high dependency care may be limited from both nursing and medical staff perspectives. It is unlikely that there will be many nurses in such areas with specific expertise in the area of critical care. Medical cover would probably be by the resident house officer. It is unlikely to have its own technical support and would be reliant on 'borrowing' such support from other areas within the hospital. Those nurses who do have critical care experience and possible additional qualifications may feel that they are not fully utilising their knowledge and skills all of the time. This could lead to frustration. They may also be expected to work most frequently in the HDU part of the ward, and this may not optimally facilitate the development of critical care skills in other nurses with less experience or fewer qualifications.

The HDU as a discrete unit

Advantages.   The unit would have its own staff resource, which would probably include a higher proportion of nurses with critical care experience than in a combined HDU/surgical area.

Disadvantages.   Staffing would be less flexible, there would be a need to maintain a core workforce at all times of medical, nursing and support staff which may not be utilised if the unit's patient turnover is not consistent or occupancy level fluctuates.

The HDU as part of an ICU

Advantages.   There is always a senior resident doctor on duty in the ICU to support staff working in the HDU area. They may have prior knowledge of patients who have stepped down from the ICU. The ICU would usually have technical support, which would be available to the staff working in HDU. There would be a skilled workforce with a large proportion of staff having expert knowledge and skills in critical care. Owing to the closeness of the two units there would be the potential for flexibility amongst staff within ICU and HDU and centralisation of equipment. All the above have the potential for economic savings.

Disadvantages.   HDU beds may be filled with ICU patients, leaving patients requiring HDU back on the wards unless a clear protocol for use of HDU beds is in place.

Staffing resources can be stretched and difficult to manage if HDU beds can become ICU beds. ICU nurses may also perceive that if they are frequently working in the HDU they are not fully utilising their knowledge and skills, which may impact on their job satisfaction/morale.

SPECIFICATIONS FOR HDUs

Designing a new high dependency area, or commissioning changes to an existing area to turn it into a high dependency unit must take into consideration both the aesthetics and functional design elements. Although functional aspects have to take priority in the development of an HDU, the importance of the more aesthetic considerations should not be underestimated. Poor design has been shown to adversely affect patient outcomes such as recovery and reliance on analgesia (Ulrich 1984, 1992).

Size

The size and throughput of an HDU is an important issue as it will have an effect upon the quality of the service that the unit will be able to offer. At present there does not seem to be a normative number of high dependency beds for a given population.

The size of HDUs in the UK varies between four and 12 beds, with the most common size being four beds (Thompson & Singer 1995). Thompson & Singer found that many HDUs in the UK in 1994 were not open to their full potential, with budgetary constraints cited as the main reason for the closed beds.

Deciding on the size of a HDU will require careful consideration of the following issues – the relative importance of each will vary depending on the position of the HDU:

- the level of other services within the hospital
- the type and level of medical cover which is required and which is feasible
- the need to meet both elective and emergency needs
- the need for certain core staff regardless of the actual number of beds
- occupancy levels, which will need to reflect both the economic use of the facility and the need to be adaptable and responsive at short notice.

Building

There is no specific literature pertaining to the physical characteristics of the building for an HDU. Building Note Number 27 (DoH 1993b) gives guidance on standards for the building of intensive therapy units and has some relevance to HDUs. It includes the following key features:

- sufficient room between beds to allow for the passage of equipment
- good quality lighting
- windows allowing natural light
- where possible, close proximity to theatres and the accident and emergency department.

Also relevant to HDUs, particularly if they are based in either a discrete area or a ward area, is Building Note Number 4 (DoH 1990). This gives guidance on standards for the building of adult acute wards. Specific points of potential relevance to the development/building of an HDU include:

- the need for natural light
- surgical wards should have easy access to theatres and ICU and preferably be on the same floor; medical wards should be within easy reach of diagnostic and treatment facilities
- colours of walls should be light so as not to distort the colour rendering of light sources
- bed spaces should not be less than 2.9 m × 2.5 m.
- centrally located toilets should be available, no further than 12 m from bed areas, and there should be shower and bath facilities
- the staff base should be positioned to see and hear the majority of patients.

Building maintenance, fire prevention and other essential services

In relation to essential services there is little literature pertaining specifically to HDUs. The following points

are, however, essential to consider and would be similar to those for an ICU.

Immediate power back-up in case of a power failure must be available. This should include the power sources of data collection equipment (DoH 1993b). Similar immediate back-up should be available in the event of medical gas failure, further supported by a supply of medical gas cylinders which are easily accessible and stored in a well-ventilated area (NHS Estates 1994). The location and design of the HDU and means of escape facilities should comply and be maintained in accordance with the requirements of FIRECODE the fire policy document and fire officers' recommendations at local level. Evacuation procedures and training should be well developed and regularly tested. The unit and building should be regularly reviewed by building and maintenance staff.

THE HUMAN RESOURCE IN AN HDU

Nursing staff

The appropriate number of nursing staff for a high dependency unit is an area that does not appear to have been examined to date. The Intensive Care Society recommends that if the average dependency weighted occupancy is 1.0 then there should be a staffing level of 6.5 nurses per bed (ICS 1990a). In theory, patients in an HDU would require close supervision, but not necessarily the continuous presence of a nurse at the bedside. In the UK, nurse–patient ratios in HDUs are at least 3 : 1, with the smaller units having a tendency to have more nurses (Thompson & Singer 1995).

In relation to staffing for HDUs not positioned within an ICU where there is a specialised workforce, there is the issue of skill mix to address. What percentage of nursing staff do you require with specific knowledge and expertise in the area of critical care?

Reflective point

What knowledge and skills would be essential for nursing personnel working in an HDU?

For HDUs that are placed within wards, it appears that the more senior staff in that area would be expected to have specific knowledge and skills in the area of critical care nursing, either through a period of working in ICU and/or having undertaken a course in ICU or HDU nursing.

Patient dependency and workload measurement are key factors to consider when establishing the ideal staffing levels for a particular HDU; however, there are many other factors that also need to be taken into consideration, and it is therefore hard to lay down absolute guidelines. Other factors influencing both skill mix and establishment include the layout and positioning of the unit, the available medical cover, the experience of the nurses involved and the level and type of technical support.

Patient dependency and nursing workload measurement systems

In the last 10 years there has been a growing interest in the UK in the rising cost of health care and efficient utilisation of resources. This has led to political and professional initiatives to explore the efficiency and cost-effectiveness of the health care service. Such issues are particularly important for critical care areas such as ICUs and HDUs where treatment is expensive and outcomes for the sickest patients remain poor (RCN 1995).

A range of mainly quantitative measurement tools have been developed, focusing initially on the severity of the patients' condition and the level of medical intervention, and more recently on nursing workload as the cost implications of high nurse–patient ratios have been realised (RCN 1995).

There are several illness severity scoring systems in use in the UK, including the Simplified Acute Physiological and Chronic Health Evaluation Score (APACHE) and the Mortality Prediction Model (MPM), which are based on physiological criteria. There are also treatment scoring systems such as the Therapeutic Intervention Scoring system (TISS) and the Intensive Care Register (RCN 1995), which also focus on medical interventions which the patients require. TISS is commonly used within the UK to 'cost' critical care services (RCN 1995).

Nursing workload scoring systems in use in critical care in the UK include GRASP, the Criteria for Care Patient Dependency Tool, and the NMS system (RCN 1995). Other systems for measuring workload in critical care are in use abroad; these include the OMEGA system and the PRN system (Miranda et al 1990). One of the original aims of the authors of TISS was that it would be used to calculate appropriate staffing levels. However, although TISS is an internationally recognised and widely adopted, research-based scientifically validated tool commonly used within the UK, there appear to be no examples either in the USA or the UK literature of it being used for the purpose of calculating nursing workload (Chelsea & Westminster ICU/NDU 1995, RCN 1995).

Systems such as GRASP and TISS are task-oriented, capture only selected nursing activity and do not acknowledge or relate to professional activity (Birdsall 1991). As a result many critical care areas have developed their own methods of measuring patient dependency and nursing requirements on a day-to-day basis. These are generally based on broad descriptions of the typical characteristics of patient categories and are quantified in hours of care per day (Birdsall 1991). Although in such systems the level of inter-rater reliability is more subjective, and they are more difficult to replicate than other systems, they are generally much simpler to use and are seen to adequately meet the needs of the individual unit or department.

As highlighted, there has been rapid development of measurement systems in the health services throughout the UK over recent years; however, this has not always been matched by a thorough understanding of the phenomena being measured and has rarely been based on any assessment of reliability or validity. There are several different approaches to measuring nursing workload (DHSS 1983):

1. Demand and/or dependency driven. Workload measurements are dependent on the dependency of patients on a certain amount of nursing care in order to perform their activities of daily living. Patients are classified into broad bands of needs, e.g. patients who are low, medium or high dependency.
2. Care plan driven. Workload measurements are dependent on very detailed data, e.g. minutes of nursing time required to carry out specific nursing interventions.
3. Consultative/professional approaches. Workload measurement is dependent on simple data which are recorded, e.g. admission and discharge together with the nurses' impressions of workload and level of care.

It is important that all HDUs have information regarding nursing dependency: to provide a patient case mix/severity of illness profile; to show the level of nursing interventions provided; to help calculate required staffing levels and skill mix; and to provide an information resource internally and externally. The decision about which system is used in any HDU needs to be made in collaboration with both medical and nursing staff, bearing in mind why the data are being collected, for what purpose they will be used, what resources are available, and how the data will be analysed.

Medical staff

Medical support will vary depending on the position of the HDU. Thompson & Singer (1995) found that only 50% of units had a designated consultant in charge. Consultants varied from surgeons, anaesthetists, physicians and intensivists. Junior medical cover was generally provided by the team on call. In an HDU there is a need for a consultant to be available to provide support to junior staff, at least by telephone, 24 hours a day.

Reflective point

What are the implications for nursing staff, particularly in relation to managing an HDU and maintaining consistent standards, if there is not a designated consultant in charge of the HDU?

Technical support

Nurses and technicians are organisationally discrete groups who come together in hi-tech care in response to technological developments (IMS 1992). A recent study showed that in England and Wales most high technology areas (ICU, CCU and renal units) do not employ a technician, and for those that do few are directly employed (IMS 1992). For those areas that do employ a technician, intensive care is the area that had most variation in nurse and technician activity, although generally the nurses' and technicians' activities complemented each other (IMS 1992).

Decisions about the need or otherwise for a technician in high technology areas rests principally with the consultant or director of the unit and/or the senior nurse manager (IMS 1992). For nurses who may be involved in commissioning a new HDU there is a need to have an understanding of the role of technicians to allow an informed decision regarding their potential value in any individual area.

Specific advantages identified of having a technician employed in ICUs, which could be applied to HDUs, include:

- The presence of technicians to undertake routine, but technical tasks allowing nurses to concentrate on nursing care.
- Technicians can be relied upon to be responsible to undertake certain activities.
- Technicians are able to provide a first-line repair service.
- Technicians are able to develop units in terms of equipment used and procedures undertaken.
- The continuous presence of a technician means that technicians are available to teach nurses about

equipment used on the unit, increasing the technical knowledge of the nurses.

- Technicians are able to deal competently with company representatives (IMS 1992).

The principal disadvantages have been identified as follows:

- There is the potential for technicians to exert too much power and to 'interfere' with the delivery of nursing care.
- Technicians undertaking technical tasks are seen by some as detracting from the overall role of the nurse in patient care and preventing nurses from acquiring necessary technical knowledge.
- Technicians tend to work only days. At night, nurses have to undertake many of the activities that technicians undertake during the day (IMS 1992).

The specific relevance of the advantages and disadvantages of technical support identified will depend on the set-up in individual areas. Through clear role descriptions and collaboration between technical staff and nursing staff there is potential for a mutually beneficial relationship. The overriding benefit of technical support is that it allows nurses to concentrate on caring for the patients and their relatives.

For HDUs that receive technical support, the level and type of technical support available will depend on the geographical position of the HDU. HDUs placed within ICUs would potentially have access to the same technical support services, support of equipment and technical expertise, that would be available to the ICU. Those HDUs which are positioned in a discrete area or attached to a general ward are less likely to have direct access to a technician and the situation regarding technical support is less clear. Such areas will need to negotiate the level and type of technical support that they require from another area, and define the nursing mix and technician utilisation. Regardless of the technical support available to an HDU, all nurses working within such an environment will be responsible for acquiring the technical knowledge necessary to ensure patient safety and to carry out the basic technical activities which need to be undertaken 24 hours a day.

Secretarial and administrative support

Each HDU should assess their requirements for secretarial and administrative support; this may be supported further by workload measurements. Such support should facilitate all staff, but particularly the nursing staff, to focus on their patient care.

In common with all critical care areas, the amount and range of data collected within an HDU can be considerable, both in terms of patient-centred and unit-centred information. Although all data collection should be carefully rationalised, and no member of staff should collect data for the sake of it, or without a clear understanding about how such data are to be used, administrative staff are an important resource in assisting with unit-related data collection in terms of maintaining consistency, if carefully trained and supported.

Interactions with other professionals

All areas within a hospital, but particularly areas such as HDUs and ICUs, which do not have their own clients, need to ensure that they have a close working relationship across all specialties using their service. The patient's GP and referring consultant should routinely be informed of the reason for the patient's admission, the treatment given, and any onward referral details.

Particularly important for an HDU is liaison with the accident and emergency department in major accident planning.

ROLE AND FUNCTION OF THE NURSE

Before considering the role and function of the HDU nurse, the nature of HDU nursing needs to be made explicit.

Critical care nursing has only existed in the UK since the early 1960s and HDU nursing since the 1980s. Possibly owing to the newness of HDU nursing, there is little literature relating specifically to the nature of HDU nursing. The nature of critical care nursing has received increasing attention in recent years. In critical care and HDU environments, because of the nature of the work, nursing and medical care is often inextricably linked, making it difficult to identify what critical care nursing uniquely is. Past work about the critical care nurse's role has mainly focused on activities that critical care nurses undertake, for example assessment and interpretation of physiological and psychosocial data and providing appropriate interventions related to this (Breu & Dracup 1982).

More recent work has recognised that human caring is an essential component of critical care nursing practice, but acknowledges that frequently the ICU environment fails to recognise the value of care (Cooper 1993) and the nurse's attention is focused away from the subjective dimensions of nursing practice by the technological environment (Henderson 1980). Walters (1995) focused on the caring aspects of critical care nurses and identified two key themes: balancing, which was seen as the ability of the nurse to manage the paradoxical relationship between the technology of ICU and the processes of caring; and being busy, which recognised the technical nature of critical care nursing.

Yet, within many critical care areas there seems still to be a preoccupation with technical competence, and technical skills are frequently seen as more important than caring.

The development of unit philosophies, which are statements of values and beliefs held about nursing and critical care nursing, is becoming more common (Warfield & Manley 1990). These explicit values and beliefs can guide nurses in their organisational approach to care, the nursing model that they choose to use, and in their overall nursing strategy. For example, in an area where staff hold beliefs about the importance of continuity of care and the development of a therapeutic relationship, primary nursing would be an appropriate and congruent way of organising care, as opposed to patient allocation, which may not facilitate continuity of care for more than one, or at the most, two shifts (Manley 1994) (see also Ch. 2).

One key difference between intensive care and high dependency care is that all patients will be self-ventilating. Although patients in an HDU may require different levels of respiratory and cardiovascular support, with the exception of those with specific medical conditions, the vast majority of patients will be conscious and able to communicate with their carers and the people that are important to them. This reinforces the even greater importance given to providing information for HDU patients.

Nursing models for HDUs

Nursing models represent 'a way for nurses to organize their thinking about nursing and then to transfer that thinking into practice with order and effectiveness' (Wright 1986). As already highlighted, the nursing model chosen should be congruent with the values and beliefs that are held about nursing. It is therefore inappropriate to advocate the use of one particular model that is appropriate for caring for HDU patients. However, there are several key questions that nurses should ask themselves when identifying which model of nursing they want to use, and these are outlined in Box 16.3.

Critical care nursing over the last 20 years has seen an increasing recognition of and emphasis on the psychological care and needs of both patients and their families. Ideally, the model chosen for any high

---

Box 16.3 Key questions to be answered in identifying what model of nursing to use (Aggleton & Chalmers 1986)

- What assumptions does the model make about people and health-related needs?
- What values does the model hold?
- What are the key concepts that the model uses?
- What relationships are suggested between these concepts?
- How does the model see the role of the nurse?
- Does the model present things in a clear-cut and understandable way?
- Does the model have something to say about nursing in the context for which its use is being considered?
- Is the model likely to lead to better care?
- Is the model likely to be used in practice?

---

dependency area will reflect such humanistic values and continue to raise nurses' awareness of the importance of these aspects of care in an area of ever increasing technology. By using a nursing model, high dependency nurses can start to begin to make explicit the nature of high dependency nursing.

Organisational approach to care in the HDU

The organisational approach to care selected in any HDU should be congruent with the values and beliefs held by staff about the nature of HDU nursing, also taking into consideration government recommendations and standards, such as the Patient's Charter (DoH 1991) and the Vision for the Future (DoH 1993a).

The benefits of primary nursing as an organisational approach to care for patients, families, nurses and the multidisciplinary team are well documented and supported by current research (Manley 1988, 1990, 1994, Schiro 1980, Thompson 1990, Worobel 1981).

Primary nursing is seen to be particularly well suited to intensive care as it identifies the relationship between the nurse and the patient as key, which also constitutes one of the central beliefs in relation to ICU nursing (Manley 1994). Manley (1994) identifies several other key points which make the practice of primary nursing in intensive care easier compared with other areas:

- more favourable nurse–patient ratios
- consistent nurse–patient ratios on all shifts, including at night
- all qualified workforce
- greater opportunities for autonomous action.

Although nurse–patient ratios are not going to be so high in an HDU, all of the above factors would appear to be equally applicable to a high dependency environment as to an intensive care unit.

Whatever organisational approach to care is chosen, the practicalities of the area, for example the position of the HDU, skill mix, shift pattern, etc., all need to be given careful consideration prior to its operationalisation, as does the approach to implementing any major change.

NURSE–PATIENT PERSPECTIVES

Within HDU nursing there are many nurse–patient perspectives that will also be common to other areas of surgical nursing. The focus of this section will therefore be on nurse–patient perspectives that are unique to, or have more relevance to, the area of high dependency nursing and which surgical nurses may not be so familiar with.

Technology and high dependency nursing

Technology in critical care and high dependency care areas exists to benefit patient care. The nurses in such areas are themselves an integral part of the technology of the area and are constantly interacting with the patients, their families and the machinery. Within their work, nurses need to achieve a balance between ensuring that the machinery is operating safely, providing optimal support to patients, and delivering nursing care of the highest standards to patients and their families.

Technology and caring

As stated earlier, there is a concern expressed by several nurse theorists that science, technology and caring are in fact incompatible and that the nurse's attention is focused away from the art of nursing by the technological environment (Hawthorne & Yurkovich 1995, Henderson 1980, Ray 1987). Caring has been described as the 'essence of nursing and the central, dominant and unifying feature of nursing' (Leininger 1981) and as the 'human mode of being' (Roach 1987). Caring is an essential component of all critical care nursing (see also Ch. 7).

Nurses in high dependency areas need to be aware of the importance of caring for their patients and their patients' families; such values should be made explicit in the unit's philosophy and reinforced through the organisational approach to care and the model of nursing used.

Yates (1983) identified two ways in which inexperienced critical care nurses respond to entry into a critical environment with its unfamiliar technology. They will either focus on the surrounding technology and fail to see the patient as their primary concern, or they focus all their attention on the patient, attempting to cope with the fear of the unknown (i.e. the technology) by ignoring it. It should be recognised that nurses need to reach a comfortable level of technical competence to gain the knowledge and skills necessary to make the right decisions about the uses and applications of technology. Having achieved a comfortable level of technical competence, the nurse can concentrate more fully on the needs of the patient and family (Ray 1987). This is supported by the observations of Benner et al (1996, p. 205) that the novice tends to give little information about how the patient looks and responds but is more likely to note changes in the heart monitor. Experts, in contrast, through 'expert mastery of technology, coupled with expert caring' tend to be much more critical of technology's value (p. 165).

The level of technical competence that individuals feel comfortable with will vary from person to person, as will the time it takes to reach this level. However, until nurses feel that they have mastered caring for the equipment around the patients, they generally are not able to focus on the psychological and psychosocial aspects of caring for the patients and their families.

High dependency nurses need to be aware of the potential conflict between caring and technology to reduce the potential impact that such a conflict could have on their caring role in such an area. It has particular implications for new staff within the environment. These staff will need mentorship and support to ensure that they develop confidence and competence in using technology and also meeting the non-technological needs of patients and their families.

Sensory perceptual alterations

The ideal environment for anyone who is ill is one that is conducive to rest. Very few areas within a hospital are able to offer such an environment, particularly high dependency/critical care areas. Patients requiring high dependency nursing are critically ill, they will require almost continuous interventions and will be exposed to a bombardment of continuous strange sensory stimuli. This can have a twofold effect: sensory deprivation where patients exhibit a variety of symptoms such as loss of sense of time, hallucinations, restlessness and presence of delusions as a result of a reduction in the degree or structure or quality of sensory input; and sensory overload where patients exhibit symptoms similar to those above but as a result of loud, continuous, strange stimuli.

Both sensory deprivation and overload adversely affect patients and have been closely linked with psychotic behaviour (Adam & Osborne 1996). High dependency nurses need to be aware of the environment in relation to sensory stimuli, e.g. lights, sounds, touch, interruptions (Helton et al 1980, Hilton 1985) and the need to maintain an environment that provides appropriate (quantity and quality of) sensory stimulation and ensures minimum disturbance to patients' sleep. This could be achieved through, for example, clustering of care to avoid continuous disturbance of the patient, controlling noise, turning lights down at night, not having the radio on continuously (Glen 1991, Turner et al 1990).

Communication

Technology has psychosocial implications for both patients and families. Patients in any critical care area are exposed to high levels of technology and are more likely to feel anxious due to a fear of dying, loss of control, a sense of loss of function and self-esteem, a sense of isolation and a feeling of helplessness (Hudak et al 1990). Descriptions of personal experiences of being a patient in intensive care highlight the noise level, alarms, feeling tied down by tubes, immobility, and fear that the machinery will break down (Asbury 1985).

Meaningful and honest communication with patients will help increase their sense of control, as will including them in decision-making, allowing choices where possible and providing some sort of order and predictability. Nurses should be aware of the potential for becoming efficient and active around patients but not actually involving them and communicating with them therapeutically. This increases the patients' sense of isolation. Scholes (1996) identified three ways in which ICU nurses brought humanity to the 'technological nightmare' of ICU. This was through humanising the patient, therapeutic presence and therapeutic absence. Box 16.4 outlines these concepts in more detail.

Nonverbal communication such as touch is also particularly important with critically ill patients to make the interaction therapeutic and minimise their isolation (Glen 1991, Scholes 1996).

Caring for the patient's family

Family members are an important part of caring for the critically ill patient (Manley 1990), with the family

---

Box 16.4 Three ways in which nurses bring humanity to the 'technological nightmare' of ICU through establishing a dialogue with a deeply unconscious patient (Scholes 1996)

Humanising the patient
- How nurses make their presence known to the patient
- How nurses maintain their presence
- Touch talking
- Closure – keeping the patient in a peaceful restful state
- Tuning in to the patient as a person

Therapeutic presence
- How nurses use themselves in a therapeutic way to calm, orient and return patients to a peaceful, restful state

Therapeutic absence
- Use of absence to ensure that the patient has adequate rest, peace and space

---

forming the critical intervening variable between society and the individual (Norris & Grove 1986). The quality of the functioning and health of the family in critical care has been closely related to the health of its members (Olsen 1970, cited in Norris & Grove 1986).

Communication with patients and relatives is vitally important and has been closely linked with both patient and relative satisfaction (Hardy & West 1994, Kleinpell & Powers 1992). Relatives have a crucial role to play in comforting and reassuring patients. Patients and their relatives need to be informed about the nature of the machines and other technology, how they function and the nature of the alarms.

The patient's admission to a high dependency unit for a serious illness causes a great deal of distress and anxiety for relatives and may result in disequilibrium within the family unit (Breu & Dracup 1978, Bouman 1984, Daley 1984, Leske 1986). Breu & Dracup (1978) identify several unavoidable consequences of having a critically ill family member:

- deprivation of social contact and major source of gratification and self-esteem
- imposed autonomy
- altered daily patterns of living
- role reversal
- dysfunctional social contacts
- relocation to an unfamiliar environment for most of the day
- interruption of personal reward system.

Reactions to such a crisis will vary from family to family, but are likely to include high levels of anxiety, denial, anger, remorse, grief and reconciliation (Breu & Dracup 1978, Kane 1988). The outcome of such an experience is partly governed by the interaction that occurs between the individual and significant others within the emotional environment (Kane 1988). Significant others within the high dependency environment would be the primary and associate nurses and other members of the multidisciplinary team caring for the patient. Primary nursing as an organisational approach to care has the potential to offer more support to families through continuity of care and the therapeutic relationship that develops with families (Manley 1990).

Nurses in high dependency units have a key role to play in facilitating effective family functioning. Nursing interventions should be aimed at helping the family regain a sense of equilibrium. This can be achieved through effective and honest communication and information-giving, allowing relatives to participate in care if they wish, open visiting hours, showing that you care about the patient, encouraging family members to verbalise their fears and feelings, allowing the family to stay nearby and meeting other needs identified as important for relatives of critically ill patients (Hudak et al 1990, Kleinpell & Powers 1992, Leske 1986, Molter 1979).

Although the main focus of supporting the families of high dependency patients has been on the role of the nurse, it is important to understand that this cannot be done in isolation. To achieve effective outcomes in terms of family support requires collaboration with all members of the multidisciplinary team, to ensure common understanding and purpose.

Ethics

Patients who are being cared for in critical and high dependency care areas today are older and sicker than they were in past years. This has been accompanied by an increase in the technology available to extend and prolong life. As a result, all nurses but particularly those working within a critical care environment, either ICU or HDU, are likely to be more involved in complex ethical situations at some point in their nursing career. Within the role of the high dependency nurse, particular aspects such as being the patient's advocate, maintaining confidentiality, and respect for persons influence moral problems and decision-making.

Beauchamp & Childress (1989) identify four ethical principles which provide a foundation for the analysis of ethical dilemmas in health care: autonomy, non-maleficence, benificence and justice. Knowledge of basic ethical principles and the ability to apply them systematically is essential to professional nursing practice; as nurses our responsibility does not end here, but lies in actively trying to understand our patient's values and beliefs. More details on ethical principles are explored in Chapter 4.

Many approaches to moral reasoning and ethical decision focus on steps in the decision-making process rather than on content. Such steps tend to include:

1. Identify the problem.
2. Identify how you feel about it.
3. Identify the patient's values.
4. Identify the ethical principles involved.
5. Determine the relevant factual information.
6. Identify who will be involved in the decision-making process.
7. Identify the values of the decision makers.
8. Examine and categorise the alternatives.
9. Rank order the various alternatives.
10. Decide on a course of action.
11. Evaluate your action in relation to the current and possible future ethical dilemmas (Tuxill 1994).

Common ethical issues that high dependency nurses are likely to encounter concern admissions to high dependency, particularly those of 'inappropriate' admission; withdrawing and/or withholding treatment; surrogate decision-making; the patient who is unable to make an informed contribution; and 'do-not-resuscitate' orders.

All of the aforementioned ethical issues have profound social, moral and economic consequences. Making decisions about such issues requires all members of the multidisciplinary team to examine their values and obligations as health care professionals, such as respect for autonomy, respect for life, respect for dignity; and their beliefs about the purpose of health care.

The 'appropriateness' of admissions to HDU

The 'appropriateness' of admission to critical care areas is a frequent ethical dilemma that both critical care nurses and high dependency nurses will have to face. Inappropriate admission can be seen as being wrong from both a moral and economic perspective. Decisions about whether or not to admit a patient will involve consideration of all information, both strategic and that concerning the individual patient. For example, in a situation where acute on chronic illness is concerned, or a very elderly person, the potential outcome of treatment must be considered in depth. Age, although an important consideration, should not be the sole reason for refusal of admission to an HDU (see also Ch. 11).

Withdrawing and withholding treatment

Withdrawing treatment refers to actually stopping treatment once it has been started. Withholding treatment refers to never initiating treatment. Both situations are often complex, both ethically and emotionally, for both health care staff and the family.

In such situations all the medical and social facts of each case need to be gathered together, for example laboratory results, prognosis, alternative treatments, assessment of the patient's normal living environment, the situation of the family/significant others, and the patient's wishes/decision-making ability. Once these data are available, the situation should be explored and analysed collaboratively using the basic ethical principles already outlined as a foundation.

Reflective point

Is it possible to create an outcome for a patient that is worse than death?

Do-not-resuscitate status

Do-not-resuscitate status is an act of withholding treatment; and as such can result in conflict between patients, relatives and multidisciplinary team members. Open communication has been identified as crucial to minimising and preventing any conflict surrounding do-not-resuscitate orders (Jezewski 1994). It is important that the readiness of families to be involved in such decisions is assessed, and that they understand the meaning of a do-not-resuscitate order. Sensitivity, support and time are needed to make a decision about withholding resuscitation if a caring, humanistic focus is to be maintained. If families are involved in such decision-making, it is important that they are supported in whatever decision they make, even if it is one that the health care team do not agree with.

Surrogate decision-making

If a patient is comatose or otherwise unable to express his or her wishes, an advocate, someone who would be able to make a 'substituted judgement' for the patient must be identified. Advocacy is the moral commitment to enhance a patient's autonomy. This is particularly important in critical care areas where patients are frequently in this position. If no advocate is available, the team need to be guided by all the information they have about the patient, as well as their moral values and obligations as health care professionals (Gadow 1989).

In the USA, and to a lesser extent in Britain, there is growing interest in and use of 'advanced directives' or living wills which express the views and values of the patient about health care should he or she lose the capacity for decision-making. Although such documents are not recognised as legal in the UK, they do provide the health care team with a clear picture of the patient's wishes (see Ch. 11).

In any ethical situation that arises, the caring component involved in reaching a decision is absolutely crucial. This will ensure that decisions which are potentially stressful are implemented in a humanistic way.

Whatever ethical situation nurses find themselves involved in, it is vital that discussions to resolve the situation involve collaboration between the patient (if possible), the patient's family and or significant other, and all members of the multidisciplinary team.

EDUCATION OF HIGH DEPENDENCY NURSES, ROLE AND COURSE DEVELOPMENT

In the future, high dependency nursing looks set to become a speciality in its own right. Today there are several academic institutions offering post-basic courses in high dependency nursing. The content, length and focus of these is very variable at present.

There is a need for nursing to try to articulate what high dependency nursing is, so as to move forward and develop courses which facilitate the development of autonomous professional high dependency nursing. Relevant education, and guided reflection on practice, through for example clinical supervision, will result in more effective and therefore higher quality of care being delivered to patients and their families (Johns 1995).

CONCLUSION

In summary, this chapter has attempted to give the surgical nurse an understanding of the main issues associated with high dependency nursing and highlighted the differences between high dependency and critical care nursing. For all nurses, but particularly surgical nurses, as surgical patients currently represent the majority of those patients requiring HDU care, there is a specific need to develop an understanding of HDU nursing, to ensure that patients requiring HDU care either in a designated HDU or in a general ward, receive high quality nursing care.

High dependency facilities are at the present time generally lacking in the UK (Thompson & Singer 1995). Within the present health care climate there is considerable interest in developing further HDU facilities. Proper utilisation of this resource could have significant implications for medical and nursing care of critically ill patients in the future. However, although there is some evidence of the advantages of HDUs, particularly in relation to cost-effectiveness and the potential impact that they can have on reducing admissions and re-admission to ICU, studies focusing on economic and client/patient benefit are urgently needed to validate this.

REFERENCES

Adam S, Osborne S 1996 Critical care nursing: science and practice. Oxford University Press, Oxford

Aggleton P, Chalmers H 1986 Nursing models and the nursing process. Macmillan, London

Asbury A 1985 Patients' memories and reactions to intensive care. Care of the Critically Ill 1(2): 12–13

Association of Anaesthetists of Great Britain and Ireland 1988 The high dependency unit – acute care in the future. Association of Anaesthetists of Great Britain and Ireland, London

Association of Anaesthetists 1989 Intensive care services – provision for the future. Association of Anaesthetists, London

Association of Anaesthetists of Great Britain and Ireland 1990 Report on high dependency units. Association of Anaesthetists, London

Beauchamp T, Childress J 1989 Principles of biomedical ethics. Oxford University Press, New York

Benner P, Tanner C, Chelsa C 1996 Expertise in nursing practice: caring, clinical judgement and ethics. Springer, New York

Birdsall C 1991 Management issues in critical care. Mosby, St Louis

Bouman C 1984 Identifying priority concerns of families of ICU patients. Dimensions of Critical Care Nursing 3: 313–319

Breu C, Dracup K 1978 Helping the spouses of critically ill patients. American Journal of Nursing 78: 50–53

Breu C, Dracup K 1982 A survey of critical care nursing practice part 3. Responsibilities of the intensive care unit staff. Heart and Lung 11(2): 157–161

Campling E A et al 1992 The report of the National Confidential Enquiry into Perioperative Deaths 1992/1993. London

Carr P 1988 Discharge planning: a critical care nurse responsibility. Critical Care Nurse 8: 78–84

Chelsea and Westminster ICU/NDU 1995 Annual report. Chelsea and Westminster Hospital, London

Cooper M 1993 The intersection of technology and care in the ICU. Advances in Nursing Science 15(3): 23–32

Crosby D, Rees G 1983 Post operative care: the role of the HDU. Annals of the Royal College of Surgeons 65: 391–393

Crosby D, Rees G, Gill J 1990 The role of the HDU in postoperative care: an update. Annals of the Royal College of Surgeons 72: 309–312

Daley L 1984 The perceived immediate needs of families with relatives in the intensive care setting. Heart and Lung 13: 231–237

Department of Health (DoH) 1990 Adult acute medical wards. Health Building Note 4. HMSO, London

Department of Health (DoH) 1991 The patient's charter. DoH, London

Department of Health (DoH) 1993a A vision for the future. DoH, London

Department of Health (DoH) 1993b Intensive therapy unit. Health Building Note 27. HMSO, London

Department of Health (DoH) 1994 The challenges for nursing and midwifery in the 21st century. DoH, London

Department of Health (DoH) 1995 Study of provision of intensive care in England. HMSO, London

Department of Health and Social Security (DHSS) 1983 Nurse manpower planning: approaches and techniques. HMSO, London

Donabedian A 1989 Institutional and professional responsibilities in quality assurance. Quality Assurance in Health Care 1(1): 3–11

Donnelly P, Sandifer R Q, O'Brien D, Thomas E 1995 A pilot study of the use of clinical guidelines to determine appropriateness of patient placement on intensive and high dependency care units. Journal of Public Health 17(3): 305–310

Gadow S 1989 Clinical subjectivity: advocacy with silent patients. Nursing Clinics of North America 24(2): 535–541

Glen A 1991 Psychological aspects of critical care. Surgical Nurse 4(3): 15–17

Hardy G, West M 1994 Happy talk. Health Service Journal 104: 24–26

Hawthorne D, Yurkovich N 1995 Science, technology, caring and the professions: are they compatible? Journal of Advanced Nursing 21: 1087–1091

Helton M, Huffman A, Gordon S, Lambert T, Nunnery S 1980 The correlation between sleep deprivation and ICU syndrome. Heart and Lung 9(3): 464–468

Henderson V 1980 Preserving the essence of nursing in a technological age. Journal of Advanced Nursing 5(3): 245–260

Hilton D 1985 Noise in acute patient areas. Research in Nursing and Health 8(3): 283–291

Hudak C, Gallo B, Benz J 1990 Critical care nursing: a holistic approach. Lippincott, Philadelphia

Institute of Manpower Studies (IMS) 1992 Nurses and technicians in high technology areas. IMS, Brighton

Intensive Care Society (ICS) 1990a Intensive care in the UK. ICS, London

Intensive Care Society (ICS) 1990b Intensive care audit. ICS, London

Jezewski M 1994 Do not resuscitate orders, conflict and culture brokering in critical care units. Heart and Lung 23(6): 458–465

Johns C 1995 Achieving effective work as a professional activity. In: Schober J E, Hinchliff S M (eds) Towards advanced nursing practice: key concepts for health care. Arnold, London, pp 252–280

Kane C 1988 Family social support: towards a conceptual model. Advances in Nursing Science 10(12): 18–25

Kilpatrick A, Ridely S, Plenderleith L 1994 A changing role for intensive care: is there a case for high dependency care? Anesthesia 49: 666–670

Kleinpell R, Powers M 1992 Needs of family members of intensive care unit patients. Applied Nursing Research 5: 2–8

Leininger M 1981 The phenomena of caring: importance, research questions and theoretical considerations. In: Leininger M, Slack C (eds) Caring an essential human need. Thorofare, New Jersey

Lenihan J 1979 The history of intensive care. Nursing Focus 1(2): 75–76

Leske J 1986 Needs of relatives of critically ill patients. Heart and Lung 15(2): 189–193

Manley K 1988 Evaluation of primary nursing in the ICU: short report. Nursing Times 84(48): 57

Manley K 1990 Intensive disagreement. Nursing Times 86(19): 67–69

Manley K 1992 Knowledge for nursing practice. In: Brykczynska G, Jolley M (eds) Nursing care. Edward Arnold, London

Manley K 1994 Primary nursing in critical care. In: Burnard P, Millar B (eds) Critical care today. Baillière Tindall, London

Mills C 1995 The lived experience of families whose family member is transferred from an intensive care practising primary nursing to a ward that is not. BSc in Nursing (Hons) dissertation. Institute of Advanced Nursing Education RCN/University of Manchester

Miranda D, Williams A, Loirat P 1990 Management of intensive care: guidelines for better use of resources. Kulwer, Netherlands

Mitchell I, Grounds M, Bennett E 1995 Availability of intensive care beds in the United Kingdom. St. George's Health Care NHS Trust, London

Molter N 1979 Needs of relatives of critically ill patients. Heart and Lung 8: 332–339

Nehre et al 1994

NHS Estates 1994 Health Technical Memorandum 2022: Design considerations medical gas pipeline systems. HMSO, London

Nightingale F 1859 Notes on nursing. Republished 1990, Churchill Livingstone, Edinburgh

Norris L, Grove S 1986 Investigations of psychosocial needs of family members of critically ill adult patients. Heart and Lung 15(2): 194–197

Ray M 1987 Technological caring: a new model in critical care. Dimensions of Critical Care Nursing 6(3): 166–173

Rennie M 1995 Strengthening the case for high dependency care. British Journal of Intensive Care 5(1): 5

Ridley S, Biggam M, Stone P 1991 The cost of intensive therapy. Anesthesia 46: 523–531

Roach S 1987 The human act of caring. Canadian Hospital Association, Ottawa

Royal College of Nursing (RCN) 1969 Intensive therapy units. RCN, London

Royal College of Nursing (RCN) 1995 Dependency scoring systems: guidelines for nurses. RCN, London

Saarmann L 1993 Transfer out of critical care, freedom or fear. Critical Care Nursing Quarterly 16(19): 78–85

Schiro A 1980 Primary nursing in critical care areas. In: Zander K (ed) Primary nursing: development and management. Aspen, Maryland

Scholes J 1996 Therapeutic use of self – how critical care nurses use self to the patient's therapeutic benefit. Nursing in Critical Care 1(2): 60–66

Singer M, Myers S, Hall G, Cohen S, Armstrong R 1994 The cost of intensive care: a comparison on one unit between 1981 and 1991. Intensive Care Medicine 20: 542–549

South East Thames Regional Health Authority 1994 Intensive therapy services service standards. SETRHA, London

Thompson D 1990 At the heart of caring. Nursing Times 86(19): 70–71

Thompson F, Singer M 1995 High dependency units in the UK: variable size, variable character, few in number. Postgraduate Medical Journal 1: 221–227

Turner J, Briggs S, Springhorn H, Potgieter P 1990 Patients' recollection of ICU experiences. Critical Care Medicine 18(9): 966–968

Tuxill C 1994 Ethical aspects of critical care. In: Millar B, Burnard P (eds) Critical care today. Baillière Tindall, London

Ulrich R 1984 View through a window may influence recovery from surgery. Science 224: 420–421

Ulrich R 1992 How design impacts wellness. Healthcare Forum Journal 35(5): 20–25

Van Maanen H 1981 Improvement of quality of nursing care: a goal to challenge the eighties. Journal of Advanced Nursing 6(1): 3–9

Walters A 1995 A Heideggarian hermeneutic study of the practices of critical care nurses. Journal of Advanced Nursing 21: 492–497

Warfield C, Manley K 1990 Developing a new philosophy in the NDU. Nursing Standard 4(41): 27–30

Worobel P 1981 Peer support in implementing primary nursing. Nursing Administration Quarterly 5(3): 33–38

Wright S 1986 Building and using a model of nursing. Edward Arnold, London

Yates L 1983 Technology in nursing. Nursing Focus 5(2): 8

17

Perspectives on major disaster nursing in the developing world

Dina Plowes   Lesley Fudge

AIMS

This chapter aims to:

- provide surgical nurses with practical insight into aspects of major disaster work in the developing world
- explore the psychological and social factors often encountered by nurses
- identify practical strategies to enable appropriate care
- encourage more surgical nurses to offer their services to overseas aid programmes.

INTRODUCTION

Experienced surgical nurses' knowledge and skills are invaluable when working within a major disaster situation in the developing world, such as war, famine, natural disasters. The nurses' specialist skills complement those of their medical colleagues. They are specialist practitioners and should not be viewed as adjuncts to medical intervention. It is not our intention to describe in detail immediate surgical nursing interventions following major disasters as these are usually dealt with by agencies, such as the Army, who respond according to the nature of the incident, using resources which have been tried and tested in a variety of settings.

It is our intention, however, to focus on our personal experiences and insights of disaster nursing in the developing world. In preparing this chapter we have therefore attempted to utilise a reflective process for nurses (Strathie & Holmes 1996) within James's (1996) transformative potential of exchanging stories of experience and practice among nursing peers. We believe that to produce accounts of our experiences reflects an enlightened approach to knowledge development of surgical nurses. Telling one's story is also viewed as a traditional approach to 'consciousness-raising' in feminist circles (Weller 1991). Indeed,

Connelly & Clandinin (1990, p. 24) assert that narrative is the study of how humans make meaning by endlessly telling and retelling stories about themselves that both refigure the past and create purpose in the future. This process is viewed by Vezeau (1994, p. 61) as aesthetic inquiry which has benefits to offer all nurses and is fundamental for caring in nursing. Caring depends on caregivers having knowledge of the general situation and aesthetic knowledge of individuals. Aesthetic knowing, as one of nursing's important patterns of knowing, was identified by Carper (1978). It encompasses the art of nursing – it is the direct apprehension of a situation, the intuitive and embodied knowing that arises from the practice/praxis of nursing (Chinn 1989). Nursing praxis reflects the moral obligation to act and the transformation of one's values into action.

INITIAL THOUGHTS

Nurses going to a war zone or to a disaster area will either be going as part of a team or will join a team of colleagues with whom they have not previously worked. The latter situation will be the more difficult for all members of that team as they will have no prior knowledge of each other's skills, personalities and, if they are a multinational team, possibly also language. The ideal situation is for teams to be formed from nurses, surgeons, anaesthetists and others who are known to each other and have worked together. This ensures a common bond before the team have to face what may well be difficult and challenging situations together. They should, if possible, meet together before departing for their destination and receive a briefing from their team leader as to what they are likely to find on their arrival and the equipment that they will be likely to need when they arrive. If the team are going under the auspices of a non-governmental organisation (NGO) such as UK Med, there will be representatives of the organisation who will have prior knowledge and be able to advise the team. There is also likely to be financial support for the purchase and export of equipment and supplies along with travelling and subsistence expenses for the team. Seven principles for humanitarian agencies have been identified (Porter 1997):

- People who work for the aid agency are integral to the effectiveness and success of the agency.
- Human resource policies aim for best practice.
- Recruitment policies aim to be efficient, effective, fair and transparent.
- Field staff are consulted when developing recruitment policies.

- Plans and budgets reflect the aid agency's responsibilities towards recruited staff.
- Appropriate training and support is provided before, during and after assignments.
- All reasonable steps are taken to ensure staff security and well-being.

Cavanagh (1977), an aid worker, describes his experiences as exciting and rewarding, yet he is cautious: 'Going anywhere to do this form of work should be a carefully thought-out decision. For your own safety it is best to apply for work through an organisation rather than arriving in a country and then beginning to look for something to do.'

Within a major disaster setting the nurse's knowledge and skills are highly valued within collaborative interdisciplinary teamwork. In the ordinary 'home' situation the nurse will be aware of all the components that go together to arrive at a safe and satisfactory outcome for the patient and staff. For example, medical staff normally arrive at an operating theatre and complete their surgery with little knowledge of the planning which has been undertaken beforehand to ensure that there are adequate supplies of all surgical, anaesthetic and housekeeping equipment for the smooth running of the department. The nurse ensures that all systems are in place to enable surgery to be performed with all the appropriate equipment to hand. The nurse's knowledge of forward planning will be much in evidence prior to the overseas visit. In consultation with team members, an inventory of all the equipment the team will need will be developed. Responsibility often rests with the nurse for ensuring that all the necessary items on the inventory are present at the time of departure.

It is all too easy for nurses who travel abroad to become the 'jack of all trades', being called upon to perform a wide variety of skills. The issue of professional accountability (UKCC 1992) must be explored, particularly if nurses are challenged to work outside of their area of expertise. It is our experience that nurses tend to find a relevant role as general daily coordinator of care, as well as practical nurse. Whilst specialist nursing knowledge and skills are valued within western society and aid agencies, nursing in the developing world is generally given little official recognition. Culturally, the profile of doctors is much higher and given more attention and weight. This can sometimes present as a very real difficulty, but we have always underpinned our practice within the universal definition of nursing by Henderson, originally published in 1958 but equally relevant today. The sentiments apply equally to working abroad as well as at home:

The unique function of the nurse is to assist the individual, sick or well, in the performance of those activities contributing to health or its recovery (or to a peaceful death) that he would perform unaided if he had the necessary strength, will or knowledge. And to do this in such a way as to help him gain independence as rapidly as possible.

PREPARING FOR THE MISSION

It is essential that nurses who travel and work in the developing world have a thorough and clear understanding of the knowledge base which underpins nursing practice, and they must be prepared to examine their own professional practice and share their knowledge, in order that others can use it as a foundation for practice. When embarking on work in the developing world, nurses should be very receptive to the local circumstances, and not attempt to enforce the standards and practices they are familiar with in their western world employment. This is not to say that all standards should be forgotten; a valid standard will travel and remain relevant if applied correctly. It is our experience that agencies who recruit nurses to work overseas may conduct an interview and examine the curriculum vitae (CV) of the nurse they are recruiting, but that CV does not necessarily reflect the individual's ability to adapt to a new, even alien, working environment. In terms of experience, agencies are wise to recruit someone with a number of years of practical surgical experience rather than an enthusiastic novice. This has been demonstrated by Suserud & Haljamae (1997) in their study of Swedish nurses acting at a disaster site, 'negative experiences, such as feelings of being inefficient ... were commonly mentioned by the inexperienced nurses'.

In considering the historical basis of overseas nursing, it is impossible to ignore one name, that of Florence Nightingale. Her work in Scutari in the 19th century and her *Notes on Nursing: what it is and what it is not*, which was originally published in 1859, can still provide significant insights. More recently published works include commentaries on the Vietnam war and shared experiences of events such as Desert Shield and Desert Storm in the Gulf (Nusbaum 1994). On a more peaceful note, writings such as 'African Diary' (Rigby 1995) provide information about working overseas in a day-to-day format. However, each nurse who is working overseas will find that it is a very personal experience. In order to prepare for this, we would suggest that nurses should research the country, culture, climate and political situation before they go. This may appear obvious, but it is not always an easy task. Information can be gleaned from previous teams' feedback, but circumstances may have changed radically in

the interim. There may not, of course, have been a previous team presence and so it is vital that the nurse has a clear idea of the team objectives. When travelling as part of an aid mission, nurses must be very careful to establish their exact roles and responsibilities. Any worthwhile aid programme should have set objectives for the mission, such as how many people will be trained, in what time scale and to what depth; if not it may be the nurses' responsibility to establish these criteria. The local people may also have their own objectives, or hopes of what they will gain from the mission. If the visiting team do not relate to or understand these objectives, then the mission is unlikely to reach its full potential.

CHALLENGING CONVENTIONAL PRACTICE AND WISDOM

The Red Cross, established in 1863 by Henry Dunant as a reaction to the horrors he witnessed following the battle of Solferino in Italy, is one of the most famous aid agencies who call upon surgical nurses to volunteer their services for working abroad. The organisation have produced booklets on the Geneva conventions which apply mainly to those working in an area of, or relating to, armed combat. These may be useful as guidelines, for example setting out the rights and responsibilities of medical personnel and patients, but they cannot begin to give the detail of circumstances which surgical nurses will find. It is a sad fact of life that surgical teams who are working abroad are likely to find themselves treating patients who have suffered their injuries as part of war or civil unrest. This work also encompasses psychological problems such as 'post-traumatic stress syndrome' and physical concerns such as exhaustion and malnourishment of both patients and staff.

It is also important to remember that life does continue even in major disaster situations. Thus patients may present with familiar conditions such as cholecystitis, appendicitis, strangulated hernias as well as the less familiar gunshot wounds and shell injuries. One of the authors, whilst part of a plastic surgical team, well remembers operating on a patient to correct 'bat ears' in a hospital in Sarajevo. The decision as to which conditions require intervention can cause much concern, but is much easier if the team as a whole understand why that decision has been reached. Local surgeons, anaesthetists and nurses may well benefit from involvement in the decision-making process and in the entire operative intervention plan.

The visiting team may well find that some principles are not universally accepted by the local teams, the classic example being that of pain relief. In times of crisis and shortage, compounded by a lack of local medical expertise, pain relief may be given scant attention by the permanent medical and nursing staff. In some countries, pain relief may not have a high profile even without the particular adverse circumstances, or it may be administered in an unfamiliar format, unknown to the visiting team. Morphine, for example, is often regarded with suspicion owing to fears of creating drug addiction, whereas ketamine, an inhalation anaesthetic, enables effective analgesia and may be regarded as an acceptable substitute. It is titrated to avoid both overdosing and encountering undesirable side-effects. Many doctors and nurses from this country are wary of or unused to this application on a regular basis, despite its inclusion in the British National Formulary (BNF 1997).

The nurse working in the developing world will be challenged in many ways. Other cultures may appear cruel to nurses who have the ethic of compassion at the centre of their standards. For example, we were initially shocked to see a patient's wound debrided without the use of a local anaesthetic, and we were unable to give him the pain control prior to treatment which we would have normally administered had we been back at home. As Sofaer (1994) states: 'All living human beings are entitled to have the moral right not to be denied help in life-threatening situations'. Nurses would expect to give patients in their home situation a much higher standard of care, but in the host country the level of help is often determined by the local economy and the amount of humanitarian aid which has been provided.

Other practices which may seem self-evident to western teams, but are not viewed with such importance in a local disaster environment, include patient dignity and privacy, confidentiality, patients' rights, nutritional needs and hygiene. In an ongoing crisis situation the local staff may not feel it appropriate to acknowledge the significance of any or all of these human needs. This perspective challenges the visiting team's conventional practice and wisdom. Yet, one of us found, whilst working in the Sudan amongst Ethiopian refugees, that privacy was considered an unusual concept, as the patients and local staff had adapted to very communal living conditions owing in part to shortage of space and facilities.

ANTICIPATING PROBLEMS

One aspect that nurses have to consider amongst many issues when they are invited or volunteer to go to a war or disaster area, is whether they have common objectives (a) with the host country and (b) with the team they are going out with or will join in the host country. Problems may well arise when a nurse's values and beliefs about the purpose of human life, the role of the nurse and standards of care are incongruent with those of the host country or colleagues. The most significant challenge to a nurse's belief system may be that of healing the wounded only to return them to the battlefield, to continue with their attempt to militarily dominate their enemy. Other problems encountered may be due to the resentment from local nurses of their foreign colleagues. The local nurses may believe that outsiders perceive them as not being capable of coping with the current situation. This may in fact be true because of the overwhelming numbers of ill or injured people involved. Nurses must remember that they are visitors and must make clear that their purpose is to help the nursing staff to achieve their objectives of caring for their people.

Reflective point

Why do you think that local nurses may be very reluctant to hand over care to a visiting team?

It is possible that local staff who have dealt with many casualties will be war-weary and in a burn-out situation. It may, though, be difficult for them to accept relief offered by foreign nurses, i.e. for them to take a rest from their efforts in order to recover their reserves of strength. Visiting nurses need to consider how they might feel if the situation were reversed. They may find it difficult to leave their ward or operating theatre in the care of a foreign stranger.

If the people have been in a siege situation, then another problem that may well be encountered is that the nurses will be as undernourished as the patients and may hold a belief that they have been abandoned by the outside world of which the visiting nurses are representatives. Consequently, anger and resentment may be shown towards the visiting nurses, which may cause them some distress as they have come to the country for altruistic reasons and find themselves apparently disliked and resented

FIT FOR PURPOSE?

Visiting nurses should take great care that they remain fit and do not allow their empathy and compassion for their hosts and patients to prevent them from looking after themselves. Aid workers should try to maintain their health, for if they should become ill they are, of course, less effective carers and are unable to achieve their primary objective which is to care for others. All visiting medical and nursing staff should be properly immunised for the country they are to visit and should be assessed as to their fitness for the role they are to play. This should not only include a physical assessment but consideration should also be given to whether staff are emotionally able to deal with the situation they will be facing. Post-traumatic stress disorder has been recognised in people who would have normally been considered emotionally capable of coping in extreme situations. Consequently, people who show existing signs of overanxiety should not be put in situations of unnecessary stress. Bassett (1995) discusses the recognition and management of post-traumatic stress disorder in general and Short-DeGraff & Endelman (1992) consider it in specific relation to those nurses involved in the after-effects of combat. The nurse may exhibit signs of irritability, lack of concentration, loss of sleep and general apathy.

IMPORTANT STRATEGIES

Adaptability and experience of decision-making and prioritising care are important assets for surgical nurses working in a crisis situation in the developing world. They will have little if any first world or peacetime supplies so will have to assess each new situation and adapt their practice accordingly. Gaining some knowledge of the language of the host country is a most useful asset. All nurses will acknowledge that personal communication provides the foundation on which to build a trusting relationship to enable support and the implementation of a treatment regime. Knowing the word for 'pain' can be very useful. Learning correct forms of address as well as an understanding of sexual taboos will prevent conflict and embarrassing situations. Very often, basic humanity is all that nurses can offer. Where appropriate, a touch, a smile together with a compassionate attitude may be all the comfort that they can give.

In Sarajevo, we planned to perform surgery on an 8-year-old child. He turned up on the morning, alone and clutching an envelope which contained his medical notes. He looked tired, frightened and confused. The local staff ignored his distress and continued to prepare the theatre for his operation. They tried to explain to us that children in Sarajevo had been through many distressing events, and as this was planned and for his own good he did not need comforting. It was distressing to us, as we could not communicate verbally with him and sitting next to him on the trolley where he had been told to wait appeared to upset him, as he anticipated that 'something' was going to be done to him by a stranger with no explanation. Just putting an arm round him and giving him a hug brought a hesitant, but relieved, smile to his face.

The services of a dedicated translator are essential. Often, we found that host doctors will try to speak English, and those who do not will get a friend to translate for them. As has already been mentioned, nursing does not have such a high status, and the local translators will be 'borrowed' by or will gravitate to the visiting doctors, because of their perceived superior status and power base. If the funding organisation is not prepared to supply a translator dedicated to the surgical nursing part of the programme, then they are effectively gagging western surgical nurses. It became very obvious to us that although one may wish to share expert knowledge and skills, if communication is only possible in a very limited fashion with nursing colleagues (or the presence of a doctor is needed for translation purposes) then the idea that nursing exists as an adjunct to, and not separate from, doctoring will be reinforced. We would suggest that nurses will find it very difficult indeed to even set, never mind meet, any nursing objectives. Nurses have much to offer the developing world, and much to share with their interprofessional colleagues in whatever circumstances, but this will prove virtually impossible if they cannot communicate and share ideas. For example, it is possible to demonstrate and role model practical skills and supervise and encourage host colleagues to perform them skilfully, but to ensure safe practice it is essential to communicate and ensure understanding of the theoretical knowledge that underpins clinical nursing practice.

Reflective point

Recall caring for a patient whose culture and language was foreign to you. How did you feel about nursing this patient? Did you feel that you communicated effectively? Was an interpreter always available? How could you improve the situation for the next similar patient?

In developed countries, in conjunction with all the emergency services, there are plans in place for major incidents. In war, famine, and natural disasters, especially those occurring in underdeveloped countries, these plans may be absent, inapplicable and inappropriate. Part of the work of the team should be to enable the people of the country to feel that they have not been taken over by foreigners. To enable them to participate in the care of their own people, their opinions should be sought when developing current and future major disaster care strategies. The focus of the visiting teams should therefore be empowerment of their hosts. Education is provided to enable them to make informed decisions. Knowledge and skills are shared so that future casualties may receive timely intervention, with life-saving outcomes. For example, many countries will not have developed a system of triage for their ill or injured. Teaching host teams to use a method of evaluating the needs of the patients will prove to be instrumental in the saving of many lives. In a war situation, casualties may arrive in large numbers with varying degrees of injury, for example following the market bombings in Sarajevo. If the receiving teams are overwhelmed, patients may die unnecessarily because of inadequate assessment. Advanced trauma life support training is a useful method of achieving effective triage and can be taught by visiting medical and nursing teams both formally and in the practical situation.

RESOURCES

It is inappropriate to use all the stocks of the host nation and, if possible, the team should try to take with them as much as they can of what they perceive they will need. Stocks or very basic equipment in the host country may not be present or be severely depleted by war or siege, and, if the visiting teams are going to perform specialist surgery, they should ensure that all the equipment they need is taken with them.

We have found that aid donated to areas perceived as 'underprivileged' or 'underdeveloped' is not always appropriate, and this is just as true of medical items. Whilst working with Ethiopian refugees in the Sudan one of the authors witnessed 'aid' being delivered. Included in the items, expensive to transport and often problematic to deliver, were broken metal retractors, cracked electrical cables and clearly out-of-date drugs. Some years later whilst in Sarajevo we saw the same types of items. The local people were less than impressed; they were just as able as we were to read that the expiry dates on antibiotics and anaesthetic agents were long passed. Their morale was not improved by being treated as a 'dumping ground' for these items. This can seriously affect the credibility of the visiting team; they may be seen to bring other people's 'cast-offs' with them. Their hosts may question the importance and validity of everything else, including the visiting team's knowledge base and expertise. As a complete contrast, state of the science drugs such as desfluorane had also been sent, but no-one had any experience of using this drug. It seemed a bitter irony that a recent drug was easily obtained yet what was really needed in the hospital was a constant supply of running water and electricity. Aid is only of use if it actually assists the process of helping or improves local circumstances in a practical and sustainable way.

What are the most useful resources needed in a developing country experiencing a major disaster? We make no apology for reiterating that a good knowledge base and understanding of basic principles is essential as is a flexible and empathetic approach to the surgical nursing of patients. When the surgical nurse is faced with compiling a checklist of essential items to take to the host country, lateral thinking is required.

Reflective point

Are disposable items, which may guarantee sterility and standardisation, really appropriate in the developing world? Where will they be disposed of? Will they readily be disposed of, or will there be the temptation to reuse them in ways which were never intended by the original manufacturer?

Do not misunderstand us: we are the first to stand in awe of the kind of nurse who can do wonders with a piece of Sleek and a pair of forceps, but the National Association of Theatre Nurses' position statement on the reuse of medical devices intended for single use (Plowes & Green 1995) refers to the misuse of single-use items. We have witnessed a life unquestionably saved by using a Foley urinary catheter and a milk bottle to make an underwater seal drainage system (invented by Ethiopian nurses). Our advice would be to include on your checklist as much and as many reusable useful items as you can. If an item is then adapted to a different use, at least it will probably be robust enough to withstand the adaptation.

As operating theatre nurses, one important item on our checklist would be swabs – good-quality, large, absorbent swabs. They do not have to have a Raytec or X-ray detectable line in them. X-rays are probably a luxury or only a theoretical concept 'out there' and scrupulously careful counting and checking should render the likelihood of leaving a swab in the wound remote. But they can be used for padding, dressings, swabs, cleaning cloths, etc. The swabs in Sarajevo were tiny, and had been deliberately cut that way by the staff in the hospitals with a view to saving limited material. We used hundreds for every case, thus defeating the object of all that careful cutting. Common sense is, and always will be, an essential part of good surgical nursing knowledge.

Arrange to take plenty of syringes and needles; these are essential items of equipment for surgical nurses, but also arrange to take sharps boxes too to ensure safe disposal. You may, however, have to bring these boxes back with you – how you get them through customs is another issue. Can you, though, justify leaving sharps boxes behind? They may be reused (with or without cleaning, disinfection or sterilisation) by medical or nursing staff, or found on tips or dumps by the people who live in the area. In some situations, families survive by combing these dumps for 'useful' items, and drug dealers and unscrupulous people do not only exist in developed countries.

Of course, the whole situation is not as simple as that. Gates (1993) details the dilemma when she speaks of the problem of using 'out-of-date' milk products because the alternative was starvation for the children they were treating. High moral and professional standards may be easily stated but are less easy to deal with in a 'life and death situation'.

It can be very irritating to discover that the team have failed to bring a very basic but very important resource, for example Elastoplast for dressings. When in Bosnia, in the outpatients clinic, one of the team who was helping with dressings used what would have been deemed to be an economical amount of Elastoplast for a bandage and was firmly shown by the Bosnian nurse that she was wasting their sparse supplies. She was shown how to cut the Elastoplast lengthways to economise. This would have been a good idea had it not been so hot and the Elastoplast so old that it did not stick. Cutting the bandage and tying it without causing constriction to the limb was the obvious answer and then the failure to bring Elastoplast no longer mattered, but we learnt from this as well as many other small but annoying omissions. It is very easy to become irritated and stressed by the situation when it is hot and you feel helpless, hungry and inadequate, but a smile and a hug can restore equilibrium quite quickly. However, as Gates (1993) discloses: 'Nurses often discover hidden resources in themselves, including an ability to respond with innovative solutions to problems that arise.'

Our ability to economise and use our practical knowledge and skills in a creative way was demonstrated on a visit to Sarajevo during the war. It was difficult to try to maintain our usual standards of care and asepsis without water, gas and electricity supplies.

Surgery was undertaken under block and local anaesthetic because there was no oxygen to give general anaesthetics. Thankfully, someone had the patience to hold a torch when the power failed during intricate surgery. It is amazing that a running tap for 'scrubbing up' can be done away with if someone is standing by with a jug of water, filled from the tank when the rationed water supply is turned on, to pour over the scrub team's hands.

Some equipment, for example complicated medical equipment, unless it has been specifically and appropriately asked for, can end up creating more problems than it solves. Developing world areas can not provide the same treatments as in developed countries because they lack resources and maintenance expertise. They can not 'match up' to the standards set by their western colleagues when using sophisticated equipment. It is a dilemma which is always present in this kind of exchange of experience. We would suggest that (a) recognising the existing skills and expertise, (b) supporting and educating the practitioners and (c) introducing proposals for expanding relevant knowledge are of more value than dazzling and undermining host colleagues with affluent, wasteful inappropriate western medical equipment.

GAINING TRUST

On arrival at the destination where the team are to work it is important for nurses to gain the trust of their nursing colleagues as quickly as possible to enable the team to begin treating patients. They should at all times remember that they are visitors and respect the fact that their hosts have worked in this situation longer than they have and may have developed very practical methods of coping with lack of supplies, electricity, water and the fundamentals which nurses take for granted at home. The host nurses may have a great deal to teach the visitors and the learning process becomes two-way. Nurses should be careful not to waste any of the precious supplies of the host country and will find that they can be very economical when they have to be. An enhanced knowledge of cost-effectiveness is acquired, a most useful asset too on returning home.

Gaining trust can be difficult both when adapting to standards of care that may be completely different and seeing the host nurses behave in a subservient way. This will be a major challenge for visiting nurses. They must remember that their standards must be universal and that they would want to uphold them in all situations. This does not mean that they should enforce others to comply with their standards. They can still uphold them and by so doing enlighten the host nurses and involve them in considering their own practice and the possibility of change. It may be impossible to discover what standards were in place prior to the disaster and whether they will be reverted to after the situation settles. Nurses may be able to ascertain what type of system was in place previously from observing current responses of the host nurses to swab, needle and instrument checks during surgery as well as observing the pre- and postoperative care of patients. Visiting nurses, without imposing their own standards, but by gaining trust over the time they are there, can demonstrate in an unassuming way the standards which they normally would use at home. It is intended that either by example or when the occasion arises by formal teaching, visiting nurses can demonstrate that standards can be maintained even in the most dire circumstances. There is a feeling of delight on both sides when host nurses demonstrate that they have adapted their practice for better outcomes for their patients.

It is important that visiting nurses do not take on roles that they would not consider doing at home and would compromise their accountability (UKCC 1992). However, they may find themselves in situations which involve them in becoming 'girl Friday' in the team. When ward rounds or outpatient sessions are taking place they may automatically become the secretary for the team, documenting patient examinations for the surgeon and compiling operating lists as there are no medical secretaries or junior doctors on hand. They may also be involved in the care of patients, both in outpatients and on the ward on a daily basis, taking down dressings for pre- and postoperative assessment of wounds. This will involve them in gaining the trust of staff in many different areas and in having the opportunity of teaching aseptic techniques by example. They will also learn many adaptations for their own techniques, either because of a lack of equipment or because the equipment available differs from that they use at home. This reinforces our previous statement that only experienced adaptable people should be part of such a team, as the inexperienced may not be able to adapt their practice. If, however, the team is large, it is possible to take less-experienced staff. Support can then be provided for those with less experience.

DIFFERING PERCEPTIONS

If we consider that the perspectives of nurse, patient, and doctor differ in the developed world, hence the need for a Patient's Charter (DoH 1991), we must be acutely aware of differing expectations in a disaster area. Visiting nurses must appreciate that many patients perceive their situation as desperate. The concept of going home may not be a relief or hoped-for outcome. Indeed, we found that for many patients a stay in a hospital was welcomed. Patients had contact with the visiting team from the 'outside world'. We were perceived to have wealth and influence. The local staff's aim, however, was to empty the bed as soon as possible to treat more cases. As visitors, we were aware that it may prove problematic to intervene, and could cause a significant division between the local and visiting nurses.

We found that many of the things we said were also unintentionally problematic and reflected our initial inappropriate interpersonal skills. For example, saying to a patient (or indeed a local nurse or doctor) 'I hope that one day you will visit me in the UK' may be wrongly interpreted as 'I will get you out of this situation'. We soon realised that we could be the cause of raised false expectations. Equally, 'I wish you could see my operating theatre suite', spoken to a foreign colleague, was seen as an invitation home with flights, papers and accommodation included (provided by us, or the relief agency). Even less positive statements, such as 'It would be nice if you could see where I work' or 'Don't worry, we have lots of these back home' can lead to false expectations and unreal hopes. We are not advocating that one says nothing, but be aware that in many cases the people to whom you are speaking are desperate to leave the situation, and are looking for any clue to help them escape.

It may be that people want to stay and do their best in the world they know, but they do look for extended help from visiting teams. It may not be possible to guarantee that a subsequent team will arrive, or that their remit will be similar. The watchword here is caution; deal with the situation as you see it, but know that what you are saying may mean more to your host than you think. If you want to go home and continue with your normal life, so do the people you are working with, but it may be that they are looking for 'one out of two' and normal life in a foreign country is more attractive than staying in a totally deprived situation. To get the visiting team out of the situation can sometimes prove difficult enough; to take a local person away can be misguided as well as difficult, however well meaning the intention behind the act.

PSYCHOLOGICAL SUPPORT

World-wide, nurses probably share similar reasons for being in the profession (this may be different in a war or disaster where people who did not join the profession but have been 'conscripted' for the duration of the crisis are part of the workforce, but they are less likely to be part of the teams in a specialist area). There is, therefore, a bond between nurses and one of the most important roles which visiting nurses can perform is the psychological and emotional support of their colleagues, who may have lost family and friends in the conflict, be burnt out by their endless care of casualties, and distressed by their lack of resources and the instability of their situation. Many will live in fear of travelling to work to care for others as they take the risk of being shot and becoming patients themselves. One important role that visiting nurses can play is to be a listening ear to their colleagues. There may be resentment of other countries not intervening to stop the situation and visiting nurses may, as previously mentioned, become targets for that resentment just because they are foreigners. Time spent in caring for host colleagues may cause great distress and a guilt feeling in visiting nurses who know that they will be returning home to a stable life when they leave the disaster area. Not every individual can deal with this situation. We felt privileged, though, to be part of our host colleagues' lives for a short time and attempted to be empathetic. Often the host nurses will just want to share their grief and pain with someone who is not involved with the situation on a long-term basis. It is widely accepted that one can sometimes share a problem with a stranger more easily than with a friend.

Surgeons will be more relaxed and able to function as they do at home when they have the nursing personnel who normally work with them as part of the team. The extra stressors of little or no electricity and water and abnormal working conditions will make surgery more of an effort than at home and much more tiring. Surgeons will also be teaching host medical staff by passing on skills to enable them to continue with effective care of their casualties after the departure of the team, and this will be an added challenge because of potential language difficulties. This, however, although hard to believe, can also be fun and every opportunity should be taken to alleviate stress by introducing humour. Snyder (1992) explores the scientific basis of humour and its use in decreasing anxiety and tension and enhancing learning. Learning the language by getting to know the basic words for instruments, being able to ask circulating personnel for supplies in their own language, and being able to say 'please' and 'thank you' can be a great source of fun, especially if the visiting nurse mispronounces some word and asks for something completely inappropriate. A sense of humour is a great asset and can

develop a common bond between the staff of both nations and also show that the visiting staff respect their nationality. Many foreigners speak English and it is well known that the British have not learnt other languages perhaps as much as they could. This can be the chance to redress the balance and can lead to new learning opportunities.

The strengths and difficulties encountered when working in a major disaster setting in an underdeveloped country provide a significant, never forgotten life experience for the surgical nurse. The situation experienced may completely change the life and attitude of the teams involved. It is the authors' experience that the bonds formed when working closely as a team last, and that deep trust and friendship can develop from sharing stressful experiences. It is important to have realistic expectations of what can be achieved and to appreciate from the start that one is unlikely to be able to change the world. It is a chance to find out about yourself. Your own basic values and beliefs may be challenged. This may be a threatening experience but should always be a positive learning experience from which to grow. Nurses may find that their principles are challenged to a degree that they find quite devastating and they may well need much support throughout this experience to rebuild their confidence in themselves and their abilities. At any time during work of this kind individual members may become overwhelmed by the magnitude of the task and it is important that members are able to share their emotions and use their colleagues as a sounding board to support them. It is possible to feel completely helpless as an individual, but by having briefing sessions it is possible for individual members to see that they are achieving a result as part of the whole team. These briefings do not have to be formal or even with the whole team. Sometimes a half an hour of rest with a drink is sufficient to lift the spirits and renew a positive attitude (see also Ch. 5).

CONCLUSION

There is a fine balance between visiting surgical nurses being perceived as working colleagues, advisors, educators and being able to empower host colleagues, and being seen as mistrusted, privileged outsiders. Past experiences regarding visiting nursing and medical teams will affect the host's attitude towards new visitors. It is important to remember that the staff who may well be 'burnt-out' may have stayed throughout the situation or conflict either through choice or because they felt that they could not leave. They often have a real sense of duty and care for their patients, who may also be their family and friends. In some situations staff will only receive food or humanitarian aid if they come to work, even though they are tired, undernourished and have lost hope for their future. It is easy in this situation to attract criticism from one's hosts as the visiting team have usually come with set objectives and a time scale for their mission. If work is not done with care and sensitivity, then the host staff will be unimpressed and resentful of other visitors from the same nation or mission. Host staff may feel uncomfortable if they are aware that the standards that they achieve are seen as unacceptable to outsiders. They will resent being watched or feel ashamed of their circumstances.

Yet, there are many opportunities for sharing surgical nursing knowledge and skills and working together for the sake of humanity. Every human emotion is experienced including much laughter. Lifelong

friendships often result. This type of life experience, though, can make one's own work on returning home seem unimportant. It can take some time to settle back again. However, your current surgical role is now your reality and it can be approached with a much deeper understanding. From our experiences of working in disaster areas in developing countries we now view the nature of life from many perspectives. We can reflect on our own work within the surgical setting with deeper insight and perform our roles with greater effectiveness and empathy when caring for patients. We have a heightened awareness of our ability to work in collaboration alongside our nursing and interprofessional colleagues. We have both personally grown and developed as individuals. Overall we recognise the value of major disaster nursing within the developing world and the need for sharing experiences to inform and support one another.

USEFUL ADDRESSES

Agencies which may be contacted about surgical nursing in the developing world include:

British Red Cross
Medical Personnel
International Aid Department
19 Grosvenor Crescent
London SW1X 7EJ

MERLIN
49 Portland Road
Holland Park
London W11 4LJ

Médicins sans Frontières
3–4 St Andrews Hill
London EC4V 5BY

UK Med
North Staffordshire Hospital
Princes Road
Hartshill
Stoke on Trent ST4 7LN

REFERENCES

Bassett C C 1995 Post-traumatic stress disorder: recognition and management. Professional Nurse 10(11): 709–710
British National Formulary 1997 British Medical Association and the Royal Pharmaceutical Society of Great Britain, London
Carper B A 1978 Fundamental patterns of knowing in nursing. Advances in Nursing Science 1(1): 13–23
Cavanagh C 1977 A world apart. Nursing Times 93 (29): 34–35
Chinn P L 1989 Nursing patterns of knowing and feminist thought. Nursing and Health Care 10(2): 71–75
Connelly F M, Clandinin D J 1990 Stories of experience and narrative inquiry. Educational Researcher 19(5): 2–14
Department of Health (DoH) 1991 The patient's charter. HMSO, London
Gates E 1993 Nursing under fire. Nursing Times 89(51): 26–28
Henderson V 1958 Basic principles of nursing care. International Council of Nursing, Geneva

James P 1996 The transformative power of story-telling among peers: an exploration from action research. Educational Action Research 4(2): 197–221
Nightingale F 1859 Notes on nursing, what it is and what it is not. Reprinted 1969. Dover Publishing, New York
Nusbaum N J 1994 Casualties abroad and at home. Journal of Community Health 19(1): 1–5
Plowes K D, Green A 1995 Use, re-use and misuse of single use items. National Association of Theatre Nurses, Harrogate
Porter R 1997 Aid-related risks. Nursing times 92(9): 14–15
Rigby D 1995 African diary. British Journal of Theatre Nursing 5(8): 25–28
Short-DeGraff M A, Engelman T 1992 Activities for the treatment of combat related post-traumatic stress disorder. Occupational Therapy in Health Care 8(2–3): 27–47

Snyder M 1992 Humor. In: Independent nursing interventions, 2nd edn. Delmar, Albany, New York, ch 35

Sofaer B 1994 Achieving a better life on the planet. Are we our brothers' keepers? Nursing ethics. Edward Arnold, London

Strathie L, Holmes C 1996 Story as a reflective process for nurses. International Journal of Nursing Practice 2: 99–104

Suserud B, Haljamae H 1997 Acting at a disaster site: experiences expressed by Swedish nurses. Journal of Advanced Nursing 25: 155–162

United Kingdom Council for Nursing, Midwifery and Health Visiting (UKCC) 1992 Code of professional conduct. UKCC, London

Vezeau T M 1994 Narrative inquiry in nursing. In: Chinn P L, Watson J (eds) Art and aesthetics in nursing. National League for Nursing Press, New York

Weller K 1991 Friere and feminist pedagogy of difference. Harvard Educational Review 61: 449–474

PART 4

Health outcomes of surgery

PART CONTENTS

Introduction to Part 4

Michael Lyon   Bernice West

In addressing the issues of health outcomes, the authors have chosen to define this part of the book in such a way that the identification of improved health care outcomes becomes a developmental opportunity and a challenge for the nursing profession.

Rather than concentrate on outcome measures which previously have been identified in the literature, we have chosen to open up the endeavour in such a way as to promote the advanced role of the nurse in developing health care. To achieve this aim, we have reconsidered the ideas underpinning procedures of methodology and the implications of these for evidence-based nursing practice. Accordingly, our pursuit of methodology is open, unified and practical – and is intended to draw together research approaches and nursing care.

The first chapter of this part of the book (Ch. 18) analyses the purposes and values of research methods, and the second chapter (Ch. 19) develops these ideas in a specific, operational, way. By sustaining these complementary concerns, a prescriptive approach to health outcomes is avoided. Instead, the authors advocate that the autonomy and discretion afforded by the scope of professional nursing practice is utilised fully by surgical nurses.

In recent years nurses have engaged in debates about how to develop (and differentiate) nursing as distinct from other aspects of health care (Gray & Pratt 1991, UKCC 1992, West 1996), and how to identify and measure specific aspects of nursing care (Balogh 1992, Harvey 1991, Koch 1992, West & Lyon 1995). The professional literature suggests that there is a mixture of current proposals about the range and scope of the nursing role.

What constitute nursing practice, care and role development have been influenced in recent years by several political developments within the British health service (NHSME 1991) and by changes in the education of nurses (UKCC 1990, 1995).

The scope of professional practice in nursing has been developed to include an impressive array of roles in clinical practice (Laurenson 1996, Read & Graves 1994). These roles now often involve nurses taking on aspects of work previously defined as the prerogative of other health professionals. Where such role extension and development has been effective (Greenhalgh & Co. Ltd 1994, Laurenson 1996, Read & Graves 1994, Touche Ross et al 1994), health and service outcomes have been evaluated and managed in a personalised way which expresses the patient-oriented approach to nursing care being provided. This last point is particularly important when considering the evaluation of health outcomes and in assessing quality of care.

Concern about the best research which can be used to determine health outcomes and quality of care may initially seem esoteric and of limited utility to the surgical nurse. Answers have been identified as problematic, particularly the validity of measurement techniques adopted (Balogh 1992, Redfern & Norman 1990). It may seem that these concerns are mainly tasks for the outside researcher who has to select the optimum method to answer a research problem. As well as matters of clinical concern there are also pressures of policy outcomes and quality. These are often aligned with non-clinical ideological interests and such values as cost and commerce, or other choice priorities over and above health outcomes. The decision to emphasise one set of outcomes, for example, may stress the alternative of a short length of hospital stay following a total hip replacement over patient mobility on admission and discharge. As our concluding section of the next chapter indicates, the policy decisions made will reflect ideological beliefs as well as practical priorities.

Where this problem becomes manifest and apparent is when there are conflicting interests operating simultaneously. In acute surgical settings there are often sicker patients who require care for an intensive, yet shorter, hospital stay. Advances in medical technology and treatment regimens place further demands on nurses to practise in an ever-changing technological environment. In such a context of health care the nurse faces three key professional challenges:

- differentiating nursing from, and then integrating it with, the care and treatment provided by other health professionals
- balancing standardised care with individualised care in order to demonstrate effective health outcomes
- reconciling cost-containment with quality of care.

We suggest that these three key challenges must be addressed by the nursing profession.

The current trend in the health service to evaluate effectiveness in clinical and cost terms requires reconsideration by nurses in order to enhance the professional health role of nurses. Rather than automatically accept the political accounts and managerial ideologies which underpin the current practices, it is essential to provide an informed basis for the professional nurse to develop health outcomes which are effective (in the broadest sense) and integrated with those of other health professionals. The next two chapters are intended to provide this informed basis.

REFERENCES

Balogh R 1992 Audits of nursing care in Britain: a review and critique of approaches to validating them. International Journal of Nursing Studies 29(2): 119–133

Gray G, Pratt R 1991 Towards a discipline of nursing. Churchill Livingstone, Melbourne

Greenhalgh & Co. Ltd 1994 The interface between junior doctors and nurses: a research study for the Department of Health. Greenhalgh & Co. Ltd, Macclesfield

Harvey G 1991 An evaluation of approaches to assessing the quality of nursing care. Journal of Advanced Nursing 16: 277–286

Koch T 1992 A review of nursing quality assurance. Journal of Advanced Nursing 17: 785–794

Laurenson S 1996 Health service developments and the scope of professional nursing practice: a survey of developing clinical roles within NHS trusts in Scotland. Scottish Office Department of Health, HMSO, Edinburgh

National Health Service Management Executive (NHSME) 1991 Junior doctors: the new deal. NHSME, London

Read S, Graves K 1994 Reduction of junior doctors' hours in Trent Region: the nursing contribution. Sheffield Centre for Health and Related Research (SCHARR) and Trent Regional Health Authority NHS Executive, Sheffield

Redfern S J, Norman I J 1990 Measuring the quality of nursing care: a consideration of different approaches. Journal of Advanced Nursing 15: 1260–1271

Touche Ross Management Consultants and South Thames Regional Health Authority 1994 Evaluation of nurse practitioner pilot projects executive summary. Touche Ross, London

United Kingdom Central Council for Nursing, Midwifery and Health Visiting (UKCC) 1990 The report of the post-registration and practice project. UKCC, London

United Kingdom Central Council for Nursing, Midwifery and Health Visiting (UKCC) 1992 The scope of professional practice. UKCC, London

United Kingdom Central Council for Nursing, Midwifery and Health Visiting (UKCC) 1995 Preparation for education. UKCC, London

West B J M 1996 Health Service developments and the scope of professional nursing practice: a review of pertinent literature. HMSO, Edinburgh

West B J M, Lyon M H 1995 Surgical nurse: principles of audit and clinical practice. British Journal of Nursing 4(17): 987–991

18

Methodology and health outcomes

Michael Lyon   Bernice West

AIMS

This chapter aims to:

- introduce the surgical nurse to a range of methodologies for developing health outcomes
- encourage an eclectic approach to methodology and the development of evidence-based nursing practice
- identify ways of applying methodology to nursing actions
- identify ways of improving nursing standards and performance through the use of research methods.

INTRODUCTION

This chapter will discuss the research basis of health outcomes along a broad methodological front, in order to provide a foundation for use in clinical nursing practice. Research has become indispensable in forming knowledge and managing change, and so complex as a tool of discovery, that this chapter begins with a brief review of the range of approaches which can be adopted and of the problems which are typically involved. Once this challenge has been outlined, and the practical procedures have been clarified, relevant answers will be offered and inspected by means of key substantive examples.

Concern for the understanding, analysis and improvement of health outcomes has become increasingly research-dependent for four persuasive reasons:

- the requirements for new knowledge
- the requirements of financial management
- the desirability of nurses carrying out nursing research
- the availability of powerful techniques.

New knowledge requirements

Reliance on research is notable when special knowledge must be found in order to deal with new situations.

Research is often called upon to be the science of change. Fortunately, the extra demands being placed upon research, as a means to informational ends, can be met because the various powers for acquiring knowledge have also expanded.

Financial management requirements

Traditionally, research in Britain has been mostly under the control of academics in terms of the training of personnel, maintaining of standards and conception of knowledge aims. The design and direction of contemporary research is either increasingly being controlled by commercial agencies and designated according to the interests of management commissioning (Jeffries, cited in Gabe et al 1992), or is following the pathways of professional self-direction. The trend in research activity is strongly influenced by financial considerations within a framework of overall policy (Bond 1996). This connection may have professional advantages since it provides a clear informational basis for evidence-based practice.

Researchers and professionals

In the contemporary health service, skilled nursing staff need to be conversant with research findings and should ideally acquire expertise to mount their own investigations. In terms of personal commitment and development, competence in research is becoming more important for developing clinical practice and for planning effective care policies at upper, managerial, levels.

In nursing terms, it is undesirable that temporary non-nursing assistants are employed for specialist research on clinical matters. In general, investigators should not be strangers to the ongoing activities and contextual knowledge where the study is actually located. Many health problems involve substantive skills and concerns. There are now whole generations of fresh concerns (for example changing organisations and improvements and ever-emerging health problems). It is suggested that professional workers are most prepared and suitable to tackle these by virtue of their special knowledge, and their responsibilities and values. Ideally, therefore, the addition of special research capability and readiness, in order to utilise – and inform – existing professional skills, provides the best preparation for conducting evidence-based practice and nursing research. The optimal combination is that research should be secured on a professional basis and become influential in developing nursing roles and in influencing the assessment and application of health care policies.

Availability of powerful techniques

More advanced modes of library search (such as CD-ROMs); a greater development of, and respect for, measurement procedures; and the widespread use of computer software means that the relationship between information-gathering and professional action has become much more hi-tech in instrumentation and more sophisticated in its analysis and application. The most useful sources for searching the literature on health outcomes are the two CD-ROMs, MEDLINE (primarily recording articles on medical research) and CINAHL (Cumulative Index to Nursing and Allied Health Literature), which covers research journal articles in nursing and other allied health professions. The Cochrane and York databases are also useful.

METHODOLOGY OVERALL: THE AUTHORS' REVIEW

We begin with the observation that there is no single research method, technique or procedure which comprehensively serves all purposes – or commands universal consent. In fact, many different types of research approaches should be taken into account. Yet each major method, or genre, of research has special aims and distinctive procedures.

It is possible to see the overall array of methods as a competition between alternatives – and to actively discount some types in searching for the most superior research method. We must declare, at the outset, that we do not consider it correct to attempt a prior judgement of the relative values of research methods here. Rather, we advocate the worth of comprehending a broad range of possible approaches, and of appreciating their distinctive meanings and designs, so that the selection, and use, of any specific type of research will be made on a basis which is most informed and fully formulated (Cormack 1996, Giddens 1976, Nachmias & Nachmias 1992, Robson 1993, Rose 1982).

This broad approach is adopted in the conviction that personal research experience should be as diverse as is practicable, but that each research project must be planned and developed according to standards which are professionally rigorous and objective. Research is a means of acquiring fresh knowledge which is, ideally, systematic and certain and which is characteristically modern in methods of discovery and modes of correction. It is important to choose widely and wisely among the many different types of research methods which can be selected and used.

The authors, whilst practising in the social and health sciences, naturally have their own subjective and working preferences as to particular methods which should be used – according to practical considerations, such as objectives, suitable procedures, and the context of the study. However, in principle, as a matter of professional impartiality, it should be stated that we hold an overall position which can be summarised according to the term and concept of 'methodological eclecticism'. We begin by accepting that a broad range of potential approaches exist, advocate that all should be recognised in principle, and argue that the selection of the ideal method(s) should be made, in practice, according to what is most appropriate, as a means to serve the end purpose(s) of the particular research at issue. This stance welcomes the fact that a variety of valuable research methods actually exist, and proposes that the resultant wealth of professional research knowledge is understood as a general resource advantage and as an opportunity to adopt the right, relevant, strategy. The existence of so many methods, or means, for accomplishing the ends of research is neither undesirable nor unmanageable. In many respects the variety of research methods that can be used is congruent with, and extends across, the range of options available in nursing practice.

The diversity of research methods should not be treated as a contradiction which invites/compels the mind to dismiss 'alternative' methods as unscientific, speculative or anecdotal – as if the correct basis for knowledge must be naturally scientific or else anti-positivistic, either monistic or pluralistic; either empirically grounded or theoretical in character.

We propose, instead, to take a fresh, and catholic, perspective by adopting an all-embracing acceptance of the diversity of research methods, as an initial and opening stance for their examination. Within this broad methodological frame of reference, we will concentrate upon those sources of evidence which seem most productive and fitting to surgical nursing and nursing practice generally.

It then becomes possible to evaluate further, and critically, the relationships between various types of research methods. This eventual purpose, of deciding with knowledge on the best method for answering a research problem, will be termed one of 'methodology'. Furthermore, the authors suggest that, in order to identify health outcomes for surgical patients, it is preferable for nurses to use a problem-solving approach which takes cognisance of the principles of methodology.

In determining health outcomes, as in research, there is an ultimate need to transcend personal preferences for any particular method, and to discover how a professional commitment to problem-solving altogether

may be selectively guided by a clear sense of design and may be decisively directed by substantive problems and the value aims of informational concern.

In short, we hold the postulate that there is a definite value, even an ethic and obligation, to begin by understanding and accepting the whole array of research methods and to proceed by promoting knowledge of their distinctive utilities and combined potentials.

In order to overview the field of research genres and their implications for different types of investigation, a schema is presented which displays two dimensions for classifying research aims and provides examples, in each quadrant, by way of illustration (Fig. 18.1).

The horizontal axis refers to a range of research orientations towards information. On the one hand these may be treated as intrinsic, instrumentally neutral and 'pure'. On the other, they may be considered as social bases – both in derivation and in usefulness – from which values are achieved. In the left-hand column investigators typically aim to be informationally complete and precise. These studies claim to be scientific and exact within their cognitive framework. The two left-hand quadrants – both researcher as reviewer (Example I) and scientific experimentation (Example II) – illustrate this informational, self-contained, type of research. Such research avoids accepting any 'external' purpose and strives to minimise value judgements as part of the technical task remit.

On the other hand (at the opposite end of the horizontal coordinate), there are research investigations which are crucially social. Being generally oriented to the social actions of others, they are designed to take into account immediate social purposes and possible policy matters. Social surveys and observational studies (Example III) clearly rely upon obtaining the perception of subjects under study. When the work of investigation includes issues of policy and evaluation (Example IV), then inference towards further, future, values and changes is also social in character – but deeper in analytical concern.

The vertical coordinate (or axis which is drawn down the page) refers to different analytical levels of enquiry: from very descriptive forms of research which begin by eliciting, and representing, existing knowledge (Examples I and III) to more sophisticated methodologies, which attempt to draw and establish logical inferences, not only within their own specific conditions of research, but also, by design, across wider conditions.

Experimental designs (Example II) and evaluative/policy research (Example IV) both provide

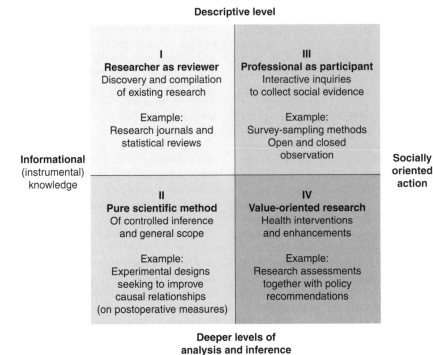

Descriptive level

Figure 18.1 Methodological overview.

instances of this inferential mode of work which aims to generalise beyond its limits.

The distinctions between genres of research are shown as coordinated positions on axes. That is, each pair of cells represents a dichotomous 'split' (or a two-way division) upon each of the two main parameters of Figure 18.1 – analytical level and data orientation. It is possible, however, to see the vertical distinction, of levels of analysis, as polar oppositions on a common dimension and to add intermediate positions to illustrate other research approaches.

In the first example, for instance, an informational description of the research literature may simply summarise the array of existing knowledge and present it as 'the facts'. It is further possible, and often desirable, however, to add a commentary to this evidence. Particularly when a research review is statistical, it is usual and advisable to carry out some secondary analysis of the numerical data in order to make findings meaningful, in prose, and to obtain a common framework of assessment from many sets of statistics. Once the secondary researcher (i.e. the reader) begins to re-work the original findings and data, the new piece of work moves on to a deeper level of connection and analysis; for the significance of the subsequent

research is then derived firmly from past recorded knowledge and can be developed as a part of the overall advancement of the field.

A similar process is carried out when the secondary researcher conducts a meta-analysis of published research papers. In this case, the data from previous studies are generally tested and commented upon in terms of analytical variation.

The grid introduced in Figure 18.1 and discussed above will now be used to structure the core sections of this chapter, namely:

- Researcher as reviewer: health, ethnicity and policy (dimension I)
- The pure scientific method: experimental design (dimension II)
- Interactive approaches: researching social values (dimensions III and IV).

RESEARCHER AS REVIEWER: HEALTH, ETHNICITY AND POLICY

A necessary (and sometimes sufficient) condition of investigating, when initially wanting to obtain information or to plan a practical project, is to establish what is already known on the topic. This preliminary check upon extant knowledge should be made into a routine precaution before commencing any research, for several reasons:

- Often the 'new' information needed exists already and only requires discovery.
- To begin collecting fresh research data, if the problem has been studied and answered satisfactorily, could be a bad practical mistake because of time and effort expended. (In any case, setting up a problem for investigation may be best conducted with some critical knowledge of previous findings, interests and problems in the research field.)
- Empirical investigation is an extremely specialising business and concentrates attention. Cutting deep into a topic is only possible if the sense of intervention is sharply defined. Therefore, the early stage of problem specification is critically important – and tends to operate by means of a progressive funnelling-down process in several stages. The sharp focusing-down of concern for future enquiry can be facilitated by reference to extant advice and admissions, failures and findings.

In order to illustrate this initial stage of research, and to demonstrate some of the skills and developments which are useful, one example of research reviewing into special health outcomes will be presented. We will search for evidence upon 'health' and 'ethnicity'. This topic, or conjunction of terms, will be addressed by describing a library search into studies reported in journal articles which are stored, and accessible, on two CD-ROMs. This search for relevant journal articles will be purely descriptive in reviewing findings.

The second question will move away from prose summaries of the literature towards findings which are essentially statistical, but which require some secondary analysis. The problem of infant mortality and ethnicity will be covered in order to demonstrate this concern. The material is more specialised in scope and more technical in treatment. However, statistical studies of this problem have been most systematic and represent a considerable sophistication in measuring health outcomes and various social differences. (Both sets of material will be reviewed according to the pattern of their findings, their research purposes and health implications.)

The topic of health and ethnicity has been selected as an illustration of literature-searching for several reasons. Information on health and ethnicity is applicable to the practice of surgical nursing. Individual or group distinctions may influence nursing care in a variety of

ways. Often the concept of ethnicity is viewed from one perspective only, namely that of your own membership group. In nursing practice, such a restricted ethnocentric perspective may result in inappropriate care or stereotypical approaches to caring for certain patients. To provide insight into the wider concepts of health and ethnicity is, therefore, important (see Ch. 10).

The best sources for good information and searches on research reports are CD-ROMs. These compact discs may be 'read-only' since the information which is stored can be received but not changed. Each represents a particular band of academic disciplines and covers research articles published in the cognate professional journals. In the past, library searching for relevant published research was a relatively tedious and time-consuming process, which involved acquiring detailed search knowledge and skills such as authoritative advice and access; repetitive checks on specialist journal issues; and trying to trace select publications from a host of bibliographical lists routinely appended to whichever research reports had been previously detected and read.

Nowadays, the electronic storage and accessing of articles published in journals means that literature searches can be directed very precisely and comprehensively, and that the state of knowledge on any topic can be ascertained in a very short time. Standard citations include the item's title, author(s), source (journal, in this case) and also an abstract of 200 words or so. All of the information may be printed as hard copy.

Electronic search-processes operate lexically, by recognising exact words for scanning. So the search term(s) given must be chosen shrewdly: to express the review purpose well; to fit the language of the literature; and be sufficiently broad in scope so as to obtain a suitable range of thematic references and a manageable amount of relevant articles. In our case, the search began with the previous 5 years of MEDLINE on the words 'ethnicity & health'.

Out of 33 items selected by the CD-ROM, reference was made to the USA (in 22 articles), UK (3), other English-speaking areas (4), miscellaneous (4). In order to inspect the publication sources and research themes, coding and breakdown of citations was confined to articles from the USA.

All selected research came from different journals – except for two pairs of articles which derived from public health reports and the *American Journal of Epidemiology*. Both titles were models for dealing with health and ethnicity in that causal relationships were identified in the public domain and used to target problematic populations. The importance of ethnicity was never defined theoretically (nor even hypothetically). The concept referred to foreign cultures generally, and especially to racial minorities. Specifically, according to scientific procedures, ethnicity was treated as one of many standard demographic measures, such as age or gender, and the research designs were devised to demonstrate which of the variable associations were statistically significant.

Returning to the original set of 33 and leaving aside five cases where information was indeterminate, the health purposes of the set of reports fall into three main categories: 12 articles on public health monitoring of periodic routines or interventionist programmes; 10 articles on abuse (substance and sexual risk); and 6 other research studies, which were mainly on health staff themselves.

Under half of the findings contained some policy recommendations for reform. An epidemiological logic in monitoring, and explaining, population risks in health was the dominant pattern. The medical science emphasis on the numerical measuring of health dangers was strong. MEDLINE research was limited, as the information-base of the ROM was drawn from medical science journals with distinctive professional and disciplinary approaches. The question then arises: 'Is the reported research from other health professionals different?'

To find out, the extra term 'policy' was added and the search was extended to CINAHL (Cumulative Index to Nursing and Allied Health Literature) for the same 5-year period. The 'slate' of periodicals was found to be different from the MEDLINE ones – but, once again, the article selection represented a complete array of research journals. In the resulting data-set of 16 articles, 14 were from the USA. The societal focus seemed similar at first sight. However, the scope of CINAHL research references proved to be wider in key respects: three citations derived from doctoral theses based on a broad investigation of health and social statuses; seven other articles took as their main tasks a review of the existing research literature and provided an average of 50 expert bibliographical references per article. Three-quarters of the articles recommended health remedial and promotional policies. Of the last sub-set of six miscellaneous reports, three dealt with health enhancement and three were concerned that ethnic language skills and values were accorded cultural respect.

The overall research literature on both CD-ROMs is clearly dominated by an American perspective on health journal concerns and problems which are perceived to be of interest. It may be that more research is published in the USA, but the present American dominance in information technology exaggerates this impression. Alternative British CD-ROMs are now becoming available. The Royal College of Nursing has recently produced a full electronic index to nursing journals, which should bring knowledge of publications and the professional concern for practical British problems closer together.

To conclude this brief section, it is important that the research reviewer should be careful in choosing the index of information, as the bases of collection produce certain biases in every literature compilation.

Secondary research analysis

Turning attention to the British case, therefore, it is most useful to pursue evidence within the same topic by examining the other main type of secondary research analysis: statistical evidence which has been derived from official records and special surveys. Better empirical evidence has recently become available. A report by Smaje (1995) aims to make sense of reported findings by assessing both sides of the minority ethnic/health equation and by reviewing British evidence on mortality and morbidity, and also on policy issues of health care and service utilisation. The basic method of analysis may be described as both scientific and secondary. On the first point, the 'positivist' type of research selected for examination always concentrates upon measuring variables and obtaining statistical results. On the last point, the report accepts the assumptions of primary researchers: their population parameters and operational concepts; their frameworks of inference and codings.

The potential for extending knowledge is, therefore, limited by the narrow conventions which have been accepted. Humanistic health concerns for interpersonal care and cultural understanding can find little support or space. In respect of infant mortality rates (as well as enquiries into specific diseases), the research searches for ethnic differentials and repeatedly finds interethnic differences which are statistically suspect and medically meaningless.

For instance, protracted discussions about ethnic explanations of infant death (Smaje 1995, pp. 33–43) are based upon data involving less than one percentage figure of variation in the rates, small cell sizes and occasional differences between particular minorities. Minute 'ethnic' differences are treated as important – though they remain insignificant and inexplicable. Another example of a pathological approach to health problems is diabetes, which – together with coronary heart and cerebrovascular diseases – is distinguished as ethnic and explained accordingly. Comparatively slight, and intermittent, differences in the diabetes rates of 'coloured' minorities, which are usually exceeded by gender and age differentials, are accepted – on the evidence of small community studies – and are attributed in theory to a peculiar environment or to hypothetical genes which resist insulin. The 'ethnic' explanation is clearly disproportionate to the slight data differences – and has no value in healing the diagnosed disease.

In the authors' view, most research into minority health conditions finds differences which are not significant empirically or theoretically. Instead of looking for health distinctions as characteristic of ethnic groups, it would be more reasonable to make the assumption that ethnicity, if devoid of status implications, is *not* significant for health: that equality of treatment (and parity in explanation) according to similar health conditions and needs is, in principle, the right standard and policy. In the ethnicity studies reviewed, one can detect a racist insistence as to who is the problem: a stance which tends to blame the victims and has failed to advance the science, and promotion, of health.

Reflective point

Consider (in relation to establishing what is already known in your area) what policies or standards exist in your place of work with regard to preoperative information-giving for patients from different ethnic groups. What if any research studies underpin them?

THE PURE SCIENTIFIC METHOD: EXPERIMENTAL DESIGN

Some research questions cannot be solved by reference to extant, available, findings. Yet, to obtain fresh evidence to answer the specific question by means of special surveys or ethnographic studies may be dauntingly difficult because of the heavy data collection costs which are necessary (in terms of the skill resources and time duration which are involved, and also because the research problem to be investigated may require cause–effect explanations to be obtained according to the strictest standards of evidence). The problem of finding a method which can best produce suitable evidence in practice may, therefore, be answered by adopting an experimental method for a designed purpose which is clear and limited in scope, neat in its problematic aims and proofs and can take advantage of surgical circumstances – involving highly controlled intervention procedures,

clinical conditions and small numbers of permanent personnel.

Experimentation must seem specially appropriate for the consequences of surgical work, for operating theatres, intensive care units and high dependency units possess many obvious resemblances to experimental laboratories. Both types of context involve conditions of enhanced (though incomplete) control wherein a preplanned change is deliberately introduced and monitored by precise, technical measures. Both types of hi-tech intervention require vital confidence and a high degree of certainty and their sets of procedures are very exact and, ideally, preplanned and well prepared. Both situations of intervention produce extreme proactive boldness – and must be capable of making wide generalisations from findings obtained in a highly specific, artificially controlled situation. Because the two contexts are analogous and surgical conditions for experimental investigation seem so suitable, we will advocate some of the most attractive features of experimental methods and suggest how to avoid potential disadvantages.

The logical advantages of experimental methods may be summarised as residing in high standards of certainty, control over comparative conditions and explicitness of procedure. It is suggested that these clear inferential advantages may be retained and utilised at different levels of logical strictness across three main types of experimental design.

In practice, however, idealised laboratory experiments entail disadvantages arising from their artificial features: namely, problems of ethics and extrapolation; the distortions of demand perspectives within, and of strict limitations of policy separation without, the social context. More suitable models for health outcome research will be proposed which are free of these disadvantages yet still offer key advantages of experimental explanation. The types of research design to be preferred will be referred to as natural 'field' or retrospective experiments.

The ideal properties of experimentation may be identified by three inferential criteria:

• the achievement of clear theoretical meaning throughout the whole research process
• the manipulation of one experimental variable and prevention of other changes
• total control over the comparative conditions of the investigation and, therefore, over the general inferences which can be firmly, and finally, drawn between them.

These three criteria for experimentation should all hold, in principle, for an explanation to be tested in the fullest sense as being demonstrably universal, verifiable and replicable.

However, these three scientific requirements are typically not attainable, as a complete combination, under research conditions within the humanistic and the health sciences. How strictly do these three defining criteria have to be observed in any practical social investigation before the research design can be recognised as being experimental?

Conventionally speaking, an absence of the first ideal standard, that pure theory is being tested, does not prevent research from being described as a recognisable 'experiment' – otherwise the accolade would be so rare as to be extraordinary in the social sciences. On the other hand, if a particular research project fails to accord with all of the three criteria, as outlined, it would be misleading to call the overall set-up 'experimental'. There are many in-between situations, of partial fulfilment, where the research designs involved may be defined as involving different types, or modes, of experimentation.

What is meant by experimental design needs to be redefined thoroughly, with both research realism and methodological clarity. In research practice, different levels or degrees of stringency in experimentation must be distinguished. Methodological standards and expectations can thus be revised accordingly, at the appropriate intermediate levels. We will, first of all, consider practical departures from the three ideal principles, in order to discuss the utility of actual experimentation for purposes of investigating health outcomes in the postsurgery context.

Theory-testing: the experiment as general verification

In scientific principle, any one clear hypothesis which is to be tested by a proposed experiment should be deductively derived from a precise universalistic theory, which will then confer a general value and significance upon the empirical findings (Popper 1972). In practice, the hypothetical propositions which require, and set up, actual experiments rarely have such secure foundations in being derived specifically from established theory.

Typically, a particular 'operational' hypothesis will be adopted which has a tight, empirical, reference so that it has a clear meaning under the conditions of study, but its explanatory potential for making strong theoretical statements of an extended, universal, scope is therefore very limited. Instead, conclusions are typically constructed from (and confined to) contingent relationships between the independent (experimental) variable and dependent (resultant) variables. Where

this is so, any demonstrated or confirmed (statistical) connection which is established may not be universal in scope; and explanatory findings may only be generalised to other identical, empirical conditions.

Of course the pivotal relationship between key experimental variables can be explored further by more extended investigation – and checked by means of replication studies using the same experimental method (a major advantage of its procedural explicitness). The researcher's strategic concern in design, and the crucial locus of proof, however, can no longer be focused on general theory testing in a hypothetico-deductive fashion. It must be operationally causal – and involve an examination of the imputed connection between the independent (experimental) variable and other dependent (outcome) variables to discover if this 'internal' cause–effect relationship is strongly significant. In default of ideal theory-testing (by deduction to hypotheses), investigative concern must turn to investigation of experimental change by bivariate analysis and aim to show that a causal (or, at least, correlative) relationship exists between the independent (introduced) and the dependent (ensuing) variables.

For example, such a design may be used to test the clinical effectiveness of a particular wound dressing on a necrotic wound. It would be intended that the application of a particular dressing-product would result in a sloughing of the necrotic tissue and the promotion of granulation tissue, with no further health detriment to the patient.

Reflective point

In the above example which would be the independent variable and which the dependent variable?

The ideal manipulative experiment: problems of design and control

In principle, the most logically certain procedure for experimental inference entails the follow-up examination of one deliberate change under known, and constant, conditions. If the conditions of causal inference actually hold true, then measurements of change on the 'resultant' dependent variable must indicate the true 'effect' of experimental change.

In practice, to follow this counsel of perfection, requiring 'pure' manipulation of all experimental conditions is extremely demanding, since several distinct requirements have to be met if simple interdependence of the 'causal' connection is to be assured.

• The experimental change must be isolated as a discrete idea or potential 'cause'.

• The independent (or 'experimental') variable should be introduced deliberately.

• Other conditions must be equal – so that 'effects' can only be attributed to the 'cause'.

Table 18.1 shows how the relationship between experimental inference and design can be ascertained and improved.

To be logically certain that the independent variable (for example the wound dressing) causes the dependent variable (i.e. the experimental outcome; for example granulation of tissue), it is necessary to prevent the possibility that other causal conditions also produce the results – by ensuring a careful design of control conditions.

Under the simple experimental hypothesis (left-hand column of Table 18.1), there cannot be complete certainty of inference that IV causes DV, because there may also be 'internal' investigation biases of testing and time between measures taken at T1 and T2. These research influences might include subject self-awareness and practice effects, or any processes where changes occur due to the passage of time, such as decay, wastage, maturation or subjective experience.

The solution to this problem of uncertain inference is to design a distinct control condition which is identical in all respects, except that the initial, independent, variable is omitted (Campbell 1957). If any effect is present under the experimental condition, and not under the control condition, then the inference that the result must originate from the independent variable is practically certain – unless an alternative 'contaminating' condition is present which cannot be eliminated and might influence the outcome.

An interesting example of using the operative situation for experimental purposes is a research study to investigate the importance of preparing patients for a planned operation – psychologically as well as physically. Here the significance of preoperative cautionary counselling was analysed against postoperative measures of pain and anxiety and the results were found to be positive. That is, verbal preparation reduced pain symptoms.

Clearly, all other operational conditions were strictly controlled to be the same between the two sets of patients. Thus the difference between patients who were given special verbal preparation (experimental subjects) and those who were not given any (control subjects) was so identical in all other respects that the result could only be due to the unique experimental condition and distinctive, preparatory cause (Hayward 1975).

This manipulative, laboratory-type experiment, however, is flawed by the artificiality of control conditions and context which are required to construct the exact inferences. This experimental artificiality has doubtful implications in respect of external validity – questioning the generality and representativeness of findings – and also in respect of its strict internal orientation, which makes subject responses peculiarly compliant to experimental demands (Rosenthal 1976), whilst the research situation and analysis becomes segregated from outside conditions and general values.

Social experimentation: retrospective analysis and controls

The ideal manipulative experiment, as described above, relies upon the fact that it is conducted with a prospective time perspective, an advanced knowledge which favours both the completeness of its design controls and the certainty of its logical inferences. The crucial change to be introduced – and the distinction between experimental and control conditions – are planned clearly beforehand and the outcome is anticipated.

In normal social circumstances (as opposed to laboratory-like contexts) researchers often find themselves interested in examining a change which has already taken place but attempting to analyse its causal origins by means of experimental procedures, because this ideal method of explanation has been most powerful, stringent and certain in the physical sciences which deal with natural matter and formulate universal laws.

In the behavioural and health sciences attention has moved away from the traditional model, which has been upheld by the physical sciences dealing with laws about matter, towards experiments involving social phenomena which have occurred spontaneously – and

Table 18.1 Relationship between experimental inference and design

Experimental hypothesis	Control condition
T1	T1
IV	
T2	T2
DV	DV

Key: IV = independent variable (the hypothesised cause); DV = dependent variable (hypothetical consequence or experimental outcome); T1 = first time (or first test) – when the experiment starts; T2 = second, and final, time – when results are measured are therefore investigated retrospectively using a different mode of experimentation.

In a historic path-breaking book called *Experimental sociology, a study in method*, Greenwood (1945) declared that the logic of physical/manipulative experiments and of social/spontaneous experiments is the same, but that a different 'field' procedure needs to be followed. He defines the key feature of an experiment as: 'The proof of an hypothesis which seeks to hook up two factors into a causal relationship through the study of contrasting situations, which have been controlled on all factors except the one of interest, the latter being either the hypothetical cause or the hypothetical effect' (p. 28).

Once this alternative type of experiment is recognised, the manipulation of key control conditions may not be physical and direct: it may become symbolic and more indirect. Typically, retrospective processes of inference rely on different devices of selection and statistics to ensure the control condition. In order to estimate the contribution of any independent causal variable, a contrasting group is created which is similar in all relevant respects, but which differs critically in not being exposed to the experimental variable.

This *retrospective* experimental design is achieved either by means of randomisation (the selection of a control population, made equivalent by virtue of statistical chance), or by matching procedures (whereby control group attributes, for each subject, are selected to ensure similarity with the experimental group). The method of allocation by group matching, upon relevant criteria, has the advantage that unexpected differences on these lines may be examined, if the variables (also) prove to differentiate the two groups. It is possible, by these techniques of group control and statistical analysis, to retain the stringent design advantages of experimentation yet to extend the scope of its natural methodology and also to enhance its practical usefulness.

Because of its laboratory origins and eminence in the history of science, the 'ideal' (or 'manipulative') experiment is hailed as a source of 'pure' knowledge, in the sense that the evidential findings and generalisations are valued as essentially analytical and not designedly applied; as separate in derivation from the 'external' context and divorced from normal practical pressures and from problems of application. In naturally occurring field experimentation this strict separation of contexts is unnecessary and undesirable.

In fact, practical field experiments provide a valuable method in the applied sciences. Applied experiments in engineering (e.g. into metal stress), and in agriculture (e.g. upon crop yields), and in medicine

(e.g. drug trials) must have their findings checked in open 'field' conditions with extreme care and rigorous controls. However, research expectations that the findings should be applied in practice is clear in the planning of these exemplary experimental designs. In these particular applied, and organic, contexts it is clear that experimental methods can be stringent, in methodological inference, and also planned to be intentionally useful.

In the case of *drug trials*, similarly, 'field' experiments involve a valuable combination of strict, statistical controls and systematic, monitored, applications of the knowledge. For they involve key experimental devices such as subject-matching (between those who have received the drug and those who have not) and placebo, or psychological, controls (between those who believe that they are receiving the drug and those that actually have).

Furthermore, the lack of theoretical direction in such trials confers the important benefit that negative and positive outcome conditions can be assessed comprehensively. In the formally ideal experiment, the significance of findings should be determined by whether the results are in accord with theory predictions. In the more empirical trials, however, it is possible (and preferable) to monitor all of the results. Whether the results are deduced from correct pharmaceutical theory is often a question of limited interest. What is important for health outcomes is to know the direct (beneficial) effects and also the unexpected 'side' effects which may be clinically undesirable – but need to be known and taken account of. For example, in setting up a trial to test the absorption rates of two synthetic polymer sutures used to close abdominal muscle, the pharmacological and biochemical interest will be in the rate of breakdown of the suture material by hydrolysis. To know that one is more slowly absorbed than the other is of value when considering abdominal wound strength during the recovery period. However, if the suture with the slower absorption rate is associated with a higher incidence of wound sinus then there is a clinical problem which must be addressed.

Where have we got to in our overview of methodology? Purely informational research (of various analytical depths) has been considered within its own terms of reference. According to the layout plan in Figure 18.1, discussion has covered the left-hand column of descriptive/informational research and dealt with the second quadrant of 'deep' experimental analysis, which does not make direct allowance for social values – either within the purposes of subjects, or according to social (health) aims and objectives – as held by patients, health professionals or wider social policies and programmes.

Reflective point

Consider which aspects of the information presented so far surgical nurses need to consider. To assist you in this exercise, focus on the following: What problems would you encounter in designing an experiment to compare the use of paracetamol, tepid sponging or the use of a fan for temperature reduction in the postsurgical patient with hyperpyrexia due to infection?

INTERACTIVE APPROACHES: RESEARCHING SOCIAL VALUES

Attention now turns to the social basis and significance of research – then towards the value this approach has for informing nursing actions and improving health outcomes. We begin with the participatory position that social knowledge and skills, empathy and commitments are not to be avoided: they constitute the basis for advancing professional meanings, clinical judgements and a self-directed sense of collective competence. In this endeavour, social objectivity is not without the social process, but part of it. Others' knowledge and values represent the basic data, or evidence for research. We therefore begin with a central perspective of sociology: that social understanding must begin in interaction with the other, for this focus is where social sharing and existence arise and where social understanding and analysis must be developed.

In origin, Continental (and especially German) philosophers have established a concern for the appreciation of social action, showing that a correct understanding of the intentions, values and perspectives of others is the sure basis upon which to build sociology particularly and social scientific research in general. This revised and extended methodology has now become accepted across the English-speaking world. A synoptic account of the process and of the major philosophical positions may be found in what Giddens calls *New Rules of Sociological Method* (1976). There are many schools of theory and variant emphases, but certain common features of the broad approach may be recognised and summarised for present purposes.

1. *Subjective* meanings of others comprise data, or evidence, for social understanding.

2. In principle, it is possible, to construct *objective* science from these materials.

3. To accomplish this epistemological *transformation*, and obtain congruence between the two levels of knowledge may involve special methods of coordination, such as theoretical application, language interpretation, data analysis and triangulation.

Several important implications follow for professionals who are conducting research.

• *Participation* is not an undesirable situation for researchers to avoid if possible: it is an indispensable cultural position for gaining knowledge and informing practice.

• The primary task is to record and complete a social *description* of phenomena. This requirement involves careful documentation of detailed social interaction.

'*Action-research*' refers to the basis of knowledge in subject-purposes and behaviour, not to the advanced intention of integrating knowledge with programmes of change. There is a risk of misinformed activism and confusion about the authority of research if the expression 'action-research' is mistakenly used in a simple interventionist sense. However, participatory, action-based research is not necessarily pure and separate. Once the distinction between the subjective basis and the practical use of research is respected, action-oriented research can lead to better-informed professional planning (see also Ch. 2).

In order to show how investigations may operate with different types of research procedure and at different levels of social interaction, we will distinguish two principal methods and illustrate their value by reference to examples of good substantive studies. The methods are social surveys, and observation research, either participatory or else clinical and case oriented. The sequence of treatment involves progressively greater interactive complexity and personal depth.

Surveys: quantitative techniques and qualitative designs

The authority of social surveys, which use questionnaires and/or interviews in order to represent public knowledge, is basically descriptive. The act of obtaining information which is already in mind, but not on record, involves a careful describing and collecting of data in the form of verbal responses from a wide sample of subjects on specific issues.

The survey as a principal method of fresh data collection possesses two major advantages in its worked-out routine techniques which are currently adopted and widely appreciated. Sampling procedures ensure the representativeness of findings, and well-structured sets of questions may elicit relevant responses for analysis in a common frame of reference. These characteristics, in respect of sampling selection and questioning organisation, operate to make research procedures clear and accountable; also to produce research findings which are comparatively reliable and capable of recording general meanings.

It is desirable that social surveys accurately 'match' the populations to be represented, both in their sampling distinctions and in the appropriateness of question-formulation. The more complex modes of sampling which stratify selection at suitable levels are much more powerful and effective in 'fitting' sub-populations and their particular concerns than sampling methods which simply rely upon the randomness of case selection to supply an impersonal assurance that there is no statistical bias in choosing respondents. In fact, a shrewd use of complex designs – at different 'levels' of sampling representation – can, in effect, permit an independent inspection of the contributory effect of crucial variables. In this way a designer sample may approximate to the field experiment, as described, in the research's degree of statistical control and sureness of inference.

Simple and complex types of sampling will be discussed and contrasted, to develop this suggestion about the advantages which can be gained by using advanced sampling designs. For details of sampling techniques, see Gilbert (1993) and Moser & Kalton (1971).

A simple sample-survey, consisting of multiple interviews (or cases) can ensure that all of the findings are rendered both 'externally' generalisable and 'internally' comparable in defining data collection along two broad lines of administrative standardisation: by choosing all cases by means of systematic random sampling; and also by making sure that the analysis of all responses, across the data-sets, is self-consistent and uniform.

However, there is a high price to pay, if purely statistical ideas of objectivity – stipulating uniformity of representation, impartiality of measurement, and degrees of uncertainty – are so narrowly conceived that other, more subjective, considerations of personal meaning and particular variation are treated as relatively unimportant in sampling. For the construction of a relevant, more complex and stratified, sampling design can be crucial to a survey's subtlety and incisiveness in entering into the social differences and meanings of subjects.

This is particularly relevant when using survey-type methods to determine the long-term health outcomes of surgical patients. For example, if nurses had identified a set of long-term health outcomes with a group of patients over a 2-year period (as would be the case for cardiac rehabilitation following coronary artery bypass grafting), then a stratified sampling process would be most appropriate. Stratification could be carried out by patients' gender, age, social class, and/or by type of surgery.

A random-sample survey consists of evidence based upon cases which are deliberately chosen by pure-chance selection in order to represent equally all members of a particular population. When sampling is thus simple – and random – in representing a social universe, it cuts right across the social interactions of sample members and their living cultural differences. In fact, actual interviews between two persons must involve a special relationship of social interaction: from both points of view – and together.

The standardisation of question-sets – both in formulation, to be structured, and in administration, to be replicable – enables the collection of data combined statistically.

The survey is a powerful, cost-effective means for collecting fresh and special social data, since it can be applied speedily to strange, and unrecorded, situations and does not necessarily require the use of skilled interviewers. However, highly structured survey schedules which presume complete social uniformity – usually for administrative reasons of statistical convenience and coding reliability – must fail to penetrate the more qualitative, and encompassing, meaning systems of the subjects and risk neglecting other cultural differences and the personal interrelationships in their lives (Field & Morse 1992).

There is a polarisation in methodology between scientific, quantification approaches to research and humanistic, qualitative approaches which is undesirable and unnecessary. (For a good review of the Continental arguments and approaches see Giddens 1976.). Those who adopt strict measurement procedures, and prefer statistical forms of analyses, frequently fail to obtain more subjective, meaningful types of evidence and often scorn such concerns as substandard, non-scientific research. The attempt to collect both types of evidence, and to enhance the advantages of each, in combination, can be inhibited by dogmatic 'scientific' methodology. In fact, the statistical requirements of both sampling and interview structuring should not be conceived so rigidly that they prevent a parallel account from being taken of sub-variations within the outline sampling framework.

The benefits of quantification in a sample survey of structured interviews need not altogether prevent sensitivity to qualitative variations. Research designs can take account of action requirements, both by discerning meaningful parameters for sampling selection and in the meaningful planning of 'open' and qualitative interviews. Interview procedures which are thematic and flexible (rather than strictly scheduled), designed to be exploratory and other-directed (not strictly pre-coded and overuniform), make it possible for interviewer questioning to elicit more complex actions and to probe deeply into personal experiences and values. For example, in asking patients about postoperative pain it may be more insightful to carry out an in-depth interview which explores the patient's personal experiences of pain management and pain relief. Such information will provide rich data about personal experiences which could be used to inform the range of potential health outcomes with regard to pain management.

Sampling and stratification

The selection of evidence in *complex* sampling too need not be crudely standardised for the sake of statistical uniformity. The method of *simple* random sampling must assume social homogeneity – because the representation of all cases is guaranteed to be even (each case having an equal chance of being chosen) and the sampling universe, or population unit, is 'the same'. By contrast, a stratified sampling procedure is capable of making a series of finer distinctions and of constructing subsamples which are defined, and designed, to be diacritical for the population and crucial to the purposes of enquiry.

One study of informal 'network' care and health outcome support around elderly people, for instance, is interesting in this connection because the complex sampling was so well stratified that the investigation could simultaneously examine the effects of age and gender, continuity (or migration) and of community integration. Wengler & Leger (1992) sampled and interviewed elderly people from eight Welsh rural communities (to obtain wide differences in their degree of residential continuity) and then followed up this study (using the same instruments and checking the first model of analysis) across three Irish urban communities: an urban village; a mixed suburb; and a peripheral housing estate.

Variations in integration between these communities were found to result in specific types of support networks. The differences were examined both quantitatively, by survey findings, and qualitatively, by local knowledge and history, to explain peculiarities.

Where continuous residence and kin support were lacking, in two Welsh cases, the elders' support networks were markedly private (conjugal or isolated) or dependent upon wider social circles and local associations. Wider community-focused support networks were associated with higher status and strong trends of incoming retirement migration.

In Belfast, these two types of support were absent. Instead cohesive urban communities gave rise to locally integrated networks or (more restricted) family-dependent networks. In respect of policy-making, the researchers suggest 'that the distribution of support networks may be a better social or service indicator than single demographic variables'.

The implications of this study for surgical nursing can be understood in terms of the social factors that may influence community care. For example, in establishing a day surgery unit, it is advisable to explore the nature of informal support for the follow-up care and discharge planning of patients, especially the elderly and socially dependent (West & Lyon 1995) (see Ch. 15).

A well-stratified sample can thus investigate a set of definite, relevant parameters and combine the strengths of a well-designed, field-experimental framework with the exploratory value of dealing with unexpected findings and special circumstances.

Observation: open and closed

The value of observational work needs to be distinguished according to its use. A researcher's role may be socially open, or effectively closed, in observation. Methodological approaches are very different for general observations which are made in unbounded contexts, where cultural participation is 'open' in scope and purpose, as against 'closed' observations which operate where perceived role-obligations and relational values are quite fixed and already known. The closed observational characteristics, of course, are typical of clinical situations, where the patient focus is firmly established and the observer's concerns are tightly related to case-care objectives. The open and closed methods will be outlined and exemplified briefly.

In anthropology, observations aim to become culturally meaningful by recording interpersonal rituals and beliefs in their entirety. The modern tendency, as untouched cultures have virtually disappeared, is to specialise in a smaller group, context or problem. For instance Sokolovsky (1990) concentrates on the position of aged people in their communities. The experiences of health and ageing are universal, but clearly the meaning given to these developments varies considerably within each particular culture (see Ch. 10).

The perspective achieved by participant observation research, according to one astute philosopher (Bruyn 1966), is obtained by coordinating three methodological bases of knowledge – coherence, consistency and consensus.

- Coherence: involves drawing out clearly the meaning of other people, as understood.
- Consistency: tests the empirical fit between operational concepts and observations.
- Consensus: supplies a general validation that those studied accept the interpretation.

The subjective meaningfulness of knowledge exploration must be checked by objectivity in evidence-recording and research procedure. One classic way of doing this is advocated by Becker (1955) who treats the method as ideal in comprehensiveness but specially difficult as regards proof, because theory is a subsequent product not a prior guide and check, and because uncritical interpretative findings are easily self-validating. His suggested solution is to progress in stages by clarifying the problematical focus and patterned findings; constructing and checking a model of analysis; and providing a lucid research history to readers – which makes the whole procedure become accountable.

Lofland & Lofland (1984) show how the social observational method of obtaining qualitative data (in values, language-use, personal styles and activities) can be transformed into quantitative evidence (procedures for recording, statistical analysis and reporting).

In conducting an audit, to explore the clinical effectiveness of named nursing, it may be that a focus group discussion of nursing values combined with direct observation of nurse–patient interactions and resultant health outcomes would produce considerable qualitative data. If the information was collected within a known conceptual framework (named nursing) then categories and themes can be identified and the resultant data made quantifiable.

The two modes of evidence are not incompatible – as if based on opposite principles. They are best considered complementary aspects of a combined analytical sequence. Modern anthropologists, such as Ellen (1984), prefer to treat the open (participant form of) observation as being only one of several, simultaneous approaches to research, which may be combined with the use of extant records and systematic interviewing.

In fact, research workers (unless artificially separated from their subjects of enquiry) do actually participate in the social meanings of their engagement, but are persuaded that these perceptions involve a different (subjective) method and often discount them. Yet, the observational aspects of enquiry need not contrast with the verbalised question-based modes of information-getting which are typical of social surveys.

Participant perception tends to concentrate 'in depth', because it entails a close, sympathetic and meticulously detailed focus on one immediate context to obtain particular, personal meanings and understandings. Survey sampling, by contrast, seeks to represent individual positions by means of elicited verbal responses 'in breadth'.

We suggest that the two approaches can be drawn together, with mutual and fruitful benefit. In research practice, of course, a complete combination of both approaches is probably excessively demanding of time and attention. To focus upon a case study, however, is inherently selective in the use of resources and contained as a personal commitment. Therefore case support, to be developed in analytical depth, may strengthen more general evidence, which has been obtained in evidential breadth. In this process of adding special exploration and personal exemplification in order to illustrate the wider social patterns, care must be taken as to which case (whether patient or nurse) should be chosen as properly representative of the more systematic survey findings.

An interesting and impressive example of clinical research which combines interview, questioning and keen observation of personal relations between nurses and patients is provided by Lawler (1991). This Australian somological study investigates how intrusive problems of the body – principally arising from sexuality – affect both nursing staff and patients, influencing their personal relations, social embarrassments and professional standards of care. The research evidence is derived from verbal staff self-reporting (on youth, training and practice) and from professional and observational knowledge as to how nakedness ('privacy') is managed on the wards.

Another example of rounded clinical observation, which is case-focused and of evident nursing interest, is given in research conducted and described by West, one of the present co-authors. Her postoperative report is given verbatim in Case study 18.1, in which a very independent, demanding lady shows where there have been special aspects of caring, whether good or bad. Such data provide information about the patient's experiences.

Reflective point

Consider conversations you may have had with a client you have recently cared for. What did you learn from these about the patient's experiences?

Case study 18.1   Experiences of care in a thoracic unit

In a study of nurses' perceptions of patients in a perioperative context West (1992, 1993) obtained detailed observational and interview data from both nurses and patients about care experiences. The study was exploring the perceptual constructs used by nurses when caring for patients. The following extract from a case study provides insight into the richness of data that can be obtained by studying the real world of nursing.

[This] patient case study is of a lady who had undergone thoracic surgery for cancer of the lung. She spent a lot of time travelling abroad, and over the past three years she had developed severe chest pain and breathing difficulties. The nurses in the ward saw her as not demanding of nursing time pre-operatively, stating that she did need some information about her operation, but not very much because she seemed to know everything that was going on. This patient was perceived as difficult to talk to because she was always complaining and always asking questions. Her progress and recovery, according to the nurses, were really quite poor and she was quite dependent on nurses in some respects, but she wouldn't actually let anyone get close to her.

This lady was in a single room in the ward and she was visited regularly by her sister. When asked about how she knew about the ward routines when moving around the environment, she said; 'I don't really know, my sister asked about visiting, I shut my room door because people are always staring in. I miss the newspapers, they [the nurses] are very lax about telling you things, I wouldn't have known about the library unless my sister, who was put out by the dragon-lady [physiotherapist] hadn't seen the ladies with the trolley [the WRVS library service]. She asked if they had any Mills and Boons, bloody awful books really, but I like to read them. They are very lax about telling you anything, also nobody introduces themselves, they just come in and take over, I always ask them though who they are and what they are going to do'.

When asked what she expected when she went to the operating theatre she replied, 'the Consultant told me some things. There are nice girls down there, very caring, one held my hand – she's special, that was nice'.

She said that she had a lot of pains since her operation: 'I told everybody about it – nurses and doctors. I've a low pain threshold, maybe not, maybe others would be screaming. I'd one horrible incident, I was having my first cup of tea in two days, when this lady comes in, pushes my tea aside and starts to pummel me. I told her this was my first tea in two days, the pain was awful, I called her the dragon-lady and told her to get out. The next day she came, the nurses gave me painkillers beforehand, one good thing though was that she [the physiotherapist], the dragon-lady, got me a ladder. When the physio first said this I thought where the hell does she expect me to climb to. It was a rope ladder for pulling yourself up the bed'.

She said she had been sleeping fairly well, but that the hospital was noisy during the night. Asked if she needed help with anything in particular, she said 'I need some help with these tubes here – chest drains. Today, I didn't though. I walked back from the X-ray myself. I gave up waiting for the porter. I have to be careful that I don't lie on these tubes'.

Her relationship with the nursing staff she described as 'very good, most of them very good and kind – they are you know, I'm not backward at coming forward to ask any questions, I just use the buzzer or I call them'.

When asked about what information she'd been given about her surgery and recovery, she stated that she felt she had been given information by the consultant whom she described as very good indeed. She also said that she felt included in conversations with doctors and nurses on the ward rounds.

'The last time I saw them, the doctor explained that my lung was expanding and that I should be ready to go home soon. I've enjoyed being in here, but now I've had enough. I know I had cancer and that I've just bought time. I'd only have six months or so if I had not had the op. I have to give up smoking, I promised my sisters that I would, but hell I think if I knew that I'd have a couple of years and go out painless, I'd continue with my cigarettes – God damn it, I like my cigarettes'.

Integrating methods

Clinical observation, a most valuable approach, includes case-study skills (in the narrow sense of concern for one patient, for example) but also extends to an assessment of wider informational issues and the main interpersonal processes which are at issue. Even more is called for than practical responses to case care and meticulousness of clinical concern. What is desirable is advanced evidence-based professionalism, which might display the following considerations:

- self-awareness in interacting – including reflections on personal developments
- sociological influences around the situation – of culture (see Ch. 10), perceptions and relations
- recording of informal but important events – especially unexpected observations
- imaginative involvement with nursing programmes and integrated care.

In order to consider the professional and policy aspects of nursing participation, attention will move, in Chapter 19, towards a discussion of evaluation research and the benefits of information analysis in dealing with health outcomes.

This section will briefly outline some of the ways in which policy-related research is being advocated and conducted within the contemporary health service. In

1983 Griffiths, in his management studies report into the NHS, wrote that 'clinical evaluation of particular practices is by no means common and economic evaluation of those practices extremely rare'. This assertion, in such an influential report which was to reshape the health service and introduce the principles of general management into the health care sector, has informed the recent developments in health service evaluation and the market quest for clinical effectiveness and cost-effectiveness.

Before proceeding with an analysis of the processes involved in investigating clinical effectiveness and cost-effectiveness in health care it is necessary to clarify the major concept of evaluation.

Evaluation

Evaluation is a type of operational research. It involves conducting a study which has a distinctive purpose. Evaluation per se is not a type of research strategy; rather the process usually attempts to assess the worth or value of an innovation, an intervention, a service or an approach. Evaluations deploy a range of research methods, for example survey, case study, interviews, meta-analysis of literature. Intrinsically it can be sensitive where the findings can be used to affect the service provision in favourable or disadvantageous ways.

Evaluations are often commissioned or sponsored by those who have a direct interest in the intervention or treatment under scrutiny. This may mean that the findings of the evaluation will influence policy. The ethical problems surrounding the study are large: whose interests are best served by the intervention; who is the real client; and how are vested interests being coped with? Political issues are also apparent: namely what type and style of evaluation is being sought; what criteria are used to carry out the evaluation; is one choice of perspective being given dominance over another?

There are many different types of and purposes for evaluation. Table 18.2 illustrates some of the most common types in use in the contemporary health service.

In any of these evaluations the important aspects are to choose the appropriate method for obtaining information about the intervention under scrutiny in order that the resultant data are useful and serve the purpose of the evaluation.

Robson (1993) has argued that 'Accountability is now a watchword in the whole range of public services involving people, such as education, health, and social services. This concern in the United Kingdom arises in part from recent political and ideological considerations, where it forms part of a drive to place public services within a framework similar to that governing private profit making businesses.' He continues: 'Irrespective of its origins, the notion that we should seek to understand and assess critically the functioning of services and programmes has much to commend it. The contentious issues are more to do with who does this, in what way and for what purposes.' (p. 171).

Understanding the clinical worth of certain aspects of nursing practice has always been of concern to the

Table 18.2 Types of evaluation

Type	Definition and purpose
Formative evaluation	A type of evaluation intended to help in the development of an intervention or treatment For example a survey of staff and patients' views of proposed changes to outpatient facilities
Summative evaluation	A type of evaluation designed to assess the effectiveness of an intervention or treatment For example the assessment of readmissions following the implementation of a new guideline on early discharge
Cost–benefit	A type of evaluation designed to assess the relationship between the use of a new treatment and the benefits expressed in monetary terms For example a comparative costings analysis of hospital stay following open herniorraphy compared with laparascopic herniorraphy as a day patient
Cost-effectiveness	A type of evaluation designed to assess the relationship between the use of a new treatment and the benefits expressed in non-monetary terms For example a survey of patients' and staff views of day case surgery for herniorraphy compared with a 3-day hospital stay service

profession. Increasingly, though, there has been a demand made with the introduction of general management principles into health care to not only ensure safety and efficacy of a particular intervention or treatment but also to ask whether the intervention or treatment is worth it in financial investment terms. This new managerial ideology of health care raises several questions in the minds of health professionals who have been concerned formerly only with the humanitarian aspects of health care.

The wider notion of evaluation must be further problematical as the process of evaluation treats the particular intervention under scrutiny as having known or fixed outcomes. Clinical practice is rarely so means–end rational in choosing selected means in order to achieve a known end. The demands of the context and interpersonal intuition often interfere in planned activities. Conducting a clinical evaluation is a diverse and difficult process which requires an open and pragmatic approach towards the health ends which may be attained. Nolan & Grant (1993) argue that in evaluating the effectiveness of a particular programme or intervention 'it is not itself sufficient for an intervention to produce the desired effects (if indeed they can be identified) but also that the fundamental purpose of the intervention should in some way be concerned with improving human welfare'. Such a definition endorses the fundamental premise of nursing care, namely to do health good.

Within nursing over the past 25 years the individuality of patient care has been emphasised through theories of nursing and in clinical practice. Since the NHS reforms in 1990 and 1992 there has been a closed-market concern with cost-effectiveness and clinical effectiveness and ways of evaluating these two unrelated set of values. These interests have encouraged a move away from individual patient care towards a more utilitarian approach to health service provision and health care practice (see Ch. 4).

It has been promulgated (Appleby et al 1995) that there is a need to 'shift the culture of health care provision away from basing decisions on opinion, past practice and precedent and towards making more use of science, research and evidence to guide decision making. It requires the evaluation of the effectiveness of interventions, the dissemination of the results of evaluation, and finally the application of those findings to practice'. We welcome this ideal and accept this new role for research. It cannot be assumed, however, that the transferability of research findings into action poses no administrative problems. Any synthesisation of re-evaluation and action requires management support in order that those required to change or modify

practice have aid mechanisms available. It also requires nurses who are research aware and who are able to critically appraise research.

Change management

The investment necessary to establish such a process must be taken seriously within the health service, for the application and utilisation of research findings in practice requires a planned programme of change management. Stocking (1992) has identified five characteristics of resistance to change, adapted from Rogers (1983) (Box 18.1) which will be redefined for the present argument in order to illustrate the importance of professional questioning of new interventions which are based on the dual dimensions of cost-effectiveness and clinical effectiveness.

Advantages and opposition. Professional opposition, even where there is clinical advantage, may be present for the following three reasons: the absence of appropriate education or training in order to enable health professionals to undertake or carry out the intervention; the need to change existing working practices; the perceived reduction in professional status.

The absence of appropriate education or training in order to enable health professionals to undertake or carry out the intervention. For example the introduction of laparoscopic surgical techniques for cholecystectomy was perceived negatively by health professionals. The various professions involved recognised that there was a need for education and training (indeed this received considerable publicity in the national media and induced a response from the Royal Colleges to ensure that practitioners were competent to practise). Theatre nurses recognised that the role of the 'scrub nurse' in laparoscopic procedures was different and that new educational programmes were required to ensure safe and competent nursing practice.

The need to change existing working practices. Where custom and practice have been long established in a particular aspect of care, then it is difficult for the professional group to change existing practices without there being a resultant effect on other aspects of work.

Box 18.1 Factors influencing resistance to change (adapted from Stocking 1992)

1. Professional advantages and opposition
2. Compatibility
3. Complexity
4. Observability
5. Trialability

In nursing there is a security in following similar procedures, yet the majority of nurses recognise that it is essential to aim to provide optimum care for all patients. For example, when the idea of 'universal precautions' (see Ch. 13) with regard to the handling of blood and body fluids became a new practice, many nurses found themselves having to change previous working practices. Special precautions used to be taken with known-status (hepatitis or HIV/AIDS) patients but other patients were not handled in the same protective way. The naiveté of the former practice may appear incredible nowadays but even the smallest of change (ensuring that the nurse wears gloves when handling blood and body fluids) had extensive ramifications (education, available resources and appropriate disposal mechanisms).

The perceived reduction in professional status. One of the best recently introduced cost-effective changes is the employment of phlebotomists to carry out venepuncture. This procedure was generally the prerogative of the junior doctor or a senior nurse. In a busy acute ward the first 2 hours' work of a junior doctor in the morning from breakfast onwards could be spent collecting blood samples from patients. Venepuncture is a skilled procedure requiring an understanding of the anatomy of veins and arteries, aseptic technique, universal precautions and laboratory testing procedures. The decision that a technician could be trained in this procedure and become expert in this one particular task initially caused some concern for the obvious reason that, whereas previously only a doctor (with all the associated university education) regularly carried out this procedure on ill patients, now an apparently less-educated person was being trained for this particular job. Today, in some trusts, this role is frequently undertaken by surgical nurses or even health care assistants.

Compatibility. Adopting a new intervention or approach to care may conflict with deeply held values and beliefs. For example, the cost limitations imposed by the new drug tariffs may mean that a patient's previous drug regime will have to be altered. Health professionals may find that this produces conflict, not only for their professional practice but also from the patient's point of view as non-compliance may be more likely.

Complexity. Some apparently straightforward changes indicated by clinical or economic evidence are very complex to implement as they may involve several departments in the hospital. For example, changing meal times in a care of the elderly situation involves the patients, the nursing staff, the medical staff, other health professionals, the portering staff and the catering staff (West & Lyon 1995).

Observability. This involves seeing evidence of the beneficial outcomes of the intervention or treatment. For example, study tours or visits to units utilising new interventions are beneficial to health professionals. Many nursing development units throughout the country have made themselves available to the nursing profession and have actively encouraged visits by professional peers (Wright 1989). This practice affords the opportunity to discuss the ideas with peers, to observe the practices and to discuss the outcomes with patients.

Trialability. This is related to observability but involves professionals trying out the intervention before committing themselves to it. If the change is based on economic evaluations, then health professionals may consider the validity of such to be questionable and therefore not worth trying. For example, in many locales there has been a purchasing decision made to restrict the range of wound dressing products available for use in the hospital. If this decision has been informed by research and accredited expert opinion as well as cost, then the new treatments are more likely to be accepted.

These are not the only issues involved in the process of change management. Other points of concern in the application of research into practice are to do with the realism of managers dictating how health professionals should deliver services. Clinical and non-clinical objectives are not always easily reconciled.

For many clinicians the question of proof and the standard of proof required before a new intervention is introduced are problematic on two fronts. Firstly, from a methodological standpoint the standard of proof advocated as reliable in the medical sciences is that of probability. This is often couched in statistical terms and involves an analysis of confidence levels. As practitioners, it is very difficult to incorporate confidence levels into clinical decision-making when faced with an individual patient. Many health professionals would question the assumption that because the level of confidence in an intervention has been shown to be 95% then it is good enough for all patients. The reliance on quantitative measures and probability theory to make generalisations raises many questions about the hierarchies of evidence which have been developed in current health policy documents (SIGN 1995).

Reflective point

Would you change your nursing practice for all patients on the basis of statistical evidence?

To carry out evaluation research, whether to assess the outcomes of a whole new service (for example nurse-led hysteroscopy service) or to assess the individual health outcomes of 10 patients undergoing surgery for repair of an inguinal hernia, requires the application of research principles to the evaluation process. Such an activity and such an approach to the evaluation of nursing interventions is as Bond (1996, p. 200) states 'An entirely different order to other approaches to evaluation which lack scientific rigour, and may amount to no more than a group of professionals sitting around a table and passing opinions.'

In conclusion, the notion of an iterative method for evaluation purposes is worth commenting upon in a little detail here. As has been suggested, evaluation of new services or interventions is often sought from within the health service. In many cases, any health intervention can be considered complicated, often elusive, certainly active. The evaluation methods deployed by the researcher must be equally subtle and sophisticated, rigorous yet dynamic to the context of study.

CONCLUSION

Having discussed four very different types of research method for present purposes, it is necessary to consider and summarise the relationship between the various methods, and suggest how the presented schema has value in selecting methodological approaches. This conclusion will, therefore, attempt to review the scope and development of the whole plan and to examine practical separations, and possible sequences, between its component parts.

The framework for research methods: questions of value

The overall schema, as presented in Figure 18.1 – and the whole chapter – consists of coordinates, which may be understood as resembling the compass directions on a map or sighting alignments in an optical instrument, such as a telescope. They are not absolute dimensions, nor even tabular parameters which set finite bounds to the internal cells. Rather, they have value in conferring relational meaning upon the field of observation. The substantive evidence offered, consisting of types of methodological approaches, cannot, in principle, 'fill the boxes' or claim to be the only examples possible. Different types of methods are placed along the coordinates in order to illustrate their relative positions and value – and to facilitate the assessment of their research purposes.

To outline and indicate the vast field of methodological possibilities does not imply, of course, that it is possible or desirable to cover the wide range of research approaches. On the contrary, a choice between methods is proposed, if only on grounds of practical limitations of resources and the need for specific clarity in defining research objectives.

How can the researcher decide between the directional alternatives so far discussed? We begin with an evaluative judgement which operates up and down the informational/instrumental axis by comparing the different levels of analysis – between the descriptive and deep levels of information processing – according to scientific standards.

A scientific hierarchy: in depth of analysis?

One very straightforward argument from the natural sciences is that the deeper, more exact and provable knowledge afforded by scientific methods, such as experimentation, is more lawful, correct and exemplary. In contrast, alternative research methods, which are not so procedurally systematic and precise in their measurement and inference – and which allow considerable subjectivity of judgement – are said to be less valuable; and, accordingly, should not be treated so seriously as truly ideal scientific methods. High astronomical knowledge, of universal certainty, is sharply contrasted in value from personal accounts, merely based on individual observations and casual reportings, which are contrasted as being limited in providing evidence and their general interest. (These different positions in credence in fact occupy poles so extremely counter-opposed that they are both 'off the map' in respect of practical (and routine) research methods.)

Table 18.3 illustrates one suggested current hierarchy of knowledge sources in use for policy development.

The high claim of science to possess the grandest, surest methodologies is epistemological (in respect of the nature of knowledge) rather than technological (being concerned with the skills and methods of applying knowledge). Yet the polarisation of philosophical positions, and the forced choice between them, seems unnecessary, since the two priorities seem to have very different, independent, values.

In research practice, there are many reasons for preferring the advanced information technology of a CD-ROM to search the literature. These include: proper preparation for research; the availability of practical resources; and speed/effectiveness of access. As an initial attack on the problem for enquiry, to find out what

Table 18.3 Hierarchy of research evidence (developed from SIGN 1995)

Level of attributed importance	Type of research
A1	Meta-analysis of randomised, controlled trials
A2	Analysis of evidence obtained from controlled studies without randomisation
B1	Analysis of evidence from quasi-experimental studies
C1	Analysis of evidence from non-experimental descriptive studies
D1	Analysis obtained from evidence produced by expert committees and/or the experience of respected clinical authorities

aspects have been dealt with – and what has been discovered already – it is the wisest introductory step. There may be no need to conduct further research, once extant answers become known. Even if the ongoing project is clearly interested in collecting and analysing fresh data, knowledge about the relevant literature – especially as published in the research journals – is an important, if not indispensable, part of the preliminary procedure of defining the problem and deciding what is the most suitable research design.

Other practical reasons for pursuing information technology (IT) reviews of previous research turn upon resources. A CD-ROM search can be conducted by one individual student and completed in hours. Elaborate experimental investigations, by contrast, involve expensive and long-term support: skilled staff and costly equipment, long deliberation and preparation, and a high-risk 'bid' that specific hypotheses will be fruitful. In a cost-effective evaluation, it is increasingly difficult to justify and support the ponderous process of experimentation, if the pragmatically better method is compared.

Finally, computer technology is now widely available and informational enquiries are no longer the preserve of a few experts. Whether an investigation will go 'deep' eventually is not always known at the initial stages. However, more people can currently start to investigate their problems of understanding than was previously possible. As research is being democratised, the range of concerns open to systematic investigation has increased. Obtaining quality information, often of a relatively descriptive kind, for the public, is of value in terms of growing knowledge and extending rationality of life.

Other, social, reasons for opposing hierarchical claims of the physical sciences must be mentioned. For social and health research operate with a distinct subject-matter, and, accordingly, adopt methods of understanding human action which are not of a sub-scientific standard but involve the pursuit of qualitatively different materials and aims.

The high-priestly 'pure' procedures of science highlighted earlier, may be appreciated, in context, without any implication that they should be mandatory or that alternatives methods are inferior. Admitting absolute status to natural scientific methodology over other forms of knowledge seems excessive. Allowing a single set of hypostacised principles to be granted the exclusive right to determine all standards of enquiry (as the philosopher Popper proposes) would distort our overall perspective on knowledge and may also operate to damage the distinctive prospects and contributions of other disciplines and discredit their different approaches to research.

Is the 'deep' experimental method always to be preferred in research to a descriptive search of the extant literature by using, for example, a CD-ROM? In some ways only.

Of course, fresh research is more vanguard in adding to knowledge than summary descriptions of extant information. Furthermore, the natural scientific ideals have universal impressiveness, but they are not, therefore, so exemplary for others that all other 'non-scientific' methods should be judged in imitative terms and held to be inferior.

On the contrary, this hierarchical idea of knowledge may be irrelevant for, and even impede, other modes of advancing knowledge. The scientific model for progress carries with it a set of assumptions which are often inappropriate for the social and health sciences and which will burden their researchers with inappropriate methodological requirements unless those available are critically examined before being selected.

Since the social and health sciences have come of age, therefore, the research methods respected and used have been extended from those conventionally used in the natural sciences towards fresh methods, such as interviewing and surveys, observation (participant and clinical), and types of action research which have been described.

In Figure 18.1 and chapter coverage, therefore, our purview of the range of methods to be advocated has been extended systematically, from the left-hand side of the figure, which refers to informational and instrumental analyses, towards broadly socially valorised research. This wider scope for methodology refers to studies which are based on the social (action) meaning of subjects and also to approaches which incorporate social end-values, professional care standards and modes of assessment, and to health outcome purposes.

In the overall research schema, there are two dimensions or directions of presentation. The vertical (or 'down') coordinate, designates depth of methodological processing, whereas the horizontal (or 'across') axis distinguishes degrees of sociality, including research that is purely informational in character (and typically instrumental in derivation) or else socially oriented.

The two coordinates, when brought together, yield a set of four quadrants as shown in Table 18.4.

If we consider the layout, in order to assess which sequences in the research process may lie between the quadrants, across positions in the overall methodological schema, then the workable direction for practical development is mainly downwards – from the surface, descriptive levels, down – and deeper – towards the more analytical and highly processed levels. This pattern, or suggested sequence, holds for both the 'Value aims' columns in Table 18.4.

Development from 1 to 2 is desirable if 2 is the objective – but is not necessary otherwise. Development from 3 to 4 is quite possible, and usual, for a great deal of staff and service knowledge is needed as preparation for professional/managerial research materials. Once again, there is no necessity for research to progress across the rows, unless the further goals are sought and there is a wish to link the two-step deepening sequence.

Though moving downwards is possible, to move upwards is extremely undesirable, if not impossible. Experimenters should not defer researching the literature until after their results are known. Infirmity of design purpose beforehand and a risk of spurious confirmations or special rationalisations afterwards make this reverse sequence unwise. In terms of the depth of information-processing and inference, therefore, the direction of analysis is downwards – towards greater depth.

With regard to the horizontal coordinate, between purely informational study and engaged, socially involved and committed work, the ontological gap is greater. It is possible to move from 1 to 3, from descriptive review of the literature towards the collection of further, fresh evidence. However, movement between 2 and 3 or 2 and 4 is virtually pre-empted by experimental conceptions of method, detachment and objectivity, which have been critically assessed and relativised.

The suggested reorientation for the research field is towards the social end of the horizontal axis. The investigation of surgical health outcomes clearly involves a value commitment and a sphere of professional knowledge and informed practice. It is towards this goal of advancing research as a means of improving analysis, practice and policy in combination that the next chapter will turn.

Table 18.4   Methodological schema

Levels of analysis	Value aims	
	Informational and instrumental	Social orientation
Descriptive data	1. Informational and descriptive	3. Social evidence and data collection
Deeper processing in analysis	2. Analytical and inferential	4. Socially valued professional scrutiny and policy guides

REFERENCES

Appleby J, Walshe K, Ham C 1995 Acting on the evidence. National Association of Health Authorities and Trusts Research paper No. 17. NAHAT, London

Becker H S 1955 Problems of inference and proof in participant observation. American Sociological Review 23: 652–660

Bond S 1996 Evaluation research. In: Cormack D F S (ed) The research process in nursing. Blackwell Science, Oxford, ch 18, pp 190–200

Bruyn S T 1966 The human perspective in sociology. Prentice Hall, Englewood Cliffs, NJ

Campbell D T 1957 Factors relevant to the validity of experiments in social settings. Psychological Bulletin 54(4): 297–312

Cormack D F S (ed) 1996 The research process in nursing. Blackwell Science, Oxford, ch 18, pp 190–200

Ellen R F 1984 Ethnographic research: a guide to general conduct. Academic Press, New York

Field J M, Morse J (eds) 1992 Qualitative health research. Sage, California

Gabe J, Calnan M, Bury M 1992 (eds) The sociology of the health service. Routledge, London

Giddens A 1976 New rules of sociological method: a positive critique of interpretative sociologies. Hutchinson University Library, London

Gilbert N (ed) 1993 Researching social life. Sage, London

Greenwood E 1945 Experimental sociology, a study in method. Kings Crown Press, New York, p 28

Griffiths R 1983 NHS management enquiry report. Department of Health and Social Security, London

Hayward J 1975 Information – a prescription against pain. RCN Nursing Series No. 5. RCN, London

Lawler J 1991 Behind the screens: nursing somology and the problem of the body. Churchill Livingstone, Melbourne

Lofland J, Lofland L H 1984 Analysing social settings. Wadsworth, Belmont, Ca

Moser C, Kalton J 1971 Survey methods in social investigation, 2nd edn. Heinemann, London

Nachmias D, Nachmias C F 1992 Research methods in the social sciences, 4th edn. Arnold, New York

Nolan M, Grant G 1993 Service evaluation: time to open both eyes. Journal of Advanced Nursing 18: 1434–1442

Popper K 1972 Objective knowledge: conjectures and refutations. Oxford University Press, Oxford

Robson C 1993 Real world research: a resource for social scientists and practitioner researchers. Blackwell, Oxford

Rogers E M 1983 Diffusion of innovations, 3rd edn. Free Press, New York

Rose G 1982 Deciphering sociological research. Macmillan, London

Rosenthal R 1976 Experimental effect in behavioral research. Irvinfor, New York

Scottish Intercollegiate Guideline Network (SIGN) 1995 Criteria for critical appraisal of national guidelines. Scottish Intercollegiate Guideline Network, Edinburgh

Smaje C 1995 Health, 'race' and ethnicity: making sense of the evidence. King's Fund Institute, London

Sokolovsky J (ed) 1990 The cultural context of aging. Bergin & Garvey, New York

Stocking B 1992 Promoting change in clinical care. Quality in Health Care 1: 56–60

Wengler G C, Leger St F 1992 Community structure and support network variations. Ageing and Society 122: 213–236

West B J M 1992 Nursing perceptions of patients in the nursing process: a study of two cardiothoracic units. PhD Thesis, University of Edinburgh

West B J M 1993 Caring: the essence of theatre nursing. British Journal of Theatre Nursing 3(8): 13–18

West B J M, Lyon M H 1995 Surgical nurse: principles of audit and clinical practice. British Journal of Nursing 4(17): 987–991

Wright S G 1989 Changing nursing practice. Edward Arnold, London

19

Health outcomes and surgical nursing practice

Michael Lyon   Bernice West

AIMS

This chapter aims to:

- introduce the surgical nurse to the key issues of audit, clinical guidelines, health economics and evidence-based practice
- encourage an integrated multiprofessional approach to the identification of health outcomes in surgical settings
- identify a system of care planning which articulates health outcomes
- promote professional nursing development.

INTRODUCTION

In recent years there have been developments within the health service which require that nurses critically audit and evaluate the nature of their working discipline. They have required the setting of current clinical standards. These standards have previously focused on issues which combined structural aspects of care with the nursing processes in order to achieve specific work outcomes. This resulted in a highly personalised care process which obscured specific health outcomes by enabling nursing outcomes to be articulated. It is contended here that nursing practice should take cognisance of wider health outcomes outside of previously circumscribed concerns in order to influence future health care policy.

This chapter builds upon the ideas which were presented in the previous one. The aim now is to address the issues of designating and documenting health outcomes which should be attained for surgical patients. The operational framework for nurses to be proposed will be called one of integrated optimal-care planning.

This approach to nursing is ideal, yet pragmatic, calling for both personal commitment and interprofessional coordination. In knowledge terms it requires a sound information base and extensive problem-solving skills. To illustrate the processes involved in producing such integrated optimal-care plans with identified health outcomes, it is necessary to address both the diagnostic aspects and the interventionist nature of planned nursing care in an acute surgical setting. Consequently, considerable attention will be given to these topics in the chapter and also to the complementary value of using research methodologies to enhance nursing practice.

To enable readers to chart the development of these ideas and to appreciate the relevance of several interrelated issues, the chapter is organised in three main sections.

The first section examines the political and strategic organisation of clinical guidelines, clinical audit and health outcomes within the contemporary health service in the UK. Next, some basic ideas underpinning evidence-based practice, nursing diagnoses, interventions and health outcomes are discussed, and examples of integrated optimal-care plans for particular surgical patients are provided. Finally, the last section concludes with an analysis of the processes required for the full development of evidence-based practice and health outcomes in nursing

CLINICAL GUIDELINES AUDIT AND HEALTH OUTCOMES

In 1986 Saltman stated that in the present financial climate there is a danger in a number of countries that political forces may seek directly to define the permissible boundaries of patient care. In the decade since this statement, and in the 1990s in particular, there has been considerable political influence on the current health service in the UK. Much of this has affected the quality of patient care (DoH 1995b, Williamson 1992); the range and type of health service provision available to the public (DoH 1989a, b); the role of health care professionals (DoH 1995a); and the structure and organisation of the former national health service (DoH 1989b). The resultant outcomes of such political influence are open to interpretation depending on how the sources of information are dealt with in the first instance and secondly how they are analysed by the interpreter. Suffice it to say, at this juncture, that a critical appraisal of the available information is essential in order to determine the utility and benefit of such to a national health service.

In recent years a new language of health care has emerged. Phrases such as clinical guidelines, clinical audit, standards, health outcomes have become conventionally honoured, even axiomatic. It is necessary to give some attention to these concepts in order that present understandings are explained reflectively and are not taken for granted.

Clinical guidelines

Clinical guidelines have been defined as systematically developed statements which assist practitioners and patients in appropriate decision-making (Clinical Resource and Action Groups of the Scottish Office DoH 1993, Duff et al 1995, Institute of Medicine 1992, SIGN 1995a).

The term 'guideline', however, has ambiguous connotations. On the one hand it may be associated with providing order in a chaotic system; on the other it has undertones of limiting freedom. In the health care setting these ambiguous connotations are of concern to health professionals in particular. Clinical guidelines have been perceived as providing a means of 'reducing uncertainty in medical practice – to assure the effectiveness, efficiency and patient-orientation of care delivery [and also as] an attempt to reduce professional and management autonomy and create mechanisms for accountability.' (Klazinga 1995, p. 11). With such ambiguous connotations it is apparent that there will be professional and ethical concerns about the deployment of clinical guidelines in the health service. In Sweden where clinical guidelines have been developed and put into practice by both the nursing and medical professions for over a decade, their value and role in developing clinical care is controversial. Different perspectives vary as to their stringency, flexibility and applicability in clinical practice, yet very few evaluative studies have been conducted (Kendell 1995).

Good clinical patient care is of paramount concern to all health professionals. The expert nurse or doctor appreciates that there is a variety of treatment options available and most will have a preferred method. Clinical practice becomes a critical concern to professional groups if these preferred methods become ritualistic, based on hearsay, ineffective over long periods of time, or are allowed to be detrimental to the well-being of patients. Clinical practice becomes additionally questionable to managerial forces when it is too costly, too slow and publicly decried. A new clinical guideline ideology has been given a central role in the campaign to achieve greater clinical effectiveness and cost-effectiveness in the health service. For these reasons it is necessary to reflect upon the methodology which has been advocated for the construction of national clinical guidelines.

'The purpose of clinical guidelines is to improve the effectiveness and the efficiency of clinical care through the identification of good clinical practice and desired clinical outcomes' (SIGN 1995a, p. 1). Working with this definition, an iterative, reflexive methodology for the development of a clinical guideline has been advocated by the Department of Health in Scotland and by the various medical Royal Colleges. Other health professionals have been more critical of the methodological requirements which have been stipulated. Some of these criticisms have been dealt with in the previous chapter. What follows now is an examination of the origins and aims of guideline administration.

In the constitution and administration of a clinical guideline there are many potential areas of bias which require addressing. The considerations and criteria which require attention include the following:

- Who has been involved in the production of the guideline?
- What evidence has been appraised to enable the construction of the guideline?
- How have the recommended actions come about?
- How will the effectiveness of the guideline be evaluated?
- Is the guideline governed by clinical or cost-effectiveness?

To address each of these questions, the methodology advocated by SIGN (1995a) will be used and developed (see Ch. 18).

The guideline development group membership

It is important that a range of health disciplines are represented in the group. These individuals should have administrative and clinical knowledge of the care proposed. In addition it is also suggested that, where possible, patient representatives should be involved. In the past, guideline development has been uniprofessional, primarily focusing on the medical, nursing or pharmacological management of a particular condition 'rather than the overall care of the patient with the condition under scrutiny' as Kitson advocates (1995, p. 86). Integrating specialist knowledge across disciplines requires considerable effort and the appointment of a skilled facilitator. Furthermore, as expert objectivity is required, it is necessary for personal and non-personal interests to be declared lest they may unknowingly influence the resultant guideline. For example, a member having a consultancy role with a major drug/product manufacturer or a unit or department supported by pertinent commercial interests should declare their interests.

The Royal College of Nursing (Duff et al 1995) carefully consider methods of incorporating patients and service users into the group. The RCN stresses that it is important to avoid tokenism and to ensure that a network of patient representatives is established. Bodies such as local health councils and The Patients' Association can be of value in establishing networks.

Critical appraisal of evidence

Systematic literature reviews are required in order to ensure that recent and most relevant research-based knowledge is incorporated into the guideline. The search strategies used on the CD-ROMs and the sampling techniques deployed in analysing the literature should be provided (see Ch. 18). Ideally a formal meta-analysis should be conducted in order to synthesise the results obtained across the sample of literature (Goodman 1993).

SIGN (1995a) building upon earlier work conducted in 1992 by the US Agency for Health Care Policy and Research (Hudgings 1995), has identified a hierarchy of knowledge from which evidence can be analysed. In accordance with the dominant research paradigm of the medical sciences, evidence gathered by means of experimentation, and in particular randomised controlled trials, is given pre-eminence. Quasi-experimental studies are considered of high value followed by non-experimental descriptive studies. The hierarchy has been summarised in the conclusion of the previous chapter.

Such a hierarchy is of value where there is a wealth of clinical trial research data and, as such, the development of a clinical guideline is relatively straightforward in that it usually focuses on pharmaceutical treatment regimes and clear-cut medical management techniques. The nursing aspects of the patient care are unlikely to have been studied by these top rating controlled methodologies, and consequently there has been a tendency in some guidelines to disregard the valuable nursing aspects of patient care. Rather it has been assumed that the nursing input is the administration of medical orders.

Reflective point

Identify any difficulties you can foresee with regard to the involvement of nurses in the development of clinical guidelines.

Recommended actions

In general, guidelines contain courses of recommended actions which have been derived from analyses of different sources of evidence. The processes involved in articulating the finished guideline must both be consensual to the group and reliable in terms of the information sources used in its construction. Furthermore, the guideline should take care to distinguish professional issues from administrative ones and clinical outcomes from managerial ones. Furthermore, within the guideline, information must be provided to allow for professional flexibility in order to cater for complicated or idiosyncratic clinical cases.

A full account of the methodology used in the guideline production is required in order that it can be scrutinised. It is suggested that critical reading of the guideline is carried out on a wide scale and the following questions borne in mind when reviewing it:

- Are the methods used to assess the strength of scientific evidence provided?
- Are there links between the evidence and recommended actions?
- Have the recommended actions been appraised by people not on the development group?

Effectiveness of the guideline

The evaluation of the clinical guideline is a two-stage process. The first stage involves the systematic review of the guideline per se and the second stage requires clinical audit to be conducted over a period of time.

For immediate evaluation of the actual guideline, an assessment covering the following issues may be used:

- clinical applicability
- clinical flexibility
- clinical benefits
- health outcomes
- patient accessibility
- clarity of expressed actions
- dissemination strategies
- implementation strategies
- audit techniques
- resource implications.

By contrast, the longer-term evaluation of the guideline requires the instigation of audit techniques which address key clinical outcomes, standards of care to be achieved, and patient health outcomes.

In 1995 a national clinical guideline on prophylactic interventions to prevent venous thromboembolism

was published (SIGN 1995b). This guideline has particular relevance for surgical nurses. A modified version of the quick reference guide to this clinical guideline is presented in Box 19.1 and Table 19.1.

Clinical effectiveness

This aspect of the guideline is most significant as the optimisation of health is the ultimate standard for the majority of health professionals. Most importantly, the guideline should provide an adequate account of the health benefits expected by such a course of clinical actions. The potential risks or harm that may result from the recommended clinical actions should also be specified.

The costs and expenditure associated with the clinical actions and the responsibilities of managers and financiers are also required to be specified. Government departments have argued that the availability of financial resources for the development of the health service is limited. In the UK there is a wish to build up primary care and contain hospital costs. Because of this marketisation of health care, any clinical guideline has the potential to restrict access to health care for certain populations, and increase selective inequalities in health care uptake. For these

---

Box 19.1   Modified clinical guideline

Standard statement.   All hospital patients who have reduced mobility due to surgery merit consideration for specific antithrombotic prophylaxis using mechanical methods and/or antithrombotic drugs.

Types of trauma and surgery
Acute trauma
- Hip fracture
- Lower limb fracture
- Spinal cord injury
- Other major trauma

Major surgery
- Hip or knee replacement
- General surgery especially for cancer
- Gynaecological surgery especially for cancer
- Urological surgery
- Cardiothoracic/vascular surgery
- Neurosurgery

Other contributing factors
- Patient's age
- Immobility
- Previous deep vein thrombosis or pulmonary embolism
- Known thrombophilia

Table 19.1 Graded recommendations for prophylactic treatments (adapted from SIGN 1995b)

Condition	Treatment				
	Low-dose heparin	Low-molecular-weight heparin	Warfarin	Dextran 70	IPC/GECS
Hip fracture or lower limb fracture	—	A	A	A	—
Spinal cord injury	B (adjusted dose)	C	—	—	C
Other major trauma	C	C	C	—	C
Intracranial neurosurgery	—	—	—	—	A
Hip replacement	A (adjusted dose)	A	A	A	A
Knee replacement	—	A	A	—	A
Other major surgery	A	A	A	A	A

Important: combinations of heparin, low molecular weight heparin, warfarin and dextran should not be prescribed.
Key: A – recommendation based on meta-analysis of randomised controlled trials; B – recommendation based on evidence from controlled studies; quasi-experimental designs and non-experimental descriptive studies; C – recommendation based on evidence obtained from clinical experts/authorities or committee reports or opinions; IPC = intermittent pneumatic compression; GECS = graduated elastic compression stockings
Note: This guideline was published in a pilot edition in 1995 and was under review in 1999.

reasons any evaluation of the guideline must include population health outcomes and parity of patient and treatment access.

Clinical audit

The definition of audit most often quoted is that of the Department of Health (1989b), namely 'Clinical audit is the systematic critical analysis of clinical care including the procedures used for diagnosis and treatment, the use of resources and the resultant outcome and quality of life for the client'. This definition enables the audit process to evaluate clinical guidelines at political, strategic and operational levels.

To explain this further, it is necessary to consider the three levels of audit which are relevant in contemporary health care settings. Table 19.2 illustrates the analytical schema.

In order to conduct an audit, it is essential that standards have been set and outcomes have been specified. Most surgical care teams need a system for planning, implementing and evaluating their own clinical management programmes in order to ensure the effectiveness of treatment and the delivery of good care for every patient.

A *performance standard* defines the quality of care and the criteria for evaluating the effectiveness of care. Ideal performance standards identify the responsibilities of the practitioner and define the nature of clinical management and the resultant patient benefits. In many respects a clinical guideline adapted to a local situation can be considered as a series of performance standards. It has been suggested that the performance standards that most accurately reflect the complexities of surgical practice focuses on the content of the performance and the health outcomes expected for the

Table 19.2 Audit schema

Type of audit	Auditor	Audit examples
Public sector	Government bodies Audit Commission	Health of the Nation targets Patient's Charter targets
External contractual	Purchasers/Stakeholders	Contractual arrangements Waiting times Patient throughput Bed occupancy Readmission rates
Internal clinical	Health professionals	Incidence of pressure sores Prevalence of hospital-acquired infections
	Service managers	Uptake of screening services Attendance rates Patient satisfaction

patient (Lyon & West 1995, West 1988). By identifying the nursing actions and the resultant effects of these on the patient's well-being, a system of professional audit can be established which utilises health outcomes.

Outcome performance standards define the resultant changes in the patient's health status following care interventions. Both positive and negative outcomes can result from care. When the care or action undertaken is appropriate to the patient's needs, the outcomes are positive, and negative outcomes are prevented. When writing down the select standards for audit purposes it is suggested that the absence of negative outcomes as well as the presence of positive outcomes should be stated. Likewise, the same principle holds in the construction of a clinical guideline.

The process of auditing generally requires a systematic approach to information-gathering and then converts this information into data by means of analyses. The knowledge and skills gained from an understanding of research methodology are essential for these processes.

Reflective point

What knowledge from research methodology is of value to the surgical nurse who is planning to conduct a clinical audit?

Much has been written about methodologies that may be used in audit (Balogh 1992, Redfern & Norman 1990). The majority of the most appropriate methodologies are not truly scientific but applied evaluations. In fact the use of such methods questions the value of audit to the development of clinical guidelines. There is a risk of health professionals finding themselves in self-fulfilling procedures by adopting a clinical guideline, evaluating its effectiveness by means of audit, and then developing the guideline on the basis of the evaluation. For clinicians who are eclectic in their approach to methodology, this is unproblematic. For those who rigidly uphold the scientific policy of audit, however, there is a double bind which has to be addressed.

To evaluate a clinical guideline such as the example given previously (prophylactic treatment for the prevention of venous thromboembolism) requires a range of methodologies to be adopted. The hierarchy of scientific method suggests that the most reliable evidence comes from randomised controlled trials. To conduct such a trial to ascertain the effectiveness of a clinical guideline poses several ethical dilemmas. In the guideline example given, it is recommended that all treatment options could be used for patients who have undergone a hip replacement. If the researcher-clinician is strongly in favour of the positivist approach to research, then to evaluate this guideline she or he will be obliged to conduct a controlled study (namely following the guideline with a sample of patients and not following it with another group). Ethically this approach would provoke the question 'is the clinician-researcher actually doing harm to patients under the guise of research?' (see Ch. 4).

Reflective point

Consider this argument and what it means for health professionals who wish to do good and do no harm to patients.

Health outcomes

For many years, gross ill-health indices have been used to provide a demographic picture of the prevalence and incidence of diseases, mortality rates and morbidity rates across populations. Much of this information has been gathered to provide epidemiological data for public health use. The overriding approach to the analysis of this information in the past has been to compare data over time. A single measurement of anything has no meaning unless there is something against which to compare the measurement. This statement suggests that inferences cannot be drawn on changes in performance outcomes unless comparisons can be made. In clinical practice, personal comparisons are being drawn regularly and inferences made. This may be two readings of vital signs or two self-report statements about pain. The methodological point being made here is that it is essential to identify the baseline measurement and the outcome measurement. As with any measurement, there are principles and practices which must be taken seriously in order to ensure the accuracy and value of the data obtained (see Ch. 18).

Selecting an appropriate outcome indicator is essential if the process of audit or evaluation is to be meaningful in clinical terms. To date, the health outcomes which have been identified and used to compare the effectiveness of NHS trusts across the UK are not refined or 'at-risk' measures, but gross indicators drawn from a range well within the normal expectations of a health service.

Recent growing trends in the use of outcome indicators in the health service raise concerns for health professionals. The outcomes are crude and general and it could be argued not always the most applicable for the intervention under scrutiny. Traditional measures of mortality and morbidity are still of importance but increasingly there has been an introduction of other measures such as readmission rates and waiting times.

Table 19.3 illustrates a range of current clinical outcome indicators used by the health service.

From Table 19.3, current health policy, government targets and outcome indicators may be examined and applied. The lack of clinical sensitivity in these outcomes questions the health benefits of carrying out such measures and auditing activity in this way. The measures take no account of the processes involved or the dynamics of the care situation. For health outcomes to be meaningful and useful in clinical practice research sensitivity is necessary.

In addition to these indicators, a range of other health-assessment devices and economic health indices have been discussed in the literature, and in many cases adopted by purchasers and providers of health services to inform contractual arrangements. For example, in order to target hospital admissions, health profiles of 'at-risk' populations have been carried out. The most notable group is the over-75-year-olds in the general population. Screening targets have been set for this group and risk assessments conducted. Some examples of health profiles in wide use are the General Health Questionnaire and the Nottingham Profile (Newell & McDowell 1987). *Health*

profiles tend to be multifaceted and designed to examine physical, psychological and social well-being.

In conjunction with health outcomes, the economic utility of interventions has become part of the evaluation process. Health economists suggest that there is 'an ethical imperative to evaluate the economic implications (costs) of achieving changes in health status (benefits or effects)' (Appleby et al 1995, p. 7). The logic behind this assertion is based on the assumption that health care resources are scarce and that the health service should be choosing treatments 'which minimise costs and maximise benefits ... The costs of not doing this will be the lost opportunity to treat more people or more generally to increase healthiness overall' (Appleby et al 1995). This assumption has metricised health care to such an extent that the narrow cost-effectiveness calculus of economics is inadequate as a guide to anyone concerned with sustaining and enabling the optimum health and well-being of people.

Different economic analyses have been developed and, in order to critically appraise these, Table 19.4 outlines the main analyses used in evaluating health outcomes.

The cost per quality adjusted life year (QALY) ratio is a relatively recent innovation which is designed to differentiate the utility of a year of perfect well-being from a year of pain, disability or disease. This index has been devised to assess the value of treatment for types of patients against a range of demographic and clinical indicators. The index has been widely criticised (Moatti et al 1995). The authors argue that

Table 19.3 Examples of health outcomes

Outcome indicator	Definition
Teenage conception	Reduction in the rate of conception amongst young girls aged 13–15 years
Therapeutic abortion	Ratio of abortion to live births; abortions per 1000 women aged 15–44; proportion of abortions performed at less than 10 weeks' gestation
Cervical cancer mortality	Death rate per 100 000 of the female population
Suicide	Deaths recorded as self-inflicted injury whether accidentally or purposefully
Inpatient stays for children with asthma	Number of inpatient episodes of 4 days or more among children under 16 years
Survival after admission for fractured neck of femur	Survival for 30 days after admission with a principal diagnosis of fractured neck of femur
Discharge home after emergency admission with fractured neck of femur	Patients discharged home (i.e. usual address) within 56 days of admission
Reoperation after transurethral prostatectomy	All patients aged 55–84 who require a further prostatectomy 1 year after the initial surgery
Emergency readmission after discharge from a medical specialty	Emergency admission as an inpatient within 28 days of discharge
Survival after admission following a stroke	Patients surviving beyond 30 days from an emergency admission with a stroke
Discharge home after admission for a stroke	All patients discharged home (usual address) within 56 days of admission
Deaths within 1 year of discharge from psychiatric inpatient care	All deaths including suicides

Table 19.4 Health economic outcome analyses

Economic analyses	Definitions
Cost–benefit (CBOA)	This compares an intervention's costs and benefits using monetary measures. When the financial benefits are greater than the costs, then the economic evaluation suggests that the treatment is worth doing. This is a complex analysis to carry out, as it involves assessing the direct costs to the health service, the costs to the patient and society and attributing overall benefits in monetary terms
Cost-effectiveness (CEOA)	This is the cost of achieving a given unit of effect by using different interventions. Known units of measurement are used to determine effect. For example: temperature range; blood pressure levels; incidence of disease; number of days in hospital
Cost-minimisation (CMOA)	The results of two or more interventions are shown or assumed to be identical and the analysis is restricted to a simple comparison of costs. For example, the use of two hydrocolloid wound dressings identical except for cost
Cost–utility (CUOA)	This has been designed to analyse situations where there is more than one effect from the intervention. Each effect is evaluated relative to the others. The most common unit of comparison is the quality adjusted life year (QALY)

QALYs are not a straightforward application of economic utility theory as the individual's preferences are important in any health assessment. They conclude that the cost per QALY approach should be abandoned in order to avoid ambiguities that could impede the development of health economics in the medical field. There are potential biases in the use of the QALY ratio in that only high-cost curative interventions will be assessed in this manner. This ultimately leads to questions of concern in health prioritisation and in the allocation of resources.

What is suggested here is that in addressing the cost–utility argument, practitioners explore the ethics of independence in terms of length of life and quality of life, examine the constant trade-offs that take place between quality and length of life and investigate the utility attributed to each coveted health state. By applying ethical principles in discourse with the patient, the optimum treatment regimen may be reached.

To conclude this section, it has been suggested that there is a risk in constructing health outcomes that are so general and gross that their clinical application is of limited value.

Reflective point

If the cost–utility thesis were to be fully applied in your area of work, which surgical procedures would be affected?

The practice of nursing involves the planning of effective health outcomes in conjunction with the patient and other health professionals. This process involves the deployment of a systematic methodology. The next section of the chapter addresses the component parts of a methodology for evidence-based practice.

EVIDENCE-BASED PRACTICE IN SURGICAL NURSING

There has been a concern in the nursing literature for over 15 years that nursing practice should be evidence-based. Authors such as Walsh & Ford (1989) have discussed the rituals of nursing practice and questioned many of the previously held assumptions about what constitutes good nursing care. It is of parallel interest that the medical profession are raising a debate about the authority-base of clinical practice and patient management (Sackett & Haynes 1995, Sackett & Rosenberg 1995 plus a series of correspondence in the *BMJ*, July 1995 et seq.).

The current debate being addressed by health professionals is about what constitutes evidence. The traditional question of how to apply research findings to clinical practice has long been recognised. Unfortunately the discussion has focused on the mechanics of dissemination of research findings (Cormack 1991, Polit & Hungler 1993) rather than on the applicability of the research to clinical practice. The extrapolation of research results into action for individual patients is not always possible. This may be for several reasons: the research was not designed in the first instance to be applied; the methodology used in the research was restricted in its techniques and no planned outcome was reached; the conditions of research investigation cannot be guaranteed in normal clinical contexts. Therefore, when we consider evidence-based practice the policy actions require more than research-based evidence. All sources of knowledge become important: experience, analysis of practice, intuition, literature and research findings.

Evidence-based practice involves moving away from decision-making based on opinion, past practice and precedence solely towards the inclusion of research and artistic evidence. It is an iterative process involving the assessment of fresh information, and the evaluation of clinical action may be at successive stages. In the psychology of decision-making this requires that the practitioner begins to optimise the decision-making process. There is evidence to suggest that traditional 'minimal' nurses only obtained sufficient information to tackle the immediate clinical issue with which they were confronted (West 1992). This process of decision-making can be termed *satisficing* (West 1992) – as sufficient unto itself – but not optimal. The alternative approach to decision-making is *optimising*. This superior process occurs where the practitioner has gathered optimal information and evidence from a variety of sources to improve all decision-making processes. Crucial to this mode is the practitioner's ability to:

- display a sophisticated use of clinical skills such as diagnosis, assessment and evaluation
- deploy a wide range of knowledge bases
- interact effectively with other professionals and patients
- analyse and evaluate practice.

Many of these optimising abilities are being incorporated into current education at pre-registration and post-registration levels (UKCC 1995). The development of specialist and advanced practitioner education and employment opportunities taps into this emphasis on evidence-based practice.

The current concern in nurse education to develop reflective practitioners who can analyse their nursing practice is a welcomed change. In the analysis of practice each stage of the caring process is deconstructed in order to be understood.

Traditional methods of nursing have not enhanced this process in the past. Recent developments which involve personalised care planning and the identification of health outcomes enable the nurse to more easily reflect upon nursing practice and the resultant clinical effectiveness.

Nursing diagnosis

We have suggested that what is required is that nurses carry out evidence-based practice. The first key point raised was that the nurse must be able to display a sophisticated use of knowledge and clinical skills. It is suggested here that the starting point for this is the nursing assessment and diagnostic process. This section will present a means of patient health assessment and identify the meaning of nursing diagnoses. It will also show how health outcomes can be reached by carrying out these procedures.

The term nursing diagnosis has many different meanings (Long et al 1995). These include:

- the identification of a physical health problem by task and authority
- the conclusion reached from a cluster of signs and symptoms
- the act of identifying and listing responses to actual or potential health problems or stressors.

For the present analysis it is suggested that the final definition is most useful in the surgical setting as it allows for an optimising approach to clinical decision-making. Nursing diagnoses provide the basis for selecting nursing interventions in order to achieve the health outcomes for which the nurse is accountable. Nursing diagnoses complement and enhance the care programmes identified by other health professionals.

In order to make an informed nursing diagnosis, it is necessary to systematically collect information from the patient. This process of taking a patient history is very different from a medical history. Nursing is primarily concerned with the human response to actual or potential health problems, whereas medicine is concerned with the identification and aetiology of a health problem. While taking a nursing history, information is elicited about individual responses to actual or potential health problems. This information, coupled with that of other professionals, provides the foundation for the nursing diagnoses and planned interventions.

Throughout this process the nurse will carry out the following:

- review the reliability and validity of the information obtained
- reflect on the information with regard to previous knowledge
- plan effective health outcomes based on good practice and patient involvement
- decide on optimum nursing interventions to enable the health outcomes to happen.

In this process, the nurse collects subjective data from the patient covering the four key domains of health (West 1992) (which are dealt with in detail below):

- somatological health: care of the body and functional activities
- social health: relational well-being and involvement of others
- psychological health: emotional well-being and coping strategies
- health maintenance activities: actions regularly carried out by the individual and health professionals to optimise health and manage illnesses.

In addition, objective data are gathered by the use of a systems approach to the human body. Each of the major bodily systems is examined and measurements are taken as appropriate. By combining such approaches, immediate, short-, medium- and long-term health outcomes can be identified in accordance with planned nursing interventions and the priorities of the patient.

The idea of patient priority is an important one. There may be a lack of congruence between the priorities of the patient and the those of the health professionals. For example, the nurse may have a priority in obtaining a particular specimen for testing but the patient may only be interested in obtaining rest. Until the patient's priority is met the nurse may be unsuccessful in meeting the nursing priority goal. At the outset, the patient's priorities and expectations must be discussed and negotiated in line with the professional priorities for optimum health.

Reflective point

How does the nursing process recommended differ from your current practice? What are the potential benefits and disadvantages of constructing nursing diagnoses?

The four domains of health and the associated sub-domains within each may be used as the basis for a nursing assessment. In everyday life healthy individuals normally care for themselves within and across these four domains. In carrying out a thorough nursing assessment upon which to form nursing diagnoses and interventions, it is essential to establish the patient's normal self-care practices. By doing so, a care plan can be developed which optimises the patient's health status and level of independence.

Table 19.5 outlines the four key domains of health and their associated sub-domains. In addition, examples of assessment queries to determine normal self-care practices are also provided.

By conducting such an assessment, the nurse will obtain a self-report account from the patient about his health and the normal management strategies deployed. In addition, a series of physical examinations and measurements may also be taken to determine the normal functioning of the bodily systems, as illustrated in Box 19.2.

In addition, a physical examination may also be carried out by means of inspection, percussion, auscultation and palpation. The information gained from these procedures can then be used alongside the assessments of other health professionals to plan health outcomes for the patient. The resultant health outcomes will be personalised yet also standardised according to nursing diagnoses. A comprehensive assessment and identification of diagnoses facilitate a holistic approach to determining socially meaningful health outcomes for surgical patients.

This approach to care planning assumes that the patient actually prefers to be involved in care and is actively seeking a return to independence. Whilst this is the ideal for many people who are unwell, it is by no means the only psychological reaction to hospitalisation or surgery. To appreciate the psychological complexity of the surgical sick role, it is worth briefly considering the concept of control and the relevance of this to contemporary perioperative nursing which generally occurs in a context of rapid patient throughput with associated short-time hospital stay.

Control

The sick role of a patient involves transferring a certain amount of control to a health care professional in order to be cared for. Having major surgery may illustrate the situation where patients may be totally helpless for some of the time but it is contended that they are never hopeless so long as they have some control (West 1992).

Table 19.5   Health assessment process

Domain	Sub-domains	Assessment queries to determine usual self-care practices
Somatological health	Elimination pattern	Description of usual bowel and urinary patterns Use of external aids Description of usual perspiration patterns Signs of itching Menstrual cycle
	Activity and exercise pattern	Description of energy requirements for normal activities, usual type of exercise and range of activities, signs of breathlessness, chest pain, palpitations, stiffness, aching muscles and weakness Ability to carry out normal functional activities e.g. feeding self, cooking, bathing and grooming, dressing, bed mobility, general mobility, toileting, home maintenance activities, shopping
	Nutrition	Typical daily food intake Use of supplements Typical daily fluid intake Weight change Appetite Discomfort associated with food Food preferences Food allergies Skin problems Healing potential Dental problems
	Sleep and rest	Usual sleep pattern Usual sleep rituals Effect of sleep on preparedness for daily activities
Social health	Role and relationship patterns	Description of normal living arrangements Description of normal processes for resolving problems Significant others' feelings about illness Description of normal social encounters and activities Effects of current illness on normal social activities
Psychological health	Coping and stress management	Causes of tension What helps alleviate tensions Recent life changes Usual problem-solving techniques Strategies for managing pain
	Self-awareness	Normal self-description Effects of illness on self-description
	Values and beliefs	General satisfaction with life Special health beliefs Special religious beliefs Any conflict between beliefs and health care treatment
	Cognitive patterns	Description of usual functioning of senses and memory Easiest way to learn things Normal communication patterns Understanding of present illness Understanding of treatments Description of usual sexual relations Effect of illness or treatments on sexuality
Health maintenance	Health perception	General state of health and reason for visit Identification of most important things done to keep healthy Current medication

---

Box 19.2   Functional assessment

General state of health
- Stature
- Speech
- Body movements
- Nutritional status

Vital signs
- Blood pressure
- Pulse
- Respirations
- Temperature

Integument
- Colour
- Lesions
- Scars
- Oedema
- Turgour
- Vascularity

If one of the key aims of nursing the acutely ill patient is to maximise health and well-being, then it is imperative that the perioperative nurse has a sound understanding of the psychology of control. There are four forms of psychological control which are important to the management of interpersonal relationships where parity of power is not apparent. Each applies equally to all parties in an interpersonal relationship. In perioperative nursing both the nurse and the patient will strive to utilise psychological aspects of control. The four types of psychological control are:

- informational control
- behavioural control
- cognitive control
- retrospective control.

It is contended that these four forms (West 1992) can be utilised to enhance patient health outcomes during and following perioperative nursing care.

Informational control.   This involves the individual learning about adverse or fearful experiences in order to manage a situation which may be a unique experience. In the case of surgical patients this includes preoperative information-giving, consultation and explanation about the nature of surgery and the expected outcomes.

Behavioural control.   This requires that the individual acts directly upon a situation. For example, aspects of control can be understood by the patient choosing to have surgery and being part of the care process. The patient is encouraged to be an active participant in care rather than a passive recipient of care. If the latter

is the case, then it is contended that nurses are exercising their behavioural control to the exclusion of that of the patient.

Cognitive control.   This requires that the individual thinks differently about a particular situation. For example, counselling, social support mechanisms or health promotion techniques can enable patients to think differently about their self-image. Following surgery, the concept of the self has been altered. An extreme example of this is the patient who undergoes a panproctocolectomy and has an ileostomy fashioned. With such a patient there is often a strong need for particular nursing interventions which enhance cognitive control.

Retrospective control.   This involves individuals in accepting that they could have controlled the adversive situation in the past and will be able to reduce the risk of future reoccurrence. For example, patients who have undergone surgery for coronary heart disease must understand the contributing risks factors which led to the need for surgery, in order to optimise their rehabilitation in the future. Discharge planning, health promotion, self-awareness training and the promotion of self-esteem are examples of some nursing processes which can be used to enhance retrospective control.

These four aspects of control are interrelated psychologically and are part of the continuum of the perioperative experience. By incorporating some of these ideas, the essentially social nature of nursing can be better understood and used to optimum health effect for the patient.

Reflective point

How important is self-control for the patients you care for? Does your current nursing practice hinder or enhance patient self-control?

Integrated optimum-care plans

Integrated optimum-care plans provide documentary evidence of the range of care being given to any one patient by the full interdisciplinary team. Using the information obtained from the assessments and other literature, outcomes are agreed with the patient. Then, by means of a multidisciplinary and patient-centred conference, interventions can be planned. Interventions will be based upon sound rationales, intuition, creativity, availability of resources and, when patients are able, according to their prerogative. At all times, however, the benefits must outweigh the disadvantages.

Nursing interventions can be considered as any direct actions performed on behalf of a patient by a nurse or appropriately designated others. Actions may be initiated by the nurse following the identification of a nursing diagnosis; from physician-initiated treatments; and from the identification of essential daily activities that the patient cannot perform or wish to perform independently.

In planning effective health care, it is the integration of all health professional activities that leads to successful health outcomes. For these reasons, it is not sufficient for the care plans to be uniprofessional but, rather, it is preferable that optimum-care plans are integrated and interprofessional. Integrated clinical practice provides the means of directing the health care team in daily activities to optimise patient health and well-being. It includes a care plan which covers the pre-hospitalisation, hospitalisation and post-hospitalisation phases. Such a system assists in the organisation of health care. Patient health outcomes and clinical effectiveness are enhanced as the activities of each professional group in each stage of the process are made explicit.

An integrated optimum-care plan outlines the clinical practice and treatment requirements of a patient at specified times throughout the period of ill health. Figure 19.1 outlines a typical framework for such an interprofessional care plan.

This chart would normally be used in conjunction with the health assessment and detailed plan of nursing interventions based on the identification of nursing diagnoses.

Integrated optimum-care plans: total hip replacement

This section will provide examples of an integrated care plan covering a particular surgical intervention. The area selected is typical of surgery performed in most surgical units.

Total hip replacement is an important and seminal advancement in reconstructive surgery. It has provided a significant relief of pain and improved physical functioning for patients with arthritis. Hip replacement is widely used in the treatment of osteoarthritis and rheumatic arthritis as well as for hip

Pathway	Outcomes Day 1	Outcomes Day 2	Outcomes Day 3	Outcomes Discharge	Outcomes Community care	Outcomes Discharge
Diagnostic studies						
Medical interventions and treatments						
Referrals						

Nursing interventions
  Elimination
  Sleep
  Role relations
  Coping and stress
  Self-awareness
  Cognition
  Health perception						

Nutrition						
Activity and exercise						
Education						
Discharge planning						

Figure 19.1 Example of health outcomes record and plan

fractures. The nursing care of the patient undergoing a total hip replacement must begin with education and the setting of realistic goals. The preparation for the surgery, the duration of hospital stay and the expected postoperative events must each be discussed with the patient and others in order that realistic and effective health outcomes can be identified. The long-term health benefits to the patient are considerably greater than the costs of carrying out the surgery.

To illustrate the process, nursing diagnoses have been identified in Box 19.3. From these an integrated care plan can be developed in conjunction with other health professionals.

Health and illness are multifaceted concepts which have as their basis subjective experiences. In helping a patient achieve a state of health the nurse must take into consideration the multiple factors involved; consequently it is suggested that, in health, outcomes must be equally refined. Health is a dynamic state which reflects an equilibrium across the four domains of health which were discussed previously.

Each patient is assessed on these domains, and commonalties based on illness can be discerned. Health, however, is often more individualised; consequently, integrated and refined health outcomes are required for the enhancement of clinical practice when the goal of nursing is to provide holistic high-quality health care.

Reflective point

Construct an integrated optimal-care plan for categories of patients. Which areas of the care plan require individualization?

THE DEVELOPMENT OF EVIDENCE-BASED PRACTICE AND HEALTH OUTCOMES

In clinical care, it is important that the professional can deliver expert care to the patient. It would be naive to assume that a nurse in a surgical setting has limitless time to make the optimal decisions or has limitless resources to conduct sophisticated research. Consequently, if a provider of health services truly wishes to accommodate health care of the highest human and technical quality, investment is necessary. This must include investment in:

- the education and training of health professionals and other health care workers
- the deployment of sufficient professionals and other health care workers

---

Box 19.3 Nursing diagnoses appropriate for total hip replacement

Specific postsurgical nursing diagnoses
Mobility
1. Impaired physical mobility related to pain, stiffness and surgical procedure
2. Reluctance, unwillingness or inability to participate in physical rehabilitation
3. Expressed fear of walking and or moving
4. Self-care deficits due to restrictions imposed by surgery
5. Expressed fear of performing normal daily routines

Infection control
1. Risk of infection related to exposure of joint during surgery
2. Risk of infection due to environmental pathogens
3. Risk of infection owing to ineffective prophylaxis

Personal safety
1. Risk of personal injury related to pain, weakness, fatigue, orthostatic hypotension
2. Risk of personal injury related to use of ambulatory aids

Patient education and involvement
1. Risk of ineffective management of care regimen owing to lack of knowledge
2. Risk of ineffective personal coping strategies owing to unrealistic expectations
3. Risk of ineffective personal coping strategies owing to inadequate support mechanisms

Specific collaborative diagnoses
1. Risk of peripheral neurovascular dysfunction
2. Risk of dislocation of prosthesis because of improper movement and/or infection
3. Risk of thrombophlebitis due to surgery and immobilisation

Examples of health outcomes to be achieved prior to discharge
- Patient has a decrease in or absence of pain as measured by a pain-assessment tool and expressed satisfaction of patient.
- Patient has sufficient muscle strength to continue an activity programme designed to optimise her walking gait as measured by clinical indicators of muscle strength devised by physiotherapist.
- Patient's mobility is restored and she is using walking aids optimally as measured by a staged activity programmed, self-assessment process and absence of postoperative complications, e.g. flexion contracture of the hip.
- Patient has healthy skin as measured by pressure area and wound-assessment tools.
- Patient is free from infection as measured by temperature photographs of wound site.
- Patient has a personal plan for managing care at home, as documented by community nurse and patient, with specified goals.
- Patient is confident of her recovery process as measured by a self-report scale covering well-being and anxiety.

- research.
- the education of patients about treatment and care options.

Evidence-based practice in nursing will influence many aspects of nursing care in perioperative settings. Such an approach could result in patients receiving optimum care. Indeed, if this rational model of clinical decision-making is endorsed and seriously upheld by clinicians, managers and politicians, then there may be many beneficial effects on health care. For example, as nurses are being asked to base their decision-making on scientific evidence, clearly the same rigour should be applied to managers and policy-makers. Appleby et al (1995) conclude by stating that in the future we could see a more scientific, evidence-based approach to defining health policies and priorities; testing and piloting options for service funding, organisation and delivery; and using the experiences of past policies to inform the future development of the NHS (p. 33).

Evidence-based health care requires a fundamental shift in the current thinking and practices of health service management. Indeed, it has been argued that there is now a need for a professional specialist who is authoritative in:

- setting up systems (and understanding the outcomes) for the coordination of information on clinical effectiveness
- matching information on clinical effectiveness and cost-effectiveness from a well-informed basis
- making access to available information easier for clinical staff
- redefining conditions of employment to take cognisance of the requirements of evidence-based practice
- questioning and redefining hierarchies of knowledge
- facilitating others in order to attain integrated clinical care (Appleby et al 1995).

The adoption of such a programme of development across professional groups would contribute to a high-quality integrated health service.

Reflective point

Reflect on who or which role would be the most appropriate for undertaking this function in your area.

To conclude this chapter there are a few points to be made specifically for nursing. Integrated optimum-care planning is the work of the advanced practitioner in nursing and as such requires the following considerations.

Advanced nursing intervention criteria

1. *The appropriateness of the nursing diagnosis.* Before any care can be planned and implemented, a health assessment and the identification of nursing diagnoses must be carried out. This process requires the sophisticated use of knowledge and clinical skills.

2. *The research basis of the intervention.* The selection of the correct intervention to achieve the optimum health outcome comes from the ability to deploy research findings in practice.

3. *Feasibility of successfully carrying out the proposed interventions.* The economics of care are taken into consideration in all clinical contexts – therefore before instigating an intervention the feasibility of doing so is considered.

4. *Acceptability of the intervention to the patient.* All interventions involve a relationship with a patient. For effective health outcomes the involvement of the patient is desirable.

5. *Capability of the nurse.* A competent nurse who has been educated and trained appropriately is required.

To summarise, this and the preceding chapter have suggested that the recent developments within the health service have required nurses to critically audit and evaluate the nature of their working discipline. This has involved the setting of clinical standards and the meeting of managerial targets. It has been suggested that nursing practice should take cognisance of wider health outcomes through the use of an iterative methodology to construct integrated optimum-care plans for use in contexts of surgical nursing.

REFERENCES

Appleby J, Walshe K, Ham C 1995 Acting on the evidence. National Association of Health Authorities and Trusts Research paper No. 17. NAHAT, London

Balogh R 1992 Audits of nursing care in Britain: a review and critique of approaches to validating them. International Journal of Nursing Studies 29(2): 119–133

Clinical Resource and Action Groups of the Scottish Office Department of Health Clinical Resource and Audit Group 1993 Clinical guidelines: a report by a working group set up by the Clinical Resource and Audit Group Scottish Office Edinburgh

Cormack D E S 1991 The research process in nursing, 2nd edn. Blackwell Scientific, Oxford

Deighan M, Hitch S (eds) 1995 Clinical effectiveness from guidelines to cost-effective practice. Earlybrave Publications, Brentwood, Essex

Department of Health (DoH) 1989a Caring for people: community care in the next decade and beyond. HMSO, London

Department of Health (DoH) 1989b Working for patients. HMSO, London

Department of Health (DoH) 1995a Research and development: towards an evidence based health service. DoH, Leeds

Department of Health (DoH) 1995b The patient's charter. HMSO London

Duff L, Keslon M, Marriott S et al 1995 Clinical guidelines: involving patients and service users. The report of a seminar held on 10/5/95, British Institute of Radiology. Royal College of Nursing, London

Goodman C 1993 Literature searching and evidence interpretation for assessing health care practices. Swedish Council on Technology Assessment in Health Care, Stockholm

Hudgings C 1995 Guideline development and dissemination programme. Agency for Health Care Policy and Research USA. In: Deighan M, Hitch S (eds) Clinical effectiveness from guidelines to cost-effective practice. Earlybrave Publications, Brentwood, Essex

Institute of Medicine 1992 Guidelines for clinical practice: from development to use. National Academy Press, Washington

Kendell R 1995 Improving clinical effectiveness: the future. In: Deighan M, Hitch S (eds) Clinical effectiveness from guidelines to cost-effective practice. Earlybrave Publications, Brentwood, Essex, pp 137–144

Kitson A 1995 The multi-professional agenda and clinical effectiveness. In: Deighan M, Hitch S (eds) Clinical effectiveness from guidelines to cost-effective practice. Earlybrave Publications, Brentwood, Essex, pp 83–91

Klazinga N 1995 Clinical guidelines bridging evidence based medicine and health service reform: a European perspective. In: Deighan M, Hitch S (eds) Clinical effectiveness from guidelines to cost-effective practice. Earlybrave Publications, Brentwood, Essex, pp 11–14

Long B, Phipps W, Cassmeyer V 1995 Adult nursing: a nursing process approach. Mosby, London

Lyon M H, West B J M 1995 London Patels: caste and commerce. New Community 21(3): 399–419

Moatti J P, Auquier P, le Coroller A G, Macquart-Moulin G 1995 QALYs or not QALYs: that is the question? Revue Epidemiologie Sante Publique 43(6): 573–583

Newell C, McDowell I 1987 Measuring health: a guide to rating scales and questionnaires. Oxford University Press, Oxford

Polit D E, Hungler B P 1993 Essentials of nursing research, 3rd edn. J B Lippincott, Philadelphia

Redfern S J, Norman I J 1990 Measuring the quality of nursing care: a consideration of different approaches. Journal of Advanced Nursing 15: 1260–1271

Sackett D L, Haynes R B 1995 On the need for evidence based medicine. Evidence Based Medicine 1(1): 5–6

Sackett D L, Rosenberg W 1995 The need for evidence based medicine. Journal of the Royal Society of Medicine 88(11): 620–624

Saltman R 1986 Designing standardised clinical protocols: some organisational and behavioural issues. International Journal of Health Planning and Management 1: 129–141

Scottish Intercollegiate Guideline Network (SIGN) 1995a Criteria for critical appraisal of national guidelines. Scottish Intercollegiate Guidelines Network, Edinburgh

Scottish Intercollegiate Guideline Network (SIGN) 1995b Prophylaxis of venous thromboembolism. A national clinical guideline recommended for use in Scotland, pilot edition (September). Scottish Intercollegiate Guidelines Network, Edinburgh

United Kingdom Central Council for Nursing, Midwifery and Health Visiting (UKCC) 1995 Preparation for education. UKCC, London

Walsh M, Ford P 1989 Nursing ritual. Blackwell, Oxford

West B J M 1988 Quality assurance: a manager's model for nursing. British Journal of Theatre Nursing 25(8): 16–22

West B J M 1992 Nurses' perceptions of patients in the nursing process: a study of two cardiothoracic units. PhD Thesis, University of Edinburgh, Edinburgh

Williamson C 1992 Whose standards? Consumer and professional standards in health care. Open University Press, Buckingham

FURTHER READING

Clinical Resource and Audit Group (CRAG) 1995 Clinical outcome indicators report. Scottish Office CRAG, Edinburgh

Department of Health (DoH) 1994 The challenges for nursing and midwifery in the 21st century. DoH, London

NHS Management Executive 1993 A vision for the future: the nursing midwifery and health visiting contribution to health and health care. Department of Health, Leeds

United Kingdom Central Council for Nursing, Midwifery and Health Visiting (UKCC) 1990 The report of the post-registration and practice project. UKCC, London

United Kingdom Central Council for Nursing, Midwifery and Health Visiting (UKCC) 1992 The scope of professional practice. UKCC, London

West B J M 1993 Caring: the essence of theatre nursing. British Journal of Theatre Nursing 3(8): 13–18

West B J M 1995 Health service developments and the scope of professional practice. Scottish Office Department of Health, HMSO, Edinburgh

West B J M, Lyon M H 1995 Surgical nurse: principles of audit and clinical practice. British Journal of Nursing 4(17): 987–991

PART 5

Key concepts when caring for patients undergoing surgery

20

Principles of preoperative preparation

Sarah Dawson

AIMS

The aims of this chapter are:

- to explore ways in which the surgical nurse provides safe, effective and consistent care for patients prior to surgery
- to encourage surgical nurses to critically analyse routine preoperative nursing practice
- to explore the potential for partnership and participation in preoperative nursing care.

INTRODUCTION

This chapter will focus on supporting the surgical nurse in the creation of a positive experience and outcome for preoperative patients and their carers. The main aim of effective preoperative nursing care is to enable the patient and their carers to understand and be appropriately prepared for the surgical experience. Within the chapter, the surgical nurse will be encouraged to consider the application of the concepts of patient participation and partnership for contemporary preoperative nursing practice. It is acknowledged that not all patients would view the nurse–patient relationship as one of partnership, or would wish (or indeed be able) to participate in their own care. However, surgical nurses need to reflect on the extent to which they engage patients in establishing, implementing and evaluating mutually agreed goals of care. To achieve this preoperatively, nurses and patients need to feel able to share their knowledge and skills and learn together as well as from one another. Key outcomes which could evolve from a partnership/participation approach to surgical care include personal growth and development for both parties, valuing and empowering the patient as an informed individual participant, reduced preoperative stress and anxiety, and patient satisfaction.

Patients should be enabled by nurses to adapt to the preoperative experience and subsequently should feel less vulnerable and more in control of their situation. Surgical nurses have to initiate and support the process. They need to be flexible and innovative to meet the individual needs of patients. Effective nursing practice should be underpinned by artistic and scientific nursing knowledge. This approach reflects the underlying philosophy of both clinical nurses and nurse theorists. The Roy Adaptation Model (Andrews & Roy 1991, Roy 1976) can provide an appropriate holistic framework for preoperative nursing practice. In this chapter, Roy's model provides the basis for the preoperative assessment approach.

PARTNERSHIP

Partnership, as a concept, has been encouraged and adopted for nursing (DoH 1994). Yet to what extent has partnership been discussed, researched, implemented and evaluated in surgical nursing practice? The NHS Executive (1996) describes partnership at the level of individual care: 'to promote individual involvement in one's own care and enable a more informed choice and decisions'. Partnership has also been described as an association with another in which risks and benefits are shared; the relationship is based upon equality and mutual commitment (Bayntun-Lees 1992). The application of this concept requires practitioners and patients to enter into a sharing relationship which empowers the patients, provides them with knowledge to make informed decisions and should enable them to actively participate in their own care. Humphris (1997) asserts that for the patient partnership to be successful the culture of the NHS must change to one in which it is instinctive for health care professionals and managers to think and act in a way which involves individuals in their care and users in service development. Coulter (1997) explores the pros and cons of shared decision-making within the medical literature. However, many of the arguments can be related to nursing practice. For example, except for emergency situations, the preferences of patients should be included in the decision-making process. Four key characteristics of shared decision-making identified by Charles et al (cited in Coulter 1997) are:

- it involves at least two participants – nurse and patient
- both parties take steps to build a consensus about the preferred approach
- information is shared
- agreement is reached on the approach to be implemented.

One example of the application of this theory in practice could be surgical nurses exploring with patients their knowledge of their forthcoming surgery and pain management and whether they would like to administer their own postoperative analgesia via patient-controlled analgesia (PCA). However, the idea that patients participate in decision-making, e.g. goal setting, is not new. The nursing process has encouraged mutual goal setting and care planning since its inception over two decades ago. Surgical nurses have had to learn and develop excellent communication skills to ensure that patients participate within the partnership, in the surgical experience.

Concerns about shared decision-making identified by Coulter (1997) include the perceived loss of autonomy (by health care professionals); worries about adverse effects of information on patients; worries about the impact on costs/time/equity. Coulter (1997) argues that these concerns may reflect a misunderstanding, as shared decision-making does not constitute an abdication of professional responsibility. She advocates the need for shared decision-making based on scientific evidence which takes account of patients' preferences, clinical effectiveness, and cost-effectiveness (p. 118). However, it is equally important to recognise that within any decision-making process there will be cultural differences in interpretation and understanding (also see Ch. 10).

PATIENT PARTICIPATION

Patient participation in care can result from an effective nurse–patient relationship. Cahill (1996) identified the following attributes from her concept analysis of patient participation:

- A relationship must exist.
- There must be a narrowing of the appropriate information, knowledge and/or competence gap between the nurse and patient using suitable modalities in different contexts.
- There must be a surrendering of a degree of power or control by the nurse.
- There must be engagement in selective intellectual and/or physical activities during some of the phases of the health care process.
- There must be a positive benefit associated with the intellectual and/or physical activity.

Loughlin (1993) states that it is generally accepted that patients respond better to treatment if they are involved in their own care and are given more information. If they know and understand about the operation, they heal faster. If the drugs are explained, patients are more likely to comply and use them appropriately (p. 163). When patients participate in their care, there should be mutual agreement as to what is expected of them and what they should expect to happen to them.

Reflective point

Do you support the views expressed above? To what extent are they reflected in your everyday practice? Is patient participation identified within the ward/unit philosophy? Is there a shared understanding of the concept between the nurses and between the interprofessional team? Is patient participation identified within the ward/unit audit criteria?

Ashworth et al (1992) provide a phenomenological account of participation. They state that participation is best highlighted by reference to situations in which it is not found, for example, on a ward round where the patient as a lay person is unable to participate in nursing and medical interaction. Another instance is when a nurse asks standard routine assessment questions without individualisation, e.g. the authors observed that an obviously mobile young adult was asked whether she could manage to climb stairs.

It would be a mistake for any doctors and nurses to assume that they know intuitively what the lived experience of any patient is like. The gap between the lay world and that of the health care professional can be surprisingly wide, even where the point of discussion seems to be a matter of common experience framed in everyday language, (Ashworth et al 1992).

Frequently patients have commented to me that their admission and surgery were not as bad as they had anticipated because they were encouraged to ask questions and were provided with appropriate information (verbal and written). Providing patients with information empowers them to be able to make choices, ask questions and helps to relieve the stress and anxiety that accompanies any hospital admission.

The experienced practitioner will be observing patients from the moment that they first meet. This involves identifying the cues, verbal and nonverbal, that the patients may be communicating about their physical and psychological state. By identifying and acting upon these cues, the practitioner enables patients to explore any issues or concerns that they may have about surgery; this enhances the nurse–patient partnership.

It should not be assumed that all patients wish to ask questions, participate in the planning of their care or indeed, are able to participate. Such patients need to be identified as early as possible so that they are not subjected to staff bombarding them with choices. All patients have a right to information and the practitioner has a duty to help provide this information at a level appropriate to the individual person. If patients decline information, this is their prerogative. However, even if patients state that they have complete faith in you and the system and just want you 'to get on with it', explanations of clinical procedures still need to be given.

The Patient's Charter (DoH 1991, 1995) has made patients aware of their rights to a consultation and subsequent surgical procedure within identified time limits. An outcome of this is to place additional pressure on the surgical nurse to ensure that the stay of patients is minimised and that they consider that they have received quality care.

One of the standards in the Patient's Charter identifies that patients have the right to be told before admission whether they will be cared for in a mixed or single-sex ward. If they prefer to be cared for in single-sex accommodation, their wishes should be respected wherever possible. This could potentially reduce bed occupancy by patients indicating that they do not wish to share a bay or ward with the opposite sex and endanger other Charter standards regarding the number of cancellations and expected time for operation (see also Ch. 14). However, one of the key aims of the recently relaunched Patients' Association is to commission new research into the cost of closing all mixed-sex wards in NHS hospitals (Smith 1997). Complaints received by the association include:

Hospital staff seem to forget that what is normal to them is far from normal to ordinary people, (G. Goodwin, in *Patients' Voices* (Patients Association 1996, p. 3).

Mixed sex wards are undesirable being contrary to the general concept of modesty and privacy (A. Sydenham in *Patients' Voices* (Patients Association 1996, p. 3).

One doesn't have mixed sex dormitories in Youth Hostels, or mixed sex hotel room sharing with strangers – it's all in the interests of money, money, money, (E. Raymont in *Patients' Voices* (Patients Association 1996, p. 3).

Reflective point

What are the views of patients in your ward? Should the economics of bed occupancy outweigh the personal preferences of patients for mixed or single-sex wards?

PREOPERATIVE COMMUNICATION

The early research undertaken by Boore (1975) and Hayward (1978) identified that information given preoperatively can reduce the stress, anxiety and pain of patients. Surgical nurses would generally support this view, although recent critiques have highlighted some deficits in these research studies (see Chs 2 and 18). As a consequence of the partnership between the patient and the surgical nurse, the patient's level of existing knowledge, interest and ability to comprehend further information can be assessed. Effective communication could, though, still prove difficult as stress and anxiety are barriers to communication (Bellman 1994). Stress interferes with a patient's ability to concentrate and learn (Abbott & Glenn 1994). Logical thinking is impaired (Atkinson et al 1993), which could lead to reduced assimilation of information. Therefore the patient, whether as a routine or as an emergency admission, will probably process far less information than is generally anticipated. This is something I always try to remember when offering explanations to patients.

Teasdale (1993) provides a different interpretation on information-giving. He considers that the nurse needs to be able to communicate with patients to enable them to gain the same meaning from the words and phrases used as the information provider places on them. An example of this is the case of a non-nursing colleague who recently underwent emergency surgery. Her surgery had to be delayed because the inferential meaning of the words 'nil by mouth' were not the same for the patient as the nurse; this scenario will be expanded upon later in the chapter.

Preoperative patient education

Preoperative teaching of techniques to reduce potential complications of surgery should help to allay the anxiety of patients and enable them to participate in their own care. Ultimately, by reducing the incidence of postoperative complications, this should reduce the length of stay of patients and help make their recovery uneventful.

Cupples (1991) suggests that the optimum time to provide patients with information about their operation is 10–14 days preoperatively. This allows sufficient time to digest the information given and the opportunity to ask any questions on admission, yet long enough prior to surgery for the information to be absorbed. Information given on the day prior to surgery is not retained as well as that given during the 2 weeks preceding operation (Nelson 1995). This

highlights the significance of the surgical nurse's role in information-giving in the pre-admission clinic and/or surgical outpatients to both potential patients and their partners/families.

Information leaflets are considered to be an effective method of providing information and teaching as long as they are backed up with one-to-one contact (Lowery 1995). Written information can be read outside the hospital environment to reinforce the information given by the staff. This also enables carers to have some insight into the expectations of forthcoming surgery.

If specific postoperative equipment or techniques are to be employed, e.g. patient-controlled analgesia (PCA), this type of information may need to be repeated and an assessment of the patient's understanding should be undertaken. An explanatory leaflet that the patient can keep helps to reinforce the information. The patient may be offered the facility of PCA, or have another analgesia process explained. Whatever the pain management policy within your unit, the patients need to be reassured that their pain will be controlled to enable mobility and independence to be restored as soon as possible (see also Ch. 24).

The use of videotapes in preoperative teaching has been evaluated positively (Nelson 1995); they are especially useful if they show patients talking about their personal experiences. As previously stated, stress and anxiety will influence how much information/teaching is assimilated. Further information regarding patient education is to be found in Chapter 3.

Informed consent

The concept of informed consent requires that all patients give their consent for surgery, having been provided with appropriate information and the opportunity to discuss the implications of the surgery with a suitably qualified medical practitioner. However, many patients are still in awe of doctors and will sign a consent form without fully understanding the surgery they are to undergo. Surgical nurses, therefore, have a responsibility to ensure that patients comprehend what is likely to happen to them. If nurses are concerned that the patient's consent is not informed they have a duty to tell the medical personnel concerned (see also Ch. 4).

The Code of Conduct (UKCC 1992) states that the nurse must always act in the patients' best interest. Therefore, as the patient's advocate the nurse has a number of responsibilities. These include ensuring that the consent obtained is indeed informed, acting in the patient's best interest, e.g. informing the medical team if a patient develops a pyrexia or cold the evening prior to surgery. Consequently, the anaesthetist and medical staff may review the patient's suitability for surgery. If the decision is made to postpone the operation because of the patient's cold, it is less stressful and distressing to do so the night before or morning of surgery rather than in the anaesthetic room.

PREOPERATIVE VISITING

Social visiting by partners, family and friends should be encouraged in the preoperative phase to enable the person to retain contact with the outside world. Preoperative visiting by the perioperative nurse can reduce patient anxiety and provide additional information for theatre staff to enable them to develop a good intraoperative care plan (Baldwin 1993, Webb 1995). The availability of staff to provide preoperative visits can be sporadic. Preoperative visits are also undertaken by staff from high dependency areas (intensive therapy/care unit (ITU/ICU)/high dependency unit (HDU)) if the patient is expected to spend some time there.

From personal experience, talking to patients following surgery, some have considered it most helpful to see a familiar face when they were being 'put to sleep', but not so much when waking as this memory often fades. However, some considered it reassuring to see the same nurse again if they were in ITU/HDU (see also Chs 14 and 16).

ELECTIVE SURGERY

Patients for elective surgery should have had time to reflect on their forthcoming admission. They should have received printed operation-specific information and commenced physical and psychological preparation as necessary. Ideally, patients would attend a preadmission clinic where they would meet their named nurse. This approach would serve to establish a therapeutic relationship early in the surgical experience.

Discharge planning

The significance of early discharge planning cannot be overestimated (Savill & Bartholomew 1994, Wiffin 1995). The average length of hospital admission has been reduced dramatically owing to the advances in technology, financial considerations and contracting requirements of purchasers; consequently, discharge planning should be initiated prior to admission (Malby 1992). If the patient has attended a pre-admission clinic, discussions about discharge should have

commenced. Patients and their families/partners need to be aware of the expected care requirements on discharge. All patients will need a degree of support at home after surgery. Even patients undergoing day surgery need a period of convalescence and recuperation (see also Ch. 15). Most patients have an approximate idea when they will be offered surgery and can therefore plan who will be available to help look after them at home. If the need for external agencies can be identified in the preoperative stage, an assessment visit from, for example, the occupational therapist can be considered and organised. If there are the resources and time for a multiprofessional assessment prior to surgery, this can facilitate and speed up the discharge process.

Other agencies involved in the provision of health care and aftercare, for example social services, also need to be involved as early as possible. The potential for patients to occupy beds unnecessarily, i.e. when considered medically fit for discharge, will increase if the hospital and social services do not agree on the funding for the continuing care of the patient. Additionally, if the person appeals against the proposed package of aftercare (because in many cases the patient and carer will have to contribute financially towards the cost) this has to be reviewed by a local arbitration panel and may entail the patient staying in hospital until a decision has been reached.

However, a word of warning! A number of patients have stated that when they first arrived in hospital, they were made to feel welcome by their named nurse yet were puzzled when very soon into an initial assessment interview they were asked, in some detail, about their discharge. This can make patients feel that they are on a conveyer belt and are to be in and out of hospital as soon as possible. Careful explanation of why such information is required at the beginning of a patient's stay would help to provide reassurance; for example, we do not wish to discharge patients until they have recovered and feel ready to go home but we need to ensure that adequate provision for discharge is available.

EMERGENCY ADMISSION

The nurse–patient relationship will need to develop with greater speed for an emergency admission than for an elective admission, as there is frequently a much shorter time for preparation prior to surgery.

The factors that may influence the patient's and carer's level of stress and anxiety, for the emergency admission, are:

- lack of time for information-giving
- reduced psychological preparation

- reduced physical preparation
- reduced time to discuss the implications of surgery with carers.

Within the emergency situation, the surgical nurse needs to make swift and accurate assessments of the patient's physical and psychological needs as well as those of the carers. The patient may be in considerable pain and discomfort or appear drowsy as a result of previously administered analgesia; consequently it may be impracticable to undertake an in-depth assessment.

PREOPERATIVE ASSESSMENT

Roy's Adaptation Model (Andrews & Roy 1991, Roy 1976) is an appropriate framework to use when developing a plan of care for surgical patients because they may experience much stress and have to make many physical, psychological and social adaptations during the pre- and postoperative period. The surgical nurse assesses if the person's coping mechanisms are adaptive or ineffective. Within the partnership relationship, the surgical nurse can help to trigger coping behaviour by, for example, offering appropriate information.

Roy's model proposes that adaptation is a process in which the person will grow and develop, and adaptation will be demonstrated in positive outcomes. Understanding the concepts of stress, coping and adaptation within Roy's model offers the surgical nurse a sound basis for providing constructive and individualised care. Pearson et al (1996, p. 124) present a case study of a surgical patient within Roy's framework (see Further reading). A nursing assessment using this model is demonstrated within Case study 20.1.

Overview of Roy's Adaptation Model

The model of choice should be congruent with and reflect the values and beliefs of surgical nursing care within the team. The use of Roy's model is particularly appropriate for those patients undergoing major surgery which can severely alter body image. David will have to undergo many adaptations, from adapting to a different physical environment (i.e. the ward) to adapting to the rest of his life without his right leg.

Reflective point

Which nursing model do you use as a framework for surgical nursing practice in your clinical area? How is it used? Is it the most appropriate choice for your type of patients?

Case study 20.1   David

The nursing assessment outlined is for a 63-year-old man, called David; he was prepared for a right below-knee amputation. David had peripheral vascular disease and had experienced severe claudication at work. His circulation has gradually deteriorated. Recently he noticed an ulcer on his right foot which had not healed and had become gangrenous. He married Nancy 43 years ago; they have a son and a daughter and three grandchildren. He and his wife live in a hilly suburb of a large town; they own a car and caravan. David now smokes 10 cigarettes a day. Before he retired he was a manager at the local canning factory.

Adaptation

All surgery requires adaptation. Patients are faced with stressors that they would not ordinarily encounter in their everyday lives. Nursing activities and interventions are therefore required to facilitate patients in making successful adaptations. Figure 20.1 illustrates how the person can be viewed as an adaptive system.

The environment provides internal and external stimuli which Roy calls stressors. Stressors provoke a response which is demonstrated in the form of behaviour. Stressors can produce adaptive responses or ineffective responses. The surgical nurse needs to identify the ineffective responses and promote adaptation through nursing interventions. Nursing interventions can either manipulate stimuli or broaden the person's adaptation zone, for example by providing appropriate information, thus assisting in adaptation. The goal of nursing in Roy's model is to promote adaptation in the four adaptive phases: physiological, self-concept, role function and interdependence. These should facilitate a positive state of health in patients, enabling them to become integrated and whole persons (Andrews & Roy 1991). The four adaptive modes are used to structure the assessment (see Fig. 20.2).

Nursing process

Roy's model encompasses six steps in the nursing process: assessment of behaviour (first level), assessment of stimuli (second level), nursing diagnosis, goal setting, intervention, and evaluation.

The first and second levels of assessment will be illustrated in detail for David in his preoperative period. The partnership that I was able to develop with David enabled him to participate in establishing appropriate nursing diagnoses. Consequently the

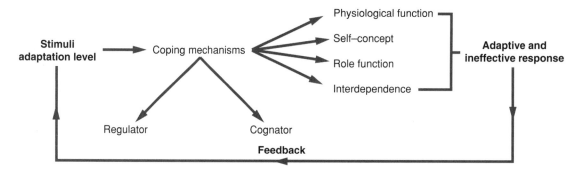

Figure 20.1 The person as an adaptive system (adapted from Marriner-Tomey 1994).

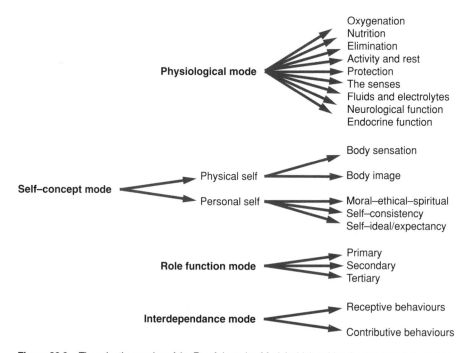

Figure 20.2 The adaptive modes of the Roy Adaptation Model which guides the assessment process.

approach to goal setting, interventions and evaluation was also undertaken in partnership with David.

First level of assessment

The first level of assessment is essential. Without obtaining the necessary information and data, an effective assessment and subsequent individualised plan of care could not be developed and agreed. Methods used to collect this data included observation of David's responses to his environment, interview and objective measurement.

Physiological mode. Because David was to undergo surgery, major stressors were exerted on his physical adaptive processes. To assess how David was coping with these stressors and in order to make an initial plan of care a comprehensive assessment was performed. Box 20.1 illustrates the physiological mode assessment for David.

The surgical nurse requires an in-depth knowledge of physiological assessment to be able to interpret the results from the assessment. Chapters 8 and 23–27 provide in-depth information related to the physiological mode assessment of surgical patients.

Box 20.1 David's assessment in the physiological mode

Oxygenation. David smokes 10 cigarettes per day; he is 'slightly' short of breath when he reaches the top of his 17 stairs (he has to rest half-way up owing to severe claudication) and when returning home from the shops up the hill. He is alert and oriented. Clinical observations are within normal limits. David is concerned that he has recently had a cold and that this may affect his anaesthetic. He does cough first thing each morning.

Nutrition. Height 170 cm; weight 105 kg. David has put on some weight since he has retired and has become less active owing to his reduced mobility. He has recently tried to lose weight by adopting a low fat and high fibre diet. He is aware that he has a tendency to put on weight as he enjoys his food. He is concerned about possible additional weight gain when he believes he will be less mobile with only one leg (and a prosthesis). He has a part top denture which enables him to chew effectively. His skin appears healthy except below his knees. This skin has a fragile, paper-like appearance and seems very friable. All pressure points are intact. David thinks that he will be starved for at least a day before surgery and that it will be a few days after his operation until he can eat normally again.

Elimination. David passes urine 3–4 times during the day and usually once or twice during the night. He has full bladder control. Urinalysis is within normal parameters. Bowels open daily, usually just after breakfast. His temperature is 36.7°C (oral).

Activity and rest. David is able to maintain his own personal hygiene and nutritional needs. His activities are restricted by severe claudication; he was able to walk 20 paces before he experienced pain. David uses a stick to help him walk. David usually goes to bed around 23.00 and gets up at 06.30; he often has a nap for an hour during the afternoon. David is concerned at his reduced mobility and the need to use a wheelchair in the early stages following his amputation.

Protection. David is able to protect himself physically. Psychologically he seems to accept that his amputation will change his life, but presents a positive approach and outlook.

The senses. David wears glasses to read and prefers to read under a bright light. He has no hearing deficit. David has decreased sensation in his left foot, but increased and heightened sensation in his gangrenous right foot. David does not anticipate having a great deal of pain after his surgery and mentioned that he has heard about phantom limb pains.

Fluid and electrolytes. David normally consumes six cups of tea per day, one cup of coffee and a hot milky drink before retiring to bed at night. David is aware that he will need to have a 'drip' immediately following his surgery; he is concerned that this may mean that he cannot get out of bed.

Box 20.1 (Contd.)

Neurological function. This appears to be intact. David responds in an appropriate manner and is oriented in time and space.

Endocrine function. This appears to be functioning normally. All clinical test and investigation results are within normal limits.

Self-concept mode. This is the first of three psychosocial modes. This mode focuses on psychic integrity, encompassing the person's self-esteem. The mode is divided into the physical self (including physical attributes, sexuality and wellness–illness status) and the personal self, which considers personal characteristics, expectations, values and worth. Box 20.2 illustrates David's assessment in the self-concept mode.

Box 20.2 David's assessment in the self-concept mode

Physical self – body sensation (how one feels about oneself). David expresses anxiety and concern at not being in control of the situation, not knowing what to expect because he has not been a patient in hospital for 20 years.

Physical self – body image (how one feels about one's body and what it looks like). David acknowledged that he will feel 'incomplete' without his right leg; however, he is hopeful that with a good prosthesis nobody will notice. He is not looking forward to being in a wheelchair initially: 'people don't talk to you or if they do they think you are stupid.' Nancy already, jokingly, calls him 'peg leg'. David did not express any worries about continuing to have a sexual relationship with Nancy, and seemed to be extremely positive about his forthcoming altered body image.

Personal self – moral-ethical-spiritual self (the individual's belief and moral system). David stated that he was a 'lapsed Catholic', he believed in God but had no desire to see the priest. He believed that he had made his disease worse by smoking and was paying the price.

Personal self – self-consistency (one's personality traits/personality). David was usually a calm person; he expressed no undue anxiety. What concerns he did have, he was able to verbalise.

Box 20.2 (Contd.)

Personal self – self-ideal/self-expectancy
(one's expectations in relation to one's capabilities).
David ultimately wanted to be able to walk with a
prosthesis and continue driving his car (he already had
an automatic). He was aware that this goal would take
months to achieve and was prepared to participate in the
physiotherapy programme to reach his goal.

Practitioners often neglect the areas of psychological and social needs (Mitchell 1994) when admitting and assessing patients. This could be attributed to the surgical nurse adopting a medical model rather than a nursing model with a key focus on physiological needs. Roy's framework clearly demonstrates the importance of exploring psychological needs. However, insufficient time to talk to patients is often the reason given for not providing psychological preparation and support prior to surgery. Benner (1984) states that expert practitioners will use their knowledge and expertise to gather this type of data in an unobtrusive and constructive way. I would suggest that all surgical nurses whatever their level of experience should develop expertise in and make time for this essential aspect of preoperative care.

Reflective point

Do you provide time to gather information about your patients' psychosocial needs? What information do you elicit? How do you interpret the information?

Role function mode. The second psychosocial mode is concerned with social integrity. We all assume a number of roles in our lives; some change with time others remain relatively static. These roles dictate, to a greater or lesser degree, how we behave. Societal expectations identify norms of behaviour and indicate where we fit into society. The role function mode is divided into primary, secondary and tertiary roles. Box 20.3 illustrates David's role functions.

Reflective point

Have you ever been a patient? How did you adapt to the role? It is interesting to ask patients how they have (or have not) adapted to the patient role. To what extent has this role adaptation been influenced by their expectations, current and past experiences?

Box 20.3 David's assessment in the role function mode

Primary role. David is a 63-year-old mature male.

Secondary role. David is a husband and parent to two children whom he sees fairly regularly. He has three grandchildren; he would like to see them more. He has many close friends in the neighbourhood where he has always lived.

Tertiary role. David had recently retired as a manager from the local canning factory. He used to enjoy travelling throughout Britain in a caravan, and is a member of the Caravan Club. He is a member of the local bridge club, playing once or twice per week.

Although David and Nancy are not used to being apart, David is not unduly concerned about Nancy having to 'fend for herself'. Although David acknowledges that he will not be complete following his surgery, he does not see that this will alter his roles. David is determined to return home as soon as possible and carry on a 'normal life' with Nancy.

Interdependence mode. The final mode focuses on relationships: the ability and willingness to accept and respond to respect, love, trust and valuing others. Box 20.4 represents the assessment of David in the interdependence mode.

Second level of assessment

The second level of assessment tries to assess the factors that have and will contribute to the adaptive and ineffective (maladaptive) behaviours demonstrated by David. The focal, contextual and residual stimuli have to be identified. Frequently, the stimuli cross more than one adaptive mode. Figure 20.3 is a diagrammatic

---

Box 20.4 David's assessment in the interdependence mode

Receptive behaviours. David has accepted the help that has been offered in the form of surgery. He is in a loving relationship with his wife and has accepted the additional help that she has given him in the last few weeks prior to admission.

Contributive behaviours. David has offered information freely to help with the admission and assessment process. He has always enjoyed looking after Nancy but has appreciated her reciprocating, in a different manner, recently. He has considered that Nancy will be helping to look after him when he returns home until he is fully 'independent' again.

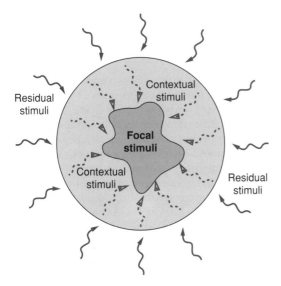

Figure 20.3 Focal, contextual and residual stimuli.

interpretation of focal, contextual and residual stimuli. Focal stimuli represent the provoking situation or event that has prompted the person to seek help. Contextual stimuli are all the other stimuli contributing to the focal stimuli. Residual stimuli are vague hunches or ambiguous factors that could be affecting the person. Box 20.5 represents David's second level assessment. This level of assessment acknowledges the importance and existence of the hunches and intuition that Benner (1984) attributes to the expert nurse.

Box 20.5 David's second level assessment

Focal stimuli (the provoking situation or event that has prompted the person to seek help). David was aware that the ulcer on his foot was deteriorating, began to smell and caused him increased pain.

Contextual stimuli (all other stimuli contributing to the focal stimuli). David's peripheral vascular disease had progressed to a state where he had very little peripheral circulation in his feet. The circulation was deteriorating and caused increasingly severe claudication. Smoking has probably contributed to/hastened the disease process.

Residual stimuli (vague hunches or ambiguous factors that could be affecting the person – once positively identified they become contextual or focal stimuli). David seemed too accepting of his situation. He would need to be observed for how he actually coped with his amputation and the bereavement process associated with the loss of a limb. David may have a 'stiff upper lip' attitude and therefore find it difficult to display his emotions and feelings.

Nursing diagnosis

David appeared to demonstrate effective coping strategies. He required support and further information about his impending surgery to prepare him psychologically and physically. From the information gathered, he was concerned about his recent cold and remained in pain from his leg.

A problem (actual or potential) will be examined in more detail for each of the four adaptive modes. The diagnosis of potential chest infection was identified from the information gathered during the first level assessment of oxygenation in the physiological mode: David stated that he had had a cold recently, smoked 10 cigarettes a day and tended to cough first thing each morning. Because of these factors, plus the effects of a general anaesthetic and reduced mobility in the postoperative period, he was at high risk of developing a chest infection. Therefore David agreed that his care plan should include referral to the physiotherapist to teach him breathing and coughing exercises, that I would reinforce and encourage him to practise these exercises regularly preoperatively and that we would continue to debate the implications of continuing to smoke.

David expressed concern at not being 'complete' once he had had his amputation. A diagnosis of loss and grieving regarding altered body image could be made in the self-concept (physical self) mode. David's care plan also identified the need to provide him with the time to express these fears and anxieties pre- and postoperatively. David agreed to meet with a past amputee who had a prosthesis. This gave him reassurance, helped to reduce his anxiety and enabled him to verbalise his concerns and discuss issues surrounding life after an amputation.

A nursing diagnosis was also made of imminent role transition and change (role function mode) in the immediate postoperative period. David, recently retired, had always been the main financial provider in the household. Nancy was slowly adapting to being the main financial support. David's care plan included referral to the occupational therapist for home assessment and discussions about adaptations required in the home. I encouraged Nancy and David to discuss how they felt about their potential change of role.

Within the interdependence mode a diagnosis of anxiety was made. Reasons for anxiety overlap with all the other modes of adaptation. David was anxious about his operation, that no complications should occur and that his amputation did not extend to above the knee. How would he adapt to his altered body image?

Will Nancy still love and care about him in the same way? How will his children and grandchildren view him? Will he be able to regain his independence and walk again? These and many other questions caused anxiety for David. I put David's care plan into action by making time and providing opportunities for him to talk about his fears, concerns, anxieties.

In conjunction with David, I was able to undertake effective first- and second level assessments, and develop a nursing diagnosis, or problem identification (Cox 1994) (see also Ch. 19). When caring for David I used my knowledge of interpersonal skills, nursing theory and nursing practice, nursing research, personal knowledge and experience, and biological and behavioural sciences. My nursing knowledge, which continues to develop and advance, enabled me to assess David, develop a nursing diagnosis, set goals, plan interventions and evaluate his adaptive or ineffective (maladaptive) behaviours.

Spiritual dimension

The use of Roy's model will enable the surgical nurse to undertake ongoing holistic preoperative assessments. Biological, psychological and sociological factors can be clearly identified. The spiritual dimension is made explicit within the self-concept mode.

All religions embrace spirituality but religion is only one way of understanding spirituality. Spirituality may be defined as a belief or personal value system that provides strength, hope, meaning. Human beings continually search for meaning in their lives. A major disruption in one's life, for example undergoing surgery, may therefore lead to spiritual distress. Surgical nurses need to acknowledge and provide support for spiritual distress in their patients. Nolan & Crawford (1997) explore how individuals experience spirituality on at least four different levels:

- First level: How I relate to myself – a healthy relationship with myself means setting alongside my achievements a clear understanding of who I am.
- Second level: How I relate to others – appreciating the worth of others; transcending without belittling the characteristics of other people as represented by their culture, language, religion, class, education, wealth or disability.
- Third level: Relationships between and within groups – social awareness, knowing what and when to give and take, understanding personal duties and responsibilities; personal growth and self-realisation are achieved through others.
- Fourth level: A relationship with that which is transcendent, whatever the transcendent may mean to

any individual. The transcendent may be defined as God or the cultural equivalent; or personal meanings of life and death and the joys and sufferings encountered during life.

Some patients may express concerns and anxiety about the outcome of their operation, but in my experience not many verbalise fear of dying. As with psychological preparation, nurses may feel ill-equipped to deal with a patient who fears death. If patients have strong religious beliefs they may require a visit prior to surgery from their spiritual representative. Surgical nurses need to explore together and with patients how they may integrate spiritual care into their everyday practice. Yet, Nolan & Crawford (1997) clearly identify the difficulties of introducing spirituality into the language of nursing:

At present it is difficult for nurses to acknowledge their own spirituality, which is essential if they are to nurture their clients. The health services are dominated by the language of the market place and this has resulted in the depersonalization of many staff. The emphasis on being a grade rather than a person is one of many symptoms of spiritual alienation suffered by nurses and expressed in the language they use about themselves and their work, (p. 293).

A nursing model, for example that of Roy, which has a spiritual dimension incorporated into the assessment phase can enhance surgical nurses' spiritual knowledge and practice. Surgical nurses need, however, to recognise and value this dimension of holistic care. If they practise or continue to practise within a medical/technical model of care they will only, from a nursing perspective, address Roy's physiological model of care (see also Ch. 9).

Reflective point

Note the difference between Roy's approach to assessment and that of another nursing model of your choice. What are the advantages and disadvantages of using Roy's two-stage assessment?

CRITICAL CARE PATHWAYS

Critical care pathways are increasingly being developed for surgical patients. They are also known under a number of other titles; these include anticipated recovery pathways and collaborative care plans (Riches et al 1994), integrated care pathway (Johnson 1994) and coordinated care (Brown & Simpson 1994). The USA has an established history of planning a patient's anticipated care requirements, with an emphasis on providing quality care in a cost-effective and efficient way. Figure 20.4 illustrates how a critical care pathway can be designed and created. This is achieved through a multidisciplinary plan of care which directs, documents and coordinates the patient's care (Johnson 1994) – assuming, of course, that the patient follows a predictable course of recovery (Riches et al 1994).

Figure 20.5 illustrates a coordinated care plan for a person undergoing an abdominal hysterectomy. The critical care pathway has the potential to eradicate duplication of information (which is both time-consuming and unnecessary for patients and staff) and foster a truly multidisciplinary team approach to care, facilitating communication between all team members. However, a note of caution should be sounded in relation to how such care pathways may affect individualised and holistic care? Walsh (1997) states that the discrepancy between expected and actual events on a critical pathway is known as 'variance'. When a deviation from the critical path is recognised, the explanation must be found and the problem rectified. However, if patients do not follow their anticipated recovery pathway, will the skills required to plan and provide their care still be available? Critical pathways reflect the current political approach to managing patient care. Evidence is required, however, which demonstrates their positive contribution to patient care without compromising the individual approach which UK nurses espouse (Walsh 1997). Also see Chapter 2.

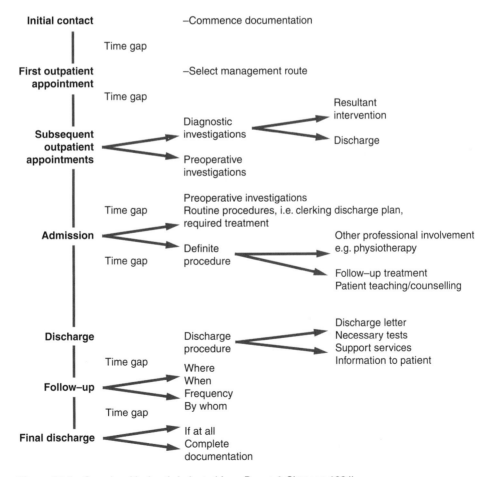

Figure 20.4 Sample critical path (adapted from Brown & Simpson 1994).

	OPD	DAY MINUS 1	OPERATION DAY	DAY 1
M E D I C A L	History, allergies, etc. Chest X-ray, ECG if indicated FBC, group & save Check smear Anaesthetist	Review medical history Physical examination & check allergies Obtain consent Complete anaesthetic sheet Prescribe antibiotic DVT prophylaxis & night sedation	Audit form Vital signs & urinary output IV regime Medication/analgesia	Review analgesia & regime Prescribe oral analgesia Check bowel & bladder function Commence oral fluids when satisfactory Check general condition & wound daily
N U R S I N G	Urinalysis & MSU Pulse & BP Admission sheet Discharge planning commenced Weight	Nursing assessment Measurement for TED stockings Order PT medication Shave Check bowel function	Prep for theatre Pre-op medication Complete check list Check valuables Check documentation BP, pulse & responses PCAS observations Observation of wound sites & drainage measurements Observe general condition	Continue 4-hourly measures TDS observations Observe wound Remove drain Commence 30 ml fluids hourly Review PCAS & IVI Vulval toilet with sterile water Check bowel & bladder function Review PV loss
P H Y S I O		Breathing exercises Post-op exercises Circulatory exercises Pelvic tilting Discuss abdominal exercises & back problems		Assess chest Breathing exercises and mobility Back care as appropriate
P A T I E N T **T E A C H I N G**	Info pamphlet to patients Admission details Health education re diet, exercise and smoking	Patient informed of surgery time Counselling pre- and post-op care Reinforce patient teaching information	Nil by mouth for 6 hours pre-op	Assist patient out of bed & encourage exercises General hygiene

Figure 20.5 A coordinated care plan for a person undergoing an abdominal hysterectomy (adapted from Brown & Simpson 1994).

DIAGNOSTIC SCREENING

Diagnostic screening is an essential part of patient preparation prior to an anaesthetic and surgery. Surgical nurses should be familiar with 'normal' test results and inform the medical practitioner if they are concerned about a test result prior to surgery, thereby acting as the patient's advocate. The term 'normal' identifies a specific range of results which are accepted as safe by the anaesthetist and surgeon. If results fall outside this range, the patient will usually be medically treated to bring them to within normal limits.

Screening ranges from the standard tests/investigations for the majority of patients to specific investigations which enhance the surgeon's understanding of the precise type and nature of surgery required. The initial investigations and tests that the surgical nurse performs will help establish a rapport with the person and facilitate the partnership.

Baseline clinical observations

There is a wealth of evidence and research to demonstrate that stress affects the cardiovascular system. The blood pressure, in particular, can be elevated as a result of stress/anxiety providing an atypical measurement for the patient (Hinchliff & Montague 1991). For this reason, baseline clinical observations of temperature, pulse, respiratory rate and blood pressure should ideally be undertaken once the newly admitted patient has had time to 'settle' into the new environment. The ward urinalysis test, routinely carried out (if not already undertaken in a pre-admission clinic) will exclude many major illnesses/diseases. Whilst surgical nurses are performing these investigations, they should explain the necessity for them and offer the results to the patients.

Laboratory tests

The standard laboratory tests performed for most patients will include a full blood count (FBC), to ensure that the person does not have an abnormal blood picture and specific medical problems, e.g. anaemia, which would hinder postoperative recovery. Patients undergoing major surgery will always have their blood cross-matched as they may require a blood transfusion. Patients for day case or minor surgery will have their blood type identified but not usually cross-matched as they are not expected, by virtue of their surgery, to require a blood transfusion. Blood urea and electrolyte (U&E) levels are checked to ensure that, amongst others, renal function is 'normal'. Surgical nurses, as an extension to their scope of practice, may undertake venepuncture. Initial test results will be used as a baseline guide for comparison with future test results.

The criteria for some preoperative screening have altered in recent years. This is due to changing ideas and practices, especially regarding cost-effectiveness. In the past, virtually every surgical patient underwent a chest X-ray and electrocardiograph (ECG) prior to their operation; NHS trusts now have different criteria and policies for those who require these investigations. Some patients considered fit and well, for example someone about to undergo vasectomy, will probably not have either of these tests performed.

Reflective point

Do you consider that in the past investigations and tests were unnecessarily performed because of traditional practice? Rationalisation of tests and investigations may be as a result of evidence-based medicine. Patient outcomes from surgery may demonstrate no significant increase in risk. Indeed, by altering the patient criteria for investigations there is not only financial saving but a significant reduction in discomfort and stress to patients.

Investigations

When undertaking major surgical procedures, surgeons use a number of investigations to enable them to assess the patient's condition and plan the surgery with greater accuracy. Arteriography/venograms are performed, in general, for patients undergoing some types of neurological, vascular, renal and cardiac surgery. These investigations will outline the blood vessels that have been injected with a radio-opaque dye (X-ray contrast) which are then identified with the use of X-rays. This will help identify the extent of occluded vessels and/or the flow of blood to that particular area.

Radio-opaque dyes are also used to outline other structures. A barium swallow through and enema will outline all of the gastrointestinal tract. This type of information could be of use to the ear, nose and throat and gastrointestinal tract surgeons. Endoscopic retrograde cholangiopancreatography (ERCP) outlines the gall bladder to facilitate assessment for gallstones and

preparation in a cholecystectomy. The use of CT (computerised tomography) and MRI (magnetic resonance imaging) scans is becoming increasingly common. The surgeon can assess, for example, the size of a tumour with the aid of a CT scan, therefore enabling better planning of the surgery. Lung function tests and stress ECGs enable the surgeon to ensure that patients are at their optimum state of health for surgery. With all the tests and investigations now available, the consequent information should enable the surgeon to provide each patient with the options available. Included in this assessment and subsequent explanation to the person, should be a discussion regarding the appropriate surgical technique, which could include keyhole or laser surgery.

The surgical nurse has an important role in clarifying and ensuring that patients understand what has been said to them and the implications of their proposed surgery. The surgical nurse needs to have knowledge of the operation and the pre- and postoperative pattern of events, to clarify to patients what the surgeon proposes, and be able to answer questions that they may have. As an advocate for the person, the surgical nurse should, as far as possible, establish that patients are aware of the alternatives that are available to them. This demonstrates partnership in care and, in particular, patient choice.

PREOPERATIVE PREVENTION OF POSTOPERATIVE COMPLICATIONS

A significant aspect of a surgical nurse's role is to reduce the risk of postoperative complications for patients. Each complication following surgery carries a potential risk to a person's recovery, as well as incurring significant financial costs. Some of the more common complications will be considered, identifying how each may be prevented.

Some of the common postoperative complications are:

- wound infection
- deep vein thrombosis (DVT)
- chest infection
- urinary retention
- urinary tract infection (UTI)
- paralytic ileus
- nausea and vomiting
- joint stiffness
- pressure sores.

Wound infection

This is one of the most common postoperative complications. Preoperative consideration should be given to three physical approaches which may reduce the risk of wound infection: skin preparation, including hair removal, and clean linen.

Freshwater (1992) advocates that organisations need to regularly review their skin preparation and hair removal policies in the light of up-to-date research. Yet, according to Llewellyn-Thomas (1990), although there is a vast literature concerning preoperative skin preparation and reduction of the risk of postoperative wound infection, the evidence is inconclusive. The objective of skin preparation is to reduce the risk of postoperative wound infection by:

- removing dirt and transient microbes from the skin
- reducing the residential microbial count to subpathogenic levels in a short period of time and with the least amount of tissue irritation
- inhibiting rapid rebound growth of microbes.

This may be undertaken by physical cleaning, including hair washing, and/or disinfection. The removal of body hair in the management of risk reduction remains controversial.

The question of whether to remove body hair from an operation site has been debated over time and been the source of much research (Alexander et al 1983, Kovach 1990, Seropain & Reynolds 1971). One side of the debate contends that the potential for infection is increased by removing body hair, either by shaving or depilatory cream. The rationale is that by removing and destroying the natural flora that occurs on the skin's surface the body's defence mechanism is weakened. Depilatory cream also destroys the body's natural barrier by its very nature of being a chemical agent. Nicking the skin when using a razor could offer bacteria the ideal environment for reproducing and therefore the risk of infection is increased. The latter point is particularly important if a preoperative shave is performed the night before surgery. Clipping or trimming with scissors may be preferred (Llewellyn-Thomas 1990).

The other side of the hair removal argument is that by leaving body hair in place it encourages the bacteria surrounding the hair follicles to be introduced to a wound because of their proximity to the operation site. The discussion therefore centres around whether the body's naturally occurring flora is indeed harmful and, if removed, whether this leaves the patient more vulnerable to wound infections (see also Ch. 13).

Wound infection may be reduced by providing clean linen for patients immediately prior to surgery. Once patients have showered or bathed they will have removed many loose skin cells. Clean linen will help to keep them and the wound site area as clean as possible. Some hospitals require patients to wear hair

---

Reflective point

In your experience, is the incidence of wound infections significantly different when body hair has (or has not) been removed? Do other factors seem to be equally significant? A guiding principle from Gauthier et al (1993) is that hair is not removed from the skin unless its presence will compromise the anaesthetic and/or surgical procedure.

---

caps. Scant evidence exists for continuing this traditional practice. However, safety rather than potential risk of infection may support this practice, as long hair could hamper intubation/anaesthesia for some patients.

Deep vein thrombosis (DVT)

This is a complication of reduced mobility which is generally preventable. With advances in surgical techniques and the changing outlook on care, patients are encouraged to mobilise during the preoperative phase and as early as possible postoperatively. Many patients are encouraged to mobilise the day following surgery. There is an ever-increasing range of drugs that can, potentially, derange the clotting mechanism. Patients do not always remember or appreciate that the medication they are taking could be influential in DVT formation. I have had several female patients who, when asked if they take medication, state 'no', yet later in the conversation reveal that they take the contraceptive pill. This is another example of Teasdale's (1993) proposition that not everyone shares the same inference about the same question/information. Many women do not consider the pill to be a medicine because they are healthy. Yet, as a healthy individual taking the pill, there is an increased risk of developing a DVT. Therefore thorough assessment of the individual is crucial.

The current trends in DVT prevention are mini-hep injection (2000 units of heparin subcutaneously twice daily) and/or wearing antiembolic stockings. Best practice for antiembolic stockings is to ensure that the legs are measured correctly, and that the stockings are worn in the correct fashion, i.e. wrinkle-free. Evans (1991) is very damning and suggests that many nurses will 'guess' the size needed by the patient. The skin must be inspected at least once daily. There have been an increasing number of incidents reported where heel necrosis has occurred as a consequence of wearing stockings. I am aware of one instance that is currently being pursued through litigation where a pressure sore developed as a result of antiembolic stockings not being removed and the heel not inspected. Sometimes the fitting and removal of stockings is undertaken by a novice nurse or the health care assistant (HCA). Surgical nurses, therefore, need to ensure that junior and unqualified staff appreciate the significance of their actions. Ultimately patients have a right to safe, ethical care, and the nurse has a legal duty to provide it. The nurse, as part of the partnership relationship with patients, should ensure that the information they receive about the purpose and significance of wearing stockings correctly is understood. The education of patients and their understanding of the rationale for wearing the stockings will help with compliance. Smith (1992) found that nearly 25% of patients thought that they had to wear the stockings to keep their legs warm. If a patient is expected to remain immobile for longer than 24 hours, the use of limb movements to promote venous return is taught by the physiotherapist and reinforced by the nurse. These exercises also help to maintain muscle tone for those who are expected to be immobile long term, for example some patients who have had orthopaedic surgery.

Chest infection

Chest infections which occur postoperatively are another potentially preventable complication of surgery. Those particularly at risk are patients who smoke, the elderly and those who have lung conditions, e.g. asthma. Surgical nurses use their knowledge and experience to make an initial assessment of the patient's respiratory performance, and to notify other members of the multidisciplinary team as necessary (see also Ch. 23).

Preoperative teaching and discussions within the nurse–patient partnership will give patients knowledge of how to help prevent a chest infection. The physiotherapist will play a major part in the teaching and postoperative care of those who are identified as being at risk, either because of their past medical history or because of the type of surgery. Deep breathing and expectoration will help reduce the risk of developing a chest infection as a consequence of the anaesthetic. Early mobilisation plays a key role in reducing the risk of occurrence. Thoracic and cardiac surgery have special risks of chest infection because patients may be more reluctant to inspire deeply as a result of their surgery and the subsequent pain caused when they cough. It also has to be remembered that a patient who is drowsy because of opiate analgesia could have a compromised respiratory rate. In addition patients have to remain hydrated, ensuring that secretions or phlegm are moist and therefore more easily expectorated (see also Ch. 23).

Urinary retention

As a postoperative complication, urinary retention is not usually predictable unless the patient has had previous surgery and experienced a similar problem. Patients who have been admitted for hernia repair, bowel or gynaecological surgery are more at risk because of the potential for touching or handling the bladder during the operative procedure.

Urinary tract infection (UTI)

This is usually a consequence of having a urinary catheter inserted. Gould (1994) states that 44% of catheterised patients develop bacteriuria within 72 hours. The patient needs to be informed prior to surgery that a urinary catheter will be inserted, otherwise this could be considered an assault on the person. The practitioner has to ensure that the person understands what a urinary catheter is and why it may be necessary. If the patient is catheterised, the procedure for keeping the catheter and perineum clean also needs to be explained. Patients may develop a urinary tract infection as a consequence of a reduced fluid intake and/or because they have been nil by mouth. Patients who are susceptible to cystitis could benefit from intravenous hydration in the immediate pre- and postoperative period to try to prevent this occurring. Refer to Chapter 26 for further information on fluid and electrolyte balance.

Paralytic ileus

This is a potential complication of surgery involving the bowel. Paralytic ileus (or adynamic ileus) occurs because the bowel has been handled during surgery; consequently peristalsis ceases as the bowel is recovering from the associated trauma. A paralytic ileus, however, can also occur as a result of anaesthetic agents. It is important for patients to be aware that they will be asked about bowel functions and flatus postoperatively, and whether they are feeling sick or nauseous.

Nausea and vomiting

Postoperative nausea and vomiting can cause patients much anxiety, especially if they have had a previous bad experience which they attribute to an anaesthetic. If nausea and vomiting are identified as problems prior to surgery, the anaesthetist should be informed and an anti-emetic should be included with the pre-medication. Excess vomiting following surgery can disturb the patient's electrolyte balance creating the potential for further postoperative complications. Vomiting also exerts excessive pressure on the wound.

Joint stiffness

Patients who, it is anticipated, will be immobile for a substantial period of time postoperatively or have known joint problems will need to be assessed and shown exercises by the physiotherapist to help reduce joint stiffness. The nurse will reinforce the exercises and techniques that have been agreed by the patient and the physiotherapist, stressing their significance and encouraging patients to participate in their own care.

Pressure sores

These are another potentially avoidable complication of bed rest and decreased mobility. In many areas pressure sores should be a diminishing problem as surgical patients are often day cases or are mobilised within 24 hours of surgery. Patients who are more prone to the development of pressure sores include:

- those who are in a poor state of health before they reach hospital
- older people and those with reduced mobility in the community
- those who have a prolonged wait lying on a hard trolley in the accident and emergency department without being moved.

Tissue viability assessment on admission by the nurse is essential. The use of a recognised tool, e.g. Waterlow, Norton or Lowthian score (Flanagan 1995), to aid pressure sore risk assessment should enable the nurse to intervene before problems develop, and help the prevention of a pressure sore by the use of appropriate pressure-relieving devices. An explanation to patients about the need to relieve pressure from specific points and their participation in the techniques employed is important. This should include those areas not always evident to the patient, e.g. ears, knees and scapular areas.

Reflective point

Which is the most appropriate pressure sore risk assessment tool for your area? Do you think that assessment scores help prevent or minimise pressure sores?

It is now considered to be traumatic to the skin if patients are turned from side to side to relieve their sacral pressure points. The most effective way to relieve pressure is by turning the patient by 30 degrees (Preston 1988). This prevents the person's body weight being transferred through the relatively small surface area over the hip/pelvis area, transferring it to the larger buttock area instead. The notion of providing a change of position every 2 hours is historical. There is no scientific evidence to support the 2-hourly turn. It is simply the length of time that it took the attendants, in one military ward, to turn all of the patients. Therefore patients will require an individualised plan of care to minimise pressure sore development.

It is well recognised that assessment, prevention and early detection will help reduce the incidence of pressure sores. Pressure sores are very painful, prolong the period of stay in hospital and are, therefore, extremely costly. Sharing information with patients regarding pressure area care and prevention of pressure sores puts them in a better position to alert the nurse at an early stage to a potential problem. More experienced surgical nurses will often subconsciously take note of pressure areas every time they provide care for patients.

The concept of individualised patient care is especially applicable to pressure area care. Once the initial assessment has been undertaken, preferably using a well-researched and documented tool, the patient's condition needs to be reassessed regularly. In the preoperative phase, therefore, individuals who are at risk of developing pressure sores because of underlying pathologies or reduced mobility, or because of the predicted time that they will be immobilised postoperatively, may require a very different regime of care. Pressure sores are not only confined to the areas traditionally considered, e.g. sacrum, heels, elbows, etc. Specialist surgery and the resultant frames, plasters, braces and other devices that patients have to endure, all carry their own risks of pressure-related problems. Plaster jackets, boots and cylinders, ill-fitting splints and braces will potentially cause pressure sores and necrosis of tissue if they are not adequately padded and fitted. The patient should be made aware of tissue viability problems and be asked to alert the nurse at the earliest opportunity.

As a final yet most important point to consider, the peripheral cannula that many patients have inserted is also a potential source of pressure. When administering intravenous drugs the top port of the cannula is frequently used. The pressure exerted on the syringe plunger can cause tissue damage, especially if the cannula is secured with a restrictive dressing or bandage.

IMMEDIATE PERIOPERATIVE CARE

Immediate perioperative care includes ongoing physical care which may seem routine to the experienced surgical nurse. Psychological support is required for this anxiety-provoking time, which may include skin and/or bowel preparations, being nil by mouth, removal of personal possessions/prostheses, cannulation. The patient feels vulnerable and is potentially powerless.

At this stage much of the preparation will have been completed. For example, some bowel preparations commence 48 hours preoperatively. (Much bowel preparation is now commenced in the patient's home before admission). In some instances, especially if a patient has a history of allergies, an iodine patch test will be undertaken. The test area will be inspected prior to surgery to ensure that the patient is not allergic to the iodine.

On the day of surgery the HCA or a novice nurse may assist the patient to prepare for surgery, helping with personal hygiene and preparing the bed area.

Reflective point

Patients often express anxieties and concerns in the period immediately prior to surgery. How may experienced surgical nurses prioritise their time to ensure that they are able to provide support?

The nurse is responsible for ensuring that patients are physically and psychologically prepared for surgery, making certain that people, who will be at their most vulnerable, will be as safe as possible whilst undergoing a general anaesthetic (or sedated if having surgery under a local or epidural anaesthetic).

Nil by mouth

Part of the preparation for all surgery is to ensure that the stomach's contents are at a minimum (except in extreme emergency situations when gastric contents are aspirated). The period of time that a patient needs to be nil by mouth has been the source of great debate. It has been suggested that 4–6 hours is a safe time since the last ingestion of food or drink (Hung 1992, Torrance 1991).

However, Chapman (1996) concludes from a search of current literature that gastric volume and pH are independent of a fluid fast beyond 2 hours, implying that patients can be offered fluids up to 2 hours preoperatively. Indeed, an oral premedication with water is often administered 1 hour prior to surgery. Yet, in reality, it is still not uncommon for a patient to be without fluid for up to 12 hours. In Chapman's (1996) research participants recorded a mean fasting time of 11 hours. This can be particularly dangerous for the elderly and children, who will become dehydrated more quickly than the average adult.

Some hospitals have protocols identifying when fluids should be withheld and when an intravenous infusion should be commenced if the period of fasting has been exceeded. Chapman (1996) concludes that the fear of a change in the order of an operating list was a major contributing factor to the adoption of routine practices which prolonged fasting times and inhibited staff from offering patients fluids 2–3 hours preoperatively.

Equally, emergency patients may be dehydrated, especially if they are in delayed shock. The surgical nurse needs to be aware of and observe for the signs of dehydration, offer mouth care to cleanse and freshen the mouth, ensure that patients understand the significance of being nil by mouth and do not become 'desperate' and eat or drink through a lack of understanding.

An illustration of such an incident happened to a non-nursing colleague recently who was admitted to a surgical ward at 7 p.m., after 4 hours in casualty, for an evacuation of retained products of conception following a miscarriage. There were three other ladies who were to undergo the same operation. One, who had been waiting for 3 hours in the ward, had a drink because she had been told not to eat anything but assumed it was all right to drink, especially as she had had no fluids since breakfast time. The list, therefore, had to be delayed for a further 4 hours to ensure that this lady was 'safe' to undergo an anaesthetic. The anaesthetist and houseman were too busy to commence an infusion so in my colleague's case it was nearly 21 hours before she was able to have fluids again.

Reflective point

We need to question why periods of fasting have not decreased with our level of knowledge about gastric emptying. How many patients in your area are put at risk because of extended periods of fluid deprivation prior to surgery? How can this situation be changed?

Cannulation

Many patients who undergo surgery will require a cannula to be inserted. For a highly anxious patient the nurse should obtain a local anaesthetic cream, which when applied and allowed to become effective, reduces the pain and possible trauma of cannula insertion. If a patient has a history of poor venous access, a glycerine trinitrate (GTN) patch may be prescribed to help dilate the blood vessels, making cannulation easier for the anaesthetist and less traumatic for the patient. Obviously, the person's medical history must indicate no contraindications to the use of GTN.

Preoperative checks and premedication

The standard checks performed by the nurse are designed to minimise mistakes and delays in surgery. It is essential that the correct patient goes to the correct theatre for the correct operation on the correct site at the correct time. Protocols and procedures vary from trust to trust and organisation to organisation, but the overriding principle is that of patient safety. Name bands are mandatory. However, the majority of patients no longer have a premedication. Some surgeons and anaesthetists, though, still prescribe a premedication, particularly for major surgery or if the person is known to experience acute postoperative nausea. Additionally, some premedications only consist of prophylactic antibiotic cover, not the relaxing and secretion-drying drugs that patients may expect. In some instances, when a person is very anxious, the nurse should discuss with the patient and anaesthetist if a sedative would be appropriate.

An anaesthetist colleague informed me that the reduced use of premedications is because patients are being considered on a far more individual basis, especially as many are discharged earlier when premedication agents can still be active. The use of premedication in day surgery is kept to a minimum because this will prolong the period of stay for a patient within the unit, and therefore has cost implications. If a sedative is prescribed as a premedication, patients may become disoriented, and must therefore be warned to stay in bed and told to summon help with a nurse call button if they require anything, even to go to the toilet. In place of a sedative premedication it is worthwhile exploring whether complementary therapies, such as burning essential oils, could be used to produce a relaxed atmosphere (Jackson 1987).

Reflective point

Does your NHS trust/organisation have a complementary therapy policy? Do surgical nurses use complementary therapies to help reduce anxiety and tension in patients, especially in the immediate preoperative phase?

Other anxiety-reducing approaches include enabling patients to retain their glasses and hearing aids (if they so wish) until they undergo the anaesthetic process. When visually impaired patients have their glasses removed they could become disoriented and suffer sensory deprivation. This equally applies to those who have removed their hearing aid and cannot hear what is going on around them or respond to the inevitable questions that they will be asked in the anaesthetic room. It can be more difficult for patients to retain their contact lenses as they may not be efficient in removing them once they have been sedated.

When considering individuality in the immediate perioperative stage, the issue of wigs, hairpieces, jewellery, dentures and prostheses is also raised. If patients are more comfortable and relaxed with their body image intact, this should be respected, as long as they are aware that the item will have to be removed in the anaesthetic room (but will be returned at the earliest possible time). Music therapy, e.g. a Walkman, could also accompany the patient to theatre. However, false nails and eyelashes must have been previously removed. A record may be kept of items to ensure that they are returned to their rightful owner.

Patients are also requested to remove make-up and nail varnish for safety reasons. The significance of being able to observe true skin colour and nail beds should be clearly explained. Patients are requested to remove all jewellery, primarily so that it does not act as a source of infection or get lost. If metal is left on the patient it can cause burns if diathermy is used during the operation. For this reason a patient who does not wish to remove a wedding band should have it covered with tape.

Escorting patients to the operating theatre

Transport to the operating theatre can be an extremely anxious time for patients. In an ideal world, they would be escorted to the theatre/anaesthetic room by their named nurse, affording each person continuity and familiarity of personnel. In some areas, theatre staff come to collect the patients from the ward and take them to the bed waiting area. This means that the ward staff do not have to spend long periods away from the ward escorting patients. However, the patients will not have met their escort unless they received a preoperative visit from the theatre nurse.

It should be recognised that there is greater potential for a breakdown in communications if ward staff do not escort patients to the operating theatre. The escort staff, unlike the ward nurse, are less familiar with the patients and problems can occur, particularly in the anaesthetic room, with the potential for oversight regarding removal of dentures, hearing aids, prostheses, etc. Some ward policies advocate continuity of care; their own staff escort patients to the theatre.

Consideration should be given to the issue of whether HCAs (health care assistants) should be trained to accompany patients to theatre. There may be both psychological and financial benefits for training a ward-based HCA to escort a patient to the theatre. The outcome should be continuity and familiarity for the patient, rather than the alternative option which is for a trained nurse to come from outside the ward environment to act as an escort. When I have discussed transportation to theatre with patients, their overall opinion seemed to be that familiarity with the escort person was reassuring – although the escort might not be their named nurse. A note of concern is that many members of theatre staff are not identifiable by name or even grade. Having been a patient too, it is considerate to know the name of the person who is caring for you.

Transportation to the operating theatre

Many patients are transported to the theatre on their own beds and re-awaken on the same bed. Once on the journey to the theatre, it used to be the practice for patients to lie supine. However, not knowing where you are going can be disorienting, especially with only strip lights flashing past your eyes. Sensory deprivation and disorientation are increased if you are lying flat on your back, possibly adding to anxiety and stress. Therefore it is suggested that, whenever possible, patients have their backrest out so that they have a better view of their journey, whether they are travelling on a bed or a trolley.

> **Reflective point**
>
> During the journey to the theatre there can be an issue of who has control of the patient. I have witnessed, on numerous occasions, the porters racing off at speed leaving the escorting nurse behind. Who is in charge of the situation and how does this affect the patient? Some patients now walk to theatres; would this be an appropriate option for some of your patients?

Reception in the operating theatre complex

Different schemes have been developed to facilitate the smooth running of a theatre suite, ensuring that the next patient is ready and available for the anaesthetist and surgeon. One scheme that I am familiar with is patient bed wait. The patients are collected by theatre staff or escorted to the bed wait area by ward staff; here they are 'handed over' to the bed wait reception staff and then taken to the anaesthetic room when the anaesthetist is ready to receive them. This system has many positive aspects for the effective and efficient organisation of the theatre complex but has distinct disadvantages for the patient. There will be at least two separate handovers of the person's details which leads to repetition of information.

> **Reflective point**
>
> Acknowledging that safety checks are vital, how many times should we expect patients to answer repetitive questions, e.g. regarding allergies, their address, or what operation they are going to have performed?

In the bed wait area Walkmans may be provided for patients to listen to music, if they so wish. Moss (1988) and Gaberson (1995) suggest that music can help reduce preoperative anxiety. The alternative to bed wait is for the surgical nurse to escort patients to the theatre complex, into the anaesthetic room and stay with them until they are unconscious. However, this can be very time-consuming and may not be the most effective use of costly nursing time, but it must be argued that this system enhances the quality of patient continuity of care.

CONCLUSION

The nurse is a key player in the surgical experience of patients in the preoperative period. The nurse enables patients to adapt to their new situation and environment. The use of a recognised nursing model, e.g. Roy (1976), can help to structure the plan of care for the patient, enable a partnership to evolve, and enhance holistic care. Many ways of knowing, including spiritual care, should be incorporated into the advancement of the art and science of surgical nursing practice. To enhance the quality of care provided, the nurse needs to be enabled to reflect on and critically review clinical practice. The use of research to underpin/evaluate practice should shape surgical nursing for the future. Surgical nurses must value, share and advance their knowledge with patients, and within the nursing and interprofessional team. Having to undergo surgery is one of the most stressful events in a person's life. The significance of the nurse's knowledge and skill in providing a safe and meaningful pre-operative experience for the surgical patient should *never* be underestimated.

REFERENCES

Abbott, D, Glenn E 1994 Patient education in a pre-admission clinic. Surgical Nurse 7(2): 5–8

Alexander J W, Fischer J E, Boyajian M, Palmquist J, Morris M J 1983 The influence of hair removal methods on wound infections. Archives of Surgery 118(Mar): 347–351

Andrews H A, Roy C 1991 Essentials of the Roy Adaptation model. In: Roy, C, Andrews H A The Roy Adaptation model: the definitive statement. Appleton and Lange, Norwalk

Ashworth P D, Longmate M A, Morrison P 1992 Patient participation: its meaning and significance in the context of caring. Journal of Advanced Nursing 17: 1430–1439

Atkinson R L, Atkinson R C, Smith E E, Hilgard E R 1993 Introduction to psychology 11th edn. Harcourt Brace Jovanovich, San Diego

Baldwin C 1993 Welcome visitor. Nursing Times 89(27 Jan): 44–46

Bayntun-Lees D 1992 Reviewing the nurse–patient partnership. Nursing Standard 6(8 July): 36–39

Bellman L 1994 Principles of educating patients. Surgical Nurse 7(1): 7–10

Benner P 1984 From novice to expert: excellence and power in clinical practice. Addison-Wesley, Menlo Park

Boore J 1975 Prescription for recovery. RCN, London

Brown J, Simpson L 1994 Co-ordinating patient care: putting principles into practice. North Allerton NHS Trust, North Allerton

Cahill J 1996 Patient participation: a concept analysis. Journal of Advanced Nursing 24: 561–571

Chapman A 1996 Current theory and practice: a study into pre-operative fasting. Nursing Standard 10(24 Jan): 33–36

Coulter A 1997 Partnerships with patients: the pros and cons of shared clinical decision-making. Journal of Health Service Research Policy 2(2): 112–121

Cox G 1994 Applying the model III. In: Akinsanya J, Cox G, Crouch C, Fletcher L The Roy Adaptation model: model in action. Macmillan, Basingstoke

Cupples S 1991 Effects of timing and reinforcement of pre-operative education on knowledge and recovery of patients having coronary artery bypass graft surgery. Heart and Lung 61: 654–660

Department of Health (DoH) 1991 The patient's charter. HMSO, London

Department of Health (DoH) 1994 Working in partnership: report of the mental health nursing review team. HMSO, London

Department of Health (DoH) 1995 The patient's charter and you. HMSO, London

Evans A 1991 Sensible stockings. Nursing Times 87(18/25 Dec): 40–41

Flanagan M 1995 Who is at risk of a pressure sore? Professional Nurse 10(5): 305–308

Freshwater D 1992 Preoperative preparation of skin – a review of the literature. Surgical Nurse 5(5): 6–10

Gaberson K B 1995 The effect of humorous and musical distraction on preoperative anxiety. Association of Operating Room Nurses Journal 62(5): 784–791

Gauthier D K, O'Fallon P T, Coppage D 1993 Clean vs sterile surgical preparation kits: cost, safety, effectiveness. Association of Operating Room Nurses Journal 58(3): 486–495

Gould D 1994 Keeping on tract. Nursing Times 90(5 Oct): 58–64

Hayward J 1978 Information: a prescription against pain. RCN, London

Hinchliff S, Montague S 1991 Physiology for nursing practice. Baillière Tindall, London

Humphris P 1997 Patient partnership strategy. Health Service Manager Briefing 20: 4–5

Hung P 1992 Pre-operative fasting. Nursing Times 88(25 Nov): 57–60

Jackson J 1987 Aromatherapy. Dorling Kindersley, London

Johnson S 1994 Patient focused care without the upheaval. Nursing Standard 8(13 Apr): 20–22

Kovach T 1990 Nip it in the bud. Today's Operating Room Nurse 12(9): 23–26

Llewellyn-Thomas A 1990 Preoperative skin preparation. Surgical Nurse 3(2): 24–26

Loughlin L 1993 Involving patients in the planning and delivery of care: working towards a common goal. Journal of Interprofessional Care 7(2): 161–166

Lowery M 1995 Knowledge that reduces anxiety: creating patient information leaflets. Professional Nurse 10(5): 318–320

Malby R 1992 Discharge planning. Surgical Nurse 5(1): 4–8

Marriner-Tomey A 1994 Nursing theorists and their work, 3rd edn. C V Mosby, St Louis

Mitchell M 1994 Preoperative and postoperative psychological nursing care. Surgical Nurse 7(3): 22–25

Moss V A 1988 Music and the surgical patient. Association of Operating Room Nurses Journal 48(1): 64–68

Nelson S 1995 Pre-admission clinics for thoracic surgery. Nursing Times 91(12 Apr): 29–31

NHS Executive 1996 Patient partnership: building collaborative strategy. Department of Health. NHS Executive Quality and Consumers Branch, London

Nolan P, Crawford P 1997 Towards a rhetoric of spirituality in mental health care. Journal of Advanced Nursing 26: 289–294

Patients Association 1996 Patients' voices. Patients Association, London, Autumn no. 1

Preston K 1988 Positioning for comfort and pressure relief: the 30 degree alternative. Care – Science and Practice 6(4): 116–119

Riches T, Stead L, Espie C 1994 Introducing anticipated recovery pathways: a teaching hospital experience. International Journal of Health Care Quality Assurance 7(5) 21–24

Roy C 1976 Introduction to nursing: an adaptation model. Prentice Hall, Englewood Cliffs

Roy C, McLeod D 1981 Theory of the person as an adaptive system. In: Roy C, Roberts S L (eds) Theory construction in nursing: an adaptive model. Prentice Hall, Englewood Cliffs

Savill R, Bartholomew J 1994 Planning better discharges. Journal of Community Nursing 8(3): 10–14

Seropain R, Reynolds B M 1971 Wound infections after preoperative depilatory versus razor preparation. American Journal of Surgery 121(Mar): 251–254

Smith J 1997 Relaunch of The Patients' Association: will it help to empower patients? Editorial, Journal of Advanced Nursing 26: 220

Smith P 1992 Compression hosiery in a surgical unit. Nursing Standard 6(26 Aug): 25–28

Teasdale K 1993 Information and anxiety: a critical reappraisal. Journal of Advanced Nursing 18: 1125–1132

Torrance C 1991 Preoperative nutrition, fasting and the surgical patient. Surgical Nurse 4(4): 4–8

United Kingdom Central Council for Nursing, Midwifery and Health Visiting (UKCC) 1992 Code of professional conduct. UKCC, London

Walsh M 1997 Will critical pathways replace the nursing process? Nursing Standard 17(11): 39–42

Webb R A 1995 Preoperative visiting from the perspective of the theatre nurse. British Journal of Nursing 4(16): 919–925

Wiffin A 1995 An assessment of procedures. Nursing Times 91(12 July): 31–32

FURTHER READING

Akinsanya J, Cox G, Crouch C, Fletcher L 1994 The Roy Adaptation model in action. Macmillan, Basingstoke

Bates J 1994 Reducing fast times in paediatric day surgery. Nursing Times 90(30 Nov): 38–39

Bridge C, Nelson S 1994 A deficit in care: the educational needs of thoracic patients. Professional Nurse 10(1): 8–13

Christensen J 1993 Nursing partnership: a model for nursing practice. Churchill Livingstone, Edinburgh

Dalayon A P 1994 Components of preoperative patient teaching in Kuwait. Journal of Advanced Nursing 19(3): 537–542

Jarrett N, Payne S 1995 A selective review of the literature on nurse–patient communication: has the patient's contribution been neglected? Journal of Advanced Nursing 22(1): 72–78

Jewell S E 1994 Patient participation: what does it mean to nurses? Journal of Advanced Nursing 19(3): 433–438

Johnson S 1995 Pathway to the heart of care quality. Nursing Management 1(8): 26–27

Johnson-Lutjens L R 1991 Callista Roy: an adaptation model. Sage, Newbury Park

King C 1994 Documentation and discharge planning for elderly patients. Nursing Times 90(18 May): 31–33

Moran S 1995 Quality indicators for patient information in short stay units. Nursing Times 91(25 Jan): 37–40

Moshy R E, Phillips C A 1989 From ward to X-ray: a practical guide. Austen Cornish, London

Oakley K 1988 A nurse's guide to radiological procedures. Edward Arnold, London

Pearson A, Vaughan B, Fitzgerald M 1996 Nursing models for practice, 2nd edn. Butterworth Heinemann, Oxford

Radcliff S 1993 Preoperative information: the role of the ward nurse British Journal of Nursing 2(6): 305–309

Rayfield J 1995 Focus on needs. Nursing Times 91(23 Aug): 42–43

Reihl J P, Roy C (eds) 1980 Conceptual models for nursing practice, 2nd edn. Appleton-Century-Crofts, New York

Roy C, Andrews H A 1991 The Roy Adaptation model: the definitive statement. Appleton-Lange, Norwalk

Ryan A 1994 Improving discharge planning. Nursing Times 90(18 May): 33–34

Trevelyan J 1993 Massage. Nursing Times 89(12 May): 45–47

Trevelyan J 1996 A true complement: a Nursing Times survey on complementary therapies. Nursing Times 92(31 Jan): 42–43

Walsh M, Ford P 1989 Nursing rituals, research and rational actions. Butterworth-Heinemann, Oxford

21

Perspectives on intraoperative care

Deena Graham

AIMS

This chapter aims to begin a wider debate so as to facilitate depth, insight and understanding of the role of the nurse in providing intraoperative care in the operating department.

The discussion will concentrate on:

- the role of nursing in the light of contemporary nursing practice
- the nurse's role in the domain of the diagnostic and monitoring function as described by Benner (1984) in relation to patients being treated in the operating department
- critical reflection specifically on the aspect of providing individualised care for the ever-increasing number of patients that are now being treated under local anaesthetic within main theatres.

The section relating to critical reflection has been structured in a manner to help facilitate nurses working in the operating department through the process of reflection and applying nursing knowledge to practice. Johns' model of guided reflection (1995) will be used to facilitate this process, and Carper's ways of knowing (1978) will then be used to consider the knowledge used, or that could have been used, to inform nursing practice.

There are many and varied texts which refer to the technical and safety aspects of the nurse's role; however, the aim of this chapter is to discuss nursing practice issues within the operating department setting and so emphasis will not be placed on these aspects.

CURRENT PERSPECTIVES AND APPLICATION TO NURSING

Nursing in the operating department is currently facing the challenge of having been dominated for too long by the medical model of practice and the philosophical challenges of mind–body dualism (Dein 1994). Contemporary nursing has identified itself as a humanistic profession with a philosophy which embraces individualism, holism, autonomy, advocacy and empowerment as necessary aspects of patient care. The allegiance of nursing is to value the individual and the complex meaning within which the individual experiences illness (Munhall 1994, Oiler 1982). This holistic view of the person respects the individual as a being for whom all things have value and significance (see also Ch. 7).

According to Brykczynska (1995), current nursing practice is based on the philosophy of humanistic values. These include such aspects as respect for the person, freedom of choice and valuing the integrity of each individual. Redfern (1996) would concur with this view, claiming that holistic individualised care is based on the concept of treating each patient as an individual. Associated with this claim is the assertion that individualised care needs to be acknowledged through individual practice. This argument is taken further, as it is also stated that there is an underlying assumption that the practice of providing individualised care is equal to the provision of high-quality care.

On the other hand, Butterworth (1996) would dispute this claim, asserting that there is little evidence to support the view that individualised care is equal to good nursing care. It is argued that patients and carers are not interested in the provision of individualised care, but that they seek a contact person who can provide understandable, up-to-date and relevant information. Accordingly, it could be maintained that this view suggests that it does not matter who undertakes task provisions, provided that they are safe and have been trained for the task (Ellis 1992). Butterworth also states that individualised care that is 'good enough' may be all that can be achieved in some areas such as short-stay and fast-turnover settings. In defining care that is 'good enough' the following attributes are mentioned: safe and attentive care, appropriate dignity, appropriate information-giving and a short period of restful recuperation. Consequently, it is argued that in such areas as the operating department, the search for meaningful and individual relationships may be unnecessary and wasteful in terms of time and resources. However, who is to define 'good enough' and appropriate care in the operating department, if not the nurses who are providing that care? As professionals, can we justify what could be argued to be second class care just because the patient's stay in the care environment is limited?

Meleis (1991) states that the domain of nursing has both theoretical and practical boundaries and encompasses knowledge of practice that is based on philosophy, common sense and research findings. The art of nursing has been described as humanistic with interaction at its core, enabling the nurse to understand the meanings and experiences of the patient. Nursing has developed and encouraged this role in nursing by expressing the need for the nurse to develop skills in assessing, planning, implementing and evaluating the holistic needs of the patient. This represents a positive person-centred application to care provision, firmly rooted in the domain of nursing, and involves much more than the biomedical approach to care.

That is not to say that there is no place in nursing practice for scientific medical research, but instead to place the evidence used in practice into the context of what nurses are trying to achieve. Therefore, there has been a shift in nursing away from the medical model of care and task allocation to a more holistic, individual and person-centred approach to caregiving (Playle 1995, Ramos 1992). The central philosophy of this paradigm shift has been the idea that each person has unique individual needs (Atkinson & Murphy 1993). In the light of contemporary nursing practice, this is the area that seems to create the most difficulty for nurses who practise in the operating department. As practitioners they believe in and aspire to the philosophy but find it very difficult to emulate in the reality of day-to-day practice.

The interventions that take place in the operating department are often complicated and the complexity of these procedures requires the nurse to work in collaboration within a wide and varied multidisciplinary team. However, there is also a clear independent role for nurses in providing nursing care. Benner (1984), in describing the domains of nursing, describes the domain of diagnostic and monitoring functions. It is asserted that these functions are central to the nurse's role and that this is a major domain of nursing practice. In the operating department the nurse's careful monitoring and early detection of problems is the first line of defence for patients. This is pertinent whether the patient is having a procedure under local anaesthetic or general anaesthetic, and is applicable to nurses working in the role of anaesthetic nurse, circulating nurse, scrub nurse or recovery nurse.

In the operating department this domain of practice can be interpreted as:

- understanding the particular demands and experiences of technical intervention
- anticipating patient care needs, identifying potential problems and observing for signs of patient deterioration
- the documentation of significant changes in the patient's condition.

Understanding the particular demands and experiences of technical interventions

The main contention levelled against nurses practising in the operating department is that they work in a framework that is predominately structured around the medical model of nursing. The work in the department is seen as task-oriented and predominately focused on getting the list done. Patients are part of a production line of tasks that have to be completed before the end of the list (Williams 1997). This perception is not enhanced by views such as those of Carrington (1991) who described the function of the theatre nurse as a person with complex technical knowledge which is required in the care and maintenance of instruments. Carrington acknowledges that the nurse has advanced technical expertise which is necessary for the rotation of stocks and supplies and the selection of appropriate instruments and sutures. Carrington also contends that part of the nurse's role is to maintain a calm and mature attitude when the surgeon encounters periods of stress. It is important that the nurse is able to concentrate and anticipate needs during long operations. Taking the technical aspects of the role further, Curry & Poole (1991) would argue that the next logical step for nurses working in the operating department is to perform surgery as a surgeon's assistant. This is seen as progression of the nurse's role towards advanced practice.

There is no doubt that in order to practise as a skilful competent nurse within the operating department, the nurse needs to develop technical skills, manual dexterity and in-depth knowledge of the anatomical and mechanical aspects of particular types of surgery. During any surgical procedure, patients may experience a wide variety of responses, e.g. hypothermia, risk of development of pressure sores or hyperextension of limbs. The nurse needs to be able to understand and interpret these responses and to respond quickly, efficiently and appropriately. It is important that the technique of the surgical procedure does not detract from the provision of individualised care. Intraoperative care must move towards personalising the operative procedure and giving attention to the principle of respect for persons (Williams 1997). However, Wicker (1987) claims that the patient's care needs are often not assessed and the nursing care received in the operating department still rotates around operations and work routines not individualised care.

Baxter (1987) attributes the provision of physical care, psychological support and a safe environment as areas of nursing that are specific to theatre nursing practice. The role has also been defined as assessing, planning, implementing and evaluating patient care. To assess the patient and plan appropriate care, it is necessary for theatre nurses to collect data with the patient, thereby assessing the patient's psychological as well as physical needs. (See Ch. 14 for the range of approaches for giving patients information.)

The National Association of Theatre Nurses (1991) put forward the perspective that theatre nurses should set standards of care, ensure a systematic approach to care and maintain continuity of that care. An integral part of the nurse's role is to coordinate patient care and lead and supervise nursing practice.

In understanding the particular demands and experiences of technical interventions for patient care, theatre nurses have a great deal of experience but may not have clarified that experience in terms of nursing knowledge. The nurse's role involves coordinating and managing a wide range of activities before, during and after the surgical procedure. This includes appropriately preparing the physical environment, transferring and positioning the patient, ensuring that there are no breaks in aseptic technique and maintaining a safe physical as well as psychological environment for each patient. The skill that is inherent in expert operating department practice is found in those individual practitioners who carry out these activities and interventions for patients in an individual holistic manner. These practitioners can be observed continually assessing the situation, and the environment, in order to respond in the most appropriate way to provide care that is safe for the individual patient. Making these types of judgement is crucial to nursing practice. However, such practitioners often have difficulty understanding and explaining how they can improve patient care and decrease the fragmentation of care delivery (Hodson 1998).

It is well known among nurse practitioners that the most critical person in the operating theatre when there is a crisis is the nurse who has the skill, knowledge and competence to interpret the situation, make nursing judgements and act promptly and appropriately. The challenge for theatre nurses is to begin to recognise and draw out the nursing knowledge that is being used in these situations and explain their actions in terms of excellence in nursing practice, not just as a reaction to a medical model of practice. Identifying a knowledge base that defines nursing in this complex area of practice needs to be developed through the systematic study of the purpose and substance of nursing in the operating department. Knowledge used in practice that needs to be defined in terms of the art and science of nursing is identified in Box 21.1.

Box 21.1 Knowledge used in practice that needs to be defined in terms of the art and science of nursing

- Pharmacology
- Anatomy and physiology
- Airway management
- Microbiology
- Anaesthesia
- Surgical procedures
- Physics and electronics
- Instrumentation
- Gas laws
- Wound healing
- Hazards in the operating department

Reflective point

How can we reconstruct the knowledge which underpins our actions in the domain of diagnosing and monitoring to define nursing in the operating department and advance nursing practice?

Anticipating patient care needs, problems breakdown and deterioration

Much of the debate about assessing and anticipating the patient's needs has been expressed in Chapter 14. However, in trying to make explicit the nurse's role and function in the intraoperative period it is important to further examine why assessing individual need is so important. Benner (1984) states that all members of the multidisciplinary team have a responsibility to present their own perspectives on the assessment process and this is particularly important in the operating department.

The process of identifying and making nursing diagnosis is crucial to acknowledging the vital role of nursing within the multidisciplinary team. The information gained from the assessment process should have a direct influence on the care planned for patients in terms of their well-being and safety throughout the surgical procedure. By identifying patient needs, nurses in the operating department are able to quantify what nursing actions will be needed to prevent problems occurring during the operative procedure. They can then decide on appropriate interventions and implement them, documenting the patient's responses and evaluating the outcomes.

On a wider scale, the operating department is well recognised as an area where risk management is important in terms of providing care which is safe and legally sound (NATN 1995). In providing appropriate

care it is important that needs are assessed and the practices that are being carried out are acceptable practices that are continually monitored and reviewed (NATN 1994). By carefully thinking through and planning care for patients before they arrive in the department, nurses will be aware of the issues which may potentially lead to problems and deterioration in the patient's care. Areas of care that need specific monitoring on a regular basis are outlined in Box 21.2.

The documentation of significant changes in the patient's condition

The nurse is responsible for documenting the nursing care that the patient has received during the intraoperative period. It is important to document and evaluate the care given in order to make a judgement about its worth or effectiveness (UKCC 1993). Good nursing records are more than just documentation of facts, they are a record which shows the diagnosis of nursing care and a response to the care that has been given.

The documentation of care given is important in forming a clear and continuous record of information for the staff in the recovery area and in the wards. Communication through clear, well-written records is just as important as any other kind of communication. Moreover, Hale et al (1997) argue that often nursing documentation does not meet this clinical standard of providing a good chain of communication.

Often in theatres, care plans are standardised and superficial and do not deal with identified individual problems. This tick-list, task-oriented approach to care is often justified as using precious time resourcefully. However, the UKCC (1993) view careful record-keeping as an integral part of care provision, not

---

Box 21.2 Areas of care that need specific monitoring on a regular basis

- Specific client groups – especially older adults
- Type of anaesthetic to be administered
- Level of anxiety
- Mobility – range of movement and/or physical handicap
- Patient transfer
- Correct positioning
- Awareness of prosthetic devices
- Risk of pressure sore development
- Infection control
- Wound management – proposed incision site
- Current tubes, drains, catheters, etc.
- Known allergies

something separate and distant. Good patient care records are an essential component of good nursing practice and accurate documentation is seen as vital in order to record changes in the patient's progress during the intraoperative period and to document the nursing actions taken.

In terms of identifying nursing actions and developing nursing knowledge in the intraoperative phase, accurate documentation and evaluation enable nurses to demonstrate a level of nursing knowledge and accountability in practice. There is a need for nurses in the operating department to clearly evaluate the effectiveness of the nursing care given and, without appropriate documentation of nursing interventions, evaluation cannot take place. In order for it to take place, nurses working in the operating department must explicitly define and explain the nursing actions that have been undertaken; this includes assessment, nursing diagnosis and the implementation of care. True evaluation of care requires a conscious effort on the part of the nurse and needs to be based on and reflect the individual care plan for the patient (Hale et al 1997).

THE NATURE OF REFLECTION AND ITS APPLICATION TO OPERATING DEPARTMENT PRACTICE

Reflection has been described as an important activity which enables people to recapture an experience, think about it and evaluate it (Boud et al 1985). Therefore reflection can be defined as an active process of exploration and discovery which enables nurses to explain and critically examine their practice world.

The process of reflection occurs as practitioners examine the outcomes of practice to consider whether the end results could have been achieved more efficiently. Consequently, reflection has the potential to allow for examination and understanding of nursing practice.

It can be argued that nurses in the operating room practise in a routine manner without enough knowledge base to explain how and why they act in the nursing domain. They have a degree of technical competence and function expertly following the biomedical model of care provision; therefore they are content with their explanations of practice. For these reasons they see little or no need for any further insight into clinical practice and may well agree with Butterworth (1996) that individualised nursing care can only be provided to a standard that is 'good enough'. They are not comfortable opening their world to the swampy lowlands of clinical practice

which would enable clarification of nursing practice issues by freeing them from habitual ways of thinking, and allowing them to develop new perspectives on experiences (Clarke 1986, Schon 1987). This new perspective would encourage and develop clinical nursing knowledge and skills and directly benefit patient care. However, by remaining in the paradigm of technical rigour with which they are familiar, actions become routine, ritualistic and alienated from the process of nursing. When this occurs, it can be argued that patients are dehumanised and are treated as cases rather than clients or patients (Jarvis 1992).

Reflection and knowledge generation

It is important for nurses, especially nurses in 'high technology areas' to be able to explain and justify the practice discipline of nursing through knowledge development in practice. Gray & Forsstrum (1992) acknowledge that clinical practice is a rich and diverse field which is more complex than empirical theory alone can define. By using reflective techniques to examine practice issues, nurses can discover and create a strong personal knowledge base of nursing theory. Accordingly, reflection can generate knowledge that is firmly embedded in action and leads to theory generation from practice. Fitzgerald (1994) states that there is a relationship between personal knowledge generated from individual experience and developed theories. Although they are derived from different perspectives, it is maintained that together they complement each other and provide a total view of the situation under scrutiny. Nurses working in the operating department have a wealth of personal knowledge which should be explored and used to develop theories relevant to this practice area. The argument is often used that contemporary nursing theories and frameworks are not applicable to the area or are difficult to use and adapt. However, if theatre nurses could begin to describe and explain practice issues related to providing individualised patient care, a contextual understanding could be developed which would generate meaning within the profession. The knowledge gained from practice could then be used possibly together with developed theories to explore and explain further practice issues in the world of nursing in the operating department.

Cox et al (1992) describe the process of critical theorising which allows nurses to grasp an enlightened understanding of the nursing world. It emphasises the development of emancipatory knowledge which permits practitioners to look at nursing from a very broad perspective including social and political elements.

Nurses are encouraged to become aware of areas and influences on practice which are unjust, contradictory or frustrating, and it can be a liberating experience. Critical theorising is important in all aspects of nursing but seems to be essential in the world of operating department practice where the boundaries of nursing practice are very much influenced by outside political policies (NHSME 1989). However, critical self-reflection can also be difficult, as practitioners may find it disturbing to face the tensions and contradictions which contribute to their practice. Therefore, it can be inferred that reflection on nursing practice in the operating department is derived from practitioners with a strong commitment to improving practice, who wish to free themselves from the constraints of their own conventional practice and ways of thinking and the sociopolitical influences which also impinge on how nursing practice is described and is therefore valued (Emden 1992) (see also Ch. 2).

Application of reflection to practice

It has been suggested that guided reflection enables practitioners to learn in a structured and supported way. It aims to develop the practitioners' thinking at a conceptual level which enables them to begin to effect change within nursing at professional, social and political levels.

Johns (1994) describes guided reflection as a combination of techniques which enable practitioners to reflect on their professional work experiences in order to develop and become more effective at therapeutic work. There are three elements to guided reflection: using the model of structured reflection, supervision and diary structure. The underlying philosophy of the model is the premise that learning is an essential aspect of the clinical development process. This enables practitioners to reflect on and challenge what constitutes desirable practice.

Atkinson & Murphy (1993) identified what they considered to be the key skills needed for reflection. These were self-awareness; the ability to recollect and describe accurately key aspects of the situation; critical analysis of the situation and synthesis of new knowledge gained with previous knowledge, in order to develop a new perspective. These skills and the fundamental patterns of knowing outlined by Carper (1978), in conjunction with Johns' model, provides a means of mapping and framing the knowledge gained from practice (Johns 1994).

I shall draw upon personal experience of being a nurse teacher with an operating department practice background and clinical links with the operating department to reflect on the notion of nursing practice in the operating department.

A description of a situation depicting the nurse's role in caring for patients undergoing local anaesthetic is given in Case study 21.1 to show how the model described by Johns (1994) was used in practice. A discussion will then follow which will describe how the experience has influenced ways of knowing about nursing practice. The debate will be in depth with support from the literature and further critical reflection.

In trying to make sense of the situation described in Case study 21.1, it was necessary to begin to unravel the knowledge that had influenced my practice and empowered me to act in the way that I did.

It would be easy to claim that empirical knowledge of preoperative anxiety (Boore 1978, Model 1987, Wilson Barnett & Batehup 1988) influenced the way I intervened and interacted in this case. However, the initial contact with the patient was based more on human interpretation of the situation than research-based informed practice. Contact was made with Mary because of my concern for her as an individual. After communication had been established, then personal knowing and empirical knowledge were used to guide and influence the care given. Therefore, in order to understand and describe the nursing knowledge that informed practice, I shall explore how my understanding of different ways of knowing as described by Carper (1978) influenced this situation.

Aesthetic knowledge

Carper (1978) describes the aesthetic experience as the direct feeling of a situation and the knowledge gained by subjective acquaintance in that situation. Aesthetic knowledge is specific and unique to each situation, as opposed to empirics which is predictable and generalisable.

The patient's behaviour is important in an aesthetic interaction, as it is the perception of the need being expressed that influences the action taken by the nurse. Therefore, it is argued that perception is more than recognition of what is happening; it includes assessment of the whole situation and evaluation of the most appropriate interaction (Carper 1978).

Consequently, the nature of aesthetic knowledge has been described as grasping the nature of the situation, interpreting and giving meaning to those involved, envisioning what the desired outcomes might be and responding with appropriately skilled action. The nurse then evaluates whether the outcomes have been achieved (Johns 1994).

Case study 21.1 The nurse's role in caring for patients in the operating department

I was visiting the operating department one morning to help with the orientation of a new staff nurse. My remit for the time I was there was to introduce her to the student nurse teaching programme, the clinical assessment profiles and the philosophy of facilitation and preceptorship used in the department.

When I had finished my session with her, I just happened to visit a student who was working in another theatre. I noticed that the list for that morning consisted mainly of day surgery cataract cases which were to be done under local anaesthetic. While I was talking to the student, I noticed that the next patient was waiting in the anaesthetic room. She had been there for a while and there was going to be a considerable wait. I was a little concerned, because although there were people in the anaesthetic room with the patient, the staff were having a private conversation at one end of the room and the patient was lying on a trolley in the middle of the room on her own.

I finished my conversation with the student nurse and went into the anaesthetic room. I introduced myself to the patient and apologised for the delay, explaining that the previous procedure was near ending and the anaesthetist would be with her soon.

Mary was a 78-year-old lady who lived locally on her own. My first impression of her was that she was very middle class, very stoic and did not want a fuss made about the procedure. Anyway I stayed and made small talk, to keep her occupied until the anaesthetist arrived, as her nonverbal cues seemed to show that she was anxious and maybe a little afraid of what was going to happen.

I am very glad I did stay. The anaesthetist came in, introduced himself and gave a very brief synopsis of how the local anaesthetic would be given. He then proceeded with the local anaesthetic. All this time Mary lay there still being very stoic and tight-lipped, with her fists tightly clenched. I impulsively reached out and touched her hand and she then held my hand in both her hands. We did not actually speak to each other but she held on to me for dear life. I stayed with her until she had been positioned on the operating table, at which time I left briefly, the intention being to get someone to stay with her throughout the procedure. As soon as I turned my back she asked the anaesthetist for her nurse – she needed her nurse to stay with her until the end. As it happened, on that morning I had the time to stay and so I stayed with her and cared for her until she was ready for transfer back to the ward.

What was I trying to achieve? I thought the patient looked frightened and I wanted to be there for her.

Why did I intervene as I did? The patient had been lying there for 10 minutes while I was in the department with no-one acknowledging her. I felt that it was no way to treat a patient.

Grasping and interpreting the situation

Johnson (1994) would contend that grasping the situation involves the process of defining a meaningful connection between the nurse and the patient. This then becomes central to the provision of care, since it is through this meaningful connection that physical and emotional support are offered and accepted. Carper (1978) suggests that empathy is an important aspect in an aesthetic interaction. Empathy is defined as 'the capacity for participating in or vicariously experiencing another's feeling' (p. 17). Thus, the empathic nurse has the ability to listen to the feelings, moods and nonverbal behaviour as well as to words.

According to Morse et al (1992), emotional empathy allows the caregiver to respond professionally to the patient. This has been described as 'implicitly knowing what to do'. The actions resulting from empathic responses are usually targeted to relieve distress and promote comfort and are of great comfort value to the patients. They usually include nonverbal actions such as touch. Consequently, when used expressively and in the correct situations, empathic insight ensures that the response given is correct for each individual patient.

In the operating department the complexity of grasping the situation and providing empathic care can be greater, as often patients are not aware or not able to articulate what their needs are. In such situations the use of nonverbal communication is paramount and, therefore, the nurse needs a heightened perception of each patient situation in order to determine when it is relevant to intervene. In this type of unit it is the nurse's artful interaction that can help to bridge the gap between the provision of individualised holistic care and the performance of technical skills (Johnson 1994).

Envisioning and responding

In any clinical situation, an appropriate and skilled response involves the ability to determine an appropriate course of action and anticipate the outcome of the intervention. In order to do this, nurses need to understand the meanings they have interpreted and be able to effectively draw valid conclusions from existing knowledge. However, the actions undertaken are not ritualistic or automatic but are grounded in understanding each specific clinical situation (Johns 1994).

In trying to respond to the clinical situation described, it was tempting to give an automatic response which might benefit the patient. Therefore, I held the patient's hand hoping to use touch to promote comfort even though the patient's verbal and nonverbal communication had not encouraged that form of interaction. At the time I felt that the act was intuitive, but further exploration of the topic has enabled me to articulate the knowledge which will inform my future practice.

Synnott (1992) would argue that touch is probably the most common and the most important nonverbal communication channel in western culture. In nursing, touch is not only utilitarian, for example helping a patient to wash and dress, but it also conveys without words a wide variety of emotions, meanings and relationships. Touch can also be seen as a behaviour that communicates comfort, security and warmth. Nurses often use touch to provide human contact when it is the only avenue of comfort and communication available (Benner 1984). However, Brykczynska (1992) would contend that the permission for touching must come directly from the patient, either by tacit approval or by overt request, as it should be the patients who give permission for the nurse to enter their personal space.

During the interaction with Mary, I had considered using touch on several occasions but it did not seem appropriate. However, it was only when the nonverbal cues became overt that human compassion made me offer touch as a means of comfort. Socially and culturally Mary and I were very different and I was always aware that she may reject that offer of comfort.

In nursing then, touching and physical contact are matters of everyday interaction and may be a prime mode of communication and, yet, it may also be strangely taboo. Touching is culturally determined with a wide variety of tactile interactive patterns and, consequently, cross-cultural communication using tactility may be difficult. Nurses need to be aware that touching someone in a caring manner can be seen as an intrusive act, entirely invading an individual's personal space. Nurses therefore need to be aware of a patient's reaction to their offers of comfort and compassion.

Knowing the patient: the nurse–patient relationship

What internal factors influenced you? I felt for the patient, for the patient's isolation within an alien environment.

What external factors influenced you? The environment and the fact that she was on her own. Something made me feel that she should not have been lying there in that situation 'on her own'.

It could be argued that patients who arrive at hospital for day surgery treatment have no expectations of the nurse apart from a skills-based competence approach to care, which means that the nurse provides the care that is necessary quickly, efficiently and in a professional manner. This task-oriented pattern of providing care allows for minimal and superficial interaction between the nurse and patient, with little space for negotiation, and is all that is necessary within this clinical environment (Morse 1991, Ramos 1992).

On the other hand, it can be argued that one characteristic of professional nursing is allowing the patient to be the focus of care. Therefore, the nurse needs to be aware of the concerns of the patient, notice the behaviour of the patient both verbal and nonverbal and be mindful of the messages that may be present. During this assessment, the nurse decides whether or not it is appropriate to enter into connected relationship. This decision should be a conscious and deliberate one which allows the patient time to decide if he or she wishes to enter into this negotiation. This period of assessment allows for the beginning of the interactive process in which the nurse begins to know the patient (May 1991, Morse 1991, Peplau 1994). While trying to interpret and give meaning to a situation, it is often tempting for a practitioner to provide an automatic response which it is felt might benefit the patient. Benner (1984) claims that this is because nurses are trained to believe that they are most effective when doing something for the patient.

While making small talk with Mary (we discussed her garden and all the things she needed to get back to do), I was constantly assessing her anxiety levels and nonverbal cues and this assessment was the reason I stayed and talked rather than just giving an explanation for the hold-up and leaving.

There are occasions when the most appropriate form of action is to be there for the patient, which has been described as presencing (Benner 1984). This allows time for the nurse to reassess the situation and begin to gain an understanding which leads to recognition of a particular form of action to provide a desired outcome. It is argued that in some situations the appropriate response is the use of touch, which relates messages of support, comfort and person-to-person contact.

This type of knowledge which informs response is not the empirical formalised textbook knowledge, but nevertheless it is central to skilled clinical judgement in allowing the patient to feel valued, human and cared for and is the type of knowledge that nurses in the operating department need to operationalise (Jenny & Logan 1992, Tanner et al 1993).

Empirical knowledge

The importance of ritualisation in the operating department

The staffing structure in the operating department is very bureaucratic and consequently hierarchical. There is no doubt that the power in the structure lies with those at the top. Consequently, surgeons often ask for patients to be sent for much earlier than necessary to prevent a hold-up in the operating list.

It is a brave theatre sister or anaesthetist who does not comply. Therefore patients often have long waits in holding areas or anaesthetic rooms before a procedure begins.

(Personal observation – on 10 years of clinical practice)

Ideas about the body, what it is, what it means, its moral value and the value of its constituent parts, the limits of the body and symbolic value vary widely from person to person and have changed dramatically over time (Synott 1993). Throughout the 20th century, constructions of the body have been in flux. Old certainties and meanings of the social construct of the body and the person are no longer secure. The body mechanical has become the dominant paradigm, particularly with the rise in biomedicine. The development of vaccines, anaesthetics, sterilisation and antibiotics have all contributed to the rise in scientific status for medicine and the line between human and machine is blurred.

According to Kirmayer (1988), the most influential metaphor used in medicine is that of the body as a mind–body machine. It is argued that biomedicine as it is understood today was founded from the Cartesian division of man into a soulless, mortal machine capable of mechanistic exploration and manipulation. This mind–body dualism has the effect of focusing medical techniques on specific problems related to specific systems in the body. The highest status and greatest public kudos in medicine today goes to the doctor who works with spectacular 'scientific' machinery (Bennet 1987).

Illness for the patient is more than the breakdown of a complex machine; it needs to be understood within the meaningful context and culture of the patient's world. The nurse, therefore, is not expected to know patients by breaking them into parts (Leonard 1994). This is particularly important in an environment such as the operating theatre which is seen as highly technical and where the depersonalisation of the person experiencing the system seems to be actively encouraged.

The theory of mind–body dualism, it is argued, devalues the relationship with patients, which relies upon contact, intimacy and trust. Stein (1990) maintains

that fragmentation, compartmentalisation and isolation are necessary to protect practitioners from disturbing thoughts and feelings that would emerge if they considered the patient as a whole. It can be argued that remaining with the biomedical theme of the body as machine allows practitioners to withdraw from patients and keep a safe distance from their inner pain, thoughts and feelings. This could be an explanation that allows practitioners to send for patients early without necessarily thinking of the consequences of their actions. In thinking of the person as the next operative procedure and not an individual there is no need to consider the person's isolation, anxiety and inner pain; these are all distant.

Rituals, according to Baumann (1992), are performances of a symbolic nature which unite members of a culture or subculture. Rituals provide a shared pursuit that displays the basic values of the culture or creates a shared world meaning. As a result, rituals perpetuate the social values and norms of that culture. The construction of a ritualised environment expresses the values and experiences of those with power upon the community. Many hospital settings are enshrined in the unwritten laws of compulsive ritualistic behaviours.

Kratz (1984) claims that ritual activity in the operating department actually contributes to the efficiency of the team by compartmentalising roles and thereby giving autonomy to the practitioners. These rituals permit the participants to engage in a particular mental set which allows them to participate in a dispassionate manner in activities they would normally view with strong emotion.

Walsh & Ford (1990) contend that ritualistic action in nursing implies carrying out a task without thinking it through in a problem-solving, logical way. In abiding by rituals, the nurse undertakes an action because it has always been done that way. Therefore, there is no need to think about individual solutions.

The operating department is an environment that values technology, and thus, skilful and compassionate caring may sometimes be overlooked. However, it is often the attitude and commitment of the nurse that is important to the patient, not the task that is being undertaken. Care provided in this type of atmosphere tends to be limited by the assumption that the nurse knows exactly what the outcomes of care should be and is only concerned with the most efficient ways of achieving these aims.

Nurses working in technical environments may lose the skills needed to form relationships with patients and so over time may only see the patient as an object or a case. They may seem to lack insight into the patient as a person who has the ability to feel pain, fear and distress. Therefore, patients being treated under local anaesthetic may find themselves in a strange environment, surrounded by unfamiliar sounds and machinery and at the mercy of strangers whose roles they do not understand. In such an environment there is a profound need to feel secure, safe and cared for (Carper 1979, Griffen 1983, Raatikainen 1989).

It is argued that such compulsive ritualistic behaviour denotes responsibility avoidance and also implies an absence of freedom to choose to do otherwise. Power in the operating department can be understood as the ability to determine what meanings are attached to ritualistic activities (Fox 1992). Fox states that in this field, the person who has the authority to define meaning and expect others to accept this definition is the surgeon, as he has been denoted an 'expert' in the field. The surgeon claims a right to autonomy of action, as it is claimed that the well-being of the patient is the primary and overriding concern of a doctor's practice.

It is acknowledged that in the operating department patients are often depersonalised into procedures, which allows them to be viewed as objects rather than complex human beings with rights to be protected. It is further contended that nurses submit to this type of authority out of feelings of powerlessness or fear of reprisal. According to Walsh & Ford (1990), the power situation between doctors and nurses is such that confronting a surgeon on an aspect of care involves making one's needs known in a self-confident manner without inviting confrontation and unjust criticism. It may be that nurses in the operating department do not feel confident to do this because of the power of the hierarchical structure.

On the other hand, if the philosophy of nursing embraces individualism, holism, autonomy, advocacy and empowerment, then it is vital that the nurses in this situation recognise and advocate the patient's basic human rights. The fundamental ideas and philosophies of nursing are changing and it is therefore time for nurses in this environment to question how they can incorporate into practice the philosophy espoused by Munhall (1994) (see also Ch. 2).

Ethical knowing

Could I have dealt better with the situation? I do not think I would have changed anything.

What other choices did I have?

- I could have not intervened – the patient was 'safe', there was no real reason for me to go into the anaesthetic room.

- I could have spoken to the staff in the anaesthetic room.
- I could have mentioned the situation to the nurse in charge.
- I suppose I could have asked the student nurse to go and stay with the patient in the first place.

What would have been the consequences of these actions? For me, speaking to members of the trained staff would have been traumatic as I think I would have been perceived as interfering – that is why I stayed with the patient. It seemed the easy option at the time; I was only going to offer the patient reassurance on my way out of the department.

According to Carper (1978), the ethical pattern of knowing in nursing requires an understanding regarding 'what is good, what ought to be desired and what is right' (p. 21). Knowledge of morality goes beyond simply knowing the norms and ethical codes of the discipline. It includes all voluntary actions that are deliberate. Therefore moral choices must be considered in terms of specific actions to be taken in specific context-related situations. Moral codes, it is argued, will provide guidelines for decision-making but do not always provide answers to moral questions, nor do they eliminate the need for nurses to make moral choices (Kushe 1993).

This moral sense of nursing is integrally connected with the notion of good embedded in practice. Consequently, it can be argued that the moral sense of caring is dominant in actual practice (Maeve 1994). According to Johns (1995), thinking practitioners do not passively apply knowledge in practice. In responding appropriately to particular situations they always interpret the situation and analyse the various sources of knowledge available to them whilst envisioning the outcome and its consequence. Therefore in any clinical situation an appropriate and skilled response involves the ability to determine an appropriate course of action and anticipate the outcome of the intervention. These actions are in response to specific clinical situations and are not automatic and ritualistic but realistic (Johns 1994).

The ethic of caring is carried out by individual self-direction, choice and commitment. This involves a sense of willingness on the part of individuals to convey their personal beliefs and values about caring and caring behaviours into the practice setting. Through a personal sense of value they take decisions, make choices and act upon them, making sense of all ways of knowing (Mulligan 1993).

The ethic of caring in a professional sense means acting out of compassion for the person who is suffering or in some kind of distress and need. This, it is argued, presupposes an awareness of the real value of the person as an holistic being (Eriksson 1994). The caring commitment involves a form of professional assurance that the nurse will always try to act in the interests of the patient. In an environment where the emphasis is placed on the accomplishment of technical skills, the nurse's artful interaction can help to bridge the gap between the provision of individualised care and skilled technical performance. This provision of artful nursing comes from an ethic of caring which is guided by a commitment to the facilitation of holistic care (see also Ch. 7).

Once a commitment is made to care for another, time and to some extent effort becomes immaterial. In the nursing context, commitment to the patient is part of the moral contract that the nurse undertakes when caring for patients. To be professionally committed requires considerable forethought and courage and even political and legal awareness. Sometimes this is manifested by standing up for patients' rights and by being a patient's advocate (Brykczynska 1992) (see also Ch. 4).

Respect is an often neglected but essential concept within nursing. Without respect, patients are dehumanised (Morse et al 1992). McGee (1994) would argue that respect is a moral obligation towards others and it is also a human right. Therefore, if respect is a moral obligation and a human right, we cannot be selective about whom we will respect. It is argued that respect is demonstrated through approaching patients as equals and trying to understand their point of view (Browne 1993).

Respect can be shown through:

- nonverbal signals such as facial expressions and gestures, courtesy and honesty
- the use of a communication style that conveys interest and avoids expressions likely to cause offence
- acting in a way that shows recognition of the patient's rights as well as privacy and dignity (adapted from McGee 1994).

I tried to respect Mary as an individual, although this was not an easy situation. We had very little in common both socially and culturally and verbal communication was difficult for me as Mary's clipped middle-class accent could have been interpreted as arrogant and condescending. However, my overriding concern was for the person as a patient and as a professional nurse this meant demonstrating respect and care for Mary as an individual.

Caring is a fundamental value or a moral ideal in nursing, the substantive base of which is nursing

preserving the dignity of patients (Eriksson 1994). Caring is the adherence to the commitment of maintaining the individual's dignity and/or integrity. Thus caring can been seen as a moral imperative that provides the basis for all nursing actions (Morse et al 1992). A great deal of today's human interaction has a social motive. Human interaction may tend to become reduced to a superficial social responsibility. We want to intervene and correct the behaviour we do not accept, but in a deeper sense we are not prepared to take care of the person; our motives are not very profound. Nurses have a professional responsibility for human needs and therefore need to be prepared to help within certain limits.

Personal knowing

Carper (1978) describes personal knowledge as the 'knowing, encountering and actualizing of the concrete self'. It is about striving to know oneself in order to interact in a relationship with another human being. Taylor (1992) maintains that humans are connected through their ordinary human identity. Consequently, nurses need to maintain their ordinariness in the context of delivering care in order to be effective in their use of therapeutic self. Nurses, it is argued, cannot be separate and detached in this type of situation. They need to pay attention to what they feel and how they interact in conveying messages through their gestures and body postures, in order to work with patients and gain invaluable observations about what patients are feeling (Johns 1994, Peplau 1987).

Benner (1984) argues that expert nurses have the self-esteem and self-confidence to see the value of their presence for their patients. The concept of 'presencing' oneself refers to a person being available to understand and be with another; therefore, while physically present with a person one is not preoccupied with other thoughts (Ersser 1991).

The significance of the opening interaction is also a consequence of the way in which the nurse's presentation contributes to the patient's definition of the situation. The manner in which the nurse initiates contact with the patient is known to be important in helping to alleviate the high anxiety often associated with hospital admission. The patient may benefit from continuing contact with the nurse and this allows the patient the opportunity to develop trust in the nurse. Caring contact can be therapeutic for clients who are helped to feel comfortable, secure, at peace and relaxed.

This interaction with Mary, which initially lasted about 10 minutes, made me reflect on many aspects of my personality and how I was reacting in the situation.

I was aware that I was trying to offer comfort to Mary in the most appropriate way that could be achieved in such a short space of time. This was the first time I can remember actively questioning the fact that there was a difference in race and culture and maybe this could have hindered our communication. As it was, this was just a passing thought and as the context of the situation moved on it was far more important that I was a professional nurse, offering a nursing service to Mary. However, for those passing seconds it was an uncomfortable thought and something I have reflected on several times since.

Taylor (1992) maintains that it is a sense of ordinariness and being oneself which enables a connection between the nurse and patient and allows a nurse to offer help and a patient to accept the offer of help. There is sometimes a sense of obligation to try to establish a context of attentiveness central to being a nurse that is not dependent upon social contracts or social context. The sharing of self comes from the respect one gives to another human being and is an important aspect of providing care and comfort at a suitable level. It could be considered unethical to know about another person's sorrow and not to demonstrate concern and care (Eriksson 1994).

Compassion is seen to encompass more than just the notions of pity or concern. As nurses, we should be able to empathise with all patients at least to some degree and this should not have to depend on our personal experiences, but rather on our level of sensitivity and common human understanding of life and life events (Brykczynska 1992). True caring is based on compassion. The nurse's ability to feel compassion emerges from personal experiences; one does not acquire compassion by advanced skills and technique because it is a natural response to the sensitivity and pain of others. Compassion, it is argued, involves an unpretentious attention to each other.

Patients look to nurses for kinds of help that are different from what they expect or receive from other helping professionals. According to Benner (1984), help seeking and help receiving are two different issues; a person can receive help without asking for it and can ask for it without being able to receive it. Some individuals with a strong need for personal control may not be able to acknowledge that they need help or even that they are being helped.

Providing comfort measures and preserving personhood in the face of pain mean that the nurse must be able to overcome the usual mind set. If our notion of science dictates that we ignore meaning, then we are cut off from practical holism and cannot facilitate the person's sense of meaning and dignity. Nurses in the operating department may feel that it is impossible to care meaningfully for all patients that come through the department and so protect themselves from becoming involved in caring relationships; in doing so, however, they avoid the anxiety and stress that this involves (Brykczynska 1992).

OPERATING DEPARTMENT NURSING IN THE HUMANISTIC PARADIGM

The personal difficulties in implementing and evaluating therapeutic practice can be great in traditional settings where the philosophy of the multidisciplinary team and the expectations of the nurses held by all the disciplines involved are at variance (McMahon 1991). Patients' problems in the operating department are often viewed as the surgeon's and/or anaesthetist's problem, or that of any other number of health care workers. This reductionist division of patients' problems into disciplinary areas is a popular but problematic practice. Indeed, the perception that the patient has separate 'medical' problems, nursing problems and other disciplines' problems is an approach that seems to lead to constant conflict due to differing expectations and theoretical frameworks.

It is easy to argue that each nurse should work for high standards of practice; however, this is simplistic unless the nature of practice and the values that underpin it are explored and defined.

In order to practise therapeutically, each nurse has to have a very clear vision of what nursing is (see Box 21.3). Therapeutic nursing must encompass the positive values of the art and science of nursing. Alternative approaches which at best tend to reduce patients to what can been seen as the production line of care, where patients are divided into a series of tasks to be completed, carried out by varying levels of staff according to status and experience, and where no-one is left to care for the patient as a whole must be challenged.

The therapeutic nurse recognises not only the value of each person but also that of nursing. For many nurses in the operating department there is still a tendency to devalue areas of their practice termed basic or menial. Instrumental skills are deemed to be more important and have greater significance attached to them. Thus it is seen that skilled nursing is usually closely associated with medical care and a high degree of medical technological intervention. That is not to say that these activities should be devalued. They should not, for they are an important and supportive part of the nurse's role, but only a part. The expressive skills lie at the centre of nursing; these are the 'high-touch' skills of nursing without which the high-tech

---

Box 21.3   Characteristics of nursing in the operating department

- Being a competent, independent and collaborative practitioner of nursing
- Being able to develop therapeutic relationships (in context) with patients and staff
- Knowing the patient
- Respecting the individual
- Presencing
- Providing individualised care
- Effective communication (verbal and nonverbal)
- Being able to articulate the intrinsic worth and value of nursing
- Setting standards of nursing care
- Being there for each other

---

skills have little meaning to the patient. Wright (1991) would argue that nurses who view themselves only as 'biological plumbers' mates' are anything but nurses.

Caring in nursing is viewed as a humanistic process which allows the nurse to respond to the needs of the patient (Leininger 1988). It can be seen to be central to effective nursing practice and be understood as the human expression of respect and value for the person. Therefore, inherent in the notion of caring is the commitment that all individuals have the right to be treated with integrity and dignity (Boykin & Schoenhofer 1990).

Accordingly, it can be considered that caring is fundamental to therapeutic nursing and involves being available for the patient and providing comfort and security. Therefore the caring therapeutic nurse has been described as taking time, listening and being genuinely interested in the patient. In order to care effectively, the nurse must respect the differences in values between the one caring and the one being cared for (Harison 1990).

According to Morse et al (1992), emotional empathy allows the nurse to respond professionally to the patient. This has been described as 'implicitly knowing what to do' (p. 17). Thus the empathic nurse has the ability to listen to feelings, moods and nonverbal behaviour as well as to words. The actions resulting from empathic responses are usually targeted to relieve distress and promote comfort and are of great comfort and value to patients. Consequently, when used expressively and in the correct situation, empathic insight ensures that the response given is correct for each individual patient.

The UKCC (1994) specify that nursing practice must develop in response to the needs of individual patients without fragmenting or compromising the care delivered to individuals. Advanced practice should be a professional model of nursing practice which is patient-centred and keeps a distinct focus on improving patient care and nursing practice. Thus, it should be accompanied by specialised knowledge and skills in dealing with all types of human responses (Calkin 1984, Manley 1993).

There has been a great deal of discussion about the role of advanced practice in the operating department. It has been claimed that nurses seek to increase their status and expertise by emphasising and developing the highly specialised knowledge and skills of biomedicine and technology, rather than caring knowledge. It is recognised that technical expertise is necessary and the range of technical expertise will change over time, but the role of the nurse is centrally one which should emphasise certain personal skills and qualities of patient care (Ford & Walsh 1994).

It seems that advanced practice in the operating department is in a state of professional uncertainty (Wichowski 1994). Consequently, nurses in the operating department are developing their technical skills to a higher level because these are highly visible and are seen to be important to the effectiveness of the team. Mundinger (1990) argues that if nursing could offer something more concrete, it might be more highly valued. Perhaps that is why nurses tend to spend time on techniques and tasks involving machines, instruments, high technology and the mystique of medicine. These are seen and are recognised as visible signs of a special service.

CONCLUSION

Nursing practice is a dynamic and changing discipline, and this has an implication for practice in the operating department. In the past, others have defined the roles they wish to see implemented in the department and imposed those on the nursing profession. It is now the responsibility of nurses to ask the questions: 'How do we want to be practising nursing in the future?' and 'How can we achieve changes in nursing and nursing practice in this specialty?' It is only by addressing these questions and actively seeking ways to implement change that we as professionals will be able to determine the future.

Russell (1991) argues that many of the changes that occur in nursing have drifted upon us, without nursing involvement. It is further argued that no other profession should decide what it is that nurses do. There are many changes and challenges in health care in the 21st century. It is the responsibility of nurses in the operating department to reflect on the notions of contemporary nursing and grasp all available opportunities to implement the philosophies of holism, individual care, autonomy and respect for the person into their daily practice.

In order to achieve innovations in practice, nurses need to feel supported and empowered to begin to make the change (see also Ch. 5). If such philosophies are not encouraged within the organisation, and nursing work is not seen as being valued and important, then nurses will lack the decision-making powers to enable them to change their practice. To become true advanced practitioners, nurses working in the operating department need to value the humanistic nature of nursing and develop role models who can demonstrate the value of advanced practice to nursing.

REFERENCES

Atkinson S, Murphy K 1993 Reflection: a review of the literature. Journal of Advanced Nursing 18: 1158–1192

Baumann G 1992 Rituals implicate 'others': rereading Durkheim in a plural society. Cited in: de Copper D (ed) Understanding rituals. Routledge, London

Baxter B 1987 Staffing of operating theatres – role of the nurse. NATN News (Oct): 21–24

Benner P 1984 From novice to expert. Addison-Wesley, London

Bennet G 1987 The wound and the doctor – healing technology and power in modern medicine. Secker & Warburg, London

Boore J R P 1978 Prescription for recovery. RCN, London

Boud D, Keogh R, Walker D 1985 Promoting reflection in learning: a model. In: Boud D, Keogh R, Walker D (eds) Reflecting: turning experience into learning. Kogan Page, London

Boykin A, Schoenhofer S 1990 Caring in nursing: analysis of extant theory. Nursing Science Quarterly 3(4): 149–155

Browne A 1993 A conceptual clarification of respect. Journal of Advanced Nursing 18: 211–217

Brykczynska G 1992 Caring a dying art? In: Jolley M, Brykczynska G (eds) Nursing care – the challenge to change. Edward Arnold, London

Brykczynska G 1995 Humanism: a weak link in nursing theory? In: Schober J E (ed) Towards advanced nursing practice. Arnold, London

Butterworth T 1996 Individualised care: a cuckoo in the teams nest? Nursing Times Research 1(1): 34–37

Calkin J D 1984 A model for advanced nursing practice. Journal of Nursing Administration 1(4): 149–155

Carper B A 1978 Fundamental patterns of knowing in nursing. Advances in Nursing Science 11: 13–28

Carper B A 1979 The ethics of caring. Advances in Nursing Science 1(3): 11–20

Carrington A 1991 Theatre nursing as a profession. British Journal of Theatre Nursing (Apr): 5–7

Clarke M 1986 Action and reflection: practice and theory in nursing. Journal of Advanced Nursing 11: 3–11

Cox H, Hickson P, Taylor B 1992 Exploring reflection: knowing and constructing practice. In: Gray G, Pratt R (eds) Towards a discipline of nursing. Churchill Livingstone, London

Curry I, Poole D 1991 The question of the operating department. British Journal of Theatre Nursing, Oct, pp 4–9

Dein S 1994 From semiotics to phenomenology: towards an anthropology of the body. British Medical Anthropology Review 2(2): 48–55

Ellis H 1992 Conceptions of care. In: Soothill K, Henry C, Kendrick K (eds) Themes and perspectives in nursing. Chapman and Hall, London

Emden C 1992 Becoming a reflective practitioner. In: Gray G, Pratt R (eds) Towards a discipline of nursing. Churchill Livingstone, London

Eriksson K 1994 Theories of caring as health. In: Gaut D A, Boykin A (eds) Caring as healing – renewal through hope. National League for Nursing Press, New York

Ersser S 1991 A search for the therapeutic dimensions of nurse patient interaction. In: McMahon R, Pearson A (eds) Nursing as therapy. Chapman and Hall, London

Fitzgerald M 1994 Theories of reflection for learning. In: Palmer A, Burns S, Bulman C (eds) Reflective practice in nursing. Blackwell Scientific Publications, London

Ford P, Walsh M 1994 New rituals for old – nursing through the looking glass. Butterworth Heinemann, London

Fox N J 1992 The social meaning of surgery. Open University Press, Milton Keynes

Gray J, Forsstrum S 1992 Generating theory from practice: the reflective technique. In: Gray G, Pratt R (eds) Towards a discipline of nursing. Churchill Livingstone, London

Griffen A P 1983 A philosophical analysis of caring in nursing. Journal of Advanced Nursing 8: 289–295

Hale C, Thomas L, Bond S, Todd C 1997 The nursing record as a research tool to identify nursing interventions. Journal of Clinical Nursing 6(3): 207–214

Harison L L 1990 Maintaining the ethic of caring in nursing. Journal of Advanced Nursing 15: 125–127

Hodson D 1998 The evolving role of advanced practice nurses in surgery. Association of Operating Room Nurses Journal 67(5): 998–1009

Jarvis P 1992 Reflective practice and nursing. Nurse Education Today 12: 174–181

Jenny J, Logan J 1992 Knowing the patient – one aspect of clinical knowledge. Journal of Nursing Scholarship 24(4): 254–258

Johns C 1994 Guided reflection. In: Palmer A, Burns S, Bulman G (eds) Reflective practice in nursing. Blackwell Scientific Publications, London

Johns C 1995 The value of reflective practice for nursing. Journal of Clinical Nursing 4: 23–30

Johnson J L 1994 A dialectical examination of nursing art. Advances in Nursing Science 17: 1–14

Kirmayer L J 1988 Mind and body as metaphors: hidden values in biomedicine. In: Lock M, Gordon D R (eds) Biomedicine examined. Kluwer Academic Publishers, London

Kratz P 1984 Rituals in the operating room. Ethnology 20: 335–350

Kushe H 1993 Caring is not enough: reflection on nursing ethics of care. Australian Journal of Advanced Nursing 11(1): 32–42

Leininger M M 1988 Care: the essence of nursing and health. Wayne State University Press, Detroit

Leonard V 1994 A Heideggarian phenomenological perspective on the concept of person. In: Benner P (ed) Interpretative phenomenology. Sage Publications, London

Manley K 1993 The clinical nurse specialist. Surgical Nurse 6: 21–25

Maeve M 1994 The carrier bag theory of nursing practice. Advances in Nursing Science 16(4): 9–22

McGee P 1994 The concept of respect in nursing. British Journal of Nursing 3(13): 681–684

McMahon R 1991 Therapeutic nursing: theory issues and practice. In: McMahon R, Pearson A (eds) Nursing as therapy. Chapman and Hall, London

May C 1991 Affective neutrality and involvement in nurse–patient relationships. Journal of Advanced Nursing 16: 552–558

Meleis A I 1991 Theoretical nursing: developmental and progress, 2nd edn. J B Lippincott, London

Model G A 1987 Preoperative and postoperative counselling. Nursing 21: 800–802

Morse J M 1991 Negotiating commitment and involvement in the nurse–patient relationship. Journal of Advanced Nursing 16: 455–468

Morse J M, Bottoroff J, Anderson G, O'Brien B, Solberg S 1992 Beyond empathy: expanding expressions of caring. Journal of Advanced Nursing 17: 809–821

Mulligan J 1993 Activating internal processes in experiential learning. In: Boud D, Cohen R, Walker D Using experience for learning. Open University Press, London

Mundinger M 1990 Autonomy in nursing. Aspen System Corporation, London

Munhall P L 1994 Revisioning phenomenology. National League for Nursing Press, New York

National Association of Theatre Nurses (NATN) 1991 A strategy for nursing in the operating department. NATN, Harrogate

National Association of Theatre Nurses (NATN) 1994 Quality assessment document. NATN, Harrogate

National Association of Theatre Nurses (NATN) 1995 Risk assessment guide. NATN, Harrogate

NHS Management Executive (NHSME) 1989 The management and utilisation of operating departments – the Bevan Report. HMSO, London

Oiler C 1982 The phenomenological approach to nursing research. Nursing Research 31(3): 178–181

Peplau H E 1987 Interpersonal constructs for nursing practice. Nurse Education Today 7(5): 201–208

Peplau H E 1994 Interpersonal relationships: the purpose and characteristics of professional nursing. In: Werner O'Toole A, Welt S (eds) Hildeguard E Peplau – selected works. Macmillan, London

Playle J F 1995 Humanism and positivism in nursing: contradictions and conflicts. Journal of Advanced Nursing 22: 979–984

Raatikainen P 1989 Values and ethical principles in nursing. Journal of Advanced Nursing 14: 92–96

Ramos M C 1992 The nurse patient relationship: themes and variations. Journal of Advanced Nursing 17: 46–56

Redfern S 1996 Individualised patient care – its meaning and practice in a general setting. Nursing Times Research 1(1): 22–33

Russell R L 1991 Are we asking the right questions? In: Gray G, Pratt R (eds) Towards a discipline of nursing. Churchill Livingstone, London

Schon D A 1987 Educating the reflective practitioner. Josey-Bass, San Francisco

Stein H F 1990 American medicine as culture. West View Press, London

Synnott A 1992 The body social. Routledge, London

Tanner C A, Benner P, Chesla C, Gordon D 1993 The phenomenology of knowing the patient. Image; Journal of Nursing Scholarship 25(4): 273–280

Taylor B J 1992 Relieving pain through ordinariness in nursing: a phenomenological account of a comforting nurse–patient encounter. Advances in Nursing Science 15(1): 33–43

United Kingdom Council for Nursing, Midwifery and Health Visiting (UKCC) 1993 Standards for records and record keeping. UKCC, London

United Kingdom Council for Nursing, Midwifery and Health Visiting (UKCC) 1994 The future of professional practice – the Council's standards for education and practice following registration. UKCC, London

Walsh M, Ford P 1990 Nursing rituals. Heinemann Nursing, London

Wichowski H C 1994 Professional uncertainty – nurses in the technologically intense area. Journal of Advanced Nursing 19: 1162–1167

Wicker P 1987 The role of the nurse in theatre. Senior Nurse 7(4): 19–21

Williams M 1997 Quality in theatre care: a critical analysis. Nursing Standard 12(3): 46–48

Wilson Barnett J, Batehup L 1988 Patient problems – a research base for nursing care. Scutari Press, London

Wright S 1991 Facilitating therapeutic nursing and independent practice. In: McMahon R, Pearson A (eds) Nursing as therapy. Chapman and Hall, London

22

Principles of postoperative care

Karrie Ward   David Morris

AIMS

The chapter aims to:

- critically appraise contemporary approaches to postoperative care
- evaluate current postoperative surgical nursing practice in the light of contemporary theoretical perspectives
- develop and enhance specialist knowledge of postoperative surgical nursing interventions
- develop awareness and understanding of the factors influencing surgical recovery
- challenge traditional beliefs and assumptions existing in postoperative surgical nursing.

INTRODUCTION

Surgery is an assault, not only on the biological individual but also on the individual's perception of self. As a process, surgery is discrete and transient in that it has a well-defined beginning and end. However, its precursors and consequences are unique to each individual.

This chapter is designed to provide the practitioner with the opportunity to review and develop knowledge and enhance the professional attitudes that are appropriate to the nurse working in surgical areas. The development of the ability to reflect critically upon practice and make sound clinical judgements based on established concepts and theories will be facilitated, thus enabling the practitioner to improve and develop clinical expertise.

The decision on how to structure the content of the chapter was a difficult one. In writing it, the view has been taken that there is no such thing as 'the typical surgical patient'. Most practitioners would probably acknowledge that the range of nursing activities surgical nurses undertake when caring for their patients is very diverse. Patients have complex physical, emotional and social needs and are influenced by different developmental and cultural factors. Consequently, we did not feel it to be appropriate to follow the more traditional medical approach for writing this text.

In a chapter of this nature, it would not be possible to address all aspects of surgical intervention such as the care of the patient following bowel surgery, thoracic surgery and so on. We acknowledge that those practitioners working in specialised areas of surgery will also need to consult more specialist literature. However, in structuring the chapter, we have chosen to emphasise what it is that nurses do when caring for postoperative patients. We feel that there are significant roles which nurses adopt in the postoperative period, and in identifying these we have been informed by the domains of nursing (Benner 1984, see Box 22.1).

Benner's domains of nursing

In the postoperative period we believe that nurses are often managing the care of patients in rapidly changing situations and an important aspect of their role is the administering and diagnosing function. The helping and coaching roles have been acknowledged as an integral part of the nurse's activities and function in this period and the text will therefore reflect this. The patterns of knowledge identified by Carper (1978), encompassing the science and art of practice allied with ethical and personal knowledge have also influenced the structure of this chapter. Furthermore, if nurses do not question or reflect on the care they deliver, there is no foundation to improve standards or to develop new approaches to nursing practice.

In acknowledgement of this view and in order to illuminate the content, we have included examples of incidents from the writers' practice in the hope that this will help to highlight the realities and complexities of nursing.

IMMEDIATE POSTOPERATIVE CARE

The post-anaesthetic recovery period requires specific skills in the administration and monitoring of the medical and nursing regimen allied with the ability to diagnose and effectively manage changes in health status. On arrival of the patient in the recovery room or area designated for recovery of postoperative patients, an immediate assessment of the patient's health status must be carried out. The nurse will obtain full patient details which will include the surgery performed, anaesthetic history and any specific postoperative instructions.

The patient is nursed in the lateral 'recovery' position, providing surgery allows, to minimise the risks of aspirating vomit and to facilitate airway management. Hip, neck or spinal surgery, for example, might require different positioning strategies. If the patient is unable to fully maintain the airway, an artificial airway should be inserted, if one is not already in situ, to facilitate the management of this crucial stage of recovery.

In addition to artificial airways, a number of other items must be readily available in case of a respiratory emergency (see Box 22.2).

Effects of general anaesthesia

General anaesthesia causes changes in normal breathing control and response (see Ch. 23). The chemoreceptors which mediate hypoxic responses are much more sensitive to the depressant effects of volatile anaesthetic gases such as halothane, sevoflurane and enflurane. This effectively reduces the functional residual capacity of the lungs, contributing to both respiratory depression and the potential for upper airway obstruction. In addition, Doyle (1998) concedes that the effects of general anaesthetic agents, the use of muscle relaxants, intrasurgical artificial ventilation and the supine positioning of the patient may contribute to the incidence of hypoxaemia and consequently have implications for the ability to maintain adequate oxygen perfusion. The nurse must monitor the level of oxygen saturation in the blood. Hypoxia, defined as low oxygen tension in the tissues, may be assumed when the

---

Box 22.1 Domains of nursing (Benner 1984)

- Helping role
- Teaching/coaching role
- Diagnostic and monitoring role
- Management of rapidly changing situations
- Administering/monitoring therapeutic interventions/regimens
- Monitoring quality process
- Organisational, work role competencies

Box 22.2 Respiratory emergency equipment

- Airways, various sizes
- Oxygen supply, disposable mask and tubing
- Suction equipment, selection of suction catheters
- Disposable gloves, gauze swabs, bowl of water and receiver
- Expired oxygen saturation monitor
- Emergency cardiopulmonary resuscitation equipment

SaO_2 falls below 90%. A non-invasive oximeter, often applied to the patient's digit, is invariably used and should indicate a level of oxygen saturation in the vicinity of 95–100% in the adequately perfused patient.

It is essential that the nurse in the recovery unit is able to recognise any signs of impaired respiratory function due to airway obstruction. These might range from a degree of restlessness and mouth breathing, noisy or laboured breathing with the exaggerated use of accessory muscles of the neck and abdomen, to the absence of breath sounds and chest movement. Agitation, confusion or aggressive behaviour are often signs of diminished oxygen levels and hypoxia. When oxygen saturation levels are lowered because of obstruction, a cyanosis of the peripheral extremities, particularly of the lips, finger and toe nails which exhibit a bluish tinge, may present. It must, however, be remembered that, in contrast, evidence of cyanosis will be absent in the case of hypovolaemic shock when the patient will exhibit increasing pallor. An increasing anoxia will lead to a centralised cyanosis seen in the tongue and surface tissues. An immediate examination of the mouth and throat must be performed to identify and remove any mechanical obstruction to breathing. An artificial airway, such as an endotracheal tube, laryngeal mask or Guedel airway, should be examined for blocked or obstructed lumens and suction equipment may be used to remove any oral or nasal secretions, vomit, or blood to ensure a clear airway.

Box 22.3 lists the causes of respiratory distress and inefficiency.

Stridor, a laryngeal obstruction resulting in a stertorous and laboured noise on inspiration, is also a relatively common occurrence postoperatively, often because of the irritant effects or incomplete reversal of the anaesthetic agent or the trauma of intubation or extubation. The patient requires a calm and reassuring approach from the nurse. The nurse must ensure there is no mechanical obstruction of the airway and should administer oxygen via an appropriate mask at a high concentration, often 10 litres a minute, or as prescribed, reducing the concentration as stridor recedes. Persistent stridor or signs of progressive airway distress will require the immediate attention of the attending anaesthetist.

Most patients admitted to the postoperative recovery unit should receive oxygen at a prescribed rate for a variable period of time, ranging from 15 minutes to several hours, depending upon individual circumstances, in a bid to improve effective oxygen exchange. Oxygen should be administered in accordance with the anaesthetist's instruction via a correctly fitted clear, soft mask that fits over the nose and mouth, or by nasal cannulae. Humidification is commonly used and is recommended to reduce the drying effect of oxygen on the upper respiratory tract. Individual assessment is crucial, and for some patients oxygen requirements may be influenced by existing pathology. As Craft & Upton (1992) state, patients with chronic obstructive pulmonary disease are likely to have lost their sensitivity to carbon dioxide, relying instead on hypoxia to trigger ventilation. Such patients may suffer potentially fatal respiratory depression if even moderate amounts of oxygen are administered.

Nurses must remain with patients until they are fully conscious, providing reassurance and support at frequent intervals, orienting patients to their surroundings and reinforcing the fact that the surgery is now over. To monitor general recovery, the patient's vital signs of blood pressure and temperature, pulse rate and volume, and respiratory rate should be recorded at 15-minute intervals postoperatively, unless otherwise instructed, until the patient's condition is stabilised (Smeltzer & Bare 1992). This is to enable the detection of any deviation in the patient's condition from the baseline observations which were established preoperatively. An awareness of the physiological implications of anaesthesia and recovery after anaesthesia is obviously essential, because despite the best efforts of the postoperative nursing team, a number of potential complications may occur in the postoperative period.

Shock

The presence of postoperative shock is a complex life-threatening process of haemodynamic dysfunction

---

Box 22.3   Causes of respiratory distress

Mechanical airway obstruction
- Blood clot
- Mucus
- Aspiration of vomit
- Surgical pack
- Dentures
- Tongue
- Oedema

Functional airway distress
- Neck position
- Inadequate reversal of muscle relaxants
- Inadequate oxygen therapy
- Pre-existing pulmonary disease
- Anxiety

which may result in diminished tissue perfusion as described in Chapter 25. The resulting deficit of cellular metabolites will lead to intracellular imbalance and cellular hypoxia promoting anaerobic cellular respiration (Clancy & McVicar 1995). If not recognised and treated appropriately, circulatory failure of this type will lead to metabolic disturbance and renal, hepatic and heart failure, irreversible cerebral damage and death. Essentially four main causative classifications of shock may be identified (see Box 22.4).

For the surgical patient a number of causative agents and processes are potential precipitating factors in the development of a shock syndrome. However, sound nursing assessment, diagnosis and management can greatly reduce the risk and effects of this process. For the surgical nurse, an understanding of the potential causes and the physiological processes involved is essential in early diagnosis of the shocked patient. Whilst the general principles for the care and management of the shocked patient will be applicable regardless of cause, the authors will refer most specifically to hypovolaemic shock, reflecting its likely incidence and observation in surgical settings. Whilst the potential for shock is greatest in the immediate postoperative period, it is essential to recognise that, dependent on cause, it may not be immediately apparent or present until some hours or even days later. Haemorrhage and loss of body fluids is probably the most significant cause of surgically associated shock. Primary haemorrhage occurring during surgery is the most likely precursor to shock.

However, reactive haemorrhage is not an uncommon occurrence. As the patient's blood pressure rises postoperatively, this leads to bleeding from vessels apparently intact during surgery. This might be a particular concern following anaesthetic procedures designed to reduce blood pressure during surgery. Anaesthesia for prostatic, gynaecological and some ear, nose and throat surgery commonly utilises this technique. As pressure rises in the vessels postoperatively, they ooze and bleed if not adequately sealed by ligature or diathermy during surgery. Secondary haemorrhage can occur days after surgery and is commonly due to the presence of infection. In the early stages of shock, compensatory mechanisms will attempt to maintain homeostasis. An increase in depth and rate of respiration and the activation of the autonomic nervous system initiated by chemoreceptors and baroreceptors may maintain blood pressure. However, if not treated, or in cases of severe blood loss, progressive organ damage ensues. Box 22.5 lists the progressive signs of shock.

Nursing care

The primary medical consideration in caring for the patient in hypovolaemic shock is to restore oxygen delivery to the tissues and to correct the underlying cause of the bleed. Medical interventions will require intravenous blood volume replacement in the form of crystalloids, whole blood, packed cells or, if not immediately available, blood plasma expander solutions. Intravenous infusion enables the patient to receive fluids by the quickest route, thus increasing intravascular fluid volume immediately in emergency situations.

Traditional management of the shocked patient has included elevating the foot of the bed or trolley as a

---

Box 22.4   Causative classifications of shock

- *Cardiogenic shock* in which there is a sudden failure in cardiac output, generally due to acute heart disease such as myocardial infarction or pulmonary embolism.
- *Vasogenic/neurogenic shock* in which there is excessive expansion of the vascular bed and subsequent loss of motor tone. Usually initiated by neurogenic causes such as spinal cord injury, anaphylaxis, toxic shock syndrome or by spinal anaesthesia. This may also be effected by sudden severe pain or a major emotional episode.
- *Anaphylactic shock* as a consequence of an allergic reaction.
- *Hypovolaemic shock* is probably the most commonly encountered shock syndrome, which may be related to either haemorrhage, trauma associated with haematology, severe injury, surgical procedure and burns or to dehydration in cases of severe vomiting or diarrhoea.

Box 22.5   Progressive signs of shock

- Pallor
- Restlessness
- Thirst
- Tachycardia – rapid and thready pulse
- Hypotension
- Air hunger
- Cold and clammy skin
- Diminished urinary output
- Extreme hypotension
- Extreme pallor/waxy complexion
- Cyanosis
- Collapse
- Coma

means of increasing the blood flow to the brain. Whilst there is a lack of definitive literature, the effectiveness of this practice could at face value be considered contrary to physiological homeostatic theories. Elevating the foot of the bed, whilst initially increasing blood flow to the brain, concurrently distends the carotid arteries. These contain the baroreceptors which form part of the blood pressure regulatory mechanism. Raised pressure detected by the baroreceptors sends messages to the brain stem which instigate peripheral vasodilatation and subsequent hypotension as a compensatory mechanism. Such an effect is obviously not conducive to the recovery of the shocked patient. In practice, however, moderate elevation of the bed is unlikely to bring about any adverse effects. For the shocked patient with an already reduced circulatory volume, the degree of distension of the carotid baroreceptors is likely to be appreciably less than for the normovolaemic patient.

The nurse's first priority is of course to assist in ensuring that the medical prescription is implemented and monitored to restore and maintain homeostasis. However, it is imperative in urgent and emergency situations that the nurse does not forget the individual undergoing the crisis. The patient in shock is likely to be anxious, distressed and even confused and disoriented. The provision of clear and appropriate information regarding the cause of the shock condition is crucial in promoting the comfort and dignity of the patient. This is allied with ongoing information and explanation as treatment continues. The worth of a calm, controlled but empathic nursing presence, with appropriate use of touch and reassurance, cannot be overestimated.

Hypothermia

The need to promote and maintain an adequate body temperature is often considered secondary to the need for surgical access. Whilst a state of hypothermia is advantageous and even induced in some surgical procedures, for the recovery nurse a reduction in body temperature of the postsurgical patient is usually viewed as a deleterious stressor. There are a number of contributory factors to body temperature reduction during and immediately after surgery, many of which might be considered to be iatrogenic in origin.

Reflective point

Identify a client in your care and, utilising your knowledge of homeostasis, anaesthesia and the process of surgery, reflect on the factors that may influence the regulation of body temperature during the perioperative period.

Both the recovery and surgical (ward) nurses must be aware of the physiological effects that non-therapeutic hypothermia may have on the patient. Box 22.6 lists the factors influencing the regulation of body temperature. There is potential for myocardial depression and central nervous system depression which may lead to an increase in recovery time. Additionally, lowered basal metabolic rate and subsequent diminished heat production may lead to reduced carbon dioxide production and depressed respiration. Dennison (1995) further emphasises how protein catabolism, hypocalcaemia, glucose metabolism and glomerular filtration may be adversely affected.

Wong (1991) recognises that the capacity for drug metabolism may also be reduced, adversely affecting the effectiveness and monitoring of analgesic regimens. Whilst all patients should be monitored and their temperature recorded at least on arrival in and discharge from the recovery unit, prevention of hypothermia requires an awareness of those most at risk (see Ch. 11) as well as an insight into the procedures and equipment available to minimise the effects.

Kurz et al (1995) carried out a prospective, randomised, clinical study to evaluate the consequences of intraoperative core hypothermia. Primarily examining effects on heart rate and blood pressure, the researchers concluded that the effects of intraoperative hypothermia are generally modest in the younger and healthier patient. However, the study also demonstrated a higher level of comparative discomfort, shivering, persistence of the hypothermic state and peripheral vasoconstriction in the experimental group. Effectively, a delayed return to normothermic state and a delayed recovery in the hypothermic patient

---

Box 22.6   Factors influencing the regulation of body temperature

- Body exposure in the theatre combined with a lack of clothing
- Loss of radiated heat through a large incision
- Muscle inactivity during surgery
- Inhalational gases and narcotic drugs causing a lowering of the hypothalamically controlled temperature norm and reduction in the basal metabolic rate and subsequent heat production
- Use of cool or cold intravenous fluids and antiseptic lotions
- Inability to shiver as a homeostatic response owing to the effects of muscle relaxants
- Peripheral vasodilatation following spinal or epidural anaesthesia

provide clear evidence for appropriate thermal management. For those undergoing long operations with large fluid or blood loss from open body cavities and those at the extremes of the life span, there is a substantially higher risk (Surkitt Parr 1992). Older patients have reduced shivering reflex ability and, when combined with the other risk factors highlighted, this represents a challenge to nursing intervention.

Although clearly an important homeostatic mechanism, shivering produces other considerations for the surgical nurse. Postoperative shivering is a common feature following anaesthesia and has been well documented over a number of years. Fotheringham (1995) provides an illuminating review of the literature and concludes that cause and management remain somewhat speculative in nature. Commonly known as halothane shakes, this episode of post-anaesthetic involuntary muscular activity which can manifest in particularly violent tremors, has been commonly linked to the use of anaesthetic agents and techniques. In particular, procedures which utilise volatile anaesthetic agents such as halothane, and to some extent regional anaesthetic techniques, have been implicated (Crossley 1992).

It is also a common consequence of urological surgery where cold fluids might be introduced into the body in the form of irrigation. Additionally, surgery which promotes radiated heat loss, such as open abdominal surgery, may contribute to this effect. Shivering greatly raises the metabolic rate (Crossley 1992) and will increase the oxygen requirements of the patient enormously, requiring oxygen intake to be greatly increased to prevent hypoxia. Consequently, the patient will require high levels of oxygen via mask or cannulae until oxygen saturation measures have reached normal levels and shivering has stopped. Interestingly, in a comparative study of shaking and non-shaking patients, Vogelsang (1991) concluded that there was no evidence to support the hypothesis that shaking is directly attributable to thermoregulatory function. Some have identified the use of pethidine, doxapram and certain opioids as potentially beneficial pharmacological interventions (e.g. Singh et al 1993); however, Fotheringham (1995) concludes that providing radiant warmth alone may be as effective in management as in combination with drug therapies.

Whilst the phenomenon of post-anaesthetic shaking may be obscure in definition and origin, there can be little doubt that maintaining an appropriate core temperature will benefit patient recovery. As in the theatre, the recovery nurse must ensure that the patient is not exposed unnecessarily, which often happens when the patient is being collected from or returned to the ward. It is imperative to ensure that ward staff are also fully aware of the hazards of the patient arriving in the theatre and arriving back in the ward cold. Intravenous fluids and topical lotions should be warmed and, if appropriate, a thermoinsulating 'space blanket' or a warming mattress utilised. Ambient temperature of the ward or unit must also be maintained at a level conducive to thermal homeostasis. The use of devices for warming urological irrigation and intravenous fluids is essential in promoting and maintaining body temperature and general homeostasis. Additionally, the shivering patient will often become very restless, requiring the nurse to ensure the maintenance of a safe environment to prevent injury to the patient.

Restlessness

Restlessness and confusion in the postoperative patient are common yet often poorly considered features which may take a number of forms and be due to many causes. Hypothermia, pain, nausea, hypoxia and orientational confusion, often leading to anxiety and agitation, are potential contributory factors in postoperative restlessness. This phenomenon is a common feature throughout the life span. Children and young adults in particular commonly become agitated and confused when first emerging from the anaesthetic. However, for the older patient, restlessness can signify a potentially more serious and certainly more prolonged state of confusion and disorientation. There are a number of contributory factors in the elderly postoperative patient (see Box 22.7).

It is vital that the surgical nurse is aware of and able to recognise the potential for this disturbance and is able to identify likely causes or influencing factors (see also Ch. 11). So often the authors have heard nurses rationalising postoperative confusion in the older patient as an inevitable consequence of advanced years and anaesthesia. A sound nursing assessment, however, is likely to identify the presence of one or more of the potentiating influences identified in Box 22.7.

Discharge from recovery unit or area

Whilst it is recognised that a number of factors, both clinical and organisational, are likely to influence local policy in the decision to transfer the patient back to the ward setting, all guidelines or criteria must reflect the necessity for safe discharge and transfer. It should

---

Box 22.7 Contributory factors to restlessness and confusion in the elderly

- Reduced respiratory efficiency
- Reduced cardiovascular haemostatic response
- Lower tolerance of heat loss
- Diminished metabolism
- Intercurrent medication
- Over-medication
- Changes in physical environment
- Sensory impairment.
- Concurrent pathology:
  - amnesia/senility
  - chronic obstructive airways disease
  - diabetes

Box 22.8 Discharge criteria from recovery units following general anaesthesia

- The patient must be able to protect his or her own airway.
- There is no evidence of haemorrhage, internal or external.
- A minimum of three stable observations have been obtained, consistent with preoperative readings and individual patient assessment.
- Body temperature is relatively normal for that individual and shows no evidence of hypothermia or pyrexia.
- No patient should be discharged from the recovery unit with a low oxygen saturation level and patients should remain in the recovery room for a minimum of 15 minutes following the withdrawal of oxygen therapy.
- The patient's pain/nausea level has been assessed and controlled with prescribed analgesia/anti-emetic/pharmacy and nursing measures.
- All patients should be kept in the recovery room for a minimum of 30 minutes following administration of opioid analgesia by any route.
- All adult patients will remain in the recovery room for a minimum of 30 minutes.
- All patients who are admitted to the recovery room still intubated will be kept in the recovery room for a minimum of 30 minutes following removal of the endotracheal tube.
- Observations of respiration, oxygen saturation level, pulse and blood pressure will be recorded at 5-minute intervals for the first 15 minutes following extubation.
- Patients having a blood transfusion will be kept in the recovery room for a minimum of 1 hour following commencement of the transfusion, and respiratory and pulse rates, blood pressure and temperature will be assessed every 15 minutes.

---

always be borne in mind, however, that the patient is more likely to be moving from a high dependency area with appropriate staff to patient ratio, to a less intensive ward situation.

Patients discharged from the recovery room will be accompanied by all completed relevant paperwork, including nursing and anaesthetic records, operation notes, and completed discharge notification where appropriate. Written prescription for oxygen therapy and intravenous fluids, where necessary, along with a written prescription for postoperative medication, should all be completed prior to transfer to facilitate communication and continuity in care. Discharge from the recovery room should be undertaken by a suitably qualified member of the recovery team and handover should only be given to an appropriately qualified member of the ward nursing staff.

Box 22.8 provides the discharge criteria from recovery units following general anaesthesia.

Vigilance is essential in ensuring safety for our patients in the immediate postoperative period. Whilst the majority of patients will continue to make a successful recovery from their operation and anaesthetic, there is the potential for sudden changes in condition at any stage of the surgical process (see Case study 22.1).

The business of the ward had meant that nurses in Case study 22.1 were dealing with what they perceived to be more acutely ill patients than Mr Rhodes. It is easy to reflect and in hindsight to say what we might have done differently. The nursing team in fact felt very guilty and negligent even though observations had been carried out according to the normal procedures. Some of the feelings expressed included disbelief in the accuracy of the observations made previously, which gave no indication of any

impending change in condition. Additionally, questioning how the patient's condition could have deteriorated so quickly was a feature of their evaluation of this incident.

These events are often unexpected and frequently add to already stressful ward situations. This experience demonstrates the speed at which a patient's condition can deteriorate and that nurses need to be aware that even perceived minor surgery such as this can have untoward consequences. It highlights additionally the need for nurses to avoid making preconceived judgements of the likelihood of postoperative complications based solely on the minor or major nature of the operative procedure performed.

Case study 22.1   Alan Rhodes

Alan Rhodes, a 51-year-old postman, was admitted for investigations of pain and poor circulation in his right leg. Mr Rhodes had gone to the X-ray department for an arteriogram and returned to the ward an hour later. His blood pressure, radial and femoral pulse observations were recorded on return to the ward and were within normal parameters, and there was no sign of any bleeding from the puncture site dressing.

It was normal practice on the ward to record these observations half-hourly for 2 hours, and to reduce the frequency of observations if no signs of complication were detected. It was also normal practice to place patients requiring close observation in clear view of the nurses' station. As Mr Rhodes' condition was not considered likely to deteriorate, he was observed at a distance from the nurses' station. Between nursing observations, the surgeon arrived on the ward to review his patient's progress. He was angry and dismayed to find Mr. Rhodes in a shocked and moribund state owing to significant bleeding from the puncture site.

Case study 22.2   Paul Hargreaves

Paul Hargreaves was a 43-year-old estate agent who returned to the ward following an emergency femoral embolectomy. He had a wife and a son of 10 years. They lived in a small village some 15 miles from the hospital. On return to the ward, Mr Hargreaves was clinically stable, although a little restless. The staff nurse responsible for his care felt a level of apprehension for his recovery, despite the absence of any logical or empirical evidence for her concern.

Mrs Hargreaves phoned the charge nurse at 7.30 p.m. and was truthfully told that his condition was satisfactory, and that he was awake and responsive. At 8.10 p.m. Mr Hargreaves' condition suddenly deteriorated, he was ashen, sweating and had great difficulty in breathing. Moments later he collapsed and a cardiorespiratory arrest was diagnosed. Despite the prompt and prolonged resuscitation efforts, Mr Hargreaves was pronounced dead due to a suspected pulmonary embolism at 8.50 p.m.

Reflective point

How do you think the nurses might have evaluated their effectiveness in managing Mr Rhodes' recovery? Would you have monitored Mr Rhodes' condition differently?

Reflective point

Are you able to identify a situation or critical incident where, despite the presence of evidence to the contrary or the assertions of your colleagues, you have felt disquiet or apprehension about the condition or progress of a patient? How valuable do you believe such insights are to the practice of nursing?

INTUITION AND PROFESSIONAL KNOWLEDGE

It is clearly essential that the surgical nurse has the ability to recognise and appropriately manage rapidly changing situations. However, most nurses will recognise that they often function in practice where the absence of any theory or scientific knowledge requires them to draw on previous experiential learning. The status of common sense as a legitimate source of nursing knowledge may rightly be considered to be a misnomer as it implies logic and possession by the majority. However, its more primal cousin, intuition, is a concept often held to be an admirable professional virtue.

Intuition is usually described as a feeling or sixth sense which provides the practitioner with an inner awareness and subsequent anticipation of an event prior to explicit or empirical confirmation; see for example Correnti (1993). Perhaps the most common description of intuitive awareness is in the detection of unfavourable changes in clinical condition (see Case study 22.2).

Whilst it is all but impossible to provide empirical evidence of the existence or non-existence of intuitive awareness, perhaps a more logical explanation might involve the recall of previous experiences. It is hard to imagine a very junior nurse or student possessing the kind of insight evident in an experienced nursing practitioner. It is indicative, perhaps, of the evidence of reflection in practice identified by Schon (1983) and characterised by the rapid analysis of professional knowledge gained through previous emotions and experience being constantly brought to bear on a new situation. Indeed, Schon suggests such a phenomenon to be a hallmark of the advanced professional or expert practitioner identified by Benner (1984).

Preventing postoperative complications continues to be an important goal in the postoperative stage. A number of complications arise in the continuing postoperative period. Clearly, a major element of the nurse's role in the postoperative period is to diagnose, monitor and intervene in rapidly changing situations. Whilst this chapter is unable to address every complication that may arise, the writers have considered those that may be most familiar to nurses working in most surgical areas.

WOUND CARE

In the immediate postoperative period, the nurse is responsible for observing the wound site at frequent intervals (see Ch. 28). If drainage from the wound is excessive, the operation site and/or drain site would need to be examined more closely and the wound dressing removed for this purpose. Some capillary bleeding from the wound is to be expected as the blood pressure returns to normal, but continued and excessive bleeding may require further medical intervention or even a return to the operating theatre.

Dealey (1994) states that several studies have shown that in wounds which heal by first intention, the dressing can ideally be removed after 24–48 hours and need not be replaced. Some nurses, however, may prefer to use a semipermeable membrane-type dressing, if appropriate, which would facilitate close observation of the wound and maintenance of optimum temperature.

Reduction in wound temperature is generally accepted to be a factor associated with delayed wound healing. In the case of more complicated wounds, lengthy or repeated dressing changes are inevitable and this may be exacerbated by cleansing with cold solutions reducing the temperature at the wound surface. This is not to suggest that frequent removal of the dressing should occur as routine practice, as repeated exposure of the wound within 48 hours of surgery increases the risk of the patient developing a wound infection (Wilson 1995).

The nurse continues to monitor and assess the wound site for signs of healthy healing or any complications such as wound infection in the postoperative period. An acknowledgement of the interrelationship between wound healing and psychological status has been articulated for a number of years. In an illuminative and experiential account, Kelly (1985) describes feelings of mutilation following bowel surgery. The patient may experience a change in body image and a profound psychological reaction to having a wound. Wound assessment should therefore incorporate exploration of the patient's emotional responses to the wound as well as obtaining perhaps more obvious information relating to the nature and size of the wound. Sorensen & Luckmann (1986), for example, suggest that the nurse should perform an assessment which acknowledges the person's total body response. This should incorporate observation and recording of

the vital signs, mental alertness, degree of anxiety, the nature and frequency of pain and the effects of analgesia prescribed. More recently, Flanagan (1997) stated that the psychological well-being of patients has both direct and indirect effects on the rate of wound healing and suggested that the following influencing factors (motivation, compliance, attitudes of patients and their carers, their knowledge and understanding and body image) could all be integrated into a holistic assessment of the patient's wound and healing response. Furthermore, psychological stress has been shown to reduce healing rates by interfering with the body's immune system (Pediani 1992). A nurse who is sensitive to the needs of patients will therefore try to understand their perceptions of having a wound and their response to this experience (see also Chs 7, 9 and 28).

The nurse in caring for the patient's wound will also need to assess the volume and nature of drainage, maintain patency of wound drainage and ensure that any equipment used to facilitate effective drainage, such as suction apparatus, is functional.

Wound dehiscence

Many patients are afraid of moving because of incisional pain after surgery. If not resolved by the nursing staff, this may lead to further complications relating to restricted mobility (pp. 432–434). Patients are frequently also frightened that their wounds will tear. Minimising the potential for wound dehiscence involves identifying the risk factors and resolving them wherever possible. Box 22.9 lists the risk factors in wound dehiscence.

Complete wound dehiscence is becoming less common with advances in surgical wound management but can be a significant postoperative problem for some patients (Perkins 1992). Dehiscence is a wound complication following surgery, resulting in the splitting open of part or all of a primary closed wound. According to Nettina (1996), it occurs most frequently in abdominal wounds. Perkins (1992) distinguishes between early wound dehiscence related to suture failure or poor surgical technique and late dehiscence related to infection. Complete dehiscence may result in protrusion of the viscera through the incision, commonly referred to as 'burst abdomen'. One of the first indications you may have that a patient's wound has dehisced is when a patient complains that the wound feels wet or complains of 'a feeling of something giving away'.

Observation and assessment may reveal a pale and anxious person with notable changes in vital signs due

---

Box 22.9 Risk factors in wound dehiscence

- Jaundice
- Diabetes
- Obesity
- Poor nutritional status
- Abdominal distension and vomiting putting a strain on sutures
- Advanced age may result in poor nutrition and delayed wound healing
- Ascites
- Distended bowel
- Coughing
- Vomiting
- Straining
- Wound or abdominal infection
- Contamination from a nearby drain or stoma
- Poor surgical technique

---

to anxiety or lowering of blood pressure if shock is present. On removal of the wound dressing, you will note that it is saturated with serosanguineous drainage, the wound edges are open and, in the case of an abdominal wound, loops of bowel may be protruding from it. It is essential that the patient undergoes further surgical intervention in order to repair the wound. The complications that arise from this situation are that the exposed wound becomes a medium for the development of new infection and septicaemia could develop.

Reflective point

Consider wound management practice on your ward and how you would care for the patient with a wound dehiscence.

Whilst advances in wound management and the use of minimally invasive techniques have made complete wound dehiscence relatively rare, it is important to know how to deal with this emergency should it arise. Advise patients who are already lying down to keep as still as possible; otherwise, patients should be helped on to the bed immediately. Since these patients are awake and are probably very frightened, it is important to stay with them, reassure them and explain that their wound has opened. Once on the bed, patients should be encouraged to lie in the recumbent position with head, shoulders and feet slightly raised. Maintaining this position will help to reduce intra-abdominal pressure and prevent any further strain on the wound, which could make the evisceration worse.

While waiting for medical and nursing assistance to arrive, a thorough assessment of the degree of the dehiscence and evisceration can be made and the patient observed for signs of shock. The patient's vital signs are monitored and recorded. Wound swabs should be taken if there is any indication of infection, so that appropriate treatment can be prescribed. The wound is then covered with sterile wound pads soaked in warm saline. This helps to keep it clean and protect any exposed bowel from drying out. It is likely that once the doctor has seen the patient, the patient will be prepared for theatre.

Carers should be informed of the change in the patient's condition and advised if further surgery is required. An intravenous infusion may be prescribed and antibiotic therapy commenced. Surgical repair is the usual course of treatment if the patient is physically well enough to undergo surgical intervention. The patient will be taken to theatre for irrigation, possible debridement and closure of the inner layers of the wound. In some instances, where infection is present or difficulties are encountered in achieving closure of the outer layers of the wound, these may be left to heal by secondary intention.

On return to the ward after surgery, the patient is monitored for any signs of wound infection developing, because such an occurrence is more likely following a second surgical intervention. The patient should be given advice regarding how to avoid putting strain on the incision, will be taught how to support the wound when coughing, and advised to ask for assistance to get out of bed. It is important that patients are reminded to use the call bell if they need assistance.

Whilst admittedly a relatively unusual occurrence, it is important to note that dehiscence may occur once patients have been discharged from the relative safety of the hospital, especially as the emphasis of contemporary practice is on short hospital stay and earlier discharge. This emphasises the need for effective liaison with community nurses. Vulnerable patients should be assessed and identified as part of the discharge process and referred to the community liaison manager.

POSTOPERATIVE CIRCULATORY COMPLICATIONS

Deep vein thrombosis

The formation of clots in the veins of the pelvis and lower extremities is a comparatively common and potentially life-threatening postoperative complication. Deep vein thrombosis (DVT) is probably the greatest single threat to successful postoperative recovery, and is the most common cause of pulmonary embolism. Autar (1996) stresses that it is a largely preventable occurrence and certainly one in which the treatment costs far outweigh the cost of prevention. Clearly, the nurse must be acutely aware of the potential for deep vein thrombosis.

Box 22.10 lists the factors which increase the risk of venous thrombosis.

Clancy & McVicar (1995) identified key physiological factors which can predispose to the formation of venous thrombosis, namely venous stasis, hypercoagulability and blood vessel damage. Autar (1996) identifies seven risk categories: increasing age, build and body mass index, immobility, special DVT risk, trauma, surgery and high-risk disease. It is also worthy of note that some surgical procedures increase the risk of thrombosis. Craft & Upton (1992) identify gynaecological surgery in women over 40 years and orthopaedic surgery as procedures representing the greatest risk. Surgical iatrogenesis may also predispose to deep vein thrombosis. Compression of pressure points caused by inappropriate positioning on the operating table combined with the effects of hypotensive anaesthetic agents and increased coagulability as a result of surgery may also exacerbate the potential for thrombosis (Tyrell et al 1995).

There are predominantly two major circulatory postoperative complications, phlebothrombosis and thrombophlebitis. The terms are often considered as interchangeable and, indeed, the latter may be seen as an extension of the former. Phlebothrombosis occurs when a blood clot forms in one of the larger veins, which may or may not give signs of inflammation or located pain. The thrombus is usually loosely attached to the vessel wall and a portion may break free and be carried to the heart, lung or brain, with the potential for causing sudden, fatal embolism. In contrast, the term thrombophlebitis is usually applied to the condition in which the clot forms a stronger attachment to

the vessel wall and is therefore less likely to enter the systemic circulation. See Box 22.11 for the common signs of venous thrombosis.

The thrombosis may be accompanied by localised pain, swelling or tenderness. Tissue overlying the affected site may be reddened and warm or hot to the touch. In superficial veins a reddened line along the vessel route may be observed. Thrombosis development in deeper vessels such as a femoral or iliac vein may predispose to the entire limb becoming swollen, tender and cool, because of arterial spasm and lymphatic obstruction. Homans' sign characterised by pain in the calf or behind the knee on dorsiflexion of the foot may be present, although Robinson & Stott (1987) suggest that this sign is too often falsely positive or negative to be of diagnostic value. They state that 70% of deep vein thrombosis reveals neither sign nor symptom. Patient education which stresses the need for the patient to report any of the problems outlined above is likely to promote speedy and potentially life-saving treatment of the disorder.

A sound nursing assessment should identify the risk factors preoperatively and be supplemented by regular observation postoperatively for subsequent signs of the occurrence of DVT.

Interestingly, Autar (1996) developed a nursing risk assessment for DVT. Whilst the limited sample in the study is acknowledged, the tool provides potential for further development.

Should the surgical nurse have any suspicion of the presence of deep vein thrombosis, it is imperative to reassure the patient and ensure that bed rest is maintained until medical diagnosis and treatment can be instigated. Additionally, the nurse must encourage the patient to keep the affected limb inactive to reduce the risk of a thrombus breaking free from the vessel wall and into the systemic circulation causing pulmonary embolism. Edmonson & Cohen (1994) state that such an occurrence will be recognised by the patient complaining of pleural pain, possible expectoration of blood-stained sputum, respiratory distress and dyspnoea, nausea/vomiting and showing probable signs of shock requiring urgent medical treatment.

Box 22.10 Factors which increase the risk of deep vein thrombosis

- Varicose veins
- Obesity
- Malignancy
- Systemic infection
- Oestrogen therapy
- Old age
- Prolonged surgery
- Pregnancy
- Peripheral vascular disease
- Impaired mobility

Box 22.11 Possible signs of deep vein thrombosis

- Localised pain or tenderness in the calf
- Puffiness or swelling around the site of DVT
- Warmer to the touch than other surrounding tissues
- Obvious redness around the site of DVT
- Pyrexia

Nursing intervention

A number of interventions have been demonstrated to be beneficial in reducing and preventing venous thrombosis and subsequent potentially fatal pulmonary emboli in the postoperative patient. The continued use of correctly measured and fitted anti-embolism stockings until full mobilisation is achieved has been shown to significantly reduce the incidence of venous thrombosis (Bright & Georgi 1994). Whilst the use of anti-embolism stockings may be contraindicated in peripheral vascular disease, poorly fitted anti-embolism stockings can pose a potential danger. Tight stockings will be constrictive and diminish blood flow. Similarly, short stockings will fail to provide the appropriate pressure gradient, limiting any benefits. Commonly, stockings are either removed by patients, who are unaware of their benefits, or fall down in the postoperative period. It is obviously essential that the nurse monitors and ensures their continued and effective use, in particular ensuring patient cooperation through adequate education. Such interventions may be implemented and monitored when assisting patients with their daily hygiene needs, allowing for the concurrent inspection of the lower limbs and stockings (see also Ch. 20).

Early mobilisation is the primary nursing goal, and should be preceded by instigation of active leg exercises as soon as possible following surgery. Passive limb exercises are imperative in those unable to comply. The patient should be encouraged to participate in regular flexion, rotation and extension exercises.

The use of heparin has been shown to reduce the incidence of deep vein thrombosis in the postoperative patient (Hopkins 1995). The nurse has a key role both in ensuring its administration and in monitoring its effects as a prophylactic measure. In particular, regular urinalysis for evidence of haemorrhage and wound assessment for similar reasons are vital observations. Evidence of such occurrences may necessitate the withdrawal of heparin and the subsequent administration of protamine sulphate as a specific antidote. In addition, the nurse must be aware of the effects of polypharmacy. The concurrent administration of alcohol or aspirin might enhance the anticoagulant effect and reduce prothrombin time and, as Edmunds (1991) recognises, some antibiotics, hormones, cimetidine and a variety of narcotics have similar effects.

DIGNITY

Whilst the nurse is involved in monitoring physiological recovery indicators, maintaining the dignity and comfort of patients is also an integral aspect of care in postoperative nursing management. Preserving or maintaining the patient's dignity is a commonly cited aim in nursing, and treating patients with respect and compassion is central to good nursing practice and is inherent within the Patient's Charter (DoH 1991). Dignity is a reflection of peoples' perception of their worth and self-respect. Failure to respect people's dignity has the effect of devaluing their individuality.

Reflective point

Reflect on your own clinical experiences and identify examples or possible reasons for loss of dignity. Identify ways in which caring can enhance the promotion of dignity.

Hospital admission and treatment often predisposes to some extent to depersonalisation of patients, which may be due to separation of individuals from their belongings and removal from their normal roles, routines and environment. Hospital admission is compounded by fear of surgery or, in an emergency, a lack of preparation increasing the sense of vulnerability. Because much of the freedom and many of the everyday experiences which we take for granted are compromised when we are ill, the dependence which is then placed on nurses deprives people of some of the control normally expected over their lives.

Loss of or reduced consciousness as a feature of anaesthesia will result in the compromise of nearly all activities of living and patients being unable to maintain their own interests. This therefore imposes reliance on surgical nurses to maintain their patients' dignity and safety. Pain, immobility, the effects of anaesthesia and of medications also increase the vulnerability and dependence of patients in the postoperative period. Invasion of patients' personal space during nursing and medical examinations and nursing admission and assessment procedures is a common reason for loss of dignity.

Intimate procedures such as vaginal and rectal examinations are often witnessed by the nurse who is in reality a complete stranger, which may only exacerbate the feelings of anxiety and loss of dignity. Under other circumstances and in most cultures, intimate self-disclosure to anyone other than loved ones would normally be overwhelmingly intrusive.

The patient's rights to privacy and dignity can be affected by allocation to mixed-sex wards (Burgess 1994, Cole 1991). For instance, a woman may not find it acceptable to find herself lying in a night-dress next to a bed occupied by a man who is also a stranger. Furthermore, most patients may expect privacy when they are in a sick and vulnerable state. The hospital attire patients are given to wear may also be a contributory factor to loss of dignity. Patients feel exposed in backless surgical gowns and may have to walk past the opposite sex in night-wear to use the toilet and washing facilities. It is the authors' opinion that nurses have a duty to bring patient dissatisfaction with accommodatory arrangements to their managers' attention and indeed to lobby politicians and those who seek to increase throughput at the expense of human dignity (see also Chs 14 and 20).

Loss of dignity may be experienced by some patients as a result of disfigurement and altered body image. In addition, a sense of being a burden on others by virtue of enforced dependence may be experienced.

In highly technical environments such as that of surgical nursing, the stress and vulnerability experienced by patients may be alleviated by the nurses' awareness of the need to address the maintenance of the patients' dignity. The emphasis on caring becomes even more important so that the potential dehumanisation of both patient and nurse can be avoided. Patients who perceive that nurses are concerned about their well-being and preservation of dignity may be better prepared to deal with the stresses of events in the postoperative period. Therefore nurses must be aware of their actions and how they are perceived by patients.

Explaining the details of postoperative procedures and giving this information in a way that patients can understand promotes dignity and increases their control over the situation. Furthermore, guidelines relating to mixed-sex wards emphasise the importance of attention to the patient's privacy and dignity (RCN 1988, 1993). In addition, the Patient's Charter (DoH 1991) supports the patients' right to have a nurse of the same sex in attendance for some intimate procedures if they so request.

The promotion of dignity and self-esteem must be uppermost in the minds of every surgical nurse. Such considerations will by their very nature extend to the care of patients with catheters, wounds and associated drainage systems, nasogastric tubes and intravenous infusions in the postoperative period.

URINARY CATHETERISATION

Anaesthesia and particularly regional blocks such as spinal and epidural anaesthesia may affect bladder tone and consequently produce difficulty in micturition postoperatively. It is essential that nurses are alert to any ensuing discomfort and are able to note the volume of urine output. On occasion a small amount of urine may be passed as overflow. In such cases any evidence of distension of the bladder suggesting an obstructive problem should be referred to a medical officer so that remedial action can be instigated. Some patients may return from surgery with a catheter in situ depending on the nature of the surgery performed, for instance to achieve bladder decompression after lower abdominal or pelvic surgery and/or to ensure accurate fluid balance management in high dependency patients. Catheterisation may be indicated specifically for the surgical postoperative patient for the relief of urinary retention when all other appropriate interventions have been unsuccessful.

The safe insertion, assurance of patency, maintenance of accurate fluid balance record and the prevention of complications such as urinary tract infection are key nursing skills. An adequate state of hydration is necessary in order to ensure a good fluid output, thus minimising the risk of urinary stasis and subsequent urinary tract infection.

The risks of structural damage to the urinary tract and/or the development of more widespread infection are minimised by the use of appropriate equipment, its proper maintenance and by preventing contamination of the closed drainage system (Jamieson et al 1997).

The nurse's helping role includes an appreciation of the patient's possible embarrassment at being catheterised as well as the more obvious functions of safe and effective catheter management. On many occasions the authors have observed the indiscreet exposure of male urinary catheters, often in full view of members of the opposite sex, and in consideration of the patient's dignity recommend that catheters are concealed where necessary, for example with the use of leg catheter bags.

NASOGASTRIC INTUBATION

The absence of peristalsis or the presence of bowel obstruction results in the accumulation of gas and gastrointestinal secretions, abdominal distension and the patient experiencing varying degrees of abdominal discomfort. Gastrointestinal intubation is commonly employed in surgical management to achieve gastric decompression through the removal of secretions and accumulated gas from the gastrointestinal tract via a tube.

Nursing activities in relation to caring for the patient with a nasogastric tube include the management of nasogastric aspiration based on the frequency and characteristics of the drainage. This sometimes utilises suction apparatus, ensuring measurement and recording on the fluid balance chart. The nurse's responsibility also extends to ensuring that infection control procedures are followed when emptying and collecting the drainage.

Securing the nasogastric tube is of utmost importance from both physiological and psychological perspectives. The use of non-allergenic tape to anchor the tube is recommended (Luckmann 1997). It is also important to affix the tube to the patient's clothing so as to avoid pull and tension on the nose. Excess tubing should be arranged to allow for the patient to turn and move in bed.

The presence of the tube may cause both physical and psychological distress to patients. Several patients that we have nursed were more concerned about their carers' reactions to the sight of such a tube, than the physical discomfort of its presence. Such observations highlight the need to appreciate how apparently insignificant perceptions of altered body image to nurses, may be of much greater importance from the patients' perspective. Patients often voice a loss in relation to the pleasures of eating and tasting food and often complain that their mouth feels very dry. Frequent rinsing of the mouth will relieve thirst and help to keep the mouth clean. The mouth and nose should also be inspected regularly and appropriate oral and nasal hygiene implemented on the basis of such an assessment.

INTRAVENOUS INFUSIONS

In the postsurgical period, an intravenous infusion may be prescribed for patients because they are either unable to tolerate oral fluids or oral fluids are withheld. Tradition has often guided practice in the resumption of oral fluids postoperatively. The routine of a substantive period without fluids postoperatively is often a ritual without foundation. On return of the cough reflex, which may be quite speedy with the use of modern anaesthetic techniques, the patient can have sips of fluid to start with and, if tolerated, progress to increasing amounts of fluid.

The patient can normally be allowed to resume oral fluids once the cough reflex returns postoperatively. Exceptions to this might include, for example, some types of oral, dental and gastrointestinal surgery, and following the use of local anaesthetic throat sprays.

Regardless of the clinical rationale for resumption of oral fluid, preoperative and postoperative fasting and the effects of the anaesthetic agents are likely to produce a very dry mouth and throat. Clearly, the use

of regular mouthwashes and oral hygiene measures can be very effective and refreshing for the patient as well as promoting general well-being.

Intravenous fluids in themselves provide little in the way of nutritional value and therefore the intravenous solution prescribed must be individual to the specific needs and requirements of the individual patient. Nausea, vomiting, hypovolaemic shock, paralytic ileus, peritonitis or prolonged diarrhoea all contribute to the risk of dehydration and electrolyte imbalance. Surgical patients who are receiving gastric or intestinal suction are also at risk because of the fluid deficit which occurs and the loss of electrolytes such as potassium and magnesium. Patients with a large draining wound or fistula can also lose excessive amounts of fluid and accompanying proteins and electrolytes. This is further complicated if the patient has any degree of sepsis and a pyrexia associated with this. The intravenous route provides access for administering medications which may not be absorbed or may otherwise be destroyed by digestive juices.

The prime responsibility of the surgical nurse in caring for the patient with an intravenous infusion is to ensure that the fluids are administered safely and in accordance with medical instruction. The fluid output as well as input is monitored and the patient assessed for signs of over- or underhydration. Circulatory overload might be identified by distension of the neck veins or the patient complaining of dizziness or shortness of breath. In addition, the assessment and monitoring of the patient's reactions to intravenous additives, such as antibiotics and electrolytes if prescribed, are essential. The intravenous cannula site should be observed for any signs of inflammation, extravasation, or infection, which might indicate the need for resiting of the infusion.

The more recent reliance on machines, ensuring accurate fluid delivery, has taken away the need for nurses to regulate the flow of intravenous infusions manually but they should still observe that any pumps used are infusing the fluid correctly. The nurse who acts as an advocate for the patient should consider the positioning of an intravenous infusion on the patient's behalf and be aware that patients may feel more in control if the infusion is sited in the non-dominant arm, thus enhancing their self-esteem and dignity.

In consideration of threats to self-image through surgery, Price (1993) suggests that wounds, tubes, drains and dressings all represent an alteration to body and self-image both real and perceived and that these issues may be overlooked in relation to the patient undergoing relatively routine surgery.

He recommends that nurses pay attention to the discreet positioning and attachment of these extensions in order to respect and promote the patient's dignity and sexuality. The nurse can help the patient to feel more positive about these extensions to the normal body image and in this sense the patient can be helped to regain more control over the situation. For instance, patients can be gently reminded that having a nasogastric tube does not mean that they cannot mobilise, and some patients may wish to be involved in such activities as keeping their own fluid balance records, which may facilitate their acceptance of the intravenous line. Also, providing patients with information as to why such lines and tubes are necessary may serve to reassure them and increase their understanding and cooperation in such situations.

NUTRITION

Adequate nutrition is required to enable patients to withstand the trauma of disease, surgery, possible infection or drug therapy (see also Ch. 27). In our experience, the provision of adequate nutrition in hospital has tended to be accorded low priority. Historically, a number of research studies have focused on the specific nutritional needs of patients who have undergone surgery. The study of Bistrian et al (1974), for example, found moderate to severe protein–calorie malnutrition in 50% of 131 surgical patients. These deficiencies were related to illness and drugs causing decreased appetite, patient discomfort at meal times, the poor quality and presentation of food, lack of nursing supervision and patients in some cases not ordering the full three-course meal which was provided. Since many modern hospitals now use plated meal systems and lack ward-based kitchen facilities, nurses may rarely be involved in the control or supervision of the nutritional intake of their patients. More recent studies have confirmed that the potential for surgical malnutrition persists (Dickerson 1995).

Reflective point

From your clinical experience, consider practices which may enhance patients' intake of adequate nutrition in the postoperative period.

As discussed in Chapter 20, surgical patients are often fasted longer than necessary and without regard for the actual time of their operation. Despite early research findings which have highlighted this practice (Hamilton-Smith 1972), more recent studies by Thomas (1987) and Chapman (1996) confirm that it still persists. The oral intake of postoperative patients is often restricted in order to help prevent gastrointestinal complications such as vomiting and the breakdown of anastomoses occurring. Patients who cannot begin oral nutrition immediately may often spend a prolonged period following surgery on intravenous infusion therapy. In addition, the use of nasogastric or intestinal aspiration necessitates that the body draws on its own reserves for energy until the gastrointestinal tract resumes normal motility.

A surgical patient whose nutritional state is neglected, or who is malnourished, will of necessity stay longer in hospital, run the risk of developing pressure sores, and have delayed wound healing. Also, increased glucose levels in the peripheral tissues form a good medium for the multiplication of bacteria; hence the increased susceptibility to wound or skin infection. Infection causes an increase in the metabolic rate and therefore the average energy requirement also rises. Thus it can be seen that the consequences of malnutrition in postoperative patients are far-reaching and the potential for this occurring is also influenced by the nutritional status of the patient on admission (see also Ch. 13).

Recommendations for good practice

As surgical patients are at risk of being malnourished during their time in hospital or may already be malnourished at the time of admission, it is essential that surgical nurses assess the nutritional status of patients on admission and obtain an accurate and complete history from either the patients or their families regarding their normal eating habits and patterns. Information of this kind is necessary in designing an individualised plan of care and to gain an appreciation of the importance food has for the patient.

The assessment includes ascertaining the patient's weight and identifying the presence of any physical discomforts such as nausea, dyspepsia and taste abnormalities. Anxiety and apprehension about the illness or operation should also be acknowledged as potential factors which might reduce the appetite. Chapter 27 discusses nutritional assessment in more depth.

For those patients who are unable to absorb or digest food or obtain an adequate nutritional intake, supplementation by either the enteral or parenteral route may be initiated so that major problems attributable to malnutrition can be alleviated if not prevented.

SLEEP

Adequate rest and sleep facilitate recovery from the trauma of surgery. The need for rest and sleep may be taken for granted until sleep is interrupted and this fundamental need warrants further attention by surgical nurses.

The potential for sleep disturbance and indeed sleep deprivation in the surgical environment may be high and can be attributed to a range of factors (see Box 22.12).

Box 22.12 Factors influencing sleep disturbance (Closs 1990, Dodds 1980, cited in McMahon 1992)

- Being in a strange environment and a strange bed
- Feeling alone at night
- Lying awake with pain or discomfort
- Difficulty in obtaining a comfortable position
- Siting of intravenous infusions, tubes or drains
- Noisier environment than the patient is accustomed to
- Nurses making frequent recordings or observations

This list is by no means an exclusive one but all of the factors identified may result in sleep fragmentation. Following surgery, patients may complain of insomnia which may be secondary to the stress and anxiety of acute illness and/or physical discomfort. It is therefore likely that instead of patients obtaining essentially all of their 24-hour quota of sleep in an uninterrupted period, it is gained in more frequent and shorter periods.

Lewis & Timby (1993) acknowledge that sleeping in a different environment is often associated with sleep disruption. In a study of 100 patients who had undergone abdominal surgery and who were interviewed about their experiences of pain and sleep, Closs (1992) reported that pain was the most common cause of disturbed sleep. Half of the patients studied felt that their pain was worse at night. More than one-third of the patients felt that tiredness accentuated their postoperative pain. One-third of the sample felt that sleep reduced pain intensity, three-quarters felt that sleep helped them to cope with their pain and almost all believed that sleep enhanced their postoperative recovery. Many other research studies have confirmed that in hospital, patients rarely meet their personal sleep requirements and that clear changes in sleep patterns often occur.

It is important to people to feel that they have slept adequately, in order to cope with the demands of the day ahead of them. Indeed, the effects of insomnia can be exacerbated by the fear of the effects of sleeplessness. The implications of loss of sleep in the postoperative period will now be considered.

Shortened bulk periods of sleep tend to result in loss of REM (rapid eye movement) sleep. According to Lewis & Timby (1993), sleep disruption is a result of early awakening and delay in getting to sleep. It is also thought that frequent awakenings are possibly more harmful than a lack of sleep, because of the disruption in the person's sleep cycles. Sleep deprivation mainly affects the central nervous system and the effects of this may be observed. They include speech slurring, memory lapses, disorientation with time, visual misperceptions, difficulty in concentrating, irritability, feeling cold and a reduced ability to perform psychomotor skills accurately.

Recommendations for best practice

The surgical nurse, using the information gained from conducting a nursing assessment about a patient's normal rest and sleep patterns, may be able to plan care which aims to minimise the factors which are known to result in sleep disturbance for that particular individual. Relevant information that is gathered on assessment may be:

- the number of hours the patient normally sleeps each night
- the time period in which this normally occurs
- if any naps are taken, when and how frequently.

A description of any particular pre-bedtime routines the patient adopts and information relating to the patient's normal sleep environment should also be obtained.

Of course there are individual differences in sleep needs which also have to be taken into account, such as changes in sleep patterns throughout the life span and a tendency towards a reduction in total sleep time and in the proportion of REM sleep with advancing age.

Rest

It is worth considering that patients who are prescribed bed rest may not actually feel rested, rest being associated with feelings of peace and relaxation. For patients to 'be at rest', they must be free of anxieties and troublesome thoughts. On the contrary, patients who are prescribed enforced bed rest may often be disturbed by their relative inactivity.

From the writers' own observations it is interesting that many wards now advocate a compulsory daytime rest period for patients. These are often of an hour or two in duration, and take no regard of the fact that not all patients may feel tired or want to rest at this time. The effectiveness of such rest periods might be open to debate unless all unnecessary nursing and medical activities do actually cease and may depend on whether the nursing staff are able to control noise within the environment and the flow of visitors to the ward area.

From the above discussion on sleep it is obvious that adequate sleep is vital to the recovery of patients. Since lack of sleep may be detrimental to the physiological and psychological well-being of patients, it is hoped that this will lead you to consider implementing changes in practice which will minimise sleep disruption and assist those patients who are experiencing problems with sleep fragmentation and disturbance.

PAIN ASSESSMENT AND MANAGEMENT

Closs (1992) asserts that pain and sleep are symbiotic and that the patient in pain is likely to suffer the effects of sleep deprivation. The management of pain is a fundamental aspect of postoperative care and is discussed in depth in Chapter 24. Patients undergo surgery with an expectation of pain and are seldom disappointed.

Numerous clinical studies in recent years (Balfour 1989, Carr 1990, Field 1996) have identified the discrepancy between the need for pain relief and its appropriate action. Patients in pain are often undermedicated, even when appropriate narcotic analgesia is prescribed and available. Failure to provide adequate pain relief produces a potential for the occurrence of postoperative complications quite apart from the humanitarian requirement for analgesia. Pain is likely to reduce mobility, making venous thrombosis more likely. Chest infections too may be a problem associated with late mobilisation, particularly when exacerbated by the fear of coughing following abdominal surgery.

Reflective point

Identify a patient you have recently nursed following surgery. What tools and mechanisms for pain assessment did you utilise and what factors influenced your assessment of this patient's pain?

Consider also how involved your patients are in the process of pain management. How might the information gathered in pain assessment influence the subsequent management of pain?

There are a number of well-reported factors which might influence the patient's perception of pain. Whilst an understanding of their potential influence is useful to the surgical nurse, it is surely more important to avoid stereotypical assumptions or subjective observation (see Case study 22.3). Pain assessment and control must be a paramount priority in surgical practice. Whilst the use of objective measures of pain has a key role to play in pain management, nurses often feel the need to verify patient pain by nonverbal signs or by physiological manifestations such as raised blood pressure or sweating. Such indicators can obviously be misleading and often modified by adaptive and coping mechanisms.

Case study 22.3   Mrs Wilson

Mrs Wilson is a 54-year-old housewife admitted with abdominal pain. A succession of scans and X-rays fail to reveal any abnormalities and leave the surgical registrar in no doubt that the lady is somewhat hysterical. He prescribes an intramuscular injection of sterile water and instructs the nurses to monitor its effect. The nurses quickly come to share the registrar's opinion and despite the obvious lack of placebo effect, are slow to administer further doses of opioid. It is only when the consultant surgeon does his round and raises the possibility that there might, despite the lack of scientific evidence, be a surgical pathology that Mrs Wilson is taken to theatre for a laparotomy.

Mrs Wilson was discovered to have a number of adhesions which had been causing intermittent colic, and indeed a segment of small bowel had to be resected because of its ischaemic state. In the light of this diagnosis, nursing staff found it hard to believe that they had been unable to accept Mrs Wilson's description of her pain.

Reflective point

What factors might have influenced nursing staff perceptions of Mrs Wilson's pain in Case study 22.3? What lessons might the nursing staff have learnt here and how could a similar situation be avoided in the future?

Failure of postoperative pain relief is often partly due to the poor understanding and utilisation of drugs available. The standard prescription 4- to 6-hourly often has little use in modern pain management. The peaks and troughs such regimens provide must only reduce the chances of activating adequate analgesia. In addition, such regimens are often inflexible, poorly prescribed and often with a significant delay between the request for and the eventual administration of the drug.

The use of pain assessment tools provides the patient with an opportunity to take an active role in pain management, promoting a feeling of being taken seriously. This participative and collaborative alliance will promote the nurse–patient relationship as well as providing an evaluative mechanism for the success of individual regimens.

The use of patient-controlled analgesia (PCA) was developed in this country and the USA as long ago as the 1960s, though primarily as a research tool. In Britain, the Working Party Report from the Royal College of Surgeons of England and College of Anaesthetists (1990), which describes the desperate state of current analgesic practice, has motivated a review of pain management and increased the use of PCA. Additional motivation was provided through the Patient's Charter (DoH 1991), which increased public knowledge and awareness of health issues and promoted a greater patient empowerment in their own pain management.

Whilst the potential benefits are discussed in Chapter 24, it is worth noting that not all patients will wish to access or benefit from this intervention. It is the surgical nurse's responsibility to assess and subsequently monitor patients and evaluate each individual's decision to either participate or reject the opportunity to use a PCA device.

Currently, nurses tend to rely on the use of pharmacological interventions in the management of pain. Certainly, the use of opioids and other drugs plays a prime role in pain control immediately following surgery. However, as the patients' perception of their pain diminishes during the recovery period, there is the potential for consideration of other strategies in the total pain management plan. The use of transcutaneous electrical nerve stimulation (TENS) machines, acupuncture, relaxation, and diversional therapies such as listening to music, massage and the use of aromatherapy, are all identified as having potential in pain relief (Watson & Long 1995).

In summary, a number of recommendations may be utilised in enhancing appropriate pain management in the postoperative period. These are identified in Box 22.13.

PROMOTING HEALTH AND PATIENT EMPOWERMENT

Much nursing research in the past 20 years has stressed the importance of patient education as an

---

Box 22.13 Strategies for achieving suitable pain relief

- Practice with the belief that pain is not an inevitable consequence of surgery.
- Understand the nature and effect of analgesia.
- Talk to your patient, listen to and respect your patient's perspective.
- Utilise appropriate assessment tools.
- Recognise that analgesia given for pain will never lead to addiction.
- Review analgesic regimens constantly.
- Consider alternative, non-pharmacological approaches in pain management.

---

element in the promotion of health. Studies have continued to report the effects of information-giving through verbal or documentary communication (Luker & Caress 1989, Redman 1993). For many years researchers such as Boore (1978) and Hayward (1975) have demonstrated how provision of information can reduce pain and anxiety, reduce postoperative complications and enhance recovery rates in surgical patients (see also Chs 2 and 18).

The involvement of the patient in care management is clearly desirable and conducive to recovery. Indeed, the informed participative and active individual is central to all modern nursing theory and the goals of equity, partnership and informed decision-making enshrined in current nursing philosophy (see also Ch. 20).

However, health promotion activity and, more specifically, health and patient education, have been less conspicuous in surgical nursing settings than in longer-term medical and community settings. Macleod Clark et al (1992) found health education to take low priority compared to general ward activities in acute units. Yet the previous Government's initiative, 'The Health of the Nation' (DoH 1992, 1993), and the proposed new health strategy 'Our Healthier Nation' (DoH 1997) both recognise hospitals, and nurses in particular, as offering unique and 'unparalleled' opportunities for health promotion for patients and their families. For the patient in a vulnerable, compromised, and often disempowered state, health promotion is a major opportunity for the nurse working in surgical care settings to enable, advise and empower (see Ch. 3).

It is commonly agreed that a major goal of health care should be to create autonomy for the client. To empower people is to facilitate them in the development of this autonomy, but there are basic conditions necessary to achieve this end. Seedhouse & Cribb

1989 identify three conditions: the ability to understand one's environment and circumstances; the ability to make rational choices; and the ability to act on these. It is evident that to achieve such goals and abilities the individual needs education, for without information and explanation or adequate understanding, informed, rational choice is not possible.

Reflective point

In your own clinical setting identify examples of health promotion, education and teaching activities provided for your patients.

You might have identified some of the following:

- How to manage a colostomy
- Caring for a 'stump' wound following amputation
- Teaching a patient to examine breast or testis for signs of recurring growth
- Giving dietary advice in ulcerative colitis or Crohn's disease.

Of course, promoting health in a surgical setting is not only about providing information. Health promotion must be perceived as an element of health care in which the professionals seek to enable their clients to take control over their own lives and health through processes of education and equitable partnerships. Principles of patient participation, freedom of choice, interagency collaboration and the pursuit of patient empowerment are fundamental to a non-coercive and facilitative approach to care.

Lay participation is also considered an integral theme of patient empowerment (Salvage 1992) and is characterised by the nurse's expressed desire to include the patient and/or family in planning and decision-making processes of health promotion. However, many patients, because of their stage of illness or unconditional faith and trust in the health professional, have little desire for involvement in decision-making processes. 'You do whatever you need to do, nurse, you know what is best' is a comment heard regularly in surgical wards. This apparent abdication of rights in participation is consistent with Waterworth & Luker's (1990) findings. They suggest that some relatives and patients prefer not to participate in care and decision-making but are often coerced as reluctant participants. Clearly, the need for nurses to consult with patients and their families on a regular

basis to assess this potential is vital in promoting a minimally stressful interaction.

Reflective point

What factors influence the potential success of health promotion activities in your care setting? How might successful patient education and teaching be better managed in your clinical setting?

Box 22.14 lists the factors influencing the potential success of health promotion.

Box 22.14 Factors influencing the potential success of health promotion

- Time
- Patient motivation
- Resources
- Perception of work/low priority of educative activity
- Nurse motivation
- Conflicting sources of knowledge
- Management commitment

Studies by Latter et al (1992) suggest that in acute settings, nurses are reported to see information-giving and coercive lifestyle change as legitimate and the predominant forms of health-promoting activity. Philosophical underpinnings of health promotion, i.e. empowerment and partnership, are often paid only lip service as nursing goals. Indeed, nursing and health promotion are often seen as distinct and mutually exclusive concepts. Such traditional health care roles involve professionals as experts with prestige, power and a monopoly in knowledge. Contemporary nursing practice rightly advocates that nurses can no longer regard their patients as passive recipients unless this is their wish. Yet because more didactic activities in teaching and advice-giving may coexist within a traditional, authoritarian model of nursing practice, many nurses persist in utilising these as a legitimate approach to patient education. Consequently, patients are seen as passive recipients, vulnerable and with few alternatives (see also Ch. 3).

These perceptions may be influential in subsequent surgical nursing practice which promotes a hierarchy of nursing activity where physical and often medically oriented routines, tasks or procedures take precedence over patients' emotional and psychosocial care or teaching.

Reflective point

Does your ward philosophy reflect a belief in the values of positive health promotion, making explicit views on the worth of patient participation, informed freedom of choice and the promotion of self-empowerment? If so, can you identify four ways in which these beliefs have been translated into postsurgical activity?

You might have identified:

- Encouraging patients to ask questions about their problems
- A structured and individually focused teaching programme
- The encouragement of family participation in care
- All staff participation in ward policy and protocol development
- Collaboration with other health professionals to provide a multidisciplinary care package
- Evaluation of patients' satisfaction with their care.

Specific examples might have included:

- Ensuring patient awareness of medication regimens
- The use of patient-controlled analgesics postoperatively
- Encouraging the patient's carer to participate fully in therapeutic activities.

Nurses should be working towards the maintenance, improvement or restoration of optimum health levels for those within their care. Traditionally prescriptive treatment should be superseded by negotiated and collaborative interaction to enable such choices to be made. For effective decision-making, the client needs a conducive environment insulated from factors which might inhibit this process. The positive encouragement of these principles should facilitate empowered patients who are informed and able to make appropriate decisions about their care and problem management. Health promotion and health education should involve making healthy choices easier choices. Arguably, changes in practice would necessitate a major philosophical and paradigm shift which addresses the knowledge, values, attitudes and associated skills of practising nurses. However, the fostering of individual responsibility for health through empowerment, collaboration and equitable partnerships is essential in achieving professional nursing excellence.

ETHICS AND MORAL ISSUES IN SURGICAL PRACTICE

The principles of consent to treatment have been discussed in Chapter 4 and similar principles are often paramount in the postsurgical period. There is a duty on health care professionals to ensure that patients are provided with significant information concerning their care and management. However, there is also a duty to withhold information deemed not to be in the patient's best interest to know. This principle of therapeutic privilege (Dimond 1995) provides the doctor with the authority to withhold information considered harmful or non-beneficial. Examples might include diagnosis of terminal disease or chronic illness. Subsequently members of the health care team are required to accept and implement this decision. Indeed the nurse who chooses to ignore the doctor's wishes might well face disciplinary proceedings. The nurse, then, cannot ignore the doctor's prescription, even if the patient is considered ultimately to have a right to know. Such situations provide the potential for enormous conflict and dissonance, not least for the surgical nurse (see Case study 22.4).

Case study 22.4   Patient A

Mr Jones is a 45-year-old police officer who is discovered, following a laparotomy, to have an inoperable pancreatic cancer. The surgeon feels that it is not in his best interest to know the diagnosis and subsequent prognosis at this time and instructs the nursing team to withhold any specific information. Mrs Jones is in full agreement with the doctor's decision to withhold information and believes that her husband's 'morbid dread of cancer' would precipitate feelings of terror and depression should he become aware. Mr Jones is informed that he has a growth on his pancreas which might be better managed through medication. Mr Jones asks a staff nurse when he might return to work and enquires about the exact nature of his 'condition and medication'.

Reflective point

An explicit philosophy or protocol which provides guidance for nurses and clinical staff concerning 'truth telling' can provide a focus for nursing activity. If such a statement is in place in your care setting, do you believe it to be of practical use and reflective of reality? If no policy or protocol exists, do you believe such a protocol could usefully be developed?

Reflective discussion

How might the staff nurse react to Mr Jones's request in Case study 22.4?

What moral, ethical and legal issues might be apparent in this conspiracy of silence and what justification can there be for withholding or providing untruthful information?

There is the potential for much soul searching and, indeed, as Dimond (1995) points out, ethical and legal conflicts in this often 'grey area'. Clearly, the nurse should not act in a manner contrary to the medical decision on disclosure but neither should she lie to the patient. Whilst she could refer any enquiry from the patient to the doctor, this is clearly not the most satisfactory solution. Essentially in our scenario Mr Jones alone has the right to insist that he receives the information he requires, yet the practitioner must consider a host of other factors when selecting the course of action. Ultimately, the use of euphemisms such as ulcer, growth, and blockage as descriptions of malignancy and cancer are likely to provide only confusion and resentment. Yet it is not at all unusual for carers to ask for the diagnosis and/or prognosis to be withheld from the patient. However, it is often debatable whether it is the patient's perceived inability to cope with the information or the relatives' inability to cope with the patient knowing which motivates this conflict.

Reflective point

In your clinical area, is the family of the patient ever informed of diagnosis or prognosis before the patient is informed? What justification might the doctor or nurse make for such a decision?

You might have recognised that in law such a situation should not have arisen. Dimond (1995) succinctly outlines the professional and ethical stances of the professional bodies. She recognises that the General Medical Council is quite clear in its views on disclosure, stating that the doctor who chooses to disclose confidential information to a third party regardless of circumstances must be prepared to explain and justify this decision.

There are implications for the nurse too. The 'Guidelines for Professional Practice' document (UKCC 1996) states that in all cases where practitioners deliberately disclose or withhold information they must be prepared to justify this action. Patients are entitled to confidentiality with respect to their medical condition, and indeed are entitled to ask for information to be withheld from their family. Ideally, the surgical setting should provide an environment conducive to truth telling and yet maintain the right of the practitioner to make considered professional judgement or therapeutic privilege. However, it is essential that the decision not to tell is made for the most appropriate of reasons. The best interests of the patient and not the staff are paramount here. Additionally, such a decision must be constantly re-evaluated. What may be right today, may not be right tomorrow. Perhaps, most importantly, there should be the forum and opportunity for all staff to be involved in discussion to raise consciousness of the issues involved and to enable clarification of the potential conflicts. It is the multiprofessional, collaborative debate which is most likely to provide the framework and support required in clinical decision-making. Whilst there is rarely a clear-cut right or wrong answer, disagreements may at least be aired and shared, and the potential for a consensus might be reached. Certainly it is in our patients' best interests to provide the most informed and considered management of this crucial area of postsurgical practice.

CONCLUSION

Most surgical texts have traditionally utilised a reductionist systems approach to the care of the surgical patient. Our approach to this chapter was not intended to compete with, but rather to complement, texts of this nature. Nurses need comprehensive explicit information on specific surgical operations, techniques and their management. However, we also believe that no nurse can be an expert in all fields of surgical nursing. Accordingly, it is unlikely that nurses will make full use of all specialist sections of such texts. In recognition of this, we have attempted to provide a springboard for reflection on practice and provide a catalyst for its examination in the light of the current knowledge and philosophy underlying surgical nursing. Benner (1984) suggested that unless nurses use reflection to gain insight and explanation of their actions, the knowledge embedded in clinical practice will remain as hidden knowledge unless it is articulated and shared. In essence we have attempted to identify sound clinical practice and complemented this with an exploration of what it is that surgical nurses do. Today there is increasing recognition of, and readiness to explore, sources of knowledge less amenable to scientific explanation. Essentially then, the 'aesthetic' (Carper 1978) or artistic qualities of nursing, utilising qualitative approaches, may equally inform nursing practice.

Surgical nurses must be able to critically assess contemporary approaches to postoperative patient care and evaluate practice in the light of these. It is hoped that this chapter may provide the reader with the desire to develop a greater awareness and understanding of the factors which influence successful surgical recovery. In turn, this should facilitate an exploration of the traditional beliefs, attitudes and assumptions which exist in relation to caring for the postoperative surgical patient.

REFERENCES

Autar R 1996 Nursing assessment of clients at risk of deep vein thrombosis (DVT): the Autar SVT scale. Journal of Advanced Nursing 23(4): 763–770

Balfour S 1989 Will I be in pain? Patients' and nurses' attitudes to pain after abdominal surgery. Professional Nurse 5(1): 28–33

Benner P 1984 From novice to expert: excellence and power in clinical practice. Addison-Wesley, California

Bistrian B, Blackburn G, Hallowell E, Heddle R 1974 Protein status of general surgical patients. Journal of the American Medical Association 230: 858–860

Boore J 1978 Prescription for recovery. RCN, London

Bright L, Georgi S 1994 How to protect your patient from DVT. American Journal of Nursing 94(12): 28–32

Burgess L 1994 Mixed responses. Nursing Times 90(2): 30–34

Carper B 1978 Fundamental patterns of knowing in nursing. Advanced Nursing Science 1: 13–23

Carr E 1990 Post-operative pain, patients' expectations and experiences. Journal of Advanced Nursing 15(1): 89–100

Chapman A 1996 Current theory and practice: a study of pre-operative fasting. Nursing Standard 10(18): 33–36

Clancy J, McVicar A 1995 Physiology and anatomy: a homeostatic approach. Edward Arnold, London

Closs S 1990 Influences on patients' sleep on surgical wards. Surgical Nurse 3(2): 12–14

Closs S 1992 Post-operative patients' views of sleep, pain and recovery. Journal of Clinical Nursing 1: 83–88

Cole A 1991 Still mixed up. Nursing Times 91(6): 14–16

Correnti D 1993 Intuition and nursing practice, implications for nurse educators: a review of the literature. Journal of Advanced Nursing 18(3): 91–94

Craft T, Upton P 1992 Key topics in anaesthesia. BIOS Scientific Publishers, Worcester

Crossley A 1992 Peri-operative shivering. Anaesthesia 47: 193–195

Dealey C 1994 The care of wounds. Blackwell Science, Oxford

Dennison D 1995 Thermal regulation of patients during the perioperative experience. Association of Operating Room Nurses Journal 61(5): 827–828, 831–832

Department of Health (DoH) 1991 The patient's charter. HMSO, London

Department of Health (DoH) 1992 The health of the nation. DoH, London

Department of Health (DoH) 1993 Targeting practice: the contribution of nurses, midwives and health visitors. The health of the nation. DoH, London

Department of Health (DoH) 1997 Our healthier nation. DoH, London

Dickerson J 1995 The problem of hospital-induced malnutrition. Nursing Times 91(4): 44–45

Dimond B 1995 Legal aspects of nursing, 2nd edn. Prentice Hall, London

Dodds E J 1980 Slept well? A study of ward activity and nurse–patient interaction at night. MSc Thesis, University of Surrey

Doyle J 1998 Recognising the signs of hypoxia. Hospital Medicine 34(7): 46–48, 54–56

Edmonson R, Cohen A 1994 The causes and management of pulmonary embolism. Care of the Critically Ill 10(1): 26–30

Edmunds M 1991 Introduction to clinical pharmacology. Mosby, St. Louis

Field L 1996 Are nurses still underestimating patients' pain? British Journal of Nursing 5(3): 778–784

Flanagan M 1997 Wound management. Churchill Livingstone, Edinburgh

Fotheringham D 1995 Post-anaesthetic shaking. British Journal of Nursing 4(15): 857–860

Hamilton-Smith S 1972 Nil by mouth. RCN, London

Hayward J 1975 Information – a prescription against pain. RCN, London

Hopkins S 1995 Drugs and pharmacology for nurses. Churchill Livingstone, Edinburgh

Jamieson E M, McCall J M, Blythe R, Whyte L A 1997 Clinical nursing practices, 3rd edn. Churchill Livingstone, Edinburgh

Kelly M P 1985 Loss and grief reactions as responses to surgery. Journal of Advanced Nursing 10: 517–525

Kurz A, Sessler D, Narzt E et al 1995 Postoperative haemodynamic and thermoregulatory consequences of intraoperative core hypothermia. Journal of Clinical Anaesthesia 7(5): 359–366

Latter S, Macleod Clark J, Wilson-Barnett J, Maben J 1992 Health education in nursing: perceptions of practice in acute settings. Journal of Advanced Nursing 17: 164–172

Lewis L W, Timby B K 1993 Fundamental skills and concepts in patient care. Chapman and Hall, London

Luckmann J (ed) 1997 Saunders manual of nursing care. W B Saunders, Philadelphia

Luker K, Caress A 1989 Rethinking patient education. Journal of Advanced Nursing 14: 711–718

Macleod Clark J, Wilson-Barnett J, Latter S, Maben J 1992 Health education and health promotion in nursing: a study of practice in acute areas. Nursing Studies Department, King's College, London

McMahon R 1992 (ed) Nursing at night: a professional approach. Scutari Press, London

Nettina S M 1996 The Lippincott manual of nursing practice, 6th edn. Lippincott – Raven, Philadelphia

Pediani R 1992 Preparing to heal. Nursing Times 88(27): 68–70

Perkins P 1992 Wound dehiscence: causes and care. Nursing Standard 6(34)(suppl): 12–14

Price B 1993 Dignity that must be respected: body image and the surgical patient. Professional Nurse 8(10): 670–672

Redman D 1993 Patient education at 25 years: where we have been and where we are going? Journal of Advanced Nursing 18: 725–730

Robinson R, Stott R 1987 Medical emergencies: diagnosis and management. Heinemann, London

Royal College of Nursing (RCN) 1988 Statement of policy on mixed sex wards. RCN, London

Royal College of Nursing (RCN) 1993 Mixed-sex wards: principles for practice. RCN, London

Royal College of Surgeons of England and College of Anaesthetists 1990 Commission on the provision of surgical services report of the working party on pain after surgery. RCS, London

Salvage J 1992 Policy issues in nursing. Open University Press, Milton Keynes

Schon D 1983 The reflective practitioner – how professionals think in action. Maurice Temple Smith, London

Seedhouse D, Cribb A 1989 Changing ideas in health care. John Wiley, London

Singh P, Dimitrou V, Mahajan R, Crossley A 1993 Double blind comparison between doxapram and pethidine in the treatment of post anaesthetic shivering. British Journal of Anaesthesia 71(5): 685–688

Smeltzer S, Bare B (eds) 1992 Brunner and Suddarth's textbook of medical–surgical nursing, 7th edn. J B Lippincott, Philadelphia

Sorensen K, Luckmann J 1986 Basic nursing: a psychophysiologic approach, 2nd edn. W B Saunders, Philadelphia

Surkitt Parr M 1992 Hypothermia in surgical patients. British Journal of Nursing 1(11): 539–545

Thomas E 1987 Pre-operative fasting – a question of routine. Nursing Times 83(49): 46–47

Tyrell M, Birtel A, Taylor P 1995 Deep vein thrombosis. British Journal of Clinical Practice 49(5): 252–256

United Kingdom Central Council for Nursing, Midwifery and Health Visiting (UKCC) 1996 Guidelines for professional practice. UKCC, London

Vogelsang J 1991 Patients who develop post-anaesthesia shaking show no difference in post operative temperature from those who do not develop shaking. Journal of Post Anaesthetic Nursing 6(4): 231–238

Waterworth S, Luker K 1990 Reluctant collaborators: do patients want to be involved in decisions concerning care? Journal of Advanced Nursing 15: 971–976

Watson J, Long B 1995 Pain. In: Long B, Phipps W, Cassmeyer V (eds) Adult nursing: a nursing process approach. Mosby, Philadelphia

Wilson J 1995 Infection control in clinical practice. Baillière Tindall, London

Wong C 1991 Physiologic responses to anaesthesia. In: Shekleton M, Litwack K (eds) Critical care nursing of the surgical patient. WB Saunders, Philadelphia

FURTHER READING

McMahon R 1992 Nursing at night: a professional approach. Scutari Press, London

Walsh M, Ford P 1992 Nursing rituals research and rational actions. Butterworth Heinemann, Oxford

Walsh M, Ford P 1994 New rituals for old nursing: through the looking glass. Butterworth Heinemann, Oxford

23

Maintaining effective breathing

Debbie Field

AIMS

This chapter focuses on the surgical nurse's important role in optimising and maintaining effective breathing for patients who require or have undergone surgery.
    The aims of the chapter are:

- to provide an understanding of the concepts of normal and disordered respiratory physiology
- to describe, give a rationale for, and analyse the importance of undertaking a thorough preoperative and postoperative respiratory assessment
- to identify and give a greater understanding of the main principles of preoperative and postoperative respiratory care, prevention of pulmonary complications and applied therapeutic nursing interventions
- to briefly describe and give a rationale for the pharmacological interventions used in the prevention of postoperative pulmonary complications
- to begin to help surgical nurses develop awareness of some of the ethical issues relating to the offer of surgery for those patients who are elderly, have a chronic pulmonary disease, or who smoke
- to stimulate surgical nurses to reflect upon and critically analyse their own practice of respiratory care in the surgical patient.

INTRODUCTION

Over the past 20–25 years many advances have been made in the preoperative, perioperative and postoperative care and treatment of surgical patients, such as new technology, refined surgical skills, keyhole surgery, day surgery and improved anaesthetic agents. However, even with these advances, respiratory complications, specifically atelectasis and pneumonia, remain the leading cause of postoperative morbidity and death (Davies 1991, Pesola et al 1990). Respiratory complications have been shown to account for about 24% of all deaths which occur within 6 days after surgery (Pierson & Branson 1992, cited in Brooks-Brunn 1995), and postoperative pneumonia has been associated with up to a 46% mortality rate (Iwamoto et al 1993). This has major implications for all surgical nurses because it requires them to have a thorough understanding of the pathophysiology, risk factors and appropriate interventions involved in the recognition and prevention of these complications. Also, nurses must have a sound working knowledge of essential nursing theories and concepts and have the ability to critically analyse current respiratory care interventions and treatments. By using their clinical wisdom and demonstrating an understanding of both the physiological and psychological response to breathing, nurses will realise that they are not just an instrument of other professions in curing the patient but rather they are uniquely significant in the patient's recovery. This is not 'in spite' of nursing care but as a direct result of deliberate decision-making in partnership with patients, their carers and the multidisciplinary team.

The central focus of this chapter, therefore, is to demonstrate that by being proactive, dynamic and creative in optimising and maintaining effective breathing in surgical patients and manipulating the patients' care in relation to their physical, psychological and spiritual well-being during the preoperative, perioperative and postoperative periods, the nurse will effect a quality patient outcome by reducing morbidity and mortality in surgical patients.

It is not the purpose of this chapter to explore specific surgery but to offer the surgical nurse a firm foundation in respiratory assessment, nurse intervention and care in order for the patient to maintain an effective breathing pattern.

Current perspectives

It is important to realise that pulmonary complications, specifically postoperative pneumonia and atelectasis, were cited as far back as 1898 (Featherstone 1924). Pasteur (1910) and Featherstone (1924) described and demonstrated the incidence of postoperative atelectasis and pneumonia, and many of their thoughts and concepts concerning postoperative management and the care of pulmonary complications are still relevant today within our current health care system and its advances in surgery. With the introduction of innovative health care initiatives the length of stay for any surgical patient has been greatly reduced (DoH 1993) in relation to both preoperative and postoperative

time. This is due to many factors such as economics, advances in both general and local anaesthetic agents, day surgery and improved surgical techniques. It has led to those patients who are elderly or acutely or chronically ill being routinely offered complex surgery which was inconceivable in the past (Brooks-Brunn 1995). However, as much of the literature demonstrates (Davies 1991, Ephgrave et al 1993, Martin et al 1984), there has not been a marked reduction in postoperative complications such as atelectasis and pneumonia. Indeed, the anecdotal evidence suggests that it is because surgery is being offered to, and undertaken on, those patients who are elderly, have a chronic pulmonary disease and are acutely ill, that there continues to be a high incidence of postoperative pulmonary complications. It is the writer's opinion and experience that other factors, such as reduced preoperative and postoperative time, the multiple cancellation of operations, and the lack of appropriate and specific nurse education, are influential on the incidence of pulmonary postoperative complications. Reducing both preoperative and postoperative time does not allow the nurse caring for the patient to maximise information-giving, patient-teaching and patient education or the development of a positive and effective nurse–patient relationship. Nursing research has demonstrated that patient anxiety levels, stress and pain can be reduced by effective preoperative information (Boore 1978, Cochran 1984, Hayward 1975, Raleigh et al 1990). Although further research needs to be undertaken in this area, reducing a patient's anxiety may result in fewer postoperative complications and therefore earlier patient discharge, which is the current and desirable economic goal (Kempe & Gelazis 1985, Nelson 1995). Surgical nurses are now in a prime position to take control over the very essence of their practice: to optimise and maintain effective breathing in their surgical patients and meet current health care challenges. The UKCC's Scope of Professional Practice (1992), has opened the door for surgical nurses to develop patient-centred initiatives such as preoperative assessment clinics (Nelson 1995), hospital at home (Elliott 1995), nurse-led day surgery (Rose 1995) and the further development of the generic clinical nurse specialist (CNS) in areas such as asthma care and chronic airway limitation.

Reflective point

How have you taken your practice forward during the past 2 years to meet changing health care demands and ensure quality nursing care?

THEORIES UNDERPINNING THE CHAPTER AND IMPLICATIONS FOR PRACTICE

For surgical nurses to optimise and maintain effective breathing in patients and demonstrate the ability to recognise and act rapidly to changing clinical events, they must have an understanding of normal respiratory function. Therefore, it is necessary to give a brief overview of the principles of normal respiratory physiology and for the reader to review respiratory anatomy and lung volumes (see Hinchliff & Montague 1988).

Normal respiratory physiology

The overall function of the respiratory system is to provide adequate oxygen to the tissues for the oxidation of respiratory substrates (carbohydrates, fats and proteins) in order to yield energy and to remove metabolites (i.e. carbon dioxide and water) produced from this process following cellular respiration (Hinchliff & Montague 1988). This is achieved by and dependent upon the complex and interrelated processes that are summarised in Box 23.1. Disturbances of any of these processes will result in the disruption of homeostasis with the risk of developing mild to severe respiratory failure.

Preoperative, intraoperative and postoperative changes related to respiratory function

It has been well documented by various authors (Knill 1988, Sykes & Bowe 1993) that general anaesthesia,

---

Box 23.1   Determinants of respiration

- An adequate air (ventilation) and blood supply (perfusion) which must be evenly matched to ensure efficient gas exchange to occur by diffusion.
- Mechanical efficiency which includes an atmospheric air–lung pressure gradient, airway resistance, muscular function, lung compliance, intrapleural pressures and neural control.
- Adequate gas exchange of CO_2 and O_2 at alveolar and capillary level by diffusion (external respiration).
- Adequate uptake of O_2 by haemoglobin.
- The transport and distribution of the oxygenated haemoglobin by the cardiovascular system to the tissues in order for cellular respiration to take place and the removal of CO_2 and H_2O back to the lungs (see Ch. 25).

---

whether through inhalation or injection, has a direct effect on ventilation and perfusion during both the perioperative and postoperative phases of any type of surgery requiring a general anaesthetic and will ultimately affect the recovery of the patient. During general anaesthesia there is approximately a 20% decrease in the patient's functional residual capacity (FRC). This is due to the effects of the general anaesthetic on the shape and position of the chest wall and diaphragm. Intravenous narcotics that are used for induction or maintenance of general anaesthesia may substantially reduce the postoperative hypoxic and hypercapnic ventilatory drive. This is especially important to note when patients who already have lung disease or are elderly are to undergo surgery. Elderly patients appear particularly susceptible to hypoxaemia postoperatively if they have received narcotics during anaesthesia.

Diaphragmatic dysfunction after abdominal or thoracic surgery may be related to a reflex inhibition of the phrenic nerve as a result of sympathetic, vagal or splanchnic receptor stimulation (Sykes & Bowe 1993).

It must also be remembered that administration of many of the premedications such as lorazepam and omnopon and scopolamine may cause respiratory depression and induce hypoxia prior to surgery. Research undertaken in patients undergoing open heart surgery demonstrates that after patients received premedication of 1 mg oral lorazepam in the anaesthetic room prior to induction, their arterial PO_2 was only 6–8 kPa (Bailey et al 1993). This, therefore, has major implications for such patients who already have decreased ventilation and perfusion of their myocardium owing to cardiac disease.

Nurses, therefore, need to question and analyse the use of premedications on certain kinds of patients who may be put further at risk. It may be more therapeutic to develop other interventions to help patients prepare for surgery rather than use pharmacological agents to make them relax. Surgical nurses could initiate research into the use of such interventions as music therapy, massage, relaxation tapes or story-telling. This would also enhance the nurse–patient relationship and may help patients become empowered, thus allowing them to take control of their situation.

At-risk patients

In order to understand the importance of optimising and maintaining effective breathing in surgical patients, it is important first to identify those patients who have an increased risk of developing respiratory complications and consequently respiratory failure during the surgical experience and the types of surgery which have the greater incidence of postoperative pulmonary complications. By identifying those patients most at risk and applying the known theory alongside their own personal and intuitive knowledge (Carper 1978), nurses will be able to plan individual nursing care strategies in order to intervene to optimise and maintain effective breathing in their patients.

Patients who have a greater risk of developing respiratory complications are identified below. This list is not exhaustive but represents many of the patients seen most often within the surgical environment.

- *Patients with chronic lung disease* – asthma, chronic airway limitation, emphysema, pulmonary fibrosing alveolitis.
- *Patients with signs of respiratory failure* – this will include patients who have chronic cardiac failure because they will develop signs and symptoms of respiratory failure due to pulmonary congestion.
- *Patients with a history of taking aminoglycosides* – these patients have a greater risk of pulmonary complications following surgery owing to the fact that aminoglycosides when combined with muscle relaxants may potentiate neuromuscular blockade. This may lead to decreased respiratory muscle function and thus decreased respiratory function in these patients if the residual effects are not recognised (McConnoll 1991).
- *Upper abdominal surgery* – the higher the incision in abdominal surgery the greater the risk of decreased diaphragmatic movement leading to atelectasis (Chunter et al 1989).
- *Chest surgery* – open heart surgery and thoracotomy are both operations which will directly interfere with the mechanical efficiency of respiration and may lead to atelectasis and pneumonia (Litwack 1995). Cardiopulmonary bypass also carries its own risk of developing postoperative pulmonary complications (Matthay & Wiener-Kronish 1989).
- *Patients requiring a nasogastric tube (NGT)* – an NGT in situ for more than 24 hours may lead to pulmonary complications. This is possibly due to an increase in reflux and aspiration of gut contents and/or decreased coughing efficacy (McConnell 1991).
- *Patients with signs of cardiovascular disease* – this, of course, will directly affect perfusion and oxygen uptake by the cells.
- *Patients whose respiratory centre is depressed* – including drug-induced depression and neurological injury.
- *Patients with respiratory muscle weakness* – including myasthenia gravis, Guillain–Barré syndrome, poor

nutritional status. Poor nutritional status, in particular low serum phosphate, will directly affect respiratory muscle strength. Phosphate is the major energy source for muscle function. To maintain and optimise respiration, the patient has to have an adequate supply of respiratory substrates, i.e. carbohydrates, fats and proteins (see also Ch. 27).

- *Patients who are immobilised* – immobilisation potentiates the risk of venous stasis which increases the risk of developing pulmonary emboli. Immobilisation also has a psychological impact on the patient which will influence respiratory function. This relates to feelings of depression, helplessness and lack of control by the patient. This may result in a lack of compliance with nursing interventions and physiotherapy regimes.
- *Patients who are over the age of 60* – Foyt (1992) demonstrated that patients who were over the age of 60 years had a decreased physiological reserve to cope with stresses. Also, studies have demonstrated that elderly patients' lungs are more prone to terminal airway closure (Seymour & Vaz 1989) (see also Ch. 11).
- *Patients who have a history of smoking* – many studies have demonstrated that even when patients stop smoking for 2 or 3 months prior to surgery their risk of developing postoperative pulmonary complications such as hypoxia, atelectasis and pneumonia remains just as high as if they had not stopped smoking (Wewers et al 1994). It appears that the risk decreases only after a cessation of 12–18 months.
- *Patients who are obese* – these patients are more inclined to develop postoperative atelectasis, hypoxaemia and respiratory acidosis owing to the decrease in respiratory muscle function.
- *Patients who have undergone non-elective surgery* – patients who undergo emergency surgery are at greater risk of developing pulmonary complications than those patients who have had elective surgery. This is due to a number of factors: there is less time to prepare the patient physically and psychologically; the patient will be stressed and the physiological response to stress will be initiated, namely sympathetic nervous system arousal. The result is that it increases the patient's heart rate and causes vasoconstriction by releasing adrenaline and noradrenaline. This results in an increase in oxygen demand and decreases perfusion of the vascular system, splenic bed and renal artery.

COMMON POSTOPERATIVE COMPLICATIONS

It is also important to identify the most common and likely postoperative pulmonary complications that may occur and for the surgical nurse to understand why these occur. These include aspiration, obstruction, shivering, hypoventilation, bronchospasm, atelectasis and pneumonia.

Aspiration

Surgical patients may aspirate foreign matter, blood or gastric contents. In most cases postoperative aspiration is caused by regurgitating gastric contents into the tracheobronchial system. Unlike vomiting, regurgitation is a passive and often silent process and is potentially a serious airway emergency (Cullen & Cullen 1975). It can occur during induction, in the operating room, recovery unit or at any point during transfer. Patients most at risk are those who are oversedated, comatose, pregnant, obese, have a tracheostomy, have neuromuscular disease or have a nasogastric tube.

Aspiration causes chemical pneumonitis. Symptoms include bronchospasm due to reflex airway closure; hypoxaemia due to a compromised alveolar–capillary membrane; atelectasis due to loss of surfactant; interstitial oedema due to loss of capillary integrity, haemorrhage and adult respiratory distress syndrome (ARDS). However, signs and symptoms depend upon the severity of the aspiration.

Obstruction

The tongue is considered the most common cause of upper airway obstruction especially in patients following anaesthetic (Cullen & Cullen 1975). Patients at risk are those with poor muscle tone and tongue swelling. Patients who are obese or have a very short or large neck are also at risk. Patients with Downs syndrome are at risk because their tongues are significantly larger than normal. Symptoms and signs include snoring and use of accessory muscles.

Laryngeal obstruction is due to partial or complete spasm of the intrinsic or extrinsic muscles of the larynx which then obstruct the flow of air in and out of the lungs (Bidwai et al 1979). Patients at risk are those who have a history of asthma, chronic obstructive pulmonary disease (COPD) or smoking. The airway may be irritated intraoperatively by an endotracheal tube or multiple attempts at intubation.

Patients experiencing laryngeal obstruction are awake and usually agitated owing to the feeling of suffocation. These patients manifest signs of acute respiratory distress, experiencing dyspnoea, hypoxaemia and hypoventilation. Partial obstruction may present as stridor.

Shivering

Shivering is a normal homeostatic mechanism which raises the body's temperature and is activated by the thermoregulating centre in the hypothalamus in response to a drop in the body's core temperature. Shivering will often affect patients immediately postoperatively owing to induced hypothermia during open heart surgery or neurosurgery or other iatrogenic factors. Shivering is a common feature following anaesthesia where volatile anaesthetic agents such as halothane are used. Shivering greatly raises the patient's metabolic rate and consequently increases oxygen demand by as much as 400–700%. Therefore, those patients who have reduced respiratory function will be unable to meet the increase in demand. Those at risk of developing hypothermia include patients who undergo long operations with large fluid or blood loss, or surgery that exposes large cavities such as abdominal surgery. The residual effects of muscle relaxants reduce patients' ability to shiver and therefore they will not be able to raise their body temperature (see also Ch. 22).

Hypoventilation

Hypoventilation decreases the transfer of oxygen between the alveoli and the atmosphere leading to hypoxaemia, specifically with a PaO_2 of less than 8.8 kPa (66 mmHg). It is characterised by a variety of non-specific clinical signs and symptoms ranging from agitation to drowsiness, and changes in the pattern, rhythm and rate of breathing.

Factors that lead to postoperative hypoventilation include residual paralysis of the respiratory muscles, respiratory centre depression, increased airway resistance, increased tissue resistance and decreased compliance of the lungs and chest wall.

Hypoventilation can also decrease the excretion of carbon dioxide from the alveoli into the atmosphere. Although carbon dioxide retention is not usually a problem, it may affect patients with advanced chronic lung disease or neuromuscular disease.

Bronchospasm

Bronchospasm is a result of an increase in bronchial smooth muscle tone which results in the closure of the small airways. Oedema in the airways builds up, which leads to increased secretions in the airways themselves (Litwack et al 1991). The patient will be wheezy, dyspnoeic and will probably be using the accessory muscles and will be tachypnoeic. Causes of bronchospasm are aspiration, endotracheal intubation, tracheal or pharyngeal suctioning, and a history of asthma and COPD.

Atelectasis

Atelectasis is defined as closure or collapse of alveoli and is caused by airway obstruction. In postoperative patients this is usually due to retained thick bronchial secretions. Atelectasis causes an altered production of surfactant which makes lung re-expansion difficult. Patients who are more at risk include the elderly, patients who are obese, have a history of smoking or have an ineffective cough or respiratory dysfunction.

Postoperatively, all patients have some atelectasis but it is usually self-limiting. However, if atelectasis persists for more than 48 hours and there is also clinical evidence, then treatment is required. Atelectasis leads to hypoxaemia due to decreased alveolar oxygen exchange and desaturated blood being shunted into the systemic circulation. The clinical significance of atelectasis depends upon the patient's respiratory and cardiac function. Common signs and symptoms include decreased breath sounds, basal crackles, cough and sputum production (Johnson & Pierson 1986, Scuderi & Olsen 1989). Pyrexia is often cited as a clinical sign but there are little data to support this. It is most likely that the pyrexia accompanying atelectasis is due to infection distal to the obstructed airway (Johnson & Pierson 1986, Robert et al 1988).

If atelectasis is allowed to progress, then the patient will present with confusion, fever, dyspnoea and coughing and will eventually develop acute respiratory distress and failure due to profound hypoxaemia and hypercapnia.

Pneumonia

Persistent atelectasis may be associated with the development of bacterial pneumonia, although there is little evidence to support this causality (Johnson & Pierson 1986, Pepper & Conrad 1990). Bacterial growth may be enhanced in atelectasis because of the decreased mucociliary transport distal to the obstruction.

Other conditions also put the postoperative patient at risk of pneumonia and include pre-existing chronic airway limitation, smoking history, dehydration, malnutrition, immunosuppression, decreased ability to cough, length of anaesthesia, nasogastric tube and mechanical ventilation (Craven et al 1991).

Signs and symptoms include dyspnoea, pleuritic chest pain, chills, pyrexia and sputum production which is rusty or purulent in colour.

These complications are considered the most frequently observed in the postoperative patient. However, the nurse working in the surgical area needs also to be aware of the other respiratory complications which patients may develop postoperatively. These are listed in Box 23.2 and discussed fully in other texts (see Litwack 1995).

What needs to be stressed is that all these complications can cause the patient to develop respiratory distress which will lead to acute respiratory failure. Therefore, meticulous attention to detail during respiratory assessment by the surgical nurse is paramount and the implementation of effective nursing interventions to prevent postoperative respiratory complications is essential. Constant nursing assessment and intervention is very important throughout the preoperative and postoperative periods.

RESPIRATORY ASSESSMENT OF THE SURGICAL PATIENT

In order for surgical nurses to identify those patients who are at greater risk of developing postoperative complications and recognise respiratory complications postoperatively, it is extremely important that they carry out and document a thorough respiratory assessment throughout each patient's admission. This will require surgical nurses to use skills of observation, communication, monitoring, and analysing and interpreting data in order to care for their patients effectively. The skill of observation, which includes sight, hearing, touch and smell should not be underestimated. It is an important method of assessing and collecting information about patients' respiratory function. From observing patients, surgical nurses will often gain an intuitive perception of their patients; how they are reacting to their impending surgery, their reaction to their environment, their response to treatment and care and their whole sense of being. This intuitive knowledge of patients is just as important (Benner 1984, Carper 1978) as the meticulous collection of empirical data in relation to patients' physiological

---

Box 23.2   Respiratory complications
• Pulmonary oedema • Sputum retention • Pleural effusion • Pulmonary emboli • Pneumothorax • Pericarditis

status and should never be trivialised in relation to its contribution to the care and treatment of surgical patients.

Preoperative and postoperative respiratory assessment

Chapters 20 and 22 explore the important principles of preoperative and postoperative assessment when caring for the surgical patient. It is important, however, to highlight those areas of patient assessment which are directly related to maintaining effective breathing, always remembering that the respiratory assessment is part of the individual holistic patient assessment and should not be seen as a separate concept.

The purpose of assessing the patient's respiratory status preoperatively is to ascertain the presence of pre-existing disease with the goal of decreasing perioperative morbidity (Litwack 1995), also to identify those patients at greater risk of developing postoperative pulmonary complications as discussed earlier. The overall aim of respiratory assessment in the postoperative period is to detect any decrease in the patient's respiratory function, recognise the signs of respiratory distress and prevent potential respiratory complications. Therefore, surgical nurses must pay meticulous attention to detail and respond rapidly to changing clinical events during their assessment of patients' respiratory function.

It is important to ask patients or their carers what their normal respiratory function is. This history will include the following areas, much of which relate to the complications of surgery highlighted earlier:

- Relevant past medical history.
- Any history of dyspnoea at rest or on exertion, for example by enquiring whether the patient's exercise tolerance has decreased recently and in what circumstances.
- Any history of coughing – productive or dry.
- Any history of haemoptysis.
- Any history of asthma – if the patient does have a history of asthma then the nurse needs to enquire about the patient's history of bronchospasm, its trigger, medication used and how frequently taken.

- Any history of smoking.
- Any recent or chronic respiratory infections – patients with upper respiratory infections are at greater risk of developing perioperative bronchospasm, laryngospasm, decreased oxygen saturations and sputum retention.
- The type of operation the patient is to undergo.
- The age of the patient.
- A history of chronic obstructive pulmonary disease (COPD) which includes chronic bronchitis, chronic asthma, fibrosing alveolitis, emphysema – these patients have a higher risk of developing postoperative pulmonary complications which include a decreased vital capacity and decreased diaphragmatic function. A study by Feeley (1990) estimated that 60% of patients with COPD develop postoperative pulmonary complications when given no special postoperative care. However, in the same study, this incidence of pulmonary complications was reduced to 22% when antibiotics, bronchodilators and chest physiotherapy were included in the routine care of these particular patients.

It is also important to note that even patients with normal respiratory function run a 6–10% risk of developing postoperative pulmonary complications.

- Relevant drug history.
- How the patient copes with stress. Stress will increase the patient's sympathetic response and therefore increase oxygen demand (see also Chs 8 and 9).
- The patient's normal sleeping pattern. How the patient sleeps. If the patient can only sleep sitting up, then care has to be directed towards meeting this need pre- and postoperatively.
- Nutritional history – whether there has been any recent weight loss or increase. Underweight patients have reduced respiratory muscle mass, which will therefore reduce respiratory muscle function. Obese patients are more prone to postoperative atelectasis. (See Ch. 27.)
- Pain strategies – how the patient copes with acute or chronic pain (see Ch. 24).

Observation of patients' physical characteristics preoperatively is important, especially in relation to their effects on patients' respiratory function peri- and postoperatively; obesity, spinal or chest deformities and overt airway deformities need to be specifically noted.

If a chest X-ray (CXR) is ordered prior to surgery, this should always be viewed by the anaesthetist. Preoperative CXRs are not always routine and will depend upon the individual patient, operation and unit policy. The CXR offers anatomical information from which pathological conclusions can be drawn when complemented by clinical data, and is an important adjunct to the patient's respiratory assessment.

In addition to taking a full preoperative respiratory history from the patient, the surgical nurse needs to also obtain baseline observations of temperature, cardiovascular status, respiratory rate and pattern, and breath sounds, all of which will be used as reference in the assessment of the patient in the postoperative period.

Depending on the patient's history, physical examination and CXR, baseline pulmonary function tests and/or arterial blood gases may be carried out.

Although pulmonary function tests may be an addition to the patient's respiratory assessment, it is not the intention of this chapter to describe the techniques or principles of pulmonary function tests. However, the following references will be of use to surgical nurses in their understanding of pulmonary function tests: Cole (1975), West (1990).

Baseline observations and their significance to respiratory function in the postoperative period

Respiratory rate, rhythm, depth and breath sounds

An increase in respiratory rate of even 3–5 breaths from the patient's normal respiratory rate at rest is significant and is an important and *early* danger sign of respiratory distress. A rise in respiratory rate initially minimises the increase in respiratory work required as the patient's lung compliance falls (Gilston 1976). Initially, it may affect patients so little that they deny that they are breathless. However, alongside the small increase in respiratory rate, the nurse's observation may demonstrate that the patient's talking becomes appreciably impaired. This is because at this stage of respiratory distress talking requires greatly increased ventilation and uses over 50% of the patient's vital capacity.

Gradually breathlessness increases, and the patient begins to show further signs of respiratory distress. Some signs are more subtle than others but just as significant. These may include the following:

Mouth opening.   This may be observed in the early stages of respiratory distress. Although it may only be slight in the beginning and therefore difficult to detect, it increases as the patient becomes more distressed. Its function is to decrease anatomical dead space and respiratory work. It is often seen in patients with pre-existing chronic lung disease.

Pursed lips.   This sign may be combined with mouth opening and acts as natural positive end-expiratory pressure (PEEP) in order to optimise alveolar ventilation, thus increasing functional residual capacity (FRC) and gas exchange.

Nostril flaring.   Flaring of the patient's nostrils is a late sign of respiratory distress in adults and is not always reliable. Nostril flaring in children is indicative of acute respiratory distress and immediate intervention is required.

Use of accessory muscles.   The use of accessory muscles will be observed in patients who develop moderate to severe respiratory distress. This demonstrates an increase in the work of breathing with a consequent increase in oxygen demand. Accessory muscle actions include suprasternal retractions, intercostal retractions and diaphragmatic breathing or abdominal breathing. Patients who have pre-existing lung disease may have chronic use of accessory muscle breathing, but this may be further exaggerated because they are experiencing respiratory distress.

Depth of breathing.   Depth of breathing is assessed as being shallow, regular or deep and is assessed alongside the rate of breathing. As respiratory distress increases, breathing will become laboured and the use of accessory muscles will become even more prominent.

Regularity of breathing.   This will also change as respiratory distress worsens, from being regular to being irregular and eventually becoming periodic where the patient exhibits periods of apnoea.

Chest wall movements.   These will also change as the work of breathing for the patient is increased. Movement of the chest wall also relates to the anatomy of the patient and whether movements are restricted by chest drains, wound drains, wound site and/or dressings.

Breath sounds/air entry.   Although 'listening to the patient's chest' was considered in the past to be the domain of the doctor's assessment, the surgical nurse will also need to master this skill in order to carry out a thorough holistic assessment of the patient pre- and postoperatively.

Breath sounds result from the noise of air passing through the larynx, and vary in loudness and rhythm depending on the position of the stethoscope. Two types of normal breath sounds can be heard: vesicular breathing and bronchial breathing.

Vesicular breathing.   A gentle rustling noise is audible all over the periphery of the lungs. It is loudest on inspiration and fades away rapidly during the early part of expiration.

Bronchial breathing.   This indicates the presence of underlying lung disease and has the following characteristics:

- it has a blowing quality
- the sound of inspiration is loud
- there is a pause between the inspiratory and expiratory sounds
- the expiratory sound is loud and prolonged.

Diminished breath sounds. This indicates that there is a barrier to the conduction of the noise of breathing to the chest wall. It can either be an acute obstruction of a major bronchus or because of pleural thickening due to chronic pathology. It can also indicate pleural effusion or pneumothorax.

Crepitations. These are fine crackling noises heard mainly during inspiration. They occur in diseases affecting the alveoli or terminal airways and often (but not always) there is an excessive amount of exudate or transudate in these regions. Crepitations will be heard in conditions such as pneumonia, bronchiectasis and pulmonary oedema.

Coarse crepitations are loud bubbling sounds due to copious secretions in the large airways and are heard during both inspiration and expiration.

Wheezes. These are musical sounds of low or high pitch that can occur on inspiration or expiration. They are due to the passage of air moving through narrowed airways at high velocity. Wheezes are commonly heard in patients suffering from chronic airway limitation or bronchial asthma when the obstruction is due to secretions and bronchospasm.

Friction rub. This may be heard as the visceral and parietal pleura rub together. The patient will usually complain of chest pain on inspiration. A friction rub is most clearly heard around the lower anterolateral chest wall and sounds like a creaking or grating sound that does not clear with coughing. It often indicates pleurisy, tuberculosis or pneumonia.

Sputum/secretions

If the patient is producing sputum, it is important to observe the colour, consistency and amount. Copious amounts of white blood-stained frothy sputum is indicative of pulmonary oedema which may be seen in some patients who develop respiratory distress. This is due to an increasing oxygen debt, anaerobic respiration and sympathetic response leading to an increase in workload on the heart and pulmonary congestion. Sputum which is yellow/green in colour is evidence of infection. Sputum which appears rusty is indicative of pneumonia. Thick and tenacious secretions may indicate that the patient is dehydrated. The patient may find it extremely difficult to expectorate such thick secretions, which may lead to the development of sputum retention. Sputum retention leads to bronchospasm and alveolar hypoventilation with the consequence that the patient will develop acute respiratory failure.

Cardiovascular status

If there is decreased perfusion for any reason during the postoperative period because of hypovolaemia or cardiac failure, it will directly affect alveolar and cellular respiration. (Ch. 26 provides a more in-depth consideration of the maintenance of adequate circulation in the surgical patient.)

Heart rate and rhythm. Poor perfusion results in an increase in heart rate because of a reflex response from the baroreceptors which activate the sympathetic nervous system. This increase in heart rate demands an increase in oxygen supply.

Hypoxia will affect coronary artery blood flow and myocardial perfusion which in turn affects the functioning of the sinoatrial node. The consequence will be rhythm disturbances, from atrial or ventricular ectopics or atrial fibrillation to more life-threatening arrhythmias such as ventricular fibrillation.

Blood pressure. Hypotension due to hypovolaemia is a late sign of poor perfusion. Hypoxia will initially cause the patient to become hypertensive but ultimately will lead to hypotension.

Peripheral perfusion. If the patient appears cold and clammy, this is indicative of poor perfusion and again is due to the sympathetic response of the nervous system. Peripheral cyanosis, however, is not indicative of arterial desaturation (central cyanosis) but reflects peripheral constriction due to activation of the sympathetic nervous system in response to a decreased cardiac output and perfusion pressure. It is significant because decreased perfusion indicates decreased cellular respiration.

Central cyanosis. This is indicative of arterial desaturation and consequently hypoxaemia. Central cyanosis can be observed in the discolouring of the patient's mucous membranes and buccal cavity only if haemoglobin levels are normal.

Temperature

Core temperature. If the patient's temperature is raised above normal on or during admission or for 24 hours postoperatively, infection is indicated. A raised temperature will cause an increase in oxygen demand. A decreased central temperature will also affect oxygen demand because oxygen will not be so readily released to the tissues from the haemoglobin molecule. Hypothermic patients will also 'shiver' to try to raise the core temperature. This increases oxygen demand by 400–700% which, if not met, will cause an oxygen debt at tissue level.

Peripheral temperature. This is an observation which is often overlooked but is an important sign in patients who are at risk of developing respiratory distress. Cooling of the extremities, with a gradient between the patient's core temperature and peripheral temperature is indicative of decreased perfusion.

Further important observations in relation to respiratory function in the postoperative patient

Neurological status

The patient's level of consciousness deteriorates as respiratory distress increases. Often the patient will gaze vacantly ahead and is apathetic. Eventually the patient will lapse into a coma if the respiratory distress is not treated. The reasons for these changes are still not completely clear because initially with a changed level of consciousness the patient's arterial blood gas is often not deranged. It is suggested that as the patient's work of breathing increases there is autoregulation of cerebral blood flow in order to protect the brain from ischaemia provided that the patient's mean arterial blood pressure does not fall below 50 mmHg (Hinchliff & Montague 1988).

Psychological status

Anxiety is one of the earliest, but most significant signs of respiratory distress. The patient will frown and the furrows of the frown can most obviously be seen at the root of the nose. Patients may also become restless and fidget to try to make themselves more comfortable. As respiratory distress increases, patients will become agitated and confused.

If a patient is agitated and confused, then the nurse must presume that the patient is hypoxic until proved otherwise and the hypoxia must be treated. Often first-line management of hypoxia is to administer supplemental oxygen.

A patient's psychological distress, which may be caused by a number of factors such as pain, anxiety, anger, fear or confusion, can initiate a pathological process leading to dyspnoea (Knebel 1991). This is demonstrated in Figure 23.1.

This cycle of events has to be interrupted if the patient is to be prevented from developing acute respiratory failure.

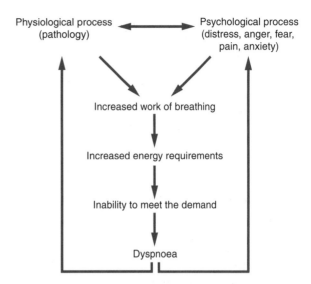

Figure 23.1 Relationship between psychological distress, pathology and dyspnoea. A negative circle of events.

Blood results

It is important that surgical nurses understand the significance of blood results in order to enhance their respiratory assessment of patients. The following blood profiles will help surgical nurses in their assessment of patients' respiratory status.

Haemoglobin (Hb). It is important that the patient is not anaemic as this will reduce the oxygen-carrying capacity of the haemoglobin molecule. This will lead to reduced O_2 uptake at cellular level.

It is important to remember that with a low Hb level the patient may still have O_2 saturations of 95–100%. But it must be stressed that the O_2 content is reduced with a low Hb. Consequently, there will be an O_2 debt at cellular level.

Haematocrit. This is the ratio of the volume of red blood cells to the volume of whole blood; in other words it is an indicator of the viscosity of the blood. The greater the percentage of red cells in the blood the more viscous the blood, which will directly affect the velocity of flow through the blood vessels. A high haematocrit reduces the flow of blood through the microcirculation and can indicate haemorrhage, anaemia and dehydration, all of which will increase cardiac workload and oxygen demand. Maximum oxygen-carrying capacity is achieved if the haematocrit is between 35–45%.

Phosphate. As previously discussed, phosphate is required for the synthesis of major high-energy compounds such as adenosine triphosphate (ATP) in order for normal aerobic cellular respiration to happen. It is a major source of energy for respiratory muscle function. Therefore, ensuring that patients' phosphate levels are within normal limits is paramount.

Urea and creatinine. If there is any derangement of these two electrolytes in conjunction with renal failure, the outcome will be the disruption of one of the body's major buffering systems. It will lead to an acid–base imbalance, either metabolic acidosis or metabolic alkalosis, both of which cause a shift in the oxyhaemoglobin dissociation curve. If not corrected, an oxygen debt will develop (See Ch. 26).

Arterial blood gases (ABGs)

These will be taken as a final assessment of a patient's respiratory status once all the other data have been extrapolated and analysed, and the doctor or senior nurse believes that they will add important and useful insight into the patient's condition and consequent treatment.

Making sense of ABGs requires the nurse to have knowledge of normal acid–base balance and experience in analysing such results. Table 23.1 gives a few examples of normal and deranged ABGs.

The first thing that the nurse should look at when analysing a patient's ABGs is the pH value. This will tell you whether the patient is acidotic or alkalotic. A pH below 7.35 is indicative of acidosis and a pH above 7.45 is indicative of alkalosis. The next step is to discover the primary cause of the acidosis or alkalosis; whether it is respiratory, metabolic or a mixture of the two. This can be deduced from analysing the PaO_2, PCO_2 and HCO_3.

If respiratory acidosis or alkalosis has been diagnosed, it is then important to find out the cause in order to direct nursing care and treatment that is appropriate for that patient.

Pulse oximetry

Pulse oximetry has established itself as the most convenient non-invasive method of monitoring arterial oxygen saturation continuously. A pulse oximeter measures the differential absorption of red and infrared light by haemoglobin and oxyhaemoglobin in the pulsatile fraction of blood under the sensor probe. It then calculates the percentage saturation of haemoglobin. However, pulse oximetry is not foolproof and it has its limitations. The pulsatile signal is very susceptible to noise, especially in association with poor peripheral circulation and movement, and this can produce a false reading (Hutton & Clutton-Brock 1993). Stoneham et al (1994) demonstrated that knowledge about pulse oximetry among medical and nursing staff was poor. The study found that both medical and nursing staff did not always realise that a pulse oximeter saturation (SpO_2) value below 90% implied that arterial partial pressure of oxygen (PaO_2) was low and that there may be critical hypoxaemia (Stoneham et al 1994). This revealed a misunderstanding of the basic physiology of respiratory failure (Davidson & Hosie 1993). Alveolar hypoventilation is the main form of respiratory failure postoperatively, as identified earlier. As arterial carbon dioxide tension rises, so does alveolar carbon dioxide tension (PCO_2); and alveolar oxygen (PO_2) falls leading to arterial hypoxaemia. If the patient is breathing room air and has an adequate pulsatile flow to the sensor, then the SpO_2 will fall early and is a good indicator of hypoventilation. However, this is very different if the patient is receiving supplemental oxygen. A normal reading of saturation in the presence of an increased inspired oxygen concentration gives no indication about the adequacy of ventilation. The alveolar PO_2 will now be much higher; therefore alveolar PCO_2 will have to rise much further before hypoxaemia is sufficient to produce measurable desaturations via the pulse oximeter.

Assessing the patient's SpO_2 must always go hand in hand with the other respiratory assessments and clinical signs and should never be relied upon as a sole indicator of respiratory function.

Chest drains

If the patient has a chest tube in situ postoperatively, the nurse must identify whether it is mediastinal or pleural. A mediastinal tube is used for wound drainage and is usually attached to low continuous

Table 23.1 Normal and deranged ABGs

	ABG values		
	Normal	Respiratory acidosis	Respiratory alkalosis
pH	7.35–7.45	7.2	7.55
PaO_2 (kPa)	12–13	5.0	8.9
$PaCO_2$ (kPa)	4.7–6.0	8.0	3.5
HCO_3 (mmol/l)	19–29	32	39
Base excess	−2 to +2	−4	+4
O_2 saturation (%)	95–100	85	95

wall suction. A pleural drain is designed to reinflate the lung and/or drain the wound. Pleural drains used for reinflating the lung are designed as an underwater seal drainage system and bubbling of the water is expected until the lung has re-expanded. If bubbling in the water-seal chamber suddenly diminishes, it is important that the nurse checks the drainage system for kinks or blockage of the drainage tubing. If this is not done, a tension pneumothorax may develop.

When assessing chest tube drainage, output should be measured every 15 minutes as haemorrhage is a potential early complication of chest surgery. If drainage exceeds 100 ml/hour, if fresh bleeding is noted, or if a sudden increase in drainage occurs, haemorrhage should be suspected and the doctor promptly informed. Decreased perfusion will lead to anaerobic respiration at tissue level and decreased alveolar ventilation.

THE ESSENCE OF CARING FOR PATIENTS

In order to care for patients in an individual effective and holistic way, the nurse needs to develop a therapeutic relationship with each patient and with that patient's carers. This requires the nurse to make patients and their carers the true centre of care (Fig. 23.2).

This involves demonstrating an atmosphere of security, freedom, love, hope and trust; it means being there for patients; empowering them and their carers by giving them back control and developing contracts of care; and communicating effectively with patients and their carers by verbal, nonverbal and touch methods. It means developing a partnership in care between the nurse and the patient which also involves mutual giving, trust, faith, intimacy and companionship. A conceptual framework of care involving these concepts can be seen in Figure 23.2 and may be used to help nurses develop such partnerships in care. This therapeutic caring relationship must go hand in hand with meeting patients' immediate physiological needs and cannot be seen as a separate domain of patient care. It is, therefore, important to integrate the physical, psychological, social and spiritual needs of patients in order for them to become truly healed (see also Ch. 7).

> **Reflective point**
>
> How do you organise your preoperative and postoperative nursing care in order to optimise ventilation and perfusion in the surgical patient? How does your philosophy of care influence your nursing interventions?

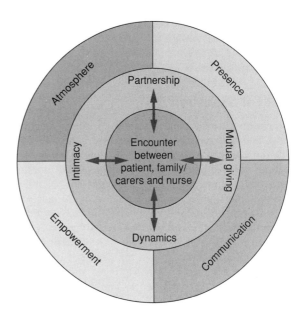

Figure 23.2 A conceptual framework for therapeutic nursing intervention.

PREOPERATIVE NURSING CARE IN RELATION TO MAINTAINING EFFECTIVE BREATHING

The overall aim of preoperative pulmonary care is to optimise the patient's preoperative pulmonary status. This includes modifying risk factors, for example by smoking cessation and weight reduction, although once the patient has been admitted to hospital it is too late to modify these risk factors in any appreciable way. However, time could be used to educate patients in smoking cessation and guide their dietary intake during their whole admission time. Further research into this area of patient education within the hospital environment and how effective it may be needs to be undertaken in the near future (Wewers et al 1994).

Preoperative pulmonary preparation also includes augmenting pharmacological therapies for those patients with pre-existing pulmonary disease (Brooks-Brunn 1995). This may include optimising bronchodilator therapy, administering antibiotics and/or steroids and focusing on methods to help secretion clearance, such as bronchodilator nebulisers or saline nebulisers along with chest physiotherapy, such as percussion and postural drainage. In the past, patients were frequently admitted to hospital a few days before their surgery in order to assess and optimise their pulmonary function. Unfortunately, with today's economic constraints and limited bed availability, these patients are managed as outpatients by their GP or are often missed, with the consequence that they may be ill prepared in relation to their respiratory status for surgery. The importance of a pre-admission assessment is emphasised therefore (see Chs 15 and 20).

Patient education

The surgical nurse plays a significant role in teaching and instructing patients on deep-breathing exercises, the importance of frequent repositioning, early mobilisation and pain-management strategies. Both nursing and medical literature support the importance of preoperative education on postoperative recovery and pulmonary function (Crawford et al 1990, Hathaway 1986). Unfortunately, although preoperative education is considered a routine and important part of preoperative care, it often becomes lost in the priorities of care or overlooked because of staff shortages and time constraints, especially in relation to the same-day admission surgery programmes. It is important, therefore, to briefly describe the rationale for teaching patients deep-breathing exercises for use in the postoperative period.

Deep-breathing exercises

A series of pleural pressure changes caused primarily by the contraction and relaxation of the diaphragm leads to spontaneous ventilation. During passive expiration there is minimal negative pleural pressure but during inspiration the pleural pressure becomes more negative owing to the contraction of the diaphragm and external intercostal muscles. Thus the main distending force of the lung during inspiration is provided by negative intrapleural pressure. This negative pressure ensures that the lungs do not collapse (Hinchliff & Montague 1988).

Anything that interferes with the generation and maintenance of increased negative pleural pressure on inspiration will decrease the distending force of the lung and lead to alveolar collapse and/or atelectasis (Wilkins 1992). In the postoperative patient this will include diaphragmatic dysfunction, altered breathing pattern and any other factor that decreases tidal volume and functional residual capacity (FRC).

Bartlett et al in 1973 (cited in Brooks-Brunn 1995) demonstrated that in postoperative situations of decreased tidal volume and FRC, deep and prolonged inspiratory efforts favour reversal of atelectasis and enhance surfactant production. For this to be truly effective, it requires the patient to take a sustained maximal inspiration for 3 seconds at least 5–10 times per hour.

Therefore, adequate analgesia and nursing strategies that enhance comfort during the postoperative period are essential if patients are to carry out deep-breathing exercises effectively.

POSTOPERATIVE NURSING CARE

The overall aim of postoperative nursing care is to prevent or limit postoperative pulmonary complications. This is achieved by effective preoperative nursing intervention, ongoing patient education, and the use of specific nursing interventions to optimise effective breathing in the patient throughout the postoperative period. These include the following:

- positioning and early ambulation
- effective coughing and deep-breathing exercises
- pain management and comfort
- oxygen administration
- non-invasive respiratory support
- pharmacological intervention.

Positioning

Although positioning appears to be one of the most fundamental and essential care elements that nurses undertake on a daily basis, it is extremely important to stress the importance of positioning postoperative patients correctly and repositioning them frequently in order to optimise ventilation and perfusion and decrease the risk of pulmonary complications.

A semi-sitting position is advocated for optimising and matching ventilation and perfusion. It also reduces abdominal pressure on the diaphragm and minimises the risk of aspiration in patients, especially those who have nasogastric tubes in situ. Turning patients from side to side at least every 2 hours is also advocated, unless contraindicated such as in patients following lobectomy or pneumonectomy (refer to other texts such as Litwack 1995), because it changes the distribution of ventilation and blood flow through the lungs and mobilises secretions. Unless the patient has chronic lung pathology, the lateral position promotes oxygenation in the dependent lung.

The cardiopulmonary effects of turning or repositioning patients have been well documented in the literature (Brooks-Brunn 1995, Gavigan et al 1990). Frequent body repositioning can be effective in enhancing oxygen transport by changing the ventilation and perfusion of the lungs through gravitational effects. Changing the patient's position also enhances mobilisation of secretions. When repositioning patients it is extremely important to monitor their clinical response to the different positions. The type of surgical procedure or if the patient has a chronic lung disease may influence the patient's cardiopulmonary response to different positioning. What has to be remembered is that repositioning patients increases their oxygen demand during the procedure.

Studies by Banasik (1987) and Shively (1988), however, are inconclusive about the effects of patients' repositioning on pulmonary gas exchange in the presence of atelectasis. Further to this, although the FRC is reduced when a patient is in a supine position, according to Banasik (1987), this does not cause too many problems for those patients who do not have pulmonary abnormalities. Thus, changing their position does not significantly affect gas exchange. There is, however, stronger evidence from the literature (Brooks-Brunn 1995) in favour of repositioning patients and enhancing ventilation and perfusion than there is against it. As nurses, therefore, it is necessary to critically analyse our practice in relation to positioning patients and begin to generate our own research.

Early and progressive ambulation of the postoperative patient is an important aspect of postoperative care and is an extension of the physiological principles of turning and repositioning the patient who is in bed. Ambulation encourages ventilation, increases perfusion, promotes secretion clearance and promotes oxygenation. Other effects of early ambulation include a decrease in venous pooling, therefore reducing the risk of thrombus formation and pulmonary emboli; improved FRC; reduced muscle wasting and deconditioning due to bedrest. What is also important for patients in relation to early ambulation is that it decreases their potential for psychological distress, such as feelings of helplessness, depression and lack of control (Wenger 1982).

When and how patients should be mobilised should be a decision made on an individual basis in conjunction with the patient, the patient's nurse, surgeon and physiotherapist. An intervention such as early mobilisation may cause patients to become quite anxious and worried about how painful and uncomfortable it may be. Therefore, it is paramount that the nurse monitors, observes and provides optimal pain and comfort strategies and interventions for the patient during this period (see Ch. 24). Alongside these strategies, educating patients and their carers in the important benefits of early mobilisation is also extremely important and allows them to build a trusting and empowering relationship with the nurse.

Specialised kinetic therapy beds can be used to facilitate the turning process and in some studies have been found to reduce pulmonary complications in different patient groups (Fink et al 1990, Gentillo et al 1988, Hess et al 1992), although these studies are small and are not convincingly conclusive. Kinetic beds are used for patients who have limited mobility with unilateral lung disease and cannot be easily positioned on one side. Although these types of beds can be useful in some circumstances, they are very expensive and are therefore not indicated for routine use or to replace quality essential nursing care.

Effective coughing and deep-breathing exercises

The time-honoured tradition of 'cough and deep breath' is often thought of as the essence of effective pulmonary care and prevention of postoperative respiratory complications. The concept can be attributed to Dripps & Waters (1941) who described three fundamental principles for patients who had or were at risk of developing respiratory complications:

- the patient must be turned
- the patient must cough
- the patient must inflate the lungs adequately with deep breaths.

They advocated that patients should be encouraged to perform these three manoeuvres every hour or half an hour depending on their physical condition (Dripps & Waters 1941). The benefits of such principles of respiratory care remain extremely important in the current preoperative and postoperative care of patients.

However, although coughing has, for a long time, been considered part of the traditional routine postoperative care, its use in this period has been questioned (Dilworth & Pounsford 1991). Encouraging the patient to cough is one method to facilitate clearance of airway secretions for those patients who have increased secretions or secretion-management problems. The majority of patients do not have excess secretions or problems with secretion management after operation. Therefore, the nurse needs to assess patients on an individual basis in relation to whether they need to be encouraged to cough as a routine aspect of their postoperative care. Surgical nurses should ask themselves:

- Does the patient have pre-existing lung disease?
- Does the patient have a history of secretion-clearance problems?
- Is there evidence of increased secretions when listening to breath sounds?
- Will the patient benefit from coughing as an intervention?

What needs to be remembered is that coughing is an expiratory manoeuvre that can cause pleural pressures to exceed airway pressure. This may result in alveolar collapse. Postoperative coughing is often contraindicated in patients having ear surgery, eye surgery, neurosurgery or repair of large abdominal hernias because of the resulting increase in pressure around or near the surgical site.

If it is decided that patients need to be encouraged to cough, then they need to be taught how to cough effectively by the physiotherapist and nurse. It is important that patients are placed in an optimal position to reduce tension on the abdominal muscles. Splinting of the wound site with a pillow, towel or crossed arms should also be encouraged.

If secretions remain a problem for the patient, or the patient has established atelectasis, then further physiotherapy interventions should be carried out by an appropriately trained person, usually a physiotherapist or an experienced surgical nurse. These may include:

• Percussion and postural drainage – these two actions facilitate the movement of secretions in the large and small airways and ease their removal by expectoration or suctioning.

• Suctioning – this is an option for intervention *only* if patients are unable to cough effectively to clear their own airways, and all other interventions have been unsuccessful. It should always be performed by an experienced member of the team, either a physiotherapist or an experienced nurse. It is a very traumatic procedure and causes patients physiological and psychological distress.

The physiological rationale for performing deep-breathing exercises has been described earlier. In order to prevent pulmonary complications during the postoperative period, it is imperative that the nurse encourages patients to take regular effective deep breaths. This requires patients to take a slow deep breath in and hold their breath for about 3 seconds at least three to six times per hour in order to prevent alveolar collapse. For such effective deep-breathing exercises to be successful it requires:

• motivation of the patient
• education of the patient
• supervision of the patient.

The nurse and physiotherapist play a pivotal role in motivating the patient to undertake the exercise, and motivation cannot just come from the patient. If there is to be a therapeutic nurse–patient relationship (Fig. 23.2) there has to be mutual giving, in this case motivation by both partners in care. It is this collaborative effort between the nurse and patient that ensures deep-breathing exercises will be effective.

Once patients have been appropriately educated in the importance of deep-breathing exercises and can perform them effectively, many do not have to be supervised continuously, although regular monitoring and encouragement by the nurse is important.

In some areas, and especially within the USA, the use of incentive spirometers is advocated to help the patient take slow deep breaths and produce a voluntary sustained maximal inspiration (SMI). They measure patient effort either in flow or volume, help maintain muscle strength and promote secretion clearance. Research into the benefits of incentive spirometry, however, has demonstrated that it has limited benefits in some patients and is only effective if the nurse continually supervises and encourages its proper use (Chunter et al 1989).

Other alternatives can also be used to prevent atelectasis, improve lung volumes and enhance gas exchange in the postoperative period, such as periodic administration of continuous positive airway pressure (CPAP) or positive end-expiratory pressure (PEEP) by face mask. However, these alternatives should only be used to treat refractory atelectasis that has not improved with other simpler techniques. They are both costly in terms of equipment and labour intensive, with numerous side-effects for the patient (see Box 23.3) (Ingwersen et al 1993).

Box 23.3 Side-effects of CPAP and PEEP

• Gastric insufflation
• Aspiration
• Hypoventilation
• Pulmonary barotrauma
• Cardiac compromise
• Patient discomfort

Pain management and comfort

Although Chapter 24 deals with the concept of pain in the surgical patient, it is paramount that pain management is stressed again when trying to maintain effective breathing in the surgical patient. It is important to remember that the most severe pain is associated with abdominal and thoracic surgery because these procedures inhibit inspiration. Abdominal pain induces voluntary and reflex muscle spasm affecting primarily the abdominal muscles and the diaphragm (Barnes et al 1991). This leads to more rapid but shallow breathing, poorly expanding the lower lobes of the lungs. Even with analgesia, many patients experience moderate to severe pain and 85–100% of patients following abdominal surgery report severe pain on movement (Acute Pain Management Guideline Panel 1992, Bonica 1990). Paradoxically, excessive analgesia for abdominal pain may also lead to hypoventilation and predispose the patient to pulmonary complications. The psychological impact of pain and discomfort will cause the patient further distress (see Fig. 23.1). Patients differ in their response to pain and to opioid analgesia and it is important to have other options and strategies to offer patients in order to manage their pain (Good 1996). These may include strategies such as those listed in Box 23.4.

Box 23.4 Alternative strategies to help manage pain

- Music
- Relaxation
- Biofeedback
- Guided imagery
- Massage
- Touch
- Transcutaneous electrical nerve stimulation (TENS)

Giving comfort to patients will also ease their physiological and psychological distress and pain. The surgical nurse is in a prime position to initiate and sustain patient-comfort measures. These should include physiological, psychological, spiritual and social comfort interventions which are listed below. All of these will lead patients and their carers to feel empowered and cared for, which will enhance the nurse–patient relationship (see Fig. 23.2).

Comfort strategies may include the following:

- adequate hydration and elimination
- adequate nutrition – to ensure wound healing and adequate immune response
- effective analgesia
- temperature control
- individual positioning
- personal hygiene
- touch
- being there for patients and their carers (presencing)
- listening to the patient
- adequate and effective sleep – to ensure wound healing, effective immune response
- presence of personal belongings
- family/carer presence (has the ward too strict visiting times? should there be such a thing as visiting times?)

- companionship
- effective communication and information
- respecting the patient as an individual.

If the nurse does not address patient discomfort then the nurse–patient relationship will be limited and patients will not be able to heal themselves.

Reflective point

What comfort do your patients receive from your nursing interventions? How can patient comfort be measured?

Oxygen administration

Supplementary oxygen is routinely prescribed by the anaesthetist immediately postoperatively to minimise the risk of hypoxaemia. Oxygen is initially given via a face mask, either by a variable of fixed-performance system. The variable system allows the nurse to manipulate the oxygen percentage delivered without having to change the mask, as the oxygen concentration is controlled by a flowmeter. In the majority of patients, those without chronic lung disease or chronically elevated $PaCO_2$, the concentration of oxygen is not too important and can therefore be given by a simple face mask or nasal cannula. With these devices, the inspired oxygen concentration varies from about 35–55% with flow rates of between 6 and 10 L/minute. Nasal cannulae are often preferred by patients because they feel less claustrophobic and allow better communication. However, if the patient breathes through the mouth for the majority of the time, then nasal cannulae are of limited use. Nasal cannulae can also cause ulceration of the nasal and pharyngeal mucosa.

There is a risk of oxygen toxicity, and lung damage can develop if the patient is exposed to too high concentrations of oxygen (55% or above) for more than 24 hours. However, *hypoxia must always be treated with supplementary oxygen at whatever percentage patients require to elevate their PaO_2 from a critical level.*

Those patients with chronic lung disease who have chronically elevated $PaCO_2$ and are exhibiting acute signs of respiratory failure must only receive low percentages of oxygen, 24–28%, because of their altered respiratory drive (see Hinchliff & Montague 1988).

If the surgical patient requires oxygen therapy for more than a few hours then it is important to humidify the oxygen. This will reduce the risk of the patient developing dry secretions and the discomfort of a horrible dry mouth.

Non-invasive respiratory support

For those patients who develop respiratory insufficiency, initiation of non-invasive respiratory support offers potential advantages over intubation and mechanical ventilation. These include:

- ease of communication
- more effective nutrition/feeding
- ability to mobilise early
- reduction in nosocomial upper and lower respiratory tract infections
- patients can be cared for within the ward environment or high dependency unit.

The term non-invasive respiratory support includes continuous positive airway pressure (CPAP), positive pressure mask ventilation and other methods such as rocking beds (Simonds 1994). There are of course a number of limitations of these techniques and therefore there has to be careful selection of the appropriate one for the patient. It requires appropriate matching of the ventilatory technique to the pathological problem. This technique may be indicated in the following situations:

- treatment of acute exacerbations of chronic respiratory failure especially preoperatively and postoperatively
- facilitation of weaning from mechanical ventilation
- to bridge patients for transplantation
- to improve cardiorespiratory status prior to surgery
- for home ventilation in patients with chronic ventilatory failure.

There are, of course, essential prerequisites for any patient who is being considered for non-invasive respiratory support. These are listed in Box 23.5.

As surgical techniques develop and surgery is offered and carried out on those patients who are at greater risk of developing pulmonary complications postoperatively, non-invasive respiratory support will continue to develop as routine clinical practice. It may facilitate earlier discharge of patients and reduce the demands on intensive care beds (Pennock et al 1994, Simonds 1994, 1996). Surgical nurses will need to develop skills within this area of respiratory care and intervention alongside their skills of respiratory assessment and care.

Pharmacological interventions

An assortment of drugs have been tried in the postoperative prevention and treatment of pulmonary

---

Box 23.5 Prerequisites for non-invasive respiratory support

- Ability to control airway
- Adequate cough reflex
- Haemodynamic stability
- Patient cooperation
- Functioning gut
- If being weaned from mechanical ventilation, the ability to breathe spontaneously for short periods.

---

complications. These include respiratory stimulants, mucolytics and surfactant stimulants, all of which have limited use and are often not indicated (Fegiz 1991, Ford et al 1993). Doxapram has been tried as a respiratory stimulant with varying results (Hollway & Stanford 1982, Sebel et al 1980). Jansen et al (1990) demonstrated that doxapram significantly reduced pulmonary complications in high-risk patients undergoing abdominal surgery compared with a control group, but further research is necessary.

Drugs such as aminophylline and β_2-adrenoceptor agonists have been demonstrated to augment diaphragm activity and prevent respiratory muscle fatigue (Ford et al 1993), but despite this there are no real data to support their routine use in reducing pulmonary complications.

Drugs such as the histamine H_2-receptor blocking drugs cimetidine and ranitidine, if administered preoperatively, can help reduce gastric acidity and volume, therefore minimising the consequence of gastric aspiration (Litwack 1995). Metoclopramide increases gastric emptying and gastro-oesophageal sphincter tone, again reducing the risk of aspiration of gastric contents (McConnoll 1991).

Currently there is little evidence to support specific drug therapies in the prevention and minimisation of postoperative pulmonary complications. However, in certain situations and for certain patients, drug intervention may be important, such as the use of a respiratory stimulant, but widespread routine clinical use of such drugs is not indicated.

It is important, therefore, for the surgical nurse to understand the implications and side-effects of any drug therapy that patients are prescribed and evaluate the usefulness of such therapy for each individual patient. For example, if the patient is prescribed a bronchodilator, it is important that the nurse measures the patient's pre- and post-peak flow and listens to the patient's air entry (in relation to wheeziness) before and after administration, to fully evaluate the drug's effectiveness.

FOOD FOR THOUGHT

As discussed in earlier sections, surgery is being offered to and carried out on an increasing number of elderly patients and patients who are at greater risk of developing postoperative pulmonary complications, such as those with chronic obstructive pulmonary disease (Artinian et al 1993, Seymour & Vaz 1989). The question here is whether these patients, who are known to have a higher incidence of postoperative pulmonary complications and who will potentially stay longer in hospital, thereby increasing health care costs, should even be offered surgery? Recently a hospital was refusing admission and routine surgery for patients over the age of 75 years, because they did not have the beds or money to care for these 'high-risk' patients. Some surgeons have refused, and continue to refuse, to operate on patients who continue to smoke even after being told of the risks involved if they carry on smoking. There is a high incidence of smoking in the nursing and medical profession, yet these are the very people who try to teach patients health education. Can we, as health care professionals, justify our position in promoting health education? With escalating health care costs and an increasing elderly population, decisions have to be made in relation to who receives treatment and care and who does not. But who should make such decisions and against what criteria should they be made? These ethical and moral dilemmas will continue far into the future (see Chs 4 and 11). There is no black or white answer to such issues but they must be debated by those health care professionals who have the knowledge and experience of caring for patients, and such important issues should not just be left to outside and casual speculation. It is the writer's belief that as health care professionals we should strive for what Hippocrates espoused and grasp the essence of our being: 'To cure sometimes, to relieve often, to comfort always.'

CONCLUSION

This chapter has provided the surgical nurse with a sound foundation in the assessment, nursing intervention and care of the surgical patient in relation to maintaining effective breathing throughout the patient's surgical experience. The surgical nurse's role is pivotal to effective pulmonary care and the prevention of pulmonary complications throughout the patient's surgical admission. In order to reduce the risk of pulmonary complications, a team approach to caring for the patient is also essential but requires the surgical nurse to be knowledgeable, proactive, dynamic and creative in all aspects of nursing care and intervention. It requires a true blending of the science and the art of nursing, allowing the nurse to become an autonomous practitioner and an effective patient advocate. The ultimate goal will be that the surgical nurse will effect a quality patient outcome by reducing morbidity and mortality in surgical patients.

REFERENCES

Acute Pain Management Guideline Panel 1992 Acute pain management: operative or medical procedures and trauma. Clinical practice guideline. AHCPR Publication No. 92-0032. DoH, USA

Artinian N T, Duggan C, Miller P 1993 Age differences in patient recovery patterns following coronary artery bypass surgery. American Journal of Critical Care 2(6): 453–461

Bailey C R, Jones R M, Kelleher A A 1993 The role of continuous positive airway pressure during weaning from mechanical ventilation in cardiac surgical patients. Anaesthesia 50: 677–681

Banasik J L 1987 Effect of position on arterial oxygenation in post-operative coronary revascularization patients. Heart and Lung 16(Nov): 652–657

Barnes W H, Pennock M M, Browne W 1991 The effect of routine vs. P.R.N. postoperative analgesia on pulmonary complications: a multicenter trial. Canadian Journal of Nursing Research 23(4): 7–22

Bartlett R H, Gazzaniga A B, Geraghty T R 1973 Respiratory maneuvers to prevent postoperative pulmonary complications: a critical review. Journal of the American Medical Association 224: 1017–1021

Benner P 1984 From novice to expert: excellence and power in clinical practice. Addison-Wesley, Menlo Park

Bidwai A, Rogers C, Stanley T 1979 Prevention of postextubation laryngospasm after tonsillectomy. Anaesthesia 51(suppl 3): 50

Bonica J J 1990 Postoperative pain. In: Bonica J J (ed) The management of pain, 2nd edn. Lea & Febiger, Philadelphia, vol 1

Boore J 1978 Prescription for recovery. Royal College of Nursing, London

Brooks-Brunn J A 1995 Postoperative atelectasis and pneumonia. Heart and Lung 24(2): 94–115

Carper B 1978 Fundamental patterns of knowing. Advanced Nursing Science 1: 13–23

Chunter T A, Weissman C, Starker P, Gump F E 1989 Effect of incentive spirometry on diaphragmatic dysfunction following cholecystectomy. Surgery 105: 488–493

Cochran R M 1984 Psychological preparation of patients for surgical procedures. Patient Education and Counselling 5: 153–158

Cole R B 1975 Essentials of respiratory disease, 2nd edn. Pitman Medical, Bath

Craven D, Steger K Barber T 1991 Preventing nosocomial pneumonia: state of the art and perspectives for the 1990s. American Journal of Medicine 91(suppl 3B): 44S–52S

Crawford B L, Blunnie W P, Elliott A G P 1990 The value of self administered perioperative physiotherapy. Irish Journal of Medical Science 90: 51–52

Cullen D, Cullen B 1975 Postanaesthesia complications. Surgical Clinics of North America 55: 987

Davidson J A H, Hosie H E 1993 Limitations of pulse oximetry: respiratory insufficiency – a failure of detection. British Medical Journal 307: 372–373

Davies J M 1991 Preoperative respiratory evaluation and management of patients for upper abdominal surgery. Yale Journal of Biological Medicine 64: 329–349

Department of Health (DoH) 1993 Targeting practice: the contribution of nurses, midwives and health visitors. The health of the nation. DoH, London

Dilworth J P, Pounsford J C 1991 Cough following general anaesthesia and abdominal surgery. Respiratory Medicine 85 (suppl A): 13–16

Dripps R D, Waters R M 1941 Nursing care of surgical patients 1: the 'stir up'. American Journal of Nursing 41: 534–537

Elliott M 1995 Providing support and care through a hospital at home. Nursing Times 91(34): 36–37

Ephgrave K S, Kleiman-Wexler R, Pfaller M, Booth B, Werkmeister L, Young S 1993 Postoperative pneumonia: a prospective study of risk factors and morbidity. Surgery 114: 185–190

Featherstone H 1924 An inquiry into the causation of postoperative pneumonia. British Journal of Surgery 12: 487–523

Feeley T 1990 The post anaesthesia care unit. In: Miller R (ed) Anaesthesia, 3rd edn. Churchill Livingstone, New York

Fegiz G 1991 Prevention by ambroxol broncho-pulmonary complications after upper abdominal surgery: double-blind Italian multicenter clinical study versus placebo. Lung 169: 69–76

Fink M P, Helsmoortel G M, Stein K L 1990 The efficacy of an oscillating bed in the prevention of lower respiratory tract infection in the critically ill victims of blunt trauma. Chest 97: 132–137

Ford G T, Rosenal T W, Clergue F, Whitelaw W A 1993 Respiratory physiology in upper abdominal surgery. Clinical Chest Medicine 14: 237–252

Foyt M M 1992 Impaired gas exchange in the elderly. Geriatric Nursing 13(5): 262–268

Gavigan M, Kline-O'Sullivan C, Klumpp-Lybrand B 1990 The effect of regular turning on CABG patients. Critical Care Nursing Quarterly 12: 69–76

Gentillo L, Thompson D A, Tonneson A S 1988 Effect of a rotating bed on the incidence of pulmonary complications in critically ill patients. Critical Care Medicine 16: 783–786

Gilston A 1976 Facial signs of respiratory distress after cardiac surgery. Anaesthesia 31: 385–397

Good M 1996 Effects of relaxation and music on postoperative pain: a review. Journal of Advanced Nursing 24: 905–914

Hathaway D 1986 Effect of preoperative instruction on postoperative outcomes: a meta-analysis. Nursing Research 35: 269–275

Hayward J 1975 Information – a prescription against pain. Royal College of Nursing, London

Hess D, Agarwal N N, Myers C L 1992 Positioning, lung function and kinetic bed therapy. Respiratory Care 37: 181–197

Hinchliff S, Montague S 1988 Physiology for nursing practice. Baillière Tindall, London

Hollway T E, Stanford B J 1982 Effect of doxapram on postoperative oxygenation in obese patients. Anaesthesia 37: 718–721

Hutton P, Clutton-Brock T 1993 The benefits and pitfalls of pulse oximetry. British Medical Journal 307: 457–458

Ingwersen U M, Larsen K R, Bertelsen M T 1993 Three different mask physiotherapy regimens for prevention of postoperative pulmonary complications after heart and pulmonary surgery. Intensive Care Medicine 19: 294–298

Iwamoto K, Ichiyama S, Shimokata K, Nakashima N 1993 Postoperative pneumonia in elderly patients: incidence and mortality in comparison with younger patients. International Medicine 32: 274–277

Jansen J E, Sorensen A I, Naesh O, Erichsen C J, Pedersen A 1990 Effect of doxapram on postoperative pulmonary complications after upper abdominal surgery in high risk patients. Lancet 335: 936–938

Johnson N T, Pierson D J 1986 The spectrum of pulmonary atelectasis: pathophysiology, diagnosis and therapy. Respiratory Care 31: 1107–1120

Kempe R M, Gelazis R 1985 Patient anxiety levels. Association of Operating Room Nurses Journal 41: 390–396

Knebel A R 1991 Weaning from mechanical ventilation: current controversies. Heart and Lung 20(4): 321–331

Knill R L 1988 Control of breathing: effects of analgesia, anaesthetic and neuromuscular blocking drugs. Canadian Anaesthetic Society Journal 35: S4–S8

Litwack K 1995 Post anaesthesia care nursing, 2nd edn. Mosby-Year Book, St Louis, Missouri

Litwack K, Saleh D, Schultz P 1991 Postoperative pulmonary complications. Critical Care Nursing Clinics of North America 3: 77–82

McConnell E A 1991 Problems. Nursing 91(Nov): 35–40

Martin L F, Asher E F, Casy J M, Fry D E 1984 Postoperative pneumonia: determinants of mortality. Archives of Surgery 119: 379–383

Matthay M A, Wiener-Kronish J P 1989 Respiratory management after cardiac surgery. Chest 95(2): 425–434

Nelson S 1995 Pre-admission clinics for thoracic surgery. Nursing Times 91(15): 29–31

Pasteur W 1910 Active lobar collapse of the lung after abdominal operations. Lancet 2: 1080–1083

Pennock B E, Crawshaw L, Kaplan P D 1994 Non-invasive nasal mask ventilation for acute respiratory failure. Institution of a new therapeutic technology for routine use. Chest 105: 441–444

Pepper E A, Conrad S A 1990 Respiratory complications of surgery and thoracic trauma. In: Frost E et al (eds) Chest medicine: essentials of pulmonary and critical care medicine. Williams & Wilkins, Baltimore, pp 453–473

Pesola G, Nashaat E, Kvetan V 1990 Pulmonary complications and respiratory therapy. In: Frost E, Goldiner P, Bryan-Brown C (eds) Postanesthetic care. Appleton and Lange, Norwalk, Connecticut, pp 63–69

Raleigh E H, Lepczyk M, Rowley C 1990 Significant others benefit from preoperative information. Journal of Advanced Nursing 158(Aug): 941–945

Robert J, Barnes W, Pennock M, Browne G 1988 Diagnostic accuracy of fever as a measure of postoperative pulmonary complications. Heart and Lung 17: 166–170

Rose G 1995 Meeting information needs of day surgery patients. Nursing Times 91(36): 28–29

Scuderi J, Olsen G N 1989 Respiratory therapy in the management of postoperative complications. Respiratory Care 34: 281–291

Sebel P S, Kershaw E J, Rao W S 1980 Effects of doxapram on postoperative pulmonary complications following thoracotomy. British Journal of Anaesthesia 52: 81–84

Seymour D G, Vaz F G 1989 A prospective study of elderly general surgical patients: II. Postoperative complications. Age and Ageing 18: 316–326

Shively M 1988 Effect of position change on mixed venous oxygen saturation in coronary artery bypass surgery patients. Heart and Lung 17: 51–59

Simonds A K 1994 Non-invasive respiratory support: intensive care applications. British Journal of Intensive Care 7(5): 235–241

Simonds A K (ed) 1996 Non-invasive respiratory support. Chapman and Hall Medical, Oxford

Stoneham M D, Saville G M, Wilson I H 1994 Knowledge

about pulse oximetry among medical and nursing staff. Lancet 344: 1339–1342

Sykes L A, Bowe E A 1993 Cardiorespiratory effects of anaesthesia. Clinical Chest Medicine 14: 211–226

United Kingdom Central Council for Nursing, Midwifery and Health Visiting (UKCC) 1992 Scope of professional practice. UKCC, London

Wenger N K 1982 Early ambulation: the physiologic basis revisited. Advanced Cardiology 31: 138–141

West J B 1990 Respiratory physiology: the essentials, 4th edn. Williams and Wilkins, Baltimore

Wewers M E, Bowen J M, Stainslaw A E, Desimone Y B 1994 A nurse-delivered smoking cessation intervention among hospitalized postoperative patients – influence of smoking related diagnosis: a pilot study. Heart and Lung 23: 151–156

Wilkins R L 1992 Assessment and management of acute atelectasis. In: Pierson D J, Kacmarek R (eds) Foundations of respiratory care. Churchill Livingstone, New York, pp 851–857

24

Postoperative pain management

*Julia Cambitzi   Mark Harries
Ella van Raders*

AIMS

This chapter aims to:

- explain the importance of effective multimodal pain control in the surgical patient
- demonstrate the application of pain assessment tools for postoperative patients
- identify and explore the most common methods of pain control for postoperative patients, particularly pharmacological interventions
- provide knowledge to empower the surgical nurse to make informed decisions regarding a surgical patient's analgesia
- provide knowledge to empower the surgical nurse to assist patients to make informed decisions regarding their postoperative analgesia.

INTRODUCTION

The subject of pain management is complex and this chapter does not aim to be a comprehensive text, but to outline the areas that the practitioner needs to consider when nursing patients who are experiencing acute pain and receiving analgesia. Policies and protocols will not be defined, rather areas of clinical importance will be highlighted, specifically in the area of pharmacological intervention.

Pain is prevalent within the population; it is one of the main symptoms that cause people to seek treatment from health care providers, yet the study of pain physiology is relatively new compared with other areas of surgical care. Despite the relative neophyte status of the science of pain, there is now a large body of knowledge concerning pain management and pain physiology; however, dissemination and application of this knowledge is not widespread within the health care system (McCaffery & Beebe 1994).

There appears to be a substantial theory–practice gap within pain management. Although there has been extensive research conducted by nurses, doctors, pharmacists and scientists into pain mechanisms and management, clinical practice does not often reflect these research findings. There is an obvious need for a strengthening of the link between theory and practice within all areas of health care (Jeans & Melzack 1992).

This is reflected in the joint working party of the Royal College of Surgeons and the College of Anaesthetists' publication: 'Pain After Surgery' which states: 'The treatment of pain after surgery in British hospitals has been inadequate and has not advanced significantly in many years.' (Commission on the Provision of Surgical Services 1990, p. IV).

This document has provided the impetus for the development of acute pain services country-wide (Cambitzi 1996) and outlines the basic principles that are important for the effective management of acute pain and the provision of acute pain services.

The Commission's opinion has been substantiated by numerous research papers over the last 15 years in both the medical and nursing press. Donovan et al (1987) found that 58% of a randomly selected medical and surgical sample of 353 patients experienced 'excruciating' pain. Seers (1989) found that 43% of an elective abdominal surgery sample (n = 80) reported 'quite a lot of pain' or more on the first day after surgery, and 86% reported 'quite a lot of pain' or more on the seventh postoperative day. Cohen (1980) reported that 75.2% (n = 109) of patients complained of moderate to severe pain after abdominal surgery.

One of the major reasons for the persistent low quality of postoperative pain relief in many hospitals has been the limited understanding of the importance of the problem amongst those who are in a position to effect change (Bonica 1990). This, combined with a persistence in using conventional, inadequate and anti-quated methods of drug administration (Mather & Ready 1994), has been fuelled by a few firmly held false beliefs:

- that postoperative pain is inevitable
- that patients may become addicted to the opioid
- that the risk of respiratory depression is greater than the risks of poorly treated pain
- that patients have less pain than they say they have
- that pain should be treated once it has occurred, not before it has occurred
- that only a single modal approach is necessary.

The beliefs listed above limit the delivery of good-quality nursing care. It is therefore important for all nurses to have appropriate knowledge regarding anal-gesia, pain mechanisms, drug selection and pain man-agement techniques in order to provide effective pain

relief for their patients. When this is the case, nursing care will and should become the cornerstone of multi-disciplinary pain management (MaCaffery & Beebe 1994).

This chapter does not explicitly address the man-agement of pain from a holistic perspective. Its aim is to focus on the more conventional approaches to pain management. The reader is therefore guided to the chapter on holism (Ch. 7), which addresses issues con-cerning complementary therapy, and also the chapter on psychological, existential and spiritual aspects of surgery (Ch. 9) to facilitate integration of other factors influencing the perception and management of pain.

DEFINITIONS

It has often been said that to treat a problem one must first define the problem. However, the definition of pain has been very problematic.

McCaffery's (1972, p. 8) often quoted and historical definition describes pain as: 'whatever the experienc-ing person says it is, existing whenever he says it does.'

The International Association for the Study of Pain (IASP), after much debate, endorsed a definition pro-posed by Merskey et al (1979): 'Pain is described as a sensory and emotional experience associated with actual and potential tissue damage or described in terms of such damage.'

The majority of postoperative patients experience acute pain. This is pain that has a recent onset, usually hours or days, and is short-lived or anticipated to be of short duration (IASP 1992).

WHY TREAT PAIN?

The benefits of effective postoperative pain manage-ment are many and far-reaching. They range from pure humanitarianism through to physiological factors and financial considerations.

The joint working party of the Royal College of Surgeons and College of Anaesthetists in their docu-ment 'Pain after Surgery' (Commission on the Provision of Surgical Services 1990, p. 3) stated: 'Treatment of pain after surgery is central to the care of postoperative patients. Failure to relieve pain is morally and ethically unacceptable'. There would be very few who could argue with this seemingly self-evident statement that pain should be treated on purely humanitarian grounds.

As mentioned in the introduction, postoperative patients experience far greater amounts of pain than medical and nursing staff generally perceive. The belief that pain should be accepted is not limited to health care professionals; it is also a belief commonly held by patients. This is supported by observation of the number of patients reporting satisfaction in their pain management regimens despite experiencing significant postoperative pain. When questioned, patients reported that they were satisfied because they were expecting pain, they knew why they had pain and that its duration would be brief (Donovan 1983).

Reflective point

As the patient's advocate, the nurse should ask the question: 'Why is effective pain management so important to the recovery of the surgical patient?'

Despite this apparent satisfaction of patients with their postoperative pain relief it is important that the practitioner is aware of the physiological effects of pain on the patient.

The physiological response to acute postoperative pain can have detrimental effects on patients' condition and significantly slow their postoperative recovery (Bromley 1993).

The under-treatment of pain following thoracic and abdominal surgery causes muscle wall splinting, where the patient takes shallow breaths to avoid the pain of normal breathing. Pain from thoracic and abdominal surgery can lead to decreased tidal volume, decreased vital capacity, decreased functional residual capacity, and decreased alveolar ventilation; in short, poor ventilation. This can lead to alveolar collapse, causing hypoxaemia and decreased oxygen delivery to organs (Breivik 1995) (see Ch. 23).

When pain stops patients from coughing, this may result in an increase in the collection of secretions in the alveoli which contributes to atelectasis and chest infections.

Pain may cause patients to remain still in an effort to avoid the pain of movement. This increases the risk to the patient of deep vein thrombosis and pulmonary embolism.

Pain is said, classically, to cause an increase in sympathetic outflow, resulting in vasoconstriction and tachycardia, which in turn raises the patient's blood pressure. However, this is an oversimplification because there are many factors which influence this response, such as age, source of pain, etc. The increase in the workload of the heart causes an increase in the myocardial oxygen requirements (Wasylak 1992). In high-risk patients with coronary artery disease, this

untreated pain situation can lead to a myocardial infarction (Watt-Watson 1992). This situation is further accentuated by the hypoxia caused by poor ventilation (Donovan 1992).

Pain also increases autonomic nervous system activity, which interferes with intestinal smooth muscle and sphincter activity. This leads to gastric and intestinal distension with the possibility of ileus formation. The interference with smooth muscle and sphincter activity can also contribute to postoperative urinary retention (Breivik 1995).

Pain accentuates the postoperative stress response that leads to catabolism of muscle mass by decreasing appetite and limiting mobilisation, and through changes in protein distribution (Kehlet 1994) (see Ch. 27).

It is generally accepted that good postoperative analgesia can reduce these responses to pain, thus leading to a safer and improved postoperative recovery (Bromley 1993).

Reflective point

Armed with this knowledge of the physiological effects of postoperative pain, reflect on the relationship between truly acting as a patient's advocate and condoning the prevalent persistent undertreatment of acute pain.

The improvement of postoperative pain management is not sufficient in itself to improve patient outcomes, such as early recommencement of diet and fluids, and early discharge. These desirable outcomes will only be achieved if the ability of the patient to mobilise and perform postoperative exercises, made possible by effective analgesia, is exploited. It is therefore essential that analgesia be used in combination with an active rehabilitation programme that increases physical activity, respiratory function and as a consequence results in an early return to a dietary intake (Kehlet 1994). Without early mobilisation, the benefits of good analgesia will not be realised.

Some indicators have suggested that the provision of good postoperative analgesia results in shorter hospital stays. This is beneficial to both patients and hospitals and has been used as a lever to obtain additional resources for acute pain services (Bromley 1993).

The motivation for effective acute pain management is further fuelled by the theory that acute and chronic pain are at either ends of a continuum, and if acute pain is not treated effectively it is likely to develop into chronic pain with associated disabilities

Table 24.1   Paracetamol

Preparations available	Dose	Route	Frequency of dose	Comments
Tablets 500 mg Dispersible tablets 500 mg Suspension 120 mg/5 ml, 250 mg/5 ml Suppositories 60 mg, 120 mg, 250 mg, 500 mg	Adults: 1g	Oral/rectal	4- to 6-hourly	Maximum 4 g/24 hours

central nervous system and so it blocks the synthesis of prostaglandins in the CNS (Amadio 1984).

Side-effects.   Paracetamol has a very low frequency of side-effects, which are usually mild, though haematological reactions have been reported (Reynolds 1996). Skin rashes and other allergic reactions occur occasionally (Reynolds 1996). Paracetamol may be administered to almost all patients irrespective of age, underlying disease or pregnancy. It is only in overdose that paracetamol can cause the life-threatening side-effect of liver damage, coma and ultimately death if not treated promptly.

An overdose of 10 g or more of paracetamol is likely to cause liver damage and, in severe poisoning, to cause liver failure leading to encephalopathy, coma and death (Reynolds 1996). Chronic paracetamol ingestion of over 5 g a day for 2–3 weeks has also been associated with liver toxicity, although most patients in those reports were exposed to other precipitating factors such as alcohol consumption (Seef et al 1986). Therefore it is important for nurses to be aware of other analgesics that contain paracetamol, e.g. co-proxamol, co-dydramol, co-codamol (see Table 24.2). The practitioner is advised to check the prescription to ensure that none of these drugs is given concurrently with paracetamol, though they can be administered alternately at the appropriate dosage intervals.

Table 24.2   Compound analgesic drugs

Generic drug (Brand name)	Constituents (per tablet/capsule)	Adult dose	Comments
Co-proxamol (Distalgesic)	Paracetamol 325 mg Dextropropoxyphene 32.5 mg	Two tablets every 4–6 hours	Maximum 8 tablets/24 hours
Co-codamol 8/500 (Panadeine)	Paracetamol 500 mg Codeine phosphate 8 mg	Two tablets every 4–6 hours	Maximum 8 tablets/24 hours. Available as a dispersible tablet formulation
Co-codamol 30/500 (Tylex)	Paracetamol 500 mg Codeine phosphate 30 mg	Two tablets every 4–6 hours	Maximum 8 tablets/24 hours. Available as a dispersible formulation. Dispersible formulation has a high sodium content, therefore avoid in renal impairment
Co-dydramol	Paracetamol 500 mg Dihydrocodeine 10 mg	Two tablets every 4–6 hours	Maximum 8 tablets/24 hours
Co-codaprin	Aspirin 400 mg Codeine phosphate 8 mg	Two tablets every 4–6 hours	Maximum 8 tablets/24 hours. Available as a dispersible formulation

Non-steroidal anti-inflammatory drugs (NSAIDs)

There are numerous NSAIDs (of which aspirin is the oldest) available for the treatment of pain and inflammatory conditions such as rheumatoid arthritis and gout. It is important to note that some NSAIDs commonly used for the treatment of postoperative pain are not licensed for this indication (see Table 24.3).

Differences in efficacy between the NSAIDs are small, but there is a variation among individual responses to the drugs, i.e. patients who do not respond to one NSAID may respond to another (Day & Brooks 1987). Therefore the practitioner can consider trying another NSAID from a different class if there appears to be a poor response to treatment. For example, diclofenac belongs to the benzene acetic acid family of NSAIDs; if it does not seem to work, it is worth trying ibuprofen instead, which belongs to the propionic acid family of NSAIDs.

The practitioner should be aware of the various routes that are available for each NSAID preparation (see Table 24.3). There is no evidence that NSAIDs given rectally or by injection perform better (or faster) than the same drug given by mouth, except for renal colic where NSAIDs given intravenously work more quickly (Tramer et al 1998). Diclofenac injection when administered intramuscularly can be painful and can cause sterile abscesses (ABPI 1998).

Therefore, the oral route is recommended followed by the rectal or injection route only when the patient cannot be administered medicines by the oral route. A useful NSAID formulation (although unlicensed for postoperative pain relief) is Feldene Melt (piroxicam in a freeze-dried tablet form) which dissolves on the tongue and can be used in patients who cannot or will not accept drugs by injection or rectally, or cannot swallow tablets (Wakeling et al 1996).

It is recommended that only one NSAID be used at a time (Orme 1990). It is important to identify less common drugs that are NSAIDs which have been prescribed for patients before admission into hospital for other conditions such as rheumatoid arthritis. It is important for the nurse to be aware that errors in prescribing can occur when, for example, diclofenac is prescribed postoperatively for patients who are already on a different NSAID (e.g. nabumetone) which the doctor failed to recognise. It is sensible in this situation to leave patients on their existing NSAID. If the NSAID is only available in an oral formulation and the patient is nil by mouth, then a different NSAID which can be administered by another route should be prescribed.

Mechanism of action.   Damage to cell membranes activates synthesis of prostaglandin from arachidonic acid. The therapeutic and adverse effects of NSAIDs are caused by inhibition of the enzyme cyclo-oxygenase (COX) which prevents the formation of prostaglandin and therefore reduces the sensitivity of the nerve endings to painful stimuli and thus relieves pain. Recent data show that the analgesic effects of NSAIDs are also partly caused by central mechanisms (McCormack & Brune 1991) which augment the peripheral effect. This may involve the inhibition of central nervous prostaglandins or inhibition of excitatory amino acids (Cashman & McAnulty 1995). However, inhibition of COX leads to a decrease in prostacyclin, which protects the lining of the gut, and decreases the level of thromboxane, which normally stimulates platelet aggregation and vasoconstriction. Therefore by blocking the production of prostacyclin and thromboxane, the risk of gastric injury and bleeding is increased (Fig. 24.2).

Side-effects.

Gastrointestinal (GI).   NSAIDs can have a direct mucosal irritant effect as well as inhibiting the production of the prostaglandins, PGE_2 and prostacyclin. Prostacyclin and PGE_2 normally have a protective effect on the stomach lining. Upper GI side-effects include dyspepsia, nausea, peptic ulceration; lower GI side-effects include small bowel enteropathy.

There are little data on the use of NSAIDs in surgery and the risk of gastrointestinal ulceration and bleeding. The relative risk of NSAIDs causing harm to the gut has been graded by the Committee on the Safety of Medicines (1994) but the data are based on long-term therapy (Table 24.4). Another study has found that ibuprofen is the safest NSAID (Henry et al 1996). One study has shown that there is a dose–response relationship between NSAIDs and upper gastrointestinal effects and that the risk of GI bleeding after 30 days of treatment is increased by 50% (Carson et al 1987). It is therefore recommended that NSAIDs should not be given to patients with a history of GI ulceration or bleeding (RCA 1998). The practitioner should check whether the patient has a history of a stomach ulcer and monitor any patient prescribed an NSAID for any signs of gastrointestinal side-effects.

Renal function. There are two ways in which NSAIDs can cause renal failure. One is by causing a decrease in the glomerular filtration rate by inhibiting the synthesis of renal vasodilating prostaglandins (Harris 1992). This effect is important in any situation where renal blood flow and/or perfusion pressure are reduced. NSAIDs will also block the prostaglandin component of renin release by the kidney (Sedor et al

Table 24.3 Non-steroidal anti-inflammatory drugs

NSAID family	Generic name (Brand name)	Preparation available	Usual dose	Route	Frequency of dose	Comments
Propionic acids	Ibuprofen (Brufen)	Tablets 200 mg, 400 mg, 600 mg Slow-release tablets 800 mg Syrup 100 mg/5 ml	*Adults:* 400 mg	Oral	t.d.s.–q.d.s.	Owing to their slow onset and offset of action, slow-release preparations are unsuitable for acute postoperative pain
	Naproxen* (Naprosyn)	Tablets 250 mg, 500 mg Suspension 125 mg/5 ml Suppositories 500 mg	*Adults:* 250–500 mg	Oral/rectal	b.d.	
Phenylacetic acids	Diclofenac (Voltarol)	Tablets 25 mg, 50 mg Dispersible tablets 50 mg (Slow-release tablets 75 mg, 100 mg)	*Adults:* 50 mg	Oral	t.d.s.	The enteric coating on diclofenac tablets may result in a slightly delayed onset of action Owing to their slow onset and offset of action slow-release preparations are unsuitable for acute postoperative pain
		Suppositories 12.5 mg, 25 mg, 50 mg, 100 mg	*Adults:* 100 mg	Rectal	16-hourly	
		Injection 75 mg/3 ml	*Adults:* 75 mg	i.m./i.v.	o.d.–b.d.	Maximum of 2 days
			25–50 mg loading dose, then 5 mg/hour	i.v. infusion	Continuous infusion	For prevention of postoperative pain for maximum of 2 days
	Ketorolac (Toradol)	Tablets 10 mg	*Adults:* 10 mg	Oral	4- to 6-hourly	Maximum 40 mg/day for for maximum of 7 days
		Injection 10 mg/1 ml, 30 mg/1 ml	10 mg (up to 30 mg)	i.m./i.v.	4- to 6-hourly	Maximum 90 mg/day (60 mg if elderly or under 50 kg) for maximum of 2 days

Table 24.3 (Contd.)

NSAID family	Generic name (Brand name)	Preparation available	Usual dose	Route	Frequency of dose	Comments
Acetic acids	Indomethacin* (Indocid)	Capsules 25 mg, 50 mg	*Adults:* 50 mg	Oral	b.d.–q.d.s.	
		Suspension 25 mg/5 ml Suppositories 100 mg	100 mg	Rectal	o.d.–b.d.	
Oxicams	Piroxicam* (Feldene)	Capsules 10 mg, 20 mg Dispersible tablets 10 mg, 20 mg Freeze-dried tablets 20 mg (Feldene Melt) Suppositories 20 mg Injection 20 mg/1 ml	*Adults:* 20 mg	Oral/rectal i.m.	o.d.	Feldene Melt formulation can be useful for patients who are nil by mouth – the freeze-dried formulation is placed on the tongue, dissolves and is swallowed in the patient's saliva.

* Not licensed for postoperative pain relief.

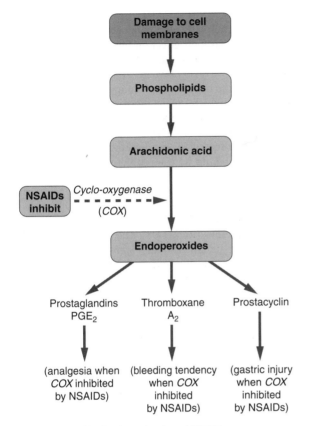

Figure 24.2 Mechanism of action of NSAIDs.

Table 24.4 Risk of GI side-effects from NSAIDs

Risk of GI side-effects	NSAID
Low	Ibuprofen
Intermediate	Diclofenac, naproxen, ketoprofen, indomethacin, piroxicam
High	Azapropazone

1986) which can lead to decreased concentrations of plasma aldosterone which in turn can lead to hyperkalaemia. Secondly, NSAIDs can cause an idiosyncratic allergic response which may lead to the development of acute interstitial nephritis.

Therefore, NSAIDs in postoperative pain treatment should be used with caution. In young and middle-aged people with normal renal function undergoing minor to intermediate surgery, NSAIDs are a safe and valuable supplement to opioid analgesics and may reduce the need for these drugs in a multimodal approach. In day surgery especially, they may contribute to an earlier discharge of the patient from the hospital (Bugge 1995) (see Ch. 15). In major surgery, there will always be a risk of bleeding and hypovolaemia and, therefore, a risk of renal ischaemia. In these cases, NSAIDs should not be used pre- or intraoperatively, but may be used postoperatively if the patient's circulation is stable and normal renal function is present (Bugge 1995). Some guidelines (Box 24.2) for the use of NSAIDs relating to possible effects on the kidney in surgery have recently been issued by the Royal College of Anaesthetists (1998).

Asthma and allergy. Aspirin and other NSAIDs can precipitate acute bronchospasm in asthmatic patients (Power 1993, Vane 1976) (Box 24.3). Aspirin-induced bronchospasm occurs in 5–10% of asthmatic people and there is evidence of cross-reactivity between aspirin-induced asthma and other NSAIDs (Bosso et al 1992) which can be fatal (Ayres et al 1987).

Haematological side-effects. NSAIDs significantly increase bleeding time by about 30%, owing to the

---

Box 24.2 Recommendations on the use of NSAIDs in relation to renal function

Avoid NSAIDs in the following clinical situations
- Renal impairment (plasma creatinine above normal)
- Hyperkalaemia
- Hypovolaemia
- Systemic inflammatory response syndrome
- Circulatory failure (hypotension and/or cardiac failure)
- Severe liver dysfunction
- During renal transplantation
- Pre-eclamptic toxaemia, eclampsia and uncontrolled hypertension

Use NSAIDs with caution in the following clinical situations
- ≥ 65 years (renal impairment likely)
- Diabetics (may have nephropathy and/or renal vascular disease)
- Patients with widespread vascular disease
- Cardiac, hepatobiliary and major vascular surgery (highest incidence of acute renal failure)
- Patients receiving ACE inhibitors, potassium-sparing diuretics, cyclosporin, methotrexate

Monitoring required
- Plasma creatinine, urea, sodium, potassium should be checked regularly in those patients for whom the use of NSAIDs requires caution (see list above) and in all patients after major surgery
- Any upward trend in creatinine, urea or potassium or decreased urine output is an indication for discontinuing NSAIDs

---

Box 24.3 Recommendations for the use of NSAIDs in patients with asthma

NSAIDs contraindicated
- Patients with aspirin-sensitive asthma
- Patients with asthma who have suffered from an NSAID allergic reaction

Use NSAIDs with caution
- Patients who have taken aspirin or other NSAIDs in the past without any worsening of asthma
- In asthmatic patients who have never taken an NSAID before, an NSAID can be administered with close monitoring of the patient

Monitoring required
- Observe and question patient for any deterioration in asthma whilst on NSAID
- Stop NSAID if deterioration of asthma occurs

---

inhibition of the formation of thromboxane A_2 which is required for the haemostatic function of platelets, but it usually stays within normal values (RCA 1998)

(see Ch. 25). Most NSAIDs exert their action on platelet function only when they are present in the circulation and so their effect on bleeding time lasts for only a few hours (Cronberg et al 1984). Aspirin, however, binds irreversibly to the cyclo-oxygenase enzyme and so has a more prolonged effect on platelet aggregation, which means bleeding time can be prolonged for several days after the last aspirin dose (Cronberg et al 1984). This is why patients who are to undergo surgery are required to stop taking aspirin (if they are taking it) a week before they have their operation.

Despite NSAIDs prolonging bleeding time, the effect of this on perioperative blood loss is less clear and it is considered that it is not significant in many clinical situations (RCA 1998). The practitioner should monitor the patient for any signs of postoperative bleeding from the wound site which could be the result of NSAID administration.

Drug interactions. NSAIDs have many interactions with other drugs. Some of the more relevant and clinically important interactions, together with their consequences, are listed in Table 24.5.

Table 24.5 NSAID interactions with other drugs

Drug interacting with NSAID	NSAID involved	Effects of drug interaction	Action to be taken
Anticoagulants e.g. warfarin, heparin	All	Damage to the mucosa of the gastrointestinal tract and inhibition of platelet aggregation by NSAIDs increase the risk of gastrointestinal bleeding in patients taking anticoagulants	NSAIDs should be avoided if possible. However, NSAIDs (except azapropazone) used in the perioperative period have little clinical effect on warfarin and so can be used but the INR (international normalised ratio) should be checked after the start or withdrawal of NSAIDs. In addition, any patients on anticoagulants who are prescribed NSAIDs should be monitored carefully for any signs of bleeding
Methotrexate (high, non-rheumatologic dose)	Probably all	Reduced clearance of methotrexate, increasing plasma methotrexate concentration and risk of toxicity	Simultaneous dosing contraindicated in high-dose methotrexate used in chemotherapy. Interaction not seen with rheumatologic doses of methotrexate
Cyclosporin	Probably all	Increased risk of renal toxicity	Avoid NSAIDs with cyclosporin
Lithium	Probably all NSAIDs except sulindac	Inhibition of renal excretion of lithium, increasing plasma lithium concentrations and risk of toxicity	Avoid NSAIDs if possible. Monitor lithium levels and make appropriate dose reduction if necessary when NSAID is used

Table 24.5 (Contd.)

Drug interacting with NSAID	NSAID involved	Effects of drug interaction	Action to be taken
Digoxin	All	Potential reduction in renal function in susceptible persons, e.g. elderly, reducing digoxin clearance and increasing digoxin plasma concentration and risk of toxicity (no interaction if renal function is normal)	Avoid NSAIDs if possible; if not, measure plasma creatinine and digoxin concentrations regularly
Aminoglycosides	All	Reduction in renal function in susceptible patients, lowering aminoglycoside clearance and increasing plasma aminoglycoside concentrations	Monitor plasma aminoglycoside and creatinine concentrations closely and adjust dose of aminoglycoside accordingly
Antihypertensive agents e.g. beta-blockers, diuretics, ACE inhibitors	Most NSAIDs	Reduction in hypotensive effect, probably related to inhibition of prostaglandin synthesis in kidneys (producing retention of salt and water) and blood vessels (producing increased vasoconstriction)	Patients on antihypertensive therapy and NSAIDs should have their blood pressure monitored closely
Diuretics	Most NSAIDs	Reduction in natriuretic and diuretic effects; may exacerbate cardiac failure	Monitor cardiac failure patients treated with NSAIDs carefully for signs of fluid retention

---

Reflective point

Consider which postoperative surgical patients may not be appropriate to receive NSAIDs.

The practitioner must assess the balance of benefits and risks of NSAID use in patients. Good analgesia can be achieved with this class of drug but one must remember that not all surgical patients postoperatively are suitable because of the potential side-effects from NSAIDs. If NSAIDs are prescribed, then the practitioner must monitor the patient for any potential adverse effect and intervene where necessary to cancel the prescription.

Nefopam

Nefopam is effective in the relief of moderate to moderately severe pain postoperatively; severe pain requires a strong opioid analgesic (Dollery 1991). Nefopam is a centrally acting analgesic but as it has no effects on opioid receptors it does not cause respiratory depression (Gasser & Bellville 1975) or constipation and there has been no evidence of abuse of the drug (ABPI 1998).

Therefore it is a useful drug to consider for patients when the usual drugs such as opioids, NSAIDs and paracetamol have been tried and an additional analgesic is required. It may be considered in addition to NSAIDs and paracetamol in patients who are considered at high risk of respiratory depression from opioids or where patients have a history of opioid drug abuse. Another situation may be a patient who is on an opioid such as dihydrocodeine or codeine but is experiencing severe constipation despite laxatives. As nefopam does not cause constipation, compared to opioid analgesics, it could be considered as an alternative together with NSAIDs and paracetamol after, for example, anorectal surgery (Dollery 1991).

It is available as a tablet and administered in a dose of 30–90 mg three times a day. An intramuscular formulation is also available and administered in a dose of 20 mg four times a day.

Mechanism of action. Nefopam inhibits neuronal uptake of dopamine, noradrenaline and serotonin (5-HT–5-hydroxytryptamine) (Heel et al 1980). Noradrenaline and 5-HT transmitter substances are thought to play a role in the descending inhibitory pathway from the brain to the spinal cord in modulating pain (Rang & Dale 1991). It is believed that inhibition of noradrenaline and 5-HT by nefopam is responsible for its pain-killing properties (Heel et al

1980). It has anticholinergic and sympathomimetic activity which is usually not noticeable unless other drugs with these properties are taken at the same time (Anon 1979).

Side-effects. Convulsions in susceptible individuals are the most serious adverse effect of nefopam (Dollery 1991). It has a high incidence of minor side-effects which include sweating, nausea, headache, urinary retention and dry mouth; these are more likely to occur after parenteral administration (Dollery 1991). Nausea and sweating occur in about 10–30% of patients (Dollery 1991). Other less common side-effects include vomiting, blurred vision, drowsiness, insomnia and tachycardia (ABPI 1998).

As it enhances motor neuron activity, it is contraindicated in patients with a history of convulsive disorders and, because of its sympathomimetic action, it should not be given to patients on monoamine oxidase inhibitors (MAOIs). Because of its anticholinergic side-effects, it should be used with caution in patients with, or at risk of, urinary retention or glaucoma (Anon 1979, ABPI 1998).

Opioid analgesics

Opioid analgesics are still the mainstay for routine postoperative pain relief, administered orally, subcutaneously, intramuscularly, intravenously or epidurally. The term opioid applies to any substance that produces morphine-like effects that are antagonised by naloxone; it includes various neuropeptides (e.g. endorphins, enkephalins and dynorphins) and synthetic analogues (e.g. fentanyl), the structure of which may be quite different from morphine (Rang & Dale 1991).

Mechanism of action

There are three receptors on which opioid drugs bind to bring about their main pharmacological effects; these receptors are termed μ (mu), κ (kappa) and δ (delta). These receptors are found in the brain, spinal cord and on nerves in the periphery. The μ-receptors are thought to be responsible for most of the analgesic effects of opioids and for some of the major unwanted effects (e.g. respiratory depression, sedation, nausea, vomiting and dependence). Most of the analgesic opioids are μ-receptor agonists.

Morphine

This is the gold standard drug against which other opioid drugs are compared either for efficacy or in terms of their side-effect profile. It is available in a wide range of formulations and has been administered by various routes including oral, parenteral (i.m., i.v. via bolus, infusion or patient controlled analgesia – PCA), epidural, topical and intra-articular routes.

Diamorphine (heroin)

Diamorphine is pharmacologically similar to morphine. Because of its greater lipid solubility it crosses the blood–brain barrier more rapidly and its onset of action may therefore be slightly faster. It is said to be less emetic than morphine but there is no evidence for this. There is no evidence that it causes less respiratory depression than morphine or differs from morphine in its liability to cause dependence (Rang & Dale 1991). It has a shorter duration of action compared to morphine.

Pethidine

Pethidine is a synthetic opioid analgesic with similar properties to morphine but has more rapid onset and shorter duration of action than morphine, which usually lasts for 2–4 hours (Reynolds 1996). The sedative and euphoric effects of pethidine may be greater than those of morphine but the evidence is conflicting (McEvoy 1998). The bioavailability of pethidine after intramuscular injection can vary as much as 30–50% after repeated administration (Austin et al 1980). This is probably the most common cause of an inconsistent clinical response to intramuscular pethidine injection.

Pethidine is metabolised in the liver to norpethidine which is an active metabolite. Norpethidine is twice as potent as a convulsant, and one-half as potent as an analgesic compared to pethidine itself (Cherny 1996). Therefore convulsions can occur and this is more likely when patients are administered large doses and/or have renal impairment where the kidney is unable to excrete the norpethidine metabolite (Pryle et al 1992, Szeto et al 1977). It has been recommended that doses exceeding 25 mg/kg per day are likely to produce excitatory effects due to norpethidine toxicity (Pryle et al 1992). In renal impairment the long half-life of norpethidine prolongs the adverse effects should they occur. Seizures have also been reported when pethidine has been used in patient-controlled analgesia (Hagmeyer et al 1993).

The practitioner should be aware of the early signs of neurotoxicity, e.g. tremors, twitching or jerking. The treatment of neurotoxicity should include discontinuation of pethidine and the prescription of a benzodiazepine, e.g. diazepam. Myoclonic seizures resulting from pethidine administration are sometimes preceded by involuntary twitching in the extremities and can be avoided by stopping the pethidine. Seizures induced by pethidine are resistant to naloxone, but respond to anticonvulsants such as diazepam and phenytoin (Koo 1995).

Pethidine is thought to cause less histamine release than morphine (although this debatable – Flacke et al 1983) and therefore it has been proposed that it may be more suitable for patients who have severe asthma or have experienced bronchoconstriction with morphine in the past. Another advantage claimed for pethidine over morphine is that it does not increase biliary pressure and so is possibly a better drug to use in patients with pancreatitis or colicky pains, although this is said not to be true (Nagle & McQuay 1990). Since the reported severity, intensity and duration of biliary pressure vary greatly, it is unlikely that any opioid has a clear advantage over another (Chisholm et al 1983).

Given the availability of alternative drugs that lack the toxicity of pethidine and its metabolite, its use in acute pain management is not recommended (Agency for Health Care Policy and Research 1992).

Reflective point

How frequently are prescriptions for pethidine written in your area of practice? Consider how many of these are justified and, knowing the disadvantages pethidine has compared to morphine, question whether morphine could be used instead. Have you noticed how the short duration of action of pethidine sometimes establishes a cycle where patients 'clock watch' until they can have a repeated dose of pethidine?

Fentanyl

Fentanyl is a very potent opioid with effects that are similar to morphine but very short-lasting. It has mainly been used in anaesthesia but may be useful for patients with renal failure as it has no active or toxic metabolites (Moore et al 1987). Owing to its high lipid solubility, it is widely used in epidural analgesia (see p. 497).

Phenazocine (Narphen)

This drug is a potent synthetic opioid which can be administered orally or sublingually in patients who are nil by mouth. It also appears not to raise biliary pressure and so, like pethidine, has been thought to be useful in patients with pancreatitis or colicky pain (Reynolds 1996).

Dextromoramide (Palfium)

Dextromoramide is a potent oral synthetic drug which is less sedating than morphine but has a short duration of action of 2–3 hours. It is a useful drug to provide pain relief before a dressing change, e.g. for burns patients.

Buprenorphine (Temgesic)

Unlike the opioids described above, which are full agonists at the μ opioid receptor, buprenorphine is a partial agonist and is used for moderate to severe pain. Its effects are only partially reversed by the opioid antagonist naloxone because the buprenorphine complex at the opioid receptor shields the receptor from naloxone (Nagle & McQuay 1990). Therefore, should respiratory depression occur, large doses of naloxone may be necessary. It appears to be safe to use in patients with renal impairment (Hand et al 1990).

It is available in sublingual tablet and injection form. Because its oral bioavailability is only 16% because of considerable first-pass metabolism by the liver (Bullingham et al 1983), the sublingual route is used. Sublingual administration of drugs bypasses metabolism by the liver. This route of administration of buprenorphine has the advantage that it can be administered to patients who are nil by mouth.

Because buprenorphine is a partial agonist, if it is administered to patients on morphine (or another strong full opioid agonist) it may result in a worsening of the pain relief. This is most likely if the patient is on a high dose of morphine because the buprenorphine competes with the morphine for the μ opioid receptors. If it binds to some of these receptors, buprenorphine will not provide as much pain relief because it has a dose ceiling as a partial agonist. Therefore, if the pain intensity is high, it will not improve pain but make it worse because it has displaced some of the morphine from the receptors.

Codeine/dihydrocodeine (co-codamol/co-dydramol)

Both these drugs are much weaker full agonists than morphine and are used for mild to moderate pain. Similar degrees of pain relief to morphine could be obtained if very high doses were administered but this is limited by the fact that the side-effects such as constipation would be intolerable.

Codeine in a low dose (8 mg) is combined with 500 mg paracetamol in the compound analgesic co-codamol, and low-dose dihydrocodeine (10 mg) is combined with 500 mg paracetamol in the compound analgesic co-dydramol. It is doubtful whether such small doses of codeine and dihydrocodeine in these compound preparations gives any better pain relief than paracetamol on its own.

Dihydrocodeine is best administered in an oral dose of 30 mg every 4 hours; this may provide better pain relief than giving 60 mg every 6–8 hours. This is because doses of dihydrocodeine above 30 mg do not usually provide better pain relief in most patients; rather it is best to give a smaller dose more often (Dollery 1991). Codeine is administered in an oral dose of 60 mg four times a day. Doses higher than this are likely to cause severe constipation.

No trials comparing the two drugs have been carried out so it is not certain whether one drug is better than another in providing pain relief. However, an analysis of separate trial data suggests that dihydrocodeine is more effective than codeine (Moore & McQuay 1997, Moore et al 1996).

Dextropropoxyphene (co-proxamol)

This drug in a dose of 32.5 mg is found combined with 325 mg paracetamol in the compound analgesic co-proxamol and is used for mild to moderate pain. Dextropropoxyphene is similar to codeine but has a longer duration of action.

Co-proxamol has recently been the subject of much discussion in relation to its effectiveness in providing pain relief (Haigh 1996, Hanks & Forbes 1998, Sykes et al 1996). It appears to be no more effective than paracetamol after single doses (Li Wan Po & Zhang 1997, Moore et al 1997) for acute pain. However, for chronic pain co-proxamol may be more helpful. This is because dextropropoxyphene undergoes extensive first-pass metabolism in the liver (Perrier & Gibaldi 1972) which means plasma levels after a single dose will be much lower than those found after the drug has been given regularly for several days.

Tramadol

Tramadol is a weak μ-receptor agonist. Its affinity for the μ-receptor is 10 times less than that of codeine and 6000 times less than morphine (Dayer et al 1994, Raffa et al 1992). Its analgesic actions also result from its inhibition of neuronal uptake of noradrenaline and enhancement of 5-HT release (Raffa et al 1992). Its actions are only partially (30%) antagonised by

naloxone (Collart et al 1993). Tramadol is as effective, and sometimes less effective, than combinations of paracetamol and codeine or paracetamol and dextropropoxyphene in acute pain patients with moderate pain (Crighton et al 1997, Stubhaug et al 1995). It is not as effective as morphine for severe pain (Houmes et al 1992).

Tramadol displays minimal respiratory effects, and seems to have a low potential for abuse and therefore is not classified as a controlled drug. It has an incidence of nausea and vomiting similar to morphine. Despite minimal respiratory depressant effects (probably due to tramadol being a weak opioid), lower doses should be used in patients with renal impairment, otherwise respiratory depression may occur (Barung et al 1997). Other adverse effects include dizziness, headache and sweating. It may cause less constipation than opioids such as codeine, but this was not shown in a trial where both drugs were administered for 4 weeks (Rauck et al 1994).

Tramadol lowers the seizure threshold and so should not be used in patients with epilepsy or in patients who are on other drugs that can lower the seizure threshold, e.g. antidepressants. Convulsions have occurred in patients at therapeutic dose and the risk may increase at doses exceeding the upper daily limit (Committee on Safety of Medicines 1996).

Tramadol seems to have a role in acute moderate pain where other equally effective agents are unsuccessful. It may be more useful in the management of chronic pain.

Table 24.6 shows the typical doses, routes and duration of the opioids described above. *Note:* The data provided give *approximate* equianalgesic doses of various opioids by i.m. and oral routes of administration.

It is sometimes required to convert patients either from one opioid to another or to administer an opioid by another route. Table 24.7 gives the conversion factors and Box 24.4 some examples to enable the practitioner

Table 24.6 Opioid drugs

Drug	Dose (mg)		Duration of action (hours)
	i.m.	Oral	
Morphine	10	20–30	4–6
Diamorphine	5	30	3–4
Pethidine	75–100	150–300	2–4
Fentanyl	0.1	N/A	1–2
Phenazocine		5–10	4–6
Dextromoramide		10–15	2–3
Buprenorphine	0.4	0.8	6–8
Codeine	130	200–375	4–6
Tramadol	100	120	4–6

Table 24.7 Opioid conversion table

Drug	Route	Total daily dose conversion factor to oral morphine
Buprenorphine	Sublingual	× 50
Codeine	Oral	× 0.08
Dextromoramide	Oral/sublingual	× 2
Dihydrocodeine	Oral	× 0.1
	Subcutaneous/intramuscular	× 0.33
Diamorphine	Parenteral	× 3
Fentanyl	Transdermal for 72-hour dose	See manufacturer's product literature
Methadone*	Oral	Switching from another opioid agonist to methadone is complex – seek advice
Morphine sulphate	Oral	× 1
	Subcutaneous/intramuscular	× 2
	Intravenous	× 2–3
Papaveretum† (formerly Omnopon)	Subcutaneous/intramuscular	× 0.67
Pethidine	Oral	× 0.125
	Subcutaneous/intramuscular	× 0.20–0.25
Phenazocine	Oral/sublingual	× 3–5
Tramadol	Oral	× 0.2
	Intramuscular/intravenous	× 0.2

* Methadone has a prolonged half-life after repeated dosing which results in accumulation of the drug.
† The factor quoted for papaveretum is derived from its constituents and is not based on any clinical data.

to calculate the conversion without loss of analgesic dose. The practitioner may consider using the pharmacist as a resource in these situations.

Side-effects

The main unwanted effects of morphine are as follows:

Respiratory depression. The effects are dose-related and may be more problematic in patients with existing respiratory problems, as the respiratory drive is reduced and hypoxia can result. One of the most important indicators for respiratory depression is sedation.

Whether or not the patient is in pain will determine if a reasonable dose of opioid will cause respiratory depression. Volunteers who are not in pain will show respiratory depression at opioid doses which will not produce respiratory depression in patients in pain (Nagle & McQuay 1990). This is probably because when a patient is in pain the respiratory centre receives stimulatory noiciceptive input which counterbalances the respiratory depressant effect of the opioid. For patients complaining of pain, in whom you might expect a previous dose of opioid to have been absorbed, it is safe to give another, probably smaller, dose (Nagle & McQuay 1990).

Physical and psychological dependence. Dependence involves psychological as well as physical factors and rarely occurs in patients given opioids as analgesics. Addiction to opioids is of concern not only to patients, but also to nurses and doctors. This concern is exaggerated, as addiction to opioids after administration is very rare. Its overall incidence is estimated at 1 in 3000 patients (Porter & Jick 1980).

Reflective point

The practitioner needs to be aware of opioid drug users who are admitted to hospital requiring surgery or in acute pain. As they are already using opioids, they will have higher opioid-dosing requirements to achieve analgesia because of a higher tolerance level established from their addiction. Careful assessment of the analgesia requirements of these patients is required. What resources are available to assist the nurse assess the daily consumption and therefore the analgesic requirements of these patients?

Reduced gastrointestinal motility. Opioids can cause reduced gut motility and smooth muscle spasm, leading to constipation and sometimes ureteric or biliary spasm (biliary spasm can make the pain of pancreatitis worse). However, it is worth noting that pain itself can cause reduced gut motility. Appropriate laxatives (e.g. senna, docusate) will need to be prescribed for the treatment of opioid constipation.

Box 24.4 Examples of conversion

Pethidine injection to morphine injection
A patient with pancreatitis has been receiving 50 mg pethidine intramuscularly every 2 hours, i.e. a total of 600 mg per 24 hours.

First convert the total daily amount of pethidine into the equivalent amount of oral morphine.

Pethidine 600 mg daily by injection; conversion factor × 0.25
  = 600 mg × 0.25
  = 150 mg oral morphine daily.

Then convert oral morphine into morphine injection.

Conversion factor ÷ 2 (morphine injection is twice as potent as oral morphine)
  = 150 mg ÷ 2
  = 75 mg morphine injection daily.

Therefore, for a 4-hourly regimen (6 doses/24 hours) of morphine injection:
  = 75 mg ÷ 6
  = 12.5 mg every 4 hours (round to 12 mg 4-hourly).

Morphine injection to oral morphine.
A patient after abdominal surgery has been receiving 10 mg morphine intramuscularly every 4 hours, i.e. 60 mg per 24 hours. The patient is now no longer nil by mouth and is able to be given morphine orally.

Morphine 60 mg daily by injection; conversion factor × 2
  = 120 mg daily of oral morphine.

To give this as 4-hourly doses (i.e. 6 doses/24 hours):

120 mg oral morphine/24 hours
  = 120 mg ÷ 6 doses
  = 20 mg every 4 hours of immediate-release morphine (e.g. Oramorph liquid or Sevredol tablets).

To give this as a 12-hourly dose (i.e. 2 doses/24 hours):

120 mg oral morphine/24 hours
  = 120 mg ÷ 2 doses
  = 60 mg every 12 hours of slow-release morphine (e.g. MST).

Nausea and vomiting. Nausea and vomiting can be as distressing to a postoperative patient as the pain, and therefore need continuous assessment and treatment. A simple nausea scale should be used with every observation recorded. An example of a nausea scale is: 0 = no nausea or vomiting; 1 = nausea without vomiting; 2 = nausea and vomiting. A score of 1 or 2 requires the administration of an anti-emetic. After an anti-emetic has been administered, further assessment using the scale will determine its efficacy. Many drugs are available to treat nausea and vomiting and they work in different ways.

It is also important to note that pain causes nausea. In patients after abdominal surgery, 59% experienced simultaneous pain and nausea but only 3.4% of morphine injections provoked nausea (Andersen & Krohg 1976). Therefore achieving good pain relief will also help reduce nausea.

Suitable drugs for the management of opioid-induced nausea and vomiting include cyclizine (an antihistamine type of anti-emetic), metoclopramide and prochlorperazine (dopamine antagonists). It is important to remember that drugs which work in different ways can be combined together and given simultaneously for an additive effect, in the same way that paracetamol, NSAIDs and opioids when combined give enhanced pain relief. Therefore cyclizine and metoclopramide can be given together. Once a response has been achieved, it is best to administer the anti-emetic regularly for 24–48 hours and then reassess the need for anti-emetics.

Histamine release. All opioids can cause histamine release. This can lead to bronchoconstriction and itching, and sometimes hypotension.

Histamine release for a given opioid seems to be dose-dependent. Fentanyl appears to produce little histamine release compared to morphine and pethidine, with pethidine causing more histamine release than morphine (Flacke et al 1983). If histamine is the main mechanism by which bronchospasm is produced in susceptible patients, then pethidine is more likely to cause bronchospasm then morphine. Whilst the risk from fentanyl would be minimal (Nagle & McQuay 1990), this is not usually found to be the case in practice.

A simple treatment for the itching most commonly seen around the head and neck is calamine lotion. If this is ineffective, an antihistamine such as chlorpheniramine (Piriton) can be used. If calamine lotion is cosmetically unacceptable, a urea cream called Eurax can be tried. The patient will need reassuring that the itching is a side-effect of the analgesic.

Opioid antagonists

Naloxone is the drug used to reverse the effects of opioids and is only available as an injectable formulation. Naloxone is best administered by drawing up 400 mcg, diluting it with 3 ml of 0.9% sodium chloride and titrating the resultant solution slowly in 100 mcg increments against respiratory rate. It is important to realise that it is a short-acting drug (half-life = 60–90 minutes) and so repeated injections or a continuous infusion may be required if the opioid has a long duration of action, to maintain the reversal of the opioid's effects until it has been eliminated from the body.

A drug called naltrexone, an oral formulation, has a longer duration of action. It is unsuitable for emergency use to reverse the effects of opioids, because of the time it would take to be absorbed from the gut into the bloodstream. At present, naltrexone has been used in the management of drug addiction.

Local anaesthetics

Local anaesthetics can be administered topically for surface anaesthesia, infiltrated into wounds, and given as nerve blocks or by the epidural route.

Surface or topical anaesthesia blocks the sensory nerve endings in the skin or mucous membranes, but to reach these structures the drug must have good powers of penetration. EMLA cream (containing lignocaine 2.5% and prilocaine 2.5%) and Ametop gel (amethocaine 4%), although used widely in paediatrics for skin anaesthesia prior to venepuncture or venous cannulation, can be useful for needle-phobic adults. Both drugs are applied to the skin and covered with an occlusive dressing prior to the procedure. EMLA cream takes about 1 hour to become effective whereas Ametop works faster, within 30–40 minutes. Lignocaine is frequently used for surface anaesthesia of mucous membranes of the throat and pharynx before intubation and bronchoscopy, whilst local anaesthetics such as amethocaine and oxyprocaine are used for anaesthetising the cornea during ophthalmological procedures (Reynolds 1996).

Infiltration anaesthesia is produced by injection of the local anaesthetic agent into and around the field of operation. Wound infiltration can be done for most wounds and is simple to perform but its effects are short-lasting.

Regional nerve block anaesthesia may include peripheral nerve blocks. This involves injection into or around the peripheral nerve or plexus supplying the part to be anaesthetised (Reynolds 1996). Examples of this type of peripheral nerve block include branchial plexus block, intercostal nerve block and paracervical block. For peripheral nerve blocks, a catheter can be inserted to allow further doses to be administered.

Epidurals should be reserved for major surgery when the potential benefits outweigh the risks (see p. 496).

An overview of the use of regional analgesia is given in Table 24.8.

Mechanism of action

Local anaesthetics work by inhibiting sodium ion conductance across the nerve membrane, thus preventing generation and transmission of impulses along nerve fibres (called C and A nerve fibres) and of painful stimuli at nerve endings (Reynolds 1996). Therefore complete pain relief can be achieved for a localised area. The effects are reversible and when the local anaesthetic wears off the pain returns. This prevention of noiciception distinguishes local anaesthetics from

Table 24.8 Regional analgesia techniques (Concepcion & Covino 1984, McQuay et al 1997)

	Indications	Advantages	Disadvantages
Topical agents	Surface surgery	Simple	Short duration
Wound infiltration	Most wounds	Simple	Short duration
Peripheral nerve blocks	Surgery to arms and legs, trauma	Catheter may be used	
Plexus blocks	Surgery to arms and legs	Catheter may be used	Nerve damage and motor block
Epidural	Major surgery: Thoracic or upper abdominal procedures Lumbar: lower abdominal surgery of the pelvis, perineum, lower extremities (legs) and obstetrical procedures	Catheter may be used; risk of thromboembolism reduced	Adverse effects (e.g. hypotension, respiratory depression, spinal cord compression), surveillance

other analgesic drugs such as morphine or NSAIDs which affect the perception of pain at a central level and inhibit the sensitisation of peripheral pain receptors respectively (Fischer 1995).

By preventing the transmission of impulses along C and A nerve fibres, local anaesthetics produce a non-selective sympathetic and somatic (sensory and motor) blockade in addition to analgesia. C fibres are responsible for pain transmission and autonomic activity, whilst A fibres are responsible for touch and pressure sensation and motor activity. In general, analgesia occurs before loss of sensory (anaesthesia) and autonomic function (paralysis) but is dependent on the concentration of the local anaesthetic (Reynolds 1996). Therefore the aim is to produce analgesia whilst minimising the side-effects.

The main drugs that are used are bupivacaine and lignocaine and Table 24.9 gives some idea of their onset and duration of action.

The local anaesthetic must penetrate the lipoprotein nerve sheath before it can act, and therefore agents with high lipid (fat) solubility have a greater potency and duration of action and faster onset of action than those with low lipid solubility (Reynolds 1996).

The duration of anaesthesia for a particular local anaesthetic can vary depending on the procedure and the site of injection of the local anaesthetic. For example the duration of action of bupivacaine after infiltration anaesthesia is 2–4 hours whilst after a major nerve block it is some 4–12 hours. The duration of action of lignocaine is only half to 1 hour for infiltration anaesthesia and 3–4 hours after a major nerve block. A more detailed description of the use of local anaesthetics for epidural analgesia is given later (p. 497).

Other factors that influence the onset and duration of action of local anaesthetics is their individual drug chemistry, their concentration and whether or not they are used with a vasoconstrictor. The use of a vasoconstrictor such as adrenaline (typically in a strength of 1 in 200 000) can extend the duration of action by slowing the uptake of the local anaesthetic into the systemic circulation. This helps maintain a higher concentration of the local anaesthetic near the neural tissue for a longer time, thus prolonging the duration of action of the local anaesthetic. However, adrenaline must not be used when producing a nerve block in an appendage, as gangrene may occur (Reynolds 1996).

Side-effects

The side-effects of local anaesthesia may be due to the drug or to errors in technique or the result of blockade of the sympathetic nervous system. Local anaesthetics may have systemic adverse effects as a result of raised plasma concentrations, e.g. after excessive dosage or accidental intravenous injection or by absorption of large amounts through mucous membranes or damaged skin or from vascular areas (Reynolds 1996).

The systemic toxicity of local anaesthetics mainly involves the central nervous system and the cardiovascular system. Local anaesthetics can readily cross the blood–brain barrier, causing signs of CNS excitation and depression, including dizziness, tinnitus, drowsiness, disorientation, muscle twitching, seizures and respiratory arrest (Concepcion & Covino 1984). Numbness of the tongue and perioral region may appear as an early sign of systemic toxicity (Reynolds 1996). Cardiovascularly, myocardial depression and peripheral vasodilatation will result in hypotension and bradycardia. Hypotension often occurs with epidural anaesthesia (Reynolds 1996).

A more detailed description of the side-effects of local anaesthetics in epidural analgesia due to the blockade of sensory, motor or autonomic nerve fibres is given on pages 497–501.

Entonox

Entonox is a combination of nitrous oxide and oxygen in equal quantities. It is the 'laughing gas' of dentist fame. Nitrous oxide is used in association with other pharmacological agents to produce anaesthesia. Mixed with oxygen, it is used to produce short-acting analgesia without corresponding loss of consciousness. It provides useful and safe analgesia for patients who are experiencing short episodes of acute pain and is often suitable for patient self-administration (Reynolds 1996). It is commonly used for obstetric

Table 24.9 Profile of local anaesthetics

Local anaesthetic	Potency	Onset (minutes)*	Duration (hours)
Lignocaine	Moderate	Fast (0.5–1)	Moderate (0.5–4)
Bupivacaine	High	Moderate to slow (5)	Long (2–10)

* Onset of action is longer for peripheral/plexus nerve blocks and epidural blockade.

analgesia, for patients in labour, and it is useful in the short-term treatment of postoperative pain, particularly dressing changes. Entonox is kept in cylinders that are black with blue and white shoulders and is administered via a valve with a mask or a mouthpiece. Positive pressure is required to initiate a breath. Breaths can be continued until the patient takes the mask from the face or removes the mouthpiece. Too many breaths of Entonox cause dizziness and disorientation which make the patient drop the mask. This effect is short-lived, lasting perhaps 1–2 minutes, after which the patient can use the mask again. Entonox is a safe technique in the short term but if used for long periods of time it can cause megaloblastic anaemia owing to its interference with vitamin B_{12} (Reynolds 1996). Therefore patients should have their vitamin B_{12} levels monitored if it is used regularly.

Antidepressants and anticonvulsants

These drugs are not usually used for acute pain but are reserved for chronic pain conditions. They are included here so that the practitioner may be aware of the role these drugs may play in pain management in particular groups of patients, such as those with vascular pain, amputees with phantom limb pain and patients with pre-existing diabetic neuropathy undergoing surgery.

Antidepressants and anticonvulsants are used in chronic pain when pain relief from conventional analgesics such as paracetamol, NSAIDs or morphine is inadequate, or when pain relief is combined with intolerable or unmanageable side-effects.

Antidepressants are helpful for neuropathic pain (pain in a numb area). Both burning pains and shooting pains respond to the tricyclic family of antidepressants (Max et al 1992). These kinds of pain have been described by patients after amputation (phantom limb pain). These drugs can be used in addition to conventional analgesics.

Older tricyclic antidepressants such as amitriptyline seem to work better than the newer antidepressants such as fluoxetine (Milligan 1997). The dose of amitriptyline should be low initially (25 mg at night or 10 mg at night for elderly patients) and increased by 10–25 mg every week up to a maximum of 75–150 mg at night. Most patients usually get pain relief from 75 mg doses; beyond this, side-effects such as dry mouth and drowsiness can become too troublesome (McQuay et al 1993). It is best to take the drug at night because the drowsiness side-effect promotes sleep. The newer antidepressants such as fluoxetine and paroxetine, which are serotonin reuptake inhibitors,

have a lower incidence of side-effects compared to tricyclic antidepressants and therefore can be worth trying in those patients who cannot take tricyclics because of adverse effects.

Anticonvulsants are also effective in the treatment of neuropathic conditions such as trigeminal neuralgia and diabetic neuropathy (McQuay et al 1995). The most common drugs used have been carbamazepine and sodium valproate. Carbamazepine is usually started in a dose of 100–200 mg twice a day and increased by 100–200 mg every week up to doses of 200–400 mg three or four times a day. The side-effects commonly seen with anticonvulsants are drowsiness, dizziness and gait disturbance, and an incidence of 25–50% has been reported (McQuay et al 1995).

Rational treatment of acute postoperative pain with analgesics

This section will aim to pull together the points made about the drugs discussed and help the practitioner to optimise the provision of analgesia for patients by selection of the right drug, by the right route in the right dose.

Selection of the right drug

Surgical patients have described their postoperative pain as moderate (47%) or severe (40%). However, almost 80% of the nurses and around 20% of the doctors who attended these patients thought that pain relief was adequate (Kuhn et al 1990). Clearly, analgesic drugs need to be used better and education is required for medical and nursing staff in how to prescribe and administer analgesia with reference to individual drug response.

Paracetamol and/or an NSAID prescribed and administered regularly, supplemented with patient-requested nurse-controlled oral or intramuscular opioid will remain the mainstay of postoperative pharmacological relief (Kehlet & Mather 1992, Rawal & Berggren 1994). Major surgery will require the use of epidural or PCA/intermittent opioid analgesia combined with non-opioid drugs. It is becoming clear that a multimodal approach is necessary to maximise the amount of pain relief after surgery (Michaloliakou et al 1996, Schulze et al 1988).

A non-opioid analgesic reduces the total amount of morphine required by up to 30% (Burns et al 1991, Delbos & Boccard 1995, Gillies et al 1987, Hodsman et al 1987, Owen et al 1986, Peduto et al 1998). Of the non-opioid analgesics, paracetamol is the safest drug for routine use. Unlike NSAIDs, it does not interfere with haemostatic mechanisms or thromboprophylactic regimens, does not cause stomach ulcers, and does not influence kidney function in elderly or hypovolaemic patients.

Paracetamol is equal to or slightly less potent than other non-opioid analgesics for postoperative pain relief, but has shorter duration of effect than, for example, ibuprofen (Morrison & Repka 1994) or diclofenac (Baer et al 1992).

Non-steroidal anti-inflammatory drugs (NSAIDs) such as diclofenac, ketorolac, naproxen, ibuprofen give good pain relief, but must be used with care in unstable postoperative patients where they can cause serious adverse effects. They should otherwise be used whenever possible in combination with paracetamol.

The Royal College of Anaesthetists (1998) have produced guidelines regarding the use of NSAIDs in the perioperative period, indicating their clinical effectiveness after different types of surgery. An outline of these is shown in Table 24.10.

Recent data have evaluated more precisely the efficacy of oral analgesics from randomised controlled trials after all kinds of surgery. Table 24.11 shows efficacy in terms of number needed to treat (NNT) – that is, the number of patients who need to receive the active drug for one patient to achieve at least 50% pain relief compared with placebo over a treatment period of 6 hours postoperatively (McQuay & Moore 1998). This method of expressing the effectiveness of a drug is a useful bedside tool that uses evidence-based medicine and puts data into a format that is relatively easy to understand.

The most effective drugs have a low NNT of about 2, meaning that for every two patients who receive the drug one patient will get at least 50% relief because of the treatment (the other patient may get relief but it does not reach 50%). For paracetamol 1 g the number needed to treat is nearly 5. Combining paracetamol with codeine 60 mg improves the number needed to treat to 3. From these data, diclofenac has the best score of number needed to treat.

Table 24.10 Use of NSAIDs in different types of surgery and clinical groups

Type of surgery	Usefulness of NSAIDs	Disadvantages
Orthopaedic	May be effective alone. Improve opioid analgesia and reduce opioid requirement. May reduce opioid side-effects	
Major gynaecological	Likely to reduce opioid requirements and side-effects. If NSAIDs used alone they are less effective than morphine in the first 24 hours	Should not be given preoperatively because of the increased risk of bleeding
Gynaecological laparoscopy	Improve opioid analgesia and reduce opioid dose. May reduce opioid side-effects. Enhanced analgesia when given with paracetamol	
General	Improve quality of opioid-based analgesia	Not to be used as sole analgesic in first 24 hours after major surgery
Oral	Effective alone after dental surgery. Preoperative administration more effective. Oral administration is effective	
Ear, nose and throat	Effective alternative to opioids after surgery	Increased bleeding has been demonstrated in some studies. Avoid in tonsillectomy patients where increased blood loss or low platelet counts pose particular risks
Postpartum pain	Effective alone after vaginal delivery. Reduce opioid requirement after caesarean section	Avoid in patients with hypovolaemia or pre-eclamptic toxaemia
Day-case	NSAIDs are drugs of choice in situations where they are likely to be effective alone (impacted molar teeth, arthroscopy). Addition of an opioid increases the efficacy	

Table 24.11 Number needed to treat (NNT) for at least 50% pain relief for single oral dose of analgesics after all kinds of surgery compared to placebo (McQuay & Moore 1998)

Drug	NNT
Diclofenac 50 mg	2.3
Diclofenac 25 mg	2.6
Ibuprofen 400 mg	2.7
Paracetamol 600 mg/codeine 60 mg	3.1
Ibuprofen 200 mg	3.3
Paracetamol 650 mg/dextropropoxyphene 65 mg	4.4
Paracetamol 1g	4.6
Tramadol 100 mg	4.8
Aspirin 650 mg/codeine 60 mg	5.3
Paracetamol 500 mg	5.6
Tramadol 50 mg	8.3
Dihydrocodeine 30 mg	9.7
Codeine 60 mg	16.7

Reflective point

Combining drugs which have low NNTs will maximise the pain relief a patient receives. Therefore it is a good idea to combine paracetamol, ibuprofen (an NSAID) and codeine or dihydrocodeine (weak opioids), drugs which all work in different ways, to provide synergistic relief for moderate to severe pain. For severe pain, a strong opioid will be necessary instead of codeine or dihydrocodeine. With this knowledge, consider how a patient could receive maximum benefit from prescribed analgesics.

Strong opioids are first-line treatment for severe acute pain. There is no good evidence that one opioid is better than another, but it is clear that pethidine has a specific disadvantage due to its metabolite, norpethidine. Pethidine is a poor choice of drug for repeated administration of doses and when renal impairment is present, owing to accumulation of the norpethidine metabolite which can cause convulsions. It also displays erratic absorption after repeated intramuscular injection (Austin et al 1980). Neither is there good evidence to suggest that the incidence of side-effects from opioids, such as nausea, vomiting, sedation, pruritus, urinary retention, respiratory depression, differs between the opioid drugs at the same level of analgesia (Nagle & McQuay 1990).

Selection of the right dose and route

The selection of the appropriate dose and route is as important as the choice of drug in pain management. The key to effective analgesia is the ability to take into account the dose and route by which the drug is administered and to titrate it correctly to minimise side-effects in addition to other factors listed below.

If a patient has a high pain score or is asking for more analgesia, then the following have to be considered:

- too little drug
- too long between doses
- lack of knowledge in analgesic pharmacology
- too little attention paid to the patient (patient does not know how or is afraid to request analgesia; nursing staff not assessing patient analgesic requirements)
- too much reliance on rigid (inadequate) regimens.

For example, if the patient is still complaining of pain after administration of an opioid, it may mean that too small a dose or too long a dose interval is being used. If you are sure that all the drug has been delivered and absorbed after administration, then it is safe to give another, usually smaller, dose. For example, more drug may be given 5 minutes after intravenous injection, 1 hour after intramuscular or subcutaneous injection, and 90 minutes after oral administration of an immediate-release formulation (McQuay et al 1997). An example of a protocol for intramuscular (i.m.) opioid analgesia is shown in Figure 24.3.

If a patient has a high pain score at rest, intravenous opioids titrated against pain score and respiratory rate should be considered. Depending on the centre, the support mechanisms may either be the acute pain team, the anaesthetist or a night sister.

Consideration of the appropriate route of administration of different NSAID preparations can be found on page 472, where it is concluded that the oral route is preferable, unless otherwise indicated.

It is inappropriate to prescribe oral slow-release formulations or transdermal preparations for acute pain as their onset of action is too slow – this is because the drug is only slowly absorbed from the gut or through the skin and so it can take several hours for adequate levels of drug in the bloodstream to be reached (Anon 1993).

Analgesic staircase for postoperative pain

The analgesic staircase or pain ladder (Fig. 24.4) is a tool devised to guide the practitioner to choose an

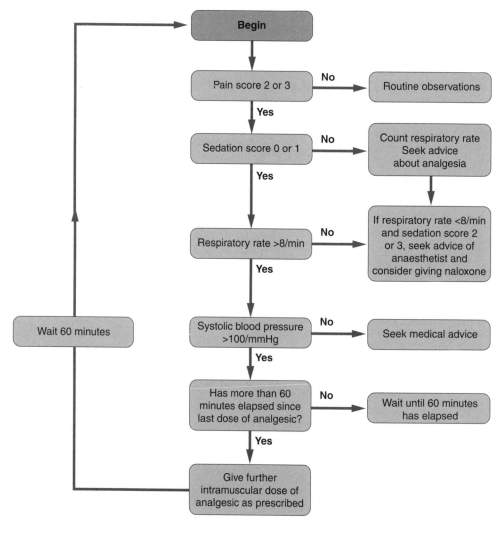

If weight less than 40 kg or more than 100 kg, then seek advice from the anaesthetist

Morphine
hourly dose intramuscularly

Weight (kg)	Dose (mg)
45–65	10
60–100	15

Every patient receiving intramuscular opioid analgesics must have an intravenous cannula in situ

Begin

Pain score 2 or 3 — **No** → Routine observations

Yes

Sedation score 0 or 1 — **No** → Count respiratory rate Seek advice about analgesia

Yes

Respiratory rate >8/min — **No** → If respiratory rate <8/min and sedation score 2 or 3, seek advice of anaesthetist and consider giving naloxone

Yes

Systolic blood pressure >100/mmHg — **No** → Seek medical advice

Yes

Has more than 60 minutes elapsed since last dose of analgesic? — **No** → Wait until 60 minutes has elapsed

Yes

Give further intramuscular dose of analgesic as prescribed

Wait 60 minutes

Key
Pain score
0 = No pain at rest or on movement
1 = No pain at rest, mild pain on movement
2 = Moderate pain at rest, severe pain on movement
3 = Severe pain at rest

Sedation score
0 = Awake
1 = Normal sleep
2 = Confused
3 = Difficult to rouse or unrousable

Figure 24.3 Algorithm for postoperative intramuscular analgesia (adapted from Gould et al 1992).

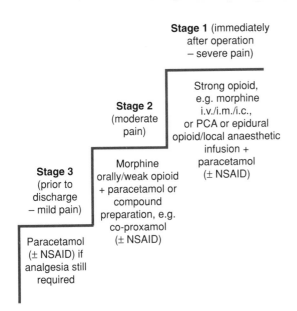

Stage 1 (immediately after operation – severe pain)

Strong opioid, e.g. morphine i.v./i.m./i.c., or PCA or epidural opioid/local anaesthetic infusion + paracetamol (± NSAID)

Stage 2 (moderate pain)

Morphine orally/weak opioid + paracetamol or compound preparation, e.g. co-proxamol (± NSAID)

Stage 3 (prior to discharge – mild pain)

Paracetamol (± NSAID) if analgesia still required

Figure 24.4   The pain ladder or analgesic staircase.

appropriate type of analgesia. The pain ladder requires a proper and full assessment of the patient's level of pain in order to choose the appropriate type of analgesia.

Although the choice of analgesia and the dosage is relevant to the type and severity of the pain to be treated, it must be remembered that there is a marked individual variability in pain perception and analgesic requirement that necessitates individual assessment of pain and titration of analgesia.

When treating postoperative pain, the analgesic staircase is used in reverse because initially the pain is severe and therefore needs strong analgesia but as the patient recovers weaker analgesia will be required.

Remember that combinations of opioids, paracetamol and NSAIDs are synergistic in the amount of pain relief they provide and help reduce opioid requirements. Regular administration of analgesics provides optimal analgesia (avoid administration 'as needed' (pro re nata – p.r.n.)).

Summary of key points to remember

- Multimodal analgesia will maximise the amount of pain relief.
- Paracetamol should always be included as part of the analgesic regimen (together with an NSAID where possible, and a weak/strong opioid depending on the severity of the pain).
- Become familiar with the analgesic drugs, their doses and side-effects, that are most commonly used

in your clinical area, e.g. for NSAIDs this could be ibuprofen and diclofenac, and for a strong opioid, morphine.

- Ensure that adequate doses of drugs are prescribed and administered.
- Analgesics should be prescribed for regular administration for maximum benefit, not p.r.n.
- The key principle for the safe and effective use of opioids is to titrate the dose against that patient's pain score and respiratory rate, thus minimising the side-effects.
- Use only one NSAID at a time – using two NSAIDs together increases the risk of side-effects without increasing efficacy.
- Consider trying another NSAID from a different class if there appears to be a poor response to treatment.
- Avoid NSAIDs in patients with known contraindications to their use – the nurse is responsible for checking for contraindications prior to administration of drugs (UKCC 1992).
- Consider using nefopam if NSAIDs are contraindicated for additional pain relief (assuming nefopam is not itself contraindicated).
- Monitor the patient for any signs of toxicity, particularly from NSAIDs (gastrointestinal, renal, haematological) and opioids (respiratory depression).
- Remember that addiction is not a problem with opioid use in acute pain.

Reflective point

Reflect on what are the most important educational factors that limit effective analgesia and what you can do to prevent this.

PATIENT-CONTROLLED ANALGESIA (PCA)

What is PCA?

Patient-controlled analgesia is now one of the most used methods of postoperative pain relief (Arfeen et al 1995). The method involves a pump that allows the patient to self-administer a predetermined dose of an opioid analgesic compound. There is a trigger for the dose, a handpiece or button, that patients can press whenever they feel they require pain relief.

PCA devices

All PCA devices have some parameters in common. These are drug concentration (the amount of drug in the solution being infused), bolus dose (the dose of the drug that is administered when demanded by the patient) and lock out time (a predetermined time between bolus doses when a demand for the drug will not result in a dose being given). Depending on the device used to administer the analgesia other features are available.

PCA devices fall into two basic categories, disposable and non-disposable.

The disposable PCA device

Disposable PCA devices (Fig. 24.5) have pre-set and non-changeable bolus volumes (e.g. 0.5 ml) and also have a pre-set and non-changeable lock out time, for example it may take 5 minutes for the reservoir to fill. They do not offer the advantage of being able to change any of the parameters should the patient's condition require an alteration in dose. However, these disposable devices have many advantages. They are fairly easy to fill and connect, as well as being small and light for the patient to carry around, and in most cases offer effective postoperative pain relief. They do not require a large capital investment but the running costs associated with them have been indicated to be higher (Arfeen et al 1995). Disposable devices typically cost approximately £25 each before they are filled; the cost of filling the device aseptically by the pharmacy department also needs to be taken into account. It is considered safer, from possible drug error and infection risk, for the devices to be filled by the pharmacy than by ward staff (Commission on the Provision of Surgical Services 1990).

The non-disposable PCA device

Non-disposable devices are essentially syringe drivers with safeguards. These include a lock on the device to ensure that the analgesic solution is not available to the patient in any way but through the device. Non-disposable PCA devices allow the practitioner to change many of the parameters of the administration of the analgesic. The size of the bolus dose can be altered, as can the lock out time, or the speed of delivery of the bolus dose. A limit to the total dose given within a set timeframe can be programmed in, as can a background infusion of the analgesia. Because all these parameters can be changed, the settings on the PCA device can be individualised to suit the patient's need. These syringe driver PCA pumps are mostly mains driven, with back-up battery, though some are battery driven only. They are usually designed for intravenous use and therefore contain pressure sensors to sound an alarm if the pressure increases, indicating an occlusion in the line (Welchew 1995).

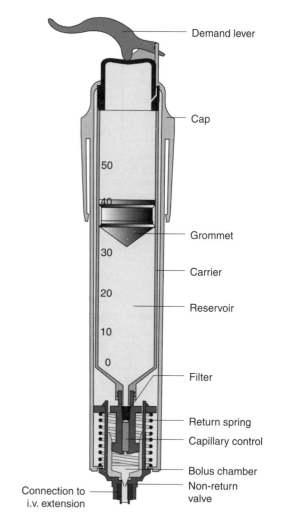

Figure 24.5 A disposable PCA device: the Vygon Freedom 5. The system is powered by a vacuum which is created when the set is filled and primed; all air must be removed from the system. The vacuum which is created in the bolus chamber pulls medication from the reservoir through the particulate filter and capillary tube into the bolus chamber. Thereafter the act of depressing the lever delivers the contents of the bolus chamber through the non-return valve to the patient. Following the release of the lever, the non-return valve closes and the bolus chamber refills ready for the next demand. The filling time is a nominal 5 minutes. (Reproduced by kind permission of Vygon (UK) Limited.)

Non-disposable PCA devices involve a large capital expenditure, but a relatively small ongoing cost (Arfeen et al 1995). Typically the PCA pumps cost around £2500.

Reflective point

Given the resources of your department or hospital, the type of surgery performed and the patient group, and the support network in place, which sort of device would allow you to offer the best service to your patients?

Drugs and prescriptions

Acute pain services within hospitals will generally have a preferred opioid, and a preferred drug regimen for delivery in the PCA device. This allows all staff in contact with the modality to become familiar with the drug regimen, thus decreasing the risk of error. The common opioids are morphine, pethidine and fentanyl. Which opioid is used depends largely on the preference of the anaesthetists in the hospital or the pain service. All have advantages and disadvantages, which are discussed at greater length on pages 478–482. Common treatment regimens for the three opioids mentioned are shown in Box 24.5.

Morphine remains the gold standard opioid analgesia for severe pain, against which other opioid analgesics are compared (British National Formulary 1998). The dosages are simple and mostly well known by nurses and doctors, thereby reducing the possibility of drug errors. It is effective for pain relief but can cause histamine release and so may be of limited value in those patients with severe asthma (see p. 479).

Pethidine can also be useful and is believed not to have the same histamine-release problem (although Flacke et al 1983 debate this), so might be useful in patients with severe asthma. It tends to be used for

patients who have an allergy to morphine although its claimed advantages in pancreatic or colicky pain are doubtful (see p. 479). Its duration of action is shorter than that of morphine, but this is not of great significance in PCA devices. Large doses of pethidine can cause accumulation of metabolites that can cause convulsions (see p. 478).

Fentanyl can also be useful in PCA devices. The dosages and the drug are less known by ward nurses and junior doctors, and this can cause some problems with the prescription and availability of the drug. Fentanyl has a very short duration, which, again, is not significant in PCA devices. Unlike morphine and pethidine, fentanyl has not been associated with clinical problems when given to patients with liver or renal dysfunction (Moore et al 1987).

Principles of PCA

The principles of PCA can be clearly demonstrated pictorially. Figure 24.6 shows a graph, with time on the x axis and blood concentration of opioid on the y axis. The y axis is divided into three zones. If the blood serum levels of opioid are too low the patient is in pain; if they are too high for that individual the patient may experience toxic effects from the drug. If the blood serum levels are at the correct level for that patient, they can be said to be in the therapeutic window for that drug. If a patient is given an i.m. injection of an opioid, the blood concentration goes from zero through the therapeutic window into the toxic band and the patient experiences a swinging effect between analgesia and pain.

There is not only a lag between the time of administration of analgesia and the time of the effect being perceived but between the patient feeling pain and receiving analgesia. This is nicely demonstrated in Figure 24.7.

With the use of PCA, patients are able to deliver a pre-set dose of opioid to themselves whenever they think that they need it, thereby keeping themselves

Box 24.5 Common treatment regimens for opioids in PCA (reproduced by kind permission of St Bartholomew's Hospital pain service)	
Drug concentration	60 mg morphine in 60 ml sodium chloride 0.9%
Bolus dose	1 mg
Lock out period	5 minutes
Drug concentration	600 mg pethidine in 60 ml sodium chloride 0.9%
Bolus dose	10 mg
Lock out period	5 minutes
Drug concentration	500 mcg fentanyl in 50 ml sodium chloride 0.9%
Bolus dose	10 mg
Lock out period	5 minutes

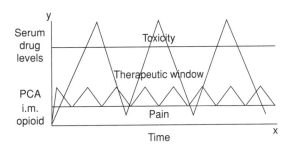

Figure 24.6 Principles of patient-controlled analgesia (from Ferrante et al Patient controlled analgesia. 1990. Blackwell Science, with permission).

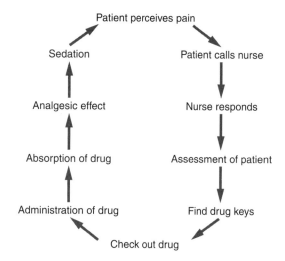

Figure 24.7 Sequence of events between perception of pain and effect of analgesia (Graves et al 1983 Annals of Internal Medicine).

within the therapeutic window and minimising the toxic effects of the opioid. It is important to realise that for this to be effective the patient needs to be in the therapeutic range when commencing the PCA. The most effective way of achieving this is for the patient to be given a loading dose of the opioid prior to setting up the PCA. The patient is prevented from administering too much opioid by the side-effect of sleep; this is a safety mechanism and the reason why it is so important that only the patient presses the button.

Why use PCA?

There can be no doubt that patients like using PCA. Collins (1994) found that 90% of patients who had previously had PCA preferred it as a method of postoperative pain relief. Patients like the feeling that they are in control of part of their clinical treatment. Nurses also like the autonomy and comfort that they feel PCA gives a patient. The advantages of PCA are discussed below. However, whatever the advantages of using this modality, the decision to use PCA must be based on the needs of the patient.

Advantages of PCA

Pain relief. As PCA delivers opioid via the intravenous or subcutaneous route to the same opioid receptors as in intermittent injection, there is little difference between efficient intramuscular (i.m.) injection and PCA (Ballantyne et al 1993). Nurse-led intermittent opioid injection requires good staffing levels to

minimise delay in the time between need and injection. Staff shortages, ward distractions and controlled drug regulations all increase the delay. PCA overcomes these logistical problems and perhaps explains why patients using PCA experienced significantly better pain control than those using an intermittent i.m. regimen (Thomas et al 1995).

Greater patient satisfaction. It has been shown that 90% of patients (n = 100) who had previously had PCA preferred it as a method of postoperative pain relief (Collins 1994).

Fewer respiratory side-effects. Respiratory side-effects have been shown to be less common with PCA than any other modality of opioid pain relief, especially if a background infusion is not used (Arfeen et al 1995).

Reduction in nursing time for administering analgesia. A research project undertaken by Koh & Thomas (1994) looked at nursing care satisfaction in 79 patients with either PCA or i.m. injection for their postoperative pain relief. The time that was taken by nursing staff to carry out pain control procedures was also investigated. It was found that using PCA showed a saving in nursing time, though the researchers stressed that this time should be used to increase patient–nurse contact.

Improved mobility therefore faster recovery. Arfeen & Owen (1995) reviewed the literature regarding the advantages and limitations of PCA. They showed studies that have indicated that improved pain management can lead to a more rapid recovery of normal ventilation, normal body temperature and mobilisation. They also indicated literature to support a trend towards shortening of hospital stays for patients with PCA.

Nursing care of the patient with PCA

Preoperative

There is much literature to demonstrate that it is vitally important that the patient receives good preoperative education regarding PCA, in order to gain the best postoperative pain relief (Williams 1996). Patients have experienced problems when they have been poorly prepared and do not fully understand how to get the best pain relief from the technique (Pediani 1998).

Reflective point

How does it work? How much should I use? Are there any side-effects? Can I give myself too much? How long will I need it for? Can I get up and walk around? Will I become addicted? These are some of the questions that patients will ask the nurse regarding the use of PCA. With your knowledge of PCA, how can you assist patients to make an informed choice concerning their postoperative analgesia?

Practitioners need to become aware of which patients need to be targeted for this PCA preoperative education. If there is doubt, one guideline is, any patient who might require more than two i.m. injections postoperatively.

Patients need to be shown the PCA device, especially the handpiece as this is the equipment they will be using, as well as instructions on how to use the equipment properly and safely. Patients are worried about overdose and addiction (Chumbley et al 1998) and these fears need to be very carefully allayed. Nurses giving preoperative information to patients will soon find their own phrases and techniques that seem to be most effective. Any preoperative instructions given to patients about PCA will need to be reiterated in the postoperative period, both immediately patients start to use the device and as they are recovering from their operation.

The following are some strategies that the authors have found useful when discussing PCA devices with patients:

- Keep it simple, without being patronising. Many patients are anxious about their surgery and will not remember a very complicated explanation. There are, of course, other patients who will want to know everything about their care and they will need a more in-depth explanation. It can be useful for some patients to back up verbal information with written information.
- It is important that patients are encouraged to use the device frequently. 'It is only a small amount of the drug that you get when you press the button, you need to use it when you are in a small amount of pain,' is a sentence that could be used to encourage the use of the PCA.
- One of the biggest fears that patients, particularly the elderly, will have about PCAs, is fear of addiction (Chumbley et al 1998). If the practitioner says to patients 'don't worry, you won't become addicted,' the word 'addicted' may be the only word that patients hear in the explanation that the nurse has given them; therefore it is better to avoid using it and related words such as 'addiction'. The patients' concerns are better alleviated by the nurse enquiring about any anxiety they may have, and saying, 'don't worry, the machine won't let you have too much', and 'the nurses will be monitoring you around the clock'.
- It is the authors' experience that it is not very useful telling patients about the lock out time specifically. PCA devices are designed to be used at any time that a patient feels pain, and if patients know that they only get the drug every 5 minutes, this may stop them pressing the button whenever they feel pain.

Postoperative

The nursing interventions required postoperatively for patients using PCA are largely centred on the monitoring and prevention of the side-effects of opioids and the monitoring of the efficacy of the analgesia system.

The complications of PCAs can be grouped into the side-effects of the opioid, mechanical problems with the pump, and operator error. All these need to be checked frequently and form the basis for the nursing interventions in the postoperative period.

The actual observations and the timing of them is a matter of hospital protocol. Figure 24.8 shows a chart used in one hospital to record all the postoperative observations in patients receiving analgesia systems.

Side-effects of the opioids:

Nausea and vomiting. One of the most evident and frequent side-effect of i.v. opioid administration is nausea and vomiting. Research into postoperative nausea and vomiting (PONV) associated with PCA generally concludes that there is essentially no difference in the incidence of emesis with the use of PCA compared with traditional drug administration methods (Albert & Talbott 1988, Ballantyne et al 1993, Berde et al 1991, Boulanger et al 1993). Despite this, it is a common belief amongst doctors and nurses that patients experience more nausea and vomiting when using PCA. The evidence for mixing anti-emetics with the opioid solution for PCAs has recently been reviewed by Woodhouse & Mather (1997), who concluded that it was controversial and a wider study was needed before its use could be supported.

There are many very effective anti-emetics available (Table 24.12) and patients should be given the option to have these drugs immediately on feeling nauseous; it is not necessary or ethical to wait until they are vomiting.

Respiratory depression. Respiratory depression is the most dangerous side-effect of opioid administration and a patient receiving PCA needs to be assessed frequently (see Ch. 23 and p. 481).

Efficacy of the analgesia system. The pain score is an indication that the analgesia device is effective. If the pain score is high then the nurse needs to review the PCA device, consider the use of adjunctive analgesia, re-educate the patient regarding the device, call the pain service or the anaesthetist, or if appropriate, consider the involvement of the surgical team if the nurse suspects a surgical complication.

Operator error. Many of the adverse events that have occurred using PCA have had an element of operator error (Fleming 1992). It is therefore necessary

NURSING GUIDE FOR USE WITH PAIN PATIENTS ONLY

UCL HOSPITALS NHS TRUST

Patient's Name

Hospital No.

Date

Ward

These guidelines and chart are to be used for monitoring of patients under the management of the pain teams and using the analgesia systems listed below. This chart is to be used in conjunction with the Epidural and PCA policies. This is not a prescription and is only to be used by nurses who have received UCLH training in the management of analgesia systems. Please tick box.

PATIENT CONTROLLED ANALGESIA

The opiate used is **morphine sulphate**. The PCA pumps will be programmed in theatre and the programme will read:—

1. Drug concentration 1 mg/1 ml
2. PCA (bolus) dose 1 mg (1 ml)
3. Dose duration Stat
4. Lock out period 5 minutes

Prefilled luer lock syringes containing morphine sulphate 50 mg in 50 ml in sodium chloride 0.9% are available from Pharmacy.

If morphine sulphate is contraindicated pethidine may be used:—

1. Drug concentration 10 mg/1 ml
2. PCA (bolus) dose 10 mg (1 ml)
3. Dose duration Stat
4. Lock out period 5 minutes

PCA DISPOSABLE SYSTEM

These are prefilled by Pharmacy with morphine sulphate 100 mg in 50 ml sodium chloride 0.9%. The concentration is 2 mg in 1 ml. The system is programmed to deliver 0.5 ml (1 mg) and this is fixed. The lock out period is 5 minutes.

EPIDURAL INFUSION

Acute pain patients: This is a mixture of bupivacaine 0.1% with or without fentanyl. If fentanyl is used it is at a concentration of 2 micrograms per ml, i.e. 500 micrograms in 250 ml. These are available prefilled.

Non-acute pain: Doses of drugs via epidural infusion will vary according to patients' needs.

Placement:

Level of Epidural _____

cm of catheter at skin _____

cm of catheter in space _____

DATE

TIME

Temp	40°C 39 38 37 36 35 34 33 32

Blood pressure and Pulse rate: 220 210 200 190 180 170 160 150 140 130 120 110 100 90 80 70 60 50 40 30 20 10

Respiration

PAIN SCORE — R (rest) M (movement)
- Worst possible pain 4
- Severe pain 3
- Moderate pain 2
- Mild pain 1
- No pain 0

LEVEL OF SEDATION
- Asleep (unrousable) 3
- Asleep (rousable) 2
- Drowsy 1
- Awake 0

RATE OF INFUSION ML/HR

PCA
- Number of Demands
- Number of Good Demands
- Total Amount of Drug Given

LEVEL OF EPIDURAL BLOCK R / L

NAUSEA SCORE
- Vomiting 2
- Nausea 1
- None 0

Figure 24.8 Analgesia systems chart (reproduced by kind permission of UCL Hospitals NHS Trust).

Table 24.12 Anti-emetics for the control of postoperative nausea and vomiting

	Dose	Maximum frequency
Metoclopramide (Maxalon)	10 mg i.m. or i.v.	6-hourly
Prochlorperazine (Stemetil)	12.5 mg i.m. 5–10 mg orally	6-hourly
Cyclizine	50 mg i.v. or orally	8-hourly
Ondansetron	4 mg i.v., i.m. or orally	8- to 12-hourly
Granisetron	1 mg i.v. or orally	12-hourly
Domperidone	10–20 mg orally	4-hourly
Domperidone	30 mg rectally	4-hourly

for all nurses and junior doctors who are involved in the care of patients using PCA to be very familiar with both the device and regimens. As part of the postoperative observations it is crucial that the nurse checks the device. If it is a syringe driver device, it is important to check the settings to ensure that they are what has been prescribed by the doctor.

Discontinuing PCA treatment

The decision to stop using the PCA device should be a joint one between the patient, the nurse and the medical team. Patients should be assured that they have access to other analgesia such as non-steroidal anti-inflammatory drugs (NSAIDs), compound analgesia or oral opioids when they require them. If more than one single dose of i.m. opioid is required, it may be necessary to reconnect the PCA and the patient needs to know that this is an option. It is important for the oral analgesia to be prescribed and administered regularly.

PCA and the acute pain service

PCA has become the cornerstone of postoperative pain control in many hospitals (Fleming 1992). It is important, however, to realise that this technique should be supported by a pain management service within that hospital. It is an important area of pain service responsibility to standardise protocols and to check that these are closely followed. If a different PCA were to be prescribed for a patient, this could confuse nursing and medical staff in the event of a complication. Many regimens are very effective, but a standard regimen is safer because of its familiarity (Pediani 1998).

The pain service will normally conduct daily rounds in order to offer support to wards with patients receiving PCA.

One of the most important responsibilities of the pain service is that of education. Fleming (1992) states that in-house education on PCA devices is essential to the safe use of the technique. Nurses need to be educated to teach the patients correctly. It is in the interests of patient safety that nurses and junior doctors are familiar with the principles of PCA and the devices, drug regimens and observations necessary in the postoperative period. This necessitates a system of continual seminars that all staff on wards with PCA are required to attend.

If used correctly by the patient, nurses and the medical staff, PCA as a postoperative pain control technique is effective and efficient.

Case study 24.1 Mrs C

Mrs C, who is 55 years old and weighs 68 kg, has a total abdominal hysterectomy. She is prescribed PCA postoperatively using the standard hospital regimen: morphine 60 mg in 60 ml saline 0.9%; 1 mg bolus; 5-minute lock out. She had no other analgesia prescribed. Initially her postoperative recovery was routine. However, 6 hours postoperatively she started to complain of itching all over her body. Pruritus caused by the morphine was diagnosed and 4 mg chlorpheniramine prescribed orally, which had some effect. She started to complain of nausea. Nurses checked the prescription chart, but no anti-emetic had been prescribed. It was the middle of the night, so medical staff needed to be called to the ward to write the prescription. Mrs C started to vomit, causing her great distress. The doctor arrived and prescribed prochlorperazine 12.5 mg i.m. This was given, but 30 minutes later it was clear that it had had no effect. Mrs C continued to feel nauseous and occasionally vomited. The doctor had left the ward again, so rather than call her back the PCA was discontinued. Mrs C's postoperative pain relief regimen was now intermittent i.m. pethidine injections, which she required every 3 hours for 2 days.

Reflective point

Read Case study 24.1 and reflect on the process. What else could have been done for Mrs C?

1. A combination of anti-emetics should have been prescribed routinely.
2. A combination of an NSAID and paracetamol could have been given, in order to reduce the opioid requirement.
3. A pethidine PCA could have been commenced.

EPIDURAL ANALGESIA

Principles

The aim of postoperative epidural analgesia is to provide analgesia over specific dermatomes for patients with moderate to severe postoperative pain. This is achieved by the administration of low concentrations of local anaesthetics and opioids via a catheter into the epidural space (Fig. 24.9). Epidural analgesia can be administered as single doses into a catheter; however, it is considered to be safer to use a continuous infusion (Dawson 1995). Epidural analgesia may also be administered as a one-off injection into the epidural space either pre- or postoperatively.

Anatomy

The epidural space is situated in the spinal cavity and skull, extending from the cranium to the sacrum. It is bound in the spine posteriorly by the ligamentum flavum and anteriorly by the dura mater.

In the cranium, the epidural space is a potential space, but in the spine it is an actual space containing connective tissue, epidural fat, arterioles, venules, nerve roots and an incomplete septum. The spinal cord is suspended in the dural sheath or sac, bathed in cerebrospinal fluid (CSF). Medial to the dura mater is the arachnoid mater and CSF fills the subarachnoid space between the arachnoid and pia mater meninges. It is this combination of fat and CSF that forms a soft protective padding around the spinal cord. The spinal cord typically ends at L1/2 and the dura and arachnoid mater extend to S2 and contain the cauda equina which is the bundle of sacral and lumbar nerves with which the spinal cord terminates. Lumbar punctures are performed below L1/2 to minimise the risk of spinal cord damage.

Drugs

The drugs most commonly used for epidural analgesia to control acute pain are local anaesthetics and opioids. They can be used singly or together. These drugs

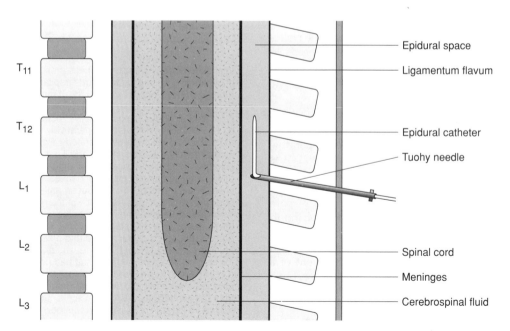

Figure 24.9 Diagrammatic representation of epidural space showing insertion of an epidural catheter. The position of the needle in the diagram is arbitrary.

have different modes of action. The local anaesthetic acts on the nerve roots that innervate the individual dermatomes, producing a transient inhibition of nerve impulses. Opioids diffuse into the spinal cord and control the pain impulses centrally by acting on the opioid receptors in the dorsal horn of the spinal cord. There is a recognised synergistic effect between local anaesthetics and opioids (Dawson 1995).

Opioids

The opioid reaches the site of action by diffusing through the dural membranes, through the CSF (where some remains), then into the dorsal horn of the spinal cord. It is this potentially large reservoir of opioid in the CSF which is carried to the respiratory centre by a process known as rostral spread, that causes the side-effect of late respiratory depression.

Rostral spread is the reason for using an opioid that is highly lipid-soluble, so that it diffuses through the dura quickly, and minimally water-soluble, so that only a small amount dissolves in the CSF, thus limiting the incidence of respiratory depression by this route. However, virtually any opioid can be used by this route. Fentanyl is the most lipid-soluble opioid, followed by diamorphine, with morphine being the least lipid-soluble. Therefore, in theory, fentanyl would be the least likely to cause late respiratory depression.

Opioids given epidurally act on the receptors in the spinal cord at the level of the surgery, producing segmental analgesia of those levels. Because the drugs act on only a small area of the body, the opioid requirement is less.

Local anaesthetics

The local anaesthetic agents act by blocking the action potential of the fine unmyelinated and scantily myelinated pain fibres (C and A delta fibres) as they pass through the epidural space (see p. 496). Thus, if the end of the epidural catheter is placed in the mid-dermatome of the wound, the local anaesthetic solution will spread over the nerve root pairs that innervate the wound, stopping the painful impulses from travelling from the wound to the brain via the pain pathways. This will produce a loss of certain types of sensation in the dermatome, commonly called a 'block'. The density of the block is related to the concentration of the local anaesthetic, while the height of the block is related to the rate of infusion. The most commonly used local anaesthetic agents are bupivacaine and lignocaine.

This method is not selective for analgesic pathways alone, which means that all fibres can be blocked, regardless of function. Heavy numb legs and buttocks have traditionally been a problem with epidural analgesia owing to high concentrations of local anaesthetic causing motor block (Bromage 1978). This is reduced by using lower concentrations of local anaesthetic, and the analgesia is optimised by increasing the infusion rate (Dawson 1995). This reduces the effect on the motor fibres, because lower concentrations of local anaesthetic are unable to penetrate the thicker myelin sheath of the motor fibres.

Reflective point

It is useful for nurses to reflect on how they feel after having a local anaesthetic injection at the dentist. Reflect on how your skin feels to the touch, if you can feel pain, if you can move your jaw and if you can sense temperature, e.g. hot tea. The concentration used by dentists is much stronger than that used to maintain epidural analgesia. Now try to relate your own experience to the concentrations used and the thickness of the nerve fibres.

Local anaesthetic blocks the small scantily myelinated fibres of the sympathetic nervous system. This causes a vasodilatation distal to the level of block, which results in pooling of blood in the limbs and abdominal viscera. This in turn reduces venous return and cardiac output, causing hypotension. It is this sympathetic blockade-induced hypotension that can lead to fluid management problems in patients who are hypovolaemic, because of preoperative fasting and/or intraoperative blood loss. This hypotension should be treated with crystalloid or colloid, not by reducing the amount of analgesia that the patient receives. The practitioner should be aware of any pre-existing renal or cardiac conditions that would restrict fluid administration (see Ch. 25).

Reflective point

Consider a hypotensive patient, whose pain is well controlled, receiving epidural analgesia via a continuous infusion where all other vital signs are stable. How should this hypotension be managed? What would be the impact on the patient's pain and hypotension of reducing the rate of analgesia? What other strategies may be more effective?

It is very important to consider carefully the cause of a patient's hypotension and to be aware of blaming the epidural prior to considering the normal postsurgical reasons.

The effect of the local anaesthetic agent on the temperature fibres is used in assessment of the level of block, because the temperature fibres are blocked shortly before the pain nerve fibres (Bruce 1992). Therefore the assumption is that patients who cannot sense cold in a particular area will also be unable to sense pain. This assumption is supported by assessment of the patient's pain score.

Measuring the height of block is done by assessing the patient's ability to sense cold on a particular dermatome (Fig. 24.10). This should be assessed on both sides of the patient as the incomplete septum in the epidural space can cause all the infusate to collect on one side of the body causing a unilateral block.

Nursing patients with epidurals

Assessment of level of block

It is important that the practitioner assesses the level of the block at least once a shift to ensure that the block has not moved too high, fallen below the wound or disappeared completely. The level of block will need to be reassessed after delivery of a bolus dose, if the patient is in pain, on return from theatre and at any change in the patient's condition.

This is usually performed with ice or ethyl chloride, because these are perceived as cold (Dawson 1995). The ice or ethyl chloride is first used on the hand or shoulder, a part of the body not normally blocked, and patients asked if they can sense the cold. It is then run down both sides of the body while asking the patient if the sensation is still cold. The dermatomes that cannot sense the cold are deemed to be blocked. It is important to remind patients to report the feeling of cold, not of touch, because they may still feel touch in blocked dermatomes.

If the level of block is below the upper aspect of the wound, and the patient is in pain, the patient will require an increase in rate or a bolus dose. If a bolus dose is given it is important that the blood pressure and respiratory rate are taken and recorded frequently, e.g. every 5 minutes for 20 minutes, and that any significant decline in the patient's level of consciousness, significant hypotension or respiratory depression is reported immediately.

If the block is only on one side of the body (unilateral), the patient should be moved into the lateral position with the unblocked side lower. This is best done before the rate is increased or a bolus dose given, so that the extra fluid delivered will bathe the nerve fibres that innervate the lower and unblocked part of the body. If this is not effective, the catheter may be withdrawn 1–2 cm if it is considered to be positioned laterally in the epidural space (Raj 1996). If the pain and temperature fibres are only blocked on one side of the body, then so are the sympathetic fibres. The nurse may observe the blocked foot to be well perfused and the other to be cold and peripherally shut down. This is much less marked for catheters placed in the high thoracic region. These are used for high abdominal or thoracic surgery, for example after thoracotomies, gastrectomies or roof top incisions for liver surgery.

However, not all centres require nursing staff to measure the height of block; the level can be assessed via an assessment of the patient's clinical picture.

Pressure areas

It is important that nurses are very aware of the patient's pressure areas, as occasionally epidurals can induce numbness and immobility of legs. Buttocks and heels are pressure areas that are at particular risk. Patients should be encouraged to mobilise with assistance when they can straight leg raise (see also Ch.20).

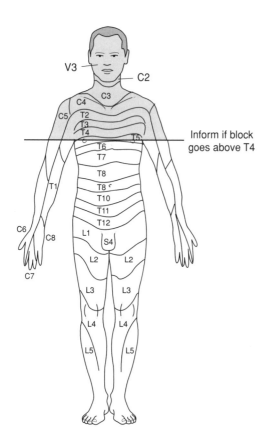

Figure 24.10 Dermatome chart demonstrating levels of block (reproduced by kind permission of UCL Hospitals NHS Trust).

Inform if block goes above T4

Nursing care in relation to complications of epidural analgesia

Opioid complications

Opioids present the same side-effect profile when given epidurally as any other route, though the intensity is reduced, reflecting the smaller dose.

Respiratory depression. A patient can experience either early or late respiratory depression. Early respiratory depression is caused by absorption of opioid into the epidural veins, which is then taken to the respiratory centre in the brain via the peripheral route. This will present within 40 minutes of the initial administration of the opioid. Late respiratory depression, caused by rostral spread of the opioid in the CSF to the respiratory centre in the brain, can present up to 12–24 hours after the administration of the opioid (Park & Fulton 1992).

It is the late form of respiratory depression that is potentially most dangerous and for this reason a patient's respiratory function should be observed closely, particularly on the first postoperative night or on the first night following insertion of the epidural catheter.

Because of the risk of respiratory depression, great care should be taken when opioids are given via any other route whilst an opioid is being administered epidurally. In some centres weak opioids such as codeine and dextropropoxyphene (co-proxamol) are routinely given to bridge the transition between epidural and oral analgesia.

Should the patient develop respiratory depression, it is the nurse's responsibility to assess the severity of the depression and instigate the appropriate treatment. Therefore the assessment of respiratory function should be performed with care. When assessing respiratory function the nurse should consider this in relation to the sedation score, the depth of respiration and the condition of the patient's airway.

A sedation score is an essential assessment tool for all patients receiving systemic or epidural opioids. It is usually a very simple scale that indicates whether the patient is awake and oriented, asleep but rousable or unrousable. Through continuous assessment the tool will show if a patient is becoming increasingly unrousable. Individual centres will have emergency procedures to follow if a patient becomes unrousable.

The procedures that the nurse would implement for a patient with respiratory depression would range from increasing the oxygen delivered via a face mask and encouraging deep breathing, to sitting the patient up to remove visceral pressure from the lung bases to allow full expansion. For a patient with a more serious

> **Reflective point**
>
> Consider, for example, two patients asleep with a respiratory rate of eight. One is rousable when called by name; the other is hard to rouse even when stimulated, respirations are shallow and the patient is snoring, which can indicate a partially obstructed airway. This example shows that simply counting the respiratory rate is not sufficient.

respiratory depression, the nurse may need to facilitate the administration of naloxone and, where necessary, respiratory support.

All nurses looking after patients receiving opioid analgesia should be familiar with naloxone, where to get it on the ward and the correct prescription dosages and administration procedures. (see p. 482).

The reversal that a patient experiences after receiving naloxone can be very profound. The patient is moved from being sedated, with well-controlled pain to being wide awake and in a lot of pain. This presents a nursing management problem as the patient's pain cannot now be managed by using additional opioid drug, only with NSAIDs or paracetamol. The reason for this is that naloxone has a half-life of 60–90 minutes, which means that the reversal effect will decline and the patient will develop a further respiratory depression The nursing implications are that this patient will need to be observed closely until all the opioid has been excreted, usually up to 4 hours but this will be extended in patients who are not excreting the drug effectively, e.g. those with renal failure. The patient will also have an elevated blood pressure owing to the effects of the drug and the effect of the pain.

To prevent this cycle occurring, the naloxone should be administered in small increments, enough to reverse the respiratory depression, but not enough to reverse the analgesia. The usual dose is 50–100 mcg. This is achieved by diluting the ampoule in 3 ml of sodium chloride 0.9%. This titration against the patient's respiratory function is a skill and, depending on hospital policy and the patient's condition, should be undertaken by suitable qualified staff, e.g. the pain service or the anaesthetists.

The potential for severe hypoxia (oxygen saturations of below 85%) may present following all types of major surgery. It is more predominant at night, within the first 48 hours, after opioid analgesia and can occur up to the fifth postoperative night (Reeder et al 1992). As this risk is increased for patients receiving opioid analgesia, it would be usual to find provision for a form of supplementary oxygen therapy within the policies of individual centres.

Pruritus. Pruritus is usually located around the head and neck, though can appear everywhere. It occurs in around 25–80% of patients (Ready et al 1991). It is associated with the ascent of opioid in the CSF into the 3rd and 4th ventricles. It can be reversed with a very small dose, 100 mcg, of naloxone (Dawson 1995) or the symptoms can be reduced with chlorpheniramine or calamine lotion.

Nausea and vomiting. The incidence of nausea for patients receiving epidural analgesia is 28–60% (Ready et al 1991). As it is the opioid that is considered to be the cause of postoperative nausea and vomiting (PONV), epidural analgesia without opioid is the method of choice for patients who have severe PONV after anaesthesia.

It is recommended that a simple nausea scale (see p. 482) is used on all patients receiving epidural opioids, and an anti-emetic offered at the first sign of nausea.

Local anaesthetic complications

Hypotension. Hypotension caused by sympathetic blockade as discussed above is treated by increasing the fluid volume with a crystalloid or colloid (Murphy 1981). In the case of a hypotension that is unresponsive to fluid and incompatible with life, an α-agonist should be available in the clinical area to produce vasoconstriction. The first choice is ephedrine as it is more pleasant for the patient than adrenaline. This is diluted to 3 mg in 1 ml with sodium chloride 0.9% and given by slow intravenous injection in doses of 3–6 mg and repeated every 3–4 minutes as required. The maximum total dose is 30 mg but doses of 9 mg are usually adequate (Reynolds 1996). Nurses should be aware of where this drug is kept in the ward. If hypotension occurs in a postoperative patient with an epidural, it is important to assess the patient holistically, and consider all possible causes of the loss of volume rather than presuming it is due to the epidural.

Respiratory depression due to ascending level of block. Respiratory depression can be caused by the blocking of the nerves that supply the respiratory muscles, the diaphragm, and the intercostal muscles. If the level of block rises higher than T4, which is nipple line, the infusion should be reviewed. There is a risk of bradycardia, respiratory depression and unconsciousness if the level of local block rises significantly above T4 (Park & Fulton 1992). For this reason patients with epidurals are never nursed head down.

Local anaesthetic toxicity. Local anaesthetic toxicity will initially present with a complaint of a circumoral tingling, a numbness of the mouth and tongue and a general light-headedness. Tinnitus and visual disturbances are other symptoms that patients may experience and will alert the nurse to local anaesthetic toxicity. The epidural should be stopped, the patient closely observed and the symptoms treated (Park & Fulton 1992).

Urinary retention. Urinary retention can develop because of the action of the local anaesthetic or opioid blocking the nerve fibres that innervate the bladder, which reduces sensory perception. It is the policy in some centres for all patients receiving epidural analgesia to be catheterised.

Catheter migration. Migration of the epidural catheter into the intrathecal space through the dura and the arachnoid mater will result in the local anaesthetic solution being infused into the CSF. Clinical manifestations may include hypotension, a change in the respiratory pattern, depression of level of consciousness and an increase in density of the block. Should this occur, the infusion will be stopped and the catheter removed.

Spinal headache. A spinal headache occurs when there is a leak of CSF through a hole in the dura, caused by accidental dural puncture during epidural insertion; this occurs in fewer than 0.5% of cases (Russell & Reynolds 1995). Though the hole is made during insertion, headaches often present after catheter removal.

The pain appears to be due to a complicated mechanism that is related to the drop in pressure in the CSF around the brain, which causes cerebral vasospasm. These headaches are characteristically frontal and occipital with associated photophobia and the pain is usually tolerable when lying flat but worsens on sitting up. A spinal headache is extremely distressing to patients and they will need a lot of reassurance and support. However, not all dural punctures cause a spinal headache.

The treatment is rehydration, up to 5 litres of clear fluid in 24 hours. Simple analgesia such as nonsteroidal anti-inflammatory drugs (NSAIDs) and paracetamol should be given, as it is important that the patient does not become constipated, because straining at stool will increase the pain. Patients will dictate what they find most comfortable; this is usually to lie flat in the dark.

The hole will resolve spontaneously; however, this may take up to 7 weeks and for this reason an autologous blood patch can be performed. This is a procedure in which 20 ml of the patient's own venous blood is inserted into the epidural space at the same level as the initial insertion site, forming a haematoma over the hole in the dura.

Spinal cord compression. This is a relatively rare occurrence and is caused by an epidural or spinal haematoma or abscess. The cord compression is caused when the collection of fluid in the spinal canal increases in size and presses on the spinal cord. The result of an untreated cord compression is paralysis. This is a clinical emergency and prognosis is improved if the cord is decompressed within 8 hours of presentation (Vandermeulen et al 1994).

An epidural haematoma is caused by bleeding into the epidural space. This can occur spontaneously but the incidence is increased if the patient has deranged clotting. The incidence of occurrence is thought to be less than 1:150 000 (Vandermeulen et al 1994).

As cord compression can develop after catheter removal as well as on insertion, it is essential that the nurse observes for signs of neurological deficit that outlasts the normal duration of the local anaesthetic. This may present as tingling and numbness in legs and motor weakness. The patient may also complain of a sharp pain in the region of the insertion site, that is radicular in nature. The diagnosis will be confirmed with computerised tomography (CT) or a magnetic resonance imaging (MRI) scan. This nursing observation is important as the prognosis is improved if the spinal cord is decompressed within 8 hours of onset of paralysis. It is important to note that these patients may be about to be discharged or be already at home. They may not be under the care of an anaesthetist or acute pain team and may not mention that they have had an epidural or spinal anaesthetic.

To reduce the incidence of epidural haematoma, the catheter is never removed from a patient with clotting abnormalities, who is heparinised or receiving warfarin. For patients receiving prophylactic heparin, the catheter can be removed 4 hours after administration of unfractionated heparin and 10 hours after low-molecular-weight heparin, and the next dose should be withheld for at least 2 hours after removal (Vandermeulen et al 1994).

An epidural abscess is caused by infection in the epidural space. There are two common routes of access for infection to enter the epidural space; one is down the centre of the catheter and the second is around the outside.

To reduce the incidence of epidural abscess, the integrity of the catheter in relation to the bacterial filter should be maintained at all times. If there is a disconnection between the filter and the catheter, the continuation of the infusion should be carefully considered, and the reconnection of the filter to the catheter performed by a suitably trained person as per hospital policy (Brooks et al 1996).

The entry site of the catheter should be observed at least once a shift for redness, pus and catheter placement. The use of a transparent dressing will facilitate observation (Brooks et al 1996). The patient should also be observed for pyrexia as this may indicate epidural infection.

Catheter removal

The catheter should be removed using aseptic technique. The patient should be in the lateral position as this reduces shearing forces that could cause the catheter to snap (Boey & Carrie 1994).

Remove the dressing and pull the catheter out slowly; if at any time during removal of the catheter the patient feels pain, the nurse should stop immediately and call the anaesthetist. After removal, the catheter must be inspected for completeness to ensure that a sheared segment has not been left in the space, and the wound covered with a small Airstrip dressing. If there is any suspicion of infection, the catheter tip can be sent for analysis.

Choice of analgesia system

This is a decision that should be made by the patient in conjunction with the anaesthetist and the ward staff. The patient should be given verbal and written information regarding the different types of analgesia systems that are suitable for that particular patient, operation and ward environment. The anaesthetist will consider the patient's medical suitably and the ward nurse will consider the skill mix and knowledge base of the staff who will be caring for the patient postoperatively. Surgical nurses will find that this becomes incorporated into their role for delivering preoperative information. It is important that practitioners do not influence patients with their personal preferences and remember that, as with all preoperative information, the patients' capacity for retention is reduced; therefore repetition and written back-up may be helpful.

REGIONAL ANAESTHESIA AND ANALGESIA

An epidural is a method of putting local anaesthetic onto nerves as they exit the spinal cord. There are several ways of blocking nerve fibres that are used by anaesthetists pre- and postoperatively to control pain. The different names of the techniques usually relate to the area of the body being blocked or the route of administration of the local anaesthetic. For example, digital nerve blocks and penile blocks will render the wound pain-free for up to 8 hours, depending on the type of local anaesthetic that has been administered. Another commonly used block is a caudal block which is an injection of local anaesthetic into the epidural space after the spinal cord has ended. It is used for analgesia after vulval and anal surgery, and is widely used in children for analgesia after circumcision, orchidopexy and herniotomy. Femoral nerve blocks are mainly indicated for analgesia following surgery to the knee and thigh. Intercostal nerve blocks can provide analgesia after thoracic or abdominal surgery.

It is common practice now for a wound to be infiltrated with local anaesthetic at the end of the surgical procedure. It is this local anaesthetic combined with an opioid and an NSAID that provides a multimodal approach to pain management (see p. 489).

The surgical nurse should be familiar with these procedures and check the anaesthetic chart immediately postoperatively to see if the patient has received a local anaesthetic block, as this may render the patient pain-free for up to 8 hours. It is advisable that the nurse observe these patients as their need for analgesia will increase as the local anaesthetic block wears off; the block may also inhibit the patient's ability to urinate.

CONCLUSION

The aim of this chapter has been to provide insight into the large subject of pain management, provide practical information and knowledge to enable surgical nurses to care effectively, and promote awareness of the factors that limit effective pain management. These are lack of knowledge regarding the pharmacology of analgesics and misconceptions about how to assess pain (McCaffery & Beebe 1994).

The most important messages from this chapter are not how to prevent respiratory depression and addiction, but to listen to and above all believe your patients. Patients have the right to make choices, to choose their method of pain relief, to decide on the intensity of their pain and the amount of pain they wish to tolerate. Pain management is a legitimate therapeutic goal and, as such, should be uppermost in our list of priorities (McCaffery & Beebe 1994). To ensure that these principles are incorporated within a holistic perspective, alternative non-pharmacological interventions to pain management need to be considered as well as the many other non-physiological factors that influence pain perception (Chs 9 and 10).

REFERENCES

Agency for Health Care Policy and Research: Acute Pain Management Panel 1992 Acute pain management: operative or medical procedures and trauma. Clinical practice guideline. US Department of Health and Human Services, Washington

Albert J M, Talbott T M 1988 Patient controlled analgesia vs conventional intramuscular analgesia following colon surgery. Diseases of the Colon and Rectum 31: 83–86

Amadio P 1984 Peripherally acting analgesics. American Journal of Medicine 77(3A): 17–26

Andersen R, Krohg K 1976 Pain as a major cause of postoperative nausea. Canadian Anaesthetists Society Journal 23: 366–369

Anon 1979 Nefopam – a new analgesic. Drug and Therapeutics Bulletin 17: 59–60

Anon 1993 Managing postoperative pain. Drug and Therapeutics Bulletin 31(3): 11–12

Arfeen Z, Owen H 1995 Patient-controlled analgesia. Current Anaesthesia and Critical Care 6: 76–80

Association of the British Pharmaceutical Industry (ABPI) 1998 Compendium of data sheet and summaries of product characteristics, 1998–1999. Datapharm Publications, London

Austin K L, Stapleton J V, Mather L E 1980 Multiple intramuscular injections: a major source of variability in analgesic response to meperidine. Pain 8(1): 47–62

Ayres J G, Fleming D M, Whittington R M 1987 Asthma death due to ibuprofen. Lancet i: 1082

Baer G A, Rorarius M G F, Kolehmainen S, Selin S 1992 The effect of paracetamol or diclofenac administered before operation on postoperative pain and behaviour in small children. Anaesthesia 47: 1078–1080

Ballantyne J C, Carr D B, Chalmers T C, Dear K B, Angelillo I F, Mosteller F 1993 Postoperative patient-controlled analgesia: meta-analyses of initial randomised control trials. Journal of Clinical Anaesthesia 5: 182–193

Barung S K, Treschow M, Borgbjjerg FM 1997 Respiratory depression following oral tramadol in a patient with impaired renal function. Pain 71: 111–112

Berde C B Lehn B M Yee J D Sethna N F Russo D 1991 Patient controlled analgesia in children and adolescents: a randomized prospective comparison with intramuscular administration of morphine for postoperative analgesia. Journal of Paediatrics 118: 460–466

Boey S, Carrie L 1994 Withdrawal forces during removal of lumbar extradural catheters. British Journal of Anaesthesia 73: 833–835

Bonica J 1990 History of pain concepts and therapies. In: Bonica J (ed) The management of pain, 2nd edn. Lea and Febiger, Kent, vol 1, pp 2–15

Bosso J V, Creighton D, Stevenson D D 1992 Flurbiprofen (Ansaid) cross-sensitivity in an aspirin-sensitive asthmatic patient. Chest 101: 856–858

Boulanger A, Choiniere M, Roy D 1993 Comparison between patient-controlled analgesia and intra-muscular meperidine after thoracotomy. Canadian Journal of Anaesthesia 40: 409–415

Breivik H 1995 Benefits, risks and economics of post operative pain managements programs. In: Breivik H (ed) Clinical anaesthesiology: post operative pain management. Baillière Tindall, London, vol 9(3)

British National Formulary (BNF) 1998 British Medical Association and Royal Pharmaceutical Society of Great Britain, London

Bromage P 1978 Epidural analgesia. W B Saunders, Philadelphia

Bromley L 1993 Improving the management of acute pain. British Journal of Hospital Medicine. 50(10): 616–618

Brooks K, Pasero C, Hubbard L, Coghlan R 1996 The risk of infection associated with epidural analgesia. Today's Operating Room Nurse (Jan/Feb): 35–37

Bruce L 1992 Epidural analgesia. Pain relief. Surgical Nurse 5(4): 4, 6–8

Bugge J F 1995 Renal effects and complications of NSAIDs for routine post-operative pain relief: increased awareness of a real problem needed. In: Breivik H (ed) Clinical anaesthesiology: post operative pain management. Baillière Tindall, London, ch 5

Bullingham R E S, McQuay H J, Moore R A 1983 A review of the clinical pharmacokinetics of opioid agonist–antagonist drugs including buprenorphine. Clinical Pharmacokinetics 8: 332–343

Burns J W, Aitken H A, Bullingham R E S, McArdle C S, Kenny G N C 1991 Double-blind comparison of the morphine sparing effect of continuous and intermittent i.m. administration of ketorolac. British Journal of Anaesthesia 67: 235–238

Cambitzi J 1996 The role of the clinical nurse specialist in acute pain management. Nursing in Critical Care 1(4): 164–170

Carroll D, Bowsher D 1993 Pain management and nursing care. Butterworth Heinemann, London

Carson J L, Strom B L, Soper K A, West S L, Morse M L 1987 The association of nonsteroidal anti-inflammatory drugs with upper gastrointestinal tract bleeding. Archives of Internal Medicine 147: 85–88

Cashman J, McAnulty G 1995 Nonsteroidal antiinflammatory drugs in perisurgical pain treatment. Drugs 41: 533–547

Cherny N I 1996 Opioid analgesics. Comparative features and prescribing guidelines. Drugs 51(5): 713–737

Chisholm R J, Davis F M, Billings J D, Gibbs J M 1983 Narcotics and spasm of the sphincter of Oddi. A retrospective study of cholangiograms. Anaesthesia 38(7): 689–691

Chumbley G M, Hall G M, Salmon P 1998 Patient-controlled analgesia: an assessment by 200 patients. Anaesthesia 53: 216–221

Cohen F 1980 Post operative pain relief: patients' status and nurses' choices. Pain 9: 265–274

Collart L, Lutty C, Dayer P 1993 Partial inhibition of tramadol antinociceptive effect by naloxone in man. British Journal of Clinical Pharmacology 35: 73P

Collins F 1994 Pain – patient in control: an evaluation of PCA. British Journal of Theatre Nurses 3(11): 9–13

Commission on the Provision of Surgical Services 1990 Report of the working party. Pain after surgery. Royal College of Surgeons and the College of Anaesthetists, London

Committee on Safety of Medicines 1994 Current problems in pharmacovigilance 20: 9–11

Committee on Safety of Medicines 1996 Current problems in pharmacovigilance 22: 11

Concepcion M, Covino B G 1984 Rational use of local anaesthetics. Drugs 27: 256–270

Cousins M 1995 The annual Magill lecture and symposium. 29 November, Charing Cross Hospital (Abstract). Charing Cross and St Thomas's Hospital Pain Management Department, London

Crighton I M, Hobbs G H, Wrench I J 1997 Analgesia after day case laparoscopic sterilisation. A comparison of tramadol with paracetamol/dextropropoxyphene and paracetamol/codeine combinations. Anaesthesia 52: 649–652

Cronberg S, Wallmark E, Soderberg I 1984 Effect on platelet aggregation of oral administration of 10 non-steroidal analgesics to humans. Scandinavian Journal of Haematology 33: 155–159

Dawson 1995 Post operative epidural analgesia. Current Anaesthesia and Critical Care 6: 69–75

Day R O, Brooks P M 1987 Variations in response to non-steroidal anti-inflammatory drugs. British Journal of Clinical Pharmacology 23: 655–658

Dayer P, Collart L, Desmeuler J 1994 The pharmacology of tramadol. Drugs 47(suppl 1): 3–7

Delbos A, Boccard E 1995 The morphine-sparing effect of propacetamol in orthopaedic postoperative pain. Journal of Pain and Symptom Management 10(4): 279–286

Depre M, Van Hecken A, Verbesselt R, Tjandra-Maga T B, Gerim M, de Schepper P J 1992 Tolerance and pharmacokinetics of propacetamol, a paracetamol formulation for intravenous use. Fundamentals of Clinical Pharmacology 6: 259–262

Dollery C (ed) 1991 Therapeutic drugs. Churchill Livingstone, Edinburgh

Donovan B 1983 Patients' attitudes to post operative pain relief. Anaesthesia and Intensive Care 11: 125–129

Donovan M 1992 A practical approach to pain assessment. In: Watt-Watson J, Donovan M (eds) Pain management. Nursing perspective. Mosby, St Louis

Donovan M, Dillon P, McGuire L 1987 Incidence and characteristics of pain in a sample of medical-surgical inpatients. Pain 30: 69–78

Ferrante F, Ostheimer G, Covino B 1990 Patient controlled analgesia. Blackwell, Cambridge

Fischer H B J 1995 Acute pain relief – the role of regional analgesia. Current Anaesthesia and Critical Care 6: 87–91

Flacke J W, Van Etten A, Flacke W E 1983 Greatest histamine release from meperidine among four narcotics. Double blind study in man. Anesthesiology 59: A51

Fleming B 1992 A survey of complications documented in a quality-control analysis of patient-controlled analgesia in the postoperative patient. Journal of Pain and Symptom Management 7(8): 463–469

Gasser J C, Bellville J W 1975 Respiratory effects of nefopam. Clinical Pharmacology and Therapeutics 18: 175–179

Gillies G W A, Kenny G N C, Bullingham R E S, McArdle C S 1987 The morphine sparing effect of ketorolac tromethamine. Anaesthesia 42: 727–731

Gould T H, Crosby D L, Harmer M et al 1992 Policy for controlling pain after surgery: effect of sequential changes in management. British Medical Journal 305: 1187–1193

Graves D A, Foster T S, Batenhorst R L, Bennett R L, Bauman T J 1983 Patient controlled analgesia. Annals of Internal Medicine 99: 360–366

Hagmeyer K O, Mauro L S, Mauro V F 1993 Meperidine-related seizures associated with patient-controlled analgesia pumps. Annals of Pharmacotherapy 27: 29–32

Haigh S 1996 12 years on: co-proxamol revisited. Lancet 347: 1840–1841

Hand C W, Sear J W, Uppington J, Ball M J, McQuay H J, Moore R A 1990 Buprenorphine disposition in patients with renal impairment: single and continuous dosing, with special reference to metabolites. British Journal of Anaesthesia 64: 276–286

Hanks G W, Forbes K 1998 Co-proxamol is effective in chronic pain. British Medical Journal 316: 1980

Harris K 1992 The role of prostaglandins in the control of renal function. British Journal of Anaesthesia 69: 233–235

Heel R C, Brogden R N, Pakes G E, Speight T M, Avery G S 1980 Nefopam: a review of its pharmacological properties and therapeutic efficacy. Drugs 19: 249–267

Henry D, Lim L I, Rodriguez L A G et al 1996 Variability in risk of gastrointestinal complications with individual non-steroidal anti-inflammatory drugs: results of a collaborative meta-analysis. British Medical Journal 312: 1563–1566

Hodsman N B A, Burns J, Kenny G N C, McArdle C S, Rotman H 1987 The morphine sparing effect of diclofenac sodium following abdominal surgery. Anaesthesia 42: 1005–1008

Houmes R J, Voets M A, Verkaaik A, Erdmann W, Lachmann B 1992 Efficacy and safety of tramadol versus morphine for moderate and severe postoperative pain with special regard to respiratory depression. Anesthesia and Analgesia 74: 510–514

International Association for the Study of Pain (IASP) 1992 Management of acute pain: a practical guide. IASP Publications, Seattle

Jeans M, Melzack R 1992 Conceptual basis of nursing practice: theoretical foundations of pain. In: Watt-Watson J, Donovan M (eds) Pain management. Nursing perspective. Mosby, St Louis, ch 2, pp 11–35

Justins D 1995 The annual Magill lecture and symposium. 29 November, Charing Cross Hospital (Abstract). Charing Cross and St Thomas's Hospital Pain Management Department, London

Kehlet H 1994 Post operative pain relief. Regional Anaesthesia (19): 369–377

Kehlet H, Mather L E (eds) 1992 The value of NSAIDs in the management of postoperative pain. Drugs 44(suppl 5): 1–63

Koh P, Thomas V 1994 Patient controlled analgesia (PCA): does time saved by PCA improve patient satisfaction with nursing care? Journal of Advanced Nursing 20: 61–70

Koo P J S 1995 Pain. In: Young L Y, Koda-Kimble M A (eds) Applied therapeutics – the clinical use of drugs, 6th edn. Applied Therapeutics, Vancouver, ch 7

Kuhn S, Cooke K, Collins M, Jones J M, Mucklow J C 1990 Perceptions of pain relief after surgery. British Medical Journal 300: 1687–1690

Li Wan Po A, Zhang W Y 1997 Systematic overview of co-proxamol to assess analgesic effects of addition of dextropropoxyphene to paracetamol. British Medical Journal 315: 1565–1571

McCaffery M 1972 Nursing management of the patient in pain. Lippincott, Philadelphia

McCaffery M, Beebe 1994 Pain: clinical manual for nursing practice. UK edition, Latham J (ed). Mosby, London

McCormack K, Brune K 1991 Dissociation between the antinociceptive and anti-inflammatory effects of non-steroidal anti-inflammatory drugs. Drugs 41: 533–547

McEvoy G K (ed) 1998 Drug information. American Hospital Formulary Service (AHFS), American Society of Health-System Pharmacists, Bethesda

McQuay H, Moore A 1998 An evidence-based resource for pain relief. Oxford University Press, Oxford

McQuay H J, Carroll D, Glynn C J 1993 Dose-response for analgesic effect of amitriptyline in chronic pain. Anaesthesia 48: 281–285

McQuay H, Carroll D, Jadad A R, Wiffen P, Moore A 1995 Anticonvulsant drugs for the management of pain: a systematic review. British Medical Journal 311: 1047–1052

McQuay H, Moore A, Justins D 1997 Treating acute pain in hospital. British Medical Journal 314: 1531–1535

Madej T, Reader M 1995 Monitoring in postoperative pain management. Current Anaesthesia and Critical Care 6: 92–97

Mather C, Ready B 1994 Management of acute pain. British Journal of Hospital Medicine 51(3): 85–88

Max M B, Lynch S A, Muir J, Shoaf S F, Smoller B, Dubner R 1992 Effects of desimipramine, amitriptyline and fluoxetine on pain in diabetic neuropathy. New England Journal of Medicine 326: 1250–1256

Melzack R, Katz J 1994 Pain measurement in persons in pain. In: Wall P, Melzack R (eds) Textbook of pain, 3rd edn. Churchill Livingstone, London, pp 339–347

Merskey H, Albe-Fessard D J, Bonica J J 1979 Pain terms: a list with definitions and notes on usage. Pain 6: 249–252

Michaloliakou C, Chung F C, Sharma S 1996 Preoperative multimodal analgesia facilitates recovery after ambulatory laparoscopic cholecystectomy. Anaesthesia and Analgesia 82: 44–51

Milligan K 1997 Prescribing antidepressants in general practice. British Medical Journal 314: 827–828

Moore R A, Hand C W, McQuay H J 1987 Opiate metabolism and excretion. Baillière's Clinical Anaesthesiology 1: 829–858

Moore A, McQuay H 1997 Single-patient data meta-analysis of 3453 postoperative patients: oral tramadol versus placebo, codeine and combination analgesics. Pain 69: 287–294

Moore A, Collins S, Carroll D, McQuay H 1997 Paracetamol with and without codeine in acute pain: a quantitative systematic review. Pain 70: 193–201

Moore A, McQuay H, Gavaghan D 1996 Deriving dichotomous outcome measures from continuous data in randomised controlled trials of analgesics. Pain 66: 229–237

Morrison N A, Repka N X 1994 Ketorolac versus acetaminophen or ibuprofen in controlling post-operative pain in patients with strabismus. Ophthalmology 101: 915–918

Murphy T 1981 Spinal, epidural and caudal anaesthesia. In: Miller R (ed) Anaesthesia, 2nd edn. Churchill Livingstone, Edinburgh, p 1081

Nagle C J, McQuay H J 1990 Opiate receptors; their role in effect and side-effect. Current Anaesthesia and Critical Care 1: 247–252

Orme M 1990 Profile of non-steroidal anti-inflammatory drugs. Prescribers Journal 30(3): 95–100

Owen H, Glavin R J, Shaw D F 1986 Ibuprofen in the management of postoperative pain. British Journal of Anaesthesia 58: 1371–1375

Park G, Fulton B 1992 The management of acute pain. Oxford Medical, Oxford

Pediani R 1998 Organising acute pain management. In: Carter B (ed) Perspectives on pain: mapping the territory. Edward Arnold, London, ch 12

Peduto V A and the Italian Collaborative Group on Propacetamol, Ballabio M, Stefanini S 1998 Efficacy of propacetamol in the treatment of postoperative pain. Acta Anaesthesiologica Scandinavica 42: 293–298

Perrier D, Gibaldi M 1972 Influence of the first pass effect on the systemic availability of propoxyphene. Journal of Clinical Pharmacology 12: 449–452

Porter J, Jick H 1980 Addiction rate in patients treated with narcotics. New England Journal of Medicine 302: 123

Power I 1993 Aspirin-induced asthma. British Journal of Anaesthesia 71: 619–621

Pryle B J, Grech H, Stoddart P A, Carson R, O'Mahoney T, Reynolds F 1992 Toxicity of norpethidine in sickle cell crisis. British Medical Journal 304: 1478–1479

Raffa R B, Frederichs E, Reimann W 1992 Opioid and nonopioid components independently contribute to the mechanism of action of tramadol, an 'atypical' opioid analgesic. Journal of Pharmacology and Experimental Therapeutics 260: 275–285

Raj P 1996 Epidural infusion and patient controlled epidural analgesia. In: Raj P (ed) Pain medicine. a comprehensive review. Mosby, St Louis

Rang H P, Dale M M 1991 Pharmacology, 2nd edn. Churchill Livingstone, Edinburgh

Rauck R L, Ruoff G E, McMillen J I 1994 Comparison of tramadol and acetaminophen with codeine for long-term management in elderly patients. Current Therapeutic Research 55(12): 1417–1431

Rawal N, Berggren L 1994 Organisation of acute pain services: a low cost model. Pain 57: 117–123

Ready L, Loper K, Nessly M, Wild L 1991 Postoperative epidural morphine is safe on surgical wards. Anaesthesiology 75: 452–456

Reeder M, Goldman M, Loh L et al 1992 Post operative hypoxaemia after major abdominal vascular surgery. British Journal of Anaesthesia 68: 23–26

Reynolds J E F (ed) 1996 Martindale. The extra pharmacopoeia. Royal Pharmaceutical Society, London

Royal College of Anaesthetists (RCA) 1998 The guidelines for the use of non-steroidal anti-inflammatory drugs in the perioperative period. RCA, Oxford

Russell R, Reynolds F 1995 Long term effects of epidural analgesia. In: Bogod D (ed) Baillière's Clinical Anaesthesiology. Baillière Tindall, London, vol 9(4), pp 607–622

Schulze S, Roikjaer O, Hasselstrom L, Jensen N H, Kehlet H 1988 Epidural bupivacaine and morphine plus systemic indomethacin eliminates pain but not systemic response and convalescence after cholecystectomy. Surgery 103: 321–327

Sedor J R, Davidson E W, Dunn M J 1986 Effects of non-steroidal anti-inflammatory drugs in healthy subjects. American Journal of Medicine 81: 58–70

Seef L B, Cuccherini B A, Zimmerman H J, Alder E, Benjamin S B 1986 Acetaminophen hepatoxicity in alcoholics. A therapeutic misadventure. Annals of Internal Medicine 104: 399–404

Seers K 1987 Perceptions of pain. Nursing Times 83: 37–38

Seers K 1989 Patients' perceptions of acute pain. In: Wilson-Barnett J, Robinson S (eds) Directions in nursing research. Scutari Press, London, pp 107–116

Stubhaug A, Grimstad J, Breivik H 1995 Lack of analgesic effect of 50 mg and 100 mg oral tramadol after orthopaedic surgery; a randomized, double-blind, placebo and standard active drug comparison. Pain 62: 111–118

Sykes J V, Hanks G W, Forbes K 1996 Coproxamol revisited. Lancet 348: 408

Szeto H H, Inturrisi C E, Houde R, Saal S, Cheigh J, Reidenberg M 1977 Accumulation of norpethidine, an active metabolite of pethidine, in patients with renal failure or cancer. Annals of Internal Medicine 86: 738–741

Thomas V, Heath M, Rose D, Flory P 1995 Psychological characteristics and the effectiveness of patient-controlled analgesia. British Journal of Anaesthesia 74: 271–276

Tramer M R, Williams J E, Carroll D, Wiffen P J, Moore R A, McQuay H J 1998 Comparing analgesic efficacy of non-steroidal anti-inflammatory drugs given by different routes in acute and chronic pain: a qualitative systematic review. Acta Anaesthesiologica Scandinavica 42: 71–79

United Kingdom Central Council for Nursing, Midwifery and Health Visiting (UKCC) 1992 Standards for the administration of medicines. UKCC, London

Vandermuelen E, Aken H, Vermylen J 1994 Anticoagulant and spinal-epidural anaesthesia. Anaesthesia and Analgesia 79: 1165–1177

Vane J R 1976 The mode of action of aspirin and similar compounds. Journal of Allergy and Clinical Immunology 58: 691–712

Wakeling H G, Barry P C, Butler P J 1996 Postoperative analgesia in dental day case surgery. A comparison between Feldene 'Melt' (piroxicam) and diclofenac suppositories. Anaesthesia 51: 784–786

Wasylak T 1992 Surgical pain management. In: Watt-Watson J, Donovan M (eds) Pain management. Nursing perspective. Mosby, St Louis, ch 15, pp 401–425

Watt-Wattson J 1992 Misbeliefs about pain. In: Watt-Watson J, Donovan M (eds) Pain management. Nursing perspective. Mosby, St Louis, ch 3, pp 36–58

Welchew E 1995 Patient controlled analgesia. BMJ Publishing Group, London

Williams C 1996 Patient controlled analgesia: a review of the literature. Journal of Advanced Nursing 5: 139–147

Woodhouse A, Mather L E 1997 Nausea and vomiting in the postoperative patient-controlled analgesia environment. Anaesthesia 52: 770–775

FURTHER READING

Carroll D, Bowsher D 1993 Pain management and nursing care. Butterworth Heinemann, London

Forrest J 1998 Acute pain: pathophysiology and treatment. Manticore Publishers, Grimsby

Lange M, Dahn M, Jacobs L 1988 Patient-controlled analgesia versus intermittent analgesia dosing. Heart and Lung 17(5): 495–498

Owen H, Ilsley E 1993 PCA devices. Current Anaesthesia and Critical Care 4: 223–228

Welchew E 1995 Patient controlled analgesia, BMJ Publishing Group, London, pp 24–48

25

Maintaining an adequate circulation

Sharon L. Edwards

AIMS

The aims of the chapter are:

- to explain the importance of maintaining an adequate circulation in the surgical patient
- to identify the many factors that can reduce the circulating volume in a surgical patient
- to demonstrate the application of a cardiac assessment in a surgical patient
- to explore the various cardiac support options
- to explain the issues in relation to continued effective observation of cardiac status in the surgical patient.

INTRODUCTION

Blood flow is essential to human life and blood is circulated to all areas of the body by the pumping action of the heart. It then flows through the arteries, arterioles, capillaries, venules and veins. Surgical patients can have problems with their circulation prior to admission for surgery, mainly from conditions such as hypertension, heart failure, peripheral vascular disease, bleeding disorders or dehydration. These patients may be on medications to control their circulation and it is therefore necessary for the surgical nurse to understand the drugs these patients may bring with them to the ward and continue to take during their hospital stay. Following surgery, complications can occur which are generally related to loss of blood or plasma, or because of dehydration. It is important, therefore, that the surgical nurse is able to assess the patient's circulation. This can be done through interview, observation and measurements. The measurements that can be undertaken to assess circulation are central venous pressure, blood pressure, urine output, blood results, urine testing, pulses, heart rate, temperature, oxygen saturation, and mental state. These factors can indicate whether there is adequate perfusion of vital organs and the extremities.

There are circulation assessment guidelines available for nurses (Braddy 1989, McGovern & Kuhn 1992, Miracle 1988, Yacone-Morton 1991). However, these assessments have mainly been developed for the elderly or coronary care patient and have yet to demonstrate their use and effectiveness in reducing circulation problems in the surgical ward setting. The more effective use of the assessment tools, documentation and an understanding of the principles of circulation could go a long way in identifying patients at risk.

If bleeding has been detected through effective assessment, treatment needs to be instigated. In this instance, whole blood, colloid or crystalloid therapy may be prescribed (see Ch. 26). All three support options have their own advantages and disadvantages and what is needed is a generation of nurses who know and understand about the controversy, arguments and counter-arguments that surround these support systems when treating hypovolaemia. It is imperative that surgical nurses up-date their knowledge and their practical skills in assessing the circulation of their patients so that the correct support can be instigated promptly and efficiently.

Knowledge of the importance of the complications that can occur from these support options is essential, whether treating bleeding, bleeding disorders or dehydration. The complication of hypervolaemia or fluid overload can occur because of circulation problems prior to admission, treatment given following surgery or for hypovolaemia, or a sluggish arterial and venous circulation as a result of continued bed rest or immobility. The complication of overload to the circulatory system can cause patients undue distress, pain and an extended stay in hospital. It is necessary, therefore, that surgical nurses understand the causes and signs of circulatory overload, so that during treatment for an inadequate circulation its complications do not occur.

Nevertheless, the most important aspect of the nursing role in maintaining adequate circulation is assessment. The nurse's role in supporting the circulation in the surgical patient will be highlighted. It is imperative that the surgical nurse's role in maintaining adequate circulation is recognised to prevent complications from a reduced or overloaded circulation.

HISTORICAL PERSPECTIVE

The heart and its role has been questioned by many ancient societies. For example, the Egyptians attributed breathing to the heart, whereas the ancient Chinese connected the action of the heart to the pulse. The Greeks thought of the heart as the region in the body in which thinking originated. However, it was the great Hellenic physician, Claudius Galen, whose view of the heart was bowed to by medicine for nearly 1400 years. Galen noted that the sides of the heart did not contract simultaneously, as he thought a pump should. He declared that blood was the agency for air, spirits, heat, and nutriment. He outlined a heart of two ventricles separated by a porous septum (which he believed joined the arterial and venous circulatory systems) that distended in active motion, and believed that the heart was the organ of respiration and heat (Bloch 1992).

However, it was not until Harvey (1578–1657) accumulated irrefutable data on the structure and function of the heart that firm foundations were established to guide further development and understanding of the anatomy and physiology of the heart.

THE CIRCULATION

The function of the circulatory system is quite simple: to deliver oxygen, nutrients, and other substances to all of the body's cells and to remove the waste products of cellular metabolism (McCance & Huether 1994). Delivery and removal are achieved via the blood vessels which are connected to a pump, the heart. The heart pumps blood continuously through the blood vessels with cooperation from other systems: the nervous and endocrine systems, which regulate the heart and blood vessels; the digestive system, which supplies nutrients; the respiratory system, which supplies oxygen and removes the gaseous wastes of cellular metabolism; and the kidneys, which remove other wastes.

The heart passages open vertically and the heart comprises two side-by-side pumps, each serving a separate blood circuit. The blood vessels that carry unoxygenated blood to and from the lungs form the pulmonary circuit. The blood vessels that carry oxygenated blood to and from all body tissues constitute the systemic circuit. The circulation and the factors that control blood flow and other related mechanisms are relevant to the assessment of the surgical patient for inadequate circulation, which will be discussed later.

The pulmonary circulation

The right side of the heart is the pulmonary circuit pump (Marieb 1995). This circuit strictly serves a gas exchange function. Blood returning from the limbs, head, chest and abdomen finds its way from a number of collecting venules into the veins and flows into the right atrium of the heart. The blood it contains is oxygen poor and carbon dioxide rich. From the right atrium, blood passes into the right ventricle, which pumps it to the lungs via the pulmonary artery. A backflow of blood is prevented by the tricuspid valve (between the right atrium and ventricle) and the pulmonary valve (between the right ventricle and the pulmonary artery). Having passed through the pulmonary artery, the blood finally reaches a fine network of very thin-walled vessels called capillaries. Through these walls, the blood exchanges carbon dioxide, which is then breathed out of the body, for fresh oxygen which has been breathed into the lungs. The freshly oxygenated blood is carried by the pulmonary veins back to the left side of the heart.

The systemic circulation

The blood vessels that carry oxygenated blood to and from all body tissues constitute the systemic circuit. The left side of the heart is the systemic circuit pump. Freshly oxygenated blood leaving the lungs is collected into the pulmonary vein (there are no valves guarding this entrance) and returned to the left atrium and, at the next heart beat, the blood passes through the mitral valve and into the left ventricle. The walls of this chamber are of very thick powerful muscle, and when they contract in turn the contained blood is forced through the aortic valve into the main distributing artery, the aorta. From there, the blood is transported via smaller systemic arteries to the body tissues, where exchange of gases and nutrients occurs across the capillary walls. The blood, once again laden with carbon dioxide and depleted of oxygen, returns through the systemic veins to the right side of the heart, where it enters the right atrium again via the superior and inferior venae cavae (there are no valves guarding these entrances). This whole cycle repeats itself continuously with every heart beat.

Factors that affect the circulation

The factors that affect the circulation are generally related to those that influence blood flow. These, in turn, are the same properties that govern the movement of simple fluids in a closed, rigid system. Blood flow is governed primarily by two factors, pressure and resistance (McCance & Huether 1994).

Pressure

Blood flow depends partly on the difference between pressures in the arterial and venous vessels that supply the organ. Fluid moves from the arterial side of the

capillaries, a region of greater pressure, to the venous side, a region of lesser pressure. The pressure exerted by the blood in the closed circulatory system is controlled by the baroreceptors, renal autoregulation and compliance.

Baroreceptors. These are major stretch receptors located in the arch of the aorta and in the carotid sinus (Marieb 1995). Baroreceptors respond to stretching of the tunica media fibres of the arteries, caused by an increased circulation. The rate of firing of the baroreceptors increases and decreases with changes in the pressure exerted by the blood in the artery (blood pressure). An increase in arterial pressure increases the rate of firing of both the carotid sinus and the aortic arch baroreceptors. This supplies sensory information to the cardiovascular centre that regulates blood pressure (BP) in the medulla of the brain. The effect of this regulating reflex is to decrease sympathetic nervous system discharge which will slow heart rate, reduce myocardial contractility and lower peripheral resistance by vasodilatation of the blood vessels (McCance & Huether 1994); the overall effect will be to reduce blood pressure to normal.

Renal autoregulation. The kidneys play a complex role in restoring extracellular fluid volume and increasing systemic blood pressure. This system is stimulated principally when there is a decrease in blood pressure. This elaborate set of interlinked processes involves the renin–angiotensin–aldosterone system, osmoreceptors and baroreceptors (Fig. 25.1) and is explained in more detail in Chapter 26 (see also McCance & Huether 1994, Ch. 32).

Vascular compliance. Vascular compliance is the ability of a vessel to increase in volume to accommodate a given increase in pressure (Marieb 1995). Therefore, compliance determines a vessel's response to pressure changes. For example, a person with normal vascular compliance could be given a very large volume of fluid and only gain a small increase in blood pressure. In this way a large volume of blood can be accommodated by the venous system. Consequently, small variations in pressure cause little or no change in the volume of blood within the arterial vessels.

The opposite of compliance is stiffness. Several conditions and disorders can cause stiffness. The most common is arteriosclerosis (Baxendale 1992). Arteriosclerosis increases the rigidity or stiffness of arterial walls, which in turn increases peak arterial pressure at a given volume of blood (Baxendale 1992). Thus, the volume of fluid in the circulation is exerting a greater pressure on the vessels, which in a patient who has a less compliant arterial system, or stiffness, will result in a much higher pressure with just a small increase in volume of fluid.

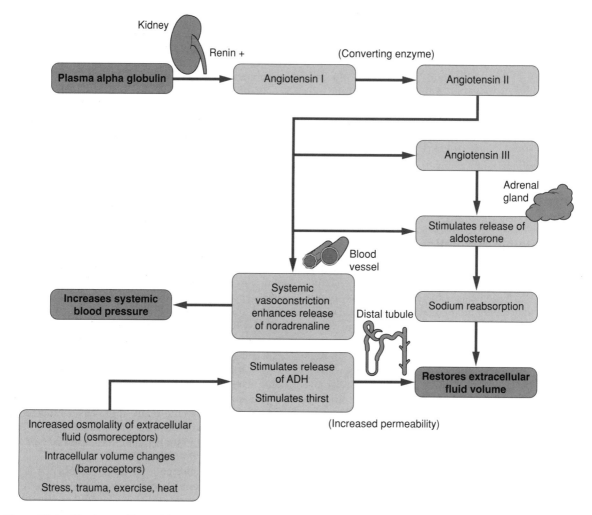

Figure 25.1 Circulatory effects of the renin–angiotensin system (reproduced from McCance K L, Huether S E 1994 Pathophysiology: the biologic basis for disease in adults and children, 2nd edn, by kind permission of Mosby Year Book, Inc., St Louis).

Resistance

Resistance is the opposition to a force (McCance & Huether 1994). In the circulatory system, most opposition to blood flow is provided by the diameter (vasodilatation reduces resistance and vasoconstriction increases it) and length of the blood vessels. Therefore, most of the changes in blood flow through an organ are due to changes in the vascular resistance within the organ. The major mechanisms causing changes in vascular resistance are blood viscosity, chemoreceptors, blood velocity, and laminar flow.

Blood viscosity. The viscosity of blood is determined by its consistency and generally depends on its

red cell content (McCance & Huether 1994). The greater the percentage of red cells in the blood, the more viscous the blood will be. This relationship is expressed as the haematocrit, the ratio of the volume of red blood cells to the volume of whole blood. Blood flow varies according to the viscosity of the fluid; thick fluids move more slowly and cause a greater resistance to flow than thin fluids.

The viscosity of blood also increases if blood flow becomes very slow or stagnates (known as anomalous viscosity). This can be observed in a number of conditions such as low cardiac output states, e.g. cardiac failure, myocardial infarction, coronary artery disease, ischaemic heart disease, cardiac valve insufficiencies; cardiogenic shock; arteriosclerosis of the peripheral arteries; or in patients with varicose veins and deep vein thrombosis, as all these affect the venous flow back to the heart, causing it to become very slow or stagnated.

Arterial chemoreceptors. There are further specialised areas within the aortic and carotid arteries which are sensitive to concentrations of oxygen, carbon dioxide, and hydrogen ions (pH) in the blood (McCance & Huether 1994). These receptors are called chemoreceptors and they transmit impulses to the centres of the brain which regulate blood pressure. A decrease in arterial oxygen concentration or pH causes vasoconstriction and, thus, a reflexive increase in blood pressure (Masasi & Keyes 1994), whereas an increase in carbon dioxide causes vasodilatation and a decrease in blood pressure. These blood pressure changes are carried out by smooth muscle layers in the vessels. The major chemoreceptive reflex is due to alteration in arterial oxygen concentration (Masasi & Keyes 1994). The effects of altered pH or carbon dioxide levels are minor.

Surgical patients are susceptible to hypoxia due to ventilation during surgery, and may be further compromised by chest problems or smoking. If hypoxia occurs during or following surgery, then patients are at risk of having an increased BP postoperatively. If they have additional circulatory problems, such as a heart condition or varicose veins, their vascular resistance and thus BP can further increase.

Blood velocity. Blood velocity is the distance blood travels in a unit of time (McCance & Huether 1994). Blood velocity is directly related to blood flow and inversely related to the width of the vessel in which the blood is flowing.

The relationship between velocity and flow can be understood by reference to vasodilatation and vasoconstriction. The volume of fluid flowing through the circulation is the same whether the blood vessel is narrow or wide. Where the blood vessel narrows, the fluid contained within it flows more quickly; where it widens out the fluid flows more slowly. Yet, in each instance, the volume of fluid moving between the vessels does not change.

In the body, as blood moves from the aorta to the capillaries, the total width of the vessels decrease causing the velocity of flow to decrease. This allows gaseous exchange to take place between the cells and the capillaries.

Laminar versus turbulent flow. Flow through any tubular system is either laminar or turbulent. Normally, blood flow through the vessels is laminar. In laminar flow, concentric layers of molecules move 'straight ahead', and each concentric layer flows at a different velocity. The molecules of blood that are in contact with the wall of the blood vessel are prevented from moving. This allows the next thin layer of blood to slide slowly past the stationary layer; the next thin layer moves slightly faster, and so on, until, at the centre, the blood velocity and therefore movement is greatest.

If laminar flow becomes obstructed, such as in arteriosclerosis or atherosclerosis, deep vein thrombosis, varicose veins or embolism, or the vessel turns owing to an obstruction, the blood then flows over rough surfaces and the flow becomes turbulent. A turbulent flow consists of whirls or eddy currents and becomes noisy, which often causes a murmur to be heard on auscultation. The resistance increases with turbulence, causing an increase in blood pressure.

AN INADEQUATE CIRCULATION IN THE SURGICAL PATIENT

An inadequate circulation can occur prior to surgery as a result of other illness or disease, and it is up to the surgical nurse to determine any past history that may influence circulation postoperatively. In addition, during and following surgery there are other problems, most notably hypovolaemia, that may affect circulation.

Factors that can affect the circulation prior to surgery

These are many, but the most common are hypertension, heart failure, vascular disease, bleeding disorders, and dehydration.

Hypertension

Hypertension is consistent elevation of systemic arterial blood pressure (McCance & Huether 1994). The generally agreed values for the upper limits of a normal BP is 140 mmHg systolic pressure and 90 mmHg diastolic pressure. However, the World Health Organization accept 160 mmHg systolic pressure as the upper limit (WHO 1992, cited in Jordon 1992). Feher et al (1992) accepted definitions of hypertension as defined by the level of diastolic blood pressure; these were: mild 95–104 mmHg; moderate 105–115 mmHg; and severe 115 mmHg and above.

Hypertension can affect the circulation by damaging the walls of the systemic blood vessels. A prolonged high pressure within these vessels, stimulates the vessels to thicken and strengthen to withstand the stress. The thickening gradually becomes sufficient to narrow the lumens of the blood vessels. This process of thickening can lead to heart disease (Fox 1996) or intracerebral haemorrhage (stroke) (Shephard & Fox 1996). Ten per cent of surgical patients have hypertension and this puts them at a higher than normal risk of cerebrovascular accident, acute renal failure, pulmonary oedema, and myocardial infarction (Nash & Jensen 1994).

The risk factors for hypertension have been identified as smoking, obesity (Froelicher et al 1995), stressful lifestyle (Engler & Engler 1995), diabetes, and eating a diet high in fat, cholesterol and sodium (Wood 1996). The treatment for a high blood pressure varies depending on its severity and can include both pharmacological and non-pharmacological methods (Griffith 1995).

Heart failure

The most common type of heart failure is left-ventricular failure (LVF), in which a proportion of the blood remains present in the left ventricle at the end of ventricular contraction (Janowski 1996). This can be caused by coronary artery disease, hypertension, idiopathic dilated cardiomyopathy and alcohol abuse (Linden 1995). The condition of LVF can continue to worsen the function of the heart. The damaged myocardial tissue, arrhythmias, or severe muscle fatigue further impairs the heart's ability to pump blood and triggers a series of events that result in congestive heart failure. This weakens myocardial contractions and all four of the heart chambers overfill during subsequent cardiac cycles (Yacone-Morton 1995). The cardiac output drops considerably and blood flow throughout the body slows down. This results in a reduction in the supply of nutrients to body tissues, circulatory stasis, pulmonary congestion and increased stress on the body (Linden 1995). This activates mechanisms that retain sodium and water, which increases circulatory congestion and vasoconstriction and further impairs the heart's pumping ability.

These are both serious conditions which can influence the patient's recovery from surgery. The patient may be on medication such as angiotensin-converting enzyme (ACE) inhibitors, digoxin or diuretics (Janowski 1996) or a combination of two or all prior to admission. While drug therapy is normally the first line of treatment, those patients with heart failure brought on by coronary artery disease or arteriosclerosis, may benefit from coronary artery bypass grafting or clot removal (Janowski 1996).

Peripheral vascular disease

The most frequent cause of diminished arterial flow is arteriosclerotic or atherosclerotic changes within the arteries (Blank & Irwin 1990). Arteriosclerosis and atherosclerosis frequently affect the peripheral arteries, which influences the survival of the body's extremities, most commonly the lower extremities. The risk factors for both of these conditions have been identified as genetic history, diabetes mellitus, and poor lifestyle habits, e.g. smoking and high fat diets (McCance & Huether 1994). However, whereas some of these factors are unchangeable, others can be altered to help slow the processes of thickening, hardening and fat or fibrin deposition present in arteriosclerosis and atherosclerosis (Blank & Irwin 1990).

Arterial occlusions are either thrombotic or embolic in nature (Luckman & Sorensen 1987). Arterial occlusions generally originate in patients with poor heart function, which diminishes the volume of arterial blood, restricting the delivery of oxygen and nutrients to the tissues, and can lead to arterial leg ulcers (Cameron 1996). Venous insufficiency is common with varicose veins in which veins become overstretched because of increases in venous pressure (Blank & Irwin 1990). This can lead to lipodermatosclerosis, which is a factor in tissue breakdown and a cause of venous leg ulcers (Cameron 1995).

Venous occlusion in the superficial and deep veins may cause a deep vein thrombosis (DVT) or a pulmonary embolism (PE). DVT has been studied extensively and can be caused by general anaesthesia with muscle relaxation, which paralyses the calf and respiratory muscle pumps; this inhibition may persist for several days following surgery (Browse et al 1988). Therefore, early ambulation is recommended to prevent the development of DVT and PE in the postoperative period (Blank & Irwin 1990). It is evident that those patients who are prone to peripheral vascular disease need to be identified prior to surgery, as they may be at risk of developing low flow states during or following surgery and may have difficulties in maintaining an adequate circulation.

Bleeding disorders

Platelet and coagulation disorders can cause or fail to prevent an internal or external haemorrhage (McCance & Huether 1994). Disorders of platelets are generally visible as a skin discoloration caused by subcutaneous bleeding (purpura), which occurs when there are not enough normal platelets to plug damaged vessels. Disorders of platelets include thrombocytopenia and thrombocytosis and can be caused by drugs, such as anti-inflammatory agents, antimicrobials, antidepressants, and adrenergic blocking agents (Contreras 1992). Coagulation disorders tend to result in more serious bleeding and are usually caused by a deficiency in one or more of the clotting factors, an insufficiency of vitamin K, liver disease (McCance & Huether 1994), or disseminated intravascular coagulation (DIC) (Bell 1992).

Dehydration

Dehydration is a common problem in hospital, especially in the elderly (Turner 1987, Martin & Larsen 1994) and may occur prior to, during or following surgery. It may be a consequence of a primary deficit of water, a primary deficit of salt, or both. A primary deficit of water leads to cellular dehydration and circulatory failure. By contrast, a primary deficit of salt leads to a reduced extracellular fluid volume, a reduced blood volume, and increasing difficulty in maintaining an adequate circulation.

Isotonic dehydration. In isotonic dehydration there are alterations in both the total body water (TBW) and electrolyte balance. It generally results from reduced fluid intake rather than increased loss, but can occur from haemorrhage, severe wound drainage, and excessive diaphoresis (McCance & Huether 1994). The most common cause of reduced fluid intake in clinical practice is the inability of the individual to take in an adequate amount of fluid (Ellerbe 1981). Water deficit causes weight loss, dryness of skin and mucous membranes, decreased urine output, and symptoms of hypovolaemia, such as a rapid heart rate, flattened neck veins, and a decrease in blood pressure. In severe cases, hypovolaemic shock can occur. Other individuals at risk of dehydration related to water deficit include infants, the elderly, and immobilised individuals.

Hypertonic dehydration. In hypertonic dehydration there is an increased concentration of extracellular sodium (hypernatraemia) in relation to water (McCance & Huether 1994). This is associated with fever or respiratory infections, which increase the respiratory rate and enhance water loss from the lungs. Severe diarrhoea also causes water loss in relation to sodium. Insufficient water intake also can cause hypernatraemia, particularly in individuals who are comatose, confused, or immobilised. In hypertonic volume depletion, the urine specific gravity will be greater than 1.030, and the haematocrit, plasma proteins and plasma osmolality will be elevated above normal (McCance & Huether 1994).

Hypotonic dehydration. In hypotonic dehydration there is a reduction in sodium (hyponatraemia) and an increase in water. This is associated with a reduced intake of sodium, continued diuretic therapy and vomiting (McCance & Huether 1994). Sodium deficits usually cause a reduction in the plasma osmolarity with movement of water into the cells. This movement will reduce the overall circulating volume and thus give the impression of dehydration.

Dehydration – a deficiency of both salt and water. This is the most appropriate term to indicate both sodium loss and water loss. A deficiency of both salt and water occurs when fluid is lost from the gastrointestinal tract (Ellerbe 1981) It is important to note that when treating dehydration a combination of normal saline, 5% dextrose and dextrose saline should be used (Martin & Larson 1994).

Factors that can affect the circulation during or following surgery

A mere glance at a surgical patient may reveal the present circulation status. For example, an ashen, restless, confused or listless patient is characteristic of a low perfusion state (Meyers & Hickey 1988). The patient's condition and the clinical setting should determine the frequency and rapidity of assessment as well as the sequence in which it should be done. For example, in a crisis situation, assessment is brief and focuses on parameters key to perfusion: the presence and quality of pulses; capillary refill; colour; and level of consciousness. The most common factor that affects the circulation is hypovolaemia due to bleeding.

Hypovolaemia and hypovolaemic shock

Hypovolaemia is defined as a diminished circulatory fluid volume (Meyers & Hickey 1988). Hypovolaemic shock is the state that results from hypovolaemia and is a further decrease in the circulating fluid volume so large that the body's metabolic needs cannot be met. The principal aetiologies of hypovolaemic shock can be classified as haemorrhage, plasma loss and dehydration. Dehydration is discussed above; therefore the variations in the different types of fluid loss discussed here will focus of the loss of blood and plasma.

The pathophysiological aspects of hypovolaemia. The decline in blood volume produced by continued bleeding, or plasma or water loss decreases venous return and cardiac output. Numerous compensatory mechanisms are activated when the circulating volume is reduced and the venous return is decreased (Meyers & Hickey 1988).

The baroreceptors become stretched to a lesser degree, decreasing their rate of discharge, which results in vasoconstriction. This will greatly increase the peripheral resistance, maintain arterial blood pressure and therefore return more blood to the heart. A decreased renal blood flow may also result in stimulation of the osmoreceptors and increase the production of antidiuretic hormone (ADH), and arouse the sense of thirst. This will also stimulate the renin–angiotensin–aldosterone system in an attempt to restore extracellular volume by conserving sodium and water. However, the continued vasoconstriction in the kidneys may cause the glomerular filtration rate (GFR) to become depressed; as a result, minimal urine is produced. If hypovolaemia is prolonged, severe renal tubular damage results, known as acute tubular necrosis (ATN). However, the continued failure of the kidneys to excrete urea causes a metabolic acidosis, with a consequent decrease in pH. The acidosis results in an impaired cardiovascular response with depression of myocardial function (Guthrie 1982) (see also Ch. 26).

These protective mechanisms will eventually cease to function and circulatory failure ensues. If metabolic acidosis or circulatory failure is not corrected or treatment instigated, death will occur in a short period of time.

Hypovolaemia caused by haemorrhage – the loss of whole blood. This is the most common cause of hypovolaemic shock. The greater the duration and severity of haemorrhage, the more pronounced the overall state of hypovolaemic shock. An acute loss of 10% of total blood volume reduces arterial pressure by 7% and cardiac output by 21%; the loss of 20% of the total blood volume reduces arterial pressure by 15% and cardiac output by 41% (Meyers & Hickey 1988). The loss of red cells decreases the oxygen-carrying capacity of the blood and contributes to hypoxia (Masasi & Keyes 1994). Hypoxaemia as well as acidosis (reduced pH) stimulates the vascular chemoreceptors. The presence of cardiovascular disease or anaemia can alter this pattern of response by critically reducing tissue oxygen availability and increasing the risk of subsequent complications.

Hypovolaemia caused by plasma loss. This is the result of an increase in capillary permeability leading to a shift of plasma fluid from the vascular space into the interstitial space. This type of hypovolaemic shock occurs most often in individuals with large partial-thickness burns, full-thickness burns, or burns over more than 20–25% of the total body surface area (Goodwin 1984). The rate and volume of plasma deficit are roughly proportional to the extent of the area burned. In other conditions of plasma loss that produce similar types of plasma deficit or fluid shifts, the measurement of loss is not easily quantified.

ASSESSMENT OF THE SURGICAL PATIENT WITH REDUCED OR INADEQUATE CIRCULATION

In this section the different skills that can be used by surgical nurses to collect data to determine the circulatory status of a patient will be considered. These are observing, interviewing and measuring.

Observation

Every nurse is aware of the crucial importance of astute and accurate observation. Florence Nightingale wrote in *Notes on Nursing* (1859): 'The most important practical lesson that can be given to nurses is to teach them what to observe, how to observe, what symptoms indicate improvement, what the reverse, which are of importance, which are of none, which are the evidence of neglect, and of what kind of neglect'. She goes on to conclude that 'if you cannot get the habit of observation one way or other, you had better give up being a nurse, for it is not your calling, however kind and anxious you may be'. As ever, Nightingale's writing is stern but the basic message is as appropriate today as it was in her time: accurate observation is an important means of collecting information about patients' cardiac/circulatory status.

Even though surgical nurses may not realise it, they begin 'to assess' and 'make observations' about patients' circulatory status, from the very moment they set eyes upon them. It might register that the patient is being admitted on a trolley or in a wheelchair or, if walking, is using a stick or has a limp or an unsteady gait. On admission of the patient, the surgical nurse automatically observes details such as facial colour, pallor, flushed or cyanosed; any respiratory difficulty, rapid or shallow breathing; cool moist or dehydrated skin; ischaemia of the eyelids, lips, gums and tongue; facial expressions; oedema; increased or decreased body weight; pulsating neck veins; posture; and dry mucous membranes.

Observations are made not only of patients' physical condition but of indicators of their psychological and emotional state too (Binnie et al 1988), for example signs of anxiety or distress, evidence of confusion, disorientation, apprehension, restlessness, agitation or calm. An important point to stress is that observation depends not just on the sense of sight, but also involves the senses of hearing, touch and smell.

Surgical nurses should remember that their initial observations about patients contribute substantially to nursing assessment. To a large extent these observations will direct the nurse's subsequent, more systematic approach to data collection and this will include further observation of specific factors.

Interview

Observational skills also play a part in interviewing because information is forthcoming from patients' nonverbal communication, in addition to what they actually say (Binnie et al 1988). Whether or not the nonverbal cues appear to support or contradict the verbal communication may be of importance. For example, a surgical patient in the postoperative ward might say to the staff nurse, 'No, I do not have any pain', but at the same time be showing facial expressions of anxiety, uncertainty and obvious pain.

Surgical nurses should not underestimate the importance of skilled verbal communication in interviewing. The admission of a patient usually commences with an interview and it is from this structured discussion that a great deal of crucial information is obtained.

To assess the surgical patient's circulatory status, a relevant health history is necessary. This includes inquiring if there is any family history of acute illnesses such as heart disease, stroke, renal disorders, bleeding disorders, cancer, peripheral vascular disease, or respiratory disease (Braddy 1989). Other areas to consider are if the patient has had any episodes of fatigue, restlessness, syncope, or confusion which may be due to oxygen deprivation and, especially in the elderly, can be early clues of congestive heart failure or myocardial infarction (McGovern & Kuhn 1992). It is always a good idea to have patients show you any medications that they are taking or sometimes take, and to check that the medications are taken as prescribed. If the patient does not have the medications on hand, ask a relative or friend to bring them in to you (McGovern & Kuhn 1992). It is necessary to determine any cardiac risk factors, such as diabetes, a high fat/cholesterol diet, whether the patient smokes or takes any exercise. Coping strategies may help to determine how well the patient copes with stress. Religious beliefs or preferences, sleeping and eating patterns might help to confirm or omit certain risk factors (Braddy 1989). The social status of the patient will help to ascertain stress levels and so questions about diet, income, family concerns and job status are necessary, as all can influence the patient's circulatory status.

A good nursing assessment relies heavily upon the nurse's skills at interviewing patients and surgical nurses need to acquire a good interviewing technique. The nurse needs to learn to ask the right questions, to know how to encourage the patient to give information, and perhaps most importantly to recognise nonverbal cues given by the patient and how to validate these.

Measurements

This term refers to data which are measurable and hence more objective, than either observation or interviewing can be (Binnie et al 1988). Obvious examples of measurements in data collection are of the patient's central venous pressure, temperature, pulses, heart rate, electrocardiograph, blood pressure, weight, urine output, urinalysis, blood results, oxygen saturation and mental state. In many instances, measurements may be carried out to substantiate information obtained from observing or questioning the patient. For example, the nurse may observe that a person looks overweight and can ascertain this fact more objectively and precisely by weighing the person and comparing the weight and height in relation to age and sex. Then, having obtained a precise measure, any subsequent change in weight (gain or loss) can be accurately compared with the baseline. This example relates to a physical factor but, increasingly, measuring instruments are being devised for psychological or emotional factors too.

Central venous pressure (CVP) monitoring

The measurement of the central venous pressure (CVP) provides important haemodynamic information to guide the therapy of patients (Potger & Elliott 1994). The adequacy of the body's blood volume, the function of the right side of the heart as a pump, vascular tone and pulmonary vascular resistance can be assessed by examining the CVP. Normally, the CVP reflects the volume of blood returning to the heart, which exerts a pressure on the walls of the right ventricle; this blood will then be circulated through the heart and lungs and around the body.

A fall in CVP can indicate moderate hypovolaemic shock in patients who are bleeding following surgery, or can be due to extreme vasodilatation, whereby the capacity of the circulation is increased but the circulating volume remains constant, as in patients with a pyrexia or from the excessive use of vasodilator drugs (Manley 1991). Potger & Elliott (1994) suggest that the CVP can be used as a guide to determine severity of loss and the fluid required to replace it. However, it is proposed that there is little or no relationship between the CVP reading and the volume of fluid needed to restore tissue perfusion to normal. This implies that CVP levels are not completely reliable in estimating fluid needs. This is because the normal CVP range is from 3–10 cmH$_2$O, yet many patients with CVP levels of 16 cmH$_2$O respond well to further fluid and blood administration. This is because the CVP monitors cardiac competence by measuring the volume that the right myocardium can manage without failing, which has been shown to differ from patient to patient. In addition, it may take nearly 24 hours for events occurring in the left side of the heart to reflect through the lungs into the right ventricle, atria, and superior vena cava, and be recorded as an increased CVP reading. Therefore, when using CVP to measure fluid replacement, the adequacy of treatment should not only be determined by the CVP but always be interpreted in conjunction with other clinical data (Manley 1991) (see also Ch. 26).

CVP measurement can also be used to determine if fluid replacement is a cause for concerns regarding overload and cardiac failure. This can be represented by an increase in CVP, where the pressure on the walls of the right atrium is augmented to bring about an increase in the CVP. This can lead to circulatory collapse, in which the left side of the heart becomes dysfunctional with the consequence that it is unable to pump blood out, giving rise to a low cardiac output and an increase in right and left ventricular filling pressures. In addition, a high CVP can represent exposure to extreme cold, e.g. following surgery which involves active cooling. This causes severe vasoconstriction, which would return more blood to the heart from the already filled veins.

In addition to measurement, the CVP catheter can also be used for rapid infusion of fluids and blood, or to withdraw blood for laboratory samples. The most common complications of a CVP line include pneumothorax, hydrothorax, ventricular arrhythmias (Darovic 1987), infection, and air embolism (Manley 1991), all of which should be observed for by the surgical nurse during the procedure

To determine an accurate CVP, the patient should be in the supine position with the backrest at an angle of up to 30 degrees (Callow & Pieper 1989) (see also Ch. 26). The most reliable external reference point used to take the CVP is the phlebostatic axis (PA). This is defined as a point in the fourth intercostal space at the mid-axilla line. The PA has been repeatedly confirmed as a valid external reference level for CVP measurements. It has been shown anatomically to be a true external point for identifying the right atrium (Kee et al 1993). The reliability of the PA for the monitoring of CVPs in various degrees of backrest elevation up to 30 degrees has been established (Callow & Pieper 1989).

However, there are attempts being made to find a reliable method of measuring the CVP of a patient in the lateral (side) position (Potger & Elliott 1994). Such a reference point would be advantageous because the patient would have longer uninterrupted periods of rest and would derive the benefits of being nursed in the lateral position, such as improved lung function and pressure area care (Jenkins et al 1988). Furthermore, there would be a reduction in the nursing time and effort spent in unnecessarily moving the patient. However, as yet, evidence is inconclusive; therefore the laterally positioned patient should be returned to the supine position for CVP measurement (Potger & Elliott 1994). The stages of measuring a central venous pressure using a water manometer are illustrated in Figure 25.2.

Blood pressure (BP)

One of the first procedures carried out when a patient is admitted to hospital is a simple blood pressure measurement. Taking the BP remains one of the most important and widely used assessment tools in hospital, as from this one test much information can be gleaned about the patient's state of health (Bardwell 1995, Henneman & Henneman 1989). Many nursing and medical staff regard this task as simple and straightforward, when in fact it is complex (Burroughs & Hoffbrand 1990). BP measurement is one of the first skills taught to nurses and one that they must master as quickly as possible. Senior students and qualified nurses are likely to accept without question their ability to take an accurate BP reading (Nolan & Nolan 1993). However, research is beginning to emerge to suggest that variations in technique of measuring BP, in equipment and between patients influence the recording in ways that are not acknowledged; neither are skills updated or knowledge checked. Consequently, BP recordings are often done poorly (Bardwell 1995).

Nurses generally record BP in the preoperative period to determine a baseline prior to operation or as a determinant of risk factors for cerebral vascular accident, ischaemic heart disease and renal disease, all of which can influence recovery from an operation (Bardwell 1995, Burnip 1991). In the postoperative period, nurses mainly record the BP to detect signs of hypovolaemic shock (indicated by a low BP) or specific 'high-risk' conditions, which are generally caused by the effects of anaesthetic or severe pain (a high BP)

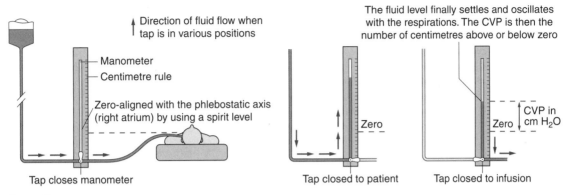

Direction of fluid flow when
tap is in various positions

Manometer
Centimetre rule

Zero-aligned with the phlebostatic axis
(right atrium) by using a spirit level

Tap closes manometer

The fluid level finally settles and oscillates
with the respirations. The CVP is then the
number of centimetres above or below zero

Zero

Zero

CVP in
cm H_2O

Tap closed to patient   Tap closed to infusion

Precautions
1. Ensure familiarity with tap as various types exist
2. Ensure intravenous fluid does not contain drug additives which may enter the patient as a bolus when measuring CVP
3. Ensure tap on manometer is below the level of patient to prevent the entrance of air when measuring CVP
4. All precautions should be taken to prevent contamination and introduction of infection

Figure 25.2 Measuring a CVP using a water manometer (adapted from Edwards & Manley 1998 Care of adults in hospital. Edward Arnold).

(Burnip 1991). The BP should be taken when a patient is admitted, postoperatively, when drugs that alter BP are taken, and when the patient's condition has deteriorated. It should also be taken when the patient is hypertensive, neutropenic, pregnant, critically ill, receiving an infusion or has an infection.

Jolly (1991) describes BP as, 'the force exerted by the blood on the walls of the arteries in which it is contained'. It is determined by a number of factors, most significantly cardiac output, peripheral resistance, elasticity of vessels and hormonal and chemical control mechanisms (O'Brien & Davison 1994). Two components of BP are evident: the systolic pressure, the pressure at which blood is forced out into the arteries at ventricular contraction; and diastolic pressure, which is the fall in arterial pressure before the next ventricular contraction (Bardwell 1995).

There are two methods of taking a BP: direct and indirect (Darovic 1987). Direct monitoring of BP is accomplished by cannulating an artery and attaching the catheter to fluid-filled tubing and a transducer, which is connected to a voltage source (Henneman & Henneman 1989). The majority of studies that compare direct and indirect methods of monitoring BP indicate that BP values obtained via direct and indirect methods are virtually never the same (see Henneman & Henneman 1989). This will be most relevant to the surgical nurse receiving a patient back from a critical care setting where BP has been monitored directly. Indirect methods of BP monitoring, which are more commonly used in surgical wards, fall into two categories: the auscultatory (manual) method and computer-assisted automatic devices.

The traditional auscultatory technique uses a pneumatic cuff and stethoscope paying attention to Korotkoff sounds (Box 25.1). Korotkoff sounds are generated by blood passing through the compressed artery under the cuff and meeting a static column of blood, resulting in turbulence and vibrations. To be detected by a stethoscope, these sounds must be at a frequency within an audible range (Rushmer 1970).

In low-flow states, such as those associated with hypotension, the auscultatory method has been demonstrated to fail, apparently as the result of the human ear's inability to appreciate low-frequency vibrations (Geddes 1970). The automatic devices have gained increasing acceptance in an attempt to solve

Box 25.1 Korotkoff sounds	
Korotkoff identified the sounds heard when blood pressure is determined by the auscultatory method. These were described in phases as follows:	
Phase 1	The pressure level at which the first clear tapping sounds are heard
Phase II	The time during inflation when a murmur and a swishing are heard
Phase III	The point when the murmur disappears and a louder and more succinct sound is heard
Phase IV	The point where there is muffling of sound
Phase V	The phase at which sound disappears

this problem, and there are now several devices which measure the BP in various ways depending on the brand used. However, their reliability has been challenged as, like the auscultatory method, many of these devices are blood-flow dependent.

Both methods of indirect monitoring of BP are subject to many sources of error, and may be unreliable in the clinical situations where they are used most (Venus et al 1985). This is mainly due to the fact that measuring and monitoring BP is frequently carried out, but often performed incorrectly. Errors in measurement may mean wrong decisions being made in BP management, thus compromising care (Nursing Times 1995). The major sources of errors are caused by the many variables associated with measuring BP (Pickering 1994). These fall into three distinct areas, the patient, the observer (doctor or nurse) and equipment (Box 25.2).

Some of the conditions/variables seen in Box 25.2 cannot be controlled, despite their impact on BP measurement giving false BP readings; however, other sources of error can be eliminated. If all nurses were taught the same method of taking a BP during their pre-registration course and continued to have updates at postregistration level, all nurses might take a BP recording in a similar way. This may serve to remove the majority of errors and make the BP recording a more reliable measurement. Recommendations on how to record an accurate BP are given in Box 25.3.

A study by Mancia et al (1983) proposed that an inaccurate BP reading is not a consequence of poor cuff application or too quick inflation of the cuff (see Box 25.2), but begins when the doctor appears at the patient's bedside. It is reasonable to assume that the doctor's visit and the expectation of having the BP measured can cause an alarm reaction in patients. Mancia et al's (1983) small study showed that 47 out of 48 subjects demonstrated a rise in systolic and diastolic BP, leading to an overestimation of BP. If nurses and doctors are measuring BP inaccurately, and the doctor's visit is causing a further increase in BP, mild hypertension (95–104 mmHg, Feher et al 1992) could be being overdiagnosed in surgical patients.

In addition, teaching is not generally updated nor is knowledge checked (Kemp et al 1994). This was confirmed in a study by Nolan & Nolan (1993), which showed that both doctors and nurses at all levels of experience had limited knowledge of the sources of error when taking a BP reading, even though prior to the test all those involved had indicated that they thought that they could take and record a patient's BP accurately. A study by Feher et al (1992) tested 80 junior hospital doctors on the practical aspects of BP

Box 25.2 The potential sources of error when taking a blood pressure reading

The observer
- Observer bias – previous recording viewed by the nurse or a preference for a specific figure.
- Cognitive deficits – inadequate education, inadequate training, no updating on the technique or principles.
- Lack of understanding of the correct procedure, e.g. incorrect positioning of the patient sitting/standing, support of the arm, positioning of the cuff bladder over the centre of the brachial artery; the equipment not level with the heart.
- Lack of concentration.

The equipment
- Incorrect cuff bladder size.
- Inadequate maintenance – BP machines should be recalibrated and assessed every 6–12 months.
- The level of mercury not at zero.
- The vent may be blocked.

The patient
- The patient may be suffering from excessive heat or cold; be wearing constrictive clothing; have a full bladder, recently exercised, been smoking, just had a meal; or there may be a distraction, all of which will serve to either increase or decrease the BP.
- Older patients may have calcified/rigid arteries or anaemia, which can all influence the BP reading.
- A patient suffering from a high temperature may have a low BP, owing to vasodilatation causing the BP to fall.
- Paediatric and pregnant women's diastolic reading should be taken at Phase IV of Korotkoff sounds, rather than at Phase V (O'Brien & Davison 1994).
- In conditions where BP is low, there may be distal vasoconstriction and it is common to underestimate the BP.
- The white coat syndrome – this is caused when doctors appear at patients' bedsides, giving an inaccurately high BP reading.
- Patients' BP can vary during the day – higher systolic readings in the evening and a low recording in the morning.
- Fear, anxiety, apprehension and pain can all raise the BP and these can be apparent on admission. It is recommended in this instance to wait at least 1 hour following admission before taking the BP.

---

measurement; 33% of those studied acknowledged no formal education on how to measure BP. These findings and others support the urgent need for further training and assessment of BP measurement for both nurses and doctors.

Very few articles mention how frequently BP readings should be taken (Toms 1993), and this is often left to the nurse's judgement. Sometimes BP is taken

Box 25.3 The recommended procedure for measuring blood pressure (adapted from Edwards 1997)

- If possible, the patient should not have eaten, exercised or smoked for at least 30 minutes before the blood pressure reading is taken.
- The patient should be sitting or lying down, in a quiet environment with the arm resting at heart level on a table or pillow (the antecubital fossa should be level with the fourth intercostal space).
    A rest period of at least 3–5 minutes should be allowed before the reading.
- Measure the circumference of the arm and use the appropriate-sized bladder. It is possible with modern BP cuffs to take an accurate BP reading even if the cuff is not an accurate size by placing the cuff over the brachial artery. The arrow on the cuff should be aligned with the patient's brachial artery before the cuff is secured.
- A gap of 2–3 cm should be left between the antecubital fossa and the cuff.
- The sphygmomanometer should be placed near to the observer (no more than 3 feet away) on a flat surface with the mercury level at zero.
- Locate the brachial artery by palpation.
- Assess the maximal inflation level that avoids causing pain by inflating the cuff and palpating the radial pulse at the same time. The maximal inflation level will be 20–30 mmHg higher than the level at which the pulse disappeared.
- The patient's legs should not be crossed, as this will give a falsely high BP reading.
- Place the stethoscope over the brachial artery, taking care not to use too much pressure, as this lowers the diastolic reading. Release the valve slowly and gently.
- The cuff should be rapidly inflated at 2 mmHg/second, and deflated slowly; a slow inflation and a rapid deflation result in inaccuracies.
- Note the systolic pressure at the onset of the first clear repetitive tapping sound of two beats or more.
- Record the diastolic pressure at the cessation of sound (Phase V). Sometimes Phase V in pregnant women and children goes down to zero and therefore cannot be read. In these instances, the muffling of sound (Phase IV) should be used and documented on the patient's chart.
- The blood pressure should be rounded up by no more that 2 mmHg.
- The procedure should not be rushed, as this will result in an underestimation of the systolic pressure and an overestimation of the diastolic pressure. It is recommended that it should take no less than 5 minutes to take a BP (Nolan & Nolan 1993).
- The measurement should be recorded on the patient's chart. If it is not possible to achieve optimum conditions, this should also be noted.
- There should be no major difference between blood pressure lying, sitting or standing in a normal healthy adult, although there is always variation in blood pressure within an individual as a function of time.
- If the reading needs to be repeated, at least 1–2 minutes should have elapsed before reinflating the cuff.

frequently in the days following admission and then the frequency is reduced haphazardly as the patient's condition improves. The rationale of nurses for recording BP in the postoperative period was investigated in a small study by Burnip (1991), which explored nurses' decision-making, knowledge base and clinical judgement in relation to the frequency and duration of BP recording. It found that nurses relied heavily on BP monitoring to detect early signs of hypovolaemic shock caused by haemorrhage and thus continued to measure BP 'just in case we miss something'.

By relying heavily on the BP, the nurse neglects the other clinical manifestations of hypovolaemic shock, e.g. pallor; cool moist skin; rapid breathing; ischaemia of the eyelids, lips, gums and tongue; weak thready pulse; and, eventually, a low BP and concentrated urine. The patient becomes apprehensive, restless and thirsty. The pulse increases, temperature lowers, respiration becomes rapid and deep as the haemorrhage progresses, cardiac output decreases and arterial and venous pressures fall. The patient may experience dots before the eyes and ringing in the ears. In addition, the intense faith given to BP measurement as an indicator of patients' progress could 'cloud' other observation skills of the nurse.

With regard to the duration of BP measurement, it is evident that it is often prolonged, perhaps unnecessarily. This emphasises the importance of understanding the physiological basis for measuring BP. Haemorrhage, for example, is either evident or concealed and can occur at the time of the operation (primary haemorrhage); during the first few hours after the operation (intermediary haemorrhage); or some time after surgery, because of slipping of a ligature, infection or erosion of a blood vessel by a drainage tube (secondary haemorrhage). This implies that BP needs to be recorded throughout a patient's postoperative stay in hospital. Nevertheless, nurses need to be able to provide a rationale for their actions (Toms 1993). If nurses are spending time making unnecessary observations, they are using time which could be spent in other patient activities. If frequent BP measurements are being made on two-thirds of patients on an average 30-bedded ward, it could take up to 2–3 hours per day of nursing time, which may be considered a waste (Walsh & Ford 1989). It was also noted that nurses were not recording factors that were likely to have adversely influenced the reading on the charts.

In addition, it is interesting to note that the importance of using the pulse as an early reliable indicator of physiological change was often overlooked. In some general surgical wards, policies have been developed to measure BP once on return from theatre and, if it is satisfactory and the patient is not in a high-risk group, only to record the pulse at regular intervals during the postoperative period. This is less invasive and less time-consuming, and the pulse is measured more accurately than BP (Burnip 1991). The rationale therefore for performing observations must be considered for each patient individually.

Weight

Taking a patient's weight is an important measurement in determining circulatory status. However, certain disease processes, such as cancer, cachexia and oedema, may affect an individual's weight, which minimises its usefulness as a measure of circulatory failure. Yet, a weight chart can be used to determine whether a patient is becoming dehydrated by losing weight or is gaining weight because of fluid retention. An increase in weight may be the first indication of heart failure, whereas a decrease in weight can be the first sign that diuretic therapy is working. Clearly, weight can be an important measurement when determining effective circulation.

Urine output

The kidney receives about 25% of the cardiac output, and glomerular filtration rate (GFR) is dependent on adequate renal perfusion. When perfusion is adequate, the production of urine will exceed 0.5 ml/kg body weight per hour. Therefore, the average urinary output should be between 30 and 70 ml or more per hour (Marieb 1995). Kidney function is monitored by a catheter; if urine output falls below 25 ml per hour, fluid administration should be increased (Dries & Waxman 1991). This is why urinary output should be measured at hourly intervals if a catheter is inserted, and accurately recorded (Christensen 1992). Interpretation of urine output should also consider overall fluid balance and the quality of urine. Thus, it is often necessary to measure urine osmolality and may also be necessary to monitor electrolyte content.

When hypovolaemia is present, there is an increase in vasoconstriction, causing the circulating blood flow to the kidneys to be reduced (Rice 1991). The overall effect is that the GFR decreases, reducing urinary output. In contrast, when there is an increase in fluid administration causing hypervolaemia, cardiac failure and pulmonary oedema may occur. In this instance kidney function may also become impaired, owing to a reduction in the pumping action of the heart, and a reduced cardiac output and blood flow to the kidneys (see also Ch. 26).

Urine testing

The kidney has a prime role in maintaining normal, healthy life, and many early changes that occur in the body may be reflected in the urine well before they become clinically obvious. Information from urine tests can aid diagnosis, assist in monitoring circulatory status and help provide valuable clues to the effectiveness of treatment (Nursing Times 1986a). In view of this it is unfortunate that urine testing is described as 'routine' and devalued (Cook 1995). This section deals with a means of simple diagnosis and detection of circulatory failure which is clearly within the area of responsibility of nurses, that of testing the specific gravity of urine.

Urine is mostly water with a variable quantity of substances dissolved in it. The concentration of these dissolved substances will depend on the body's state of hydration and the amount of waste products to be excreted (Marieb 1995). Therefore, measuring the specific gravity (SG) of urine can be one way to determine if hydration is adequate. Even though inpatient monitoring of fluid balance with intake and output charts is essential, loss of water through the breath, sweat and faeces is not so easily measured (Nursing Times 1986a). The SG of urine, therefore, will give a good indication of the net fluid balance and is of particular value in patients where there is an unquantifiable loss, such as in burns cases or breathing difficulties.

In healthy adults, SG varies between 1.005 to 1.035 (pure water is the standard, with an SG of 1.0). Since it depends on the state of hydration, the first specimen of the morning will tend to have a higher SG then one after the subject has had a drink. Therefore, an isolated assessment of SG is of little value and the test should be repeated on samples taken at known times or interpreted in conjunction with fluid balance studies (Nursing Times 1986b). Urine with a persistently low SG is suggestive of diabetes insipidus or renal damage – owing to the normal concentrating power of the kidneys being lost, the urine passed will tend to be rather dilute (Lloyd 1993). An increase in specific gravity will indicate dehydration, perhaps due to bleeding, vomiting, diarrhoea, reduction in fluid intake or fever.

The traditional method for measuring SG was by using a glass hydrometer. A popular and widely used method now is the reagent strip which measures the ionic strength of a urine sample and expresses this as a colour change. The colour changes on the reagent strips are easier to read than the gradations on the narrow stem of the hydrometer, and thus the method is less prone to errors (Nursing Times 1986b).

Blood results

Blood tests can aid diagnosis, assist in monitoring circulatory status and help provide valuable clues to the effectiveness of treatment (Christensen 1992). Taking a blood sample is often the remit of the doctor, but the results of blood tests such as haemoglobin level, plasma osmolarity and haematocrit determination can be used by surgical nurses if they suspect hypovolaemia or circulatory failure.

Haemoglobin level. Haemoglobin is contained in the cytoplasm of erythrocytes and is primarily responsible for carrying oxygen to, and carbon dioxide from, the body's tissues. The haemoglobin (Hb) level is related to the number of red blood cells in the blood, which plays a major role in blood viscosity (see p. 510).

The normal concentration of Hb in the blood is between 12–15 g per 100 ml of blood. A low Hb level will indicate that red blood cells are being lost. When considering Hb level it is important to include the patient's age, general state and the rate of fall of the Hb concentration (Contreras 1992). An Hb concentration that has fallen suddenly, such as in acute blood loss, is not well tolerated by the body and a transfusion is required to improve the delivery of oxygen to the tissues. However, a slow reduction in Hb, taking place gradually over weeks or months, is better tolerated as the body has time to adapt. This occurs in iron deficiency anaemia, megaloblastic anaemia, renal failure and anaemias associated with chronic disorders (Contreras 1992).

In addition to determining Hb levels, other signs may be present to confirm findings. For example, in white skin the colour of the haemoglobin shows through the epidermis as a pinkish tinge as the blood circulates through the dermal capillaries (Marieb 1995). When haemoglobin is poorly oxygenated, both the blood and the skin of white people appear blue (cyanosis). In black people, cyanosis of the skin does not appear, but can be observed in the mucous membranes and nail beds. The surgical nurse may notice cyanosis in a patient before the physiological parameter (Hb) is actually measured. However, it is necessary to consider cyanosis in relation to the total clinical picture because it occurs in other conditions such as respiratory diseases and heart failure.

Plasma osmolarity. Osmolarity is a measure of the number of milliosmoles per litre of solution, or the concentration of molecules per volume of solution (McCance & Huether 1994). When solute is added to water, the volume is expanded to include the original amount of water plus the volume occupied by the solute particles (e.g. sodium, potassium, calcium, etc.). So, by monitoring the plasma osmolarity the volume of water in relation to solutes can be determined. When there is an increase in osmolarity there has been a reduction of water in relation to the solutes contained within it; this is seen in dehydration when there is a lack of fluid but the solute content has not changed.

The osmolarity of intracellular and extracellular fluid tends to equalise and so provides a measure of body fluid concentration and thus the body's hydration status. The normal osmolarity of body fluids is 280–294 mOsm/l (Christensen 1992). Thus, a serum osmolarity less than 280 mOsm/l will generally indicate an excess of fluids in the vessels, indicating overhydration or hypervolaemia. An increased serum osmolarity, greater than 295 mOsm/l, indicates a loss of fluid; there are thus more solute molecules in relation to fluid and dehydration or hypovolaemia is present (Christensen 1992). With an increase in osmolarity, thirst and a dry mouth are often experienced. This may alert the nurse to consider finding or suggesting a measurement of the patient's plasma osmolarity.

Haematocrit levels. The haematocrit determination is the percentage of a given volume of blood that is occupied by erythrocytes. A high haematocrit indicates increased blood viscosity (see p. 510) and reduced flow through the blood vessels, particularly the microcirculation (arterioles, capillaries, and venules). Conditions in which the haematocrit is elevated, for example dehydration, haemorrhage, anaemias, leukaemias, cyanotic congenital heart disease or polycythaemia, can lead to increased cardiac work as a result of increased vascular resistance.

The haematocrit is a useful guide for determining if whole blood or some other intravenous fluid should be used for volume replacement in the haemorrhagic shock patient. Maximum oxygen-carrying capacity is achieved with a haematocrit between 35–45%.

Temperature

Body temperature can affect the circulation if it is abnormally low or high. If the temperature is high, as in infective states, the hypothalamus initiates dilatation of arterioles and veins in the skin. This causes shunting of blood to the skin to enable heat to be lost by convection, conduction and evaporation from the skin surface (McCance & Huether 1994). However, the dilatation of the peripheral vasculature causes a reduction in cardiac output and BP and an increase in heart rate.

When the body's core temperature decreases below normal, surface blood vessels constrict to shunt blood to the vital organs and prevent excess heat loss from the skin (Marieb 1995). A decrease in body temperature is often observed in patients who have just returned from theatre following surgery and in the elderly. The body's circulating volume does not change, but the constriction of the peripheral vasculature causes a decrease in oxygen consumption and heart rate, and an increase in BP. Even though the changes in peripheral vasculature caused by changes in the body temperature do not necessarily affect circulating volume, a redistribution of the circulating volume is effected, thus influencing circulation.

Pyrexia. It is often assumed that the majority of pyrexias have an infectious aetiology, but this is not always the case (Cunha et al 1984). Certain drugs that are commonly used in surgical patients have been associated with drug pyrexias, e.g. diuretics, antiseizure therapy, analgesics, anti-arrhythmics and antibiotics (Cunha & Tu 1988). Other non-infectious causes of pyrexia include neoplasms, surgery, central nervous system problems which do not respond to antipyretic therapy (Gurevich 1985), acute myocardial infarctions, haemolysis (seen in reactions to blood transfusions) and thyrotoxicosis (Krickler & Dodge 1987).

The consequences of pyrexia can be beneficial to the patient and it is described as an important host defence mechanism (Hart & Dennis 1988). A body temperature of 40.9°C will kill some pneumococci and gonococci and the spirochaetes that cause neurosyphilis. A reduction in serum levels of iron, zinc and copper will inhibit the replication of some microorganisms (Cunha 1985, Gurevich 1985). Pyrexia increases the body's production of interferon, which enters non-infected cells to inhibit viral infiltration. In addition, a pyrexia will break down lysosomes in infected cells, thereby destroying them and preventing viral replication. The activity of phagocytes and leukocytes is increased at temperatures between 38–40°C, thus improving the infection-fighting ability of the immune system (Bruce & Grove 1992, Howie 1989).

Nevertheless, the outcomes of a pyrexia can be detrimental (Hart & Dennis 1988). A patient with a pyrexia will have an increased basal metabolic rate, causing depletion of glycogen stores in the liver and leading to nitrogen wastage. If prolonged, this may result in debility, impaired healing of tissue damage and delirium (Kunel 1986). In surgical patients who have compromised cardiopulmonary function, the effects of increased metabolic rate, heart and respiratory rate can be quite dangerous. They can lead to an increase in carbon dioxide production and oxygen consumption (Enright & Hill 1989). Dehydration may result from fluid loss during sweating and from the

lungs because of increased respiratory rate, leading to potential problems of hyovolaemia and electrolyte imbalance (Bruce & Grove 1992). In addition, an increased temperature influences gas solubility in blood. Pyrexia shifts the oxyhaemoglobin dissociation curve to the right, resulting in lower oxygen saturation and hence blood oxygen content for any given partial pressure of oxygen (Fisher & Raper 1987). There seem to be a number of contradictions in what authors advise regarding the management of pyrexia. They centre on:

- letting a pyrexia take its course as the physiological benefits are more important than patient comfort
- putting patient comfort first
- treatment by antipyrexial drugs
- treatment by cooling methods.

Hart & Dennis (1988) remark that instead of routinely eradicating high body temperatures they should be allowed to run their natural course, as long as no detrimental effects are felt by the patient. Cunha et al (1984) advise not treating the pyrexia unless there are cardiopulmonary problems or the temperature exceeds 41°C. They maintain that the most compelling reason not to lower the body temperature is because doing so may deprive the patient of an important defence mechanism. They go on to suggest that the reason temperatures are lowered is to reduce medical personnel's apprehension rather than anything to do with the patient. Cunha (1985) added guidelines about when to give treatment to a pyrexial patient: if the patient is extremely uncomfortable, the temperature reaches 41°C or above, and in the presence of cardiopulmonary problems. McCarron (1986) takes a similar view and suggests that treatment should only be given when the hazards outweigh the benefits.

It could be argued, however, that there are no real advantages to the pyrexial response and that patient comfort is paramount. Should nurses therefore relieve patients' discomfort by giving an antipyretic (such as aspirin or paracetamol) and/or tepid sponging? Antipyretics should be used when the temperature reaches 41°C or greater or when the patient is experiencing cardiopulmonary problems. If it is decided that the patient needs an antipyretic, Bruce & Grove (1992) point out that there is the potential problem of reducing the temperature too rapidly. To avoid this, when giving antipyretic drugs, the temperature should be treated to achieve approximately 38°C and not the normal of 37°C.

Treatment by cooling methods such as tepid sponging or fanning have been criticised. Bruce & Grove

(1992) propose that cooling methods are ultimately of no use, because they will result in a compensatory response by the hypothalamus which will produce heat-generating activities like chills and shivering. These may compromise unstable surgical patients by depleting their metabolic reserves and can create a new temperature spike, which is as high as, or higher than, the original one, showing an intermittent pattern. They state that this response will further compromise, and may even increase, the patient's temperature and thus should be avoided.

Krickler & Dodge (1987) also advise against the use of cooling methods such as fanning or tepid sponging as they make patients feel weak, especially during the early stages when the temperature is still rising. This view is not supported by Fisher & Raper (1987) who suggested that physical methods of cooling (e.g. tepid sponging) are often useful as they lead to vasoconstriction which is often associated with patient comfort. Agreeing with this stance, Howie (1989) advised that cooling methods should be used before the onset of the temperature spike, i.e. before 38.5°C. However, it is argued that when we experience a pyrexia we may reach a point at which we feel cold (a rigor) and want to apply extra clothing – a contradiction.

These conflicting viewpoints can be confusing and it becomes difficult to decide what to do in the best interest of the patient. On the one hand, a high temperature is a normal body response and so should not be treated. On the other, this natural response is detrimental to the circulation, so the temperature should be treated. Yet, treating the temperature by cooling and tepid sponging can only serve to increase the temperature further and cause the patient discomfort and possible harm. It is recommended that the best way to treat a high temperature is by the use of antipyrexial drug therapy (Bruce & Grove 1992).

Hypothermia. Hypothermia is a marked cooling of core temperature and produces vasoconstriction, alterations in microcirculation, coagulation, and ischaemic tissue damage. In a controlled situation, such as a surgical procedure, most tissues can tolerate temperatures as low as 7°C. In severe hypothermia, ice crystals forming on the inside of the cell cause cells to rupture and die. Tissue hypothermia slows the rate of chemical reaction (tissue metabolism), increases the viscosity of the blood, slows blood flow through the microcirculation, facilitates blood coagulation, and stimulates profound vasoconstriction (McCance & Huether 1994). Hypothermia can be accidental or therapeutic.

Accidental hypothermia, defined as a temperature of below 35°C, is generally a result of sudden immersion in cold water or prolonged exposure to cold environments. This is often seen in the elderly and is more often a medical problem. Therapeutic hypothermia is used to slow metabolism and thus preserve ischaemic tissue during some types of surgery or limb reimplantation (Mravinac et al 1989). In addition, major surgery often induces significant hypothermia through exposure of body cavities to the relatively cool operating room environment (Morley-Forster 1986, Morris & Wilkey 1970, Rich 1983). The elderly are at a greater risk of suffering from hypothermia following surgery (Moddeman 1991).

Other mechanisms that contribute to intraoperative hypothermia include irrigation of body cavities with room temperature solutions, infusion of room temperature intravenous solutions, use of drugs that impair thermoregulatory mechanisms, and inhalation of unwarmed anaesthetic agents (Shaver et al 1984).

In acute hypothermia, peripheral vasoconstriction shunts blood away from the cooler skin to the core in an effort to decrease heat loss (McCance & Huether 1994). This peripheral vasoconstriction produces peripheral tissue ischaemia. When this occurs the hypothalamic centre stimulates shivering in an effort to increase heat production. Severe shivering occurs at core temperatures of 35°C and continues until core temperature drops to about 30–32°C. Thinking becomes sluggish and coordination is decreased at 34°C. As hypothermia deepens, the hypothalamic control of vasoconstriction is lost and vasodilatation occurs with loss of core heat to the peripheries. The hypothermic individual, therefore feels suddenly warm and begins to remove clothing. At 30°C the individual becomes stuporous, heart rate and respiratory rate decline, and cardiac output is diminished. Cerebral blood flow is decreased. Metabolic rate declines, further decreasing core temperature. Sinus node depression occurs with slowing of conduction through the atrioventricular node. In severe hypothermia (core temperature of 26–28°C) pulse and respirations may be undetectable.

Rewarming should proceed at no faster than a few degrees per hour. Short-term complications of rewarming are rewarming shock; dysrhythmias, deep-ended hypothermia; acidosis. Long-term complications include congestive heart failure, hepatic and renal failure, abnormal erythropoiesis, myocardial infarction, pancreatitis, and neurological dysfunctions. The surgical nurse needs to be aware of patients who have been subject to cooling while in theatre and alert to the potential problems caused to the circulation by hypothermia.

Taking the temperature. The most common place to take the temperature in the surgical ward is sublingually for 1 minute or in the axilla for 2–3 minutes. Fisher & Raper (1987) suggested that the temperature of the hypothalamus is best reflected by the rectal temperature, which is proposed to be more accurate. Rectal temperatures are useful as long as the probes are placed correctly, but taking rectal temperatures on surgical wards is unrealistic. Fulbrook (1993) argued that rectal temperatures are inaccurate as they are affected by heat generated by faecal bacteria, whereas Hinchliff & Montague (1995) disagree saying that rectal temperature gives a much closer approximation to the body's core temperature because of the heat produced in the rectum from the waste substances of metabolism. Nevertheless, as long as surgical nurses are aware that oral temperature is about 0.5°C, and axillary temperatures up to 1°C, below the closer approximation of core temperature (rectal temperature), oral and axillary temperatures are recommended as the most effective way to take a temperature in the surgical ward.

The technique for taking a temperature reading may seem simple, but variations do exist. Erickson (1980) examined 50 febrile and 50 afebrile patients to investigate the exact placement of the thermometer and how it affected the reading. The findings indicate that for the greatest accuracy, the bulb of the thermometer should be placed sublingually to the right or left, and not in the area in the middle of the tongue. Other variables also affect oral temperature readings. These include the ingestion of hot or cold substances, recent bathing, recent physical exertion, and smoking. All of these must be taken into account when taking oral temperature readings in the surgical ward.

The use of different equipment may influence the temperature reading. The most common thermometers in use are glass thermometers containing mercury and electronic thermometers. Single-use chemical thermometers are also available. These utilise a chemical which changes colour with increasing temperature. It has been suggested that they may be particularly useful in infectious disease units to reduce the potential risk of infection spread by thermometers. Glass thermometers are cheaper but require disinfection after use and may take longer to use. It seems that the accuracy of glass thermometers declines with increased use or long-term storage (Abbey et al 1978). In addition, errors can occur with cleaning and resetting glass thermometers, and they are likely to break, potentially exposing people to mercury vapour. Electronic thermometers are more expensive, use disposable cover slips over the probe and give a digital reading. A signal indicates when the maximum temperature has been reached, to prevent premature removal of the thermometer. The debate continues as to which type of thermometer is most appropriate for use on surgical wards.

Moorat et al (1976) studied the use of the three types of thermometer to find out which was most cost-effective and concluded that electronic thermometers were preferable. A study undertaken by Takacs & Valenti (1982) was similar but larger, comprising 1246 readings over 12 months in seven clinical areas. They found that electronic thermometers may take less time to use, but nurses often did other tasks rather than wait for the thermometer to register. This is suggested to be because nurses are used to waiting for up to 3 minutes for an accurate temperature reading with a glass thermometer and often do other tasks in the meantime. A study by Pugh-Davies et al (1986) showed that large variations existed between glass mercury and electronic thermometer readings. This could have important clinical significance.

These studies advocating the use of electronic thermometers are between 10 and 20 years old; however, the glass thermometer is still mostly used in surgical areas for taking temperatures. Brislen et al (1976) commented 'how odd it was that nurses should still cling to using glass thermometers'. Yet, it is often not nurses who are 'clinging' to the old glass thermometers, but their use being dictated by resources and the lack of finance to support the application of new, up-to-date equipment.

How long a glass thermometer should be in the mouth is often debated. Nichols & Kucha (1972) concluded that the average time required to take an accurate temperature in 90% of patients was 8 minutes for men and 9 for women at room temperatures of 18–24°C. However, in a more recent study, Pugh-Davies et al (1986) found that there was no clinical advantage in using a longer reading time than 3 minutes. Unfortunately, nurses are likely to cut down the time involved anyway, often using only 1 minute or less when the ward is busy. The accuracy of the readings may then be in doubt.

The best time of day and the frequency of temperature recording has also been studied. For example, there is diurnal variation in body temperature in humans owing to circadian rhythms, and this will affect readings. Temperature is most likely to be elevated at the peak of the circadian cycle which is between 5 p.m. and 7 p.m. Angerami (1980) studied axillary temperature recordings over a period of 15 hours in a total of 255 adult patients from a range of hospital wards. The results indicated that the time at which body temperature should be taken is between 7 p.m. and 8 p.m.; this is the time at which pyrexia, if present, is most likely to register. It appears that readings for pyrexia are better undertaken in the evenings and that temperature-taking in hospital has become ritualised in nursing and it is not necessary for it to be done so frequently. It is also suggested that when recording a temperature, it is important to mark down on the ward charts sufficient information about hypothermia or pyrexia (Closs et al 1986, Heidenreich & Giuffre 1990).

There is one other method that can help surgical nurses to determine a patient's circulation – measuring the toe temperature. When a patient's circulation is impaired, there are changes to the circulation to the body's extremities. This will be reflected in the peripheral skin temperature. Most research in this area has been undertaken in the critically ill patient; however, studies indicate that the gradient between toe and body temperature provides a valuable, inexpensive and non-invasive monitor of tissue perfusion. Therefore, surgical nurses may wish to measure toe temperature as part of their overall assessment of the patient's circulation.

The elderly in relation to temperature control. The elderly require special attention to maintenance of body temperature. The elderly have poor responses to environmental temperature extremes as a result of slowed blood circulation, structural and functional changes in the skin, and overall decrease in heat-producing activities (Moddeman 1991). Other factors affecting thermal regulation in the elderly include decrease in the shivering response (delayed onset and decreased effectiveness), slowed metabolic rate, sedate lifestyle, decreased vasoconstrictor response, diminished or absent sweating, desynchronisation of circadian rhythms, undernutrition, and decreased perception of heat and cold (Fellows et al 1985) (see also Ch. 11).

Heart rate

The volume loss from haemorrhage augments the heart rate through reflex and hormonal mechanisms (Marieb 1995). As bleeding continues, the BP decreases and the heart rate increases to over 100 beats per minute. This is an attempt by the heart to maintain the cardiac output at a normal level. However, the cardiac output may increase when the heart rate is augmented. This does not always hold true, as an increase in heart rate may actually diminish cardiac output owing to the reduction in diastolic filling time which will reduce the stroke volume. This might be observed in patients with a heart rate above 120, as the heart has less time to fill, so filling volume and subsequent

stroke volume fall. The signs include tachycardia (progressing to arrhythmia), narrowing pulse pressure (progressing to hypotension), cool to cold skin, diminished to absent bowel sounds, and mental state alteration ranging from restlessness to coma.

Conversely, a drop in heart rate will not necessarily reduce cardiac output. A decrease in heart rate prolongs diastole and increases filling volume. But a significant drop in heart rate will reduce cardiac output, resulting in hypoperfusion (Dennison 1994). In some instances, heart rate may be raised by sympathetic nervous system stimulation from exercise, fever, pain, anxiety, hypovolaemia or hypervolaemia, and most other physiological or psychological stressors. It can be lowered by heart block or from parasympathetic (or vagal) stimulation caused by the Valsalva manoeuvre, coughing, suctioning, or vomiting.

If an altered heart rate does not produce signs of hypoperfusion, it is not necessary to treat it, but if the patient does show such signs, immediate treatment is indicated. This may include drug therapy or non-pharmacological measures, such as the Valsalva manoeuvre or carotid sinus massage performed by the physician (Dennison 1994).

The electrocardiogram (ECG)

The ECG records the electrical activity of the heart. Cardiac cells are specialised and, unlike many other cells in the body, each cell can initiate its own electrical impulse. The positively and negatively charged ions contained within cardiac cells conduct electrical potential differences that can be detected by bipolar or unipolar electrodes placed on the right shoulder, left shoulder and the left or right foot. This forms Einthoven's triangle which places the heart in the centre and gives a triaxial reference point for the detection of an ECG rhythm known as PQRST waves. The ECG can give information about the heart rate and rhythm, the effects of electrolytes or drugs on the heart and the electrical orientation of the cardiac muscle (McCance & Huether 1994).

In a normal heart the cardiac electrical impulse is inaugurated by the sinus (SA) node, situated in the right atrium. The sinus node is often called the cardiac pacemaker as it beats the fastest, between 60–100 beats per minute (b.p.m.). Following discharge of the SA node, waves pass through specialised conducting pathways in the atria, each cell acting as stimulus to the next. This process causes atrial depolarisation (which leads to atrial contraction) and is represented on the ECG as the P wave (Fig. 25.3). The impulse then reaches the atrioventricular (AV) node, passes through

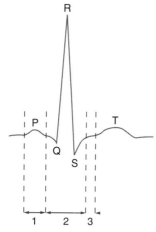

Paper speed
When recording ECGs, the paper speed should be set at 25 mm/s then: 1 mm (1 small square) = 0.04 s
5 mm (1 large square) = 0.20 s

Important landmarks
Baseline between
T wave and P wave: isoelectric line indicating no electrical activity
P wave: atrial depolarisation
QRS complex: ventricular depolarisation
T wave: ventricular repolarisation

Important intervals/segments
1. P–R interval 0.12–0.20 s
   Represents time taken for impulse to reach the ventricular myocardium from the sinoatrial node
2. QRS interval 0.08–0.12 s
   Represents time taken to depolarise the ventricles
3. S–T segment
   Deviation of this segment above or below the isoelectric line may indicate myocardial ischaemia or injury

ECG terms
Sinus rhythm: Normal ECG where the impulse originates in the sinoatrial node
All waves are present. All intervals are normal rate 60–100/min. Complexes are regular (i.e. distances between consecutive R waves are constant)
Sinus tachycardia: Complexes are normal but occurring 100/min to 160/min
Sinus bradycardia: Complexes are normal but occurring more slowly than 60/min

Figure 25.3 The electrocardiogram (reproduced by kind permission from Edwards & Manley 1998 Care of adults in hospital. Edward Arnold).

the bundle of His and down the right and left bundle branches to finally arrive at the Purkinje fibres. The time it takes an impulse from the SA node to reach the Purkinje fibres is represented as the P–R interval (significant in some heart blocks). The Purkinje fibres give rise to ventricular depolarisation (which leads to ventricular contraction), represented on the ECG as the QRS complex. The T wave soon follows which reflects repolarisation of the ventricles (i.e. the heart returning to its resting phase).

The whole PQRST sequence portrays the electrical activity related to the systolic phase of the heart's activity. The space between beats is known as repolarisation or diastolic phase (resting phase) of the heart, in which the arteries of the body are perfused and oxygen is exchanged for carbon dioxide at cellular level.

The sequence of the ECG can be affected prior to, during or following surgery. The rate of discharge of the SA node can increase because of disease (heart failure, hypertension), blood loss, pain, stress or anxiety. The SA node may reduce its rate of discharge as a result of overprescription of certain drugs (digoxin) or a lack of oxygen supply. Abnormal rhythms can occur from heart failure, coronary artery disease, myocardial infarction, arteriosclerosis, fluid overload, fluid and electrolyte imbalance.

Pulses

There are many points on the body at which an artery surfaces over a bony protrusion and where a pulse can be felt. The main pulses are apical, radial, carotid, femoral, brachial, aortic, popliteal, dorsalis pedis (Braddy 1989). By feeling these pulses, a surgical nurse can determine if a pulse is present, absent or irregular, strong and equal or faint and equal (Braddy 1989). Any weakness or abnormal sounds, a bounding feeling as if there is a great pressure within the artery, whether the pulse is fast, slow or irregular will all give the nurse indications as to whether the circulation of an area is inadequate or oversupplied.

Oxygen saturation to determine hypoxia

As previously mentioned, a decrease in oxygen (hypoxia) can cause vasoconstriction of blood vessels and thus redistribute the circulating volume. The nurse is frequently the first to observe the presence of hypoxia and the one who can intervene to correct the problem with oxygenation (Masasi & Keyes 1994). Cells require oxygen to survive, function correctly, and maintain tissues. Hypoxia can be due to a reduced blood flow as in arteriosclerosis, the loss of red blood cells as in haemorrhage, or the inability to get oxygen into the circulation as in patients with impaired respiratory function.

A surgical nurse can observe for hypoxia in a number of ways. There may be changes in behaviour and level of consciousness. The brain needs a steady supply of oxygenated blood and is a sensitive indicator of a patient's perfusion status. Very early signs of cerebral underperfusion are the inability to think abstractly or perform complex mental tasks, restlessness, apprehension, uncooperativeness, and irritability. Short-term memory may also be impaired. A family member may need to be called upon for documentation of the patient's normal personality and intellectual status. In addition, there may be changes in BP, pulse, colour of mucous membranes (Masasi & Keyes 1994). This may lead the surgical nurse to extend the assessment for hypoxia by obtaining an oxygen saturation measurement to determine the amount of oxygen that the cells are receiving. The measurement of oxygen saturation in surgical patients is becoming more frequent and it is recommended for all patients for a short time following surgery. This may be unrealistic, however, owing to the lack of resources and availability of equipment.

Mental state

Apart from oxygenation causing a deterioration in mental state, haemorrhage is a potent stimulus to adrenal medullary secretion. Circulating noradrenaline is increased, owing to the increased discharge of sympathetic adrenergic neurons. The resultant increase in circulating catecholamines may contribute to the generalised vasoconstriction in haemorrhagic shock, and may lead to stimulation of the brain's reticular formation, which regulates respiration, BP, heart rate and consciousness, and modulates sensory input. This stimulation may be responsible for some patients in haemorrhagic shock being restless and apprehensive. The restlessness increases motor activity, respiratory movements and the muscular and thoracic pumping of venous blood, which may help to compensate for the continued reduction in cardiac output from continuous bleeding. However, other patients are quiet and apathetic and their senses become dulled, probably as a result of cerebral ischaemia and acidosis.

SUPPORTING THE CIRCULATION IN A SURGICAL PATIENT

When considering support for the circulation in a surgical patient, it is necessary to ascertain whether the

---

Reflective point

You may like to reflect on the following questions:

1. Why are cardiac observations so important to the surgical patient?
2. What are the factors that can cause a reduction in circulating volume in the surgical patient?

---

patient is taking any medications that are already involved in supporting the circulation. If damage to the circulation has occurred during or following surgery, there needs to be effective clinical management of bleeding, to ensure the rapid establishment of fluid volume replacement and maintenance, and the control of haemorrhage. The immediate restoration of an effective circulating blood volume through the use of blood, a balanced salt solution, colloid solution, or all three, to minimise or reverse hypovolaemic shock, is needed.

The current concepts of fluid resuscitation are complex and full of controversy. There are constant discussions about whether whole blood, colloid or crystalloid therapy should be given in hypovolaemic shock. It might be easy to just propose that blood be given for haemorrhage, colloids be given for plasma loss and crystalloid for dehydration. However, even though it can be argued that this is rational and logical, it is much too simplistic. In this discussion, the objective is not to be conclusive one way or another, but rather to elucidate for the surgical nurse the current theories surrounding different types of fluid replacement therapy.

Drug therapy

The most common drugs used to support the circulation are angiotensin-converting enzyme (ACE) inhibitors, diuretics and digoxin.

Angiotensin-converting enzyme (ACE) inhibitors

Angiotensin-converting enzyme inhibitors are recommended for all patients who have left ventricular failure, unless a specific contraindication exists (Janowski 1996). ACE inhibitors work by relaxing blood vessels, thus making it easier for the heart to pump blood. If a patient on a surgical ward is prescribed any of these drugs (e.g. captopril, enalapril) the nurse should be aware that it may cause hypotension and coughing, and also that it should be administered 1 hour before meals, as food decreases its absorption (Yocone-Morton 1995). Despite the benefits of ACE inhibitors, Konstam & Dracup (1994) found that they are often under-used or prescribed in inadequate dosages because of clinicians' concerns about lowering BP too drastically and their lack of knowledge about the positive effects of these drugs on survival. Nevertheless, if given at optimal doses they can be very effective in patients who present with fatigue or mild breathlessness on exertion but no other symptoms of volume overload (Janowski 1996).

Diuretics

Diuretics help to remove excess fluid and sodium from the body and ultimately reduce the stress on the heart. They may be necessary because of heart failure or owing to fluid overload following intravenous (i.v.) therapy. Thiazide diuretics are indicated for mild volume overload and loop diuretics for more severe volume overload (Janowski 1996). The dosage should be based on the patient's age, size, renal function, sodium intake, and degree of oedema (Cuddy 1995, Fox 1996). The nurse's role in administering these diuretics is to check laboratory reports for abnormalities in sodium and potassium levels, as certain thiazide (chlorothiazide, chlorthalidone) and loop diuretics (bumetanide, frusemide) do not spare sodium and potassium, and levels can become depleted. Observe for arrhythmias, muscular pains or cramps. With diuretics that are potassium-sparing (e.g. amiloride, spironolactone) it is important to observe for hyperkalaemia, and therefore any subsequent irregularities in heart beat, numbness or tingling in hands or feet, shortness of breath or unusual tiredness (Konstam & Dracup 1994). With all diuretic therapy the nurse should monitor the patient for signs of dehydration, dry mouth, increased thirst, confusion or irritability (Yacone-Morton 1995).

Digoxin

Digoxin improves myocardial contractility by enhancing the strength (inotropic action) of cardiac contractions (Yacone-Morton 1995). In this way, less blood remains in the ventricles during diastole, and more is pumped into the coronary arteries. This increases the oxygen and nutrients reaching the heart's muscular walls. Digoxin is the most commonly prescribed of the inotropic agents, and the one surgical nurses are most likely to encounter. In addition to being used for heart failure, digoxin is given to control tachycardias, such as those seen in atrial fibrillation (Oh 1990). In patients with severe heart failure, digoxin should be started immediately; in severe cases ACE inhibitors and diuretics may be added.

Prior to giving digoxin, the nurse should monitor:

- the patient's heart rate to ascertain that it is above 60 b.p.m.
- for any signs of digoxin toxicity (e.g. confusion, agitation, gastrointestinal upset, loss of appetite and arrhythmias)
- potassium levels.

The potassium level is important for if it is lower than normal the digoxin dosage can have twice the effect (Cuddy 1995). This is specifically important if the patient is on a thiazide or loop diuretic in addition to digoxin.

It is important to note that prior to, during and following surgery the patient's drug therapy may be discontinued. Despite its being resumed as soon as possible afterwards, there are certain risks involved that the surgical nurse needs to keep in mind, for example raised BP if the patient is on antihypertensive drug therapy, atrial fibrillation in patients on digoxin, chest pain in patients on cardiac drugs, etc. If at any time medication is withheld, it is the surgical nurse's role to monitor the patient closely (Nash & Jensen 1994).

Blood transfusion therapy

The human cardiovascular system is designed to minimise the effects of blood loss. However, the body can compensate for only so much blood loss. Losses of 15–30% cause pallor and weakness; a loss of more than 30% of blood volume results in severe shock, and can be fatal (Marieb 1995). To treat haemorrhage during or following surgery, whole blood should be used as routine, especially when blood loss is substantial. Packed red cells (whole blood from which most of the plasma has been removed) are generally only used to treat anaemia (Marieb 1995). Fresh-frozen plasma (FFP) should never be used as a volume expander in this situation (Glover & Powell 1996). It is better to use FFP for patients with bleeding disorders in which there is a deficiency in platelets or clotting factors, e.g. in disseminated intravascular coagulation (DIC), warfarin overdose, trauma or thrombotic thrombocytopenia. Table 25.1 provides a more detailed account of blood products.

Blood groups

There are many blood group systems, but clinically the most important of these are the ABO, rhesus and human leukocyte antigen systems.

Table 25.1   Current blood products – each donation of blood can provide some or all of the following

Product	Comments
Whole blood (510 ± 45 ml)	Use is restricted to situations where red blood cells as well as plasma proteins are needed, i.e. where there is extensive blood loss. Therefore, it is ideal in hypovolaemic shock, since it both increases oxygen-carrying capacity and expands circulating volume
Packed red cells (280 ± 60 ml)	This is whole blood from which most of the plasma has been removed. Thus, it has half the volume of whole blood, and contains less sodium, potassium, albumin and citrate. However, it does contain some white blood cells and platelets. It is ideal in chronic anaemia, sickle cell disease, thalassaemia and renal disease. It is not recommended in iron deficiency and vitamin B_{12} or folate deficiency. These should be treated with the appropriate supplement, e.g. iron tablets
Washed packed cells	These are packed red cells with all the white blood cells, platelets and plasma removed. They are used for patients who have a long history of transfusion reactions
Fresh-frozen plasma (FFP) (200–300 ml)	This is a blood product which is nearly always frozen. It contains all the coagulation factors; thus it is used for the treatment of coagulation deficits. It should not be used as a volume expander, except in certain neonatal conditions
Cryoprecipitate (20 ± 5 ml)	This is prepared from FFP and contains mainly clotting factors (factor VIII and fibrinogen). It is used to treat haemophilia or AIDS patients
Platelets (50 ± 10 ml)	These are produced from the residue left over from the production of plasma and leukocyte-depleted red cell concentrates. Indications for use are thrombocytopenia, when the platelet content of blood is reduced by bleeding or diluted following massive transfusions, in acute leukaemias, aplastic anaemia, DIC or sepsis

The ABO system. The ABO system is the most common blood grouping system (Campbell 1993). In it, blood is divided into four main groups: A, B, AB, and O. The blood group of a person is determined by the presence or absence of A or B antigen on the red cells (Glover & Powell 1996). Group O, in which there are no antigens on the red cell, is the most commonly occurring blood group in the UK.

The rhesus system. The rhesus system, the second common blood grouping system, uses an antigen identified in the 1940s in the blood of rhesus monkeys (Campbell 1993). The red blood cells, in addition to the A and B antigens, express a D antigen. This factor is present or absent and is termed Rh D positive or negative. The Rh D positive strain comprises approximately 85% of the western population (Glover & Powell 1996). The rest of the population who are Rh D negative have no antigen and therefore have no naturally occurring Rh D antibody. This antibody, however, can be produced after exposure to the Rh D antigen, following a blood transfusion of Rh D positive blood to a person who is Rh D negative, or during pregnancy, when the mother is Rh D negative and the baby is Rh D positive (Glover & Powell 1996).

Human leukocyte antigen (HLA) system. White blood cells also have inherited antigens on their surface. This system of human leukocyte antigens (HLA) is more complex than the ABO system and is used, in addition to the ABO system, for 'tissue typing' to determine compatibility for bone marrow or organ transplantation (Glover & Powell 1996). Antibodies to HLA can be produced by some recipients of multiple transfusion, causing transfusion reactions (Prichard & Mallett 1993).

The changes that occur in stored blood

At present, blood is collected from a donor under strict aseptic conditions in a plastic vacuum container and then mixed with an appropriate anticoagulant solution, such as citrate phosphate dextrose (CPD) or oxalate salts, which prevents clotting by binding with calcium ions (Ala 1988). The blood can then be stored under refrigeration for up to 3 weeks at a temperature of 1–6°C until it is needed for transfusion.

Various changes occur in blood as a result of its removal from the body. These changes, which begin within 24 hours of storage, and continue throughout the entire storage period, are many and varied, and have implications for nursing practice.

Acid–base changes.   Because blood is stored in an air-free container, aerobic metabolism cannot take place, but anaerobic metabolism does occur, with the end products of lactic and pyruvic acids. Therefore, the longer a unit of blood is stored, the greater will be the amount of acid end-products it contains. The CPD solution used as an anticoagulant adds another acid component to banked blood, immediately reducing a normal body pH of 7.4 to about 7.0. Then, the accumulation of metabolic acids decreases the pH of stored blood to about 6.6–6.8 after 14–21 days of storage (Ellerbe 1981).

Alterations in electrolyte concentration.   When blood is stored, the sodium and potassium concentrations change. It can be expected that a unit of stored blood will contain approximately 75–80 mEq of sodium and 5–7 mEq of potassium (Contreras 1992). Patients with normal cardiac and renal function are more likely to be able to handle such an increase in sodium and potassium. However, in patients with profound cardiac and renal dysfunction, the sodium and potassium content of stored blood may have profound effects.

During blood storage there is also a progressive loss of red cell viability and the red blood cells tend to take up water (Marieb 1995). This can cause a leftward shift in the oxyhaemoglobin dissociation curve and cause transfused red cells to be less capable than normal cells of releasing oxygen to the tissues. While the data are by no means complete, it can at least be seen that there is the need for concern about the ability of transfused stored blood to deliver oxygen to the tissues in an efficient manner.

The microaggregate load in stored blood.   Another significant change that occurs in blood during storage is an increased aggregation of platelets and leukocytes. This phenomenon has been recognised by practitioners for many years, and blood has been filtered through 170-micron filters to remedy it. However, electron microscope studies have now clearly identified the formation of microemboli that are considerably smaller than 170 microns (Ellerbe 1981), which has implications in adult respiratory distress syndrome (ARDS). For this reason, microfilters with pore sizes ranging from 20–90 microns have been developed and tested. However, because those conditions which require massive blood transfusions are generally emergencies, it is extremely difficult, if not impossible, to prove that the use of microfilters during massive blood transfusions decreases the development of ARDS. Nevertheless, until clinical data are available, it is recommended that microfilters be used when large quantities of blood are being administered to patients, especially those with compromised pulmonary or cardiac status, as well as in infants and small children (Contreras 1992). If it is decided not to use a microfilter during transfusion, the surgical nurse must carefully assess the respiratory status of all patients receiving blood, and quickly report any changes.

Depletion of clotting factors.   Stored blood is deficient in most of the factors necessary for normal coagulation; it is specifically deficient in factors V, VIII, IX, and platelets (Ellerbe 1981). However, the depletion of platelets and clotting factors varies widely from patient to patient. Because of this, it is recommended that the patient's clotting screen and bleeding status be closely monitored during transfusion, and platelets and fresh-frozen plasma administered when required.

The temperature of stored blood.   Blood is stored at a temperature of between 1–6°C which is considerably colder than human blood. The infusion of large quantities of cold blood can cause patients to become hypothermic. This compromises the patient's heart rate, BP, cardiac output, and coronary blood flow. The first organ to be exposed to a stream of cold blood is the heart. In addition, hypothermia impairs the metabolism of citrate and lactate, and increases the patient's risk of a metabolic acidosis, it increases the affinity of haemoglobin for oxygen, may impair clotting, and impairs the possibility of detecting a major transfusion reaction.

In response to these findings, warming coils and controlled-temperature baths have been developed to warm blood safely. It is important to point out that when blood is given over the normal 3- to 4-hour period, it will probably warm sufficiently to prevent complications. However, for infants and small children, patients with pre-transfusion hypothermia, patients paralysed or anaesthetised or for some other reason unable to maintain their own body temperature, even a single unit of blood should be passed through a warming coil (Contreras 1992).

Blood transfusion reactions

When mismatched blood is infused, a transfusion reaction occurs and the donor and recipient's red blood cells are attacked by the recipient's immune system. This can occur with the infusion of as little as 10–15 ml of incompatible blood (Gloe 1991). The red blood cells are consequently destroyed by the body's own immune system. This causes a reduction in the capacity of red blood cells to carry oxygen. Obstruction to blood flow can also occur as result of agglutination of red cells, causing organ damage which is lethal (Brozovic 1988). Transfusion reactions can also cause fever, chills, nausea, vomiting and general lethargy, but these are rarely lethal (Marieb 1995). As is commonly known, reactions do not occur immediately against the foreign antibody, but on the second encounter there is a typical transfusion reaction.

Because the administration of blood and blood products is an area of nursing practice, the surgical nurse has to be vigilant, both in checking the correct blood group and Rh D antigen factor and in observing for any signs of transfusion reactions. Frequent observations will enable the nurse to detect reactions at an early stage; signs include discomfort, flushing, rash or pain (Glover & Powell 1996).

Colloid versus crystalloid therapy

Despite blood transfusions being valuable, they are at times scarce, expensive or frustratingly slow to appear in times of crisis (Napier 1988). In addition, there are many complications associated with blood transfusion (see above) and the more recent problems of contracting viral infections such as hepatitis B and HIV/AIDS (McCelland 1988). Even though many surgeons still prefer to replace blood loss with equal volumes of whole blood, there are others who prefer to take a more rational approach to treatment. It is suggested that by doing this the patient's defined needs are met more efficiently, safely and economically (Ala 1988). Therefore, other therapies and treatments have become widespread, but with them also dissension. The conflict generally arises from the use of colloid solutions (human albumin solution, Gelofusin, plasma protein fractions, salt-poor albumin, Haemacel and Hespan) or crystalloid solutions (5% dextrose, normal saline, dextrose saline). For a more detailed description of these products see Table 25.2.

The purpose of using colloids in haemorrhage is to achieve the overall primary goal of restoring plasma volume, therefore improving or maintaining oxygen transport (Ramsey 1988). According to this principle, haemodynamic stability is achieved by increasing the blood volume with plasma expanders, and thus providing adequate oxygen and nutrients which are needed for the maintenance and restoration of cellular function. This is regarded as imperative, because inadequate circulatory blood volume causes pooling of blood in the microcirculation, the major effect being a marked decrease in venous return and a diminished cardiac output (Winslow 1997). Therefore,

by administering plasma expanders there is an improvement in oxygen availability, oxygen consumption, circulating volume, haemodynamic status and tissue perfusion.

However, these views are not supported by Ellerbe (1981) who found equal evidence to support the argument for giving crystalloid in haemorrhage. The main rationale for this is that during and following hypovolaemic shock, sodium leaks into the surrounding cells and carries with it extracellular water (Meyers & Hickey 1988); therefore there needs to be a balanced use of a salt solution to restore extracellular fluid volume. A failure to do so will increase the mortality and morbidity of shock due to injury. Nevertheless, it is argued, that irrespective of how and why sodium leaks into cells during shock, the restoration of normal cellular function requires the action of the energy-dependent adenosine triphosphate (ATP) to generate the sodium pump, which can only be achieved by administering colloids (Ala 1988).

If crystalloids are to be used as the primary resuscitative agents following shock, the volumes required to achieve normal haemodynamic values are from two to four times those required with colloids (Ramsey 1988). Furthermore, it is suggested that massive crystalloid fluid resuscitation predisposes the patient to acute respiratory distress syndrome (ARDS) or pulmonary oedema, which is alleged to be negligible with colloid therapy. This is confirmed by Winslow (1997) who suggests that resuscitation with crystalloid alone dilutes the plasma proteins, thereby reducing osmotic pressure, encouraging fluid to shift from the intracellular to the extracellular compartments and predisposing to the development of pulmonary oedema. However, there is evidence emerging that appears to indicate that the use of albumin also puts the patient at risk of developing pulmonary insufficiency and ARDS.

Considerable controversy continues to surround the choice of colloids or crystalloid for resuscitation from hypovolaemic shock and injury states in surgical patients. Each of the fluids identified for use has physiological advantages and disadvantages. However, to make sense of this complex set of arguments and counter-arguments, it is necessary to have an overview of the sequence of shock. It appears that in shock there is a reduction in circulating volume; this stimulates the release of noradrenaline, which decreases the supply of fluid to the muscle beds by vasoconstriction, causing hypoxia. Hypoxia decreases ATP production within the cell, without which the cell membrane sodium pump is disarmed. This shifts extracellular water and sodium to intracellular water and sodium, which in turn further reduces circulating volume. With

Table 25.2 The colloid and crystalloid infusions available (Edwards 1998)

Product	Comments
Colloid infusions	All function in the same way. They add fluid with a higher osmolality to the extracellular fluid. This draws water from the intracellular fluid to reach a new equilibrium, which serves to further increase extracellular volume
Human albumin solution (HAS)	This comes in two concentrations, 4.5% solution available in 50 ml, 100 ml and 500 ml bottles and a highly concentrated 20% solution available in 50 ml and 100 ml bottles. The HAS 4.5% solution has an osmotic pressure of 26–30 mmHg and is used as a plasma expander. The HAS 20% solution has an osmotic pressure of 100–120 mm Hg and is used in cases of hypoalbuminaemia due to renal disease, liver disease, acute pancreatitis and sepsis. 100 ml of 20% albumin solution loads the patient with no more than 16 mmol of sodium and is useful when sodium restrictions are necessary. Human albumin solution is manufactured from blood plasma and so is more expensive than the synthetic alternatives
Haemacel	3.5% solution of gelatine. It is much cheaper, more stable and has a longer shelf life than HAS and salt-poor albumin. There are generally no adverse reactions or adverse effects on coagulation. It contains calcium and therefore cannot be given in the same line as blood because it will cause coagulation in the line
Gelofusin	Similar to Haemacel, but does not contain calcium; therefore it can be run through with blood in the same line
Dextran	This comes in two solutions – Dextran 40 and Dextran 70. It is a polysaccharide, and is stable, non-toxic and non-pyrogenic. Its use is limited as it has several problems: it can interfere with haemostasis by reducing platelet adhesiveness; can cause disseminated intravascular coagulation (DIC); anaphylactic reactions can occur; and it can cause blockage of the renal tubules resulting in acute renal failure
Hespan	This is a 6% starch solution produced from hydrolysis of corn. It is similar to Dextran 70 and has the same problems with its use. In addition, it can block the reticuloendothelial system for months following infusion
Perfluorocarbons (synthetic blood derivatives)	These are unrelated to blood, but are able to transport oxygen in solution and are being investigated as an oxygen-carrying substitute. They will be valuable in patients who refuse human blood transfusion, carbon monoxide poisoning and sickle cell crisis
Crystalloid infusions	These work in different ways to maintain osmotic equilibrium
0.9% sodium chloride (normal saline)	Contains sodium and chloride; it has no calories at all. It has approximately the same osmolality as both intracellular and extracellular fluids, therefore it will increase mainly extracellular volume with no significant increase in intracellular volume
5% dextrose	Contains only 200 calories per litre. It adds water to the extracellular compartment and thus reduces the osmolality of extracellular fluid. This allows water to pass into the intracellular fluid to reach equilibrium. There is no real effect on the extracellular volume as the dextrose solution does not stay in the circulation
4% dextrose 0.18% sodium chloride	Contains a combination of both of the above

the cellular nutrient transport mechanism of the extracellular fluid impaired, biochemical disruption and cell death ensues. Therefore, in shocked states, it seems necessary to administer a combination of colloids and crystalloid. In addition, it should not be forgotten that it is also imperative that the patient's cardiopulmonary dynamics be monitored in a way that is reliable to determine physiological trends and responses to whichever therapy is finally chosen (see also Ch. 26).

Reflective point

What are the different options available to maintain adequate circulation in a surgical patient?

AN OVERADEQUATE CIRCULATION IN THE SURGICAL PATIENT

Following fluid therapy, the patient is in danger of becoming overloaded with circulating fluid. This can be due to whole blood transfusion, fresh frozen plasma, plasma expanders (e.g. human serum albumin, Gelofusin, dextran) or aqueous solutions (e.g. normal saline, dextrose saline, 5% dextrose).

Reflective point

Revisit the assessment criteria suggested earlier in relation to reduced or inadequate circulation on page 514 and consider how they will be different in a surgical patient with overadequate circulation.

The pathophysiological aspects of hypervolaemia

In all cases of hypervolaemia there is an increased volume in the circulation. This causes pressure on the chemoreceptors and vasodilatation takes place. The BP at this point may be either normal or slightly elevated. As volume continues to increase further, the action of the chemoreceptors can no longer initiate further vasodilatation (McCance & Huether 1994). The BP may initially increase, but eventually as the signs of an overloaded circulation begin to show, together with cardiac failure, this also may fall. If this becomes severe, cardiogenic shock may ensue.

Hypervolaemia due to an overload of blood products

The consequences of overloading the circulation in this way are that the blood velocity reduces and blood flow becomes slow. This in turn causes pooling of blood in the peripheries, lungs, liver, kidneys and possibly the brain. The heart can no longer pump the increasing volume around the circulation. As the signs of heart failure increase and the kidneys become swamped with fluid and start to receive a lower blood supply, renal failure ensues. The complications of pulmonary oedema, cardiac failure, renal failure, ascites, cerebral oedema and peripheral oedema can be very serious if not treated quickly.

In the majority of cases when a blood transfusion is being administered, a diuretic is given either with each unit or with alternate units. A diuretic is even more necessary in patients who are susceptible to problems with maintaining an adequate circulation, to prevent complications with circulatory overload.

Hypervolaemia caused by water overload

Straightforward fluid overload with normal saline and 5% dextrose can cause similar problems but for different reasons. When the body is functioning normally, it is almost impossible to produce an excess of total body water. However, this can occur during i.v. treatment with normal saline or 5% dextrose, either during or following surgery. It can also occur, even though rarely, in some individuals with psychogenic disorders from compulsive water drinking (McCance & Huether 1994). The effects can be an overload of both salt and water (isotonic volume excess) or just salt (hypertonic volume excess) or a dilutional low sodium concentration (hypotonic volume excesses).

Isotonic volume excess

Isotonic volume excess is most commonly the result of excessive administration of a combination of intravenous fluids, culminating in an overload of both salt and water. As the circulating volume increases, the symptoms of hypervolaemia develop. There will be weight gain and a decrease in haematocrit and plasma proteins caused by the diluting effect of the excess volume. The neck veins may distend, and the increased BP leads to oedema formation. If the circulating volume is big enough, pulmonary oedema and heart failure may develop. This can lead to circulatory collapse, in which the left side of the heart becomes dysfunctional with the consequence of the heart becoming unable to pump blood out, giving rise to a low cardiac output and an increase in right and left ventricular filling pressures (Yacone-Morton 1995).

Hypertonic volume excess

Hypertonic volume excess is most commonly the result of an inappropriate administration of hypertonic saline solution (e.g. sodium bicarbonate or normal saline). A primary increase in extracellular sodium causes an osmotic attraction of water and intracellular dehydration ensues. The symptoms of oedema, weight gain and of general hypervolaemia occur, convulsions and pulmonary oedema being the most serious.

Hypotonic volume excess

Hypotonic volume excess generally occurs when there has been a replacement of fluid loss with intravenous 5% dextrose in water. This is known as a dilutional hyponatraemia (low sodium) and can cause weight gain, oedema, ascites, and jugular vein distension.

THE NURSE'S ROLE IN MAINTAINING ADEQUATE CIRCULATION IN A SURGICAL PATIENT

This chapter has focused on the surgical nurse's role in maintaining an adequate circulation. However, there are a few implications that have not yet been mentioned – those concerning documentation and patient education.

Documentation

Ongoing assessment, awareness and knowledge of those patients at risk from circulation disorders are essential. Even if an individual appears to have no circulation problems at the initial assessment, it is necessary to be always aware of the potential for circulatory disaster (e.g. bleeding disorders, hypovolaemia, dehydration). If the patient is showing signs of circulatory failure (see p. 511), referral to the doctor is essential. By observation and continuous documentation, a pattern may appear which may serve to prevent a severe case of circulatory failure. The problem can be identified early and treatment instigated quickly and efficiently.

If the patient's fluid intake becomes inadequate or low, or nausea, vomiting, diarrhoea or constipation occurs, then reasons for these changes should always be investigated. It may be simply that the patient does not like the water, the analgesia prescribed is causing nausea or the patient has not been to the toilet following operation. Whatever the cause, identifying it will give a pointer to the solution. All these factors should be recorded in the patient's nursing care plan to prevent serious cases of dehydration.

Documentation of BP, heart rate, temperature, urine output, urinalysis, etc. should be made and attention paid to the patient's peripheral pulses. The specific gravity of urine should be analysed, and fluid balance carefully monitored, documenting all i.v. fluids, urine output and other drainage from wound drains or wounds. There may seem to be a great deal of information in relation to the circulation to write down. However, the right amount of documentation and updating required is a judgement which involves a balance between what can be achieved and the priorities set. The nursing record is a professional document and the nurse is expected to maintain records to professionally acceptable standards. These carefully kept records are necessary for communication and continuity of care, especially where more than one nurse is involved with a patient's care.

Patient education

Surgical nurses are increasingly seeing for themselves a role as health promoters within their practice. A survey undertaken by Maidwell (1996) showed that surgical nurses saw part of their role as involving health promotion. This role is considered important and essential to nursing in surgical settings (see Ch. 3).

In addition to maintaining adequate circulation, nurses can also play an important role in helping patients with circulatory problems, whether such problems existed prior to surgery or developed as a complication of the surgery performed. As soon as the patient is admitted, education can start (Janowski 1996). As patients can sometimes wait for up to a year for elective surgery, Maidwell (1996) suggests that some of the time spent waiting should be used in a constructive way to improve their knowledge and skills about a healthy lifestyle. This might help prevent the occurrence of disorders of the circulation in the future. Many studies have documented how preoperative teaching can help to relieve patients' fears and anxieties, decrease their stress levels, enhance their psychological well-being, and promote their postoperative recovery (Chansky 1984, Moss 1986, Rabb 1986, Simms 1988). Both the patient and the family can be informed about drug regimens, dietary restriction, e.g. of sodium, exercise, the complications involved and the prognosis.

Reflective point

If you were negotiating for future-oriented education provision for surgical nurses in the area of both patient education and direct care linked to circulatory problems, what specifications would you require from education providers?

CONCLUSION

Problems with the circulation are being seen with increased frequency in health care settings today. It is imperative that surgical nurses have a clear understanding of peripheral and systemic circulation and the mechanisms that influence them, as well as the pathophysiological changes that accompany common diseases of these systems. The surgical nurse uses assessment to determine whether a problem with the circulation is present, establish if it is acute or chronic in nature, monitor progression, plan care and document findings. It is imperative that, if a problem is identified, intervention and treatment are instigated immediately. The role of the nurse is then to assess and evaluate the response to treatment and prevent complications. This process is ongoing and is an important role for the surgical nurse in order to preserve function, life, and limb in patients with circulatory problems.

REFERENCES

Abbey J, Anderson A, Close E 1978 How long is that thermometer accurate? American Journal of Nursing 78(8): 1375–1376

Ala F A 1988 Red cell components – plasma proteins and albumin: current transfusion cocktails. Care of the Critically Ill 4(4): 14–21

Angerami E 1980 Epidemiological study of body temperature in patients in a teaching hospital. International Journal of Nursing Studies 17(2): 91–99

Bardwell J 1995 For good measure. Nursing Times 91(27): 40–41

Baxendale L M 1992 Pathophysiology of coronary artery disease. Nursing Clinics of North America 27(1): 143–151

Bell T N 1992 Coagulation and disseminated intravascular coagulation. In: Huddleston V B Multisystem organ failure: pathophysiology and clinical implications. Mosby, St Louis

Binnie A, Bond S, Law G et al 1988 A systematic approach to nursing care: an introduction. The Open University, Milton Keynes

Blank C A, Irwin G H 1990 Peripheral vascular disease. Advances in Physical Assessment 25(4): 777–793

Bloch H 1992 Historic development of circulation. Heart and Lung 21(5): 411–414

Braddy P K 1989 Cardiac assessment tool. Critical Care Nurse 9(9): 71–72, 74, 76–81

Brislen W, Smart G I, Collins A 1976 Assessment of a single-use clinical thermometer. Nursing Times 72(6): 235–237

Browse N L et al 1988 Diseases of the veins: pathology, diagnosis and treatment. Edward Arnold, London

Brozovic B 1988 Non-haemolytic transfusion reactions – prevention and management. Care of the Critically Ill 4(4): 6–8

Bruce J, Grove S 1992 Fever: pathology and treatment. Critical Care Nurse 12(1): 40–49

Burnip S J 1991 Why do nurses take blood pressures postoperatively. Surgical Nurse 4(2): 15–19

Burroughs J, Hoffbrand B I 1990 A critical look at nursing observations. Postgraduate Medical Journal 66: 370–372

Callow L, Pieper B 1989 Effects of backrest on central venous pressure in paediatric cardiac surgery. Nursing Research 38: 336–338

Cameron J 1995 Venous and arterial leg ulcers. Nursing Standard 9(26): 25–30

Cameron J 1996 Arterial leg ulcers. Nursing Standard 10(26): 50–53

Campbell J 1993 Making sense of shock. Nursing Times 89(5): 34–36

Chansky E 1984 Reducing patient's anxieties. Anaesthetic and Operating Room Nursing Journal 40: 375–377

Christensen B 1992 Haemodynamic monitoring: what it tells you and what it does not: part 2. Journal of Post Anaesthesia Nursing 7(5): 338–345

Closs S J, Macdonald I A, Hawthorn P J 1986 Factors affecting peri-operative body temperature. Journal of Advanced Nursing 11(6): 739–744

Contreras M 1992 ABC of transfusion, 2nd edn. BMJ Publishing Group, London

Cook R 1995 Urinalysis. Nursing Standard 9(28): 32–37

Cuddy R P 1995 Hypertension: keeping dangerous blood pressure down. Nursing 25(8): 34–43

Cunha B 1985 Significance of fever in the compromised host. Nursing Clinics of North America 20: 163–168

Cunha B, Tu R 1988 Fever in the neurosurgical patient. Heart and Lung 17: 608–611

Cunha B, Digamon-Beltran M, Gobbo P 1984 Implications of fever in the critical care setting. Heart and Lung 13: 460–465

Darovic G O 1987 Hemodynamic monitoring: invasive and noninvasive clinical application. W B Saunders, Philadelphia

Dennison R D 1994 Making sense of haemodynamic monitoring. American Journal of Nursing 94(8): 24–32

Dries D J, Waxman K 1991 Adequate resuscitation of burn patients may not be measured by urine output and vital signs. Critical Care Medicine 19(3): 327–329

Edwards S L 1997 Recording blood pressure. Professional Nurse Study Supplement 13(2): S8–S11

Edwards S L 1998 Hypovolaemia: pathophysiology and management options. Nursing in Critical Care 3(2): 73–82

Edwards S L, Manley K 1998 Care of adults in hospital. In: Hinchliff S M, Norman S E, Schober J E (eds) Nursing practice and health care, 3rd edn. Edward Arnold, London

Ellerbe S (ed) 1981 Fluid and blood component therapy in the critically ill and injured. Churchill Livingstone, New York

Engler M B, Engler M M 1995 Assessment of the cardiovascular effects of stress. Journal of Cardiovascular Nursing 10(1): 51–63

Enright T, Hill M 1989 Treatment of fever. Focus on Critical Care 16: 96–102

Erickson R 1980 Oral temperature differences in relation to thermometer and technique. Nursing Research 29(3): 157–164

Feher M, Harris-St John K, Lant A 1992 Blood pressure measurement by junior hospital doctors – a gap in medical education. Health Trends 24(2): 59–61

Fellows I W, MacDonald I A, Bennett T 1985 The effect of undernutrition on thermoregulation in the elderly. Clinical Science 69(5): 523–532

Fisher M, Raper R 1987 Fever in the intensive care unit. British Journal of Hospital Medicine 38(2): 109–111

Fox K 1996 Hypertension and heart disease. Nursing Standard 10(23): 52

Froelicher E S, Berra K, Stepp C, Saxe J, Deitrich D E 1995 Risk profile screening. Journal of Cardiovascular Nursing 10(1): 30–50

Fulbrook P 1993 Core temperature measurement in adults: a literature review. Journal of Advanced Nursing 18: 365–369

Geddes L A 1970 The direct and indirect measurement of blood pressure. Year Book Medical Publishers, Chicago

Gloe D 1991 Common reactions to transfusions. Heart and Lung 20(5): 506–514

Glover G, Powell F 1996 Blood transfusion. Nursing Standard 10(21): 49–54

Goodwin C W 1984 Burn shock. Clinical Surgical International 9: 71

Griffith C J 1995 Hypertension: evaluation and management … recertification series. Physician Assistant 19(9): 25–28

Gurevich I 1985 Fever: when to worry about it. Registered Nurse 12: 14–17

Guthrie M (ed) 1982 Shock. Churchill Livingstone, New York

Hart L, Dennis S 1988 Two hyperthermias prevalent in the intensive care unit. Focus on Critical Care 15: 49–55

Heidenreich T, Giuffre M 1990 Post operative temperature measurement. Nursing Research 39(3): 153–155

Henneman E A, Henneman P L 1989 Intricacies of blood pressure measurement: reexamining the rituals. Heart and Lung 18(3): 263–273

Hinchliff S, Montague S (eds) 1995 Physiology for nursing practice, 2nd edn. Baillière Tindall, London

Howie J 1989 How and when should I respond to post operative fever? American Journal of Nursing 89(7): 984–986

Janowski M J 1996 Managing heart failure. Registered Nurse (Feb): 34–38

Jenkins S C, Souter S A, Moxham J 1988 The effects of posture on lung volumes in normal subjects and inpatients pre and post coronary artery surgery. Physiotherapy 74: 492–496

Jolly A 1991 Taking a blood pressure. Nursing Times 87(15); 40–43

Jordon S 1992 Reducing hypertension. Nursing Times 88(21): 44–47

Kee L L, Siminson J S, Stotts N A, Skov P, Schiller N B 1998 Echocardiographic determination of valid zero reference levels in supine and lateral positions. American Journal of Critical Care 2: 72–80

Kemp F, Foster C, McKinley S 1994 How effective is training for blood pressure measurement? Professional Nurse 9(8): 521–524

Konstam M, Dracup K 1994 Heart failure: management of patients with left-ventricular systolic dysfunction. Agency for Health Care Policy and Research, Rockville

Krickler J A, Dodge G H 1987 What to do about temperatures. Nursing Standard 14(25): 37–38

Kunel D 1986 The toxic emergency. Emergency Medicine 18: 126–139

Linden B 1995 Severe heart failure: focus on the quality of care. Nursing Times 91(33): 38–39

Lloyd C 1993 Making sense of reagent strip urine testing. Nursing Times 89(48): 32–36

Luckman J, Sorensen K C 1987 Medical–surgical nursing: a psychophysiologic approach, 3rd edn. W B Saunders, Philadelphia

McCance K L, Huether S E 1994 Pathophysiology: the biologic basis for disease in adults and children, 2nd edn. Mosby, St Louis

McCarron K 1986 Fever: the vital cardinal sign. Critical Care Quarterly 9: 15–18

McCelland D B L 1988 Virus infections following transfusion – preventive measures and risk assessment. Care of the Critically Ill 4(4); 9–13

McGovern M, Kuhn J K 1992 Cardiac assessment of the elderly client. Journal of Gerontological Nursing 18(8): 40–44

Maidwell A 1996 The role of the surgical nurse as a health promoter. British Journal of Nursing 5(15): 898–904

Mancia G, Grassi G, Pomidossi G et al 1983 Effects of blood pressure measurement by the doctor on patients' blood pressure and heart rate. Lancet 8(8352): 695–700

Manley K 1991 Central venous pressure: what, why, how? Surgical Nurse 4: 10–13

Marieb E N 1995 Human anatomy and physiology, 3rd edn. Benjamin/Cummings, California

Martin J H, Larsen P D 1994 Dehydration in the elderly surgical patient. Anaesthetic and Operating Room Nursing Journal 60(4): 666–671

Masasi R S, Keyes J L 1994 The pathophysiology of hypoxia. Critical Care Nurse 14(4): 55–64

Meyers K A, Hickey M K 1988 Nursing management of hypovolaemic shock. Critical Care Nursing Quarterly 11(1): 57–67

Miracle V A 1988 Get in touch and in tune with cardiac assessment – part 2. Nursing 18(4): 41–47

Moddeman G 1991 The elderly surgical patient – a risk of hypothermia. American Operating Room Nursing Journal 53(5): 1270–1272

Moorat D S 1976 The cost of taking temperatures. Nursing Times 72(May 20): 767–770

Morley-Forster P K 1986 Unintentional hypothermia in the operating room. Canadian Anaesthetic Society Journal 33: 516–527

Morris R H, Wilkey B R 1970 The effects of ambient temperature on patient temperature during surgery not involving body cavities. Anaesthesiology 32: 102–107

Moss R 1986 Overcoming fear: a review of research on family/patient instruction Anaesthetic and Operating Room Nursing Journal 43(5): 1107–1112

Mravinac C, Dracup K, Clochesy B 1989 Urinary bladder and rectal temperature monitoring during clinical hyperthermia. Nursing Research 38(2): 73–76

Napier T 1988 Blood transfusion in ITU: a risk or a benefit? Care of the Critically Ill 4(4): 5

Nash C A, Jensen P L 1994 When your surgical patient has hypertension. American Journal of Nursing 94(12): 39–44

Nichols G A, Kucha D H 1972 Oral measurements. American Journal of Nursing 72(6): 1091–1092

Nightingale F 1859 Notes on nursing: what it is and what it is not. Blackie, London

Nolan J, Nolan M 1993 Can nurses take an accurate blood pressure? British Journal of Nursing 2(14): 724–729

Nursing Times 1986a Focus on urinalysis – Part 1. Nursing Times 82(17): 1–6

Nursing Times 1986b Focus on urinalysis – Part 6. Nursing Times 82(32): 1–6

Nursing Times 1995 Professional development: blood pressure. Nursing Times 91(15): 5–8

O'Brien D, Davison M 1994 Blood pressure measurement: rational and ritual actions. British Journal of Nursing 3(8): 393–396

Oh T E (ed) 1990 Intensive care manual, 3rd edn. Butterworths, Sydney

Pickering T G 1994 Blood pressure measurement and detection of hypertension. Lancet 344(2 July): 31–35

Potger K C, Elliott D 1994 Haemodynamic monitoring. Heart and Lung 23(4): 285–299

Prichard A P, Mallett J (eds) 1993 The Royal Marsden Hospital manual of clinical nursing procedures, 3rd edn. Blackwell Scientific Publications, Oxford

Pugh-Davies S, Kassab J, Thrush A, Smith P A 1986 A comparison of mercury and digital clinical thermometers. Journal of Advanced Nursing 11(5): 535–543

Rabb D 1986 Patient education relieves pre-operative fears. Health Care Journal 27: 38–40

Ramsey G 1988 Intravenous volume replacement: indications and choices. British Medical Journal 296(6634): 1422–1423

Rice V 1991 Shock, a clinical syndrome: an update. Part 3. Critical Care Nurse 11(6): 34–41

Rich J 1983 Hypothermia in surgical patients. British Journal of Nursing 1(11): 539–435

Rushmer R F 1970 Cardiovascular dynamics. W B Saunders, Philadelphia

Shaver J, Camarata G, Taleisnik A, Gazzaniga A B 1984 Changes in epicardial and core temperatures during resuscitation of haemorrhagic shock. Journal of Trauma 24(11): 957–963

Shephard T J, Fox S W 1996 Assessment and management of hypertension in the acute ischaemic stroke patient. Journal of Neuroscience Nursing 28(1): 5–12

Simms G 1988 Emotional stress and the surgical patient. Surgical Rounds Orthopaedic Journal 2: 37–41

Takacs K M, Valenti W M 1982 Temperature measurement in a clinical setting. Nursing Research 31(6): 368–370

Toms E 1993 Vital observation. Nursing Times 89(51): 32–34

Turner J 1987 Problems of recognising dehydration in hospital patients. Nursing Times 83(51): 44

Venus B, Mathru M, Smith R, Phain C 1985 Direct versus indirect blood pressure measurements in critically ill patients. Heart and Lung 14: 228–231

Walsh M, Ford P 1989 Nursing rituals: research and rational actions. Butterworth-Heinemann, Oxford

Winslow R M 1997 Blood substitutes. Science and Medicine 4(2): 54–64

Wood M H 1996 Current considerations in patients with coexistent diabetes and hypertension. Nurse Practitioner 21(4): 19–20

Yacone-Morton L A 1991 Perfecting the art: cardiac assessment. Registered Nurse 54(12): 28–35

Yacone-Morton L A 1995 First-line therapy for CHF. Registered Nurse (Feb): 38–43

26

Fluid and electrolyte balance

Hilary Fanning

AIMS

The aims of this chapter are to enable the surgical nurse to:

- describe the physiological mechanisms of fluid and electrolyte balance
- appreciate the factors contributing to disturbance of fluid and electrolyte balance in the surgical patient, and the manifestations of these disturbances
- identify nursing interventions pertinent to the management of patients with fluid and electrolyte disturbances.

INTRODUCTION

The effect of injury on fluid and electrolyte balance significantly contributes to morbidity and mortality following trauma or surgery. Disturbances of fluid and electrolyte balance include changes in *volume, osmolality* and *electrolyte concentrations* (Goodman & Gilman 1980). In the clinical situation, mixed disturbance of these parameters is usual.

Nurses' need for knowledge of physiological principles on which to base practice has long been recognised, as evidenced by a considerable body of literature on the subject of fluid and electrolytes (Cullen 1992). In the main, the focus of this literature has been to explain the principles of fluid and electrolyte balance, the pathophysiological processes which alter normal homeostatic mechanisms, and the factors which influence fluid and electrolyte therapy. Anecdotal evidence suggests that nurses' direct observation of the patient not only determines efficacy of fluid and electrolyte therapy, but can importantly influence medical decision-making. The extent of this nursing contribution to multidisciplinary care appears to be unexplored in the literature.

Reflective point

Consider the following: On a ward round you are asked for your opinion regarding one of your patient's ability to ingest fluid 2 days postoperatively. This individual has been intermittently nauseated following surgery, and your stated opinion is that he will not be able to tolerate more than 1 litre orally. He is subsequently prescribed parenteral fluid administration. On what was this decision based?

PHYSIOLOGY OF FLUID AND SOLUTE BALANCE

Homeostatic mechanisms have evolved to conserve the volume and composition of body fluids, thereby maintaining the complex internal environment essential for the normal physiology of higher organisms.

Body water

The principal component of all body fluids is water. Body fluids are complex aqueous solutions, in which biochemically distinct compartments are divided by the plasma membrane (between the intracellular and extracellular compartments) or by specialised cell layers (between the intravascular, interstitial and transcellular compartments). Body water accounts for between 50–70% of an adult's total body weight, varying with sex, age and degree of adiposity. Water is gained through ingestion, either as a liquid or as a component of solid foods. Additionally, oxidative metabolism gives rise to endogenous production of water, accounting for some 200–300 ml per day. The normal routes of fluid loss are via the kidneys, gastrointestinal tract, respiratory tract and skin. In the healthy adult, the kidneys excrete approximately 1500–2000 ml of fluid daily, depending on intake. Faecal loss amounts to some 300 ml of fluid per day and losses from the skin and respiratory passages account for approximately 600–1000 ml daily.

Body fluid compartments

There are two major compartments in which body water is present, the intracellular and extracellular compartments, which are divided by the plasma membrane (see Fig. 26.1). In an average male, intracellular and extracellular water constitute approximately 40% and 20% of total body weight respectively.

There are three subdivisions to the extracellular compartment. The intravascular and interstitial compartments, which are separated by capillary endothelium, and a third, quantitatively minor, subdivision, the transcellular compartment. The transcellular compartment is a collection of biochemically distinct fluids including cerebrospinal, synovial, pleural, pericardial, intraocular and peritoneal fluids and digestive

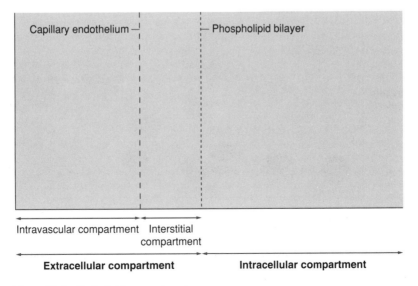

Figure 26.1   Body fluid compartments.

secretions, which have the collective characteristic of being separated from the interstitial compartment by a layer of epithelium. The specialist nature of different epithelia maintain the distinct and often variable composition of these fluids (e.g. gastric epithelium, small intestinal epithelium). This compartment is of small volume compared with the intravascular, interstitial and intracellular compartments; however, it can be greatly increased in certain pathological conditions which the surgical nurse may encounter. These include the development of gastrointestinal obstruction or of ascites. These 'hidden fluid losses' can significantly contribute to fluid and electrolyte depletion in the surgical patient.

Solute composition of body fluid compartments

The solute compositions of the extracellular fluid (ECF) and intracellular fluid (ICF) compartments are shown in Figure 26.2. The major solutes are electrolytes, i.e. products of ionic compound dissociation in solution. Cations carry a positive charge, and anions carry a negative charge. The concentration of electrolytes is measured in milliequivalents per litre (mEq/l) and this is identical to the concentration in millimoles per litre for any substance which is fully ionised in solution. Non-electrolytes are also present, i.e. molecules such as glucose or urea which are uncharged in solution.

The solute compositions of the extracellular and intracellular fluids are markedly different. The main cation of the ECF is sodium (Na^+) whereas the main cation of the ICF is potassium (K^+). The main anions of the ECF are chloride (Cl^-) and bicarbonate (HCO_3^-), and those of the ICF are proteins (which are predominantly negatively charged at physiological pH) and organic phosphates.

Several factors contribute to and maintain the differences in solute composition between the ECF and ICF. In order to pass between the ECF and ICF, a solute must cross the plasma membrane. Free diffusion through the plasma membrane is restricted to those solutes which are non-polar and therefore lipid soluble (for example carbon dioxide, CO_2). The movement of solutes by free diffusion across the phospholipid bilayer of the plasma membrane is driven by concentration differences. The majority of solutes which cross the plasma membrane require some form of assistance to do so. Transmembrane proteins provide this assistance. These proteins passively enhance permeability to a given substance by providing a channel, or pore, for easy passage of water-soluble/lipid-insoluble molecules. Alternatively, a transmembrane protein, for example Na^+/K^+ adenosine triphosphatase (ATPase) can actively transport solutes across the plasma membrane. The energy required for this latter form of transport is derived from the cleavage of a high-energy phosphate bond from adenosine triphosphate (ATP) with adenosine diphosphate (ADP) formation.

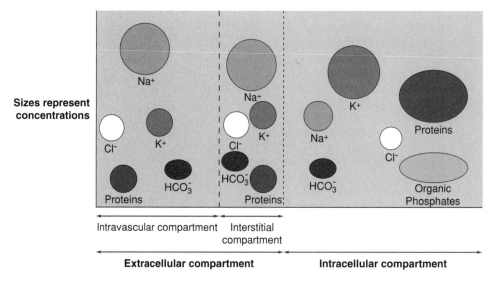

Figure 26.2 Solute composition of body fluid compartments: the sizes of solutes represent their concentration.

The maintenance of stable differences in the concentration of a given ion between extracellular and intracellular compartments requires the expenditure of energy (a consequence of the third law of thermodynamics). This is most easily appreciated in the active transport of Na^+ out of the cell and K^+ into the cell which generates the aforementioned differences in solute concentration as shown in Figure 26.2. This active transport has an equally important secondary effect: as a consequence of the markedly different permeabilty of the plasma membrane to Na^+ and K^+, a transmembrane electrical potential is generated as shown in Figure 26.3A, B and C. The 'resting

membrane potential' has an important role in transducing energy generated by the Na^+/K^+-ATPase, thereby maintaining other transmembrane concentration differences (e.g. Cl^-, Mg^{2+}, Ca^{2+}). The resting membrane potential may also become transiently reversed as a consequence of short-lived changes in ion permeabilty. This is the 'action potential', i.e. a wave of depolarisation seen in nerve cells or muscle cells crucial to their normal function. The action potential can be disrupted by changes in the concentration of relevant ions, most commonly extracellular K^+. Abnormal extracellular concentrations of potassium result in markedly abnormal responses in nerve and muscle

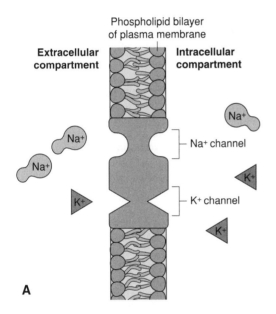

A

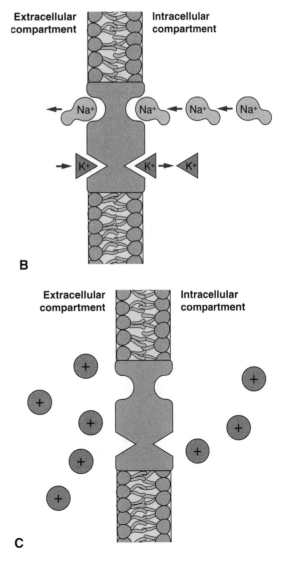

B

C

Figure 26.3 (A) Na^+/K^+-ATPase – a transmembrane protein. (B) Transport of Na^+ and K^+ across the plasma membrane by Na^+/K^+-ATPase. Three Na^+ are transported out of the cell for every two K^+ transported into the cell. (C) Generation of the resting membrane potential. The active transport of $3Na^+$ out of the cell for every $2K^+$ transported into the cell generates a difference in electrical charge across the cell membrane, whereby the inside of the cell is slightly less positive (i.e. negative) in relation to outside the cell. This is the resting membrane potential.

cells to electrical stimulation. Common manifestations of such disruption include, for example, cardiac arryhthmias or altered intestinal motility.

The electrolyte concentrations of the intravascular and interstitial divisions of the ECF are, in contrast, very similar, since the capillary endothelium which separates them allows free passage of water and low molecular weight substances. Movement of larger molecular weight substances such as proteins is restricted by size and electrical charge, as discussed below.

OSMOSIS AND OSMOLALITY

Osmosis is the term used to describe the movement of water through a membrane which is permeable to water but not to solutes, from an area of low solute concentration to one of high solute concentration. If, for example, pure water in a beaker is separated from a highly concentrated water and salt solution by such a membrane, water will flow across the membrane into the salt solution (Fig. 26.4).

Osmotic pressure is the force, measured in osmoles, required to oppose the flow of water along this osmotic gradient. The osmotic pressure generated in a solution is proportional to the number of discrete particles per unit mass of solvent. *Osmolality* is thus a measure of the osmotically active particles in solution for a given unit of mass. *Isosmolal* (or *isotonic*) solutions

will have equal concentrations of osmotically active particles in solution. *Hypo-osmolal* (or *hypotonic*) solutions will have a lower concentration of osmotically active particles than isosmolal solutions, and a *hyper-osmolal* (or *hypertonic*) solution will have a higher concentration of osmotically active particles than an isosmolal solution.

In the example given there will be a large osmotic gradient between the two solutions because of the difference in solute concentration. Therefore, a large osmotic pressure will be required to oppose water movement. It is the concentration of osmotically active solutes in the fluid compartments, and the osmotic pressure which they generate that determines distribution of body water. Solutes which cannot freely move between the fluid compartments generate an effective osmotic pressure within the compartment in which they are contained, and thus influence the movement of water both into and out of that compartment.

REGULATION OF WATER BALANCE

The mechanisms which maintain water balance in the body include hypothalamic regulation of thirst, and regulation of renal excretion of water via hypothalamic–pituitary axis secretion of antidiuretic hormone (ADH). Neural control centres for thirst are closely associated with those that regulate ADH secretion.

The primary stimulus for release of ADH from the posterior lobe of the pituitary is elevation of plasma osmolality; a secondary stimulus is depletion of plasma volume. In addition to these, there are a number of other stimuli which result in ADH release, of which the most clinically relevant is the stress response described in Box 26.1 (see also Ch. 8). Osmoreceptors, situated centrally in the hypothalamus monitor fluctuations in plasma sodium concentration, mediating pituitary response to changes. Stimulation of volume receptors, situated in the right atria, in response to circulating volume depletion, can also ultimately result in ADH release, even in the presence of a normal or low plasma osmolality (Rose 1994). (This latter response contributes to the expansion of the extravascular fluid volume seen in pathological conditions such as nephrotic syndrome, hepatic cirrhosis, and congestive cardiac failure.)

In the kidney, the effect of ADH is to cause maximal tubular reabsorption of 'free' water. The result of ADH activity on the kidney is thus reduction in urine volume and an increase in urine osmolality (Valtin & Schaefer 1995).

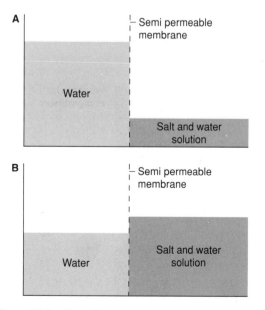

Figure 26.4 Osmosis.

Box 26.1 Hormonal mediators of fluid and electrolyte imbalances postoperatively: ADH and aldosterone

Surgery stimulates the release of ADH, a response apparently mediated by pain afferents, which results in an elevation of plasma levels of this hormone postoperatively which can persist for several days. Nausea and vomiting also stimulate ADH release. ADH increases reabsorption of water in the kidney, decreasing urinary volume. The consequence of this for the surgical patient is an increase in extracellular fluid volume with a dilution of sodium content, that is, a dilutional hyponatraemia.

Increased levels of aldosterone secretion in response to trauma are mediated by adrenocorticotrophic hormone (ACTH) secretion from the hypothalamic–pituitary axis. Aldosterone contributes to sodium retention, and a consequent fall in urinary sodium excretion.

Stimulation of 'thirst' is a response to reduction in total body water. The threshold for this is loss of 1–2% of total body water. In a 70-kg adult, a 2% loss is approximately 700 ml of water. This loss of body water will also result in an increase in plasma osmolality, the normal range for which is 287–290 mOsm/kg, and consequent ADH release.

The renal response to ADH provides an example of physiological limitation with respect to a homeostatic mechanism. Plasma increments of 1 pg/ml of ADH are matched by increments in urinary osmolality of 100 mOsm/kg. However, the kidney is unable to concentrate urine beyond an osmolality of 1000–1200 mOsm/kg. This corresponds to a plasma ADH concentration of 10–12 pg/ml (Trachtman 1995).

It is of interest to note that the experience of thirst does not occur until maximal urinary concentration under the influence of ADH has occurred and the action of ADH on the kidney is no longer sufficient to maintain water balance. The act of drinking suppresses both the thirst sensation and the release of ADH. This response is apparently mediated by oropharyngeal mechanoreceptors stimulated by swallowing (Rose 1994).

Alterations in these homeostatic mechanisms as a consequence of ageing have been described (McLean et al 1992). These include: blunting of the thirst response (Phillips et al 1984); alterations in ADH release consequent to changes in plasma osmolality; and an increase in abnormalities in serum sodium concentrations in the elderly (Lye 1985).

REGULATION OF SODIUM AND POTASSIUM

Regulation of sodium balance is achieved by the interaction of a number of neurohormonal systems which influence renal tubular handling of sodium, resulting in increased reabsorption or excretion of this substance. The regulation of potassium is closely tied to that of sodium. The renin–angiotensin–aldosterone regulatory system is the best described and will be dealt with here. Box 26.2 provides a brief consideration of other mechanisms.

Release of the enzyme renin into the circulation from cells of the juxtaglomerular apparatus (JGA) in the kidneys is stimulated by a number of factors. Among those factors proposed are reduction in plasma sodium ion concentration; an increase in chloride ion concentration; and reduced rate of luminal flow in the distal convoluted tubule of the nephron.

Renin release is also stimulated by other autoregulatory mechanisms within the kidney that are concerned with maintenance of adequate renal perfusion (for example sympathetic nervous system responses). Loss of extravascular fluid volume is sensed by nerve endings in the afferent and efferent arterioles. One of the responses to this is renin release from the JGA.

The action of renin is to split *angiotensinogen*, a substrate present in plasma, into *angiotensin I*, a decapeptide. Angiotensin I undergoes conversion by further

---

Box 26.2 Regulation of sodium balance: actions of atrial natriuretic peptide and urodilatin

There is now evidence that a number of other substances may contribute to body handling of sodium. Among these are atrial natriuretic peptide (ANP) and urodilatin.

Atrial natriuretic peptide
This substance is released from cardiocytes in the atria, and also to a lesser extent from the ventricles, in response to volume expansion of the ECF. It is vasoactive, having a direct vasodilatory effect. In the kidney, ANP has been shown to increase renal excretion of salt (Na^+) and water. However, the overall physiologic role of this substance in terms of salt and water balance in humans remains inconclusive.

Urodilatin
This is a peptide hormone, similar to ANP, which appears to be synthesised primarily in the kidney. Its principle effect appears to be increased renal tubular excretion of Na^+. The mechanisms which control its release within the kidney are as yet unknown.

peptide cleavage, to the physiologically active octapeptide *angiotensin II*, primarily in the lungs but also at other sites in the body. The conversion of angiotensin I to angiotensin II is mediated by angiotensin-converting enzyme (ACE).

In addition to its vasoconstrictive action, angiotensin II stimulates the release of aldosterone, a steroid hormone which influences renal tubular uptake of Na^+. Aldosterone is synthesised in the zona glomerulosa of the adrenal cortex and, in common with other steroid hormones, exerts its effects at an intracellular level. Na^+ reabsorption in the renal tubules is enhanced by aldosterone. Aldosterone causes increased tubular cell permeability to Na^+, and upregulation of Na^+/K^+-ATPase activity. There is also evidence that enhancement of oxidative metabolism by aldosterone increases mitochondrial production of ATP, thereby increasing its availability as the energy source for the Na^+/K^+-ATPase (Valtin & Schaefer 1995).

Aldosterone enhances K^+ excretion through mechanisms similar to those which result in Na^+ retention. Stimulation of aldosterone release occurs following dietary intake of potassium and consequent increases in intracellular concentrations of potassium ions. Increases in serum concentrations of potassium also stimulate aldosterone release. Segmental renal tubular responses to increases in potassium concentration secondary to aldosterone activity include:

- increasing cell membrane permeability to potassium ions
- facilitating secretion of potassium ions into the tubular lumen
- increasing Na^+/K^+-ATPase activity.

STARLING'S FORCES IN THE CAPILLARY

Exchange of water, nutrients and the waste products of cell metabolism takes place across the single-celled endothelial layer of the capillary beds. Bulk flow of water and solutes between the intravascular and interstitial compartments in this region is governed by differences between capillary hydrostatic pressure and the oncotic pressure exerted by protein, primarily albumin. At the arterial end of the capillary, hydrostatic pressure tends to drive water and solutes out of the intravascular compartment into the interstitium, and is of sufficient magnitude to overcome the osmotic pressure exerted by the plasma proteins, which acts to oppose this movement. The situation is reversed at the venous end of the capillary because hydrostatic pressure decreases along its length. In this region, the

plasma osmotic pressure exceeds hydrostatic pressure, and water and solutes move from the interstitium into the vascular bed (see Fig. 26.5).

Disruption of Starling's capillary forces results from alterations in hydrostatic pressure, plasma protein concentrations, interstitial fluid oncotic pressure, and vascular endothelial permeability, as shown in Box 26.3.

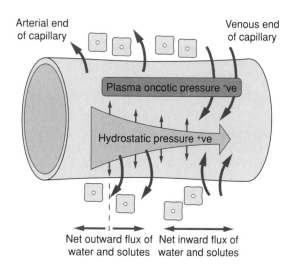

Arterial end of capillary

Venous end of capillary

Plasma oncotic pressure ⁻ve

Hydrostatic pressure ⁺ve

Net outward flux of water and solutes   Net inward flux of water and solutes

Figure 26.5 Flow of water and solutes between intervascular and interstitial compartments in the capillary bed.

Box 26.3 Factors contributory to disruption of Starling's capillary forces

Hydrostatic factors
- Hypervolaemia
- Hypovolaemia
- Congestive cardiac failure
- Venous thrombosis/occlusion
- Drugs, e.g. nifedipine

Oncotic factors
- Hypoalbuminaemia
- Secondary to nephrotic syndrome
- Hepatic failure
- Malnutrition
- Protein-losing enteropathies

Vascular endothelial factors
- Septicaemia
- Toxaemia of pregnancy

THE RELATIONSHIPS BETWEEN MAINTENANCE OF EXTRACELLULAR VOLUME, CARDIAC OUTPUT AND BLOOD PRESSURE IN THE SURGICAL PATIENT

The neurohormonal mechanisms which maintain extracellular volume by means of salt and water homeostasis are intimately linked with those which contribute to the conservation of cardiac output and blood pressure (see Fig. 26.6). Physiologically adequate function of these control systems, and intact activity at their target sites, for example the kidneys, heart and vascular bed, contribute to maintenance of circulating blood volume, blood pressure, and hence organ perfusion.

Assessment of the surgical patient's ability to maintain or regain homeostasis must take into account complicating factors in which there is cardiac, renal or vascular dysfunction.

CALCIUM AND PHOSPHATE BALANCE

Normal homeostasis of calcium is intimately linked to that of phosphate. Calcium storage in the bones accounts for approximately 99% of body calcium. Ionised calcium accounts for approximately half of the remaining 1%, and calcium bound to plasma proteins accounts for the other half. It is ionised calcium which plays a role in blood clotting, nerve signal transmission, and the coupling of nerve excitation to contraction necessary for normal musculoskeletal

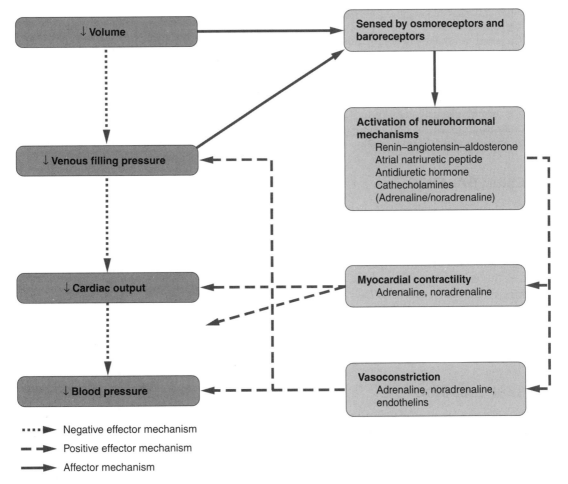

Figure 26.6   Relationship between the mechanisms that maintain extracellular volume and those that conserve cardiac output and blood pressure.

activity. Alterations in extracellular concentrations of ionised calcium have profound effects on neuromuscular excitability (for example tetany). The ionised calcium to protein-bound calcium ratio is affected by changes in plasma pH. Alkalotic states favour the binding of ionised calcium to plasma proteins, thereby reducing the plasma concentration of ionised calcium. Acidaemic states have the opposite effect. Rapid and injudicious correction of acidosis can for this reason precipitate tetany, secondary to a reduction in extracellular ionised calcium.

Extracellular levels of calcium are regulated primarily by parathyroid hormone (PTH) released from the parathyroid glands. This is an example of a negative feedback mechanism, whereby low levels of circulating ionised calcium stimulate release of PTH. PTH exerts its effects at the following levels:

• In *bone* by upregulating osteoclast activity, which results in release of Ca^{2+} and phosphate (PO_4^{2-}) from the bone into the blood.
• In the *small intestine*, where Ca^{2+} absorption is enhanced following PTH stimulation of active vitamin D_3 release from the kidneys.
• In the *kidneys*, where active renal tubular reabsorption of Ca^{2+} is enhanced, while renal reabsorption of PO_4^{2-} is simultaneously reduced. Thus, renal retention of calcium leads to enhanced excretion of phosphate, and vice versa (Marieb 1992).

MAGNESIUM BALANCE

In addition to its role in neuromuscular functioning, magnesium (Mg^{2+}) is necessary for normal carbohydrate and protein metabolism, where it functions as a cofactor in enzymatic reactions. The normal daily challenge to magnesium homeostasis is one of excretion of excess, since it is a relatively abundant ion in the diet. In the kidney, magnesium reabsorption is primarily driven by concentration gradient differences. PTH and calcitonin (produced by the thyroid gland) can also enhance renal reabsorption of magnesium (Yucha 1993).

ACID–BASE BALANCE

Acids are substances capable of donating a proton, another term for a H^+ ion. Bases are substances capable of accepting a proton. Strong acids, for example hydrogen chloride (HCl), are those which dissociate completely in solution. Weak acids, for example carbonic acid (H_2CO_3), dissociate partially in solution. Likewise strong bases, for example sodium hydroxide (NaOH),

dissociate completely in solution, and weak bases, for example sodium bicarbonate ($NaHCO_3$), only partially dissociate in solution.

$$HCl \longrightarrow H^+ + Cl^-$$
(hydrochloric acid) (hydrogen ion and chloride ion)

$$H_2CO_3 \longrightarrow H^+ + HCO_3^-$$
(carbonic acid) (hydrogen ion and bicarbonate ion)

$$NaOH \longrightarrow Na^+ + OH^-$$
(sodium hydroxide) (sodium ion and hydroxyl ion)

$$NaHCO_3 \longrightarrow Na^+ + HCO_3^-$$
(sodium bicarbonate) (sodium ion and bicarbonate ion)

pH

pH is the negative log_{10} of the concentration of *free* hydrogen ions ($- log [H^+]$). Strong acids, which dissociate completely or near completely, will contribute more free hydrogen ions to a solution than will a weak acid, which only dissociates partially. This also holds true in the case of basic, or alkaline, substances. Hydrogen ion concentration can be expressed in micromoles per litre, or nanomoles per litre.

A substance with a pH of 10^{-7} is neutral. This is given as 7 on the pH scale since minus log 10^{-7} equals 7. A substance with a pH of less than 7 will be acidic, by definition having a greater concentration of hydrogen ions than a neutral solution. A substance with a pH greater than 7 will be basic, or alkaline, having a lower concentration of hydrogen ions than a neutral solution (see Fig. 26.7).

In the normal course of events, the body regulates the balance of acid to base within a very small, slightly alkaline range, pH 7.38–7.42. Enzymatic activity and cell metabolism are highly influenced by the pH. Even relatively small changes in pH can result in serious functional derangements. Daily acid production in the body, a result of oxidative metabolism and thus CO_2 production, is considerable (approximately 13 000–20 000 mmol of CO_2). The carbonic acid formed in the body from CO_2 is a 'volatile acid'. In the steady state, metabolic production of this acid will equal its pulmonary excretion, resulting in no overall gain or loss of H^+.

The daily production of 'non-volatile acids', organic and inorganic acids not derived from CO_2, is related to dietary intake. In the UK, the average daily intake of protein is 95–100 g, mostly from meat. Under certain circumstances, for example highly catabolic states, and anaerobic exercise, endogenous production of non-volatile acids rises.

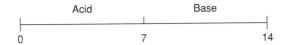

Figure 26.7 The pH scale.

The body counters the effect that volatile and non-volatile acids have in raising the hydrogen ion concentration, and thereby lowering the pH, in three ways: physicochemical buffering; respiratory compensation; and via the renal contribution to the excretion of acid load, whereby H^+ ions are excreted and HCO_3^- is replenished. Physicochemical buffering and respiratory compensation cannot contribute to the excretion of non-volatile acids, and act as temporary compensatory responses to acute changes in acid load. Buffering and respiratory compensation will return the pH toward normal but not to normal. It is the renal component which achieves this latter by excretion of acid and consequent replenishment of the buffering systems.

Physicochemical buffering systems

The function of the body's physicochemical buffering systems is to prevent large changes in the concentration of hydrogen ions in the face of an acid or base load, either endogenously produced or ingested. Effective buffer systems in the body consist of weak acids and their conjugate bases, or weak bases and their conjugate acids.

All of the body's buffer systems work in essentially the same way. Buffer systems will combine with the hydrogen ions liberated by the dissociation of a strong acid in solution to form a weaker acid which only partially dissociates in solution. Alternatively, the buffer systems will combine with the hydroxyl anions liberated by the dissociation of a strong base in solution to form a weaker base which only partially dissociates in solution. Each of the body's physicochemical buffer systems has a pH at which it will be maximally effective.

The bicarbonate buffer system

This consists of carbonic acid (H_2CO_3), a weak acid, and sodium bicarbonate ($NaHCO_3$), a weak base. It is the principal physicochemical buffer system in the plasma. The rapidity of action of this system is dependent on the ratio of carbonic acid to sodium bicarbonate. This is normally 1:20, or alternatively expressed, for each acid component of this system there are 20 basic components.

Addition of a strong acid to this system results in:

$$H^+ + HCO_3^- \longrightarrow H_2CO_3$$

Addition of a strong base to this system results in:

$$OH^- + H_2CO_3 \longrightarrow HCO_3^- + H_2O$$

The phosphate buffer system

This system consists of the weak acid NaH_2PO_4 and the weak base Na_2HPO_4. Addition of a strong acid to the system will result in the following:

$$H^+ + Na_2HPO_4 \longrightarrow NaH_2PO_4$$

The H^+ ions liberated by the strong acid will combine with the basic component of the system to form a weaker acid.

Addition of a strong base will result in the following:

$$OH^- + NaH_2PO_4 \longrightarrow Na_2HPO_4 + H_2O$$

The OH^- ions liberated by the strong base will combine with the acidic component to form a weaker base.

Activity of the phosphate buffer system is of particular importance in two sites in the body, the renal tubules and the intracellular fluids. That this is so is a reflection of the high concentration of phosphate found there.

The protein buffer system

It has been estimated that approximately three-quarters of the buffering capacity of the body fluids is intracellular and attributable primarily to the buffering capacity of proteins. Since proteins are present in the plasma, they also act as buffers at this site. Intravascularly, haemoglobin, also a protein, has a substantial buffering role. The capacity of proteins to act as buffers is related to their molecular structure. This buffer system has a H-protein weak acid component and an Na-protein weak basic component.

The respiratory contribution to acid–base balance and its control

Respiration makes a considerable contribution to the regulation of pH in the body. The carbonic acid formed by physicochemical buffering is converted to carbon dioxide and water, and this CO_2 is excreted via the lungs. Consider the following, where the H_2CO_3 has been formed because of physicochemical buffering following an acid load consequent to oxidative metabolism:

$$H^+ + HCO_3^- \longleftrightarrow H_2CO_3 \longleftrightarrow H_2O + CO_2 \text{ (liberated via the lungs)}$$

Removal of carbon dioxide by the lungs will drive this reaction to the right. Thus in order to re-establish equilibrium, bicarbonate will combine with additional H^+ ions to form carbonic acid, which will in turn dissociate to form CO_2 and H_2O. The effect of this in the body will be to restore the pH toward normal. However, in doing so the concentration of the main extracellular buffer, HCO_3^-, will be diminished.

Chemosensitive areas in the respiratory centre of the medulla oblongata are highly responsive to changes in the concentration of H^+ ions and CO_2 in the body fluids. Increases in the concentration of these result in increased alveolar ventilation, a response which increases respiratory excretion of CO_2. Conversely, decreases in the concentration of H^+ ions or CO_2 in the body fluids result in decreased alveolar ventilation and subsequent retention of CO_2. Peripheral chemoreceptors in the carotid and aortic bodies sensitive to changes in H^+ ion and CO_2 concentrations in arterial blood also contribute to this ventilatory response mediated by the respiratory centre.

Renal contribution to acid–base balance

The renal contribution to acid–base balance includes excretion of fixed-acid hydrogen ions which cannot be removed by the respiratory ventilatory response, and replenishment of the body stores of bicarbonate (HCO_3^-). While the physicochemical buffering systems work on a minute-to-minute timescale, renal regulation of acid–base balance requires hours to days (Rose 1994).

The physiological processes involved in the renal response are, bicarbonate reclamation and bicarbonate regeneration. The process of bicarbonate reclamation involves the return of bicarbonate, filtered from the glomerulus into the nephron's tubular lumen, back into the plasma. Bicarbonate regeneration couples secretion of hydrogen ions into the tubular lumen with bicarbonate generation. In the tubular lumen the hydrogen ions become 'trapped' by the basic components of the ammonia (NH_3^{2+}) or phosphate (HPO_4^{2-}) buffer systems. This trapping results in the formation of the acidic components of these systems (NH_4^+ and $H_2PO_4^-$), which are then excreted in the urine.

FLUID REPLACEMENT THERAPY

Fluid and electrolyte replacement may be administered either orally or parenterally, or by a combination of these two routes. The volume of replacement required, specific electrolyte needs, and the rate necessary to restore the individual to a euvolaemic state will influence the choice of route. Box 26.4 summarises the principles governing fluid and electrolyte replacement.

While not always possible, the oral route is preferable, not least because it avoids exposing the individual to complications associated with accessing the venous circulation for parenteral fluid administration. Thrombophlebitis and septicaemia are complications associated with venous access (MacFarlane et al 1980). Maintenance of the venous access site is an established nursing responsibility (Goodinson 1990) and, increasingly, insertion of peripheral cannulae is becoming an accepted part of the nurse's remit.

There are a number of commercially available solutions for intravenous infusion, which vary in composition.

Crystalloid solutions

Crystalloid solutions are ionic, since they contain electrolytes in solution. Those that are available for parenteral infusion contain water and sodium chloride (saline), or water, sodium chloride and additional electrolytes.

Saline solutions

- Isotonic
- Hypotonic
- Hypertonic

Isotonic saline has a sodium content approximately equivalent to that of the plasma. Administration of this solution will expand, or replace fluid and solute loss in

---

Box 26.4 Principles of fluid and electrolyte replacement

Correction of fluid and electrolyte imbalances must necessarily be based on the specific clinical needs and condition of the individual. The factors which govern choice, route, and rapidity of replacement therapy may be summarised as follows:

1. The ability of the individual to contribute to the replacement of loss
2. The site of fluid and electrolyte loss
3. The magnitude of fluid and electrolyte loss
4. The presence or absence of intact homeostatic system functioning – this includes renal and cardiovascular function
5. The presence or absence of factors which may alter capillary fluid dynamics.

the intravascular and interstitial subdivisions of the ECF.

Hypotonic saline has a sodium content usually half that of isotonic saline. Administration of 1 litre of this solution is equivalent to 500 ml of isotonic saline and 500 ml of free water.

Hypertonic saline has a concentration of sodium greater than that of the plasma (Rose 1994). The use of this solution to correct hyponatraemia needs careful consideration, particularly in view of the potentially catastrophic consequences of rapid elevation of plasma Na^+ concentration (Ledingham 1992, Rose 1994).

Polyionic solutions

- Hartmann's
- Ringer's lactate

These solutions contain calcium and potassium at physiological concentrations, in addition to sodium and chloride. The advantage of these substances over isotonic saline is unproven, and in some situations, for example where the individual has a lactic acidosis (lactate) or renal impairment (potassium), may be hazardous (Rose 1994).

Non-crystalloid solutions

Dextrose solutions

- 5%
- 20%
- 50%

5% dextrose solutions contain 5 g of glucose, a non-electrolyte, in every 100 ml of water. Once infused, the glucose is quickly metabolised to carbon dioxide and water. For this reason, the administration of this solution is equivalent to giving a litre of water. Following administration, this water will be distributed across both the ECF and the ICF fluid compartments (see Fig. 26.2). In addition, each gram of glucose will provide approximately 4 kcal of energy.

Colloid solutions

Colloid solutions contain large molecular weight substances such as protein, polysaccharides or starch molecules. Where vascular endothelial permeability is intact, colloids act as effective osmoles in the intravascular compartment, influencing water movement from the extravascular spaces into the vascular bed. Thus, administration of colloid solutions will expand the intravascular subdivision of the ECF. Colloid solutions commercially available for intravenous administration include albumin, the polysaccharide dextran (Dextran 70, Macrodex, Pharmacia), and gelatin preparations (Haemacel, Behringwerke AG).

Blood and its components are also colloidal. Administration of blood as a replacement fluid will depend on a number of factors which include the extent of blood loss, and consequent diminution of oxygen-carrying capacity in the body, and availability.

Colloid versus crystalloid fluid replacement

The relative merits of colloidal over crystalloid fluid replacement and vice versa remain controversial, with limited evidence to support the use of one as opposed to the other (Skowronski 1990). Ley et al (1990) reported that colloid resuscitation following coronary artery bypass surgery or valve replacement was superior to crystalloid resuscitation, measured by reduced fluid requirements and greater haemodynamic stability. This study was, however, small (n = 21), and individuals who had had previous cardiac surgery, renal failure, bleeding disorders, or who had had combined coronary artery bypass and valve replacement, were not included.

Fluid resuscitation protocols following thermal injury have also been a focus of consideration within this context. Loss of vascular endothelial integrity associated with burns may militate against the use of colloidal solutions, at least in the first 6–8 hours following injury. Crystalloid replacement may thus be the initial replacement fluid of choice (Milner et al 1993) (see also Ch. 25).

ASSESSMENT AND MONITORING OF FLUID AND ELECTROLYTE BALANCE

The individual's ability to contribute to maintenance of fluid and electrolyte homeostasis will be affected by conscious level, age and clinical condition. Concomitant chronic disease states, such as renal failure, hepatic failure or endocrine dysfunction, will increase the potential risk for fluid and electrolyte disorder, irrespective of the reason for admission to the surgical ward.

With reference to the section on physiological control of fluid and electrolyte homeostasis in this chapter and the experiences of your colleagues, can you account for these differences? Have you observed situations in which the postsurgical period for an individual with concomitant chronic disease has been complicated by fluid and electrolyte imbalance? What factors do you think contributed to this?

Reflective point

Consider for example, the differences in preoperative and postoperative multidisciplinary care that you may have observed in the following settings:

1. A healthy adult admitted for repair of a non-incarcerated femoral hernia
2. An adult on maintenance haemodialysis for end-stage renal failure admitted for a total hip replacement
3. An adult who is an insulin-dependent diabetic admitted for cataract removal and lens implant.

Preoperative assessment of ability to maintain fluid and electrolyte homeostasis should also take into account potential difficulties which may be encountered by the individual in the postoperative period. Knowledge of the operative procedure, its potential effect on fluid and electrolyte homeostasis, and the probable pattern of postoperative care are key prerequisites for this process. Thus, for example, one can anticipate the potential need for calcium replacement following total parathyroidectomy, or potential fluid volume with sodium and potassium electrolyte replacement where fluid and electrolyte losses from the gastrointestinal tract are considerable.

Monitoring fluid intake and fluid loss

Monitoring fluid intake and loss is a nursing responsibility and one which would appear to be not entirely unproblematic. Despite the fact that the majority of nurses in their study rated fluid balance charts as 'very important' in fluid management, Daffurn et al (1994) found inaccuracies in the volumes recorded. Of the nurses who took part in the study, 55% scored 5 or above on a Likert scale of 1–7, which was used to indicate the frequency with which they had fabricated volumes. An additional finding reported was that medical staff appeared to have little confidence in the quality of the charted records. This study also found that nurses did not rate the accuracy of fluid balance charts highly.

Accuracy of fluid intake and output measurement is facilitated when the individual is receiving parenteral fluids controlled by fluid pump (Leggett 1990a,b) and where all losses (with the exception of skin and respiratory tract loss) are draining or can be drained into measuring receptacles. Since this latter may be neither necessary nor practicable for many surgical ward inpatients, the apparent problem of maintaining accurate records requires consideration.

Reflective point

Are fluid balance charts necessary in all cases, or would recording of daily weight be as effective? If individuals were to be encouraged and supported in maintaining their own records (where appropriate), would this improve accuracy? These clinical practice issues warrant investigation.

Physical assessment

Body weight

Measurement of body weight is a cheap and accurate means of assessing both fluid and solute balance (Valtin & Schaefer 1995). Acute changes in body weight over a 24-hour period which are not ascribable to loss of flesh weight will be due to fluid loss or gain. Each 500-g change in weight is the equivalent of 500 ml of fluid. Where possible, the individual should be weighed daily, at the same time, and wearing similar clothing. Many specialised beds, for example air-fluidised systems, now incorporate weighing scales, which can be utilised for weighing the non-ambulant individual.

Arterial blood pressure

Measurement of the blood pressure reflects cardiac function, venous system filling pressures and systemic vascular resistance (see Box 26.5) (see also Ch. 25). Fluid status may be further assessed by monitoring supine and standing blood pressures, where this is applicable. An incremental rise in systolic pressure of between 10–20 mmHg should be observed in the individual on movement from a supine to a standing position. A decrease in systolic pressure on standing (postural hypotension) may indicate hypovolaemia. When using supine and standing blood pressures in this way, nurses should be alert to the following:

• Disease processes may alter this normal physiological response. An example of this is diabetic neuropathy. Thus postural hypotension in an individual with diabetes may not necessarily indicate hypovolaemia.
• Alterations in vascular tone may result from prolonged periods of bed rest, and postural hypotension in the surgical patient may be a reflection of this rather than hypovolaemia.

Peripheral perfusion

Assessment of peripheral perfusion by monitoring skin temperature at the extremities will also provide

---

Box 26.5 Blood pressure

Blood pressure is determined by cardiac output and peripheral resistance.

BP ∝ Cardiac output × Peripheral resistance

Cardiac output is stroke volume multiplied by heart rate.

Cardiac output = Stroke volume × Heart rate

The stroke volume is a function of ventricular filling pressure/venous return and ventricular contractility. This is the relationship described by the Frank–Starling Law of the heart (Berne & Levy 1995, Guyton 1986).

---

qualitative information about fluid balance. Peripheral vasoconstriction mediated by sympathetic nervous system activity is a response to a decrease in extracellular fluid volume, and may be observed prior to observation of hypotension. The practice of monitoring skin temperatures has been utilised as an adjunct to monitoring fluid volume status in such diverse settings as paediatric haemodialysis, following burn injury (utilising a non-affected peripheral site), and during the rewarming process following induced hypothermia for cardiac surgery.

Capillary refill

The speed of capillary refill may be assessed by applying sufficient temporary pressure to elicit blanching of a nail bed. Following release of this pressure, the speed at which capillary flow re-establishes the normal pink colour of the nail bed indicates sufficiency or insufficiency of arterial flow, and hence tissue perfusion. Normally, the rate of capillary refill is under 2 seconds (Swearingen & Keen 1995).

Central venous pressure measurement

Measurement of central venous pressure (CVP) is achieved by means of a catheter inserted into the superior vena cava. This measurement enables a distinction to be made between hypotension and circulatory failure due to cardiac failure (resulting in a high venous pressure), and hypotension secondary to depletion of the extracellular compartment or systemic venous dilatation (low venous pressure) (Moran Campbell et al 1984). It thus gives an indication of the volume of the extracellular compartment and, in particular, the volume of the intravascular compartment. Serial measurements of the CVP provide the most useful

information about the individual's response to, or need for, fluid replacement, thereby providing a basis for alterations to a replacement regime. (See Ch. 25 for CVP normal range.)

CVP measurements may be taken when the individual is supine, or alternatively with the individual lying at an upright angle. The choice of position when taking this measurement must take into account comfort and the clinical condition of the individual. Thus, the supine position may not be suitable following neurosurgical procedures, nor in the presence of pulmonary oedema (Cline & Gurka 1991). Comparative analyses have been conducted (Callow & Pieper 1989, Cline & Gurka 1991, Driver 1972) to assess alterations in central venous pressure readings associated with position changes. These reports suggest that alterations in position from 0–30 degrees of elevation have little significant effect on the pressure reading. However, it should be borne in mind that the determination of degrees of elevation for these studies was achieved with the use of a protractor. Without the use of such an instrument, it is doubtful whether consistent accuracy in angle of elevation could be achieved.

The reference point for alignment of the water manometer from which the pressure measurement is read is the right atrium. Alignment of the water manometer with the right atrium may be with reference to either the sternal angle, or the fourth intercostal space in the mid-axilla. Whichever patient position and point of alignment are used, all subsequent CVP measurements should be performed using the same parameters (Woodrow 1992).

Where the central venous access is also being utilised for fluid infusion, it is generally common practice to stop the infusion briefly while the CVP measurement is being recorded, and recommence it on completion of the measurement. The rationale for this is that concomitant fluid infusion may adversely affect the accuracy of the pressure reading. The evidence to support this practice is anecdotal. Additional factors should be borne in mind whilst performing these measurements. The CVP measurement will only give information about filling pressures on the right side of the heart, and will not necessarily be an accurate indicator of left-sided heart filling pressures. Defective right ventricular function, as for example with valvular disease, may give rise to a measurement which indicates fluid overload, whereas in fact, a fluid deficit may exist. Within the context of septicaemia, a lower than normal central venous pressure may be necessary for the individual because of the potential for low (central venous) pressure pulmonary oedema which is frequently associated with this condition.

Skin turgor

Turgor, the elastic property of the skin, depends to some extent on interstitial fluid volumes. Assessment of interstitial fluid volume status may be performed by gently pinching the skin on the forehead or back of the hand. In the euvolaemic person, the skin will flatten quickly once the pinch is released. Volume depletion is indicated where the skin flattens slowly after the pinch is released. As with all methods of assessment, it is necessary to consider other characteristics of the individual in order to make deductions. The elasticity of the skin decreases with age and therefore reduced turgor may not be an accurate indicator of volume depletion in the elderly person. Similarly, obesity may mask changes in skin turgor. Assessment of hydration of the tongue and mucous membranes will also provide information about overall fluid balance status (Rose 1994).

INTEGRATED PROBLEM-SOLVING AND NURSING INTERVENTIONS

The chapter so far has provided you with insight into the physiological mechanisms of fluid and electrolyte balance. It should have enabled you to review your knowledge and enhance your practice. The following three reflective points and associated case studies should enable you to further link knowledge from the chapter to caring for patients in surgical nursing practice.

The observations given in Case study 26.1 should have led you to consider that Mr Perez is hypovolaemic. He is hypotensive, peripherally vasoconstricted and has a negative central venous pressure. In addition to this, his urinary output is minimal. Did you consider that the rate of fluid replacement for this gentleman was adequate?

Restoration of this gentleman's circulating volume is a priority. Fluid replacement can be titrated according to hourly volume losses, both urinary and nasogastric, and incremental changes in the central venous pressure. Mr Perez's current rate of fluid and electrolyte replacement is inadequate. Short time intervals between measurements of vital signs may be required to assess Mr Perez's response to fluid resuscitation.

A urinary output of 0.5 ml/kg per hour in a 70-kg man, translates as 35 ml per hour, or 840 ml in 24 hours. In the initial postoperative period this may be the maximum volume of urine excreted because of the activity of ADH and aldosterone. Assessment of urine osmolality, using a reagent strip to measure specific gravity, may provide evidence to support this inference (specific gravity of 1.025–1.030). However, adequate filling pressures, reflected in return to

---

Case study 26.1   Mr Perez

Mr Perez, a 45-year-old gentleman, has had an emergency abdominal resection following presentation to the accident and emergency department. He has returned to your ward postoperatively. On his arrival you note the following:

Blood pressure:	90/60 mmHg
Pulse rate:	100 b.p.m.
Temperature:	
Core	36.8°C
Peripheral	35.0°C
Central venous pressure (measured at the sternal angle):	-4 cm

Mr Perez has a nasogastric tube in place on free drainage; you empty the drainage bag and measure 500 ml of gastric aspirate. This gentleman has also had a urinary catheter inserted which is attached to a collecting bag with an integral urinometer. You note that there is 50 ml of urine in the measuring receptacle. The central venous catheter has a triple lumen. Attached to one of the limbs is 1-litre bag of saline, which is being infused through an intravenous fluid pump at a rate of 100 ml per hour.

Reflective point

Consider Case study 26.1 and outline the possible reasons for the recorded observations. What nursing interventions will you plan for Mr Perez?

---

normotension, peripheral warmth, and a rise in central venous pressure, should result in an hourly output greater than this.

If you noted the discrepancy in Case study 26.2 between what Mr Patel said he weighed, and the weight given, well done! However, what does this tell

---

Case study 26.2   Mr Patel

Mr Patel has been admitted for a total parathyroidectomy. He has hyperparathyroidism refractory to conservative management as a consequence of end-stage renal failure. Mr Patel receives renal replacement therapy in the form of haemodialysis. On admission, Mr Patel says that he weighs 63.5 kg.
  On admission:

Weight	65 kg
Potassium (K^+)	5.8 mmol/l
Calcium (Ca^{2+})	2.9 mmol/l

you? You know that Mr Patel is in end-stage renal failure and requires haemodialysis. Fluid weight gains between dialyses are usual. In the absence of renal function, a normovolaemic state can only be achieved by fluid removal across dialysis. The weight that Mr Patel stated as his was in fact his 'dry' or euvolaemic weight following a dialysis session. Similarly, potassium homeostasis is not possible in the absence of renal function. The weight gain and increase in serum potassium noted should lead you to suspect that this gentleman requires haemodialysis preoperatively.

Mr Patel and his family should be aware of his haemodialysis needs, and minimum questioning should elicit how many times a week he dialyses (usually three times per week), for how long, and when he was last dialysed? Further questioning should focus on what Mr Patel's daily fluid and dietary restrictions are, and whether or not he has any residual urinary output. Generally, individuals on haemodialysis are restricted to 500 ml of fluid daily plus the volume of any residual urinary output. If, for example, Mr Patel has a residual output of 200 ml in 24 hours, then his *total* daily fluid allowance will be 700 ml, both pre- and postoperatively. Following your assessment, you should ensure that provision has been made for him to receive haemodialysis. You should also contact the hospital dietitian, or diet bay, to ensure that he receives a low-potassium, reduced-sodium diet. In the absence of any unforeseen event, it is unlikely that Mr Patel will require parenteral fluid replacement following his parathyroidectomy.

You should additionally have noted that Mr Patel's serum calcium is above the normal range. In individuals with end-stage renal disease hyperparathyroidism contributes to renal osteodystrophy. Furthermore the secretion of this hormone may become independent of the serum calcium, resulting in hypercalcaemia, which has a number of important adverse effects.

Removal of Mr Patel's parathyroids will result in rapid movement of ionised calcium from the plasma into the bone, reducing plasma ionised calcium levels. This will give rise to postoperative tetany if plasma ionised calcium levels are not monitored and corrected as appropriate with intravenous calcium administration. Mr Patel should be informed that he will have venous blood samples drawn pre- and postoperatively

Case study 26.3   Mrs Johns

Mrs Johns was admitted 5 days ago for repair of a penetrating abdominal stab wound. At the time of operation she had formation of a defunctioning colostomy. On admission she weighed 60 kg. Currently she is receiving total parenteral nutrition, and has required insulin infusion to maintain normoglycaemia. You are taking care of this lady following morning handover, and note the following:

Blood pressure: 80/40 mmHg
Peripheral temperature: 39°C
Central venous pressure: -7 cm

You also note that Mrs Johns is flushed and warm to touch, and that her legs are oedematous. You quickly check Mrs Johns' most recent blood results and find the following:

Potassium (K^+):   3.0 mmol/l
Serum creatinine: 180 µmol/l

to monitor serum calcium levels, and that intravenous calcium may be given. The nursing care plan you devise should make reference to interventions which monitor Mr Patel for signs of latent tetany postoperatively. These include circumoral tingling, and a positive Trousseau's or Chvostek's sign.

Like Mr Perez, Mrs Johns is also hypotensive, and has a negative central venous pressure. However, you will have noted that there are certain dissimilarities between them.

Mrs Johns has had traumatic injury to her bowel, which required repair, a potential cause of bacteraemia related to release of bowel contents. In addition, she is currently being fed parenterally via central venous access, another potential site for bacterial entry to the systemic circulation (see Ch. 27). She is now peripherally dilated, pyrexial, and profoundly hypotensive. These findings can be related to the physiological effects of septicaemia. Toxic substances released into the blood by bacteria, and the resultant stimulation of immune system activity, exert an effect on the vasculature, heart and other organ systems. The negative central venous pressure can be related to arteriolar and venous dilation; increased capillary endothelial permeability; and consequent movement of fluid and solutes from the intravascular compartment into the interstitium (see p. 544). Defective ventricular function will also contribute to hypotension in this lady.

A serum creatinine of 180 µmol/l in a 60-kg woman is indicative of markedly compromised renal function (see Box 26.6). You will also have noted that the serum potassium is below the normal range at 3.0 mmol/l. This finding may be related to the transport of K^+ into the cells, secondary to insulin infusion to ensure glycaemic control with TPN administration. It would be unusual for K^+ replacement to be given

---

Box 26.6 Implications of raised serum creatinine levels

The glomerular filtration rate (GFR) and thus renal function, can be estimated by measurement of the serum creatinine level. Creatinine is endogenously produced by skeletal muscle metabolism. In the kidney, it is freely filtered from plasma across the glomerular membrane into the nephron tubule, from where it is excreted in the urine. A decrease in renal function will result in a rise in serum creatinine. The GFR is also related to the body surface in m^2, and a normal GFR is approximately 120 ml/minute. The normal range for serum creatinine is approximately 60–120 µmol/l.

---

within this context, particularly in view of diminished renal function.

Again, restoration of circulating volume is a priority, and there is an urgent requirement for collaborative care with medical colleagues. Parillo (1995) asserts that aggressive resuscitation of hypovolaemia related to sepsis may be detrimental, arguing for inotropic support and titration of fluid replacement according to the response to this.

CONCLUSION

A complex interplay of several physiological control systems maintains fluid, electrolyte and acid–base homeostasis. Where the activity of these systems is disrupted, or where intact functioning of these systems' effector organs is diminished, fluid and electrolyte imbalances occur. The nurse's role with respect to assessment and monitoring of fluid and electrolyte balance is well established. There are, however, a number of aspects of current clinical practice identified in this chapter which arguably deserve objective consideration in the future. Future practice with respect to fluid and electrolyte balance may conceivably extend beyond assessment, monitoring and securing vascular access for intravenous fluid administration, toward protocol-bound nurse prescription of intravenous fluids.

REFERENCES

Berne R M, Levy M N 1995 Cardiovascular physiology, 6th edn. C V Mosby, St Louis
Callow L B, Pieper B 1989 Effect of backrest on central venous pressure in pediatric cardiac surgery. Nursing Research 38(6): 336–338
Cline J K, Gurka A M 1991 Effect of backrest position on pulmonary artery pressure and cardiac output measurements in critically ill patients. Focus on Critical Care AACN 18(5): 383–389
Cullen L 1992 Interventions related to fluid and electrolyte balance. Nursing Clinics of North America 27(2): 569–596
Daffurn K, Hillman K M, Bauman A, Lum M, Crispin C, Ince L 1994 Fluid balance charts: do they measure up? British Journal of Nursing 3(16): 816–820
Driver E 1972 The effect of elevating the head of the patient's bed while obtaining the central venous pressure measurement. Circulation 26(11): 241
Goodinson S M 1990 Keeping the flora out: reducing the risk of infection in IV therapy. Professional Nurse 5(11): 572–575
Goodman L S, Gilman A 1980 The pharmacological basis of therapeutics, 6th edn. Macmillan Publishing, New York
Guyton A C 1986 Textbook of medical physiology, 7th edn. WB Saunders, Philadelphia

Ledingham J G G 1992 Regulation of water metabolism, thirst, and plasma sodium concentration. In: Raine A E G (ed) Advanced renal medicine. Oxford University Press, Oxford
Leggett A 1990a IV infusion pumps. Nursing Standard 4(28): 24–26
Leggett A 1990b IV infusion pumps (continued). Nursing Standard 4(30): 29–31
Ley S J, Miller K, Skov P, Presig P 1990 Crystalloid versus colloid fluid therapy after cardiac surgery. Heart and Lung: Journal of Critical Care 19(1): 31–40
Lye M 1985 The milieu interieur and ageing. In: Brocklehurst J C (ed) Textbook of geriatric medicine and gerontology, 3rd edn. Churchill Livingstone, Edinburgh
MacFarlane J T, Ward M J, Banks D C, Pilkington R, Finch R G 1980 Risk from cannulae used to maintain intravenous access. British Medical Journal 281: 1395–1396
McLean K A, O'Neill P A, Davies I, Morris J 1992 Influence of age on plasma osmolality: a community study. Age and Aging 21: 56–60
Marieb E N 1992 Human anatomy and physiology, 2nd edn. Benjamin Cummings, Redwood City
Milner S M, Hodgetts T J, Rylah L T A 1993 The burns calculator a simple proposed guide for fluid resuscitation. Lancet 342: 1089–1091

Moran Campbell E J, Dickinson C J, Slater J D H, Edwards C R W, Sikora E K (eds) 1984 Clinical physiology, 5th edn. Blackwell Scientific Publications, Oxford

Parillo J E 1995 Pathogenic mechanisms of septic shock. New England Journal of Medicine 328(20): 1471–1477

Phillips P A, Rolls B J, Ledingham J G G 1984 Reduced thirst after water deprivation in healthy elderly men. New England Journal of Medicine 311: 753–759

Rose B D 1994 Clinical physiology of acid–base and electrolyte disorders, 4th edn. McGraw-Hill, New York

Skowronski G A 1990 Hypovolaemic shock. In: Oh T E (ed) Intensive care manual, 3rd edn. Butterworths, Sidney

Swearingen P L, Keen J H 1995 Manual of critical care nursing: nursing interventions and collaborative management. Mosby Year Book, St Louis

Trachtman H 1995 Sodium and water homeostasis. Paediatric Clinics of North America 2(6): 1343–1363

Valtin H, Schaefer J A 1995 Renal function, 3rd edn. Little Brown, Boston

Woodrow P 1992 Monitoring central venous pressure. Nursing Standard 6(33): 25–29

Yucha C B 1993 Renal control of phosphorus and magnesium. American Nephrology Nurses Association (ANNA) Journal 20(4): 447–450

FURTHER READING

Birne M H, Penney D G 1990 Atrial natriuretic peptide: a hormone with implications for clinical practice. Heart and Lung: Journal of Critical Care 19(2): 174–185

Bohony J 1993 9 common IV complications and what to do about them. American Journal of Nursing 93: 45–49

Bove L A 1994 How fluids and electrolytes shift. Nursing 94(Aug): 34–40

Gasparis L, Murray E B, Ursamanno P 1989 I.V. solutions: which one's right for your patient? Nursing 89(Apr): 62–64

Goodinson S M 1990 Good practice ensures minimum risk factor complications of peripheral venous cannulation and infusion therapy. Professional Nurse 90: 175–177

Heidenreich T, Giuffre M, Doorley J 1992 Temperature and temperature measurement after induced hypothermia. Nursing Research 41(5): 296–300

Hinwood B 1993 Chemical interactions. In: A textbook of science for the health professions, 2nd edn. Chapman and Hall, London, ch 6

Jones D H 1991 Fluid therapy in the PACU. Critical Care Nursing Clinics of North America 3(1): 109–120

Lundgren A, Jorfeldt L, Ek A 1993 The care and handling of peripheral intravenous cannulae on 60 surgery and internal medicine patients: an observation study. Journal of Advanced Nursing 18: 963–971

McVicar A, Clancy J 1992 Which infusate do I need? Professional Nurse 7(9): 586–591

Memmer M K 1988 Acute orthostatic hypotension. Heart and Lung: Journal of Critical Care 17(2): 134–141

Metheny N M 1990 Why worry about IV fluids? American Journal of Nursing 90(8): 50–55

Oliver S K, Fuessel E 1990 Control of postoperative hypothermia in cardiovascular surgery patients. Critical Care Nursing Quarterly 12(4): 63–68

Osguthorpe, S G, Tidwell S L, Ryan W J, Paull D L, Smith T L 1990 Evaluation of the patient having cardiac surgery in the postoperative rewarming period. Heart and Lung: Journal of Critical Care 19(5)(part 2): 570–574

Presig P 1994 Renal acidification. American Nephrology Nurses Association (ANNA) Journal 21(5): 251

Settle J 1986 Fluid therapy in burns Part 2. Care of the Critically Ill 2(5): 188–190

Sommers M 1990 Rapid fluid resuscitation: how to correct dangerous deficits. Nursing 90(Jan): 53–59

Vaska P L 1992 Fluid and electrolyte imbalances after cardiac surgery. AACN Clinical Issues in Critical Care Nursing 3(3): 664–671

Wilkinson R 1991 The challenge of intravenous therapy. Nursing Standard 5(28): 24–27

27

Maintaining optimum nutrition

Sharon L. Edwards

AIMS

The aims of the chapter are:

- to explain the importance of adequate nutrition in the surgical patient
- to identify the many sources of malnutrition seen in surgical wards
- to demonstrate the application of nutritional assessment in a surgical patient
- to explain the issues in relation to continued effective nutrition in the surgical patient
- to explore the various nutritional support options.

INTRODUCTION

Recently, there has been a renewed interest in nutrition and nutrient requirements of disease, especially the changes associated with bypassing the gut (Raper & Maynard 1992). This has highlighted the continued occurrence of malnutrition and the subsequent problems it causes to the recovery of surgical patients. The term 'malnutrition' tends to be the preferred term used to encompass undernutrition, nutrient deficiencies, and imbalance due to disproportionate intake. This chapter is concerned with malnutrition, since it is an agreed area of concern for all nurses.

The answer to the problems of maintaining optimum nutrition and preventing malnutrition in the surgical patient, both within the community prior to admission and in the hospital setting, is not completely clear. A recent report by the King's Fund (1992) concluded that 'doctors and nurses frequently fail to recognise undernourishment because they are not trained to look for it'. The problem is not merely a lack of education; it is also a lack of interest (McWhirter & Pennington 1994).

However, with the increased advances in nutritional knowledge and assessment, community care, and health promotion, no patient need become further malnourished in hospital. Yet, the advances in nutritional assessment guidelines available for nurses (Garvey et al 1994, Thomas 1994, Williams 1994), which take into consideration cultural, social and psychological as well as physical factors, have yet to demonstrate their effectiveness in reducing malnutrition in either community or hospital settings. A more effective use of the assessment tools and documentation, and the understanding of the modern methods of nutritional support of patients with special feeding problems, could go a long way in identifying patients at risk. Once identified, increased oral diet, total parenteral nutrition (TPN) or nasogastric tube feeding (NGF) may be necessary. However, where increased oral diet cannot be tolerated, nasogastric feeding to protect gut function and prevent sepsis occurring is preferred. What is needed is a generation of nurses who know and care about their patients' nutrition. It is imperative that surgical nurses up-date their knowledge, reflect upon their attitude toward nutrition, and enhance their practical skills in nutritional assessment and support of their patients. This chapter is a step in that direction.

HISTORICAL PERSPECTIVE

The importance given to diet in nursing care has had its ups and downs. However, the importance of nutrition in promoting health was fundamental in the 18th century (Arbuthnot 1731). A widely known example is the administration of lime juice to British sailors as prophylaxis for scurvy (scorbusis), which led to the term 'limey'. The active ingredient in citrus fruits was only isolated during this century. Florence Nightingale emphasised proper nutrition, and believed that it was the nurse's responsibility to feed the patient. She devoted two chapters to nutrition in her book, *Notes on Nursing: what it is and what it is not* (1859).

As early as the 1870s, nursing students were taught to prepare and serve food for sick patients (Englert et al 1986). At that time the focus was on teaching nursing students the art of preparing food for the sick, and acquired knowledge of nutrition and diet therapy principles (Lee & Corbett 1992). The same could not be said for food suppliers, for the hygiene and consistent handling of food, particularly meat, at this time was a large problem (Thomas 1994). Because of unhygienic food handling practices, a committee was set up in 1875 and the Sale of Food and Drugs Act was subsequently passed. In the early 1900s, specialist courses in food, nutrition and diet therapy were offered to nurses, and the nutrition content in nursing curricula increased (Stotts et al 1987). Health professionals were also becoming aware of the need for special diets for patients with specific diseases.

During the same period, the general population were not encouraged to understand the importance of a balanced diet or food hygiene. This lack of awareness was aggravated further by social, environmental or economic restraints (Thomas 1994) which became evident when many young men were recruited for the Boer War and were found to be seriously undernourished. This prompted the introduction of school meals for school children, giving them at least one balanced meal per day and improved nutritional standards in the general population (Garrow 1994). Benefits were observed during the First and Second World Wars. In the 1930s, just before the start of the Second World War, most of the vitamins were discovered, and these were shown to be therapeutically effective during rationing (Garrow 1994). Following these discoveries, the importance of nutrition began to decline as a priority in modern health care. Nutritionists concluded, complacently, that malnutrition was something of the past. The lack of interest in nutrition and understanding of its importance to the recovery of patients in hospital continued for over 40 years, for it was only two decades ago that a renewed interest in the importance of nutrition in hospitalised patients began to develop. Articles by Bistrain et al (1974) and Hill et al (1977) identified a high incidence of protein–energy malnutrition in surgical patients.

In 1977, at the beginning of this period of renewed interest, the 33rd World Health Assembly was held, in which attainment of health for all was promoted as the main social target of governments and the World Health Organization in the remaining years of the century (Downie et al 1991). This strategy developed and became known as 'Health for all by the year 2000' (WHO 1985). Although primarily focusing on health promotion and disease prevention, it is of major relevance to surgical nurses, in that it centres on certain key principles, e.g. equal opportunities for all, and satisfaction of basic needs which include food. Since the inception of the health for all strategy, the use of the term 'health promotion' began to gather momentum (Downie et al 1991). The interest in health promotion focused on the role of minerals and micronutrients, dietary fibre, cholesterol and other lipids, food additives, 'complex' carbohydrates and salt (Booth 1993). Some of these have been linked to major preventable diseases, such as cardiovascular disorders and malignancies. The specific preventive programmes were aimed at those 'risk factors' which could be reduced by eating a healthy diet.

This has implications for surgical patients admitted to hospital, for despite the healthy eating campaigns in the community and the 'Health for All by the Year 2000' strategy, malnutrition is still prevalent in patients prior to admission for surgery. This indicates that nutrition in the 1990s is influenced by other factors, such as psychological/mental state, social/economic status, religious/cultural issues and the state of physical fitness prior to admission to hospital (Thomas 1994).

In addition to the community as a source for potential malnutrition, recent studies have reported that malnutrition and the adverse changes that can occur continue to be reported in hospitalised patients (Dickerson 1995, Garrow 1994, McWhirter & Pennington 1994). Pinchocofsky & Kaminski (1985), Windsor & Hill (1988) and Reilly et al (1988) highlighted the serious complications of malnutrition in hospitalised patients. They suggested that malnutrition is associated with apathy, depression, fatigue, loss of will to recover, loss of muscle power with the consequent effects on respiratory function, impaired immune function with the increased susceptibility to chest infection, and reduced cardiac function. These complications cause patients unnecessary suffering, a lengthened stay in hospital at substantial extra cost, and can result in increased morbidity and mortality (Robinson et al 1987).

The malnutrition seen in hospitals today may be compounded by changes in health service provision and food legislation (Thomas 1994). A number of administrative changes have been identified that make it more difficult to ensure that ordinary patients get proper meals (Garrow 1994). Tendering of catering services has encouraged the use of 'cook freeze', 'cook chill' and 'cook conserve' to encourage cost-effectiveness. If control of these processes is poor, they can become microbiologically unsafe and the nutritional value of the food is diminished. Catering services are now supplied on tightly budgeted contracts and extra, informal meals require a special referral to the dietitian. As a result, nurses are not allowed to prepare any cooked food in most ward kitchens. Nurses have lost control of food, and meals are often given out by contracted staff who may be poorly trained. No wonder malnourished patients continue to lose weight in hospital.

The first Sale of Food and Drugs Act (1875) has been amended many times, most recently by the Food Safety Act 1991 (DoH 1991), which resulted in the first major review of food legislation since the 1940s. The most relevant change in the law relates to the environment in which food is prepared in hospitals. Prior to the Food Safety Act 1991, National Health Service (NHS) hospital premises were exempt from closure if food hygiene was considered to be a public health risk. Although the Act has strengthened the pre-existing out-of-date legislation and addressed food safety issues at all stages of the food chain, it has done little for the NHS trusts in relation to food supply, for without adequate food, hospital trusts cannot remain in 'business'.

It appears then that nutrition has fluctuated in importance, from being very highly rated in the 1870s to being almost forgotten by the 1930s. But despite a growing interest in nutrition since the 1970s within the community and hospitals, malnutrition with its associated morbidity and mortality is still a problem which continues to go largely unrecognised.

NUTRITION

Knowledge of nutrition builds on nursing knowledge, life sciences, psychology, sociology, dietetics and medicine (Garvey et al 1994). All these help to identify how nutrition relates to physical health and individual well-being in a unique pattern interwoven to form the human being. The energy supply of the body is obtained from nutrients to carry out vital functions to sustain life, to form new body components or to assist in the functioning of various body processes, such as breathing and physical activity. To produce a constant supply of energy, the body must be constantly replenished with food to sustain physical life.

Food contains nutrients, which are chemical substances that are digested by enzymes. The release of digestive enzymes is controlled and regulated by hormones. There are six principal classes of nutrients: minerals, vitamins, carbohydrates, fats, proteins and water. Minerals are inorganic substances and perform functions essential to life. Vitamins are organic nutrients which are required in minute amounts to maintain growth and normal metabolism. Vitamins do not provide energy or serve as building materials. The essential function of minerals and vitamins (micronutrients) is the regulation of physiological processes. The energy-yielding nutrients are carbohydrates, fats and protein or macronutrients (Williams 1994). These provide primary and alternative sources of energy. Water is the overall vital nutrient sustaining all life processes. It is important to remember that nutrients are often separated for study purposes, but are always interacting as a dynamic whole to produce and maintain the human body, providing energy, building and rebuilding tissue, and regulating metabolic processes (Williams 1994).

Guidance on the adequacy of nutrition of populations is required for many purposes, and standards have been devised against which measured intakes can be compared. These are published by most governments (e.g. National Research Council 1989) and can be found in many nutrition textbooks such as Williams (1994) and Thomas (1994). These standards have come to be known as recommended daily amounts (RDA).

In 1991, the dietary reference values were updated by the Department of Health in a publication known as the COMA (Committee on Medical Aspects of Food Policy) report. The report considers the issue of dietary reference values (DRVs) including: estimated average requirement (EAR); reference nutrient intake (RNI); lower reference nutrient intake (LRNI); and safe intake. The relevance of DRVs to surgical nurses is as a practical and positive guide during nutritional education following different types of surgery, where changes in diet are recommended. They are not intended to be used in evaluating the adequacy of an individual's daily diet as we do not need to eat the DRV of every nutrient every day (Daniels 1991). Rather than saying 'no' to a wide variety of foods, it is important to teach patients what they can eat.

MALNUTRITION

The maintenance of health in an individual depends upon the consumption and absorption of appropriate amounts of energy and all the necessary macro- and micronutrients. Too little of some over a period of months may lead to malnutrition. Therefore, malnutrition indicates that there is insufficient nutrition. When nutrition ceases during periods of fasting, there is a loss of energy stores and malnutrition will ensue. This can occur prior to, during or following surgery.

The physiological effects of malnutrition

Carbohydrates are the first source of energy utilised by the body (glycolysis) and are needed to maintain a normal blood glucose level. In the absence of carbohydrates directly from the gut as a source of energy, the body can utilise nutrients already stored elsewhere. This is generally in the form of glycogen which is stored in the liver. During approximately the first day of fasting, low glucose levels stimulate glucagon secretion by the pancreas. As a result, glycogen is converted to glucose (glycogenolysis) and released from the liver. This restores blood glucose levels to normal. However, these mechanisms cannot maintain blood glucose levels for very long. Once glycogen stores are depleted the primary energy source for most body cells is glycerol which is produced from fat breakdown.

This requires a major body adjustment, as all other body tissues must reduce their oxidation of glucose and switch over to glycerol as their energy source (except the nervous system which does not adapt well to using any other nutrient, e.g. ketones, as a source of energy). Fats are broken down and fatty acids are released into the blood (lipogenesis). As the liver metabolises the fatty acids, ketone bodies are produced in large quantities. These are oxidised by the body into carbon dioxide, water and adenosine triphosphate (ATP). As a result of these mechanisms for glucose sparing and fat utilisation, an individual can fast for several weeks, provided water is consumed.

If fasting continues, the body undergoes two adaptive processes (Harvey 1993). First, the brain, having become deprived of glucose derived from glycogen stores, gradually adapts to the use of ketone bodies as the major source of energy. However, since body cells are limited in the amount of ketone bodies they can metabolise, excess ketone bodies accumulate in the blood, resulting in ketosis. This, in turn, leads to metabolic acidosis and, together with the brain cells' use of ketone bodies as a source of energy, can result in depression of the central nervous system and may lead to coma. Second, there is a fall in the basal metabolic rate (BMR) which reduces energy requirements of the body. The BMR is defined as the energy output of an individual under standard conditions of rest, 12–18 hours after a meal in a neutral thermal environment. Therefore, the basal metabolic rate represents the energy required by a person to perform essential physiological processes at rest.

When fat reserves are depleted, which is primarily determined by the amount of stored fat in the body, large quantities of muscle protein are broken down to release amino acids as a source of energy to maintain cellular functions. These amino acids are converted by the liver into glucose (gluconeogenesis). Large amounts of amino acids can be released for conversion to glucose in the liver by gluconeogenesis; also amino acids may be oxidised directly. It is estimated that once protein stores are depleted to about half of their normal level, death results. During fasting, amino acids contribute to blood glucose only after liver glycogen and fat stores are depleted. A more detailed account may be found in Martini (1998). Malnutrition can manifest in the surgical patient either within the community or during a period of stay in hospital.

Malnutrition prior to surgery

Nutritional reserves fortify the patient for the demands of surgery. Where there is preoperative malnutrition, a poor postoperative outcome is often the result (Campos et al 1992). Thus, when surgery is planned, it is important for the patient to have a well-balanced diet. However, there are circumstances which act as barriers to maintaining optimum nutrition at home.

Psychological disturbances

Psychological disturbances can influence nutrition in many ways and for many people are the strongest influence over eating behaviour (Thomas 1994). Eating for some people can be a way of finding comfort during periods of insecurity, depression, loneliness and boredom. Anorexia nervosa can be a way of coping with hate or anger towards a parent or fear of maturity (McCarthy 1990). This of course can affect an individual's mood state and motivation to maintain a satisfactory nutritional status. These people can become vulnerable to external influences which may impair their nutritional needs in favour of their psychological and social needs (Garvey et al 1994).

In addition, changes in roles within a family or society can cause psychological disturbances, for the roles people take within society are become integrally bound up with individuals. Thus identity and functioning in a social setting can have an influence on nutrition and might involve passive or active neglect of nutritional needs (Garvey et al 1994). For example, the recently bereaved who is now alone, may not wish to bother to cook for just one, so does not bother and nutritional requirements may suffer as a result (Parkes 1985). Reactions to a stressful situation can lead to a decrease in nutritional requirements, for example a depressed mother at home who eats convenience foods owing to lack of time, or a busy secretary who does not have time to eat (Garvey et al 1994). These groups, and others, could be potentially at risk from being undernourished or malnourished prior to being admitted to hospital for surgery.

Social and economic status

In 1980 the Black Report indicated that ill health was more prevalent among people with low incomes in our society and that they were more likely to die prematurely (DHSS 1980). Research undertaken 10 years later by Davey-Smith et al (1990), Malseed (1990), Cole-Hamilton (1991) and National Children's Home (1991) concedes that the situation has not improved. In fact, the social class differences in mortality are said to be widening (Garvey et al 1994). In low-income families food concerns are often of a low priority, as surviving in very poor housing in deprived areas and on a very low income tends to take greater precedence (Thomas 1994). In addition, families often have other financial problems, e.g. being behind in paying their bills or other payments, which compound the problem of finding enough money for food. In these circumstances food is often the first item to be cut back when cash is short. Surgical nurses need to be aware of patients admitted for surgery who may be undernourished because of a low income.

Nutrition related to religion and social customs

Eating patterns may be influenced by a number of factors such as religious beliefs or other strongly held principles, cultural background, ethnic origins, and the availability of traditional foods (Thomas 1994). Whatever a person's ethnic and cultural background, food not only plays a role in maintaining good health, but it will often have an important social or religious significance as well. Some religious or cultural diets ban certain foods and have festivals which require strict fasting (Cruickshank & Beevers 1989). The fasting periods are generally observed in the older more traditional groups and, thus, not all multicultural groups will observe their traditional fasts. However, some religious beliefs and eating practices may, over a period of time, affect an individual's nutritional requirements and may lead to undernutrition (Thomas 1994). Therefore, it is important for surgical nurses to have a knowledge and understanding of the diverse cultures currently resident in Britain and take their different nutritional practices into account (see also Ch. 10).

Vegetarians are also at risk from malnutrition if they do not pay attention to a well-balanced diet (Thomas 1994). The types of vegetarian eating patterns range from simply avoiding red meat to those which are more restrictive. Variations in strictness are considerable and are largely dependent on the individual's beliefs and reasons for adopting vegetarianism. This may be for a variety of personal, philosophical, ecological and economic reasons. It is the more restrictive vegetarians where the likelihood of nutritional deficiency is higher (Dwyer 1988). Therefore, surgical nurses need to acquire sound knowledge and understanding of the diet, religious beliefs, cultural habits, lifestyle and attitudes of their patients. This assessment will ensure that patients are not undernourished prior to surgery and that dietary instruction whilst in hospital fits in with their own traditional customs and eating habits.

Elderly people

The majority of the elderly population in the UK are based in the community and many are in need of nutritional support (Thomas 1994). Sound nutritional principles apply to all age groups, but the elderly are at greater risk of poor nutrition (Cotton 1996), as they can become anxious over issues concerning diet, become ill or disinterested in food, confused or forgetful and commence completely inappropriate diets (RCN 1993, Tierney 1996). Davies (1981) identified 10 main risk factors to help nurses to recognise those in need of nutritional support in the community, e.g. Meals on Wheels or other services.

Illness, e.g. physical disability, depression or loneliness, is generally the most common cause of a reduced nutritional intake in the elderly as it affects appetite, nutritional requirement and nutrient absorption (Tierney 1996). However, poverty, restricted access to food, or shopping difficulties also need to be considered (Herbert 1996). When four or more of these risk factors are evident, an individual is likely to be malnourished (Thomas 1994). The surgical nurse admitting elderly patients for surgery therefore needs to be aware of these in order to prevent malnutrition and its complications occurring while patients are in hospital and to ensure adequate dietary intake throughout the recovery period (see also Ch. 11).

Malnutrition acquired in surgical wards

Many surgical patients may be admitted to hospital from the community, suffering from malnutrition, but patients in hospital continue to be at risk of developing malnutrition.

Malnutrition is associated with severe discomfort to surgical patients with the consequence of an increased length of stay in hospital, and increased expense. The malnutrition observed can be due to a lack of education and interest in nutrition, not only by nurses but by other members of the multidisciplinary team. However, the malnutrition observed is often a direct result of hospital practices.

Feeding not a high priority

The need for feeding or nutritional supplements is only identified after surgery or when the patient has been stabilised (Tredger 1982). This has generally been suggested to be at around 48–72 hours after surgery. At the end of this period, fat stores may have become depleted and a third of the brain's energy may now be derived from ketones (Wallace 1993). Surgical nurses should be aware that this period is crucial, as the body is trying to protect itself by the catabolism of fats to raise serum glucose levels. This can seriously hinder patients' recovery and lengthen their stay in hospital by increasing their risks of respiratory failure, infection and delayed healing.

Nutrition must be seen as a priority in a surgical patient's treatment, as the success of all other treatments may depend upon the nutritional status of the individual (Wallace 1993). Surgical nurses need to consider patient feeding as one of their priorities, to ensure that an essential component of their patients' care is not neglected. However, Hunter (1988) acknowledged that no single group of professionals can provide a food service on their own, or should be held responsible for feeding patients. Thus, all members of the multidisciplinary team must be held accountable for the malnutrition currently observed in surgical patients.

Stress of surgery

It is well documented that patients undergoing surgery will suffer from stress, which in turn increases their BMR (Cerrato 1991). Hospital staff should be immediately aware of the implications of an increased BMR. Studies show that a well-nourished man weighing 77 kg, entering the operating room for a colostomy, would expect to lose 2.3 kg over the next 4 days. Any added physiological or psychological stress following surgery would further increase the BMR, resulting in an increased demand for energy, which if it is not met will further increase weight loss. The additional complications from surgery, such as pyrexia caused by infection, or hypoxia which causes extra effort to breathe, all further increase BMR and weight loss, and decrease the patient's resistance more quickly (see also Ch. 8).

Preoperative fasting

For a surgical patient, the current process of surgery involves periods of prolonged starvation (Schilling 1976). Preoperative fasting times are necessary to reduce the risk of aspiration of gastric contents into the lungs during procedures (Chapman 1996). Preoperative fasting was described by Hamilton-Smith as early as 1972 as a 'traditional and ritualistic based practice with many patients being deprived of food and fluid beyond the accepted maximum fasting time of 12 hours'. Recent studies suggest that a patient prior to theatre only needs to be fasted between 4–6 hours (Chapman 1996, Hung 1992, Thomas 1987). Yet, there remains a difference in fasting times from hospital to hospital, with patients enduring inordinately long periods of starvation and fluid deprivation far in excess of recommended practice (Hung 1992). This prolonged fasting will result in a degree of dehydration and depletion of carbohydrate and possibly fat stores, compromising the condition of patients presenting for theatre.

The most frequent reason given for the length of time patients are expected to fast prior to theatre is the difficulty of foretelling the exact time of any operation (Hamilton-Smith 1972, Thomas 1987).

In the surgical ward environment, it should be noted that a patient who is 'nil by mouth' from midnight, in reality may have been fasted since the previous evening meal and regard should be given by surgical nurses to the possibility that the patient they have just received back from theatre, may now have been fasting for as long as 24 hours. In addition, theatre may be cancelled and patients may go without food until the evening meal. Occasionally this scenario can carry on for several days until surgery is finally undertaken, but the signs of malnutrition are neither observed nor documented. The continued practice of prolonged fasting acts against the optimal nutritional state and is neither acceptable nor justifiable (Chapman 1996) (see also Ch. 20).

The use of 5% dextrose

Some surgical patients may go without food for a number of days. However, the practice of maintaining often seriously ill individuals on intravenous 5% dextrose solution preoperatively, and sometimes for longer, promotes malnutrition (Young 1988). One litre of 5% dextrose solution contains 170 kcal; thus, a patient receiving 3 litres per day is expected to survive on 600 kcal/day (Doekal & Zwillich 1976). Fluid requirements may be met but there will be a gross shortfall in nutritional requirements. 'The well nourished post operative patient without complications requires at least 1500 kcal/day for maintenance' (Young 1988). Sepsis or other complications may increase caloric requirements by as much as 50–100% (Say 1997). Clearly, the use of 5% dextrose to maintain optimum nutrition is inadequate.

The common administration of 50% dextrose solution is also not construed as adequate, since increased carbon dioxide production from excess glucose oxidation elevates the respiratory workload and promotes respiratory acidosis (Majors 1988, Marvin 1988). Such consequences emphasise the essential need to commence adequate and effective nutritional support rapidly and early in the surgical patient's stay.

Postoperative fasting

Maynard & Bihari (1991) and Raper & Maynard (1992) tackled the age-old practice of maintaining postoperative fasting until the bowel sounds return. Raper & Maynard (1992) based their work on the long-established theory identified by Tinckler & Kulke (1963) and Wells et al (1964). This is that small intestinal motility and function are maintained in the postoperative period; it is only the stomach and the colon which are affected by a reduction in motility. Thus, the assessment for commencement of enteral feeding cannot be solely based on the auscultation of bowel sounds. The majority of recent studies demonstrate that enteral feeding can be safely initiated in the immediate postoperative period, and that there is no need to wait for the return of bowel sounds (Adam 1994, Maynard & Bihari 1991, Raper & Maynard 1992, Moynihan 1994).

Not knowing previous nutritional status

Doctors and nurses frequently fail to document any information regarding nutrition. This means that patients 'at risk' of malnutrition go unrecognised, as previous nutritional status is not documented. A recent study of 200 cases of malnutrition by McWhirter & Pennington (1994) showed no improvement in documentation of nutritional status on admission. They found that less than half of the 200 involved in the study had had any nutritional information documented and very few had had their weight or height recorded on their hospital admission notes. In addition, research is very limited into how many patients who were originally well nourished become undernourished following surgery, owing to the lack of documentation to determine the patients' previous nutritional status.

> **Reflective point**
>
> What do you consider are the main potential sources of malnutrition in the surgical patients in your care?

The adverse effects of malnutrition in the patient undergoing surgery

The length of stay of patients in hospital can be increased by complications due to malnutrition. A number of these are now considered.

Respiratory failure

Malnutrition before or after surgery may reduce pulmonary function and increase the risk from the surgical procedure itself (Moynihan 1994). The control of breathing is mediated by the respiratory centre in the brain stem; as early as 1976, Doekal & Zwillich noted a decrease in respiratory drive associated with malnutrition. Sustaining respiratory function is further hampered by the effect of protein and fat metabolism in the catabolic person which directly damages the parenchyma of the lung. However, the evidence of altered lung parenchyma is almost exclusively derived from animal studies, and therefore it is questionable whether similar events occur in humans. Majors (1988) suggested that reductions in levels of surfactant and tissue elastic recoil as well as increases in compliance occur in the malnourished patient. In addition, the loss of pulmonary diaphragmatic muscle mass and strength, seen in malnutrition, has been shown to coincide with a decrease in vital capacity and breathing strength (Aora & Rochester 1982). Factors such as a reduced respiratory drive, damage to the parenchyma of the lung, reduced levels of surfactant and tissue elastic recoil, and a reduction in pulmonary diaphragmatic muscle mass and strength, may predispose the patient to suffer from atelectasis or respiratory infection.

Reduced immune response

Research into malnutrition suggests that immunocompetence is compromised in the underfed individual (Majors 1988, Oh 1997, Young 1988). Proteins are the primary construction elements in the immune system. An anabolic state and maintenance of a positive nitrogen balance enables the body to produce a functioning immunological complement as the defence against invading infections (Hudak 1990). Changes in phagocytes and in the levels of complement circulating are associated with undernourishment. A study by Belghiti et al (1983) successfully improved the immune complement of eight malnourished patients (who were free from infection) by providing adequate nutrition, thereby indicating a definite linkage between malnutrition and immune abnormalities. Other nutrition elements have been identified as essential for a fully functioning immune system. Vitamin E, for example, assists in stimulating immunoglobulin production, enhancing humoral and cellular immunity, and copper is also important in maintaining lymphocyte functioning (Watkins et al 1994).

Delayed wound healing and increased risk of pressure sores

Hospital malnutrition commonly occurs in the surgical patient, which contributes to delayed healing and an increased risk of pressure sores (Cerrato 1991). The delivery and assessment of adequate nutrition is one aspect of management which is necessary for any type of surgical wound to heal effectively, but nutritional assessment and support in wound management is often undervalued (Wells 1994). Poor nutrition does not directly cause tissue breakdown in surgical wounds or cause pressure sores. Tissue breakdown occurs when adverse factors such as malnutrition combine with the predisposing condition. It is then that healing may be impaired or tissue becomes unable to maintain its integrity. Unless adequate nutritional support is administered, rapid weight loss will occur and fewer nutrients will be available for wound healing (Goodinson-McClaren 1992).

An inadequate protein intake has implications for both wound healing and pressure sore development (Wells 1994). A low serum albumin affects the osmotic pressure of the circulation and allows fluid to seep out, resulting in oedema. This in turn will prevent the passage of nutrients to the damaged tissue. In addition, amino acids are required for cell division and body repair; a reduction in these vital proteins will inevitably delay wound healing. Ek et al (1991) demonstrated that a low serum albumin, which can be indicative of a poor nutritional status, is nearly always present before the development of pressure sores. In general, pressure sores do not heal until the low serum albumin is corrected (Holmes & Dickerson 1987).

In the surgical patient, malnutrition can lead to a reduction in intake of vitamin C. Experimental studies have demonstrated the adverse effects of vitamin C deficiency upon wound healing (White 1990). However, the need for supplementation in surgical patients is still open for discussion (Goode et al 1992). The general consensus appears to be that benefits to healing can be gained from the use of vitamin C supplements only in deficient individuals. In addition to reduced vitamin C intake, malnourished patients may also suffer deficiencies in zinc and iron. Zinc is implicated in wound healing as it plays a role in the immune response and is required in DNA/RNA synthesis. Iron deficiencies will result in anaemia, with the consequent decrease in the transport of oxygen to damaged tissue, and may therefore delay healing. Low serum haemoglobin levels have also been reported in patients with established pressure sores, with levels improving significantly on healing (Holmes & Dickerson 1987).

The rejuvenation of a wound requires a variety of nutrients, and research shows that adequate intake of vitamins is particularly essential for the promotion of granulation. Not all wounds can be prevented or predicted, but there is increasing evidence that, for some people, nutritional status is a factor in the prevention or prediction of wound complications and pressure sores. The key to identifying the presence of such factors is assessment.

Reflective point

Consider any patients you have cared for during the past 6 months who have experienced delayed wound healing. Reflect on the extent to which malnutrition may have been influential.

ASSESSMENT OF NUTRITION IN THE SURGICAL PATIENT

Nurses are culprits in the mal-assessment of a patient's nutritional status. Hickey (1986) reviewed nursing care priorities and reported a high priority being placed on management of the physiological measurements, e.g. blood pressure and pulse, but other areas of care such as nutritional adequacy were of low priority. It appears that in conjunction with prioritising care issues, there is the shortfall involved in the assessment and determination of nutritional status.

However, most nurses are familiar with the use of assessment forms and protocols, including pressure sore management and risk assessment scales such as Waterlow (1988) and Norton (Norton & Exton-Smith 1962). Many of these scales have a nutritional assessment component and can be an important first step in identifying potential nutritional problems in at-risk patients. The use of these scales is an example of how a simple tool employed at an early stage of patient contact can optimise care to produce the best outcome. Nutritional assessment can be as simple or as complicated as desired, but should involve both subjective and objective elements. Information needs to be based on the nurse's observations of the patient and on the collection of an essential core of material, e.g. patient history, psychological and social status, physical examination, diet history and appraisal of current nutritional intake, anthropometric measurements, biochemical and laboratory data.

Patient history, psychological and social status

A concise patient history is a simple and effective method of gathering information and provides the first clues about existing or potential malnutrition (Wells 1994). Factors which would need to be ascertained would include whether the patient has had a recent bereavement, bad experience, or been ill at home for a long time, the patient's age, whether the patient is on income support, the type of accommodation the patient lives in. Physical aspects of patients would need to be considered, for example whether the patient looks thin, the appearance of the skin in terms of colour and condition, whether clothes are loose, whether dentures fit properly. These all provide warning signals to the trained eye that a problem with nutrition may exist, and may also give information about any recent loss of weight.

Physical examination

A physical examination should include areas such as: the oral cavity, as a sore mouth or dysphagia may cause difficulty in chewing and swallowing; any physical difficulties with feeding; the presence of nausea, vomiting, diarrhoea or constipation, as any of these problems will affect nutritional intake (Wallace 1993). Nausea, vomiting and diarrhoea result in reduced absorption and often a reduced appetite, whereas constipation can lead to a feeling of fullness, discomfort, depression and confusion, thereby reducing food intake.

Simple respiratory function tests can be recorded, such as vital capacity, maximum inspiration and maximum expiration, to determine respiratory muscle strength.

Diet history

A diet history should consist of questions about likes and dislikes, changes in weight, and in type, quantity and texture of food eaten since the onset of illness, as disease often alters appetite (Wallace 1993, Wells 1994). Changes in taste and the ability to obtain and prepare food should also be enquired about. All these factors should be noted and recorded in the patient's assessment and nursing care plan (Lennard-Jones 1992). Table 27.1 illustrates one approach to taking a diet history, with principles and rationale.

Anthropometric measurements

One of the most important anthropometric measurements in determining nutritional status is weight.

Table 27.1 Assessing diet history (adapted from Garvey et al 1994 and The Dairy Council Book 1)

Principle	Possible action	Rationale
Establish details of client's lifestyle	Obtain (either from case notes or by asking client) details of age, marital status, religion, medical history, nationality, work shifts, eating out and socioeconomic background	Lifestyle factors are extremely important when considering nutritional intake
Identify an appropriate time for interviewing client	In hospital wards, avoid the time of ward rounds, when the patient is undergoing tests or treatment, meal times, visiting times (unless information is required from a relative or friend). Convenient appointment times may need to be made for clients seen in the community	An assessment is less likely to be reliable if the individual is emotionally upset, distracted, in pain, hungry, etc.
Establish dietary intake and normal eating patterns	Take the client through the previous 24 hours or a normal day as appropriate. Include details of meal times, snacks and drinks	Only through assessing normal patterns can goals and interventions be planned with the client
Establish amount of food eaten	Compare with household measures, e.g. matchbox-size piece of cheese, tablespoons, packet size	An idea of the quantity eaten will give an indication of appetite and how much the dietary regime needs to be altered to meet dietary advice
Establish further details about specific types of food preferred	Ask client to identify the type of milk, bread, spread (e.g. butter, margarine, low-fat spread), breakfast cereal, etc. used	Specific details will give an idea of where changes should be made, e.g. increase fibre intake by including more wholemeal bread instead of white bread
Establish reliability of assessment and client's knowledge and understanding of what constitutes a dietary intake	Clients may not give information on sweets, snacks, and drinks (including alcoholic drinks) without prompting. A direct question may be necessary	Clients may not freely offer details about foods they regard as 'naughty' or they may not consider such foods as an integral part of their food intake
Establish additional details about eating habits	Ask client about the frequency of eating out, having fish, eating red meat, going to the pub, etc. For example: 1. How many times is red meat eaten during the week? This could highlight a nutritional deficiency of iron in someone who is anaemic 2. How often are fruit and vegetables included in the diet? This may highlight a problem with constipation (low-fibre diet or poor nutritional intake of vitamins and minerals). Also, how many drinks are taken during the day?	Encouraging the client to talk about nutrition in general will provide additional information. A question on 'eating out' may indicate more 'high calorie' meals than is at first obvious – an important fact if the patient is overweight

However, certain disease processes, such as cancer, cachexia and oedema, may affect an individual's weight, which minimises its usefulness as a measure of nutritional status. Ideal weight charts must be used with caution, as they do not take into account the effects of dehydration and fluid retention on weight. Also, the charts are designed for the younger population and take no account of variations in weight because of illness or age (Ireton-Jones & Hasse 1992).

Nevertheless, changes in body weight do give an indication of the severity of malnutrition. Ireton-Jones & Hasse (1992) advocate the determination of percentage of usual weight, a loss greater than 10% being indicative of malnutrition and a loss of 6–10% being potentially significant. Watson (1994) proposed that nurses should aim to measure body weight more often and give less significance to interpreting blood nutritional levels from laboratory reports.

Height can also be used to determine malnutrition, but it is not always possible to measure height in hospitalised patients, and may not be an adequate guide in elderly patients. It is sometimes easier to ask patients how tall they are – most people have a good idea and this is better than nothing. Height and weight measurements can be used to determine BMI and together they are the most important measurement when determining nutritional status (Lennard-Jones 1992). MacKay (1995) recommended the use of BMI tables to help confirm if an individual is of a healthy body weight or underweight. BMI is calculated as: weight in kg divided by the height in metres squared, the normal range is 19–25 kg/m² (Wallace 1993). Figure 27.1 illustrates a typical quick reference chart for determining BMI.

Garrow (1994) proposed that a BMI of less than 20 kg/m² could be a serious risk to health. The King's Fund report (1992) argued that more use should be made of the BMI. However, Jenson et al (1982) believe that the single use of such a ratio is a reason for the failure to recognise malnutrition, and urge a more global approach. Despite the reservations of Jenson et al (1982), the BMI is a useful tool for assessing nutritional status and should be included in the nutritional assessment. However, its use in isolation is somewhat limited.

More complicated anthropometric measurements can be used to gain more accurate information and can be useful in oedematous or dehydrated patients where body weight figures are meaningless. Body fat content is quickly and easily estimated from skinfold thickness measurements. Most commonly used is triceps skinfold thickness (TSF), which in combination with mid-upper-arm circumference (MUAC) can be used in the following equation to calculate mid-arm muscle circumference (MAMC) as an absolute index of muscle mass: $MAMC = MUAC - 0.3142 \times TSF$ (Wells 1994).

These measurements can be compared with standards (Bishop et al 1981) and, if performed serially, will reflect a change in body tissue. It is often noted that these measurements are only reliable if undertaken by a trained operator and are not always accurate or a true prediction of changes in body mass in overweight or elderly patients (Burr & Phillips 1984).

There are also prediction equations and formulae for determining basal metabolic energy expenditure. This may be of some use in predicting calorific needs when the resources are available. However, multiple factors affecting the metabolic rate can make estimations inaccurate (Say 1997). Sepsis and pain increase metabolic demands and factors such as the presence of oedema or malnutrition may mask the degree of activity (Harvey 1993, Majors 1988). Weissman & Hyman (1987) in a study of postoperative patients found that estimations of metabolism were often inaccurate by 50% or more. Perhaps future research should be directed towards developing prediction formulae that incorporate mitigating factors into equations to provide a more reliable estimation of metabolic demands.

Biochemical measurements

Despite Watson's (1994) suggestion regarding laboratory results, biochemical measurements can be used by surgical nurses to determine nutritional status. The most common is serum albumin, where a level of less than 35 g/litre is indicative of protein–energy malnutrition. The use of albumin as an index of nutritional status can be inaccurate as conditions such as stress, nephrosis and burns also exhibit hypoalbuminaemia. This makes the measurement often misleading and not altogether reflective of nutritional deficiency in the short term. In the chronic situation, serum albumin remains a simple and reliable indicator of malnutrition. Serum transferrin levels can be considered a better marker of acute nutritional depletion. Interpretation of serum levels is complicated by factors such as iron deficiency, which directly affects transferrin production, and they may not be wholly appropriate as a predictor of malnutrition (Majors 1988). Serum haemoglobin measurements will highlight the presence of anaemia, which has been correlated with pressure sore development (Holmes 1993). Anaemia can occur for a variety of reasons, but may be directly related to dietary inadequacy and this should always be followed up by questioning on dietary intake. Promising results have been demonstrated when nutritional assessment has resulted in initiation of preoperative feeding regimes. This method of identifying high-risk patients prior to surgery results in an optimisation of their nutritional status and may help to ensure an uneventful recovery. An outline of an 'at risk' assessment tool to determine nutritional status, using similar indices, is given in Figure 27.2.

Barriers to the introduction and maintenance of effective nutritional assessment for the surgical patient

Keeping up to date and teaching

A report by the King's Fund (1992) stated that 'emphasis in basic nurse training tends to be placed on the importance of healthy eating rather than under-nutrition, its

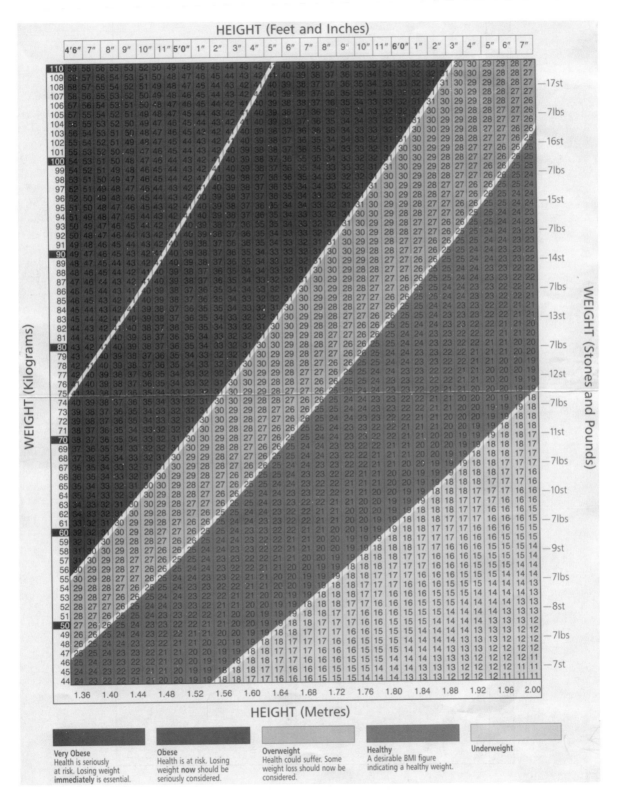

Figure 27.1 Body mass index ready reckoner. (© Servier Laboratories Limited 1991. Reproduced with permission.)

INITIAL OBSERVATION — Yes / No

Is the client:
- Thin?
- Pale?
- Wearing ill-fitting clothes?
- Elderly?
- Suffering from a condition that affects diet intake?

STATE OF MOUTH — Yes / No

Do the clients:
- Dentures fit?

Is the mouth:
- Sore?
- Dry?
- Red?
- Ulcerated?
- Infected?

PHYSICAL CONDITION — Yes / No

Is the client suffering:
- Nausea?
- Vomiting?
- Constipation?
- Diarrhoea?
- Are any of the above due to drug therapy?
- Dysphagia?
- Swallowing difficulties?

Disabilities:
- –holding utensils?
- –feeding self?
- Weight loss?
- Pain?
- Pain severity assessment scale:

PSYCHOLOGICAL — Yes / No

Is the client suffering:
- A recent bereavement?
- A bad experience?
- Confusion?
- Dementia?
- Depression?
- Eating disorder?

SOCIAL — Yes / No

Is the client:
- Having difficulty preparing food?
- Having difficulty obtaining food?
- On income support?
- Receiving Meals on Wheels

CULTURAL — Yes / No

Is the client:
- A vegetarian?
- Vegan?
- Practising religious fasting?

DIET HISTORY — Yes / No

Is the client suffering:
- Changes in diet?
- Changes in likes and dislikes?
- Alterations in appetite?
- Changes in taste?
- Approximate length of duration

MEASUREMENTS

State client's:
- Height
- Weight
- BMI
- TSF
- MAUC
- MAMC
- Serum Albumin
- Hb

OVERALL ASSESSMENT

Is the client:
- Undernourished? ☐
- High risk? ☐
- Moderate risk? ☐
- Minimal risk? ☐

BMI–body mass index, TSF–triceps skinfold thickness, MUAC–mid-upper-arm circumference, MAMC–mid-arm muscle circumference

Figure 27.2 'At risk' assessment for nutritional status: BMI – body mass index; TSF – triceps skinfold thickness; MUAC – mid-upper-arm circumference; MAMC – mid-arm muscle circumference (Edwards 1996, unpublished).

assessment, method of nursing intervention and monitoring'. This problem may be tackled by using the expertise of a registered dietitian to present nutrition content where and when it can most effectively enhance the education of nursing students. However, with the current movement of nursing colleges away from clinical practice into higher education it may be a problem to encourage trusts to allow practising dietitians to travel to higher education institutions, and back again, during work time.

Since it appears that nurse education does not include adequate information about nutritional requirements during illness, it could be argued that it is the responsibility of surgical nurses to remain up to date about issues relating to maintaining optimum nutrition for their patients and attend postgraduate study days. There is much written about the value of attending study days on caring for patients receiving total parenteral nutrition (TPN) and nasogastric feeding (NGF) (Lee 1987). There is evidence to suggest that the attendance at study days by nurses can be cost-effective for hospital trusts. Lee (1987) demonstrated that attendance of nurses at nutritional study days can contribute to a decrease in the complication rates of TPN, an increased awareness of problems associated with TPN and an increase in compliance with protocols (e.g. the number of catheter tips sent for culture was 47% in 1981 compared to 71% in 1986).

Stotts et al (1987) recommended that study days were of little benefit as they did not relate effectively to what was going on in clinical practice. They advocated increasing the clinical time spent in nutrition-related activities, such as history taking, caring for patients receiving enteral and parenteral nutrition, and dietary counselling of patients on special diets. However, this relies on senior clinical staff having some knowledge of nutrition to be able to support such teaching in clinical practice. Thus, these staff will need to attend study days which they could then use to educate other staff in the clinical area.

However, the content of nutrition study days can be complex as there is no comprehensive view of the knowledge necessary to reduce the incidence of malnutrition. Is it vital that nurses appreciate the importance of recording a patient's height and weight carefully on admission and of monitoring serial weight and food intake in the plan of care, and are also aware of the various scientific methods used to assess a patient's nutritional status? Alternatively, study content may be better focused on: valuing and encouraging the humanistic skills, which could result in patients getting fed, and strategies for health education or negotiating individual diets appropriate for

each patient following discharge. The latter strategy would certainly serve to counteract the misguided belief that a high-fibre diet is appropriate for all patients (Taylor 1988). Therefore, should study days centre around the efficiency of the mechanical or physiological functioning of the gastrointestinal tract, or the efficiency of TPN or enteral feeding techniques? Also, should they be raising awareness of the organisational issues by exploring the organisational structure by which food is delivered and circulated to patients?

Reflective point

What do you consider are the main educational issues for surgical nurses with regard to their role in maintaining optimal nutrition in their patients?

Whatever content is decided, it is the responsibility of those delivering the nutritional study day to ensure that the material used is interesting, motivating and related to clinical practice. The lack of interest in nutrition in both nursing and health care could have been partly due to the traditional methodologies used to teach nutrition and diet therapy principles to students and graduates (Lee & Corbett 1992). Holol et al (1984) suggested that more creative, effective teaching of nutrition theory within nursing curricula would improve attitudes about nutrition.

Any study days need to be creative and use different teaching methodologies to make them interesting and valuable to nurses. The study days can be varied and include fun quizzes, pre-tests to assess the knowledge of the participants, lectures on central line placements for TPN, compositions of TPN solutions and nursing responsibilities and procedures. Journal articles and case studies can be provided that require practitioners to take clinical action, to promote discussion and encourage the sharing of nutrition information. To evaluate such study days post-tests may be included to assess knowledge attained (Lee 1987).

Computer programs and board games are also available to enhance student learning in nutrition. Computer programs on nutrition provide reinforcement to students about the concepts of nutrition and their importance in the nursing care of clients (Goodwin et al 1988). Board games have been a successful innovative, dynamic and stimulating format to incorporate as an educational strategy. Using games to reinforce nutrition knowledge provides active student involvement, increased student interest and motivation and a non-threatening environment for learning and student interaction (Corbett & Lee 1992). These teaching strategies and study days should influence knowledge acquisition and a positive attitude toward nutrition in nursing to enhance clinical practice; but the facilitation of theory to practice by lecturers would enhance classroom-based learning.

Better medical cooperation

It seems that there is a deficit in nursing nutritional education, but evidence that doctors qualify knowing little about the detrimental effects of nutritional depletion has existed since studies were undertaken by Hill et al (1977) and Bistrain et al (1974). Parker et al (1992) showed that a lack of knowledge continues in relation to nutrition in medical clinical practice, where there is poor prioritising of nutrition and its related risks. More recently, McWhirter & Pennington (1994) suggested that this is still found in medical practice today and that there is a need for a continued improvement in undergraduate and postgraduate medical education in relation to clinical nutrition.

Nutritional care not a high priority

Nutritional support should be seen as a positive contribution to patient care. Holmes (1991) suggested that its success or failure depends on the nurse's interest and understanding. Horwood (1990) stated that 'nurses have a responsibility to promote awareness of the need to feed patients as soon as possible'. If this is not occurring, an essential component of the patients' care is being neglected.

However, Bladen (1986), Dickerson (1995), Goodinson (1987), Taylor (1989) and Wallace (1993) all state that nurses cannot be solely responsible for initiating and prioritising nutrition. They need the cooperation of a number of people, e.g. doctors, dietitians and pharmacists. This was acknowledged by Hunter (1988) who stated that 'no single group of professionals can provide a food service on their own, or should be held responsible for feeding the patient'. All members of the multidisciplinary team must be held accountable for the malnutrition currently occurring in surgical patients. However, the doctor often relies on the nurse to suggest the commencement of nutrition, and the dietitian also relies on referrals by nurses. So, often, the responsibility of prioritising nutrition does appear to be that of the nurse, although the nurse–dietitian interaction should be collaborative and not merely one of referral.

The nurse's responsibility does not start and end with a recommendation to the doctor to commence nutrition, or the referral of a patient to the dietitian, but remains dynamic within the provision of nutritional care. The nurse's role in nutritional care is that of giving it high priority in total patient care, the prevention and early detection of complications, and initiating treatment in partnership with other members of the multidisciplinary team.

Protocols

The introduction of protocols to help prevent malnutrition both in the community and in hospitals has been widely documented (Adam 1994, Chapman et al 1992, Finnegan 1989, Reilly 1996). They are essential in any clinical practice to identify at-risk patients in need of further intervention, and to reduce the risk of complications associated with TPN or NGF. A catheter care and NGF protocol can identify at-risk patients through assessment (Reilly 1996), and reduce the incidence of catheter sepsis (Finnegan 1989) and the discrepancies that can occur between prescription and delivery of NGF (Adam 1994). It has been shown that there is a greater percentage of delivery of prescribed feed in wards which do have a protocol than those which do not have a protocol (78% with a protocol, 66% without a protocol). This is supported by a study of 113 hospital patients where caloric goals achieved a mean of 3 days earlier using a standardised protocol (Chapman et al 1992). A standard protocol has been designed by Raper & Maynard (1992), which if not directly applicable could be adapted. However, unless protocols are performed uniformly throughout clinical practice by knowledgeable staff, their value is dubious. It is therefore important that in-service staff education is carried out.

The nutritional nurse specialist and nutrition teams

A new role of nutrition nurse specialist (NNS) has been developed over the past 15 years (Fawcett & Yoeman 1991, Taylor 1988). The NNS is an expert in nutrition and functions in both the community and in hospitals as a teacher, researcher, advisor and coordinator between multidisciplinary teams. The role has often been compared with that of the clinical nurse specialist (Hennessy et al 1990). Both roles place a strong emphasis upon clinical competence, education of staff and patients, patient advocacy, interdisciplinary team consultation, and research. Some hospitals have found that employing a specialist nurse has improved the overall standard of care for a patient receiving TPN. One survey reported a direct association between the reduction of catheter infection and the employment of a nutrition nurse (McCannon 1983). One regional centre has shown that employing a nutrition nurse has proved to be cost-effective (Keohane et al 1983). This appears to be because cost saved by reducing complications outweighs the cost of employing a specialist nurse.

It will be interesting to observe whether the development of a specific nursing nutritionist role, with access to recognised protocols, might help provide a focus of responsibility among surgical nurses. However, there are arguments as to whether the NNS role can survive in an environment with increased cost restraints (Hennessy et al 1990). Nutritional nurse specialists need to demonstrate carefully how their interventions provide quality care and cost containment to ensure continued growth and evolution of their specialty practice.

'It is widely acknowledged that the optimum care of patients receiving parenteral nutrition is best achieved by a team approach' (McCannon 1983). It is evident that many regional hospitals have established nutrition teams. These include a clinician, a pharmacist, a biochemist, a dietitian, and an NNS. The role of the team is to assess and manage all nutritional aspects of care, insertion and care of the feeding lines and review of the patient's nutritional status (Atkins 1989).

With nutritional teams, protocols for patient care can be developed, and it appears that this has helped to reduce the problems associated with parenteral nutrition. The King's Fund Report (1992) claims that 'many surveys have shown that the incidence of catheter sepsis can be reduced to about 3% by staff training, preferably by a specialist nursing sister, and by the creation of a nutrition team'.

Continued assessment and documentation

Ongoing assessment and awareness of those at risk is essential. Even if an individual is eating adequately at the initial assessment, it is necessary to be ever aware of the potential for nutritional disaster (e.g. depression in the long-stay patient, surgical intervention, or recurrent investigations).

Hospital food is not to everyone's taste and meal times are not always suitable. If the patient is shown to be eating negligible amounts or nothing at all, referral to the dietitian is essential. If intake is inadequate, for example only half meals are eaten or odd meals are missed, the reasons for this should be investigated. It may be simply that the patient has been unavailable at meal times because of clinical investigations, or is having difficulty cutting up food or chewing. Whatever

the cause, identifying why a patient is eating poorly will give a pointer to the solution. All these factors should be recorded in the patient's nursing care plan, especially periods of fasting and those where little food is taken.

Documentation should continue body weight and triceps skinfold thickness measurements, which are a good indicator of fat reserves. Attention should be paid to the patient's continued oral hygiene. Urine should be analysed for glucose and ketones, and fluid balance carefully monitored, documenting all i.v. bags, feeds, urine output and other drainage from catheters. Calcium phosphates, creatinine and magnesium should be measured together with substances such as vitamin B_{12}, folate, iron, and zinc (Banerjee 1988).

NUTRITIONAL SUPPORT OPTIONS FOR THE MALNOURISHED SURGICAL PATIENT

Successful support of the malnourished surgical patient requires a specialised team working with the patient and family to meet individual needs. The nurse together with other specialised therapists carries the nutritional care responsibility for each undernourished patient. Individual nutritional assessment is initially required to determine which nutritional therapy will be the most beneficial to meet fundamental nutrient and energy requirements. These include:

- improving dietary intake
- total parenteral nutrition
- nasogastric feeding.

Improving dietary intake

'Nutrition should be regarded as a positive contribution to treatment. Its success or failure is largely dependent on the nurse's interest, knowledge and understanding' (Holmes 1993). Improving dietary intake will depend on individual nurses' motivation, skill and knowledge. This may serve to prevent further invasive treatments, e.g. total parenteral nutrition or nasogastric feeding, to improve nutritional intake.

To improve dietary intake a thorough nutritional assessment needs to take place (see Fig. 27.2). Next, an individual personal food plan must be agreed in partnership with the patient (MacKay 1995). This would encompass:

- basic nutritional needs in increased amounts to meet additional metabolic demands (Thomas 1994).
- 'comfort foods' or familiar ethnic dishes and well-liked foods

- the patient's cultural, religious beliefs, likes and dislikes, appetite and motivation
- variety in food texture, colour, and flavour.

In addition, build-up foods may be negotiated with the patient and added in between meals. Documentation of the patient's eating must be recorded and a strict record of all food offered and eaten. It is important to evaluate the personal food plan to determine whether there is a need for further changes or adjustments to the diet or knowledge base of the patient.

There is a move towards complementary therapies in nursing, and nutritional therapy is no exception (Booth 1993). Interest in nutritional therapies is growing, despite their receiving only a passing mention in the recent British Medical Association report (1993) on complementary therapies. Nutritional therapy considers three possible diagnoses:

- allergy either to food or environmental factors
- toxicity from metals, chemicals
- deficits of nutrients because of insufficient intake, malabsorption or 'special needs' (Booth 1993).

More detailed information regarding nutritional therapies can be found in Olsen (1989), Yetiv (1988) and Holford (1992).

In addition, nurses may need to discuss with patients changing eating habits and attitudes to food as a result of surgery or illness (MacKay 1995). This may be very complex and difficult to accomplish owing to some of the issues previously discussed, e.g. culture, religion, socioeconomic status, age and physical disability, or psychological problems. However, attempts by surgical nurses should be made to discuss dietary matters with their patients and strategies which will help them maintain an adequate diet following discharge from hospital. It is highlighted that few hospital settings provide nurses with the structure, resources or appropriate opportunities to be effective at health education (Taylor 1988). However, discussions by the National Advisory Committee on Nutrition Education (1983) and the Committee on Medical Aspects of Food Policy (1984) guidelines are a step in the right direction (Daniels 1991).

Total parenteral nutrition (TPN)

TPN is 'the provision of all nutritional requirements via the intravenous route' (Mitchie 1988). Instead of food being fed into and absorbed from the gastrointestinal tract, nutrients are infused directly into the venous circulation, thus bypassing the gut. TPN is administered using an aseptic technique into a central line which is situated usually in the subclavian or internal jugular vein. Despite the recent advances in nutritional science, TPN remains a complex and hazardous procedure, with many potential complications. Atkins (1989) stated that: 'all nurses caring for patients receiving parenteral nutrition require specialist knowledge, skills and understanding'; they are then in a position to prevent some of the possible physical problems associated with TPN.

Despite the possible hazards, Raper & Maynard (1992) suggest that there are still patients whose condition warrants TPN. Banerjee (1988) states that this method of feeding is particularly valuable in patients following trauma, postoperative patients with prolonged ileus, short bowel syndrome, burns patients, patients with severe pancreatitis with fistula formation, and patients with hepatic or renal failure. It could therefore be established that TPN still has a part, if but limited, to play in the patient's well-being and recovery. However, Finnegan & Oldfield (1989) argue that 'parenteral nutrition is only indicated in patients who cannot absorb enough water, nutrients and minerals due to intestinal failure', which they suggest is very rare.

The recent literature highlights the problems associated with TPN and encourages enteral feeding as a safer alternative (Adam 1994, Harvey 1993, Maynard & Bihari 1991, Raper & Maynard 1992, Sedenvall & Ek 1993, Wallace 1993). It seems that TPN should not be undertaken unless it is impossible to feed the patient by any other route. The complications of TPN are catheter placement, sepsis, mechanical problems, and metabolic derangement, each of which occurs in 5–10% of cases (Raper & Maynard 1992). According to Wolfe et al (1986), death due to complications of TPN occurs in 0–2% of patients.

Catheter insertion

Administration of TPN involves the insertion of a central line into the subclavian vein by experienced medical staff. According to Finnegan & Oldfield (1989), 'complications are less common in the hands of those who have carried out 50 or more placements'. The potential problems from catheter insertion are air embolism, pneumothorax, haemothorax, brachial plexus injury, subclavian artery puncture, catheter misplacement, catheter infection and sepsis. The most common of these is pneumothorax, which occurs in approximately 3% of cannulations by experienced personnel (Finnegan & Oldfield 1989). To recognise the complications early, the surgical nurse must closely monitor the patient during the insertion of a central line, ensuring that the patient is positioned head down, observing for signs of pneumothorax, e.g. dyspnoea, chest pain, increased respiratory rate and reduced air entry. A chest X-ray must be ordered and taken to check the position of the catheter prior to infusion commencing.

Catheter blockage and accidental removal

Blockage of the catheter lumen can result from blood clotting or infusions of lipid. The catheter situated in the superior vena cava is a potential source for a thrombosis. If blockage does occur, difficulty will be observed in the fluid infusion and there will be swelling to the face on the side of the catheter site. These problems can be prevented by ensuring continuous infusions are administered to each lumen. Surgical nurses must be aware of these problems as they could result in the catheter being removed and another being resited, which may result in discomfort for the patient. Occasionally the catheter may slip out of the vein because of traction on the line, incorrect positioning or an insecure dressing. This may cause an air embolism, especially if the patient is sitting up, or cause fluid to leak and accumulate in the surrounding tissue. To avoid accidental catheter removal, the surgical nurse must ensure that the catheter is well secured to the patient with a dressing and that traction from the administration set is avoided. Suturing of the line to the patient is not recommended, but is often undertaken.

Sepsis

This is the greatest hazard of TPN. Sepsis can be caused as the catheter is inserted, the most common infecting organisms being *Candida albicans* and *Staphylococcus epidermidis*, both of which compromise normal skin flora. Sepsis may also be caused by contamination of the TPN solution, which is an ideal medium for bacterial growth. To minimise catheter infection, devised protocols must be adhered to. Finnegan & Oldfield (1989) stated that: 'infection is almost totally preventable and occurs due to a breach in protocols'. All care of the feeding line must be aseptic; the catheter must be used for feeding only, not for taking blood or drug administration (Finnegan & Oldfield 1989). Sepsis can be treated by the use of antibiotics, which are usually effective, although patients who contract septicaemia from a TPN line often have their stay in hospital prolonged. If the septicaemia becomes severe or goes unnoticed, the hospital stay may include some time in intensive care.

The non-physiological practice of bypassing the gut and delivering nutrition directly into the blood can affect the absorptive/immunological function of the gut, causing translocation of bacteria and toxins (Elia 1995, Meakins & Marshall 1989). There is growing evidence of the major role the gut plays, not only in the digestion and absorption of nutrition, but as a protective barrier against the translocation of bacteria and endotoxins to the bloodstream (Adam 1994). The theory of bacterial translocation was first proposed by Meakins & Marshall in 1986. Bacterial translocation from the gut refers to the migration or leakage of organisms from the lining of the gut to the mesenteric lymph nodes and systemic circulation. It occurs on a small scale at any one time, but may become the trigger for sepsis and multiple organ failure.

Laboratory work in rats has found contradictory results in relation to bacterial translocation rates (Adam 1994, Barber et al 1990, Spaeth et al 1990). However, enteral nutrition is thought to have a positive effect on reducing the incidence of bacterial translocation and maintaining the integrity of the gut mucosa (Ephgrave et al 1990, Maynard & Bihari 1991). While the majority of current published works support the theory of bacterial translocation in animals, they do not establish the occurrence of bacterial translocation in humans. The difficulty of extrapolating animal data to humans is self-evident, as is the difficulty of investigating the problem in surgical patients. However, it continues to be recommended that enteral nutrition can support gut function and mucosal integrity (Adam 1994), and may prevent the increased risk of sepsis and multiple organ failure if the gut remains inactive (Deitch et al 1987). The commencement of enteral nutrition is desirable as soon as possible and amounts as small as 10–30 ml per hour may be effective in preventing translocation of bacteria during the administration of TPN.

Metabolic derangements

Hyperglycaemia Hyperglycaemia is more common during overfeeding and generally occurs together with glycosuria. This is usually caused by a too rapid infusion rate of TPN. Overfeeding with excess carbohydrates can lead to excess carbon dioxide production, which can precipitate respiratory failure in patients following surgery (Elia 1995). With overfeeding there is generally a huge increase in sepsis owing to the fact that glucose (hyperglycaemia) favours bacterial growth. The patient may complain of thirst, vomiting and drowsiness. Regular blood sugar analysis and urinalysis should be carried out for patients having TPN.

If it is thought that the hyperglycaemia and glycosuria is caused by too high an infusion rate, the rate should be reduced and further measurements of blood glucose levels and urinalysis carried out. However, in most cases an insulin infusion is administered to assist in the digestion of the excess glucose.

Hypoglycaemia. After prolonged TPN, hyperinsulinism may result from excessive pancreatic islet cell stimulation. This is due to a rise in serum insulin which occurs with a carbohydrate infusion. Therefore, a sudden cessation of the infusion could result in hypoglycaemia. The surgical patient receiving TPN may complain of fuzziness in the head, shakiness, giddiness and light-headedness. This may be treated by administering a bolus injection of 50% dextrose, followed by a slow infusion of 20% dextrose if required. Monitoring of blood glucose should be carried out regularly, together with the physical signs above. This will enable the surgical nurse to detect hypoglycaemia early, as deterioration in the patient's condition can occur very quickly.

A reduction in trace elements and vitamins. Delivering nutrition directly into the blood, as in the case of TPN, has important consequences for the requirements of trace elements, such as iron, manganese and aluminium. When the gut is bypassed, excessive amounts of trace elements may enter the circulation and there is no effective way that they can be absorbed and controlled (Elia 1995). For example, the major regulation of iron takes place in the gut; thus, in parenteral nutrition, iron cannot be absorbed effectively, so excessive loads of iron in the circulation may lead to iron overload. A problem occurs with the trace element manganese, as it is excreted in bile. Many patients receiving parenteral nutrition have a low bile secretion because of a low oral fat intake. The excess manganese gets deposited in the basal ganglia of the brain and is associated with parkinsonian-type symptoms (Mirowitz et al 1992). Therefore, they may be at risk of manganese toxicity. Another danger of bypassing the gut is the toxic effects of aluminium (encephalopathy and bone disease). This danger is generally from the unintentional administration of aluminium in the parenteral nutrition solution, or it may be present in parenteral additives (Klein et al 1991).

A committee of the American Medical Association (1979) recommended a daily intake of most vitamins for patients on intravenous nutrition of two to three times those recommended for oral intake in normal subjects. This is suggested to cater for an inadequate previous intake, the need for new tissue synthesis and for the presumed increased requirements of disease (Elia 1995). However, there is little supportive information to suggest that patients suffering various different illnesses, who are on parenteral nutrition, have such high vitamin requirements.

However, there is evidence to suggest that the amount of vitamins infused into a patient receiving parenteral nutrition may be less than half of that added to the original mixture (La France & Miyagawa 1991). For example, many studies have shown that the loss of vitamin A during a 24-hour infusion of TPN can be 40–98%, as sunlight causes rapid degradation of vitamin A (the most photosensitive vitamin) but fluorescent light does not (Howard et al 1980). Therefore a bag of TPN placed near a window during the day will deliver much less vitamin A into the patient than a bag placed away from a window. In addition, the plastic of polyvinyl chloride bags absorbs vitamin A. Such positioning and absorption problems can severely reduce the amount of vitamin A that the surgical patient actually receives from TPN.

In the delivery of TPN the activity of other vitamins such as thiamine, vitamin E, riboflavin, pyridoxine, and vitamin C may also be reduced (Elia 1995). Thiamine availability may be reduced by 0–90% depending on the solution used, temperature, pH, and presence of sulphite. As much as 30–35% of vitamin E may be lost (La France & Miyagawa 1991) and more than half the riboflavin and pyridoxine may deteriorate in sunlight (negligible under fluorescent light). Fifty per cent or more of vitamin C may degrade over 24 hours in parenteral nutrition mixtures, especially in the presence of oxygen and copper, which catalyses the reaction (Allwood et al 1992). Additionally, parenteral nutrition lacks other nutrients such as glutamine and phosphate, which are present in the normal diet. These nutrients can be delivered in large quantities as synthetic dipeptides.

Nasogastric feeding (NGF)

There is clear evidence that long periods of time without enteral nutrition can produce detrimental gastrointestinal responses and serious complications in the surgical patient (Moynihan 1994). There is now a new area of research that advocates the use of enteral feeding early, rather than TPN, when oral diet is insufficient. Early enteral feeding immediately following any type of surgery is possible (i.e. within 6 hours of insult) and is only suggested to be contraindicated in complete gut failure, which is apparently very rare.

Enteral feeding includes any method of delivering nutrients for absorption by the gastrointestinal tract

(Bladen 1986, Taylor 1988). This generally involves feeding via the nasogastric route, even though this type of feeding can be achieved through the nasoenteric route (i.e. the tip of the catheter is placed in the duodenum or jejunum). Surgical nurses are faced with a wide choice of approaches to feeding, all of which claim to meet the specialist need of administering enteral formula to the patient.

Nasogastric versus nasoenteric route

The advantages of a gastric placement are easy access and the possibility of tolerating higher feeding rates. The disadvantages are that in common with the colon, the stomach is the first area of the gastrointestinal tract to develop dysfunction. Gastric tubes are also associated with a high incidence of feed regurgitation and possibly aspiration pneumonia (Adam 1994).

The small intestine is less sensitive than other regions of the gut and is likely to continue to absorb feed long after the stomach or colon have ceased to do so. Feeding directly into the small intestine (jejunal feeding) is considered to be less prone to regurgitation and there is a significantly increased caloric intake. Therefore, feed is more likely to be tolerated. In addition, there is a lower rate of pneumonia in those fed jejunally (Adam 1994). However, this is not supported by Strong et al (1992) who found equal aspiration rates in enteral and jejunal feeding with no significant difference in incidence of pneumonia and no improvement in the time it took to reach a desired caloric intake. These differing results may reflect the difference in the two study populations.

However, there is a risk of aspiration pneumonia and a recorded intolerance with nasogastric feeding. Therefore, it may be that, in some patients, jejunal feeding may make a difference. The major difficulty in feeding via the jejunal route is finding an effective and reliable method of bedside placement. One technique involves passing a nasogastric tube, removing the wire introducer, bending it, replacing it, and advancing the introducer, plus tube, while rotating it until the pylorus has been located, requiring considerable skill and dexterity. It seems unlikely that this technique would be useful on most wards. The most reliable method of jejunal placement is under endoscopic direct vision. However, this subjects the patient to an uncomfortable and invasive procedure and usually requires a waiting period while the endoscopy is arranged. If a suitable bedside method can be developed, then jejunal feeding may be highly beneficial in the feeding of surgical patients.

The wide-bore versus the narrow-bore tube

Traditionally a wide-bore tube was used for the purpose of enteral feeding, but in recent years narrow-bore tubes have been introduced (Bladen 1986). Fawcett & Yeoman (1991) argue that a narrow-bore tube should be used as a wide-bore tube causes the patient discomfort, oesphagitis, and gastric reflux. Wide-bore tubes are made of polyvinyl chloride (PVC) and can only be left in situ for 1 week, as they become hardened and cracks can occur in the tube itself. The patient is then given the added trauma of requiring another tube to be passed each week for the provision of enteral feeding. Small-bore tubes, depending on the substance from which they are made, can be left in situ for 30 days (Woods 1992).

Bladen (1986) and Sands (1991) state that the small-bore tube is softer, more pliable and more comfortable for the patient. Ulceration and erosion are also reduced when a small-bore tube is used. Despite these advantages, Bladen (1986) stated that the small-bore tube can block easily and has a tendency to collapse when aspirated. According to Sands (1991), the advantage of the wide-bore tube is that it does not block easily and fluid can be aspirated with ease.

Sands (1991) demonstrated that pulmonary aspiration is decreased with the use of a wide-bore tube, and according to Bladen (1986) there may be a tendency for the narrower fine-bore tube to dislodge into the trachea. These studies seem to contradict other studies, which suggest that the risk of gastro-eosophageal reflux is generally greater with wide-bore tubes than with fine-bore tubes. However, Mullan et al (1992) demonstrated no difference in incidence of gastro-oesophageal reflux between wide-bore and fine-bore tubes. The debate over the use of wide- and fine-bore tubes leaves a dilemma for clinical practitioners.

However, it is recommended that initially a wide-bore tube be passed to allow easy assessment of gastric contents. Assessment should include aspiration of the nasogastric tube 4-hourly to determine gastric content and pH. Feeding should be commenced and aspiration continued until it is evident that the patient is absorbing successfully. The wide-bore tube (Ryle's tube) should then be replaced by a small-bore tube. A small-bore tube collapses when aspirated and is therefore not suitable during the initial assessment stage, but has many benefits following effective assessment. Thus, when feeding a surgical patient enterally, a balance must be made between the advantage of ease of assessment and the long-term delivery of food.

Bolus versus continuous feeding

The method of administration of nasogastric feeding has traditionally been by bolus. Recently, however, there has been a move towards continuous feeds.

Kocan & Hiskisch (1986) state that bolus feeding 'more closely simulates normal eating patterns and allows periods of rest for the gastro intestinal tract'. However, according to Farley (1988) this is not tolerated well by patients, as it causes bloating, cramps, nausea and diarrhoea. Bladen (1986) disagrees with this and shows that diarrhoea is not necessarily caused by bolus feeding. Continuous feeds have been found to produce less abdominal distension and allow greater time for absorption in the surgical patient. Kocan & Hiskisch (1986), Farley (1988) and Bladen (1986) agree and say that there are fewer gastrointestinal side-effects when continuous feeding is implemented.

Despite the benefits of a continuous feed, there are some disadvantages. Continuous feeds need to be interrupted to allow gastric emptying prior to positioning and intense physiotherapy, owing to the risk of pulmonary aspiration. This can then reduce the nutrition that the patient receives (Kocan & Hiskisch 1986). Continuous feeds are not suited to all types of patients, i.e. restless or confused patients, as the tube may become displaced and the patient is at risk of pulmonary aspiration (Kocan & Hiskisch 1986). Bolus feeding may be indicated in these situations.

Complications of enteral feeding

Despite the benefits of enteral feeding, there are complications which can arise. Most of these complications can be prevented and easily recognised if the surgical nurse understands and anticipates the potential problems. There is evidence to suggest that some of these complications can cause discrepancies between prescription and delivery of the enteral feed (Adam 1994).

Pulmonary aspiration. This is the major risk in enterally fed patients, because of the reduced rate of gastric emptying and the presence of the nasogastric tube (Bernard & Forlam 1984, Sands 1991). However, none of the traditional methods of checking the placement of the tube is considered 100% reliable. Checking is more difficult with fine-bore tubes as they cannot be aspirated, and there are problems with the accuracy of detecting oscillating air via a stethoscope in both types of tube (Methany et al 1991). Testing gastric pH is considered a reliable method of checking placement, although it is possible to obtain false negatives in situations where gastric pH has been altered (as, for example, in the administration of H_2 antagonists, etc.). The only absolutely reliable method of checking tube placement, according to Bladen (1986), Bernard & Forlam (1984) and Adam (1994), is by X-ray examination. In some institutions a chest X-ray is mandatory following fine-bore tube insertion. In addition to checking the site of the tube to prevent pulmonary aspiration, Bladen (1986) recommended that during feeding the head of the bed should be raised at least 30–60% to aid draining of the feed into the stomach. Varella (1989) emphasised that aspiration may go undetected and recommended the addition of a blue dye to all feeds in order to facilitate rapid awareness of pulmonary contamination. Bokus (1991) and Farley (1988) consider the possibility of using the jejunal route if the risk of aspiration is judged to be high.

Nausea and vomiting. Many patients experience nausea and vomiting while receiving nasogastric feed. Taylor (1989), Farley (1988) and Bladen (1986) all recognised that this is due to a rapid infusion rate of the feed. It may also be attributed to the high fat content of the feed. Farley (1988) considers that the odour of the formulas contributes to nausea and vomiting. It is advised that the rate of the feed should be reduced and an anti-emetic, e.g. metoclopramide, given to reduce the nausea and increase gastric motility (Farley 1988). If lactose intolerance is thought to be the cause of nausea and vomiting, a lactose-free formula may be recommended by the dietitian (Bladen 1986, Farley 1988).

Diarrhoea. Diarrhoea appears to be the most common problem of enteral tube feeding. It results in loss of valuable nutrients and may contribute to pressure area breakdown and psychological distress to the patient. Food intolerance is very rarely regarded as the cause of diarrhoea and treatment should aim not at stopping enteral nutrition but at treating the symptoms and identifying the true source. There are a number of possible causes of diarrhoea (Anderson 1986, Bokus 1991, Farley 1988, Kendil et al 1993).

Diarrhoea is often blamed on the feed itself, although there is little evidence to support this. Kendil et al (1993) found that diarrhoea did not appear until feed rates had reached greater than 275 ml per hour. This is far faster than patients on continuous feeding are ever fed and it thus seems unlikely that feed alone is the cause of diarrhoea.

If a rapid infusion rate or fat intolerance appears to be the cause of the diarrhoea, Farley (1988) and Bladen (1986) agree that the infusion rate should be decreased or the type of formula changed to a low fat content. Raper & Maynard (1992) argue that the rate of the feed should only be decreased if medical staff think that it is highly likely that feed intolerance is the cause of the diarrhoea. When the rate of the feed is decreased, it should be remembered that patients do not receive their nutritional requirements, defeating the aim of preventing the effects of malnutrition.

Contamination of feeds and feeding equipment can lead to diarrhoea. In order to reduce the risk of food contamination, Raper & Maynard (1992), Bokus (1991), Anderson (1986) and Farley (1988) all stressed the importance of asepsis. This area is most important when caring for surgical patients as they are susceptible to infection (Farley 1988). Organisms from contaminated feeds may colonise the gut and cause sepsis. Farley (1988) showed that contamination occurred during preparation of the feed and equipment, or during the hanging time of the feed. Taylor (1989) agrees and also attributes contamination to poor handling technique in the preparation of the feed. The recommendations to prevent contamination are quite specific. They include a maximum hanging period for formulas of 8 hours and daily changing of giving sets and feed containers. New feed should not be added to old feed and all open containers of formula should be discarded when not in use as they provide excellent medium for growth of organisms. Williams (1992) compared incidence of infection in home-produced feeds and commercially produced feeds and concluded that, with the above precautions, commercially prepared feeds carry less risk of infection. It is therefore recommended that ready-made feed be used wherever possible.

Cold feeds are often believed to be a cause of diarrhoea (Bladen 1986, Farley 1988). It has therefore been suggested that warming feeds to room temperature can decrease the risk of diarrhoea (Farley 1988). However, Holmes (1989) suggests that there is a danger that this may promote the growth of bacteria, which can cause diarrhoea. Most of the newer ready-made feeds are stored at room temperature and do not require refrigeration.

Taylor (1989) identified drug administration such as broad-spectrum antibiotic treatment as causing diarrhoea. Taylor recommends that, if possible, broad-spectrum antibiotics, which are generally poorly absorbed, should be replaced by more specific and better-absorbed antibiotics. She also stated that the benefits of antibiotic treatment must be weighed against the disadvantages of preventing enteral feeding. The effect of antibiotic therapy may have detrimental effects on the normal gut flora. When diarrhoea occurs, nutrition should be continued and, when possible, the drug therapy stopped or changed for an alternative. However, most surgical patients require

some antibiotic cover. It appears impractical to discontinue this for the sake of enteral feeding. Perhaps in this instance parenteral nutrition will need to be considered, with a small amount of enteral feeding to prevent gut atrophy and translocation of bacteria from the gut to the bloodstream causing sepsis (Taylor 1989). The issue has been raised that surgical nurses possibly are not always accurate in their diagnosis of the cause of diarrhoea. It is interesting to consider that we may be unnecessarily stopping or reducing enteral tube nutrition just because the patient has developed diarrhoea.

The administration of live yogurt when diarrhoea occurs during NGF has been shown some interest, but the benefits to patients on NGF with diarrhoea have not been clearly substantiated by any formal research.

The only disagreement arising in the treatment of diarrhoea relates to the approaches taken regarding antidiarrhoeal drug therapy. Farley (1988) tentatively suggests the use of antimotility drugs as a last resort and stresses the need for regular monitoring of bowel sounds. Anderson (1986), however, highlights the importance of treating diarrhoea and provides a comprehensive list of drugs that could be used for this purpose. Raper & Maynard (1992), on the other hand, warn quite forcefully against giving antimotility drugs to a patient whose diarrhoea has been caused by antibiotic therapy, as a build-up of bacterial toxins could result from a sluggish gut. These inconsistencies have implications for drug management and appear quite serious. The subjects of live yogurt, drug therapy and enteral tube feeding could all benefit from further research.

Blockage of the tube. Since the diameter of the nasogastric tube is small, it may become blocked. According to Bladen (1986) the use of dense formulas can be a cause, and if so, the formula should be diluted. This will, however, decrease the nutrients the patient will receive and is thus not recommended. It is better in this instance to consult the dietitian. Raper & Maynard (1992) suggest that tube clogging is more related to the number of insufficiently crushed medications given via the nasogastric tube. Taylor (1989) and Raper & Maynard (1992) suggest that liquid medications should be used as often as possible and the tube flushed with 10–20 ml of water before and after each feed.

Discomfort, ulceration of the nose, trauma. Care needs to be taken when a nasogastric tube is in position to prevent discomfort to the patient and ulceration of the nose. As already discussed, the use of a narrow-bore tube will reduce the incidence of trauma occurring to the nose. The importance of secure fastening of the tube in order to reduce friction and pulling or the accidental removal of the tube is also highlighted. Proper taping of the nasogastric tube will help reduce discomfort to the nose (Farley 1988).

Adequate oral and nasal hygiene is also important to relieve the discomfort of a nasogastric tube (Farley 1988, Taylor 1989). Mouth dryness may develop during nasogastric feeding, owing to obligatory mouth breathing and the lack of oral stimulation. The incidence of sore throat and psychosensory deprivation due to nasogastric feeding have not received much attention. Whilst it would be interesting to learn more about patients' psychological reactions to taste and smell deprivation, it would also help to compare their emotional state with patients receiving parenteral nutrition. Where long-term nutritional support is required, and where ulceration and trauma to the nose may be difficult to prevent, the use of alternative enteral routes such as gastrostomy or jejunostomy should be considered.

The development of large residual volumes. Large residual volumes occur in the stomach when there is inadequate absorption of nasogastric feed and may be one of the main reasons patients are switched from enteral feeding to parenteral nutrition. The accepted maximum residual volume varies from 50–200 ml, illustrating a fairly wide range. The development of large residual volumes can be hard to treat and result in the need to greatly reduce nutritional input. The factors contributing to large residual volumes are proposed as bolus feeding and malnutrition, leading to malabsorption of feed (Anderson 1986). In such instances, bolus feeding should be stopped and continuous feeding implemented to allow less feed per hour, giving more time for the absorption of nutrients (Farley 1988, Williams 1994).

When large residual volumes occur because of malnutrition, it is generally because undernourishment reduces the gut's ability to absorb nutrients and destroys the mucosal lining. It is recommended in this instance that feeding should stop for 1 hour and the residual volume be rechecked. This would continue until there was evidence of absorption. Gastric emptying problems should usually resolve within 2–8 hours (Farley 1988). This procedure should continue and the enteral feeding be reduced, to allow the lining of the gut time to repair and to prevent translocation of bacteria. Under no circumstances should the enteral feeding be stopped entirely. However, a patient who is severely malnourished may only be able to regain gut function with increasing amounts of NGF and the assistance of parenteral support.

Overfeeding. Cerrato (1991) documented that patients undergoing surgery will suffer from stress, which in turn increases their BMR. This would result in an increased demand for energy, which if not satisfied will increase weight loss. Thus, with an increased BMR there is a higher energy expenditure, which requires a higher carbohydrate and fat intake. Excess carbohydrate and lipid intake can cause hepatic steatosis and abnormal liver function. Lipid may also be deposited in the lung and impair diffusion of gases, producing infusional hyperlipidaemia (Elia 1995). Overfeeding with excess carbohydrate can lead to excess carbon dioxide production, which can precipitate respiratory failure. However, Elia (1995) has shown that the energy requirements of disease have often been overestimated. The recommendation that more energy should be provided to take into account the effects of pyrexia (13% of basal metabolic rate per degree centigrade rise in temperature) is now suggested to be inappropriate (Elia 1995). It is also recommended not to account doubly for the energy cost of breathing; the resting energy expenditure of a patient with acute respiratory distress may increase by only 20–30% rather than 50%, whereas that of a normal subject with no respiratory problems would only increase by 2–3% (Elia 1992).

It appears that the energy requirements of patients who are unwell are usually similar to or less than those of healthy subjects. The reason is that the basal hypermetabolism often seen in patients in hospital disease is offset by the decrease in physical activity. The normal daily energy expenditure in adults is generally 1700–2500 kcal (30–35 kcal/kg) (1 kcal = 4.184 J). It is recommended that hypocaloric feeding should be the current practice in hospital feeding regimes, especially in the early stages of injury (e.g. 1500 kcal/day for up to a week). This would reduce the risk of liver and lung complications, and metabolic instability and their consequences. This does appear to be logical, in that a patient who is malnourished may have a reduced BMR, and therefore, if given a normal or higher calorie intake, may be at serious risk of developing some of the problems identified with overfeeding. An increase in calorie intake would take place in the recovery phase, when the nutrition level was normal and the patient was no longer at risk. This regime to reduce the prescribed energy intake initially in patients with acute illnesses and/or malnutrition is irrespective of whether the patients are preoperative or postoperative, receiving parenteral or enteral nutrition or are in intensive care units. An appreciation of these effects could restrict the overprescription of energy.

CONCLUSION

It appears that nutrition has had various degrees of importance, from being very highly rated in the 1870s to being almost forgotten by the 1930s. Despite a growing interest in nutrition, there is still a problem with malnutrition, which continues to go largely unrecognised, and can occur prior to, during or following surgery. The consequences for the patient are severe: psychological distress, increased risks of complications, and possibly a lengthened stay in hospital.

It is suggested that malnutrition in hospitals will only be reduced when the problem is recognised, when health professionals receive adequate education and when the multidisciplinary team accept nutrition as an essential part of the treatment of the patient. The most overwhelming conclusion must be the need for better nutritional assessment and organisation of nutritional support. The potential benefits warrant no further discussion, but must be recognised as a key challenge for the surgical nurse.

REFERENCES

Adam S K 1994 Aspects of current research in enteral nutrition in the critically ill. Care of the Critically Ill 10(6): 246–251

Allwood M C, Brown P W, Ghendini C, Hardy G 1992 The stability of ascorbic acid in TPN parenteral nutrition admixtures stored in a multilayered bag. Clinical Nutrition 11: 284–290

American Medical Association, Department of Foods and Nutrition 1979 Guidelines for essential trace element for parenteral use. Journal of the American Medical Association 241: 2051–2054

Anderson B J 1986 Tube feeding: is diarrhea inevitable? American Journal of Nursing 86(6): 704–706

Aora N S, Rochester D F 1982 Effects of body weight and muscularity on human diaphragm muscle mass, thickness, and area. Journal of Applied Physiology 52(1): 64–70

Arbuthnot J 1731 Essay concerning the nature of aliments. Tonson, London

Atkins S 1989 Parenteral nutrition – the nurse's role. Surgical Nurse 1(2): 13–17

Banerjee A 1988 Total parenteral nutrition in the intensive care unit. Care of the Critically Ill 4(5): 8–11

Barber A E, Jones W G, Minei J P et al 1990 Glutamine or fibre supplementation of a defined formula diet: impact on bacterial translocation, tissue composition and response to endotoxin. Journal of Parenteral and Enteral Nutrition 335–343

Belghiti J, Goldfarb G, Gautero M 1983 Impaired in vitro bactericidal power of polymorphonuclear leucocytes in patients with protein calorie malnutrition. Surgery, Gynaecology and Obstetrics 156: 489–492

Bernard M, Forlam L 1984 Complications and their preventions: enteral and tube feeding. W B Saunders, London

Bishop C W, Bowen P E, Ritchley S I 1981 Norms for nutritional assessment of American adults by upper arm anthropometry. American Journal of Clinical Nutrition 34: 2530–2539

Bistrain B R, Blackburn G L, Vitale J, Cochran D, Naylor J 1974 Protein status of general surgical patients. Journal of the American Medical Association 230: 858–860

Bladen L M 1986 Enteral nutrition. Nursing 8: 281–284

Bokus S 1991 Troubleshooting your tube feeds. American Journal of Nursing 91(5): 24–28

Booth B 1993 Nutritional therapies. Nursing Times 89(37): 44–46

British Medical Association 1993 Complementary medicine: new approaches to good practice. Oxford University Press, Oxford

Burr M L, Phillips K M 1984 Anthropometric norms in the elderly. British Journal of Clinical Nutrition 51: 165–169

Campos A C L, Meguid M M 1992 A critical appraisal of the usefulness of perioperative nutritional support. American Journal of Clinical Nutrition 55: 117

Cerrato P L 1991 Surgery, stress and metabolism. Registered Nurse 54(8): 63–65

Chapman A 1996 Current theory and practice: a study of pre-operative fasting. Nursing Standard 10(18): 33–36

Chapman C, Curtas S, Meguid M 1992 Standardised enteral orders attain colorific gains sooner: a prospective study. Journal of Parenteral and Enteral Nutrition 16: 149–151

Cole-Hamilton I 1991 Poverty can seriously damage your health – a response to the green paper 'The Health of the Nation'. Child Poverty Action Group, London

Committee on Medical Aspects of Food Policy 1984 Diet and cardiovascular disease: report of the panel on diet in relation to cardiovascular disease. HMSO, London

Corbett R, Lee B 1992 Nutriquest: a fun way to reinforce nutrition knowledge. Nurse Educator 17(2): 33–35

Cotton E 1996 A nutritional assessment tool for older patients. Professional Nurse 11(9): 609–612

Cruickshank J K, Beevers D G 1989 Ethnic factors in health and disease. Butterworth, London

Daniels L 1991 The changing face of nutrition. Practice Nurse 4(7): 394–397

Davey-Smith G, Bartley M, Blane D 1990 The Black report on socio-economic inequalities in health ten years on. British Medical Journal 6748(301): 373–377

Davies L 1981 Three score years … and then? Heinemann Medical Books, London

Deitch E A, Winterton J, Berg R 1987 The gut as a portal of entry for bacteremia: role of protein malnutrition. Annals of Surgery 205: 681–690

Department of Health (DoH) 1991 Dietary reference values for food energy and nutrition for the United Kingdom. Report No. 41. HMSO, London

Department of Health and Social Security (DHSS) 1980 Inequalities in health: report of a research working group. HMSO, London

Dickerson J 1995 The problem of hospital induced malnutrition Nursing Times 91(4): 44–45

Doekal R, Zwillich C 1976 Clinical semi-starvation: depression of hypoxic ventilatory response. New England Journal of Medicine 295(7): 358–361

Downie R S, Fyfe C, Tannahill A 1991 Health promotion: models and values. Oxford University Press, Oxford

Dwyer J T 1988 Health aspects of vegetarian diets. American Journal of Clinical Nutrition 48: 712–738

Ek A C et al 1991 The development and healing of pressure sores related to the nutritional status. Clinical Nutrition 10: 245–250

Elia M 1995 Changing concepts of nutrient requirements in disease: implications for artificial nutritional support. Lancet 345(8960): 1279–1284

Englert D M, Crocker K S, Stotts N A 1986 Nutrition education in schools of nursing in the United States: the evaluation of nutrition in schools of nursing. Journal of Parenteral and Enteral Nutrition 10: 522–527

Ephgrave K S, Kleiman-Wexler R L, Adair C G 1990 Enteral nutrients prevent stress ulceration and increase intragastric volume. Critical Care Medicine 18: 621–624

Farley J M 1988 Current trends in enteral feeding. Critical Care Nurse 8(4): 23–27

Fawcett H, Yeoman C 1991 A tube to suit all nasogastric needs: an evaluation of fine bore nasogastric tubes. Professional Nurse 6(6): 324–329

Finnegan S 1989 Mechanical complications of parenteral nutrition. Parenteral Nutrition (Apr): 325–327

Finnegan S, Oldfield K 1989 When eating is impossible: TPN in maintaining nutritional status. Professional Nurse 4(6): 271–275

Garrow J 1994 Starvation in hospital. British Medical Journal 6934(308): 934

Garvey A, Hibbert A, Manley K 1994 Nutrition and nursing. RCN, London

Goode H F, Burns E, Walker B E 1992 Vitamin C depletion and pressure sores in elderly patients with femoral neck fracture. British Medical Journal 305(6859): 925–927

Goodinson S M 1986 Assessment of nutritional status. Nursing 7: 252–258

Goodinson-McClaren S 1992 Nutrition and wound healing. Journal of Wound Care 1(3): 45–55

Goodwin S, Skaggs B J, Renshaw S 1988 Student assignments using nutrition programs. Nursing Educators Microworld 3(1): 4

Hamilton-Smith 1972 Nil by mouth. RCN, London

Harvey J 1993 Malnutrition: manifestations and treatment. Primary Health Care 3(5): 20–21

Hennessy K, Orr M, Curtas S 1990 Nutrition support nursing: a specialty practice: historical development. Clinical Nurse Specialist 4(2): 67–70

Herbert C 1996 Assessing nutrition in elderly patients. Nursing Standard 10(17): 35–37

Hickey J 1986 The clinical practice of neurological and neurosurgical nursing. J B Lippincott, London

Hill G L, Pickford J, Young G A et al 1977 Malnutrition in surgical patients: an unrecognised problem. Lancet 18013(13): 689–692

Holford P 1992 Optimum nutrition. ION Press, London

Holmes S 1989 Careful food handling reduces the risk of listeria. Professional Nurse (Apr): 322–324

Holmes S 1991 Nutrition and the surgical patient. Nursing Standard 5(44): 30–32

Holmes S 1993 Building blocks. Nursing Times 89(21): 28–31

Holmes S, Dickerson J W 1987 Malignant disease: nutritional implications of disease and treatment. Cancer Metastases Review 6(3): 357–381

Holol C, McIntosh E, Girad D 1984 Nutrition education and nursing students. Nurse Educator 9(3): 29, 36

Horwood A 1990 Malnourishment in ITU, as high as 50%: are nurses doing enough to change this? Intensive Care Nursing 6: 205–207

Howard L, Chu R, Feman S, Mintz H, Ovesen L, Wolfe B 1980 Vitamin A deficiency from long-term parenteral nutrition. Annals of Internal Medicine 93: 567–577

Hudak C M, Gallo B M, Lohr T 1990 Critical care nursing: a holistic approach, 5th edn. J B Lippincott, Philadelphia

Hung P 1992 Pre-operative fasting. Nursing Times 88(48): 57–60

Hunter M 1988 Feeding the patient in hospital. Senior Nurse 8(2): 19–20

Ireton-Jones C S, Hasse J 1992 Comprehensive nutritional assessment: the dietitian's contribution to the team effort. Nutrition 8(2): 75–81

Jenson J E, Jenson T G, Smith T K, Johnston D A, Drurick S J 1982 Nutrition in orthopaedic surgery. Journal of Bone and Joint Surgery 63: 1263–1272

Kendil H E, Oper F H, Switzer B R et al 1993 Marked resistance of normal subjects to tube feeding diarrhea: the role of magnesium. American Journal of Clinical Nutrition 57: 73-80

Keohane P P, Jones B, Attrill H, Northovers J 1983 Effects of catheter tunnelling and a nutrition nurse on catheter sepsis during parenteral nutrition: a controlled trial. Lancet 2(8364): 1388–1390

King's Fund 1992 A positive approach to nutrition as treatment. King's Fund, London

Klein G L, Alfrey A C, Shike M, Sherrard D J 1991 Parenteral drug products containing aluminium as an ingredient or as a contaminant: response to FDA notice of intent. American Journal of Clinical Nutrition 53: 399–402

Kocan M J, Hiskisch S M 1986 A comparison of continuous and intermittent enteral nutrition in NICU patients. Journal of Neuroscience Nursing 18(6): 333–337

La France R J, Miyagawa C I 1991 Pharmaceutical considerations in total parenteral nutrition. In: Fischer J E (ed) Total parenteral nutrition, 2nd edn. Little Brown, Boston

Lee B 1987 Total parenteral nutrition. Nursing Times 83(31): 58–59

Lee B T, Corbett R W 1992 Nutritional pursuit: a learning module. Journal of Nursing Education 31(6): 283–284

Lennard-Jones J E 1992 A positive approach to nutrition as treatment. King's Fund, London

McCannon G 1983 A specialist unit. Nursing Mirror (Feb): 50–55

McCarthy M 1990 The thin deal, depression and eating disorders in women. Behaviour Research and Therapy 28(3): 205–215

MacKay L 1995 The nurse's role in giving nutritional advice. Professional Nurse 10(7): 427–572

McWhirter J P, Pennington C R 1994 Incidence and recognition of malnutrition in hospital. British Medical Journal 6934(308): 945–948

Majors M 1988 Nutritional support of the mechanically ventilated patient. Critical Care Nursing Quarterly 11(2): 50–61

Malseed J 1990 Bread without dough: understanding food poverty. Horton Publishing, Bradford

Martini F M 1998 Fundamentals of anatomy and physiology, 4th edn. Prentice Hall, Upper Saddle River, New Jersey

Marvin J 1988 Nutritional support of the critically injured patient. Critical Care Nursing Quarterly 11(2): 21–34

Maynard N D, Bihari D 1991 Postoperative feeding. British Medical Journal 303(6809): 1007–1008

Meakins J L, Marshall J C 1989 Multi-organ failure syndrome (MOF): the gastro-intestinal tract, the motor of MOF. Surgery 121: 196–208

Methany N, Eisenberg P, Spies M 1991 Monitoring patients with nasally placed feeding tubes. Heart and Lung 20(4): 285–286

Mirowitz S A, Westrich T J 1992 Basal ganglial signal intensity alterations: reversal after discontinuation of parenteral manganese administration. Radiology 185(2): 535–536

Mitchie B 1988 Making sense of total parenteral nutrition. Nursing Times 84(20): 46–47

Moynihan P 1994 Special nutritional needs of surgical patients. Nursing Times 90(51): 40–41

Mullan H, Roubenoff R A, Roubenoff R 1992 Risk of pulmonary aspiration among patients receiving enteral nutrition support. Journal of Parenteral and Enteral Nutrition 16: 160–164

National Advisory Committee on Nutrition Education 1983 A discussion paper on proposals for nutritional guidelines for health education in Britain. Health Education Council, London

National Children's Home 1991 Poverty and nutrition survey. NCH, London

National Research Council 1989 Recommended dietary allowances, 10th edn. National Academy Press, Washington

Nightingale F 1859 Notes on nursing: what it is and what it is not. Blackie, London

Norton D, Exton-Smith N 1962 An investigation of geriatric nursing problems in hospital. National Cooperation for the Care of Old People, London

Oh T E 1997 Intensive care manual, 4th edn. Butterworth, Sidney

Olsen K 1989 The encyclopaedia of alternative health care. Piatkus, London

Parker D, Emmett P M, Heaton K W 1992 Final year medical students' knowledge of practical nutrition. Intensive Therapy Clinical Monitoring 9: 239–246

Parkes C M 1985 Bereavement. British Journal of Psychiatry 146(Jan): 11–17

Pinchocofsky G D, Kaminski M V 1985 Increasing malnutrition during hospitalisation: documentation by a nutritional screening program. Journal of the American College of Nutrition 4: 471–479

Raper S, Maynard N 1992 Feeding the critically ill patient. British Journal of Nursing 1(6): 273–278

Reilly H 1996 Nutritional assessment. British Journal of Nursing 5(1): 18–24

Reilly J J, Hull S P, Albert N, Waller A, Bringardener S 1988 Economic impact of malnutrition: a model system for hospitalised patients. Journal of Parenteral and Enteral Nutrition 12: 372–376

Robinson G, Goldstein M, Levine G M 1987 Impact of nutritional status on DRG length of stay. Journal of Parenteral and Enteral Nutrition 11: 49–51

Royal College of Nursing 1993 Nutrition standards and the older adult. RCN Dynamic Quality Improvement Programme, London

Sands J 1991 Incidence of pulmonary aspiration in intubated patients receiving enteral nutrition through wide and narrow bore nasogastric feeding tubes. Heart and Lung 20(1): 91–94

Say J 1997 Nutritional assessment in clinical practice: a review. Nursing in Critical Care 2(1): 29–33

Schilling J 1976 Wound healing. Surgical Clinics of North America 56: 859

Sedenvall B, Ek A 1993 Long-term care patients and their dietary intake related to eating ability and nutritional needs: nursing staff interventions. Journal of Advanced Nursing 18(4): 565–573

Spaeth G, Specian R D, Berg R D, Deitch E A 1990 Bulk prevents bacterial translocation induced by the oral administration of TPN solution. Journal of Parenteral and Enteral Nutrition 14: 442–447

Stotts N A, Englert D, Crocker K S, Bennum N W, Hoppe M 1987 Nutrition in schools of nursing in United States: the status of nutrition education in schools of nursing. Journal of Parenteral and Enteral Nutrition 11: 406–411

Strong R M, Condon S C, Solinger M R et al 1992 Equal aspiration rates from postpylorus and intragastric-placed small-bore nasoenteric feeding tubes: a randomised, prospective study. Journal of Parenteral and Enteral Nutrition 16: 59–63

Taylor M 1988 Food glorious food. Nursing Times 84(13): 28–30

Taylor S 1989 Preventing complications in enteral feeding. Professional Nurse 4(5): 247–249

Thomas B (ed) 1994 Manual of dietetic practice, 2nd edn. Blackwell Science, Oxford

Thomas E A 1987 Pre operative fasting – a question of routine? Nursing Times 83(49): 46–47

Tierney A J 1996 Undernutrition and elderly hospital patients: a review. Journal of Advanced Nursing 23(2): 228–236

Tinckler L F, Kulke W 1963 Post operative absorption of water from the small intestine. Gut 4: 8

Tredger J 1982 Feeding the patient – a team effort. Nursing 2(4): 92–93

Varella L D 1989 Nutrition in the critically ill: nutritional support and head trauma. Critical Care Nurse 9(1): 28–34

Wallace E 1993 The effects of malnutrition in hospital. British Journal of Nursing 2(1): 66–71

Waterlow J A 1988 The Waterlow card for the prevention and management of pressure sores: towards a pocket policy. Care – Science and Practice 6(1): 8–12

Watkins J, Bevan S, Hardy G 1994 Aspects of nutrition and immunocompetence: inter-relationships between the two disciplines. British Journal of Intensive Care 4: 55–63

Watson R 1994 Nutrition standards and the elderly adult. Journal of Advanced Nursing 20(2): 205–206

Weissman C, Hyman A 1987 Nutritional care in the critically ill patient with respiratory failure. Critical Care Clinician 3: 185–201

Wells C, Tinckler L, Rawlinson K, Jones H, Saunders J 1964 Postoperative gastrointestinal motility. Lancet 1(7323): 4–10

Wells L 1994 At the front line of care. Professional Nurse 9(8): 525–530

White M J 1990 Oxygen-free radicals and wound healing. Clinical Plastic Surgery 17: 473–484

Williams S R 1994 Essentials of nutrition and diet therapy, 6th edn. Mosby, California

Windsor J A, Hill G L 1988 Risk factors for post operative pneumonia: the importance of protein depletion. Annals of Surgery 17: 181–185

Wolfe B M, Ryder M A, Nishikawa R A, Halsted C H, Schmidt B F 1986 Complications of parenteral nutrition. American Journal of Surgery 152: 93–99

Woods S 1992 Clinical enteral nutrition: an RCN nursing update. Nursing Standard 6(33): 3–8

World Health Organization (WHO) 1985 Targets for health for all. Copenhagen, WHO

Yetiv J 1988 Sense and nonsense in nutrition. Penguin, Harmondsworth

Young M E 1988 Malnutrition and wound healing. Heart and Lung 17(1) 60–67

28

Principles of wound drainage, healing and management

Mark Collier

AIMS

This chapter aims to:

- introduce and discuss the anatomy of human skin in relation to wound management
- describe the process of normal wound healing related to holistic patient assessment
- consider the effect of wound drainage – both normal and abnormal – on healing
- classify the methods employed to facilitate wound healing
- critically analyse the optimum wound healing environment and factors which may affect it
- examine the properties of a variety of wound dressing materials and understand their role when used to control wound drainage
- critically appraise a number of wound drainage systems and indicate their practical clinical use.

INTRODUCTION

Caring for patients with wounds involves all practitioners and can be a very challenging and complex aspect of their work, as wounds, however caused, are found in people of all ages. This chapter reflects a dynamic approach to dealing with the many patient care aspects related to wound management, as not only does it revise the basic principles underpinning current practice but also discusses their practical application in the clinical setting before introducing the reader to recent innovations which have benefited both patients and carers alike.

It could be argued that this dynamic approach to wound management is essential for current and future surgical nursing practice. The author has gleaned from the Wound Healing Research Unit at Guy's Hospital, London, that rather than the number of patients requiring specific wound management interventions decreasing, it is likely to increase because of the number of people in the UK who are living longer. This will result in particular in an increase in the number of chronic wounds requiring treatment – pressure ulcers, leg ulcers and a variety of non-healing wounds – all of which may be seen by the nurse working within a surgical setting.

Not only will this increase have practical implications for the nurse working in these settings, but it will also have severe financial implications. Currently the associated costs of managing these patients has been reported as between £60 and £321 million per annum (DoH 1993) and this does not take into account any potential litigation or compensation costs to patients with wounds which were deemed preventable or which might have been better managed (Silver 1987).

If nurses are familiar with advances in the principles of all aspects of wound management, it could be argued that not only will the potential increase in costs be minimised but, significantly, there will be both enhanced quality of patient care and surgical nursing practice.

Generally, the principle of moist wound healing is well accepted. A moist wound surface (interface) has been shown to increase the rate of epidermal resurfacing (Winter 1962), and therefore speed up wound healing rates by as much as 40%, and improve the cosmetic appearance of wounds when compared with those that are left exposed to the air or covered with traditional dressings such as filamanted gauze-type materials (Eaglstein 1985, Thomas 1990, Winter 1975).

As a result, many types of interactive wound dressing materials have been developed during the last decade with the purpose of ensuring that a moist wound healing environment is maintained. Nevertheless, despite the increasing use of these materials, wounds which produce a large amount of exudate and/or which require long-term drainage can still present a challenge to all health care professionals. In the author's opinion it is, therefore, vital that today's practitioners ensure that the balance between keeping the wound surface moist and controlling excess exudate is considered an important assessment and management priority.

Wound exudate and drainage is normally composed of body fluids (water and electrolytes) and in the majority of cases will not pose a problem. The proportion of body fluid contained within the human body is influenced by age, sex and body fat content. In general, younger people have a higher percentage of body fluid than older people, and men have proportionally more body fluid than women. Typically, an adult will be composed of 60% fluid, approximately two-thirds of which is in the intracellular spaces, such as in the skeletal muscle mass, and one-third is in the

extracellular spaces, between the cells and in the plasma (Brunner & Suddarth 1992))(see also Ch. 26).

When caring for patients with heavily exuding or draining wounds, the treatment objectives governing nursing management should include the following:

- controlling drainage
- protecting the patient's skin surrounding the wound/drain
- controlling any associated odour
- maximising patient comfort and mobility
- optimising the patient's healing potential and being cost-effective.

In order to ensure appropriate patient care, it could be argued that all health care professionals involved in managing patients with either a heavily exuding or draining wound need to have a comprehensive but practical knowledge of the normal anatomy of the skin; the natural healing process; the factors which might affect the healing process, i.e. a holistic perspective; the importance of issues related to wound drainage, and the properties and range of products available to help minimise its effects.

THE SKIN

Structure of the skin

The skin is one of the largest organs of the body and despite its simple appearance (Fig. 28.1) is a very complex structure.

In the average adult this organ occupies a surface area of approximately 2 square metres – the size of a hospital bed; weighs approximately 3 kg – nearly twice the weight of the human brain; and ranges in thickness from 0.5 cm on the palms of the hands and soles of the feet to 0.5 mm at the eyelids and scalp.

Structurally, the skin can be divided into two main parts – the epidermis and the dermis – although these can be further subdivided into distinct regions of differing cells, all of which have a part to play in the process of natural wound healing.

The epidermis

The epidermis is composed mainly of stratified squamous epithelial tissue and contains four major cell types: keratinocytes, melanocytes, Langerhans cells and Granstein cells.

Keratinocytes produce keratin, which helps to waterproof the skin and underlying tissue and assists the process of immunity. Melanocytes produce melanin, which is responsible for a person's skin colour. This is important in relation to the visibility of

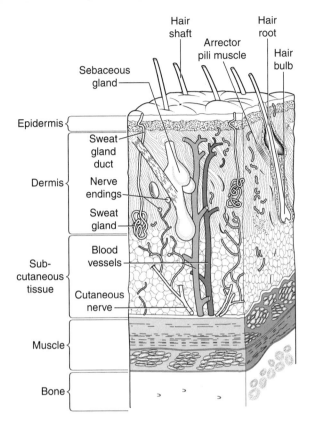

Epidermis {
  Dermis {
  Sub-cutaneous tissue {
  Muscle {
  Bone {

Hair shaft
Arrector pili muscle
Hair root
Hair bulb
Sebaceous gland
Sweat gland duct
Nerve endings
Sweat gland
Blood vessels
Cutaneous nerve

Figure 28.1   Cross-section of the skin.

'scar' tissue because, if the function of melanin is impaired as a result of the nature of the injury, there may be a permanent reminder of the patient's wound, even if it is 'healed'. Langerhans cells originate in bone marrow and invade the epidermis. Together with the Granstein cells, they assist with the process of immunity.

The number of cell layers of the epidermis will depend upon its location in the body. For example where exposure to compression forces is at its greatest (the palms and soles) five layers may be identified as follows (from superficial to deepest):

1. The *stratum corneum* – consists of 25–30 rows of dead cells filled with keratin. Continuously shed and replaced (in fact this whole layer is replaced every 24 hours and constitutes the majority of household dust particles), the stratum corneum serves as a barrier against bacteria, light and heat waves as well as many chemicals.

2. The *stratum lucidum* is normally only found in the soles of the feet and palms of the hand and is composed of clear, flat dead cells which contain a substance known as eleidin which serves to cushion surface impacts.

3. The *stratum granulosum* consists of flattened cells which are involved with keratin formation. The nuclei of these cells are at various stages of degeneration and as they break down and are no longer capable of performing metabolic actions, they die.

4. The *stratum spinosum* (also known as the prickle cell layer) consists of 8–10 rows of polyhedral cells all joined together. If this layer of the skin is permanently damaged in any wound management scenario, then the colour of the patient's scar tissue may be different from that of the surrounding skin, as it is here that melanin is produced.

5. The *stratum basale* is a single layer of cuboidal to columnar cells, which as they multiply push upwards towards the surface of the skin and become part of the layers previously described. This region of the skin plays a vital role in the germination of new cells (fibroblastic activity) essential for the process of natural wound healing.

The dermis

The dermis is composed primarily of connective tissue containing collagenous and elastic fibres. Other structures which can be found in this region of the skin are blood and lymph vessels, sensory nerve endings, sweat glands and ducts, hair, hair roots and follicles, sebaceous glands and arrectores pilorum – involuntary muscle attached to hair follicles.

The collagenous fibres in the dermis give new healing tissues their strength. Initially they are laid down in a random fashion. However, over time in the healing wound (approximately 3 weeks), these fibres will striate to lines of tension; this is especially evident on the palmar aspect of the fingers. These lines of tension are of particular interest to a surgeon, as a surgical incision parallel to the collagen fibre should heal with only a fine, minimal scar. The strength of healing tissues is further increased by the presence of longitudinal protein fibres which run across the collagenous striations in order to facilitate maximum flexibility, whilst ensuring that the structure (the skin) remains intact.

Beneath the dermis is a fatty layer known as the subcutaneous layer, which is attached to underlying organs by structures such as muscle and bone. The female has more adipose (fatty) tissue than her male counterpart and for this reason will always be assessed as being at greater risk of pressure ulcer development because of the resultant increased internal body temperature, the subsequent increase in metabolic activity, and relevant hormonal influences (Tortora 1988).

Functions of the skin

When intact, the skin essentially forms a barrier between the external and internal environments of the body. Its principal functions can be summarised as follows:

* protection
* perception of stimuli
* absorption
* synthesis of vitamin D
* maintenance of body temperature
* excretion of waste products
* waterproofing and maintenance of water balance (Tortora 1988).

Protection

The skin protects the body against invasion by bacteria and foreign matter. The palms of the hands and soles of the feet provide the tough covering required to maintain skin integrity, despite the constant pressures which are exerted on these areas during normal activities of living.

Sensory function

Normal stimulation of the receptor nerve endings in the skin enables constant monitoring of the external environment, such as the perception of changes in temperature, the recognition of pain and the differentiation of light or heavy touch. Different nerve endings are responsible for responding to each of the different stimuli. Although these nerve endings are distributed over the entire body, they are more concentrated in some areas (fingertips) than in other, larger anatomical regions (the skin covering the back).

Absorption

The structure of the skin allows certain topical compounds such as drugs (e.g. hydrocortisone) to be absorbed through it into the local surrounding tissues. Care must be taken, however, to ensure that as a result of overuse the patient's skin does not become desensitised to the beneficial effects of the compound being used.

Synthesis of vitamin D

Vitamin D refers to a group of closely related compounds synthesised naturally from a substance present in the skin as a result of direct exposure to ultraviolet (UV) radiation, such as from sunlight.

Temperature regulation

Heat, which is continuously produced by the body as a result of metabolic activity, is primarily dissipated through the skin. This is facilitated by one of three processes: radiation – the ability of the body to give off its heat to another object of a lower temperature; conduction – the transfer of heat from the body to a cooler object in contact with it; and convection – the movement of warm air molecules away from the body.

Normally the internal temperature of the body is considered to be maintained at a constant 37°C. Heat loss from the body via the skin can also be controlled by the blood supply to the skin. An increased blood flow to the skin results in an increased surface temperature and therefore a greater loss of heat from the body, whereas a decreased blood flow decreases the skin temperature and so helps to conserve body heat. Sweating is another process by which the body can help regulate heat loss.

Water balance

Under normal circumstances, the skin forms a barrier to prevent the loss of body fluid from the internal environment whilst at the same time preventing the subcutaneous tissues from drying out. If the skin is damaged, large amounts of fluid may be lost rapidly, resulting in complications for the patient such as circulatory failure, shock or even death. A small amount of fluid is lost each day (approximately 500 ml in a normal adult) through evaporation and this is termed insensible perspiration. The amount of insensible perspiration may vary depending upon the patient's skin and/or internal body temperature (Brunner & Suddarth 1992).

Normal flora of the skin

The skin has been described as a vast empire in which contrasts of terrain and climate are as varied as the earth itself (Skinner & Carr 1976). In the healthy adult patient, the skin remains inhospitable to pathogenic organisms.

The most common inhabitants of the skin are bacteria such as *Staphylococcus epidermidis* (coagulase-negative Gram-positive cocci), micrococci and diphtheroids. Gram-negative species may also be present in small numbers. Resident flora live on or within the superficial layers of the epidermal stratum corneum and also in the upper parts of the sweat glands and hair follicles. These bacteria are distributed all over the surface of the skin but are found in the highest numbers in the scalp and moist areas of the body.

The majority of resident organisms are, in the main, harmless but may become pathogenic in nature if allowed to penetrate through the skin via a wound, during surgery or other invasive procedures. For example *Staphylococcus epidermidis* can cause problems if introduced into the body via implanted material such as replacement heart valves or acetabular replacements for hip surgery.

Other organisms which do not generally multiply on healthy intact skin may be acquired transiently. They may be acquired from other sites on the person's own body, from another person or from the external environment. Transient organisms include coagulase-positive staphylococci such as *Staphylococcus aureus*, which can colonise the perineal region of approximately 10% of all healthy individuals.

Skin squames are continually shed and replaced and it is this mechanism which may also contribute to the dispersal of a number of bacteria, the most common of which is again *Staphylococcus aureus*. The rate of bacterial dispersal in this manner will be increased when the patient has a skin condition such as psoriasis where the epidermal turnover is in itself increased.

Gram-negative organisms – for example *Escherichia coli* and *Pseudomonas* – may also be acquired transiently on the skin, especially on the hands. In this location the organisms can survive for several hours unless effectively washed off. Additional problems can also be encountered if anaerobic organisms such as *Clostridium perfringens* colonise areas of the skin around the thighs and buttocks; hence the need for appropriate skin preparation prior to orthopaedic surgery of the lower limbs. Homeostasis of the skin is maintained through the acid and fatty acid content of secretions which serve as bactericidal agents, as do the antimicrobial substances produced by many of the resident flora. Organisms cannot penetrate the 'horny' keratin layer of the skin if it remains intact.

In summary, the normal flora of the skin plays a vital part in maintaining a fine microbial balance which can easily be disrupted, resulting in the invasion of superficial tissues by opportunistic organisms or pathogenic species, creating an imbalance in the system (Collier 1994a) (see also Ch. 13).

Assessment of the patient's skin condition

An individualised systematic approach to the assessment of a patient's skin condition should be adopted, to include the scalp, hair, skin creases, spaces between the digits, eyes and ears. This, as well as a protocol for the maintenance of skin condition, has been previously described by this author (Collier 1994a). Nursing staff in particular are in an ideal situation to undertake this assessment process as they often have the closest contact with the patients in their care.

THE NATURAL HEALING PROCESS

Before the healing process can begin there must be a defect or a wound in the external covering of the body. For the purposes of this chapter a wound may be described as a loss of continuity of the skin or mucous membrane, which may involve soft tissues, muscle, bone and other anatomical structures. All wounds, however caused, may be classified as mechanical, burns or chemical, or chronic in nature (see Box 28.1).

Following damage to tissues, the ideal situation would be that of primary healing with minimal scarring. However, complications may occur leading to the need for healing by secondary intention (see below) and the increased possibility of a poor cosmetic result. In general, the healing process of skin is a normal reaction to surgical interventions – the best results should be achieved in healthy individuals.

Ideally, wound healing should occur as a uniform process in all connective tissues, involving the formation of new epithelium and a contraction of underlying healthy granulation tissue to form scar tissue. The natural healing process has been classified as being achieved by primary (first), secondary (second) or tertiary (third) intention (Brunner & Suddarth 1992). In addition, the use of skin grafts and flap formation by, for example, plastic surgeons is also often identified as a classification of wound healing.

Healing by primary intention occurs when the skin edges are brought together with the aid of sutures or clips, for example as with intentional (surgical) wounds, or by the use of butterfly plasters or steristrips as in a minor trauma. In this situation, granulation tissue is usually invisible and scar formation should therefore be minimal.

Healing by secondary intention means that the skin edges are deliberately not brought together because it is not surgically practical to do so – as in a pressure

---

Box 28.1   Classification of wounds

- Mechanical: traumatic, surgical
- Burns: chemical or otherwise
- Chronic: pressure ulcers, leg ulcers, fungating lesions, or any other wound type which is failing to heal as anticipated 6 weeks after 'injury'

ulcer – and the wound therefore is encouraged to fill with granulation tissue from its base. This form of healing is most common in the management of chronic wounds whatever the cause.

Healing by tertiary intention occurs when a wound which has not been primarily closed surgically is sutured, or when a wound which breaks down is resutured at a later date, with two opposing granulating surfaces being brought together. The result is usually a deeper and more pronounced scar, a situation which may be noted following surgical debridement of a wound, or when pronounced wound infection is not effectively treated by systemic antibiotic therapy.

Phases of wound healing

The natural healing process has been described as encompassing four or five stages (Milward 1988). However, it is now widely accepted that it primarily consists of three major phases which merge into a continuous process – each phase overlapping and merging with the next (Seton Healthcare 1993). The three phases of the wound healing process have been identified as the inflammatory, the regenerative and the maturative stages (see Fig. 28.2). A number of cells are involved in this complex process, but it is the macrophage which has been identified as the key player, as it functions throughout all phases of the normal wound healing cascade (Tortora & Anagnostakos 1987).

The inflammatory phase

When tissue is damaged, blood vessels are also injured and a blood clot forms in the wound, loosely uniting the wound edges. Damaged cells release histamine, causing vasodilatation and increased permeability of the blood vessels, leading to the delivery of neutrophils and monocytes to the wounded area. The resultant increased oedema and engorgement of the tissues accounts for the characteristic inflammatory appearance, which can last for anything from 0–3 days following injury. As the blood clot (the platelet plug) dries, it forms a 'scab', local blood vessels dilate and the microcirculation slows down. Polymorphs and macrophages migrate to the area ready to ingest any wound debris and begin the process of repair (Milward 1988, Seton Healthcare 1993, Tortora & Anagnostakos 1987).

The regenerative phase

Blood vessels near the edge of the wound become porous allowing any excess moisture to escape.

Macrophage activity stimulates the formation and multiplication of fibroblasts which migrate along fibrin threads, resulting in the laying down of a ground substance (epithelial cells migrating beneath the scab) and beginning the synthesis of collagen fibres. This fibrous network traps other blood cells and damaged blood vessels begin to regenerate within the wound margins (angiogenesis). The resultant tissue filling is referred to as granulation tissue and the process of wound contraction begins. This phase of wound healing is identified as lasting from 0–24 days (Seton Healthcare 1993).

During this phase of healing, signs of inflammation should subside although the wound will often remain red in colour and to some degree 'raised' in relation to its surrounding tissues.

The maturative phase

Once the wound bed is filled with granulation tissue and the process of contraction is almost complete, the process of re-epithelialisation begins – vascularity decreases, fibroblasts shrink and collagen fibres alter red granulation tissue to white avascular tissue. The wound 'scab', essential to and part of the natural healing process, should now slough off – because of an autolytic process – as the epidermis is restored to its natural thickness. Ideally, wound 'scabs' seen during the process of wound cleansing should not be removed; this is especially important at the early stage of the natural healing process. Connective tissues reorganise themselves subsequently (Seton Healthcare 1993). In total, this phase of wound healing can last anything from 21 days through to 2 years after injury depending upon the nature of the injury, the physical and mental state of well-being of the patient at the time, and the interventions of the practitioners involved in the patient's care.

Epithelial cells migrate and proliferate from the wound edge and the remnants of hair follicles, hence the characteristic 'island' appearance on the wound surface which may be seen on closer examination of the healing wound. Nevertheless they can only migrate over viable tissue with a 'leap-frogging' action until similar cells from the opposite edge of the wound are met. Migrating cells differentiate and lose their ability to divide. When migration is complete, the epithelium thins. Hair follicles are not replaced. The optimum environment for the natural wound healing process to be activated is warm, moist and non-toxic, as highlighted in detail by previous authors (Thomas 1990, Winter 1975).

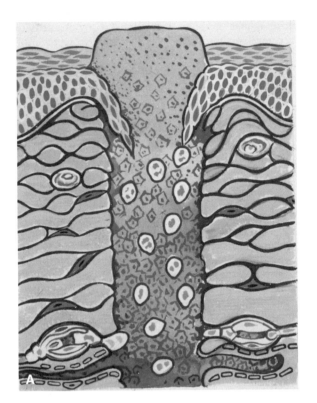
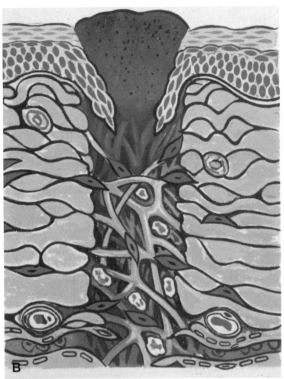
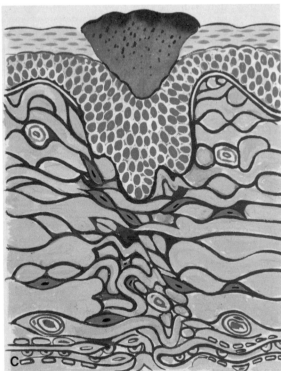

Figure 28.2   The healing process: (A) inflammation; (B) regeneration; (C) maturation (reproduced with kind permission of Seton Scholl Healthcare).

Reflective point

Identify a patient you have recently cared for. Discuss with a colleague how a greater knowledge of the structure and function of the skin and the natural healing process may have enhanced your assessment and subsequent management of that patient's wound.

BEST WOUND HEALING APPROACH – A HOLISTIC PERSPECTIVE

Undertaking a holistic assessment of a patient with a wound can be difficult; however, there is evidence that the use of a nursing model as a framework can be both helpful to the nurse and beneficial for the patient in identifying the optimum level of intervention and planning appropriate care (Bale & Jones 1997) (see also Ch. 7).

Before nurses choose a nursing model as a framework for assessment and care planning, it is important that they (a) understand the model and (b) share congruent values and beliefs about nursing which reflect the philosophical assumptions and concepts of the model.

For the purposes of this chapter, the Roper, Logan & Tierney model (Roper et al 1996) has been chosen in order to illustrate how factors that might enhance the natural wound healing process have been identified. In this author's experience, the model has been particularly helpful for ongoing patient assessment and assistance with the identification of the patient's problems/needs. Indeed, the model could be used by all members of the multidisciplinary team to plan, structure and implement quality interventions designed to have a positive impact on the patient's current and future lifestyle.

The Roper, Logan & Tierney model focuses on patients as individuals, who throughout their life span move from states of dependence to independence, according to age, circumstances and environments. The main ideas underlying the model can therefore be summarised as:

- the progression along a life span
- a dependence/independence continuum
- activities of living which are influenced by physical, psychological, sociocultural, politico-economic and environmental factors.

A patient assessment framework, structured by the influencing factors of the 12 activities of living should aim to establish what the patient can and cannot do independently. The patient and practitioner should discuss each one in turn, identifying the patient's normal level within each activity and any obstacles to accomplishment of the norm and therefore to independence. The following example reflects wound management for the management of Miss Smith's wound (see Case study 28.1).

Activities of living

An immediate assessment of the situation with regard to Miss Smith's wound highlighted the following.

Maintaining a safe environment

Allow drainage of the pus onto a wound dressing or via a drainage system in order to reduce the risk of systemic infection and to reduce the effects of the wound infection locally. This will also reduce the risk of any cross-infection to other patients, as the infection will be contained and, as long as practitioners follow local guidelines on handwashing during wound management procedures, the chance of the infection being spread should be minimised. Identify and treat appropriately the causative organism.

Wound infection has been shown to interfere with elements of the tissue repair process (Irvin 1981). Collagen, the fibre which provides both strength and flexibility to new tissue, can be weakened by infection. This weakening can lead to complete wound breakdown. Non-infected wounds may also break down under excessive stress either internally – the presence of ascites (the build-up of fluid within the abdominal cavity) – or externally as a result of strenuous activity or movement.

Case study 28.1   Miss Smith

Miss Smith is an 18-year-old student who has a long-standing history of asthma and who was recently admitted for the removal of an inflamed appendix. Following surgery, all appeared to be progressing as anticipated, despite the fact that Miss Smith's temperature had been 38°C since the open procedure, until 4 days postoperatively when the wound suddenly dehisced (suture line ruptured) and copious pus poured out.

Communication

Elicit Miss Smith's positive and negative views regarding the wound and wound pain (see also Ch. 24). Answer all questions appropriately and show Miss Smith her written nursing documentation to reinforce the wound management information and to elicit patient participation in care. Provide any relevant patient information leaflets regarding general wound management and wound healing principles and, whenever possible, provide specific information regarding the current wound infection (see also Ch. 3).

Breathing

Ensure that Miss Smith's asthma is treated appropriately and is not allowed to exacerbate as a result of her present wound condition. Adequate ventilation helps maintain a rich oxygen supply to the wound. Normally, this can be altered by pulmonary or circulatory disease as well as the ageing process.

When reviewing the literature related to the role of oxygen in wound healing, the evidence can often appear contradictory. Tissue hypoxia can seriously inhibit wound healing; however, the resultant lactoacidosis stimulates angiogenesis. Silver (1972) concluded that although angiogenesis and the formation of granulation tissue are increased by a moderately elevated PO_2, further increases in oxygen tension may reduce fibroblastic activity and thus delay healing. Later studies, undertaken in relation to the role of hydrocolloid dressings indicated, however, that the low PO_2 produced underneath Granuflex, for example, was responsible for the increase in formation of vascular tissue and that, therefore, along with other factors, this increased the speed of the wound healing process (Cherry & Ryan 1985, Eaglstein 1985) (see also Chs 23 and 25).

Eating and drinking

Ensure that Miss Smith receives all her identified nutritional requirements (either orally or via an intravenous infusion) as malnutrition, however caused, will deprive the wound of essential nutrients such as protein, vitamins (A, B_{12}, C), minerals (zinc and iron), and carbohydrates. Additional losses may also occur as a result of the wound 'exudate' currently draining from the operation site.

The primary aims of nutritional support are to maintain lean body mass and normal organ functions, promote healing, and improve the body's ability to respond to pathogenic organisms. Following injury, glucose provides a vital energy substrate for cellular infiltration of leukocytes and macrophages, both of which have a crucial role in stimulating the growth of fibroblasts and the synthesis of collagen. Protein, along with vitamins A, C, E and K, has also been indicated positively for optimum wound healing in addition to the trace elements zinc, iron and copper (Pinchcofsky-Devin 1994) (see also Ch. 27).

Elimination

Ensure that Miss Smith is enabled to perform all bodily functions in as natural an environment as is possible, in order to reduce the risk of complications such as stress incontinence or constipation. Constipation may delay wound healing as a result of abnormal pressures being experienced by the damaged tissues from within and the inability of the patient at the time to absorb nutrients from her diet as normal.

Personal cleansing and dressing

Ensure that Miss Smith is able to have frequent washes – either independently or assisted – and has clean nightwear and bed linen provided every day, in order to deal with any excessive perspiration and to optimise her feelings of comfort.

Ensure that either the appropriate absorbent wound dressing materials or wound drainage system is maintained and changed, the frequency of which should be dictated as a result of the ongoing assessment of the wound (Collier 1994b). Excoriation of the skin surrounding a wound is a common complication of excessive wound exudate/drainage, because of the 'toxins' which are released, which will lead to maceration of the skin, tissue breakdown and possibly wound infection unless adequately controlled. Stagnant exudate/drainage can also present a problem, and as such also needs to be dealt with by the use of absorbent dressing materials, as it has been associated with offensive odours reported in connection with the wound (Thomas 1990).

Maintaining body temperature

Hypothermia will delay the healing process (Collier 1990) and pyrexia may be an indication of infection (Collier 1994b). Ensure all prescribed systemic antibiotics are given as directed and take practical environmental measures to help reduce Miss Smith's temperature to 37°C or below.

In addition to the patient's body temperature, the temperature at the wound interface is also a vital consideration in optimising a patient's wound healing potential. The ideal wound interface temperature has been identified as 37°C (Turner 1985). Reduced interface temperatures may inhibit the activity of phagocytic cells and significantly affect cell mitosis. It has been reported that after the process of wound cleansing it took 40 minutes for the wound to regain its original temperature and 3 hours for mitotic and leukocytic activity to return to normal (Myers 1982) (see also Ch. 25).

Mobilisation

Ensure that during her prolonged period of hospitalisation Miss Smith is encouraged to mobilise as much as is practicable. Mobilisation will increase delivery of oxygen to the wound and reduce the risk of complications associated with immobility, such as deep vein thrombosis, chest infection and pressure ulcers.

Expressing sexuality

Enable Miss Smith to express any fears or feelings related to her own body image. She may express a wish not to view her own wound and/or worry about any potential long-term social effects if a scar remains visible once the lesion has 'healed'.

A disfiguring wound or one that has healed with a poor cosmetic appearance may lead to increased patient anxiety because of an altered body image (Topping 1992). Feelings experienced by the patient can range from embarrassment – 'nobody will want to talk to me' – through to depression (see also Ch. 9).

In addition, feelings of isolation can be experienced by patients with malodorous wounds: 'any wound assessed as being offensive by either the patient, practitioner or both' (Neal 1991). Odour can often be associated with infected wounds or ones that produce large amounts of stagnant exudate (Thomas 1990).

Working and playing

Discuss with Miss Smith realistic identified aims of wound management as agreed, and appropriate time perspectives of when the wound might heal and when she should be able to return to college and undertake normal activities associated with her active lifestyle. This would include relevant information on how best to protect the 'healed' wound following discharge from hospital and whilst the wound is still in the maturation phase of normal healing. She should, however, be able to return to all her previous sporting activities within a couple of months of her discharge from hospital.

Sleeping

Encourage and facilitate as much rest as is possible for Miss Smith during her period of hospitalisation, especially during the hours of darkness. Sleep has been shown to be an essential factor in tissue regeneration as it encourages the release of testosterone, prolactin, somatotrophin and growth hormone (Torrance 1990) (see also Ch. 22).

Fear of dying

This fear is usually allayed following recovery from surgery; however, it is important to allay any fears that Miss Smith may have because of the pus being produced from the wound and her general fever. Answer all questions with honesty and be practical about any advice given, for example 'once the amount of discharge decreases from the wound this should also result in a decrease in the associated odour and speed up the wound healing process'.

'Following assessment appropriate objectives for wound management should be set' (Collier 1994b).

Reflective point

Discuss with a colleague your recent wound management activities. Endeavour to highlight any wounds that you might now consider to have been cleaned unnecessarily or which were left exposed without a suitable dressing material for a prolonged period of time, for whatever reason. A definition of a suitable wound dressing material would not include a 'sterile' dressing towel. Identify the potential consequences of your actions.

Other factors which affect the natural healing process

The factors indicated below also need to be considered during a patient wound management assessment.

Patient's age

The older the patient the more friable the tissues and the more likely that the patient is to have had treatment with drugs for another condition or to have a systemic disease which can also interfere with the healing process. The inflammatory and immune responses may not be as effective as a result of prescribed drug therapy, and vascularity of the skin may be impaired generally (Bale & Jones 1997) (see also Ch. 11).

Drug therapy

The followings drugs significantly influence wound healing (University of Dundee 1993):

- Steroids may mask the presence of infection because they can suppress the patient's normal inflammatory response to injury.
- Cytotoxic drugs also suppress both the inflammatory and immune responses of the human body;

thus the patient may be more susceptible to the onset of infections.

• Anticoagulant drugs may cause haemorrhage and therefore adversely affect the perfusion of the patient.

Wound perfusion

If the patient should haemorrhage from and into the wound, the accumulation of blood within its margins will create dead spaces, as well as leave dead cells behind. These must be removed, as the new tissue that is laid down (granulation tissue) is unable to fill these dead spaces (Brunner & Suddarth 1992, Buckley 1992, Winter 1975).

In addition, it has been indicated by Rodheaver et al (1974) that many traumatised patients suffer from a severe loss of blood (hypovolaemic shock), which unchecked will lead to a reduction in blood flow and diminished tissue perfusion. This will seriously compromise the viability of the damaged tissues. Untreated, it will result in a progressive condition of cardiac failure, decreased cardiac output and inadequate delivery of nutrients (including oxygen) to meet the metabolic demands of the body (Buckley 1992) (see also Chs 25 and 26).

pH of the wound interface

This also needs to be considered when discussing conditions likely to be conducive to improved rates of healing. From the evidence available to date, it would appear that dressings that directly or indirectly reduce the pH of wound fluid – such as those which create a more acid rather than alkaline environment – may help to prevent infection and thereby positively affect wound healing (Thomas 1990).

Foreign bodies

The presence of foreign bodies in a wound, such as grit or non-biodegradable fibres from a wound dressing material such as gauze and clothing, have been shown to significantly affect the rate of wound healing. Therefore, if present, these foreign bodies should be removed as soon as possible in an appropriate manner which may include surgical debridement (Rodheaver et al 1974).

Reflective point

Reflect on a patient assessment you have recently documented, which included the management of a draining wound. Having read the above sections, identify any additional information that would be included in the future.

WOUND DRAINAGE

A draining wound may be defined as an abnormal opening in the skin that produces exudate or drainage and may be caused by disease, trauma or surgery.

Patients with heavily exuding or draining wounds present an enormous challenge to the health care team, although it should be pointed out that in the majority of cases it does not cause a significant delay in the patient's discharge from hospital, as care can be facilitated in the same way by community nursing staff, especially if conservative management of the problem has been decided upon.

Draining wounds secondary to wound dehiscence, infection or malignancy, require care objectives to be identified, highlighting containment of the exudate; reducing the effects of the infection; protection of the integrity of the surrounding skin; and control of any offensive odours, with appropriate care measures taken afterwards.

There are two commonly used methods for the management of draining wounds: (a) the use of absorbent interactive dressing materials; and (b) the use of collection pouches such as stoma bags, in order to collect and control the exuding body fluids. The decision regarding which type of management technique to employ should be based upon assessment of the nature and quality of the drainage.

A wound which is draining copious amounts (more than 50 ml of fluid in 24 hours) would ideally be managed by the use of a collection pouch in order to facilitate measurement of the fluid. The pouch should also reduce the risk of excoriation of the surrounding skin and prevent the need for frequent dressing changes, which take up valuable nursing time and may cause additional distress for the patient. Whenever possible, all wound drainage should be accurately measured and recorded either on a wound assessment chart or in appropriate patient documentation.

Application of a drainage pouch

Following cleansing of the skin around the wound with a normal saline solution, a protective skin barrier (stoma wafer, paste or topical application) should be applied around the wound in order to protect the skin from any 'toxins' in the wound fluid/exudate. After removal of the backing from its adhesive surface, the stoma bag/drainage pouch should then be pressed down onto the skin for approximately 30 seconds.

Management of the drainage pouch

The drainage appliance should be removed when it is one-third full of fluid, so that the weight of the contents does not cause the bag to separate from the adhesive flange, resulting in spillage. This would also be done in an effort to control the build-up of associated odours. Occasionally, commercially available deodorisers may be put into the drainage pouch, or aromatherapy may be utilised within the patient's immediate environment.

Removal of the drainage appliance

Once the patient has been made comfortable, usually in a sitting position, dependent upon the site of the wound, the skin surrounding the wound should be gently pushed down and away from the adhesive flange whilst at the same time pulling the drainage bag up and away from the wound.

A summary of the principles of wound drainage care is to be found in Box 28.2.

Surgical drainage

Surgical drainage may be used either as a method of treatment (therapeutic) or in order to prevent complications associated with the operation site/wound (prophylactic). As has been previously reported, a surgeon's philosophy may be identified as 'when in doubt, drain' (Lawsen Tait (1845–1899), cited in Westaby 1985). Nevertheless, the morbidity and mortality rate associated with enterocutaneous fistulae – associated with major bowel surgery – has been well recognised (McIntyre & Ritchie 1984).

Therapeutic drainage

Surgical intervention is often indicated for the relief of both local and systemic symptoms associated with the development of abscesses – enclosed collections of pus resulting from an acute inflammatory reaction in response to local infection.

Some common sites of abscess formation are in the skin (boils/carbuncles), on the appendix and in the peritoneal (pelvic, subphrenic or paracolic) and pleural body cavities (empyema). In the latter situation surgical drainage involving the placement of drainage tubes can prove life-saving (Westaby 1985). In all cases of abscess formation there is a closed tissue space or part of a body cavity where pus accumulates under pressure. Progressive enlargement of the abscess may result in disturbances of vital functions as a result of this increased pressure. However, whereas it was previously common to utilise multiple drainage sites – especially in the situation of diffuse peritonitis – there is now evidence that this practice is largely discontinued, as it is understood that much of the peritoneal exudate provides a protective function. Therapeutic drainage in this case then would only be advocated if an area of abscess formation had become established (Westaby 1985).

For the nursing staff involved with the care of patients requiring therapeutic drainage, the prime objectives governing their actions should include the following:

• Ensure the patient's well-being (holistic perspective).
• Reduce the risk of complications such as wound infection associated with the drainage device being used.
• Ensure the appropriate use of any interactive wound dressing materials being used.
• Optimise the patient's healing potential. Discourage any activities and minimise the effects of any factors known to delay the normal wound healing process.

Prophylactic drainage

This is usually indicated whenever physiological fluid is expected to collect following a surgical procedure or intervention, or if it is thought that an anastomosis – surgical joining of two anatomical components – may leak. After surgical drainage of cysts, such as those involving the pancreas, it is often thought prudent to insert a drain in order to prevent the reformation of the cyst.

Prophylactic drainage is also widely used in order to rest a new suture line, thereby 'diverting' natural body fluids along an alternative route for a period of time. Examples of this would be as in T-tube drainage of the common bile duct and diversion of urine via a nephrostomy or suprapubic catheter.

> **Box 28.2** Summary of the principles of wound drainage care
>
> • Reassure the patient and make the patient comfortable.
> • Collect and contain wound drainage.
> • Assess the type and amount of drainage and replace lost fluids and electrolytes.
> • Maintain adequate nutrition, vitamin and mineral replacement.
> • Cover the wound to preserve the patient's dignity and control any associated wound odour.
> • Protect the wound and surrounding skin from irritation, maceration and breakdown.

Most commonly, however, prophylactic drainage is initiated postoperatively in order to prevent the formation of wound haematoma and wound infection – such as with a closed vacuum system – thereby helping to minimise the risk of wound infection and/or dehiscence.

Common types of surgical drainage

Corrugated strips of rubber or plastic. These are used in general surgical situations to drain fat layers and the subcutaneous tissues of a contaminated wound and occasionally to assist with drainage of the peritoneal cavity (Fig. 28.3). These drains guide exudate into surface absorbent wound dressing materials (the major types of which will be reviewed later). However, these drains can be messy and lead to maceration of the surrounding skin if not observed closely or inappropriate wound dressing materials are used. They may also leave a conduit for the access of bacteria if wound dressing materials are left off for prolonged periods of time.

Tubes and catheter-type drains. These are generally the most efficient type of drain as they can in some circumstances be connected to a closed drainage bag so that the escape route of both exudate and pus may be managed in a more controlled fashion.

Examples of these drains are Portex drains (used occasionally following paediatric surgery); Shirley drains (used after liver transplantation to assess/contain bleeding); Sterimed drains (following minor orthopaedic surgery); silicone drains (following laparotomy or bowel resection procedures) and Yate's drains (following hysterectomy) (Fig. 28.4).

Suction drainage systems. Although all of the above drains are still commonly used, in this author's experience the most popular drainage systems are those involving a closed suction system (Fig. 28.5). These are ideal for the removal of blood and serous fluid from both superficial and deep wound incisions without significantly increasing the risk of postoperative wound

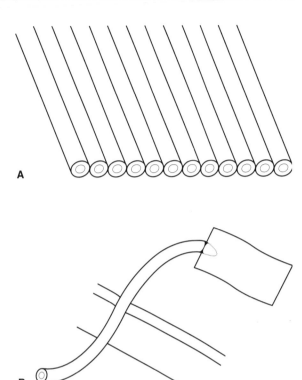

Figure 28.4 Tubular drains: (A) Yate's drain; (B) closed silicone drain.

infection. The main examples of these systems are the Dre-vac drain (often used following laparotomy and cholecystectomy procedures), Porto-vac drains (often used following plastic surgery) and Redivac drains (often used following hip surgery).

Disadvantages of drainage

- Drains may act as conduits through which skin contaminants gain entry to the wound and predispose the patient to the risk of wound infection.
- The presence of the drain may in itself impair the resistance of the tissues to the effects of local infection.
- Abdominal drains in particular may impair wound healing as the drains are 'foreign bodies' thereby adversely affecting the normal healing process.
- Drains brought out through original incisions can result in a weakness in the scar tissue which, if on the abdomen of the patient, may result in the development of an incisional hernia.
- Wound fluid/exudate brought out onto the surface of the patient's skin, if not adequately controlled

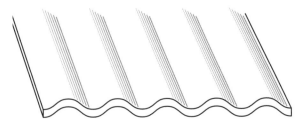

Figure 28.3 Corrugated drain.

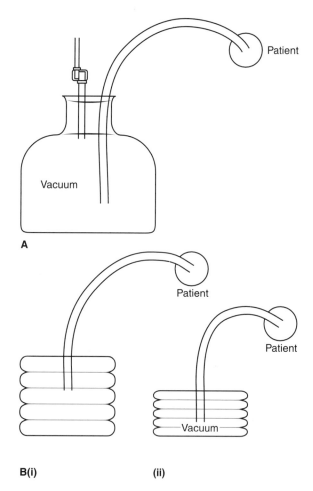

Figure 28.5 Suction drains: (A) Redivac drain; (B) Porto-vac drain.

by the appropriate use of absorbent interactive wound dressing materials, may result in maceration of the skin surrounding the drain site.

When should I remove a drain?

Drains should only be removed under the direction of a qualified nurse practitioner or, if unsure, as directed by the clinician responsible for the overall management of the individual patient in question. Notwithstanding this statement, the following may also be referred to as general guidelines for the removal of a drain:

• When the drain no longer performs the function for which it was intended, such as the drainage is minimal or has stopped (corrugated, tube and catheter types).

• When the amount of drainage recorded has fallen to below 50 ml in a 24-hour period (suction drainage systems).

• When an abscess cavity has closed. If unsure as to the complete nature of closure, radiographic investigations – involving the use of contrast medium – may be required to assist in assessment. These would need to be ordered by a clinician.

• When repair is complete, such as after the use of a T-tube drainage of the common bile duct.

• When there is a risk of drain-related complications such as wound infection and/or haemorrhage due to pressure on and erosion of local blood vessels.

WOUND DRESSING MATERIALS

The wound dressing materials discussed in this section are either used in conjunction with a variety of surgical drain types or are considered appropriate to cover the 'wound' following removal of the drain.

In order to ensure best clinical practice it is essential that all practitioners involved with the management of drainage sites and the resultant wounds have an up-to-date knowledge of the structure of the skin and the natural healing process. In addition, the surgical nurse should also be able to recognise the various stages of wound healing and be able to classify them (Collier 1994b). This theoretical and practical knowledge, together with knowledge of differing wound dressing materials, should enable the surgical nurse to undertake an accurate wound assessment and identify positive outcomes for the patient.

'Your wound assessment should have an impact':

Inspect
Measure (if appropriate)
Prevent – complications/further injury
Assess
Clean
Treat (Collier 1996).

The best dressing

There is a variety of reasons why a surgical dressing product is applied (Box 28.3). The main objectives for the use of a product over or around a wound drain site – indicated by your assessment – are likely to be absorption and control of exudate, keeping the absorbed exudate/body fluid off the surrounding skin and therefore reducing the risk of maceration, and ultimately optimising the patient's healing potential. As a result of both research and a great deal of observational activities related to modern interactive wound management products, a number of authors would agree that the 'ideal' dressing product should ensure that the wound remains:

- moist with exudate but not macerated
- free from clinical infection and excessive slough
- free from toxic chemical particles or fibres released from the dressing
- at an optimum temperature for healing to take place
- undisturbed by frequent or unnecessary dressing changes
- at an optimum pH value (Collier 1996, Thomas 1990, Winter 1975).

Classification of wound dressing types

There are many wound management products currently available. A useful approach to consider when trying to identify a practical wound management protocol (for the appropriate use of wound dressing materials in association with surgical drains and drainage systems) is to identify a product by its classification rather than its specific product name. In this way surgical nurses still have the ability to choose the most appropriate dressing, by knowledge of a group rather than of a single dressing product.

In the opinion of this author, this enhances the ability of a protocol to facilitate continuity of wound management between hospital and community care settings, as it allows for different individual products to be used – for example hydrocellular foam dressing materials – without altering the identified objectives of the patient's overall wound management. This approach also ensures that unless otherwise clinically indicated, such as an unanticipated reaction, the principal reasons for the use of the dressing remain unchanged. It is important to remember that many wound dressing materials that are available in hospitals are not on prescription – Drug Tariff, FP10 – in the community. Whatever your situation, if a dressing is not available it is of no use. However, with so many similar dressings on the market, an appropriate

alternative can usually be identified (Miller & Collier 1996).

Wound dressing products may therefore be classified by their primary functions (see Box 28.4), as belonging to one of the following groups:

- Film membranes
- Foams
- Particulates
- Hydrogels
- Hydrocolloids
- Alginates
- Enzymes
- Low-adherent.

The technology involved with the development of wound dressing materials is evolving all the time, in that dressings incorporating a mixture of materials are now available and the incorporation of growth factors along with dressing materials is actively being researched. Readers would therefore be encouraged to be aware of reported developments through relevant literature – in particular journals and research reports – as well as liaising with nurse specialists, particularly tissue viability/wound care nurses, infection control nurses, Macmillan nurses and stomatherapists. In addition, wound care company representatives can be contacted to provide regular and updated information.

Factors affecting the choice of wound dressing

Following the surgical nurse's assessment of a patient's wound, and in the light of the information contained within this chapter, the choice of dressing materials to be used should follow the 'answering' of four questions, whatever the wound scenario. The questions to ask yourself are:

- What am I looking at? (structure of the wound)
- How would I assess the wound? (using a relevant classification tool such as one based on the clinical appearance of the wound)
- What is my primary treatment objective? (may include those identified in Box 28.3)
- What dressing will I use in order to endeavour to achieve the identified objective?

It is important to note that as the condition of the drainage site or ultimate wound changes, it may be necessary to alter the type of dressing used. Reassessing the drainage site/wound at regular intervals and using relevant researched-based findings to influence practice is essential (Collier 1994b).

Box 28.3   Reasons for applying a dressing

- To control exudate
- To control bleeding
- To ease related pain
- To clean and debride the wound
- To protect newly formed tissue
- To optimise the healing potential

Box 28.4 Primary functions of dressing products by classification (Collier 1996, Thomas 1990)

Film membranes
- Permeable to water vapour and oxygen
- Impermeable to water and microorganisms
- Provide a warm, moist environment
- Comfortable
- Convenient
- Permit constant observation

Examples: Opsite,* Tegaderm,* Cutifilm,* BioClusive,* Opraflex*

Foams
- Provide thermal insulation
- Do not shed particles
- Maintain a moist environment
- Gas permeable
- Non-adherent
- Absorb significant amounts of exudate
- Easily removed

Examples: Allevyn,* Cavi-Care,* Lyofoam,* Dermasorb,* Tielle*

Particulates
- Clean and debride
- Absorb fluid
- Reduce the number of microorganisms at the wound interface

Examples: Iodosorb,* Debrisan*

Hydrogels
- Rehydrate wounds
- Debride and clean
- Painless to apply and remove
- Soothing

Examples: Gelliperm,* Granugel,* 2nd Skin,* Intrasite Gel*

Hydrocolloids
- Provide a warm, moist environment
- Impermeable to moisture vapour
- Impervious to liquids and bacteria
- Promote angiogenesis
- Promote granulation
- Protect the wound

Examples: Comfeel,* Cutinova,* Granuflex,* Tegasorb*

Alginates
- Provide moist wound healing environment
- Absorb significant amounts of exudate
- Easily removed by irrigation techniques
- Comfortable
- Haemostatic properties reported

Examples: Comfeel,* Kaltostat,* Sorbsan,* Tegagel*

Enzymes
- Cleaning and debriding
- Stimulate the patient's own healing potential

Example: Varidase*

Box 28.4 (Contd.)

Low-adherent
- Generally now used as a secondary dressing; however, may be used primarily when the wound is under an orthopaedic casting material, e.g. Gypsona*

Examples: Melolin,* Release*

* Registered trade name.

Nevertheless, it is acknowledged that other factors do still influence nurses' choice of dressing used (Collier 1995). These can be summarised as the availability of dressings – particularly those on prescription (Drug Tariff, FP10) and therefore readily available for use in community settings; education regarding dressing products – both informal and formal or from company representatives; ritualistic practice; locus of control; a practitioner's previous experience and personal preference.

Having reviewed wound dressing materials as a whole, it is now important to look in a little more detail at those dressing products most likely to be used in association with wound drains and drainage systems when the prime objectives are as previously identified: absorption and control of exudate; prevention of maceration and optimising the patient's wound healing potential.

The classification of dressing products most likely to be indicated by assessment are the alginates, foams, hydrogels (ensuring that the wound site remains hydrated, for the removal of slough and general cleansing of the wound), and occasionally hydrocolloids.

Alginates

The clinical use of calcium alginates has been investigated since the 1940s; however, despite a number of early successes in a variety of clinical settings their use in wound management declined until the mid-1980s when interest was reawakened by a number of papers that described the use of Sorbsan in the treatment of 'problem' wounds (Gilchrist & Martin 1983, Thomas 1985) – a term often used to describe wound drainage sites, in the experience of this author.

Alginate dressings have been shown to be of use for filling cavities and sinuses and therefore for use around and over wound drainage sites. One study compared the use of Sorbsan with gauze soaked in proflavine in patients with acute abscesses or localised collections of pus in surgical wound sites (Gupta et al 1988). The results of this study indicated that those wounds dressed with alginate contained fewer organisms and healed at a faster rate than those dressed with proflavine-soaked gauze. It was also reported that patients receiving the alginates experienced significantly less pain and required less analgesia.

Other authors have indicated that the use of calcium alginate in the management of a number of wound management scenarios, including wound drainage sites, has consistently resulted in both dramatic and cost-effective wound healing (Fanucci & Seese 1991).

Alginates absorb exudate and serous fluid, reacting chemically with it to form a hydrophilic gel, the exchange properties of which depend upon a number of factors which include the relative proportion of mannuronic and guluronic acid residues and the method used to sterilise the final dressing material. Alginate dressings vary in absorbency but typically will take up 15–20 times their own weight of exudate. Those made from predominantly mannuronic acid fibres (e.g. Sorbsan) form soft amorphous gels that will partially dissolve or disperse in solutions such as normal saline, whereas dressings rich in guluronic residues (e.g. Kaltostat) tend to swell in the presence of sodium ions whilst retaining their basic structure. In both cases the gelled product has been identified as providing a moist covering of the wound surface that is generally believed to enhance normal wound healing processes (Thomas 1992a).

Foams

As a group, foam dressing materials include a number of desirable properties, but in particular when used for the management of wound drainage sites they do not shed fibres or particles; are easily cut or shaped around the relevant wound drainage system; help to maintain a moist environment at the wound interface (surface); and are able to absorb significant amounts of exudate (Thomas 1993).

Allevyn consists of a hydrophilic polyurethane foam backed with a moisture-vapour-permeable polyurethane membrane. The hydrophilic foam is capable of absorbing and retaining large volumes of fluid even when subjected to pressure.

Lyofoam consists of a soft, hydrophobic, open cell polyurethane foam sheet. The wound contact surface of the product is modified by the application of heat to collapse the cells of the foam, thus allowing them to take up liquid by capillary action.

The dressing is freely permeable to gases and water vapour but resists the penetration of liquids owing to the hydrophobic nature of the unmodified back. The aqueous component of the absorbed fluid therefore evaporates into the larger cells in the back of the dressing and is lost as water vapour to the environment.

Spyrosorb consists of a thin sheet of polyurethane foam coated with a layer of hydrophile adhesive. The outer surface of the dressing is covered with a polyurethane film, the permeability of which increases as the dressing absorbs water.

Tielle is made up of a central island of foam which gently expands as exudate is absorbed. Excess moisture is drawn away from the drain/wound site, helping to reduce the risk of maceration. Moisture then evaporates through the back of the dressing as previously described. This island dressing provides a moist wound healing environment which allows granulation to proceed – as applicable – under optimum conditions.

Hydrogels

Hydrogels, or water polymer gels, are three-dimensional networks of hydrophilic polymers which interact with aqueous solutions by swelling to an equilibrium value and retain significant proportions of water within their structure. They are insoluble in water (Turner 1985), e.g. Geliperm. In addition, there is a second group of products known as amorphous hydrogels, which unlike the previous group do not have a fixed macro-structure. When these materials absorb fluid they progressively decrease in viscosity and generally take up the shape of the wound or vessel in which they are contained. Amorphous hydrogels will continue to absorb fluid until the gel loses all its cohesive properties and simply becomes a dispersion of the polymer in water (Thomas 1990). The clinical value of hydrophilic polymers has been recognised since 1960 (Wichterle & Lim 1960).

Hydrogels would be indicated for the management of wounds around drain sites, or wounds following the removal of a drain, primarily if the wound appears to be:

- discoloured or necrotic – to rehydrate and preserve tissues or to debride necrotic tissue gently as a result of an autolytic process (natural degradation of devitalised tissue)
- yellow/sloughy – to deslough and remove the unwanted material whilst at the same time protecting any underlying healthy granulation tissue.

At present there are no known contraindications to the use of hydrogels, although it should be noted that the use of the amorphous hydrogels would not ideally be recommended for a heavily exuding wound, primarily because of the potential problem of maceration of the surrounding skin by large amounts of stagnant fluid – containing a number of 'toxins' – remaining on the skin between dressing changes.

Hydrocolloids

The final major group of wound dressing materials that may be considered either prophylactically around drain sites or for the management of drain wounds is the hydrocolloids. This group of products developed from Orabase – a gel-forming paste – first used in wound management to prevent excoriation of the skin surrounding stomas, fistulas and wound drains.

Hydrocolloid dressings take up wound fluid to form a gel that produces a moist environment on the wound surface in order to facilitate healing, without predisposing to maceration of the surrounding skin. The majority of these dressings are backed with a continuous plastic film that renders them impervious to liquid and bacteria. In general use, hydrocolloids are relatively easy to use, require infrequent changing and do not cause trauma on removal (Thomas 1992b).

In the experience of this writer most hydrocolloids can be cut or shaped to fit areas that are difficult to cover, or to go around and underneath wound drains, as they have previously been reported to provide a protective function: (a) by protecting the skin surrounding the drain site from the 'toxins' contained within the leaking exudate/body fluid; or (b) by preventing drain/wound contamination from external sources.

Other wound-management products such as gauze, absorbent pads, wool pieces and gamgee may occasionally be observed in use in association with a variety of wound drainage systems. However – in the opinion of this author – it should be stressed that these materials should be used only as secondary wound dressings and in the majority of cases never as a primary dressing (placed directly against the patient's skin), especially if the drain has just been removed or if the resultant wound has been identified. If used in the final maturative phase of wound healing, these materials may result in trauma at the time of dressing change and ultimately delayed wound healing (Wood 1976).

Reflective point

Consider, in the light of what you have read so far, how in the future you are going to update your own and your colleagues' knowledge of wound dressings related to the principles of wound management.

THE TISSUE VIABILITY/WOUND CARE NURSE

A key role of the tissue viability/wound care nurse is to support nurses in surgical settings to maintain the quality of wound management interventions in relation to an individual patient's care. In the experience of this author, they are seen as an invaluable resource who maintain a number of valuable roles which may be summarised as follows:

1. Practitioner – assist the surgical nurse to assess patients comprehensively and objectively, in order to develop care plans based on advanced knowledge and expertise. Act as a role model for the surgical nurse.
2. Educator – ideally placed to educate patients, carers, nursing staff and other members of the multidisciplinary team about various aspects of wound management in both formal and informal settings.
3. Consultant – either in a formal or informal manner, but most successful if the tissue viability/wound care nurse is highly visible and available to all members of the health care team.
4. Researcher – able to initiate and undertake relevant research as well as have the ability to disseminate and implement research-based findings into current clinical practice.
5. Change agent – should be a catalyst for change within an organisation such as an NHS trust and should promote positive communication between all members of the multidisciplinary team in order to change ritualistic wound management practices (Walsh & Ford 1989). In addition, they should seek to maintain improvements in quality patient care related to the various aspects of wound management by highlighting both the need for change and the positive effects of change through the audit process.

POTENTIAL COMPLICATIONS OF POOR OR INEFFECTIVE WOUND DRAINAGE

Although there is the potential for many complications associated with 'open' draining wounds and 'closed' wound drainage systems, in the experience of this author the main complications identified are those of haematoma (haemorrhage), excoriation of the surrounding skin as a result of fluid leakage, and infection, which if poorly treated may predispose to generalised sepsis and in extreme cases septicaemia.

Haematoma (haemorrhage)

When a drain is in situ it is important for the nurse in particular to note the amount, type and nature of drainage, reporting any excessive blood loss to the appropriate personnel. Occasionally bleeding within a wound/drain will be concealed and result in the formation of a blood clot beneath the skin. If this clot is small, it will usually be reabsorbed and no further interventions will be required; however, sometimes this is not the case and the clot will need to be removed or evacuated. If this is not undertaken at an early stage, delayed wound healing may be the unwanted outcome.

Wound/wound drain infection

The nature of a patient's skin surrounding the wound or wound drain may indicate the presence of clinical infection, the signs of which can vary depending upon the host's (patient) resistance and the pathogen involved (see Box 28.5).

It could be argued that almost all wounds/wound drains will be colonised by some organism – most commonly the host's *Staphylococcus aureus*. However, bacterial colonisation may not in itself be of any clinical significance. It is important to be able to distinguish between the presence of bacteria (transient organisms detected in small numbers – not multiplying) and colonisation (organisms present that have not only multiplied but have also become established) (Cooper & Lawrence 1996).

Wound infection, therefore, may be defined as the presence of colonising organisms resulting in the appearance of distinctive patient signs. Before a diagnosis of clinical wound infection is made, a combination of clinical signs should be observed as well as taking account of the 'evidence' obtained from a wound swab. Clinical signs may include the production of excessive exudate (body fluid discharged through pores, incisions, wounds and wound drains);

copious pus which may be green, yellow or grey in colour; systemic patient pyrexia and tachycardia; wound dehiscence (the rupturing or bursting open of a wound) and offensive odour. A wound swab should only be taken when two or more of these clinical signs are evident, in order to confirm the diagnosis of the suspected wound infection and also to identify the drug sensitivity of the organism. It could be argued that the practice of routinely swabbing wounds is neither cost-effective nor beneficial to the healing process.

Remember that the presence of bacteria or slough alone in a wound does not necessarily mean that the wound/wound drain is infected. Chronic wounds, in particular, can often be colonised without these organisms causing additional tissue damage (Ayliffe et al 1992). Acute infections caused by pathogenic organisms such as haemolytic streptococci or *Pseudomonas* can certainly delay wound healing and should be treated by the appropriate use of systemic antibiotic therapy as prescribed (Thomas 1990) (see also Ch. 13).

Reflective point

Think of three patients you have recently been involved with who were diagnosed and treated as having a wound infection. Having read the above, identify the clinical signs or factors noted which you believe resulted in the diagnosis. Do you think that those patients were treated appropriately? Why is it important to ensure that systemic antibiotic therapy is only indicated when a diagnosis of wound infection has been confirmed?

RECENT ADVANCES IN THE MANAGEMENT OF PATIENTS WITH DRAINING WOUNDS

Despite the plethora of wound dressing materials currently available, not all are suited to all wound types and, in particular, to the treatment of non-healing wounds or copiously draining wounds, especially in patients who are also poor surgical candidates. Now there is a further wound management product available which can be of particular benefit in just such situations – the VAC, produced by KCI Medical Ltd. (see Fig. 28.6).

The VAC is a closed system which provides for a non-invasive, active therapy through the use of negative pressure – a concept which was first indicated for the identified wound types by Professor Louis Argenta in the USA in 1988.

Negative pressure therapy has been shown through a number of preliminary studies to increase

---

Box 28.5   Potentially pathogenic bacteria commonly found in wounds (after Cooper & Lawrence 1996)

Staphylococcus aureus
Streptococcus pyogenes
Bacteroides
Klebsiella
Pseudomonas aeruginosa
Escherichia coli
Enterococcus faecalis
Clostridium perfringens
Anaerobic cocci
Acinetobacter anitratus
Proteus species
Enterobacter aerogenes

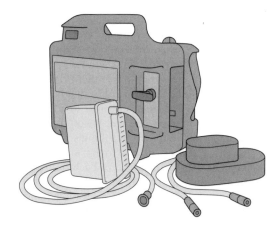

Figure 28.6 Vacuum-assisted wound (VAC) closure system.

the effectiveness of the local circulation in the wounded area; actively remove excessive exudate – thereby helping to reduce oedema and the incidence of haematoma formation; assist with the control of wound leakage – thereby reducing the risk of skin excoriation; and promote angiogenesis (the growth of new blood capillaries into the wound) (KCI 1996).

The main objectives for the use of VAC therapy are:

- to provide an occlusive protective covering over the wound/draining wound to reduce bacterial contamination and reduce the risk of wound infection
- to provide a negative pressure for improving tissue perfusion, removal of wound drainage and to facilitate mechanical desloughing/debridement
- to promote a moist wound healing environment.

However, precautions should be taken regarding: (a) patients on anticoagulants; and (b) patients experiencing difficulty with wound haemostasis.

Evidence of the effectiveness of VAC

The VAC applies a negative pressure uniformly to draw the wound closed – the therapeutic range being between 50 mmHg and 200 mmHg. The usual working pressure is around 125 mmHg; however, this pressure can be adjusted by the operator as can the on/off times when the unit is in the intermittent mode. Negative pressure applies non-compressive mechanical forces to the tissues that allow the arterioles to dilate and increase blood flow.

Evidence for the effectiveness of the VAC drainage system has been reported by Morykawas et al (1994) who state that laboratory and clinical data demonstrate

a measurable increase in adjacent vascularity, proliferation of granulation tissue, decrease in bacterial contamination and progressive wound closure. The authors also found that 'bacterial colonisation was decreased by 1000 times compared to non-negative pressure exposed wounds after four days of treatment' (Argenta et al 1993). A number of clinical studies undertaken in both the USA and the UK further demonstrate the positive effects of the therapy (Argenta & Morykawas 1994).

In summary, VAC therapy is both simple and easy to use. It is a system which, in the opinion of this author, should certainly be considered when other more conventional conservative methods of wound management/wound drainage have failed.

Reflective point

With regard to the major headings of this chapter, write down brief notes relating to the care of a patient with a wound drain in situ with whom you have recently been involved, identifying your actions/interventions. When you are next involved with the care of a patient with a wound drain repeat the exercise using the same framework. Compare your notes. Reflect upon what you have written and try to identify the rationale for any differences in the care given to your chosen patients.

CONCLUSION

Although in many circumstances wound drains and drainage systems may appear relatively 'simple' to look after compared with the other needs of patients, it could be argued that today's practitioners require a wealth of knowledge in order to ensure that the patient's care is optimised and the risk of associated complications reduced.

This chapter has therefore highlighted the need for all practitioners to have an up-to-date working knowledge of the normal anatomy of the skin, the natural wound healing process and the factors affecting it (an holistic perspective). The nature of wound drainage; why it is important; methods and equipment used to control it – including wound-management materials; and potential complications associated with poor or ineffective drainage have also been discussed. It is therefore anticipated that all readers should now be able to fulfil all the chapter aims as identified and adopt a dynamic, evidence-based approach to wound management. Practitioners in whatever surgical settings should be able to claim to be safe, knowledgeable and the patient's best advocate. Accountability rests with the need to continually update both knowledge and skills appropriate to all aspects of wound management as nursing advances into the 21st century.

REFERENCES

Argenta L, Morykawas M 1994 Case study reports. KCI Medical, Oxon, UK

Argenta L, Rouchard R, Morykawas M 1993 The use of negative pressure to promote healing of pressure ulcers and chronic wounds in seventy five consecutive patients. Paper presented at the Joint meeting of Tissue Repair Society/Wound Healing Society, Amsterdam

Ayliffe G A, Lowbury E, Geddes A M, Williams J D 1992 Control of hospital acquired infection – a practical handbook, 3rd edn. Chapman and Hall, London

Bale S, Jones V 1997 Wound care nursing – a patient centred approach. Baillière Tindall, London, ch 1

Brunner L, Suddarth D 1992 Textbook of adult nursing. Chapman and Hall, London, p 52

Buckley R 1992 The management of hypovolaemic shock. Nursing Standard 16(41): 25–28

Cherry G W, Ryan T J 1985 Enhanced wound angiogenesis with a new hydrocolloid dressing. In: Ryan T J (ed) An environment for healing: the role of occlusion. International Congress and Symposium Series 88. Royal College of Surgeons, London

Collier M 1990 Wound assessment: making informed choices. Practice Nursing (Nov): 17–18

Collier M 1994a Anatomy of the skin and the natural healing process. Educational Leaflet 2(1). Wound Care Society Northampton

Collier M 1994b Assessing a wound – RCN nursing update unit 29. Nursing Standard 8(49)(suppl): 3–8

Collier M 1995 'Spells, potions and rituals' – an enquiry to identify the major influences governing the use of wound cleansing solutions in clinical practice at a large London teaching hospital. In: Papadopoulos I, Lee H (eds) Research for practice and education. Research series vol 2. North London College of Health Studies, London

Collier M 1996 Principles of optimum wound management. Nursing Standard 10(43): 47–52

Cooper R, Lawrence J 1996 Micro-organisms and wounds. Journal of Wound Care 5(5): 233–236

Department of Health (DoH) 1993 Pressure sores a key quality indicator. HMSO, London

Eaglstein W H 1985 The effect of occlusive dressings on collagen synthesis and re-epithelialisation in superficial wounds. In: Ryan T J (ed) An environment for healing: the role of occlusion. International Congress and Symposium Series No. 88. Royal Society of Medicine, London

Fanucci D, Seese J 1991 Multi-faceted use of calcium alginate. Ostomy/Wound Management 37: 16–22

Gilchrist T, Martin A 1983 Wound treatment with Sorbsan – an alginate fibre dressing. Biomaterials 4: 317–320

Gupta R, Foster M, Miller E 1988 Calcium alginate in the management of acute surgical wounds and abscesses. Journal of Tissue Viability 1: 115–116

Irvin T 1981 Wound healing: principles and practice. Chapman and Hall, London

KCI 1996 Data on file. KCI Medical, Oxon, UK

McIntyre P, Ritchie J 1984 Management of enterocutaneous fistulas – a review of 132 cases. British Journal of Surgery 71: 293–296

Miller M, Collier M 1996 Understanding wounds. Booklet. Macmillan Journals, London

Milward P 1988 The healing process. Educational Leaflet 1. Wound Care Society, Northampton

Morykawas M, Argenta L, Rouchard R 1994 Vacuum assisted closure – a new method for healing chronic wounds. Paper presented at the American Association of Plastic Surgeons Annual Meeting, USA

Myers J A 1982 Modern plastic surgical dressings. Health and Social Services Journal (18 March) 336–337

Neal K 1991 Treating fungating wounds. Nursing Times 87(23): 85–86

Pinchcofsky-Devin G 1994 Nutrition and wound healing. Journal of Wound Care 3(5): 231–234

Rodeheaver G, Pettry D, Turnbull V, Edgerton M T, Edlich R F 1974 Identification of the wound infection potentiating factors in soil. American Journal of Surgery 128: 8

Roper N, Logan W, Tierney A 1996 The elements of nursing, 4th edn. Churchill Livingstone, Edinburgh

Seton Healthcare 1993 Wound care today – tradition or innovation. Seton Healthcare Group, Oldham

Silver I A 1972 Oxygen tension and epithelialisation. In: Maibach H I, Rovee D T (eds) Epidermal wound healing. Year Book Medical Publishers, Chicago

Silver J 1987 Letter. Care, Science and Practice 5(3): 30

Skinner F A, Carr J G 1976 The normal microbial flora of man. Academic Press, London

Thomas S 1985 Use of calcium alginate dressing. Pharmaceutical Journal 235: 188–190

Thomas S 1990 Wound management and dressings. Pharmaceutical Press, London

Thomas S 1992a Alginates – an update. Journal of Wound Care 1(1): 29–32

Thomas S 1992b Hydrocolloids – an update. Journal of Wound Care 1(2): 27–30

Thomas S 1993 Foam dressings. Journal of Wound Care 2(3): 153–156

Topping A 1992 The trauma of burns. Wound Management 2(3): 8–9

Torrance C 1990 Sleep and wound healing. Surgical Nurse 3(3): 16–20

Tortora G, Anagnostakos N P 1987 Principles of anatomy and physiology, 5th edn. Harper and Row, London

Tortora G 1988 Introduction to the human body. Harper and Row, London

Turner T D 1985 Hydrogels and hydrocolloids – an overview. In: Turner T D, Schmidt R J, Harding K G (eds) Advances in wound management. Wiley, Chichester

University of Dundee 1993 The wound handbook. Centre for Medical Education, University of Dundee

Walsh M, Ford P 1989 Nursing rituals. Heinemann, London

Westaby S (ed) 1985 Wound care. Heinemann, London

Wichterle O, Lim D 1960 Hydrophilic gels for biological use. Nature 185: 117–118

Winter G D 1962 Formation of the scab and the rate of epithelialization of superficial wounds in the skin of the young domestic pig. Nature 193: 293–294

Winter G 1975 Epidermal wound healing. In: Turner T D, Brain K R (eds) Surgical dressings in the hospital environment. Proceedings of a Conference. Surgical Dressings Research Unit, Welsh School of Pharmacy, Cardiff

Wood R A B 1976 Disintegration of cellulose dressings in open granulating wounds. British Medical Journal 1: 1444–1445

FURTHER READING

Risk assessment tools

Waterlow J 1985 A risk assessment card. Nursing Times 89(27): 49–51

Norton D, Smith A, McLaren R 1975 An investigation of geriatric nursing problems in hospital. Churchill Livingstone, Edinburgh

Wound assessment charts

Flanagan M 1990 Wound assessment. Education Leaflet No. 5. Wound Care Society, Huntingdon

Morrison J M 1987 Wound assessment. Professional Nurse 2(10): 315–317

Wound care journals

Journal of Wound Care, EMAP, London, 10 editions per annum

Journal of Tissue Viability, Tissue Viability Society, Salisbury, quarterly

Journal of Wound Care Nursing, Supplement within Nursing Times, EMAP, London

29

Safer handling in a surgical unit

Danielle Holmes

AIMS

The aims of this chapter are:

- to discuss the amount of back injuries sustained by nursing personnel when handling patients and other loads
- to explain the importance of the EC Directive on Manual Handling of Loads and its translation into the Manual Handling Operations Regulations 1992 in providing a safe system of work in all workplaces including the health services
- to discuss the role of the employer and the surgical nurse as an employee concerning these regulations
- to explore how safe systems of work can be devised
- to show how the requirements of the regulations can be met and how this is to the benefit of both nursing staff and patients.

INTRODUCTION

The manual handling of patients in a surgical area is often not seen as a priority. It must be recognised that poor handling of patients injures both patients and hospital staff. Safe handling is a subject that must be properly studied. It is at the core of all effective nursing care.

The handling of patients is an unusual skill. Unless they are fortunate enough to be properly trained, people do not know that they are unskilled in handling patients until they are injured doing a dangerous lift. The skills needed to allow someone to handle safely must be learned just the same as any other skill.

The unsafe handling of patients is the cause of many injuries to nurses and other caring professionals. This chapter deals in some depth with the causes of these injuries and with the equipment and techniques that exist to prevent injury. The chapter also looks at the law that is designed to protect all workers, including nurses, from injury in handling tasks. In the process of examining patient handling to make it safe for nurses something else was realised: most patient-handling techniques are bad for patients. This chapter therefore also shows how handling that is effective for the patient is also safe for the nurse.

THE SIZE OF THE PROBLEM

The Manual Handling Operations Regulations 1992 (SI 1992 No. 2793) identify the percentage of injuries caused by handling. The data show that manual handling problems are widespread and not just the prerogative of the health care setting. However, the problem is most severe amongst medical, veterinary and other health service workers. This group suffer the most manual handling accidents.

There have been a number of epidemiological studies that have looked at back pain in nurses. Some have been concerned with back pain in nurses compared to other hospital workers (Hoover 1973, Hickman & Mason 1994, Leighton & Riley 1995, Raistrick 1981, Stubbs 1983) whilst others have compared nurses with other occupations away from nursing (Crust et al 1972, Magora 1970).

Professor David Stubbs produced a report in 1986 that analysed the level of back injuries in the nursing profession. He identified that 764 000 working days were lost owing to nurses taking sick leave for back pain. He also noted that at the time of his survey 1 in 6 nurses had back pain. The situation does not seem to have improved since he did his original work. Improvements in equipment and techniques seem to have been offset by increases in the level of dependent patients.

The heaviest part of a nurse's work is the lifting of patients. This accounts for some 78% of reported back injuries in the health services (HSAC 1984). The RCN survey by Seccombe & Ball in 1992 confirmed an even higher level of injuries. This study showed that 1 nurse in 4 had suffered back pain.

Other studies have looked at other issues in back-injured nurses. Osborne (1979, unpublished work) showed a relationship between the nurse/patient ratios and the level of back injuries. Where the ratio was high (greater than 3:1) there were practically no reported back injuries. Where the ratio was low (less than 1:1) there was a sevenfold increase in reported back injuries.

There are many ways of handling patients. One of the better-known texts on this subject, by Lloyd et al, has been published since 1981 and is now in its fourth edition (revised 1998). This publication not only identifies handling techniques but also dangerous lifts.

These dangerous lifts are not only dangerous for the nurse but also for the patient.

There have been no detailed studies of injuries to patients. However, there are many indications that significant numbers of patients are suffering upper limb injuries from handling events. Patients also suffer from loss of confidence and fail to mobilise as a result of poor handling techniques that are routinely used in many hospitals and community settings.

WHY HANDLING INJURES NURSES

The spine is made up of a series of vertebrae (Fig. 29.1A). These vertebrae resist most of the compressive forces on the spine when the spine is vertical. The vertebrae are interspersed by intervertebral discs (Fig. 29.1B) that allow some movement of the spine and also resist compression. These discs have an outer fibrous ring (annulus fibrosis) and an inner nucleus (nucleus pulposus) (Fig. 29.1C). The annulus fibrosis can be damaged by asymmetrical bending and compression causing the inner nucleus pulposus to prolapse causing pain. The amount of twist and bend is limited by the apophyseal joints, thereby protecting the discs from shear and rotational forces. These joints will also resist the forward shearing forces on the lumbar spine.

The vertebrae are held in place by the ligaments. These ligaments provide the spine's resistance to flexion and extension. Therefore rapid bending movements will predispose the discs to high levels of mechanical loading. The surrounding musculature protects the spine.

Most of the compressive forces that act upon the lumber spine are exerted by the muscles. The vertebral bodies resist most of the compressive force, providing that it is down the long axis of the spine.

When handling loads, the weight is in front of the spine. The effective force of a load on the discs is proportional to the distance between the load and the base of the spine.

When discussing the effect of lifting on the spine, there are two loads to be considered. The weight of the lifter's upper body and the weight of the load being lifted. When lifting in an upright posture, the weight of the upper body is 5–6 cm in front of the base of the spine. A load held close to the stomach is about 10 cm in front of the base of the spine. Bending forwards to handle a load increases both of these distances.

In patient handling, it is common for the centre of gravity of the upper body to move up to 25–35 cm from the front of the spine. This increases the effective weight of the upper body of the nurse by up to sixfold. The average male weighs 76.3 kg (12 st.) and the average

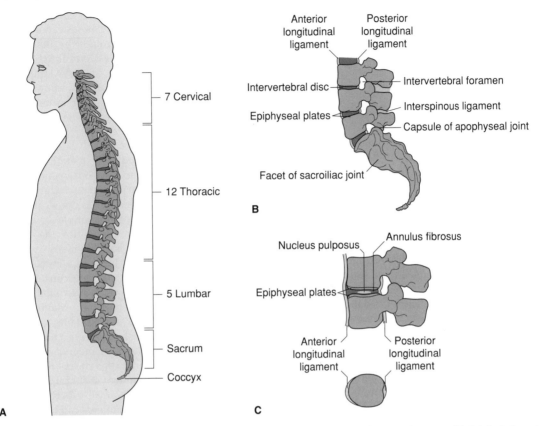

Figure 29.1   The vertebral column: (A) the main divisions of the vertebral column and its natural curves; (B) detailed view of the sacrum and lower part of the lumbar section of the spine; (C) section and plan view of an intervertebral disc.

female weighs 64.5 kg (10 st. 2 lb.) (Pheasant 1996). The upper body weighs 68.6% of body mass. Thus the upper body of a male is 52 kg and the upper body of a female is 44 kg. Therefore, the effective weight of the person's own body may be increased to 312 kg in the case of a man and 264 kg in the case of a woman.

The effective weight of the patient being lifted is also similarly increased. In a typical lifting situation the patient is being lifted some 60–70 cm in front of the nurse's spine. If a patient weighs some 63 kg (10 st.), the weight is then multiplied six or seven times. If two nurses are lifting and each lifter is taking half of this load, then the effective load on the base of the spine of each nurse would be between 190–220 kg (30–35 st.). This means that the effective forces on the base of the spine are up to half a ton.

In addition to the damaging effects of the direct loads discussed above, it has been recognised that twisting whilst handling a load increases the damage. Twisting can increase the effects on the spine by 10–20% (HSE 1992a). Almost all patient-handling techniques involve some degree of twist.

The majority of patient-handling-related injuries suffered by nurses are to the lower spine. However, there are also other injuries that do occur. The second most common site for injuries is in the area of the shoulders. These injuries usually occur because of lifting in a forward-bent posture. The load is applied at right angles to the plane of the shoulder. This creates a shearing force at right angles to the line of the spine. An examination of the bones and muscles in this area shows that the structures are not designed to take large loads in this direction. The actual site of injury varies between the shoulder muscles and joints and the vertebrae in this area.

A smaller number of handling injuries occur in the wrist. They are usually caused by the hand being trapped as a patient collapses or because the nurse has tried to lift using the wrists rather than the more powerful leg muscles.

Injuries in other joints do occur but are relatively rare.

The whole of the body is at risk in patient handling. For example, I am aware of two cases where the nurse suffered a prolapsed uterus.

THE LAW

The UK legal framework

The European Community set out a set of health and safety directives which were to be translated into the health and safety law of all member states. The enabling legislation allowing the directives to be implemented in the UK is the Health and Safety at Work etc. Act 1974.

There were six directives that were implemented on 1 January 1993 (Table 29.1).

There is a 'Code of Practice' explaining the implementation of the Management of Health and Safety at Work Regulations (HSE 1992c). Each of the other Regulations has an associated 'Guidance' produced by the Health and Safety Executive to assist the employer in their implementation (HSE 1992d,e, 1995).

Of these the Framework Directive (89/391/EEC) (CEC 1989a) was known as the mother directive and all the other directives were to be read in light of it. The Framework Directive became the Management of Health and Safety at Work Regulations 1992. These regulations require employers to make a suitable and sufficient assessment of all the risks to the health and safety of their employees while at work. If a particular hazard is defined, then that hazard must be eliminated. The Regulations govern the lifting and handling that is done by workers in the health services, which includes lifting and handling of patients.

Under the Health and Safety at Work Act 1974 the Health and Safety Executive (HSE) have powers to ensure that the Regulations are enforced. A breach of any provision in these regulations can ultimately lead to a prosecution being brought by the HSE. Several authorities and trusts have been subject to prohibition notices for infringement of the Manual Handling Regulations. These notices usually allow the employer 3 months to get things in order. After that time the employer will be prosecuted. There have been successful prosecutions under the Manual Handling Operations Regulations 1992.

The Manual Handling Operations Regulations require the employer to carry out a general assessment to establish if there are potentially hazardous handling operations being carried out in the work area. Where such risks are identified, the employer is required to take steps to remove or reduce the hazard. The Council Directive did not provide any definition of what was a hazardous lift. The view seems to have been taken that all lifting is dangerous. However, it is useful to have some definition as to what is dangerous. The UK guidance on the Manual Handling Regulations (HSE 1992a) contains advice on the process of assessing risk. There are a number of factors to be considered in the assessment of a load. These are the task, the individual (this means the handler), the load, and the environment including the equipment (TILEE). The factors cover all aspects that affect the ease of handling a load. Patients can be seen to be dangerous 'loads' under many of these assessment criteria. However, it is often simplest to look at the weights that have to be lifted. The guidance on the regulations contains information in the form of a figure showing how much can be safely lifted by 95% of the population (Fig. 29.2). Paragraphs 6–9 of Appendix 1 of the guidelines state:

6. The guidelines for lifting and lowering operations assume that the load is easy to grasp with both hands and that the operation takes place in reasonable working conditions with

Table 29.1 CEC Directives implemented on January 1 1990

Council Directives (CEC)	Regulations
Framework Directive (CEC 1989a)	Management of Health and Safety at Work Regulations 1992 (SI 1992 No. 2051). Replaced by Management of Health and Safety at Work (Amended) Regulations 1994 (SI 1994 No. 2865)
Manual handling of loads (CEC 1990a)	The Manual Handling Operations Regulations 1992 (SI 1992 No. 2793)
Workplace (CEC 1989a)	Workplace Health, Safety and Welfare Regulations 1992 (SI 1992 No. 3004)
Work equipment (CEC 1989c)	Provision and Use of Work Equipment Regulations 1992 amended June 1998 (SI 1998 No. 2306)
Personal protective equipment (CEC 1989d)	Personal Protective Equipment Regulations 1992 (SI 1992 No. 2966)
Visual display screen equipment (CEC 1990b)	Display Screen Equipment Regulations 1992 (SI 1992 No. 2792)

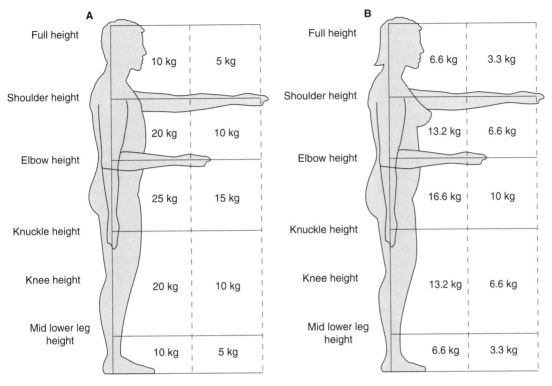

Figure 29.2 Safe lifting weights at different heights for 95% of (A) men and (B) women (HSE 1992a; Crown copyright is reproduced with the permission of the Controller of Her Majesty's Stationery Office).

the handler in a stable body position. They take into consideration the vertical and horizontal position of the hands as they move the load during the handling operation, as well as the height and reach of the individual handler. For example if a load is held at arm's length or the hands pass above the shoulder height, the capability to lift or lower is reduced significantly.

7. The basic figures for identifying when manual lifting and lowering operations may not need a detailed assessment are set out in Figure [29.2]. If the handler's hands enter more than one of the box zones during the operation, the smallest weight figures apply. It is important to remember, however, that the transition from one box zone to another is not abrupt; an intermediate figure may be chosen where the handler's hands are close to a boundary. Where lifting or lowering with the hands beyond the box zones is unavoidable, a more detailed assessment should always be made.

8. These basic guideline figures for lifting and lowering are for relatively infrequent operations – up to approximately 30 operations per hour. The guideline figures will have to be reduced if the operation is repeated more often. As a rough guide, the figures should be reduced by 30% where the operation is repeated around once or twice per minute by 50% where the operation is repeated around five to eight times per minute and by 80% where the operation is repeated more than 12 times per minute.

9. Even if the above conditions are satisfied, a more detailed risk assessment should be made where:

(a) the worker does not control the pace of work;
(b) pauses for rest are inadequate or there is no change of activity which provides an opportunity to use different muscles;
(c) the handler must support the load for any length of time.

The notes that accompany Figure 29.2 say that women can lift two-thirds of the capacity of men and that two people lifting together can lift two-thirds of their combined capacities.

This means that in the area close to the lower body:

one man can lift	25 kg
two men can lift	33.33 kg
one woman can lift	16.6 kg
two women can lift	22.22 kg.

Most patients weigh more than these values so they can be clearly seen as hazardous loads. These weight guidance figures can also be used to identify other potentially hazardous loads such as instrument trays and equipment.

The guidance points out that these values should not be treated as an indication that loads below them are automatically safe. Lighter loads can be dangerous for a number of reasons, e.g. the lifter has a particular weakness; the load may be awkwardly shaped and be difficult to get hold of; the lifter is required to hold a load for an extended period, etc. An example of the latter is holding a patient's leg by the foot whilst the leg is prepared for surgery.

There is no single test that will identify how much weight a person can safely lift. X-ray examination may show a narrowing of the disc space but is not indicative of actual or potential back pain. The only effective way of protecting staff is to reduce handling to a point where most people will be safe. The weight limits in the guidance on the Manual Handling Operations Regulations are thought to be safe for all but 1 in 20 people. Even these levels leave millions of people at risk if they handle the weights given in the guidance.

The guidance on the Regulations also gives advice on the amount that can be pulled or pushed by people. This advice is that a maximum force of 25 kg should be used to get the load moving and that the maximum force to keep the load moving should be 10 kg. This has implications for the types of lateral transfer systems that call for the nurse to push and pull the patient and when nurses are moving patients in beds, trolleys, wheelchairs and hoists. (There is no advice on differing limits for women or multiple handlers. However, it would be reasonable to assume that the same reductions in capacity should be applied as are recommended for lifting.)

Having identified a risk, the employer should follow a three-stage hierarchy of measures:

1. Avoid manual handling operations involving a risk of injury, so far as is reasonably practicable.
2. Provide equipment to allow the handling operations to be carried out without risk.
3. Reduce the risk of injury so far as is reasonably practicable.

The meaning of the phrase 'so far as is reasonably practicable' needs to be understood. The meaning was judicially determined in *Edwards* v. *National Coal Board* (1949). Lord Justice Asquith stated:

'Reasonably practicable' is a narrower term than 'physically possible' and seems to me to imply that a computation must be made in which the quantum of risk is placed on one scale and the sacrifice involved in the measures necessary for averting the risk (whether in money, time or trouble) is placed in the other; and that if it be shown that there is a gross disproportion between them – the risk being insignificant in relation to the sacrifice – the defendants discharge the onus on them. Moreover, this computation falls to be made at a point of time anterior to the accident.

This means that the employer must assess the risk of injury to the worker. The employer can then decide to leave the risk unchanged only if the cost of removing the risk can be shown to considerably exceed the cost of potential injury. This must be written down before the accident. It is not acceptable for the employer to simply see a risk but say there is no money to buy the equipment required to remove the risk, so the risk is left unchanged.

In practice the cost of action is significantly less than the cost of inaction. Therefore it is unlikely that an employer could successfully use the excuse that action was not reasonably practicable. Two examples serve to show this:

• In 1998 one community trust settled two back injury cases out of court for damages totalling £$\frac{1}{4}$ million. This was the money received by the injured persons; it does not take into account the hidden costs and legal fees. These costs vastly exceeded the amount the trust would have had to spend to protect all of their staff.
• A trust put in equipment costing £100 000. Their annual audit showed a reduction of 84% sickness absence, showing a saving of £400 000 (RCN 1996).

All assessments must be reviewed at appropriate intervals. In the case of individual patients this could be as often as several times in a day. However, with most patients, assessments will not be required so frequently. Even with long-term patients, assessments should always be formally reviewed at least every 6 months. If an injury occurs, the assessment must be reviewed. This review must be carried out on the assumption that the existing assessment or the solutions identified are at fault.

Emergencies

Under the Regulations all employers are exempt in an emergency. This means that if the handling is in an emergency situation the employer might not be responsible for any injuries. However, to be eligible for this clause the situation must be unforeseeable. There are virtually no patient-handling situations that are not foreseeable. Even the work of ambulance staff is largely foreseeable. The majority of their work involves simple, regularly repeated situations such as taking collapsed patients out of their homes. In nursing, the handling situations that are to be faced are wholly foreseeable. The nurse can expect to deal with situations such as cardiac arrests, collapsing patients, evacuation of buildings, etc. The employer has a duty to plan for the handling in these situations to be carried out safely.

Implications of the Manual Handling Operations Regulations for employees

The Manual Handling Operations Regulations set out the duties of employees. Employees are to comply with Section 7 of the Health and Safety at Work Act (1974).

It shall be the duty of every employee while at work:

a. To take reasonable care for the health and safety of himself and of other persons who may be affected by his acts or omissions at work; and

b. As regards any duty or requirement imposed on his employer or any other person by or under any of the relevant statutory provisions, to co-operate with him so far as is necessary to enable that duty or requirement to be performed or complied with.

Staff must:

1. *Use the safe systems of work designed by management.* If a piece of equipment is provided then it must be used. If the assessment shows that a hoist is to be used then the employee cannot go back to a manual procedure.

2. *Cooperate with the assessment.* The patient assessment is to be done in conjunction with the nurse looking after the patient. The nurse must adopt a positive attitude to the assessment and assist in minimising the handling risk.

3. *Report defects.* Nurses are to report any piece of equipment that is not working. It is common for bed brakes not to work efficiently. Beds whose brakes do not work should not be used. Nurses are often overheard to say that the brakes are not efficient and that they brace themselves against the bed. Such situations must be reported in writing to appropriate management. The equipment must be taken out of service until it has been repaired. Any piece of equipment that is dangerous because of some design defect is to be reported to the Medical Devices Agency.

4. *Be involved in training.* It is essential that staff attend training made available to them. It is also essential that staff apply the information that they are given in such courses. It is not acceptable to say: 'I was taught that the technique was dangerous but I thought it would be quicker to do it that way.'

The duties explained in this section can protect the employer from liability if a nurse is injured by ignoring instructions. However, the employer should be aware that there may be limits to this protection. If the employer knew that the employee routinely failed to use a piece of equipment, it may be thought by the court that the employer had accepted this failure. It is essential that the employer supervises staff handling of patients. If the staff fail to use specified safe techniques, the employer must be prepared to use full disciplinary procedures in the same way as they would be applied to other disciplinary matters.

Implications of the Manual Handling Operations Regulations for managers

The Manual Handling Operations Regulations set out the manager's specific responsibilities; they are management responsibilities and cannot be given to others. Essentially the manager is required to provide a safe system of work. There are several different aspects to be considered in the creation of a safe system of work:

- implementing a safe handling policy
- carrying out proper assessments of the handling risks of the workplace
- provision of appropriate equipment
- safe handling instructions for loads that have to be handled
- adequate training
- supervision by people who are competent
- provision of a safe place of work
- investigation of accidents that do occur.

Implementing a safe handling policy

The Health and Safety at Work etc. Act 1974, Section 3.1, obliges employers to have a health and safety policy for their employees in which there must be a section on manual handling. Health and safety policies and codes of practice on safe patient movement and manual handling of loads are a way of ensuring that all staff are aware of the dangers of lifting and are given guidance.

A proper handling and lifting policy creates a climate of awareness of the risks to the nurses' and carers' backs. Nursing problems are approached with the attitude that the danger of injury must be avoided.

Carrying out proper assessments of the handling risks of the workplace

The employer is required to carry out assessments to identify the handling risks in the workplace and to establish safe solutions to protect the staff from injury. The process of carrying out assessments is described in some detail below (pp. 615–618).

Provision of appropriate equipment

The employer must provide an adequate range of equipment to allow the nurse to handle patients safely.

This is not a simple matter of buying a hoist and leaving the staff to get on with using it. There is a wide range of equipment that is available to help nurses in the handling of their patients. Depending upon the specific patients and conditions being cared for on a ward there ought to be:

- standard sling-type hoist (Fig. 29.3)
- stretcher fittings for hoists
- standard hoists
- hard sliding boards (Fig. 29.4)
- fabric sliding systems
- profile, turning and stand-up beds.

The precise equipment needs of the ward/department will be identified by the assessments of the handling risks. The generic assessments will provide information on the equipment that is needed on the ward/department at all times. Specific assessments of individual patients may indicate that additional equipment is needed.

It is the management's responsibility to provide the equipment or to make a decision that patients who need this type of equipment will not be treated in the ward/department.

Safe handling instructions for loads that have to be handled

In a safe system of work there must be clear instructions to the staff on how they must work to ensure their safety. It is not adequate to rely simply on the member of staff's knowledge or training. The instructions need to be detailed enough to enable the member of staff to identify the method to be used. They do not need to describe in detail the way in which the procedure is to be carried out. Thus:

- 'Move from bed to wheelchair' is inadequate in that the method is not specified.
- 'Move from bed to wheelchair using the ABC hoist' will usually be adequate.

It is not necessary to tell normal staff how they are to use a hoist. Additional detail would only be required if the patient needed a special sling or to be handled in some special way to avoid a specific risk.

In normal circumstances the instructions will be provided in the form of care plans.

Adequate training

All nurses must be involved in training. It must be remembered that experience in nursing does not equate with being up to date in manual-handling techniques. All nurses should be updated on a yearly basis and as standards change.

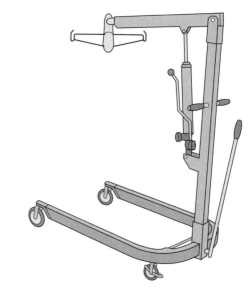

Figure 29.3   Standard sling-type hydraulic hoist.

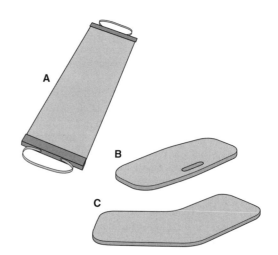

Figure 29.4   Hard boards: (A) board used for transfer from bed to trolley; (B) straight transfer board; (C) curved transfer board.

The RCN Back Pain Advisory Panel in 1988 advised that student nurses should have a minimum of 25 hours of training in manual-handling techniques. This is supported by the HSAC recommendations in 1998 that suggest that 3–5 days of training are required to train staff who have had no previous experience in manual handling.

Staff who have not been given update training since their original training will need significant periods of training to bring them up to date. For example, nurses who were originally trained in the 1970s and who have been working in an environment where all patient handling is manual will require at least 2–3 days to bring them up to date. Even those who have had no training since the introduction of the Manual Handling Operations Regulations on 1 January 1993 may require as much as 2 days to allow them to understand safe handling.

Training people in handling techniques alone is not effective. Several studies have shown that training in techniques alone did not stop staff from having injuries (Chaffin et al 1986, Dehlin et al 1981, Hale & Mason 1986, Pheasant 1991, Pheasant & Stubbs 1992, St Vincent et al 1987, St Vincent & Tellier 1989, Scholey 1983, Snook 1978, Stubbs 1983). **All training must be followed by an opportunity to put the techniques into practice.** Where student nurses are assigned to wards/departments for work experience, the lecturers must ensure that the handling practices on the ward are safe and that the students will therefore reinforce the safe techniques that they have been taught.

The training must include warning the students to avoid the use of condemned lifts. However, on its own a warning is of no value. The lecturer must provide the students with safe alternatives.

Lecturers. The person who is instructing a nurse in the handling of patients must also be trained and up to date. It is not adequate for the manager to say that the person volunteered to be a trainer. There are many people who currently train in this area but who have not kept themselves up to date.

The manager employing the person must make detailed enquiries to ensure that the potential trainer is sufficiently experienced and committed to safe handling.

Numbers of delegates. The number of delegates that are on a course is important. Where the course includes an opportunity to practise the techniques, the lecturer must have time to supervise each delegate in the practice sessions. The Chartered Society of Physiotherapists have guidance for those physiotherapists who are training others (CSP 1993). It is suggested that there must be no more than six delegates per lecturer for practical sessions. Attempts to teach groups that are greater than this size are likely to be unsafe.

Availability of training. The training must be offered in a way that makes it reasonable for members of staff to be able to attend, and alternatives must be offered for those who cannot attend. Staff who refuse to attend must be instructed to do so.

Staff who are on permanent night shift present special problems. If they are to attend training in the day time, they will need to take a minimum of 2 nights off to enable them to be awake for the training and awake for their next night shift. Training during the night shift is not usually practicable as the staff do not have sufficient time to leave their work to attend training.

Training records. Records must be kept of:

- who was trained, with their signatures to confirm attendance
- when the training took place, including time spent on training and dates
- name of trainer and signature with a copy of the content of the sessions of the course. This should be a detailed account of the content. It is not adequate to say that the students were taught to move a person in bed. The records must show what actual techniques were taught.

Records must also be kept to show that all staff have attended training; any who have not must be made to attend a session.

Supervision by people who are competent

A safe place of work cannot be created simply by teaching the junior staff to handle safely. These are often the people who do most of the handling but the senior staff set the standards and therefore they must also know how to handle safely.

Senior staff must monitor handling practices to ensure that safe standards are followed and that dangerous practices do not creep in. Supervisors must be prepared to insist on safe practice. This must include disciplinary action if poor practices continue.

Where nurses are working away from direct supervision, as in the community, extra care must be taken to ensure that they are supervised. Supervisors must make an extra, positive, effort to observe their staff in their work.

Provision of a safe place of work

The manager must ensure that the place of work is safe. In general, buildings used by the health services are structurally safe. However, there are often problems that reduce the safety for staff handling patients. The most important aspect is to ensure that there is sufficient space to handle the patients safely, for example:

- Is there enough space for nurses to work in the operating theatre or beside the bed?
- Is there enough space to operate and move a hoist?
- Is there enough space for two nurses to walk with a patient?
- Is the shower large enough?
- Are the toilets large enough?

The series of books entitled 'Health Building Note' produced by NHS Estates provide detailed guidance on the safe spaces needed in the health care setting. Health Building Note 40, Volume 1, *Common Activity Spaces*, provides information on the areas needed in most nursing applications. However, there are also Notes covering operating theatres (Health Building Note 26 1994) and other relevant areas (Health Building Note 27 1994, *Intensive Therapy Unit*, etc.).

If the space is too small, then it must not be used for handling patients.

Investigation of accidents that do occur

The Reporting of Injuries, Diseases and Dangerous Occurrences Regulations 1985 (RIDDOR; SI 1985 No. 2023) places a duty on the employer to report accidents that result in absences of 3 days or more from work. These regulations have now been updated to include the effects of violence (RIDDOR; SI 1995 No. 3163).

A safe system of work would ensure that all back injury accidents are reported. Once reported, these accidents must be investigated (HSAC 1984, 1986, 1992, 1998). Accident reporting exists for two reasons that are reflected in reactive and proactive actions. In the reactive phase, steps are taken to ensure that the injuries and damage caused by the accident have been dealt with; in the proactive phase the manager takes steps to ensure that the accident will not happen again.

Handling injuries are often not immediately recognised to be serious enough to report as accidents. It is thought that the injury is some minor strain and that it will resolve itself without problems. Whilst staff should always be encouraged to report accidents immediately, it must be recognised that some will not be reported for some days until the extent of the injury becomes apparent. Staff must never be told that it is too late to report an accident. Even accidents which are reported late must be properly investigated.

Case study 29.1 shows the importance of proper investigation. The initial form seems to say that the injury arose from some inexplicable source. It seemed to have been caused by some weakness of the nurse or because of some fault of her own. The accident form had been signed off by the nurse's manager without comment. A full investigation revealed a very different story. The nurse had been part of a group carrying out a very dangerous procedure. Retraining was given to all of the staff including, in particular, the surgical ward sister who had been responsible for the choice of technique.

Case study 29.1   Injury to a student nurse

A student nurse in her final year of training reported on her accident form:

Hurt my back whilst changing the patient's bottom sheet.
The time of the accident was 2 p.m.
There were nine staff on duty.

The investigation revealed:

The patient
The patient was a lady of some 72 years who had sustained a fractured neck of femur. She was in bed in traction. She was waiting to go to the operating theatre for fixation of her femur. Her bed sheet needed changing as it was soiled.

Number of staff involved in the lift: 5

Equipment used: patient-handling slings

Method of moving the patient
The nurses stood on each side of the bed. They placed a handling sling under the patient's thighs and under her shoulders. Each nurse had hold of a handle of one of the handling slings. The fifth nurse was looking after the traction.
   The student nurse who was injured was holding one of the handles of a handling sling. As she was holding the sling with one hand she was bending and twisting to reach under the patient to wash the patient's bottom and change the sheet.

Problems with this procedure
Patient-handling slings are pieces of thick flexible plastic with hand holds at each end. They can be passed under the patient and then used to lift the patient. The use of slings does improve the lifter's posture by reducing the amount of forward bending that would occur if they were not used, but these slings do not reduce the absolute weight of the patient. If the patient is too heavy to be lifted manually, then the slings will not make her light enough to be lifted manually.
   The student nurse who was injured was, like all four nurses, carrying an unsafe load. However, her posture was made worse by bending and reaching under the patient. This additional postural stress seems to have caused her injury.
   There was poor training of nurses. The patient was too heavy to be lifted manually. It is also well known that nurses should not undertake a second procedure whilst handling a patient.
   (It should also be noted that the use of patient-handling slings would not be appropriate for a patient who had suffered a fractured neck of femur. The lift that was carried out would have caused distress and pain to the patient.)

Safe solution to the handling need
Ideally the patient ought to have been lifted using a hoist with a slatted or scoop stretcher attachment.

Case study 29.1   (Contd.)

Alternatively the patient could have been log rolled to change her sheet. This can be acceptable with this type of patient provided the nurses give analgesics before doing the procedure. When doing this the patient should only be log rolled onto the affected hip.

Conclusions
This was an accident that need never have happened. If the nurses had been trained that patients are not to be lifted and if they had been told to log roll, the student would not have been injured.

The manoeuvre carried out by the nurses was also detrimental to the patient.

RISK ASSESSMENTS

Assessment

The assessment of manual handling situations is a two-stage process. The first stage is to identify the risks in the situation(s) being assessed. In patient handling the main risks are that the patient is too heavy to be lifted or that the patient will in some way collapse whilst being handled. However, there are other criteria to be considered such as: Will the patient be hurt by the lift and therefore react against the nurse? Will the patient react in some other way against the assistance that the nurse is giving? Is there some feature of the injuries etc. that will affect the handling of the patient?

Having identified the risks, the second stage is to identify a way of handling the patient which avoids the risk. These solutions or 'controls' must then be checked to ensure that they have not brought in new risks, e.g. a hoist would present risks with a patient who was known to struggle. Such risks must in themselves be controlled.

The chosen solutions must be recorded and made available to all staff. A date must be established for a formal review of the assessment. The period before the next review may be between a few hours and 6 months.

Generic assessments

The guidance on the Manual Handling Operations Regulations (HSE 1992a) tells employers that generic assessments can be undertaken. The objective of generic assessments is to look at the handling events that normally occur in the workplace and identify safe solutions that can be applied to control the risks that are identified. The existence of an effective generic assessment can greatly simplify the assessment of each individual handling event that is required under the Regulations.

The activity of identifying suitable subjects for generic assessments is important. The tasks that are identified need to be relatively common but also they need to have a relatively stable set of handling situations.

There are two strategies to be considered:

- assessments for specific procedures
- assessments of specific tasks.

Assessments for specific procedures

It can be useful to provide standard assessments for the handling tasks and their associated risks throughout a particular procedure such as a total hip replacement. Such an assessment will recognise that the handling needs of the patient change significantly throughout the procedure, being different at different stages. As a minimum standard, assessment of a hip replacement procedure would cover handling:

- before the operation
- during the operation
- in the recovery phase
- initial mobilisation
- development of mobility
- preparation for discharge.

At each of these points there would have to be variations for different types and weights of patients. Many of the stages would also require instructions for handling in a variety of situations such as moving to a chair, moving in bed, toileting, bathing, walking, etc.

A standard assessment for a specific procedure must be used with caution as the individual patient may not comply with the expected model. Nevertheless, a well-designed standard assessment, properly used, is valuable where a procedure is carried out regularly. This is particularly the case for situations such as hip operations where specialised equipment may be required.

Assessments of specific tasks

In other circumstances it can be more convenient to consider the separate handling events that occur in the care of patients. In this approach, the assessor identifies all of the events and a 'kit bag' of solutions that can be applied to specific patients. Typical handling events to be assessed are:

- moving the patient to and from a theatre trolley
- moving the patient in bed

- moving the patient out of bed
- taking the patient to the toilet
- taking the patient into the bathroom
- helping the patient to walk.

The assessor must look at each of these tasks to decide the risks that arise with patients of differing abilities. The assessor must then consider the solutions available and consider their application to the task. If equipment is needed to allow safe solutions, then appropriate orders must be placed as soon as possible.

A look at the generic assessment of just one task will make the process clearer. If we consider transfers from bed to trolley, there are essentially two classes of patients: those who can move themselves and those who need to be moved. (There is no safe way of manually 'helping' a person across.) Those who need to be moved across may be slid across using one of a variety of horizontal transfer methods. However, some patients will be too heavy or otherwise too awkward to be moved; these patients must be moved using an appropriate hoist. Thus the assessment for the move from bed to trolley (and vice versa) should be written down in a form such as in Table 29.2

If there is no hoist that is suitable for a stretcher transfer, the manager must be advised that patients who qualify for this type of transfer cannot be moved between trolley and bed until one is made available. (NB: Many Ambulift hoists are model D. These can be adapted from bath work to sling work. This type of hoist will take a stretcher attachment. This is often not known on the ward – check yours.)

The completed generic assessment

The full assessment of the generic handling risks of a ward will identify a common need for solutions to handling risks that occur throughout the work of the ward. The definition of controls to these risks will identify the need for a range of equipment. Some of this equipment will be in place; other items will need to be obtained. The assessment will produce a consolidated list of equipment that needs to be obtained to make the ward safe. This list must be presented to management together with an explanation of the importance of the equipment. Managers must be advised of those handling situations that will have to be avoided until the equipment is obtained. They must also be provided with a cost–benefit analysis of the reduction in risk achieved by obtaining the equipment.

There may well be an associated list of physical changes that need to be made to the environment to allow for safe handing. This list will need to be processed in the same way as the list of equipment.

Individual assessments

The Manual Handling Operations Regulations 1992 require every load to be separately assessed. This requirement presents special problems in the health services. In industry a load can be the same every time it is handled. A single assessment will serve for every time that the item is moved in a particular situation (separate assessments may still be required for the same load in different situations). People are not so

Table 29.2 Moving from bed to trolley

Condition of patient	Method to be used	Notes
Self-mobile	Allow patient to move himself	Beware of risks of assisting
Patient weighing less than *nn* kg*	Use XYZ lateral transfer system	Log roll to position transfer system
Patients weighing more than *nn* kg*	Use ABC hoist with stretcher attachment	Log roll to position stretcher canvas
Patients unable to log roll (size or special problems external fixators, etc.)	Use ABC hoist with scoop attachment	Scoop stretcher attachment available from 123 Ward

* The weight '*nn*' to be applied in deciding between patients will depend on the recommended limits supplied by the manufacturer of the transfer system.

Notes:
1. There is also a transfer trolley called the AT 2000 or Mobiliser. This can be especially useful in transferring spinal patients, transferring patients in the operating department, and in difficult situations such as transfers on to and off scanner tables.
2. Arrangements to share equipment are potentially dangerous in that people are discouraged from actually fetching the equipment. Such arrangements should only be made where the equipment is only needed very infrequently.

convenient. Patients vary in almost every way that is possible. There are great physical differences in size, weight and abilities. Patients' abilities change over time. This is particularly important on a surgical unit where many patients go from self-mobile to completely dependant back to self-mobile over a period as short as a few days. With some procedures this is compressed into as little as a few hours. Even patients who have relatively stable abilities will change in a regular pattern through the day. A patient with arthritis will find it hard to get going in the morning, move reasonably well in the middle of the day and be dependent again in the evening. The use of drugs to assist patients to sleep at night can of course make such cycles even more extreme.

Patients must be assessed separately to identify the way in which each individual will be handled in a variety of everyday situations. The list must be chosen to suit the needs of the patient. Depending on the patient, the assessment should cover:

- moving in bed
- transfers from bed to trolley, operating table, etc.
- transfers from bed to chair/wheelchair/commode
- toileting
- support in walking
- bathing.

The assessment is done in the same way as all assessments: identify the risks; select the handling solutions needed to make the handling task safe.

The results of the generic assessment can be used to provide an appropriate solution for the patient. However, the assessor must be prepared to define new solutions for individuals who present special needs not covered by the generic assessment.

The results of the assessment must be written up and made available to everyone who is likely to care for the patient. If at all possible, the handling assessment should be on one piece of paper, placed at the front of the patient's file or by the bed.

The handling instructions must be clear and unambiguous. Traditionally, patient handling instructions simply said 'move with two'. This could mean anything. It was often taken to mean 'use the drag lift'. The instructions do not need to be long-winded but they must be clear. A sentence such as 'Toilet on a commode using the Standaid to transfer; ensure that the safety buckle on the Standaid belt is used.' may be sufficient for a patient with no special problems.

All assessments must bear a date by which the patient's needs must be reassessed. With patients in long-term care the reassessments must be not more than 6 months apart. However, it is important to resist the temptation to simply sign the previous assessment off for another 6 months. Nurses must positively review patients to ensure that any slow or slight changes in their condition are identified.

Whenever something goes wrong whilst a patient is being handled the assessment must be reviewed. The prudent nurse will expect any patient to collapse. However, if a patient has collapsed, the handling plan must be altered to take into account the increased danger that it will happen again with this patient.

> **Reflective point**
>
> Consider just one of your patients who you know well. If you were to be called to attend to this patient without any verbal briefing, would you be able to find out how to handle this patient from the information in the documentation?

The philosophy of assessment is as important as the mechanism. Assessors must act to protect the nurses and other carers from injury. They must also seek to act in the interests of the patients. In the past it has been thought that the best interests of patients were for them to be lifted manually. This is, of course, counter to the best interests of the nurses, in that lifting patients puts them at risk of injury. It is now recognised that manual lifting of patients does not promote their well-being. It is now known that safe handling will improve mobility and reduce injuries and pain from handling. This means that the objectives of protecting the nurse and acting in the best interests of the patient are not in opposition.

Discharge from hospital

The discharge of patients from hospital into the community may present special difficulties for nurses in creating safe handling. The patient is to leave the hospital to either return home or go to a new nursing or care home. The district nurses or the nurses in the care home know little of the patient's mobility. They rely on the nurses in the hospital to provide them with safe advice as to the care needs of the patient. There are often problems in defining and obtaining the equipment needed to allow the patient to be cared for outside hospital. Much of the problem is due to organisational and funding problems that are outside the scope of this book. However, nurses can make a difference by ensuring that realistic written assessments are produced.

Nurses in the hospital must take care to give best advice on the patient's condition. They must resist any temptation to give too good a picture of the capabilities of the patient. Nurses outside the hospital must resist the temptation to be too optimistic about their abilities to cope with the patient's needs.

It is essential that a careful assessment is made of the patient's discharge needs. This assessment must take into account the environment into which the patient will be sent. The assessors must recognise that there is a great difference between the well-lit ward with clear spaces and hard floors and the home situation where there may be clutter and tight spaces with soft furnishings.

Where equipment is needed to allow the patient to be cared for, it must be provided before discharge, not after the patient has been left in an armchair by the ambulance staff.

DANGEROUS LIFTS

Long-condemned techniques

There are three lifts that have long been condemned as unsafe. They are so unsafe that they cannot even be used with patients who are lighter than the weight guidance in the Regulations. These techniques can and do cause injuries to nurses even when used with babies and small children.

The drag lift

This lift is any attempt to move patients by lifting them under the armpits. There are usually two nurses but sometimes one nurse will carry out a one-sided lift. The nurse's arms are usually inserted from the front but they can be put in from the back (Figs 29.5 and 29.6).

The lift is dangerous to nurses and to patients (Stubbs 1983, Stubbs et al 1980). The nurse is carrying out the lift in a forward-bend posture. All such lifting is dangerous. If anything goes wrong, the nurse may be forced to bend even further forward to lower the patient to the floor. Because of the under-arm grip the nurse can be trapped by patients closing their arms to hang on to the nurse. If this happens, the nurse is unable to let go and has to follow the patient all the way down. This can cause an even greater amount of forwards lean, resulting in even more dangerous loads on the base of the spine.

The effects of this lift on patients are also severe and can feed back to place increased loads on the nurses:

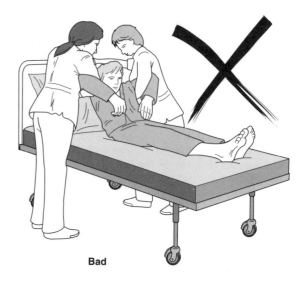

Bad

Figure 29.5 Drag and lift up the bed (reproduced by kind permission from Lloyd et al 1998).

- The lift under the armpits is dysfunctional. That is to say that it so alters the shape of the patient's body that he finds it hard to stand up. If the patient has some residual ability to stand, a lift under the armpits will mean that he is unable to use it. He will have to rely on the nurses to lift him to his feet. These effects mean that the nurses will be taking the whole of the patient's weight even though he has some ability to stand by himself.
- The lift is also painful as the force from the nurse's arms traps nerves in the patient's armpit. This pain can cause the confused patient to strike out at the source of the pain. When a patient struggles in this way, the lift can become unbalanced and throw the entire load onto one nurse.
- The lift under the armpits is one that the human body is not designed to cope with. There is evidence to suggest that many elderly people suffer dislocated shoulders from the effects of the drag lift. The pain from such dislocations is again likely to cause the patient to react against the nurse.

Sometimes the nurses using this technique will argue that they are only assisting the patient. It can be seen from the points made above that this is not the case and that even when assisting the patient the nurse can be exposed to the full weight of the patient.

The drag lift is known by many different names. However, the comments above cover all lifts where the main lifting force is applied under the patient's armpits, regardless of the name of the lift.

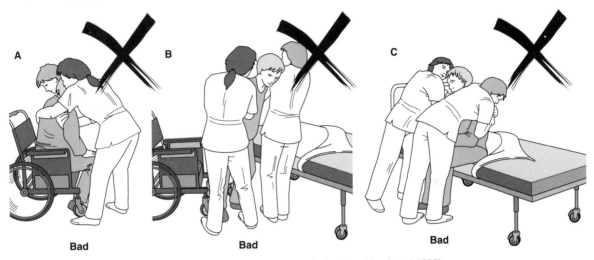

Figure 29.6 Drag lift from chair to bed (reproduced by kind permission from Lloyd et al 1998).

The dangers of the drag lift also apply to a number of different lifts known as the through-arm lift. (There seem to be as many as five different lifts with this name.) All of these lifts involve similar forces to the drag lift. Some of them have the additional risk of soft tissue damage or breakages to the patient's arms.

The orthodox lift

This is the lift where one nurse stands on each side of the patient. They bend forwards and link arms underneath her to lift her up the bed. With smaller patients, such as children, nurses sometimes do a one-person lift in the same posture (Fig. 29.7). Both versions are dangerous in that the nurse is lifting in a forward-bent posture, placing the weight of the patient at a considerable distance from the base of the spine (Stubbs 1983, Stubbs et al 1980).

This lift is sometimes called the cradle lift. The name change does not make the lift any safer.

Lifting with the patient's arms around the lifter's neck

It used to be quite common practice to carry out front transfers or standing transfers with the patient's arms round or close to the lifter's neck (Fig. 29.8). All such lifts are unsafe because the patient can hang on the lifter's neck. The whole weight of the patient is applied at a considerable distance from the base of the spine.

Other lifting techniques

Most other manual lifts are now recognised to be dangerous. They would be unsafe because the patients are

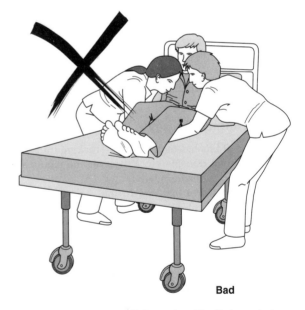

Figure 29.7 Orthodox lift (reproduced by kind permission from Lloyd et al 1998).

too heavy to be lifted manually, but on examination there are other reasons for condemning them. All manual lifts of people by people involve the use of unsafe postures and/or obstruct or interfere with patients' ability to move themselves. This is a complex subject and the detailed explanations of the faults in each lift are long. It would not be productive to reproduce them here. If more information is required, refer to Chapter 22 of *The Guide to the Handling of Patients* (Lloyd et al 1998).

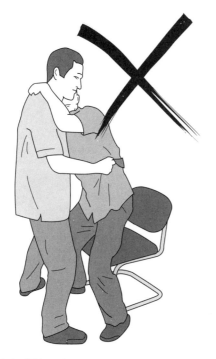

Figure 29.8   Lifting with arms around the patient's neck.

Front transfers (Fig. 29.9)

This group of lifts has many names – rocking transfer; bear hug, pivot transfer, etc. Whatever the name, all front transfers suffer from two faults:

1. The lifters are exposed to the majority of the weight of the patient. This is, as in all lifting situations, too great a load to be lifted by the nurse.

2. The lifts are dysfunctional. This is because the lifter blocks the natural standing motion of the patient. This forces the patient to try to stand with her body too far back. In this position she is going to need more lifting help to get her up, thus forcing the nurse to take a greater part of her weight.

Many nurses are injured every year using front transfers to move patients. The dysfunctional nature of the lift also means that it is of no therapeutic value to the patient. This group of lifts should not be used (Gagnon et al 1986, Smedley et al 1995).

Reflective point

How will you introduce and ensure safe handling in your surgical area

---

SAFE HANDLING

The weights given in the guidance on the Manual Handling Operations Regulations (HSE 1992a) are very convenient for the health services. Virtually all patients weigh more than the figures given in the guidance. Therefore we are not faced with the problem of deciding which patients can be lifted manually and which will need to be moved by some other means. With the exception of babies and very young children, we can simply say that people cannot lift people. Therefore we can say that nurses must not be put in any position where they can be exposed to even a significant part of the weight of a patient.

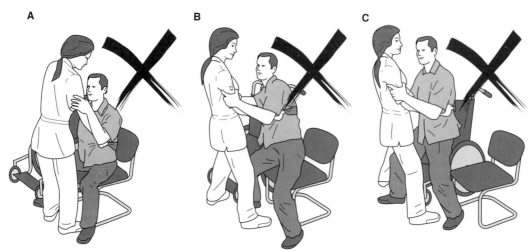

Figure 29.9   Front transfer.

That is not to say that all patients must be moved with hoists at all times. There are five main approaches to be considered:

- getting patients to move themselves
- assisting the patient (without exposing the nurse to the risk of supporting unsafe loads)
- sliding the patient from one place to another
- using a mechanical device
- leaving patients where they are.

Getting patients to move themselves

This approach is closely linked with rehabilitation which is dealt with separately in this chapter (p. 629).

It has been recognised that many lifts and transfer methods are dysfunctional. These lifts interfere with patients' abilities to move themselves. This is particularly true of the drag lift and the front transfers. If patients have been regularly moved using one of these methods, they may have learned that they cannot move themselves. They may have to be retaught that they can get themselves from bed to chair.

All manual lifts or lifts with equipment deprive patients of an opportunity to attempt to move themselves.

In the past, nurses have been injured using manual lifts on patients who could move themselves. For example there have been cases where nurses were injured using the shoulder lift to move patients up in bed even though the patients were capable of moving themselves.

Nurses using manual lifts on such patients argue that it is easier; more caring; nicer for the patient; etc. Nurses must recognise that if they physically lift patients by any means they are depriving them of their independence. Therefore they should only lift patients who cannot move themselves.

Enabling patients to move themselves is a rewarding experience for everyone involved. It is not a simple matter of telling patients to move and walking away. Nurses need to assess their pain level, talk quietly to them, and explain how to go about the move. The patients need verbal support and encouragement throughout the move until they become confident and can do it by themselves.

There are four main moves that patients can be asked to do:

- move in bed
- transfer from one seated position to another
- bathing
- getting up from the floor.

In all of these situations there is one overriding rule. Nurses must never try to assist patients physically. They should even be careful in placing their hands on a patient, as they could become trapped if the patient does collapse in the middle of the move. If a patient does collapse, the nurse must not support the patient and stop the fall. Wherever possible, the patient is lowered to the floor or back into the chair.

Guiding the patient to move in bed

The need for a patient to move in bed is greatly reduced if the patient is in a four-section profiling bed. This should now be the standard bed for patients who need nursing care. However, even with these beds, the patient does need to get to and from the edge of the bed when getting in or out. With all beds, the patient may need to be persuaded to change position in the night or to allow the nurse to change the bedding.

After the nurse has first assessed their pain level, patients should be encouraged to attempt to do any move in bed themselves. Consider the use of simple aids such as bed blocks and rope ladders to assist the patient in a move. Lifting poles (also known as monkey poles) are quite popular in hospital but they are difficult to get into the right position so that they can help the patient throughout the move. (Have you ever lain on a bed and tried to use a lifting pole? You may be surprised to find it less easy than you think, particularly in the postoperative period.) Lifting poles can be more effective for bridging when a bed pan is being inserted (Fig. 29.10).

Patients who have been manoeuvred onto a sliding sheet may be able to move themselves up the bed.

Think about the natural movements that you use yourself in similar situations. For example, even fit people find it difficult to sit up from the supine position. Most people will naturally roll to one side and push themselves up into a sitting position.

Patients transferring themselves from one seated position to another

In these transfers the important thing is to think through the move. Consider the standing process. Even normal people carry out the process in a specific way. People will only be able to stand if their centre of gravity is over their feet. This is achieved by a set of strategies:

- Ensure the patient is pain-free.
- Feet are positioned one in front of the other with the trailing heel slightly under or against the bottom of the chair.

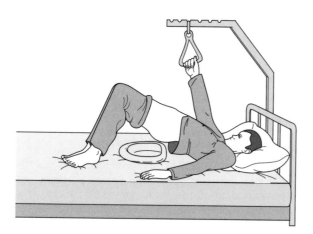

Figure 29.10   Lifting pole – useful for inserting a bed pan.

• The body is leant forward. In deep chairs the person may shuffle forward.

• The person then lunges forward to stand. This is sometimes accomplished in one go but quite often people rock once or twice to stand.

• People often use the arms of the chair to push up. In the absence of arms they push up on the seat.

When asking patients to stand by themselves do not expect them to be able to do better than a fully fit person could do. They will not be able to stand if they are not correctly positioned and properly prepared (Schultz et al 1992). Plan the stand-up. Help patients to recognise how they will go about standing. One of the best ways of improving standing abilities is to make sure that patients are sitting in the right form of chair. In other words, plan where your patients are to sit so that they will be able to stand.

If patients are going to stand and are out of bed, they should be in a firm chair that is not too low and which has arms to push down on.

It is common practice to place a Zimmer frame in front of the patient. It seems that nurses expect patients to pull on the frame to get themselves up. This does not work; a Zimmer frame is very unstable and should never be used to assist a person to stand or move position. The Zimmer frame should be kept to one side and brought in front once the patient has stood up.

The only way of extracting a patient who has been placed in a deep chair for the day is with some type of a hoist. Do not try to pull the patient out by the arms and do not consider the drag lift.

If patients cannot stand they may still be able to move themselves using a sliding board. Again, planning the move will be assisted by studying how you would do the move yourself. Straight boards can only be used for sideways transfers. Curved boards can be used for transfers through any angle up to 180° (Fig. 29.11). Hand-holds are useful to assist the patient. However, even with curved boards the arms of the chair or wheelchair may be in the way. If possible, the adjoining arms of the wheelchair and chair should be removed to make it easier for the person to move.

Allowing patients to bath themselves

Getting in and out of the bath is one of the first areas in which people need assistance. Most wards have bathing hoists. This is one of the few areas where there is usually relatively easy acceptance of the use of equipment in the handling of patients. However, a hoist may not always be necessary. People's independence can be much extended by the use of simple aids to make it easier for them to move themselves. Proper placing of hand-holds and the use of the vast range of equipment for use in the bath can greatly extend the independence of patients. The provision of a firm seat outside the bath and level with the top of the bath can also make it much easier for patients to get in and out of the bath independently.

Although many people prefer a bath, it may be safer to use a wheel-in shower. Patients may only need to be wheeled into the shower area on an appropriate wheelchair. Once there they may be able to wash themselves with minimal help.

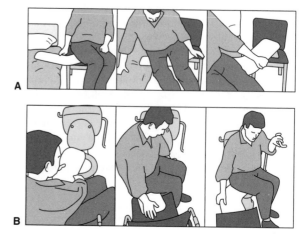

Figure 29.11   Use of a curved board for unassisted transfer: (A) commode to bed; (B) wheelchair to toilet.

Getting up from the floor

Patients may be on the floor as a result of a fall or a collapse. They may also have been placed on the floor for some form of activity or therapy.

There is no way that a person can be manually lifted from the floor by any number of people.

Before doing anything, check that the patient is not injured. Only proceed to ask him to get himself off the floor if he is uninjured. If you are in any doubt, use a hoist to get the patient off the floor and seek medical advice.

If the patient is able to get himself off the floor, he will need to be guided up. The first stage is to calm him and explain that you cannot assist him because you might both be hurt if anything goes wrong. Assure him that this way he will get up safely and will be able to do it if he ever falls again.

First get the patient to roll onto his hands and knees. Then place a stool so that he can put his hands onto it. Next he can progress to put his hands on the seat of a dining chair. From this position he should be able to turn himself to sit in a chair or wheelchair (Fig. 29.12). Let the patient rest before attempting to stand or attempt any further transfer.

Assisting the patient

Giving assistance to a patient is one of the most dangerous activities available to a nurse. Many nurses are injured every year when they are unable to separate themselves from a collapsing patient or when the assistance builds up to the point where they are lifting a significant part of the patient's weight.

With the exception of helping a cooperative patient to sit up, it is not generally possible to assist a person to move in bed. It is also dangerous to try to assist a person to get into and out of a bath.

There are only two areas where nurses can regularly assist a patient to move. These are assisting a person to stand and providing guidance in walking.

Assisting the patient to stand

The golden rule of assisting a person to stand is to stop and lower the patient if the amount of weight being supported becomes at all significant. The maximum weight that a female nurse can take when assisting someone from a chair is about 9–10 kg. This is not very great. It is about the weight of a box of copier paper. If she finds that more assistance than this is required to move the patient, then a new assessment must be done to identify a safer way of doing the move. (Male

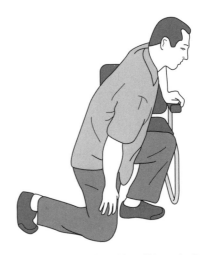

Figure 29.12 A patient lifting himself from the floor.

nurses' capacity may be a few kilograms more, but if they are taller they may have to bend further to assist the patient. The increased bending needed may negate their extra capacity.)

The second rule of assisting someone to stand is that the nurse must ensure that the assistance does not obstruct the natural body movements. Thus, if the nurse is assisting a patient to stand, the nurse must stand to the side of the patient not in front.

A handling belt is essential to provide a safe way of holding the patient. The types with external loops are best in that the nurse can let go if the patient collapses. Belts without hand-holds must be treated with care as nurses can be pulled down with patients if they are unable to disengage their hands.

The basic technique for standing a patient using a handling belt is the same as for the patient who is to stand independently (as above). The nurse is going to provide a bit of extra force to help the patient up. Therefore the nurse must not get in the way of the natural standing movement. The nurse stands to the side of the patient and, facing the patient, grasps the handles of the handling belt with both hands. She places her feet well apart so that she can rock her body from one foot to the other as the patient stands. The objective is for her to have her hands in front of her body when the patient is seated and, as the patient stands, for her to rock onto the other foot and still have her hands in front of her body. When properly carried out, this technique will avoid all twisting in the lifter.

The nurse prepares the patient by assisting him to position himself on the edge of the seat. She then takes up her position. She explains that the stand will be coordinated by the words 'Ready, steady, STAND'. They carry out two preparatory rocks and on the word 'STAND' the patient stands with assistance from the nurse.

If the nurse feels any doubt about the ability of the patient to stand up, or to balance once standing, she must protect both the patient and herself by immediately putting him back down into the seat or lowering him to the floor.

If the patient is seated in a place where the nurse cannot get into the right position to assist him to stand, he must be got to his feet by some other means such as a hoist.

When the patient is to stand from a bed, it is sometimes possible for him to be assisted to his feet using the mechanism of the bed (Fig. 29.13). The patient sits on the edge of the bed with his bottom only partially on the bed. The bed mechanism is then operated to raise the surface of the bed. The patient effectively slides off into a standing position. This method is best used with electric profiling beds as the head end of the bed can be raised to provide support and the electric mechanism gives a smooth lifting action. The method can be used with a hydraulic bed but it is less comfortable and usually requires two nurses.

Walking with a patient

It is common practice for nurses to provide support in walking during the early stages of recovery. This is a dangerous practice and many people are injured doing it.

It is explained in the section on rehabilitation (p. 629) that patients should initially gain confidence using some device that will provide support without putting the nurses at risk. However, once patients have regained some mobility and can be relied on to walk, nurses may accompany them on short walks.

Even when patients have gained some mobility, nurses must recognise that there is always a risk that any patient will collapse when being walked. If a patient does collapse, there is no way in which the nurse can safely support the patient. If he tries to do so, there is a significant risk that he and the patient will be injured.

When walking with a patient, the nurse should be on the patient's weaker side. If the patient's left side is the weaker, because for example he has an i.v. infusion in situ, the nurse goes to the left-hand side of the patient. He then holds the patient's left hand with his left hand. The patient is asked to keep her arm straight and push straight down onto the nurse's hand.

If the patient understands instructions, it is best to use the palm-to-palm thumb grip. However, if the patient is confused, it will be safer to use the grip without interlocking thumbs.

The nurse can place his other hand on the patient's elbow to keep the arm straight or he can place his other hand round the patient's waist. If the nurse is going to provide support in this way, the patient

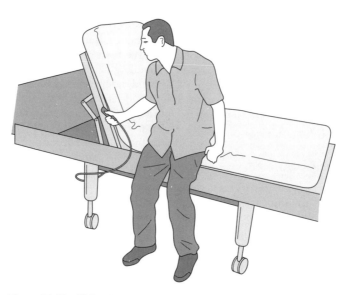

Figure 29.13 Using the bed mechanism to raise the patient to his feet (reproduced by kind permission from Lloyd et al 1998).

should have a handling belt placed around his waist. The nurse should grasp the loops on the handling belt or, in the absence of loops, he should place his hand into the belt from the lower edge of the belt. (Putting the hand into the top of the belt can lead to the nurse's hand being trapped if the patient collapses.)

Always ensure that there is room for the patient and the nurse(s) to walk without bumping into walls or furniture. If the nurse has to change his grip to get past some obstruction, he may find that he loses control of the patient and is unable to offer proper support at a critical moment.

The patient can now be gently encouraged to walk. Do not try to kick the patient's feet through. This is unsafe.

If the patient starts to collapse, the nurse may be able to supply enough correcting force to allow him to regain his balance. However, nurses must never try to support a patient who is collapsing. Therefore if the patient does not immediately regain her balance, she must be lowered to the floor. The nurse simply steps behind the patient and, releasing his grip on the patient's hand, he allows the patient to slide down his body to end sitting on the floor in front of the nurse. Thus the nurse does not allow the patient simply to fall. Instead he guides the patient to the floor without putting himself at risk of severe injury by taking the weight of the patient.

Sliding the patient from one place to another

There is a lot of equipment available to enable a patient to be slid from one place to another. The devices can be classified into six main groups:

1. Sliding boards. Boards are available for both seated and supine transfers. The key to the use of most boards is that, in general, the board itself does not move. The board stays still and the patient slides over the slippery upper surface. There are a few boards which are designed to move with the patient on the board. In these, the patient must be rolled or slid onto the board before being slid across from one place to another.

Generally, sliding boards are used where the transfer involves moving across a gap between one place and another, e.g. bed to trolley, chair to wheelchair, etc.

2. Sliding sheets. These are loops of slippery fabric that can be used in a variety of transfers in bed. They can also be used in conjunction with transfer boards to make the transfer easier (Fig. 29.14).

3. Padded transfer systems. These are similar to sliding sheets; however, they have an element of padding that allows the patient to be transferred over small gaps. These can be used, for example, to transfer from a bed to a trolley without the need for a sliding board (Fig. 29.15).

4. Turning aids. Larger fabric slides, both sheet types and padded types, can be left permanently under patients who need to be turned. The patient can then be turned simply by pulling on the sheet (Fig. 29.16).

These may not be suitable for some patients; for example, patients who have fits could fall out of bed.

5. One-way sheets. These are fabric sheets that will slide in one direction only. This is useful when positioning a person in a chair. The patient can be pushed back into the chair but will not slide out again. If patients do slip or shuffle down in the chair, they can be pushed back again with a minimum of force.

Larger sizes of one-way glides are available for use with supine patients. These can be particularly useful on A&E trolleys.

6. Turntables. Hard turntables have been used for some time. They are intended to be used to turn patients in a standing position. The problem is that in bringing patients to a standing position, their feet are too close together for a natural standing movement. Patients may also feel the turntable move and feel themselves to be unsafe as they stand. Once standing, their feet are still too close together and they are therefore unstable.

There does not seem to be a safe way of using these devices in standing turns; therefore they should not be purchased for this purpose. (Hard turntables can be

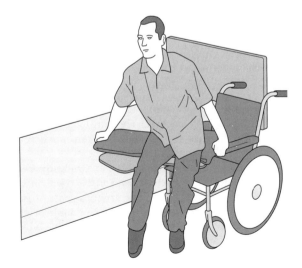

Figure 29.14 Use of fabric slide in conjunction with transfer boards.

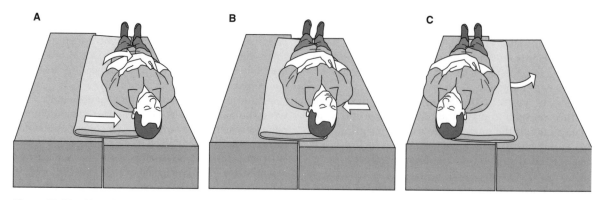

Figure 29.15 Use of a padded transfer system to move a patient over a small gap.

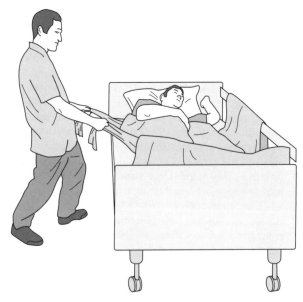

Figure 29.16 Turning a patient with a fabric slide (reproduced by kind permission from Huntleigh Technology PLC).

used with sliding systems when transferring from one seated position to another. The turntable is placed under the patient's feet so that they can move automatically as the patient slides across.)

A number of soft turntables have recently been brought onto the market. These can be used on the floor. They are most useful in turning a patient in a seated position such as turning to face a table or getting into a car. The person sits on the turntable which is then used to swing the feet round into the proper position.

There is such a wide range of sliding devices on the market that it is not possible to give a full explanation

of the best way of using each device. However, a few ground rules can be applied generally.

1. Position the device by log rolling a supine patient or rocking a seated patient. It may seem obvious but if nurses manually lift someone onto a handling device, they have destroyed the point of having it.

2. Most boards only need to be partially under the patient. Fabric sheets should be rolled up like a bed sheet and the patient rolled back to allow the sheet to be pulled through.

3. Padded sheets generally only need to be partially inserted, as with a board.

4. When the patient is wet, a towel may need to be placed between the patient and the sliding device.

5. Once on a sliding sheet, the patient is very mobile, for example beware of patients sliding off the edge of a bed.

6. Some patients may be too heavy for the sliding system. There is not enough information to enable limits to be suggested but beware of having to provide more than 20–25 kg of force to move the person (this range is for male nurses – reduce this force to 16.6 kg for female nurses). If it is difficult to move the person on a sliding system, stop and use a mechanical device. In some systems the weight limit for patients on sliding systems may be 102 kg (16 st.) or even lower.

7. Beware of pushing up hill. This can significantly increase the effort required and can make the manoeuvre unsafe.

8. Do not reach too far to push a person or reach too far to pull someone towards you. For example, when moving a patient from bed to trolley, one person should initiate the move and the person on the receiving side should not take up the effort until the patient is in easy reach. The nurse's reach can be extended by the use of sheets between the patient and the sliding device or by the use of extension straps.

9. When the move is completed, the sliding device is usually removed. Hard sliding devices can usually be pulled out because the patient has travelled to the far edge and has effectively come off the end. The patient may need to be rolled to facilitate the removal. Sliding sheets are most easily removed by reaching through the inside of the loop and pulling them inside out.

Using mechanical devices

If patients cannot move themselves and are unsuitable for sliding systems the only way of moving them is with mechanical devices. Primarily this means sling hoists. However, there are other devices that should be considered when moving patients. The nurse should have access to an appropriate range of patient-handling equipment:

- sling and stretcher hoists
- bathing hoists seats and related devices
- Standaid hoists
- beds and trolleys.

Nurses are quite often faced by a refusal to use equipment. They must never accept such a refusal where the equipment is needed for their own safety. The patient's natural fear of handling equipment can be encouraged by a diffident attitude on the part of the nurse. When preparing to use equipment it is important to do so with the same confidence as the nurse would employ when giving an injection or doing any other surgical nursing procedure.

The insertion of a sling must of course be done without lifting the patient. The exact technique will depend on the sling to be used. The easiest slings to apply are toileting and other general purpose slings (Fig. 29.17). These are put down the back of the patient and the leg pieces are led under the patient's legs. There are some slings that do not have leg pieces. Effectively the sling is a square sheet with a lifting point at each corner. These cannot be fitted in the normal way. They can only be positioned by log rolling the patient in bed.

The removal of the sling should follow a similar pattern to the application of the sling. As a general rule, the sling should be removed if possible. Where a patient has been moved to an armchair for the day, whole body slings may be left in place as it is too hard to remove them. This can present problems as the sling is now unavailable for other patients. This type of sling should only be purchased if the patient's condition demands it. (NB: Leaving the patient on a sling will probably increase risks of pressure sores.)

Getting the patient into the right position in a seat is important. If the patient is excessively reclined in the sling, he may have been lifted wrongly in the first place. Proper positioning of the sling should bring the patient into a reasonably upright sitting position. Correct sling positioning will minimise the need to adjust him as he comes down into the chair. Many slings have loops that allow the patient to be positioned differently. Nurses should make a careful study of the slings available on the ward. They should practise with the slings to find how they can be used to assist in controlling the patient's posture.

Some slings have handles at the back. These can be used to pull the patient back as she is lowered into the seat. However, the value of these handles is limited as the nurse will have to either reach over the back of the chair or reach in from the side. Either of these positions is potentially dangerous as the stresses are being applied awkwardly. It is better to push the patient's knees to push her back into the chair. Another technique is to tilt the chair back and lower the patient into the 'V' of the seat and the back. This is quite safe as the patient cannot fall even if the chair were to tip over. The brakes are left off on the hoist and as the patient is lowered the hoist is pushed naturally away from the chair. The chair comes down and the patient is neatly installed at the back of the seat.

Although patients can be moved from one place to another in mobile hoists, excessive pushing around with the patient in the hoist is best avoided. It is disorienting for the patient and the pushing forces needed to move the hoist are themselves a risk to the nurses. If patients are to be moved long distances, they should be lowered into a wheelchair and the hoist brought along separately to take them out at the other end of the journey.

There are now some hoists that will lift very heavy patients. There is at least one that will lift patients weighing up to 267 kg (42 st.). Great care should be taken with a hoist containing such a heavy patient. It will probably be better to treat the hoist as a fixed object once the patient has been lifted. For example, in a transfer from bed to commode, lift the patient from the bed, move the bed away and replace it with the commode, then lower the patient.

Reflective point

Would you like to be moved in the way in which you move your patients? (If you have not been moved in this way how can you know that it is comfortable?)

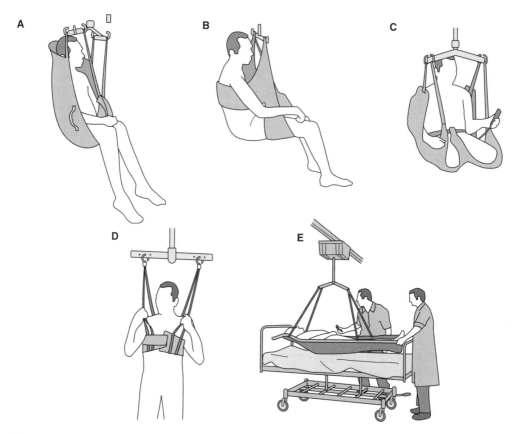

Figure 29.17 Different types of slings: (A) general purpose sling; (B) toileting sling or dressing sling; (C) amputee sling; (D) walking harness; (E) stretcher sling.

Leaving patients where they are

There is an assumption that patients have to be moved. Nurses must recognise that if it is not safe to move patients, they must be left where they are until appropriate equipment is available or until they are able to move themselves. Depending on the situation, patients may have to be left for anything from a few minutes to, in the most unfortunate of circumstances, a few days.

If a patient is in the community and there is no equipment in the home, it may be necessary to nurse the patient in a bed or reclining chair until equipment can be obtained. (Efficient ordering and delivery systems must be developed to reduce such delays wherever possible. For example, many bed manufacturers are willing to make agreements to deliver beds at short notice.)

The need to leave patients where they are is particularly an issue where a patient has fallen to the floor. The reaction of everyone involved is as though it is felt that a patient on the floor makes the place look untidy and he must be removed immediately. In fact it is often best to leave a patient where he is until he has been properly assessed. If the patient cannot get himself off the floor, a hoist (Fig. 29.18) or some other mechanical device must be fetched to lift him. Ensure that your hoist will lift from the floor. Some older models will not come down far enough. An alternative to the use of a hoist is an inflatable device (Fig. 29.19). These are more portable than hoists, so can often be brought to the patient more quickly. However, they are not suitable for all patients.

- It is not possible to manually lift a person from the floor.
- Such lifts are not safe with any number of people.
- Lifting sheets or nets do not make such lifts safe.

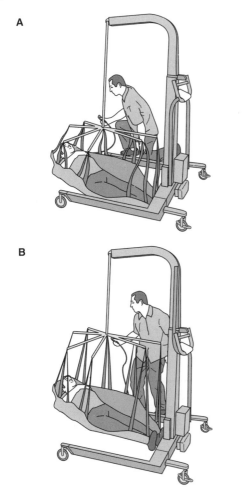

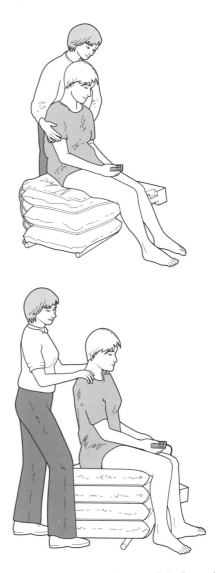

Figure 29.18 Lifting a patient from the floor (reproduced by kind permission from Liko (UK) Ltd).

Figure 29.19 Getting a patient up off the floor using an inflatable device (reproduced by kind permission from Mangar International).

REHABILITATION OF PATIENTS

It is common practice for the doctor to write 'to be rehabilitated' in the patient's notes. The extent of the rehabilitation to be achieved is rarely mentioned. Many nurses are injured trying to get patients walking when a proper analysis of the patient would have shown that this was not a realistic target. Patients are subject to falls during rehabilitation. Falls often discourage the patient from further attempts to walk.

The rehabilitation of a patient must be planned and several questions need to be asked. Is the person to be got walking again? If so, how far? Would it be enough to be able to stand to transfer from bed to wheelchair? Would the ability to do a sliding transfer on her own be enough? Is the patient mentally capable of being mobile? Is the patient to be got walking again just so that he can break the other leg?

The multidisciplinary team need to get together and plan the objectives of the rehabilitation. All in the team must agree on the target. The patient must be involved. If the patient does not believe in the objectives then the plan will not work. However, the patient needs to know his limitations and must not believe that he can do more than his abilities will allow.

In some cases it will be sensible to have a target of the patient walking unaided to the local or hospital shop. However, in other cases it may be more appropriate to simply aim to allow her to transfer herself from bed to commode using a sliding system. It is important to plan to handle the patient in ways that will avoid falls and thus avoid demotivating the patient.

The objectives of rehabilitation can be discussed under three main headings:

- reconditioning of muscles and mind
- getting the patient into a standing position
- walking the patient.

The following paragraphs assume that the patient is to be got walking again. If the rehabilitation has a different objective, different considerations will need to be applied.

The objectives and the plan must be written down. They must be reviewed and monitored as the patient progresses from one stage to another.

Getting the patient into a standing position

Saying 'the patient can stand' is fraught with danger. Does this mean that the patient can get himself into a standing position or does it mean that the patient can balance on his feet once he has been lifted there?

If patients are to stand, the rehabilitation plan will show how they are to be assisted. At first, patients may be brought into the standing position using a piece of equipment such as a hoist.

There is a Standaid hoist that will bring a person into the standing position using the normal pattern of standing, i.e. it first brings the patient forward, then up. This hoist will also reduce the amount of effort provided, thus forcing patients to use their own muscles.

Walking the patient

Patients will not learn to recommence walking if they are unable to stand. At first they may be fearful of falling, particularly with a surgical wound and possibly an i.v. and accompanying drainage tubes! They need to have confidence that they are going to be able to stay upright when they walk. There are some hoists that allow patients to be walked. These hoists will allow patients to be held firmly at first and then more flexibly as they progress. However, should patients fall, they will still be held and not injured.

Another point to remember is the time of day when patients are to practise walking and if they need to go to the toilet. Abilities will vary through the day. Choose times when patients are pain-free. If a patient is to go to the toilet, it is advisable to take her there in a wheelchair, for example, and then let her walk back from the toilet when she is more comfortable.

When planning a walk with a patient, the nurse has to also consider:

- whether there is enough space to walk alongside the patient
- whether the doors are wide enough to walk two or three abreast
- whether, when the patient is to be sat down at the end of the journey, there will be enough room for the patient with the supporting nurse(s) to turn around and sit down
- if the walk is to the toilet, whether there is enough space in the toilet for the nurses to assist the patient. (If there is not then the patient may need to be sat on a toileting chair and pushed into the toilet.)

Once walking, the patient may progress from Zimmer frame, to sticks, tripods, etc.

At first the nurse may follow behind the patient with a wheelchair. Patients can then sit down if they decide that they cannot go on. (Some nurses use a light chair instead of a wheelchair. This should be avoided as patients may sit down some way from their beds and will need to be moved off the chair.)

As always, the nurse must beware of a collapse. All patients must be treated as though they might collapse.

Discharge

The problems of assessment at discharge have been mentioned above. The state of progress in rehabilitation is an important aspect of that assessment. The plan must be up to date and clearly stated in a form that can be taken up by the nurses who will care for the patient in the community.

EQUIPMENT

The subject of equipment has already been mentioned at various points through this chapter. There is no doubt that there is a wide range of equipment to meet most handling needs. It is the employer's duty to provide equipment (HSE 1992b) and the employee's duty to use it. There is no excuse for failing to use equipment simply because the patient does not like it. A competent nurse will explain the importance of safe handling and overcome objections.

However, the choice of equipment is not simple. The first and most important need is to be aware of the options that exist. If you do not know that something is available, you cannot choose to use it. Keeping up to date and seeking advice are essential in allowing the nurse to know what is available to help in a specific situation.

The second need is to evaluate the equipment and be sure that it will help and be safe.

An example of these two points is turntables. It has been explained (see p. 626) that the hard turntables, which are better known, may not be safe, whilst the soft turntables, which are less well known, may be of value in new ways. It is clear from these considerations that equipment is not good just because it has been around for some time. Equally, do not think that every new idea is right.

Some equipment will be right for some people. Nurses must develop a skill in identifying the right equipment for a particular case. They must be ready to try out different solutions until the right one is found.

Familiarisation with the equipment

Do not try to use equipment to move a patient until you have become familiar with using it to move a colleague. Learn the ins and outs of the equipment before you find out with the patient. If something goes wrong, evaluate what happened to identify how it can be avoided in the future. Go back to the manufacturer to get help in solving the problem. If you have found a fundamental problem in the equipment, discuss it with your colleagues and ensure that everyone who will use the equipment is aware of the problem. (You should also consider reporting the problem to the Medical Devices Agency so that they can issue warnings if appropriate.)

Beds

Putting the patient on the right bed will go a long way to solving the handling needs of a patient who is going to need to be handled.

The standard flat King's Fund bed with the back rest in the headboard is badly out of date as a bed for patients with limited mobility. The bed of choice for patients in need of handling should be a four-section profiling bed. Patients with greater needs should be cared for in one of a range of beds designed to meet these needs.

- Patients in need of regular turning can be nursed in turning beds. This will enable patients to be moved much more frequently than the standard 2-hourly turn.
- Patients who are in need of pressure avoidance can be in beds with low-air-loss mattresses or in air-fluidised beds.
- Patients who have difficulty in standing may need to use stand-up beds. These are particularly useful for patients who have just had a hip replacement.

Hoists

The range of hoists to be considered can be divided into four main groups:

- bathing hoists
- overhead hoists
- mobile hoists
- Standaids.

Bathing hoists

The classic bathing hoist is the Arjo Ambulift. These hoists were installed in many hospitals long before it was recognised that hoists were needed in other situations.

Many of the hoists that were purchased were capable of being used to lift patients in slings as well as in the plastic chair attachment. These model D hoists were often supplied with two 'band' slings that were kept in a black plastic box attached to the mast of the hoist. (The slings have often been 'lost' and the box is used as a convenient place to store shampoo and other washing materials.) The band slings are now recognised to be unsafe (see below). However, the hoist can still be used with one-piece slings for patient lifting. It is also worth noting that a stretcher attachment is available for this hoist.

A further feature of this hoist is that a chassis can be attached to the chair. This allows patients to be transferred to the chair at the bedside. They are then wheeled to the bathroom where the chair is attached to the hoist mechanism. The chassis is then removed. In many cases, the chassis has been lost or pushed to the back of the sluice. It is worth getting them back into use if you can find them, as the use of the chassis can save two handling events on each bathing.

There is now a range of hoists available for bathing. Patients can also be bathed using standard mobile hoists and appropriate slings.

Overhead hoists

Overhead hoists can be easier to use in many circumstances. They do not need floor space, so there is no need to move things to provide access or move other equipment. This can be particularly important in HDUs and ITUs where the patient may be surrounded by monitors, drips, etc.

Overhead hoists can be on single tracks over the places where patients may need to be lifted. However, an X-Y system where one hoist can sweep the whole room by travelling on beams fixed to the sides of the room is more versatile.

Although they look expensive, a simple overhead installation will cost about the same as one of the more expensive mobile hoists.

Mobile hoists

The standard mobile hoist with a one-piece sling is the hoist that most people think about when the subject is raised. There is a vast range of hoists available. Prices range from a few hundred to two or three thousand pounds.

It is beyond the scope of this book to review the full range of hoists. However, the following considerations are important when selecting hoists.

Manual versus electric. There is a tendency to think that manual things are more reliable than electric things. This is not really true for hoists. Both types must be maintained. If they are properly maintained they will provide reliable service.

Manual hoists are generally cheaper to purchase. However, they may be more expensive to use. Manual hoists usually need two people to operate; one works the mechanism while the other adjusts the patient's position. With an electric hoist, the person adjusting the patient's position can also control the descent of the patient with the remote control. People are much more expensive than the difference in costs.

There is one important consideration in the selection of electric hoists. Is there an emergency lowering facility on the body of the hoist? Occasionally the remote control of the hoist becomes damaged. It also can happen that the hoist will run out of power whilst the patient is in the sling. In both cases, an emergency lowering facility may be needed to get the patient down. Nurses have been injured trying to lift patients from hoists that have become inoperative.

Mechanical hoists can also become jammed with the patient in them. However, the only answer in this case is to bring another hoist to lift the patient from the first hoist. Fortunately these things only happen very rarely in both types of hoist.

Slings. Manufacturers offer wide selections of slings to suit different sizes of patients and different needs. There are toileting slings, slings designed for amputees (see Fig. 29.17) and slings that offer extra head support. Some manufacturers offer bigger spreader bars and/or hangers to reduce compression where the patient is too delicate for the normal spreader bar.

Where a hoist is to be used by one individual, care must be taken to select the right slings. Where the hoist is to be used on a ward there must be a sufficient range of slings to suit the patients to be cared for. It is too late to try to buy a sling when the patient arrives on the ward. It is important that a system is established to hang or store the slings in one place where it can easily be seen if one is missing.

There must be sufficient slings to allow for some being in the laundry.

It has been noted above that 'band' slings are unsafe. At least two patients have been killed when they fell through these slings. Many nurses have been injured trying to save patients from falls. These slings must not be used under any circumstances (MDA 1994).

Standaids

These are hoists that are designed to bring patients to a stand for a transfer from one seated position to another. In general, patients stand on a small platform throughout the transfer. They are lifted by a single sling placed around the body. This means that they can be lifted, pulled away from one place and lowered in a new place.

It has been suggested that patients must be brought to a full standing position in the Standaid. It is argued that if patients only come to a position where they are leaning in the sling, they will become dependent and will be unable to regain a full standing position.

The more modern slings have straps which fit around the body to prevent patients falling through the sling if they lift their arms. Older designs of Standaids tended to lift patients under the armpits; this is undesirable as it mimics the effects of the drag lift.

Care should be taken to choose the right Standaid for the patient.

Sliding systems

Sliding systems offer ways of moving people that are less invasive than hoists and other machinery. They may even give a measure of independence to people who were previously being lifted by their nurses.

There is a large variety of sliding systems on the market. Almost every product has its own unique feature(s). In terms of materials there are:

- hard sliding boards (see Fig. 29.4)
- padded fabric slides
- loops of single-thickness fabric
- sheets of single-thickness fabric.

In terms of purpose, sliding systems are designed for:

- supine transfers
- turning supine patients in bed
- transferring from one seated position to another.

Each different sliding aid needs slightly different techniques. Study the manufacturer's guidance on the use of each piece of equipment.

Imoturn

This is a unique device that is designed to turn a patient with a broken hip or following hip replacement. The Imoturn is available in pairs, one for each side. The device is inserted on the non-affected side and the patient is then rolled towards that side.

I am aware of two incidents where patients who have experienced the use of an Imoturn when they had one hip replaced have refused to have the other hip done unless an Imoturn was available.

Unsafe equipment

There are two types of equipment in common use that are fundamentally unsafe. These are all forms of stretchers and carry chairs. Both of these devices involve the lifters in taking excessive loads, often in poor postural positions. They should not form part of any handling plan.

Patient-handling slings

Patient-handling slings are often found in hospitals. It has been explained above that they do have the advantage that they improve the posture of the lifter but they do not reduce weights to a point where the lift is safe. Therefore, they should not be used for lifting patients. The manufacturers of these slings also recommend their use for front transfers. All front transfers block the natural mechanisms of the patient and, again, the patient's weight is not reduced to a safe level; therefore this use should also be avoided.

Reflective point

Is there handling equipment on your ward/unit that is not being used or is in need of repair? (Look in particular for ancillary equipment for Ambulift and other hoists.)

FINANCE

There is often a reluctance to ask for equipment because the costs are seen as too high to be afforded by the trust or other employer. In fact the costs of implementing a safe-handling environment, including the purchase of patient-handling devices, are quite low. I have already pointed out the costs of litigation in respect of injuries to nurses. This is not the only cost that should be considered when looking at the costs of safer handling (HSE 1993).

The booklet 'Introducing a Safer Patient Handling Policy' (RCN 1996) shows that the costs of a safe-handling environment can be justified on the basis of savings in sickness time and associated costs.

One of the effects of the recent changes in the health services is that there has been a much greater awareness of costs. Nurses should use this information to their advantage in justifying expenditure. A typical junior staff nurse may be costing £200 a day. (This is pay plus all the overheads.) A hospital bed costs between £200 and £500 a day – possibly even more. Cost cases that show savings of even a few days of nursing time can easily justify the purchase of a hoist. Better care of patients can quickly save on valuable bed costs.

AUDIT

Just as with any other aspect of work, it is essential that positive audits are carried out to ensure that safe handling standards are being maintained. Regular audits should be carried out into every aspect of handling described in this chapter. The audit can be carried out by the staff of the unit or ward working on their own or it can be carried out by external auditors. There are advantages in both approaches. When auditing safe patient handling it would be desirable to include at least the back care advisor as well as the 'local' staff.

There should be audits of:

- The safe handling policy
  - Are names of individuals or departments correct?
  - Does it reflect current best practice?
  - Are subsidiary procedures in place and up to date?
  - Has everyone seen a copy of the policy?
- Generic assessments
  - Are they of an adequate standard?
  - Have they been reviewed when they should have been?
  - Have the actions identified been taken?

– Are any constraints identified in the assessment being applied? (e.g. Are managers applying limits on handling very heavy patients because of lack of facilities?)
– Is the assessment safe?
- Individual assessments
  – Are they written to an adequate standard?
  – Have they been reviewed at appropriate intervals?
  – Is the handling specified safe and appropriate for the patient?
- Handling practices
  – Are the actual handling practices being used on the ward or in the unit safe? (NB: Checking in the community is more difficult but this too must be positively audited.)
- Training
  – Is it up to date?
  – Are the trainers keeping themselves abreast of developments?
  – Has everyone received training and or updates?
  – Are agency staff being trained to the same standards?
  – Are all staff able to demonstrate appropriate knowledge? (e.g. Do they know the weight limits to be applied?)
- Equipment
  – Can all equipment belonging to the unit or ward be found?
  – Is all equipment in working order?
  – Has all equipment been properly maintained?
  – If equipment is unserviceable, has it been clearly marked and taken out of service?
- Accidents
  – Have any accidents occurred?
  – Have the causes of accidents been properly established?
  – Have changes been made to ensure that accidents do not re-occur?
- Patients
  – Are patients accepting the use of handling equipment?
  – Has there been a change in the rate of bedsores, sore shoulders and any other injuries that may be handling related?
  – Has safe handling affected the number and severity of falls?
  – Are rehabilitation objectives being achieved?

This list should be useful in establishing an audit of patient handling. However, it is not exhaustive. Careful thought will identify many more points to be considered. It is a useful part of the audit process for the auditors and the staff from the surgical area to be audited to consider the format of the audit. Such a group can be given the above list as a starter to provoke debate and assist them in identifying the other questions to be asked in the audit. This process will itself make the audit more effective.

CONCLUSION

The philosophy often exists amongst health care workers that it is more caring for the patients if nurses lift them manually. I have shown at several points in this chapter that this is not the case.

Much lifting directly injures patients by lifting them under the armpits or in some other way applying excessive forces to delicate bones or skin. Manual handling often blocks the natural movements of the body, thus obstructing rehabilitation.

A safe lifting approach to patient care ought to speed recovery. However, in order to overcome potential objections, this must be explained to the patient. Some hospitals have found it useful to have a small pamphlet that is given to patients on admission explaining that they will be lifted in hoists and handled in other ways for their good and for the well-being of the nurses. This approach seems to have reduced resistance to the use of equipment.

Manual lifting of people by people is dangerous to both parties. No amount of technique or training will change that fundamental fact. The equipment and associated techniques exist to enable patients to be handled and moved safely in all circumstances. There is no excuse for failing to implement a safe system of work.

Reflective point

How will you overcome objections from those who prefer to lift manually?

REFERENCES

Chaffin D B, Galley L S Wooley C B, Kuciemba S R 1986 An evaluation of the effect of a training program on worker lifting postures. International Journal of Industrial Ergonomics 1: 127–136

Chartered Society of Physiotherapists 1993 Standards of physiotherapy practice – for trainers in moving and handling. CSP, London

Commission of European Communities (CEC) 1989a Council Directive 89/391/EEC on the introduction of measures to encourage improvements in the safety and health of workers at work. Official Journal of the European Communities No L 183/1-9, Brussels

Commission of European Communities (CEC) 1989b Council Directive 89/654/EEC on the workplace. (First individual directive within the meaning of Article 16(1) of Directive 89/391/EEC) Official Journal of the European Communities No L 393, Brussels

Commission of European Communities (CEC) 1989c Council Directive concerning the minimal health and safety requirements for the use of work equipment by workers. (Second individual directive within the meaning of Article 16(1) of Directive 89/391/EEC (89/655/EEC)) Official Journal of the European Communities No L 393/13-17, Brussels

Commission of European Communities (CEC) 1989d Council Directive 89/656/EEC on personal protective equipment. (Third individual directive within the meaning of Article 16(1) of Directive 89/391/EEC) Official Journal of the European Communities No L 393, Brussels

Commission of European Communities (CEC) 1990a Council Directive (90/269/EEC) on the minimum health and safety requirements for the manual handling of loads where there is a risk particularly of back injury to workers. (Fourth Individual Directive within the meaning of Article 16(1) of Directive 89/391/EEC) Official Journal of the European Communities No L 156/9-13, Brussels

Commission of European Communities (CEC) 1990b Council Directive (90/270/EEC) on the minimum safety and health requirements for work with display screen. (Fifth individual directive within the meaning of Article 16(1) of Directive 89/391/EEC) Official Journal of the European Communities No L 156, Brussels

Crust G, Pearson J C G, Mair A 1972 The prevalence of low back pain in nurses. International Nursing Review 19: 169–179

Dehlin O, Berg S, Andersson G B, Grimby G 1981 Effect of physical training and ergonomic counselling on the psychological perception of work and on the subjective assessment of low-back insufficiency. Scandinavian Journal Of Rehabilitation Medicine 13: 1–9

Gagnon M, Sicard C, Sirois J P 1986 Evaluation of forces on the lumbo sacral joint and assessment of work and energy transfers in nursing aides lifting patients. Ergonomics 29: 407–421

Hale A R, Mason I D 1986 L'evaluation du role d'une formation kinetique dans la prevention des accidents de manutention. Le Travaille Humain 49: 195–207

Health and Safety at Work etc. Act 1974 HMSO, London

Health and Safety Executive (HSE) 1992a Manual handling guidance to regulations (L23). HMSO, London, App. 1, p. 43

Health and Safety Executive (HSE) 1992b Provision in use of work equipment regulations – guidance on regulations. HMSO, London

Health and Safety Executive (HSE) 1992c Management of health and safety at work regulations – approved code of practice. HMSO, London

Health and Safety Executive (HSE) 1992d Personal protective equipment at work regulations 1192 – guidance on regulations. HMSO, London

Health and Safety Executive (HSE) 1992e Workplace health and safety welfare regulations. HMSO, London

Health and Safety Executive (HSE) 1995 A guide to the reporting of injuries, diseases & dangerous occurrences regulations 1995 (RIDDOR). HSE

Health Services Advisory Committee (HSAC) 1984 The lifting of patients in the health services. HMSO, London

Health Services Advisory Committee (HSAC) 1986 Guidance on the recording of accidents and incidents in the health services. HMSO, London

Health Services Advisory Committee (HSAC) 1992 Guidance on manual handling of loads in the health services. HMSO, London

Health Services Advisory Committee (HSAC) 1998 Manual handling in the health services. HSE

Hickman M, Mason V 1994 The prevalence of back pain: a report prepared for the Department of Health by the Office of Population Censuses and Surveys, Social Survey Division, based on the omnibus survey March April June 1993. HMSO, London

Hoover S A 1973 Job-related back injuries in a hospital. American Journal of Nursing 73: 2078–2079

Leighton D, Riley T 1995 Epidemiological aspects of back pain: the incidence and prevalence of back pain in nurses compared to the general population. Occupational Medicine 45: 263–267

Lloyd P, Fletcher B, Holmes D, Tarling C, Tracey M 1998 The guide to the handling of patients, revised 4th edn. NBPA/RCN, London

Magora 1970 Investigations of the relationship between low back pain and occupation 1. Industrial Medicine 39(11): 31–37

Medical Devices Agency (MDA) 1994 Patient hoists – band slings. Risk of fatal or serious injury. Hazard (94)18. MDA, London

NHS Estates 1994 Operating department. Health Building Note 26. HMSO, London

NHS Estates 1994 Intensive therapy unit. Health Building Note 27. HMSO, London

NHS Estates 1995 Common activity spaces. Health Building Note 40. HMSO, London, vol 1

Pheasant S 1991 Ergonomics work and health. Macmillan, London

Pheasant S 1996 Bodyspace anthropometry, ergonomics and the design of work. Taylor and Francis, London

Pheasant S, Stubbs D 1992 Back pain in nurses: epidemiology and risk assessment. Applied Ergonomics 23(4): 226–232

Raistrick A 1981 Nurses with back pain – can the problem be prevented? Nursing Times 77(14): 853–856

RCN Advisory Panel in Back Pain in Nurses 1988 An instructors syllabus for the handling and moving of patients. RCN, London

RCN Advisory Panel in Back Pain in Nurses 1996 Introducing safer patient handling policy. RCN, London

St Vincent M, Tellier C 1989 Training in handling: an evaluative study. Ergonomics 32(2): 191–210

St Vincent M, Lortie M, Tellier C 1987 Training in safe lifting: are the methods taught used by workers? In: Buckle P (ed) Musculoskeletal disorders at work. Taylor and Francis, London, pp 159–164

Scholey M 1983 Back stress: the effects of training nurses to lift patients in a clinical setting. International Journal Nursing Studies 20(1): 1–13

Schultz A, Alexander N, Ashton Miller J 1992 Biomechanical analyses of rising from a chair. Journal of Biomechanics 25(12): 1383–1391

Seccombe I, Ball J 1992 Back injured nurses – a profile. A discussion paper for the Royal College of Nursing. RCN, London

Smedley J, Egger P, Cooper C, Coggon D 1995 Manual handling activities and risk of low back pain in nurses. Occupational and Environmental Medicine 52: 160–163

Stubbs D 1983 Back pain in the nursing profession II. The effectiveness of training. Ergonomics 26(8): 767–779

Stubbs D 1986 Back pain in nurses. Summary and recommendations. Ergonomic Research Unit, The Robens Institute, University of Surrey, Guildford

Stubbs D A, Rivers P M, Hudson M P, Worringham C J 1980 Patient handling and truncal stress in nursing. Proceedings of the conference organised by the Nursing Practice Research Unit, Northwick Park Hospital, Back Pain Association and DHSS, pp 14–27

FURTHER READING

Health and Safety Executive (HSE) 1993 The costs of accidents at work. HSE

NHS Estates Health Building Notes Nos 1–54 (various subjects). HMSO, London

RCN Advisory Panel in Back Pain in Nurses 1996 Manual handling assessments in hospitals and the community – an RCN guide. RCN, London

RCN Advisory Panel in Back Pain in Nurses 1996 RCN code of practice for patient handling. RCN, London

Glossary

Academic credits: Numerical values given to learning achievements, e.g. level 1 credits (certificate level), level 2 credits (diploma level), level 3 credits (degree level).

Acculturation: The process by which an outsider, immigrant or subordinate, assimilates and adapts to the dominant group or culture to become culturally and socially indistinguishable.

Acidotic: State of abnormally high hydrogen ion concentration in the extracellular fluid. The oxyhaemoglobin curve is shifted to the right, increasing the amount of oxygen available for the tissues.

Action learning: An approach to learning where a small group of individuals meet frequently to reflect on and analyse their actions at work, for the purpose of becoming more effective in their work. Group members provide high challenge and high support to each other through a mutual trusting relationship to help each other reflect formally on their actions and to commit themselves to future action.

Action research: An approach to research which is based in practice and focuses on issues/problems occurring in practice. It involves individual practitioners or groups who are committed to exploring their own practice, developing greater insights into their own practice and sharing transferable principles from this exploration with others. The focus is always on practitioners' actions as practitioner–researchers. Like other approaches to research, the purpose of action research is to contribute to the public theory base, but additionally, it has two further equal purposes: to improve practice, and to enable practitioners to develop.

Acute tubular necrosis (ATN): The most common cause of acute renal failure, but differentiated in that it is caused by ischaemia, most frequently following surgery. The ischaemia is generally caused by sepsis, obstetric complications, severe burns, or a severe episode of hypotension generally associated with hypovolaemia.

Adaptation: The positive response to a changing environment. Changing to enable the individual to cope with internal and external stimuli. Roy (1976) considers the goals of adaptation to include survival, growth, reproduction and mastery.

Adaptive modes: Classification of functions that can be used as part of assessment and evaluation, identifying if an individual is making effective adaptive responses to stimuli. There are four adaptive modes: physiological; self-concept; role function; and interdependence.

Adenosine triphosphate (ATP): Organic molecule that stores and releases chemical energy for use in body cells.

Age-related diseases: Health problems that occur almost exclusively in older age groups.

Agonists/antagonists: Drugs acting on receptors may be agonists or antagonists. Agonists activate the receptor when they occupy it. Antagonists cause no activation of the receptor when they occupy it and can block or reverse the effects of agonist drugs. Full agonists can produce maximal effects from a tissue (high efficacy), i.e. the bigger the dose the greater the response. Partial agonists can only produce

submaximal effects (intermediate efficacy), i.e. there comes a point where an increase in the dose will not produce a bigger response. The effects of a partial agonist are only partially reversed by an antagonist.

Airway resistance: The relationship between the pressure difference between the mouth and the alveoli and the flow of gas into the lungs. Airway resistance is due to friction between molecules of the moving gas and between the gas molecules and the walls of the bronchi. During quiet breathing, airflow in the normal bronchi is streamlined, but because the bronchi have an irregular surface and branch frequently the flow of gas becomes turbulent during rapid breathing, requiring a greater pressure difference to produce a given rate of flow. Factors which increase airway resistance are narrowing and irregularity of the airways such as chronic bronchitis and bronchial asthma.

Alkalotic: State of abnormally low hydrogen ion concentration in the extracellular fluid. The oxyhaemoglobin curve is shifted to the left, decreasing the amount of oxygen available for the tissues.

Aminoglycosides: Antibiotics derived from *Streptomyces* species; they are polycationic compounds of amino sugars. Aminoglycosides interrupt bacterial protein synthesis by inhibiting ribosomal function. Examples are streptomycin, neomycin, gentamicin.

Angioplasty: The dilatation of a blocked blood vessel, usually an artery, using a balloon catheter.

Antecedents: Events/circumstances that happen before other events can take place.

Anthropology: As the study of mankind, deals with 'other' cultures and is primarily concerned with personal worlds and small-scale events.

Antibiotic: A substance which is toxic for certain microorganisms.

Anticholinergic: Refers to the reduction or blockade of cholinergic transmission either by acting on acetylcholine receptors or by affecting the release or destruction of endogenous acetylcholine.

Antiseptic: A solution containing a chemical substance which has antimicrobial properties.

Arteriosclerosis: A chronic disease of the arterial system distinguished by abnormal thickening and hardening of the vessel walls.

Atelectasis: The collapse of lung tissue.

Atherosclerosis: A form of arteriosclerosis in which the thickening and hardening of the vessel walls are caused by deposits of fat and fibrin that eventually harden over time. It is thought to be the leading contributor to coronary artery and cerebrovascular disease.

Atrial fibrillation: An extremely rapid and disorganised pattern of depolarisation in the atria. The rhythm is irregularly irregular, that is to say the ventricular response has a marked irregularity. If atrial fibrillation is sudden in onset, the patient will be haemodynamically compromised.

Autolytic process: The natural degradation of devitalised tissue from healthy tissue.

Autonomic nervous system: The part of the nervous system responsible for the control of bodily functions that are not consciously directed, e.g. beating of the heart, intestinal movements, salivation. The autonomic nervous system is subdivided into the sympathetic and parasympathetic nervous systems.

Autonomy: The right of the individual to self-determination and rule. Respect for personal independence (Beauchamp & Childress 1989).

Autoregulation in the kidney: A local mechanism which controls the rate of blood flow through the kidneys and thus keeps the glomerular filtration rate (GFR) fairly constant over a range of arterial pressures.

Background infusion: A continuous infusion of a drug to help maintain plasma levels of the drug.

Bacteraemia: Presence of bacteria, mostly transient and of low pathogenicity, in the bloodstream without clinical consequences.

Basal crackles: Listening to breath sounds may detect brief crackling sounds that are probably produced by opening of previously closed bronchioles, and their timing during breathing is of significance. Early inspiratory crackles are associated with diffuse airflow limitation. Late inspiratory crackles are characteristically heard in pulmonary oedema, fibrosis of the lung and bronchiectasis. They may be described as fine or coarse but this is of no significance.

Beneficence: A principle that states that one should act in such a way as to do good and promote that which is good (Beauchamp & Childress 1989).

Bivariate analysis: Involves examining the statistical connection between two variables, e.g. to compare weight with height, the results may be shown in a table of figures.

Blood plasma expander: A substance that is administered intravenously, the purpose of which is to increase the oncotic pressure in a patient in cases of hypovolaemia, haemorrhage and dehydration. Such solutions usually contain water, polysaccharides, and often electrolytes. An example is dextran.

Bronchial breathing: High-pitched, loud pause between inspiration and expiration, expiration equals inspiration and in normal breathing can only be heard over the trachea. If bronchial sounds can be heard elsewhere over the lungs, it indicates the presence of underlying lung disease. Bronchial breathing results when pathological changes in the lung cause increased conduction of sound from the large airways to the periphery.

C and A nerve fibres: Names given to subgroups of nerve fibres which have different functions. C fibres are responsible for pain transmission and autonomic activity whereas A fibres are concerned with touch and pressure sensation.

Case study: Involves the thorough in-depth analysis of an individual, group, institution or other social unit.

Catecholamines: Hormones secreted from the adrenal medulla; adrenaline and noradrenaline.

Caudal block: Injection of local anaesthetic into the sacral canal, for analgesia or in order to perform surgery. The perineal area is affected.

CE mark: This mark is an EC requirement for all types of things sold in the Community. All new handling goods will bear this mark. The presence of the mark indicates that the product has been made to the correct standards. However, the mark should not be taken to mean that the equipment is safe to use. For example, it is possible to put a CE mark on a carry chair to show that it is properly made, but this will not make the carry chair safe to use in carrying a patient down stairs.

Chronological age: Simply refers to the number of years that have passed since birth.

Clinical audit: A special accounting examination which is designed to evaluate clinical procedures according to quantitative and qualitative criteria.

Clinical effectiveness: A good standard for intervention, when health aims are achieved.

Clinical guidelines: Official documentary advice to promote good operative practices.

Clinical reality: The meaning that a clinical (surgical) procedure, investigation or consultation has for those involved.

Cohort: A group of people born during specified years (the people are about the same age), for example the 'baby boomers' born between 1946 and 1964.

Commensal: Microorganisms that live on a host with no evidence of benefit or harm.

Complement: A group of blood-borne proteins which, when activated, are responsible for the membrane alterations that occur during immunological injury, e.g. increased permeability, dilatation of blood vessels and increased blood flow.

Computerised tomography (CT) scan: A scanning technique which uses high doses of radiation. It takes millimetre slices through the body outlining dense structures.

Contextual stimuli: 'All the environmental factors that present to the person from within or without, but are not the centre of the person's attention and/or energy' (Andrews & Roy 1991).

Coping: 'Operating to produce adaptive responses, ... routine, accustomed patterns of behaviour to deal with daily situations as well as the production of new ways of behaving when drastic changes defy the familiar response' (Roy & McLeod 1981).

Correlative relationship: Where measures used are known to be related to one another – usually by means of a statistical formula and a significant level of certainty.

Cost–benefit: A measure of the effectiveness and efficiency of a process in terms of the benefit obtained weighed against the cost of providing the process.

Cost-effectiveness: A modern business formula which combines an assessment of means/ends efficiency with an estimate of the associated economic cost values.

Counselling psychologist: A psychologist who has undergone further training in counselling. Likewise, a **clinical psychologist** is a psychologist who has undergone further training in clinical application. Both of these may be referred to as Chartered. It must also be noted that using **counselling skills** is an integral part of any helping role. This does not make any of us a counsellor; it is suggested that you read the British Association of Counselling Guidelines (1992) for the use of counselling skills if you wish to explore this further.

Credit accumulation and transfer scheme (CATS): A system which facilitates the accumulation of academic credits and allows holders to use their currency towards other courses or programmes of study.

Critical care: The wide spectrum of high-technology/high dependency care, encompassing intensive care, high dependency, coronary care and renal units.

Crystalloids: Crystalloids can be defined as substances that in solution can diffuse through a semipermeable membrane. They are commonly used for restoring tissue perfusion in situations of hypovolaemic shock or severe burns.

Culturally sensitive care: Care which may be delivered to ethnically, linguistically and culturally diverse groups of patients.

Culture: The ways in which we live and the meanings we attach to our behaviours.

Cytokines: A generic term for chemicals which mediate interaction between cells, chiefly of the immune system.

Deduction: A logical inference as to what follows from a premiss or first position.

Demography: The statistical study of the population.

Deontological theory: A moral concept that moral obligations and rights may be independent of the concept of good. Immanuel Kant was a notable deontologist (Beauchamp & Childress 1989).

Dependency: The degree of help that an individual requires to undertake 'normal' activities of living.

Dependent variable: The resultant change, or calculated outcome, in the analysis.

Dermatome: The area of skin innervated by the branches of a single spinal nerve.

Diaphragmatic breathing: Paradoxical inward movement of the abdomen during inspiration is seen in respiratory distress and is a sign of diaphragmatic weakness or paralysis.

Disseminated intravascular coagulation (DIC): A process in which there is activation of the clotting cascade following injury. This can lead to activation of excess clotting factors within the vascular system. Overstimulation of the clotting cascade can cause bleeding to occur elsewhere, e.g. from body cavities, wound sites, intravenous insertion sites or internal haemorrhage. Therefore, DIC is a paradoxical condition in which clotting and haemorrhage occur within the vascular system simultaneously.

Draining wound: An abnormal opening in the skin that produces exudate or drainage.

Drug concentration: Describes the amount of drug dissolved in a given volume of solution, e.g. 10 mg in 1 ml.

Dualism: The separation of the mind and body.

Early adulthood: The period between 22 and 44 years of age.

Education purchasing consortium: Body made up of trust and health authority representatives which purchases education for their local workforce.

Efficacy: Describes the effectiveness of a drug or treatment.

Efficiency: A relation between means and ends which is tight, powerful and economical.

Emic: Insider understanding or view of culture, or behaviour common to a cultural group. This might be a health behaviour which is taken for granted as acceptable to a certain cultural group and understood by them.

Empirical research: Research devised from a statement or theory which can then be tested using vigorous scientific quantitative methodologies.

Empowerment: The transfer or sharing of power and control; to have ownership over decision-making; an enabling process.

Enculturation: The process by which an individual learns to become a member of a group.

Endoscopic retrograde cholangiopancreatography (ERCP): An examination of the pancreas and bile ducts. The patient is sedated and an endoscope is inserted into the duodenum; X-ray contrast medium is then injected down the endoscope. Using X-rays, the pancreas and bile ducts can be seen and any abnormalities, e.g. gallstones, detected.

Endoscopy: The visualisation of the interior organs and cavity of the body with an endoscope. Endoscopy can also be used to obtain samples for cytological and histological examination.

Enterocutaneous fistula: An abnormal connection between the bowel and skin.

Enteropathy: Disease of the small intestine.

Epidemiological: A scientific approach concerned to explain the origins of diseases.

Erythrocytes: Red blood cells.

Ethnicity: The concept of belonging to a people or tribe. This includes sharing one or more of the following: an origin or social background; culture and traditions that are maintained through generations and lead to a sense of identity; a common language or religious tradition.

Ethnocentrism: Studying and making judgements about other societies in terms of one's own cultural assumptions and biases.

Ethnography: A qualitative research methodology which collects, then describes and analyses the ways in which human beings categorise the meaning of their world. It attempts to learn what knowledge people use to interpret experience by participating in the everyday lives of the people within specific cultural systems.

Etic: Outsider understanding of a health behaviour common to a cultural group. Etic view may be a nurse's understanding of a heath behaviour which is outside her own culture.

Evaluation: Aims to assess the contribution of research knowledge or clinical procedure.

Evidence-based practice: Where criteria for evaluating the best practical procedures are based on research and are not simply traditional or authority-derived.

Excoriation of the skin: Damage to the outer layer of the epidermis caused by the prolonged abnormal presence of normal body fluids, such as urine.

Extrinsic: Outside or external to the human host.

Exudate: Body fluid discharged through pores, incisions, wounds and wound drains.

Fidelity: The rule of fidelity is rooted in respect for autonomy and is the obligation that promises will be kept. It speaks to a covenant relationship between patient and health care provider. This principle is most eloquently presented by the moral theologian P Ramsey (Beauchamp & Childress 1989).

First level assessment: Gathering information and data in the four adaptive modes.

Focal stimulus: 'The internal or external stimulus most immediately confronting the person; the object or event that attracts one's attention' (Andrews & Roy 1991).

Functional residual capacity (FRC): The FRC is the combined residual and expiratory reserve volume and represents the amount of air remaining in the lungs after a tidal expiration.

Functionalist/structural–functionalist: Beliefs from this tradition in sociology emphasise the importance of social structures in determining human behaviour and how these structures interrelate to make society function.

Glucocorticoids: Hormones secreted from the adrenal cortex, such as cortisol, cortisone and corticosterone. Cortisol is secreted in significant amounts in humans.

Gluconeogenesis: A process which occurs in the liver where formation of glucose from non-carbohydrate sources such as amino acids and fatty acids occurs.

Gluconeogenic enzymes: Enzymes which catalyse the steps of gluconeogenesis in the liver.

Glucose: The principal blood sugar.

Glycerol: A sugar alcohol; a building block of fats.

Glycogen: The main carbohydrate stored in liver and skeletal muscle cells; a polysaccharide.

Glycogenolysis: The breakdown of glycogen to glucose.

Glyconeogenesis: The formation of glycogen from non-carbohydrate molecules.

Grounded theory: A complex qualitative research methodology which looks at ways of investigating questions concerned with the lived experiences of patients and their families.

Half-life: Time taken for the concentration of a drug in the body to halve.

HCO_3: Bicarbonate ions (a base).

Health education: A communication activity aimed at enabling individuals and groups to achieve positive health in social and lifestyle issues. Empowerment is a fundamental concept and health education addresses physical, mental, spiritual and social well-being.

Health outcome: May refer specifically to the perioperative situation or, more generally, to health conditions which require systematic explanation.

Health promotion: An umbrella term encompassing political, societal, environmental activities in which education is a composite part.

High dependency unit: An area for patients who require more intensive observation, treatment and nursing care than can be provided on a general ward but are not sick enough to require admission to intensive care.

Homogeneous behaviour: Behaviour which is common to a social or cultural group.

Hypercapnia: High levels of carbon dioxide will cause a condition referred to as hypercapnia which causes reversible deterioration in cerebral function and peripheral vasodilatation and leads to clinical signs: drowsiness, intellectual impairment, disorientation, coma; headache; pulse of large volume with warm sweaty extremities. Hypercapnia is always accompanied by hypoxia but hypoxia may occur in the absence of hypercapnia.

Hypothermia: Core body temperature below 35°C, usually secondary to a concomitant disease or disability that renders the patient more susceptible to the cold.

Hypothetical cause and effect: In order to examine evidence about cause and effect, a supposition is formulated to explain the relations, and tested accordingly.

Hypovolaemic shock: A form of circulatory shock in which there is inadequate tissue blood flow for cellular homeostatic requirements (Clancy & McVicar 1995). Hypo = low, volaemic = blood volume. Most common causes include severe haemorrhage, fluid loss in burns cases and severe diarrhoea and vomiting.

Hypoxia: A lack of sufficient oxygen.

Ideology: Advances a body of ideas to make the beliefs appealing and influential. It is typically interested in changing society, not in testing the ideas.

Idiosyncratic allergic response: Describes an unexpected or unpredictable sensitivity of an individual to a drug or food resulting in an allergic reaction.

Incidence: The rate of occurrence found, for any event, behaviour or observation.

Incubation period: Period between the invasion of microorganisms and development of symptoms of infection.

Independent variable: A measure either artificially introduced or treated as a cause.

Inference: Refers to good procedure in argumentation and seeks to imply (and show) that logical propositions are precisely derived and reached with certainty.

Integrated optimal-care planning: A proposed ideal way of maximising the overall benefits of planned, and coordinated, nursing care.

Intensive care unit: A specialist unit for the management of patients with acute life-threatening conditions.

Interactive wound dressing: A dressing which interacts with the wound to provide an environment that promotes wound healing.

Intercostal retractions: Intercostal muscles are seen moving inwards on expiration when a patient's work of breathing has increased in relation to respiratory distress.

Interdependence: The close relationships between people; their ability and willingness to respond to and give love, respect and value others.

Interdisciplinary: Involving two or more disciplines.

Interferons: A group of proteins produced by lymphocytes which promote natural killer cell activity and play a role in inhibiting viruses.

Interleukins: Cytokines produced by lymphocytes, particularly T cells.

Internal market: The creation of a market-driven service in which the concepts of competition and choice are applied to the provision of health care services.

Interprofessional team: How two or more people from different professions communicate and cooperate to achieve a common goal. The goal is usually a positive outcome for a patient.

Intrinsic: Relating or belonging to the human host.

Justice: A moral principle which states that fairness should govern resource allocation and distribution and claims of entitlement. This principle is best illustrated in the works of John Rawls (Beauchamp & Childress 1989).

Keratin: A waterproofing protein found in the top layer of the epidermis.

Laser: A source of intense radiation in the visible, ultraviolet or infrared portions of the light spectrum. The electrons emit very narrow beams of light all of one wavelength and parallel to each other. Lasers are used in surgery to divide or to cause adhesions or to destroy or fix tissue in place.

Late adulthood: The period of one's life over 65 years of age.

Lipodermatosclerosis: The clinical brown staining of the skin observed around the area of venous leg ulcers. It is caused by incompetence of the venous valves which allows a backflow of blood from the deep to the superficial veins, resulting in a high venous pressure. This pressure is transmitted to the capillaries, causing leakage of the proteins and of haemosiderin from the red cells throughout the capillaries into the interstitial space.

Lipolysis: Breakdown of fats.

Loading dose: The dose of a drug administered to achieve a therapeutic level immediately.

Lock out time: A predetermined time between bolus doses when a demand for the drug will not result in a dose being given.

Logical empiricism: The philosophy underlying the traditional scientific approach.

Lung compliance: The ease with which the lungs can be expanded – their distensibility – is referred to as lung compliance.

Lymphocyte: A mature white blood cell that arises from bone marrow and becomes functionally mature in the lymphoid organs of the body.

Lymphokines: Chemicals released by lymphocytes, mainly T cells.

Maceration of the skin: Damage to the outer layer of the epidermis caused by prolonged contact with exudate containing many toxins.

Magnetic resonance imaging (MRI): A scanning technique which uses magnetism and radio-frequency waves to identify structures; it does not use radiation. It can take images in more than one plane. This technique is especially useful for patients who have to undergo frequent scans where radiation build-up could be problematic and in neurological and soft tissue examinations.

Mass media: A generic term used to describe a variety of communication activities designed to reach a mass audience to raise awareness of health issues. They include audio-visual and printed material and involve resources such as patient education leaflets, posters, radio, television and advertisements.

Mechanical devices: This phrase is used to cover the vast range of equipment that is available to use to assist in the moving of patients. Most of the devices in this category are powered in some way by electricity, hydraulics, springs, gas struts or the counterbalancing of weights.

Medical Devices Agency (MDA): This government agency is responsible for advising all areas of health care about the safety of the various devices that are used in caring for people. Their work covers many things in addition to patient-handling equipment. The MDA will issue warning notices when equipment is found to be dangerous in some way. They also carry out comparative evaluations of some types of equipment.

Medical model: The basic paradigm of medicine and the principal form of explanation in scientific medicine.

Mentor: A qualified and experienced nurse who works with a student on clinical placements, ensuring he or she receives the appropriate experience.

Meta-analysis: Works at a high level of operation in bringing together general ideas about research knowledge with an awareness of the relevant evidence.

Metabolic acidosis: A state in which the pH of arterial blood is less than 7.35. A systemic increase in hydrogen ion concentration.

Methodology: Deals with the relations between the methods of investigation, as practical means, and the overall state of research design, proof and knowledge.

Methods: A term for research practice – refers to, and prescribes, particular procedures such as experimenting or sampling.

Middle adulthood: The period between 45 and 65 years of age.

Mixed economy of care: The provision of health and social care services from all sectors: statutory, voluntary, independent and private.

Modernisation: A process of social change by which societies become more complex. Associated with the functionalist school of thought in sociology.

Module (learning): A period of study during which a particular aspect of the course is introduced, taught and assessed. Each module has a certain number of academic credits associated with it. A module is usually 12–15 weeks in length.

Morbidity: States of ill health and the study of their nature and incidence.

Mortality: The frequency of deaths, especially in proportion to populations.

Multicultural society: A society which has different cultures and ethnic groups. Cultural variety is emphasised.

Multimodal analgesia: Describes the use of a combination of drugs which work in different ways to achieve a better quality of pain relief.

Multiple organ failure: The progressive failure of two or more organ systems after a very severe illness or injury.

μ-receptor agonists: Name given to the group of drugs which stimulate the μ (mu) receptors in the body.

Muscle relaxants: These drugs should only be used in conjunction with adequate sedation to avoid the terror of conscious paralysis. They are used for the facilitation of endotracheal intubation, assistance in the use of certain mechanical ventilatory modes, prevention of activity associated with high levels of oxygen consumption (e.g. shivering) in patients with very poor respiratory function and high FiO_2, reducing muscle spasm with tetany. Examples of muscle relaxants include atricurium and vecuronium.

Naturalistic inquiry: A qualitative research methodology.

Nerve penetration: Describes how well the nerve is penetrated by, for example, a drug.

Neurotoxicity: The quality of being poisonous or harmful to nerve cells.

Nociception: Nerve (fibres) endings or pathways that are concerned with the condition of pain.

Non-maleficence: A principle which states that one should do no harm and avoid situations that might promote harm (Beauchamp & Childress 1989).

Normal ageing: The changes – biological, sociological or psychological – that are inevitable and occur as the natural result of maturation or the passage of time.

Nosocomial: From Latin *nosocomialis* = originating in hospital.

Nosocomial infection: Acquired infection from invasive devices, environment-related problems, cross-infection, overuse of antibiotics, and in immunosuppressed patients.

Nursing diagnosis: A clinical judgement, made by nurses, about an individual, family or community group which relates to their health problems or life process. It may be either an actual or a potential diagnosis that nurses can identify by virtue of their education and experience, and following diagnosis are able to treat. It then provides the basis for the nurse to prescribe nursing interventions to achieve desired outcomes, to maintain the health-state or to reduce, eliminate or prevent alterations. For all this the nurse is accountable. The process of nursing diagnosis incorporates data analysis through gathering information about patients and their families by individual assessment, and then pulling together the data to make a diagnosis.

Ontology: The study of pure being (a branch of metaphysics).

Opiate: This is an older term than opioid and means morphine-like drugs with a chemical structure similar to morphine. It thus excludes peptides and many synthetic analogues.

Opioid: Applies to any substance that produces morphine-like effects that are antagonised by naloxone.

Opportunistic: Microorganisms capable of causing infection when the person's immune system is impaired.

Osmolality: A measurement of osmotically active solutes in a given mass of solution.

Osmosis: This is the movement of water through a membrane permeable to water but not to solutes, from an area of low solute concentration to one of high solute concentration.

Osmotic pressure: The amount of hydrostatic pressure required to oppose the osmotic movement of water within the body cells, cavities and circulation. It is determined by the thickness of the plasma membrane, the size of molecules, the concentration of molecules or the concentration gradient, and the solubility of molecules within the membrane.

Outcome: The result of a health care intervention for the patient, client or family.

Oxidation: The process of substances (e.g. haemoglobin) combining with oxygen or the removal and transfer of a pair of electrons (the breakdown of glucose and formation of ATP).

Oxygen debt: The volume of oxygen required after exercise to oxidise the lactic acid formed during exercise. An oxygen debt will also occur when demand exceeds supply. This can be caused by a decrease in either ventilation or perfusion or both due to a disease process.

Pain management techniques: Methods or treatments that are used to control pain.

Pain mechanisms: Pathways or substances that are concerned in causing pain.

Parenteral: Describes drugs given by either the intravenous, intramuscular or subcutaneous route.

Pathogenic: Disease producing.

PCA bolus dose: The dose of the drug that is administered when demanded by the patient. The size of the dose can be varied but is much smaller than that administered by traditional intramuscular bolus injection.

PCA pump: The device used to administer the analgesia.

pCO_2: Partial pressure of carbon dioxide

Pensionable age: The age at which an individual can claim the State Pension, currently 65 years for a man and 60 years for a woman in the UK.

Performance standard: A statement about the fulfilment of professional tasks which stipulates minimum requirements and their value objectives.

Perioperative: The combined preoperative, intraoperative and postoperative phases of the patients' care.

Peripheral nerve block: Describes inhibition of action of peripheral nerves (i.e. those lying outside the central nervous system – brain and spinal cord) involved in pain by, usually, the administration of a local anaesthetic.

Peritoneum: The serous membrane which lines the whole of the abdominal cavity.

pH: The measure of the relative acidity or alkalinity of a solution: the negative logarithm of hydrogen ion concentration in moles per litre.

Phagocytes: The white blood cells which engulf and digest foreign or dead cells (phagocytosis).

Pharmacodynamics: The study of changes in the effects of drugs with time. Age-related impairments of homeostatic mechanisms result in exaggerated responses to some drugs while there may be a decline in receptor and cellular sensitivity to drugs.

Pharmacokinetics: The fate of a drug in the body, encompassing absorption across the gut wall, first-pass metabolism in the gut wall and liver, protein binding, distribution throughout the body and elimination by the kidney, liver or other routes.

Phenomenology: A qualitative research methodology which looks at ways of investigating questions concerned with the lived experiences of patients and their families.

Phlebitis: Inflammation of the veins.

Plasma membrane: The cell membrane. This is a phospholipid bilayer, with hydrophobic and hydrophilic components.

Pneumonitis: Inflammation of the alveoli which can lead to pneumonia.

Pneumothorax: The presence of air or gas in the visceral or parietal pleura, which line and surround the lungs; caused by spontaneous rupture or trauma.

pO_2: Partial pressure of oxygen.

Policy: A principle or guideline, usually in written form, that determines the nature of activity and that employees or members of an organisation or institution are expected to follow.

Polycythaemia: An excessive amount of erythrocytes in the blood.

Positive end-expiratory pressure (PEEP): The resistance to expiration exerted by the pharynx and upper airways which limits alveolar collapse is normal physiological PEEP. PEEP can be given to a patient via mechanical ventilation or non-invasive respiratory support.

Positivism: The scientific doctrine that knowledge is based on sense-evidence alone – and that strict observations are required if generalisations are to be possible.

Practice development: Creating and sustaining a culture for change, personal effectiveness and professional development, for the ultimate benefit of patients.

Preceptor: A first-level nurse, midwife or health visitor with a minimum of 12 months' experience in the same field as the practitioner requiring support, who acts as a guide and source of professional advice during the first months following registration or re-entry to practice after a break of 5 years or more.

Pressure gradient: Movement of a solution or gas from a region of higher hydrostatic pressure to a region of lower hydrostatic pressure.

Prevalence: The frequency with which a set condition can be said to hold, in practice.

Principle: A general and fundamental moral exhortation that serves to justify a moral rule (Beauchamp & Childress 1989).

Probability theory: Explanatory approach which begins with the ideas of chance and risk.

Professional/clinical supervision: The mechanism by which nurses as individuals or groups explore their practice and become more effective in their practice. This involves helping nurses to think about and reflect on their practice in a structured and guided way. The supervisor's role is to provide high challenge and high support through the vehicle of a trusting professional relationship. Group supervision is similar to action learning.

Protocol: A written plan, usually formulated collectively by team members, specifying procedures to be followed with regard to a specific activity.

Psychiatry: That branch of medicine which is primarily concerned with the prevention and treatment of mental illness. Psychiatrists are medically qualified.

Psychology: The scientific study of human behaviour and experience (Caws 1975) and is a discipline in its own right, with its own awarding body, the British Psychological Society, which has within it divisions such as Clinical Psychologist, Counselling Psychologist. Psychology is made up of many different areas, for example cognitive (memory, attention, learning, perception), developmental, experimental, physiological, health, pharmacology, genetics, social, to name but a few.

Psychotherapist: Someone who has undergone extensive training in his or her chosen approach but is not necessarily medically trained. A **counsellor** will also have undergone substantial training. At the current time, however, anyone can call themselves a counsellor or psychotherapist as there is no legal requirement for training or registration, although this is being called for and developed. It is always advisable to check someone's training and experience as he or she may have little. **Psychoanalysis** is one particular approach to psychotherapy.

Pulmonary fibrosing alveolitis: Widespread involvement of the lungs by fibrosis, which particularly affects the alveolar walls, produces a typical clinical picture and functional disturbance characterised by increasing breathlessness in exertion and progressive reduction in lung volumes and impairment of gas transfer.

Pulmonary oedema: In many patients with respiratory failure, alveolar–capillary permeability is increased and there is a leakage of water and proteins into the alveolar space which leads to pulmonary oedema.

Purpura: Diffuse internal haemorrhage that is visible through the skin and causes a discoloration.

Race: A term which describes the division of humankind by physical characteristics.

Radicular: Relating to a root, e.g. a nerve root.

Reconditioning (of muscles): The process of rebuilding muscle tone and strength before attempting to get the patient to stand up.

Recovery room: A designated environment, usually purpose-built/converted for specific use in the recovery of postoperative patients.

Reductionistic: Whereby the body or other systems are reduced to their parts, and the whole is the sum total of all those parts.

Rehabilitation: A part of care in which the aim is to regain a measure of independence for the patient. This is a complex process that is often ill-defined.

REM sleep: Stages of the sleep cycle are named according to whether they are associated with rapid eye movements (REM). Dreams are thought to occur within REM sleep and REM sleep is important because of its function in the processing of information and recollection of events from the day. REM sleep alternates with NREM (non-rapid eye movement) sleep and occurs after stage four of the NREM sleep cycle.

Research sensitivity: The investigator's awareness, and development, of personal skills and qualitative judgements which are important in obtaining fresh evidence and in writing reports.

Reservoir: A source of infection.

Resident microorganisms: Microorganisms generally carried on or in a person's body; also known as endogenous organisms or normal body flora; the resident microorganisms protect the body from colonisation by more harmful bacteria.

Residual stimuli: Factors that may possibly affect the patient's ability to adapt. These factors may be unclear, not easily measured or validated. They include attitudes, values and beliefs.

Retrospective experimental design: Also known as the field experiment, as the outcome is natural (not contrived) and the direction of explanation is 'backwards': to find, and measure, the causal influence after it has been produced.

Role function: The performance of duties and roles within society. Primary role considers developmental level, e.g. middle-aged woman; secondary considers social standing, e.g. mother. The tertiary role(s) are chosen and not permanent, e.g. member of a club.

Rostral spread: Describes the movement of a drug up the spinal cord through the CSF. This is more likely to happen with water-soluble drugs.

Second level assessment: Identification of the focal, contextual and residual factors that are influencing the patient.

Secondary research: Conducts analysis upon statistical data already collected by others.

Selective committee: A cross-party committee set up by the Goverment to investigate and report on a particular issue. These committees often invite experts and stakeholders to give evidence.

Self-concept: The beliefs and feelings that are held by the individual. It is divided into physical self which examines body image and sensation and personal self which concentrates on the moral-ethical-spiritual, self-consistency and self-ideal/expectancy.

Sensitivity: The susceptibility of certain microorganisms to specific agents.

Septicaemia: The presence of bacteria, usually pathogenic in nature, in the bloodstream accompanied by clinical symptoms such as fever, rigor, low blood pressure.

Serosanguineous fluid: Fluid containing both clear serum exudate (sero) and blood (sanguine). Serum is the clear fluid portion of blood that remains after the corpuscles and fibrin have been removed.

Serum transferrin level: Transferrin is a glycoprotein synthesised primarily by the liver and assists in the transport of iron. The circulating serum transferrin level will determine how much iron is being delivered to erythroblasts in the bone marrow to make red blood cells.

Skin squames: Skin cells which have migrated to the level of the stratum corneum prior to being shed.

Sliding systems: A means of moving a person without lifting. The patient is slid from one place to another on a fabric or hard surface that has been designed for the purpose. To be effective the surface must be very slippery. Care must be taken with the use and cleaning of these systems to ensure that they continue to be effective. It should be noted that patients cannot be slid on ordinary sheets. In these circumstances the patient must be lifted to overcome friction.

Social engineering: The process of using information campaigns and social policies to promote environmental awareness and enable behaviour change for individuals.

Social policy: Refers to Acts of Parliament, central goverment and local goverment directives as well as the operationalisation of decisions. It also encompasses the values and beliefs that underlie the development and use of social institutions which affect the distribution of resources, status and power between different individuals and groups in society.

Socioeconomic status: A way of classifying individuals, families or households in terms of occupation, wealth, income or education. One of the major classification systems is that of social class measures introduced by the British Registrar General in 1911.

Sodium ion conductance: Describes the movement of sodium ions across, for example, a nerve membrane.

Somatic blockade (block): Refers to the inhibition of movement or sensation in skeletal muscle, e.g. administration of local anaesthetics can result in an inability to move/lift the legs or feelings of numbness in the legs.

Standaid: A hoist that will lift the patient to a standing position.

Stimulatory nociceptive input: Describes when messages are sent or received from nerve endings that are concerned with the condition of pain.

Stimulus: 'That which provokes a response' (Andrews & Roy 1991). Stimuli can be either internal or external.

Stratification: Represents socially structured differences of status, class and power.

Stridor: Harsh, strident breathing which is due to narrowing of the large airways.

Suprasternal retractions: Muscles around the clavicles and suprasternal notch are seen moving inwards on inspiration when a patient's work of breathing has increased in relation to respiratory distress.

Surfactant: A lipoprotein secreted by certain cells of the alveolus. It coats the inner surface of the alveolus and reduces the surface tension of water molecules. This facilitates the expansion of the lungs during inspiration and prevents the collapse of the alveoli after each expiration.

Surgical debridement: Removal of dead tissue from a wound by a surgical technique.

Susceptible: A person readily open to a risk of infection; this may be due to illness, treatment or genetic factors.

Sympathomimetic: Activity of a drug that has the effect of stimulating the sympathetic nervous system. The actions of sympathomimetic drugs are adrenergic (resembling those of noradrenaline and adrenaline).

Synergistic: A drug that interacts with another to produce increased activity which is greater than the sum of the effects of the two drugs given on their own.

Systemic: Involving the whole body.

Tachypnoea: Increased rate of breathing above the normal.

Technology: Complex, technical equipment required for interventions in and continuous monitoring of critically ill patients.

Tension pneumothorax: Pneumothorax is the presence of air in a pleural cavity causing the lung on that side to collapse. It has been postulated that a valvular mechanism may develop through which air can be sucked in during inspiration but not expelled during expiration. The intrapleural pressure remains positive throughout breathing, the lung deflates further, the mediastinum shifts, and venous return to the heart decreases, with increasing respiratory and cardiac embarrassment. This is known as a tension pneumothorax which requires immediate treatment to release the pressure. Tension pneumothorax is rare unless the patient is on positive pressure ventilation.

Therapeutic nursing: An approach to nursing where the centrality of the relationship between the nurse and the patient to the practice of nursing is a prime feature. This relationship is acknowledged as being of benefit to the patient over and above other specific interventions the nurse may provide.

Therapeutic window: Describes a drug concentration which achieves the clinical response required whilst minimising any potential toxicity.

Thrombocytopenia: A low platelet count, generally below 100 000 platelets per cubic millimetre of blood. A count of 50 000 or fewer increases the potential for haemorrhage caused by only a minor injury.

Thrombocytosis: A higher than normal platelet count, generally more than 400 000 per cubic millimetre of blood. Thrombocytosis is usually asymptomatic until the count exceeds 1 million/mm^2, causing intravascular clot formation (thrombosis), haemorrhage, or other abnormalities.

Thyrotoxicosis: Condition attributable to excess production of thyroid hormone.

TILEE: This is the acronym for the aspects to be considered in the mobility assessment process for handling patients. It stands for: task; individual; load; environment; and equipment.

Titrated: Used to describe the gradual increase or decrease in the dose of the drug being administered.

Toxin: Any poisonous substance produced by a living organism, especially a microbe.

Transcultural: Universal and specific features of cultures. Leininger (1985) has argued that transculturalism may be used to study care. Care is universal but different cultures care in different, culturally meaningful ways.

Transduce: To transduce means to change variations of one quantity into another, for example a measure of pressure into voltage.

Transfer systems: These are systems that are designed to move a patient from one piece of hospital equipment to another, for example from bed to trolley. Where the phrase is used in this chapter, it refers to the movement of the patient a distance of about 2–3 feet from one surface to another. It does not refer to systems such as the trolley itself or an ambulance that may be used to transfer the patient over some distance.

Transformational leadership: An approach to leadership which focuses on developing everyone's leadership potential and involving everyone in developing a shared vision. This is in contrast to a more traditional view of leadership where leadership is invested in one charismatic person whose vision is implemented by a band of followers who may relate to the leader's vision.

Transient microorganisms: Microorganisms originating from the environment, contact with patients and items of equipment during patient care activities, and other parts of the body, e.g. anus; also known as exogenous organisms.

Transmembrane proteins: Structures situated in the plasma membrane which facilitate transport of solutes across the plasma membrane.

Transudate: Fluid which has a protein content of less than 30 g/l and the lactic dehydrogenase is less than 200 i.u./l. Can cause pleural effusions.

Ultrasound: Sound waves at the very high frequency of over 20 000 vibrations per second. Ultrasound has many medical applications including fetal monitoring and imaging of internal organs.

Utilitarianism: A theory which states that the moral rightness of an action is determined by the maximum value of its positive consequences (Beauchamp & Childress 1989).

Ventricular fibrillation: Ventricular fibrillation is rapid ineffective quivering of the ventricles and is fatal without immediate treatment, i.e. defibrillation and advanced cardiac life support.

Veracity: Truth and truth-telling. A principle that exhorts the moral agent to tell the truth (Beauchamp & Childress 1989).

Vesicular breathing: This is a gentle rustling noise that is audible all over the periphery of the lungs. It has a characteristic rhythm, being loudest during inspiration and dying away rapidly during the early part of expiration.

Virulence: The ability of microorganisms to cause disease.

Vital capacity: The maximum amount of air that can be expelled from the lungs by forcible expiration after the deepest inspiration.

White Paper: A statement of goverment policy intent preceding an Act of Parliament.

Wound: A loss of continuity of the skin which may involve other anatomical structures.

Wound dehiscence: The breakdown of a closed wound converting it to an open wound.

Wound infiltration: Can be used to describe, for example, the administration of a local anaesthetic into a surgical wound.

REFERENCES

Andrews H A, Roy C 1991 Essentials of the Roy Adaptation model. In Roy C, Andrews H A The Roy Adaptation model: the definitive statement. Appleton and Lange, Norwalk

Beauchamp T L, Childress J F 1989 Principles of biomedical ethics. Oxford University Press, Oxford. Definitions in this glossary have been adapted.

British Association of Counselling Guidelines 1992. BAC, Rugby

Caws A G 1975 Introduction/preface. In: Altschul A Psychology for nurses. Baillière Tindall, London, p. i

Clancy J, McVicar A 1995 Physiology and anatomy: a homeostatic approach. Edward Arnold, London

Leininger M M 1985 Transcultural care diversity and universality: a theory of nursing. National League for Nursing, New York

Roy C 1976 Introduction to nursing: an adaptation model. Prentice Hall, Englewood Cliffs

Roy C, McLeod D 1981 Theory of the person as an adaptive system. In: Roy C, Roberts S L (eds) Theory construction in nursing: an adaptive model. Prentice Hall, Englewood Cliffs

Index